Veterinary Nursing

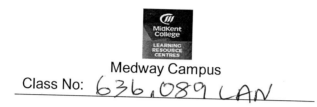

Medway Campus

Class No: 636.089 LAN

Return on or before the date last stamped below:

For renewals phone 01634 383044

TITLES OF RELATED INTEREST

LANE D. R. & GUTHRIE S.
Dictionary of Veterinary Nursing
0 7506 3615 7

THE COLLEGE OF ANIMAL WELFARE
Multiple Choice Questions in Veterinary Nursing
Volume 1: 0 7506 3611 4; Volume 2: 0 7506 3612 2

THE COLLEGE OF ANIMAL WELFARE
Veterinary Surgical Instruments: an illustrated guide
0 7506 3613 0

OUSTON J.E.
Veterinary Nursing: Self-Assessment Questions and Answers
Book 1: 0 7506 3731 5; Book 2: 0 7506 3732 3

KASSAI T.
Veterinary Helminthology
0 7506 3563 0

STEWART M.
Companion Animal Death
0 7506 4076 6

LANDSBERG G., HUNTHAUSEN W. & ACKERMAN A.
Handbook of Behaviour Problems in the Dog and Cat
0 7506 3060 4

GOLDSCHMIDT M. & SHOFER F.
Skin Tumors of the Dog and Cat
0 7506 4269 6

LABER-LAIRD K., SWINDLE M. & FLECKNELL P.
Handbook of Rodent and Rabbit Medicine
00804 2504 6

Veterinary Nursing

Second Edition

Edited by

D. R. LANE
Leamington Spa, Warwickshire, UK

and

B. C. COOPER
College of Animal Welfare, Wood Green Animal Shelter, Huntingdon, UK

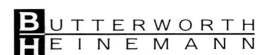

OXFORD AUCKLAND BOSTON JOHANNESBURG MELBOURNE NEW DELHI

Butterworth-Heinemann
Linacre House, Jordan Hill, Oxford OX2 8DP
225 Wildwood Avenue, Woburn, MA 01801-2041
A division of Reed Educational and Professional Publishing Ltd

℞ A member of the Reed Elsevier plc group

First published 1994
Reprinted with corrections 1995
Reprinted 1996, 1997 (twice), 1998
Second edition 1999
Reprinted with corrections 1999

British Library Cataloguing in Publication Data
Veterinary nursing.   2nd ed.
    1. Veterinary nursing
    I. Lane, D. R.   II. Cooper, B.
    636′.089′073

Library of Congress Cataloguing in Publication Data
Veterinary nursing/D. R. Lane and B. Cooper. – 2nd ed.
    p.   cm.
    Includes bibliographical references and index.
    ISBN 0 7506 3999 7
    1. Veterinary nursing.   2. Pets – Diseases – Nursing.   I. Lane, D. R.
    II. Cooper, B.
    SF774.5.V48   99–18294
    636.089′073–dc21   CIP

ISBN 0 7506 3999 7

DISCLAIMER
Whilst every effort is made by the Publishers to see that no inaccurate or misleading data, opinion or statement appear in this book,
they wish to make it clear that the data and opinions appearing in the chapters herein are the sole responsibility of the contributor
concerned. Accordingly, the Publishers and their employees, officers and agents accept no responsibility or liability whatsoever for
the consequences of any such inaccurate or misleading data, opinion or statement.

Drugs and Dosage Selection: The Authors have made every effort to ensure the accuracy of the information herein, particularly
with regard to drug selection and dose. However, appropriate information sources should be consulted, especially for new or
unfamiliar drugs or procedures. It is the responsibility of every veterinarian to evaluate the appropriateness of a particular opinion in
the context of actual clinical situations, and with due consideration to new developments.

Composition by Genesis Typesetting, Rochester, Kent
Printed and bound by MPG Books Ltd, Bodmin, Cornwall

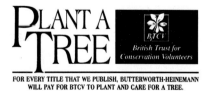

Contents

Foreword

This new edition of *Veterinary Nursing* will prove a welcome addition both to the bookshelves of veterinary nurses and to the libraries of the many practices undertaking veterinary nurse training. The new format in a single volume is to be applauded and the contents have been reworked in accordance with the demands of the modern training requirements. In acknowledgement of their increasing importance to the pet-owning public, increased emphasis is placed on the nursing and general care of exotic animals. Veterinary nurses now routinely play an important role in the maintenance and monitoring of general anaesthesia in practice. This enlarged area of responsibility is acknowledged by the inclusion of recent advances in a revised chapter covering all aspects of general anaesthesia.

The British Small Animal Veterinary Association is proud to be associated with this new edition and fully supports its use as an integral part of veterinary nurse training.

John F. R. Hird
President BSAVA
1999

Preface

It is not said often enough that veterinary nursing has significantly improved the care of all animals. We are proud to have been involved in the recent editions of *Veterinary Nursing* and believe that this new edition, where we are again joint Editors, continues the tradition of a caring profession preparing well for the future. The new assessment system, with a further emphasis on practical work recorded in a Portfolio presentation for assessment as a National Vocational Qualification, will make an increased contribution to veterinary nurse education into the 21st century.

This new edition, emphasising the importance of exotic pets in the syllabus, has brought in an additional author from Jersey Zoo to provide new material in the chapter on Exotic pets and wildlife. New contributors for animal handling, nutrition and anaesthesia add to the book's strength. Ultrasound and other forms of diagnostic imaging are covered as an innovative part of the radiography chapter. Bacteriology and fungal infections are dealt with in the same chapter for the first time with the help of an additional contributor. The decision to have all the information in a single volume allowed the Editors a regrouping of chapters so that medical nursing is followed by a chapter on medical disorders. The surgical nursing subjects are also placed together so that the book has a more logical sequence. The final chapters on Behaviour problems and their management and on Bereavement counselling bring another source of information for veterinary nurses to apply on a day-to-day basis in their work.

This text has attempted to meet the new veterinary nurse syllabus learning objectives whilst recognising that there is a requirement to refer to other texts – in particular Human First Aid and current legislation pertaining to Health and Safety.

At a time when animal owners are growing in knowledge and expectations, the 2nd edition of *Veterinary Nursing* will provide a reference source for all those involved in animal care and nursing.

D. R. Lane BSc, FRAgS, FRCVS
B. C. Cooper VN, CertEd, LicIPD, DTM,
Hon. Assoc. RCVS
February 1999

Contributors

Dr P. A. Bloxham, MVB PhD MRCVS, Robins Roost, Windward Lane, Holcombe, Dawlish, Devon EX7 0SQ

Mr D. C. Brodbelt, MA VetMB DVA DipECVA MRCVS, Highfield Veterinary Surgery, Broxbourne, Hertfordshire EN10 7PZ

Mr R. Butcher, MA VetMB MRCVS, 196 Hall Lane, Upminster, Essex RM14 1TD

Ms S. Chandler, VN DipAVN(Surg), University of Cambridge, Madingley Road, Cambridge CB3 0ES

Professor J. E. Cooper, BVS DTVM CBiol CertLAS FRCPath FIBiol FRCVS, Jersey Wildlife Preservation Trust, Les Augrès Manor, Trinity, Jersey, Channel Isles JE3 5BP

Mrs R. Dennis, MA VetMB DVR DipECVDI MRCVS, The Animal Health Trust, Lanwades Park, Kentford, Newmarket, Suffolk CB8 7UU

Mr C. J. Dutton, BSc BVSc MSc MRCVS, Jersey Wildlife Preservation Trust, Les Augrès Manor, Trinity, Jersey, Channel Isles JE3 5BP

Dr J. Elliott, MA VetMB PhD CertSAC MRCVS, Department of Veterinary Basic Sciences, Royal Veterinary College, Royal College Street, London NW1 0TU

Dr G. C. W. England, BVetMed PhD DVetMed CertVA DVReprod Diplomate ACT FRCVS, Department of Farm Animal & Equine Medicine & Surgery, Royal Veterinary College, Hawkshead Lane, North Mymms, Hatfield, Hertfordshire AL9 7TA

Mrs M. Fisher, BVetMed CBiol MIBiol MRCVS, Brentknoll Veterinary Centre, 152 Bath Road, Worcester WR5 3EP

Mrs S. Hiscock, BVetMed MRCVS, 16 Hill Place, Bursledon, Southampton, Hampshire SO31 8AE

Dr S. E. Long, BVMS PhD MRCVS, Department of Clinical Veterinary Science, University of Bristol, Langford House, Langford, Bristol BS40 5DU

Dr S. McCune, VN BA PhD, Waltham Centre for Pet Nutrition, Freeby Lane, Waltham-on-the-Wolds, Melton Mowbray, Leicestershire LE14 4RT

Ms D. McHugh, VN DipAVN(Surg), 65 High Street, Stetchworth, Cambridgeshire CB8 9TH

Dr C. May, MA VetMB CertSAO PhD, MRCVS, Grove Veterinary Hospital, 1 Hibbert Street, New Mills, Stockport SK12 3JJ

Mrs C. B. Mills, VN, Lenten House, West Willoughby, Nr Grantham, Lincolnshire NG32 3SN

Mr D. S. Mills, BVSc MRCVS, De Montfort University, Faculty of Applied Sciences, Caythorpe Campus, Caythorpe, Lincolnshire NG32 3EP

Dr H. E. Moreton, CertDHTC BSc PhD, Hartpury College, Hartpury, Gloucester GL19 3BE

Mrs S. Morrissey, CVPM, The Cromwell Veterinary Group, 36 St Johns Street, Huntingdon, Cambridgeshire PE18 6DD

Dr M. R. Owen, BVSc BSc PhD CertSAS MRCVS, Glasgow University Veterinary School, Bearsden Road, Bearsden, Glasgow G61 1QH

Mrs A. J. Pearson, BA VetMB MRCVS, Radnor Courts Veterinary Practice, 89a Cherry Hinton Road, Cambridge CB1 4BS

Mr A. R. W. Porter, CBE MA DVMS(hc) Hon Assoc RCVS, 4 Savill Road, Lindfield, Haywards Heath, Sussex RH16 2NX

Ms J. S. Seymour, VN CertEd, 19 Wheatcroft Close, Penkridge, Staffordshire ST19 5JS

Mr J. W. Simpson, BVM and S SDA MPhil MRCVS, Department of Veterinary Clinical Studies, Royal (Dick) School of Veterinary Studies, Easter Bush Veterinary Centre, Roslin, Midlothian EH25 9RG

Mrs C. A. van der Heiden, VN, The Bush, Edinvillie, Aberlour, Banffshire AB38 9NA

Ms T. Webb, VN, Animal Care, De Montfort University, Caythorpe Campus, Caythorpe, Lincolnshire NG32 3EP

Dr E. Welsh, BVMS PhD CertVA CertSAS MRCVS, Department of Veterinary Clinical Studies, Royal (Dick) School of Veterinary Studies, Hospital for Small Animals, Easter Bush Veterinary Centre, Roslin, Midlothian EH25 9RG

Miss K. A. Wiggins, VN DipAVN(Surg), 64 The Brache, Maulden, Bedfordshire MK45 2DS

1

Handling and control

T. A. Webb

A veterinary nurse should be familiar with the handling and positioning of animals that may require treatment or examination. Knowledge of behaviour and the characteristics that a breed or species of animal may exhibit is essential. Animals in pain, in a strange environment or being handled by unfamiliar people may well demonstrate behaviour that is out of character for the breed or species. A veterinary nurse should always pay attention to the 'body language' displayed (Fig. 1.1).

Restraint

Patients in a veterinary practice may be restrained by either physical or pharmacological means. Indications for restraint include (Fig. 1.2):

- Preparation for physical examination.
- To enable diagnostic procedures to be carried out.
- The administration of oral, parenteral or topical drugs.
- The application of bandages and/or dressings.

Other methods of restraint are illustrated in Figs 1.3–1.8.

> **WARNING**
>
> A muzzled dog should never be left unattended. There is a risk of asphyxiation if vomiting occurs.

A dog-catcher (Fig. 1.4) may be used for particularly nasty dogs but should always be removed as soon as some other

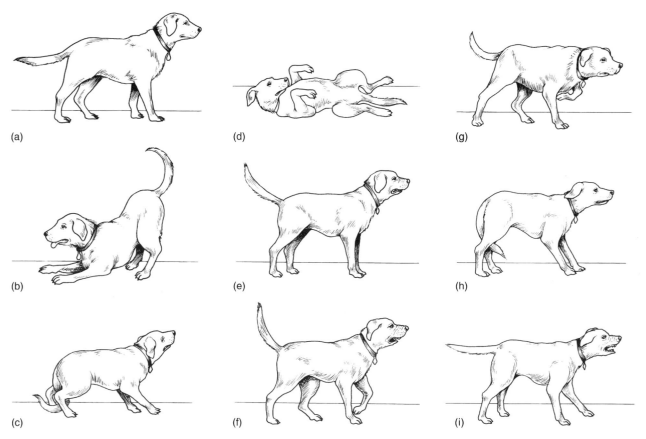

(a)　(d)　(g)

(b)　(e)　(h)

(c)　(f)　(i)

Fig. 1.1 Body language of the dog. (a) Normal. (b) Play bow: invitation to play – often seen in young dogs. (c) Active submission: gaze averted, dog crouches down, ears back, tail lowered, may urinate. (d) Passive submission: dog rolls on side, displaying inguinal region, may urinate. (e) Dominance: dog meets gaze, ears forward, tail up, hairs on neck may be raised, lips forward, may growl or attempt to bite. (f) Aggression: ears normal or forward, tail held high, body geared for action, usually growling or barking, hairs on back of neck may be raised. (g) Arousal: ears normal or forward, tail either wagging or normal, body exhibiting interest – reaching forward, may raise one front leg (i.e. 'point'). (h) Fear: ears back, tail curved between the back legs, body lowered and backing away (cringeing), often trembling. (i) Fearful aggression: ears back, body slightly lowered and backing away, growling or barking, tail level or lowered.

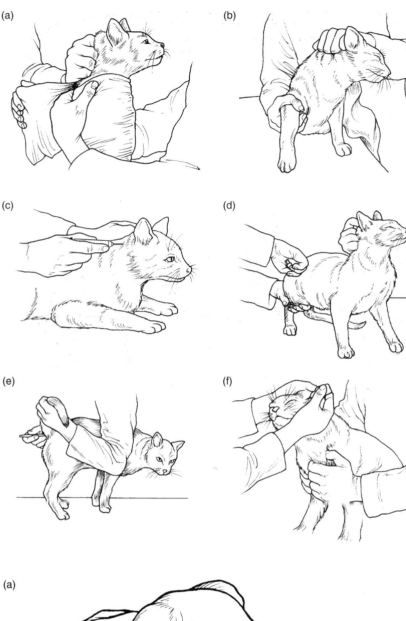

(a) (b)

(c) (d)

(e) (f)

Fig. 1.2 Different methods of restraint. (a) If a cat is particularly fractious, it is advisable to wrap the animal securely in a towel. Individual limbs can be extracted if necessary. For examination of the head, the whole body can be wrapped in the towel. (b) Venepuncture requires firm restraint. Movement during this procedure is the most common cause of painful and unsightly haematomas. Blood may be collected from either the jugular vein or the cephalic vein but if large quantities of blood are needed, the jugular vein is best. In kittens under 6 weeks, the jugular is the vein of choice. In cats, the cephalic vein is the most convenient way to give an intravenous injection. (c) Subcutaneous injections are easily given single-handedly. (d) Restraint by the scruff is usually sufficient for intramuscular injections. However, if a cat is fractious, this type of injection can be given through the mesh of a crush cage. (e) Clinical examination of the cat often involves taking the rectal temperature with a thermometer. If necessary, this can be carried out by one person as illustrated. (f) method of restraint for the administration of ear drops. If only one person is available, the scruff of the neck should be firmly grasped (with the cat facing away), the head tilted and the medicine administered. Additional restraint can be supplied by using the forearm and elbow to press the cat against the body.

(a)

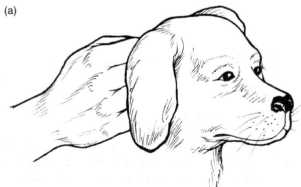

(b)

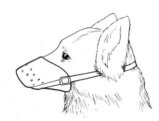

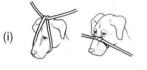

(i)

(ii)

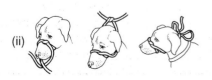

Fig. 1.3 (a) Holding a dog ready for muzzling. Although a good dog muzzle must offer safety, it should also have enough space to allow for panting and drinking. (b) Various types of muzzle: Baskerville, box, nylon and tape. A simple tape muzzle can be created from 2 cm (3/4 inch) wide bandage or tape: (i) make a loop with a single knot and slip over the dog's nose, pulling tight, and (ii) cross the free ends under the lower jaw and tie behind the back of the head. Use a quick-release bow to allow for emergency removal of the muzzle. **NB: It is difficult (or even impossible) to muzzle brachycephalic breeds such as boxers and bulldogs. They should never be restrained by the scruff of the neck because of the risk of prolapse of the eyes, so a useful method of restraint is to wrap a rolled-up towel or blanket around the animal's neck. This will prevent the dog from turning round to bite.**

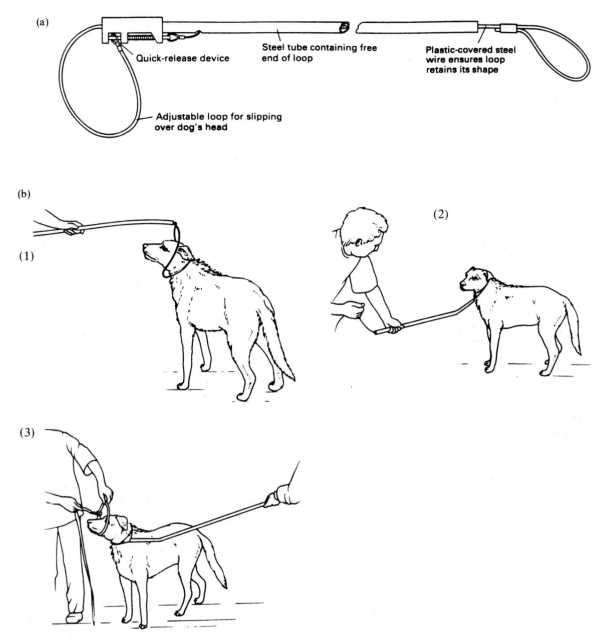

Fig. 1.4 The dog-catcher. (a) Labelled cross-section of a dog-catcher. (b) Examples of the dog-catcher in use. Can be used either for catching an aggressive dog or for removing a dog who is guarding his kennel.

means of restraint has been applied. The dog-catcher is an implement with an adjustable loop of cable at the far end which is slipped over the dog's head. The cable passes through an aluminium handle thus ensuring a safe distance between the handler and the dog. The loop is drawn tighter manually and can be locked in position by a single twist action. There is a small fixed loop at the handler's end of the tube which can be hitched over a hook or other tether to allow a muzzle and lead to be put on the dog.

> ### WARNING
>
> A cat recovering from sedation or anaesthesia should never be placed in an enclosed carrier. Airway obstruction or haemorrhage may occur and this could remain unobserved.

Chemical restraint

The veterinary surgeon may choose to use a drug to restrain a patient. Drugs commonly used to sedate an animal may include acepromazine, medetomidine, xylazine, etc.

Factors to consider before carrying out restraint:

- Ensure that all equipment is ready.
- Check that the environment is 'escape proof'.
- Use minimal restraint where appropriate.
- Use safe lifting techniques.
- Assistance should be available if necessary.
- Assess the animal's behaviour, e.g. will the animal behave with the owner present or should they be out of sight; will darkening the room help.
- Adopt a calm but confident manner – voice levels should be gentle and quiet.

Moving, transporting and lifting animals

Moving patients

In order to prevent injury to the handler, animal, owner or other members of staff, restraint is essential when moving animals from one place to another. Consideration should be given to:

- The type of animal (smaller animals should be transported in a cage, carrier or box).

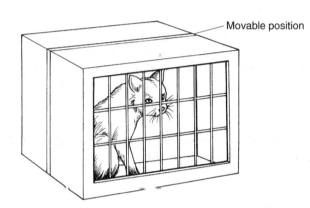

Fig. 1.5 Cat crush cage: a movable partition pushes the cat up against the wire mesh front of the cage, immobilising the animal and making the administration of medication easier.

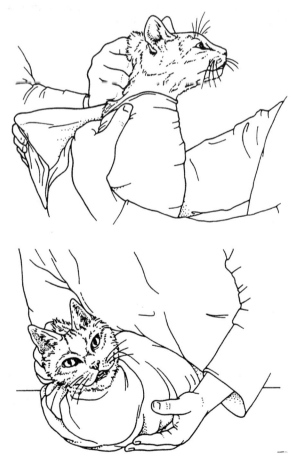

Fig. 1.6 Cat restraining bag. These are usually waterproof and made from strong nylon. The cat is placed in the bag which is zipped up, leaving only the head showing. Individual limbs can be extracted for either examination or treatment through one of the four zipped openings. This bag is also useful when performing cephalic venepuncture procedures.

- The nature of the injury and the medical condition of the animal.
- The number of staff available – will help be needed with drips, etc?
- The environment – do any obstacles need clearing, doors opened, etc?
- The behaviour of the animal, e.g. is it in pain and therefore aggressive?

Never carry a cat from one place to another in your arms: it may become frightened and bolt (often causing injury in the process). Always ensure that dogs are wearing a collar and lead if they are out of their kennel.

When moving animals that are unable to walk, a trolley or stretcher should be used unless they can be transferred to a wire box or basket in which they can still be observed. See also pp. 24 and 25.

Transporting animals

Safety is the prime consideration when transporting animals either to or from the veterinary practice. It is essential that they are properly restrained in order to:

- Avoid further injury to the patient.
- Avoid any injury to the handler or other persons.
- Prevent a driving accident.
- Prevent escape.

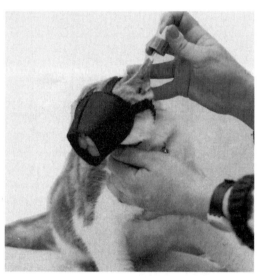

Fig. 1.7 A cat muzzle: a soft fabric muzzle covers the whole face. It is used to subdue the cat and can be useful when administering ear medication.

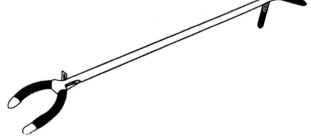

Fig. 1.8 A cat-grabber grasps the cat around the neck to allow capture. It pins the animal down so that it can be moved to a safer environment, e.g. a cage, and is useful when dealing with feral or frightened cats that cannot be approached. Do not lift a cat using the grabber alone.

It is often helpful to suggest that a cat cage be covered with a blanket or towel. This helps to calm the cat.

Lifting animals

When lifting animals, correct lifting techniques should always be followed (Fig. 1.9):

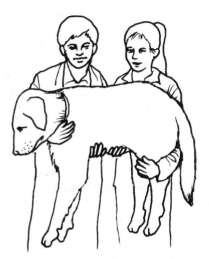

Fig. 1.9 Safe lifting techniques. Remember that when lifting animals their load can suddenly shift. Large dogs should be lifted by two people of similar height. Small or medium-sized dogs may be lifted by one person.

- Back straight.
- Knees bent.
- Legs slightly apart.
- Palms facing upwards.
- Animal held close to body.

Large breeds of dog that cannot be lifted by two people should be examined on the floor.

WARNING

Never lift a large, injured dog onto or off the table without assistance (see Chapter 3, Handling and transport of the injured animal, p. 23)

Health & Safety guidelines provide additional information on safe lifting techniques (p. 101).

Further reading

Anderson, R. S. and Edney, A. T. B. (1991) *Practical Animal Handling*, Pergamon, Oxford.
Sonsthagen, T. F. (1991) *Restraint of Domestic Animals*, American Veterinary Publications, Santa Barbara.

2

Observation and care of the patient

J. S. Seymour

Observation

During the course of a working day veterinary nurses will come into contact with a range of patients. They will have to deal with healthy animals of many species and temperaments and care for in-patients whose needs will vary from basic tender loving care to intensive treatment and nursing procedures. They must recognise the normal and abnormal appearance and behaviour patterns of those in their care, and report all relevant information to the veterinarian. The nurse's observations can give valuable input to the case history of the patient and may assist the veterinary surgeon's diagnosis and treatment. All observations should be noted and any abnormalities reported immediately.

Dogs and cats in the hospital environment

It should be remembered that every patient is different. What would be considered normal for one patient may be abnormal for another. It is necessary, therefore, to become familiar with each animal and to recognise its normal appearance and behaviour patterns.

The veterinary hospital is not a normal environment for dogs or cats. They will be surrounded by faces, smells and sounds unfamiliar to them, and therefore may be expected to behave in an abnormal fashion. Normally placid animals may become nervous and exhibit signs of aggression or submission. Outdoor cats confined to cages may be reluctant to use a litter tray and therefore become constipated.

Fear and anxiety are not conducive to a smooth and speedy recovery. The veterinary nurse should do everything possible to alleviate stress in the hospitalised patient.

The following guidelines for stress reduction should be followed:

- Wherever possible avoid placing animals in cages where they can see and be seen by other patients. If necessary, cover the cage with a blanket, but ensure that regular observation of the patient is maintained.
- Direct eye contact may be perceived by a dog as a challenging gesture and one that demands an aggressive response. This should be avoided.
- Noise levels should be kept to a minimum and any sudden loud noises should be avoided. Barking dogs should be isolated if practical and returned home as soon as possible.
- Ample provision should be made for urination and defecation. Animals easily become agitated if this is not allowed and often are mortified if they soil their kennel.

- Male dogs can become extremely agitated if kennelled in close proximity to a bitch in season. It is advisable therefore not to admit bitches in oestrus to the veterinary hospital unless absolutely necessary.
- Ideally, each patient should be monitored and cared for by a specific nurse. This will provide continuity and allow mutual trust to develop.

Normal appearance of the dog and cat

A normal, healthy dog or cat will exhibit the following signs:

- Keen reflexes with sharp reaction to stimuli.
- Clear, bright eyes that are free of discharge.
- Clear nasal orifices with no discharge.
- Clean and odour-free ears.
- Glossy coat with skin that is supple and free of wounds and parasites.
- Suitable weight for breed and size with no signs of obesity or wastage.
- Free limb movement with no signs of stiffness or pain.
- Temperature, pulse and respiration within the normal range, although these may increase slightly under the stress of hospital conditions.
- Pink mucous membranes with a capillary refill time of 1–2 seconds (Fig. 2.1).
- Clear, yellow urine passed without pain or difficulty.
- Firm, brown faeces passed freely without undue straining or pain.
- Interest shown in food if offered, with an ability to eat and drink comfortably.

Abnormal appearance of the dog and cat

Any abnormality, however minor, will be significant to the case history of the patient and therefore to the veterinary surgeon in charge. It is vital that all abnormal signs are reported by the veterinary nurse as soon as possible. It is recommended that hospital charts are utilised for all patients and that vital signs are monitored and recorded routinely.

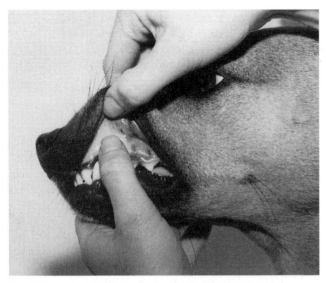

Fig. 2.1 Assessing capillary refill time by applying pressure to the mucous membranes of the gum. Photograph courtesy of Roy Hancocks and Rachel Meredith.

Abnormal signs and their possible significance

Appetite changes

Many animals, especially cats, have a normal capricious appetite. However, alterations in feeding patterns may occur in the hospital situation as a result of a change in environment or diet.

Loss of appetite is often the first sign that an animal is unwell. This may be due to a number of factors, including:

- Mouth ulcers.
- Nasal congestion, causing impaired olfactory function.
- Infectious diseases and pyrexia.
- Metabolic diseases.

Voracious appetite with subsequent loss of weight and condition may be a symptom of pancreatic insufficiency or worms. **Pica** (craving for unnatural foodstuffs) may occur as a result of dietary imbalance, but is often merely an undesirable habit. **Coprophagia** (eating of the faeces) is an example of this condition.

Changes in urination patterns

Polyuria (increased urine production) and **polydipsia** (increased thirst) are symptoms of many diseases, including:

- Nephritis.
- Diabetes mellitus.
- Diabetes insipidus.
- Pyometra.

Dysuria (difficulty in passing urine), **anuria** (total inability to pass urine) and **haematuria** (presence of blood in the urine) are potentially emergency situations and may be caused by:

- Cystic calculi.
- Feline urological syndrome.
- Prostatic enlargement.

All changes in urination patterns should be monitored and water intake and urine output accurately measured. (The normal urine output for a dog is 2 ml/kg/hour.) The colour, smell and consistency of the urine passed should be assessed and reported.

Unless otherwise instructed by the veterinary surgeon, clean, fresh water should be available to patients at all times.

Changes in defecation patterns

Constipation (the failure to evacuate faeces which may cause straining) may be caused by a number of factors, including:

- Ingestion of foreign material such as bones or fur balls.
- Tumours in the rectum or colon.
- Environmental factors such as soiled litter trays or confinement.
- Enlargement of the prostate gland.
- Dehydration.
- Key–Gaskell syndrome in cats.

Diarrhoea (the frequent evacuation of watery faeces from the bowel) may be caused by:

- Canine parvovirus.
- Bacterial infections including Leptospirosis.
- Distemper.
- Feline panleucopenia.
- Colitis.
- Tumours of the intestine.
- Intussusception.
- Endoparasites.
- Unsuitable diet.
- Ingestion of placental membranes by post-parturient bitch.

The volume and frequency of faecal material passed should be monitored and recorded. The faeces should be assessed for colour, smell and texture and examined for the presence of blood, mucus or parasitic worms. Microscopic examination may also be carried out.

Vomiting

This is the emission from the mouth of stomach contents and may be caused by:

- Ingestion of foreign material such as poisons, decaying food or small prey.
- Diabetes mellitus.
- Nephritis.
- Pancreatitis.
- Pyometra.
- Foreign body in digestive tract such as plastic or stone.
- Endoparasites.
- Viral infections (hepatitis, canine parvovirus, feline panleucopenia, feline infectious peritonitis).

The volume and frequency of vomitus should be monitored and recorded and the specimen examined for blood, mucus or evidence of poisons. The incidence of vomiting related to feeding patterns is of great relevance and should be monitored, with recording of the times that sickness occurs.

TYPES OF VOMITING

The veterinary nurse should be able to recognise the various types of vomiting that may be seen in the cat and dog. These include:

- **Projectile vomit** – forceful vomiting of stomach contents usually without retching.
- **Regurgitation** – the backflow of food from the oesophagus.
- **Stercoraceous vomit** – vomit containing faeces.
- **Haematemesis** – vomit containing blood.
- **Bilious vomit** – vomit containing bile.
- **Cyclic vomiting** – recurring acts of vomiting.
- **Retching** – ineffectual attempts to vomit. (This may be confused with coughing, especially in cats.)

Nasal discharge

This is commonly accompanied by sneezing and may be caused by:

- Foreign bodies such as grass seeds, tumours or polyps.
- Distemper.
- Feline calicivirus.
- Feline viral rhinotracheitis.

The nasal passages should be examined for any evidence of foreign bodies and the discharge examined for presence of blood or pus. Patients, especially cats, may be reluctant to eat when their nasal passages are congested due to diminished olfactory function.

Aural discharge

This is most commonly seen in long-eared breeds such as the spaniel and is often accompanied by vigorous head shaking and frantic scratching of the ears. It may be caused by:

- Foreign bodies such as grass seeds.
- Ear mites.
- Infection.

The ears should be examined for evidence of obvious foreign body. The use of an auroscope may be required.

Ocular discharge

This can cause considerable distress to a patient and signs such as pawing at the face and rubbing the head against the floor may be seen. This may be a symptom of:

- Distemper.
- Feline upper respiratory tract infection.
- Foreign body such as grass seed.
- Abnormal eyelid or eyelash structure.

The eyes should be examined carefully, taking care not to touch the surface of the cornea.

Vaginal discharge

This is associated with the reproductive cycle of the bitch or queen and may be normal or abnormal. Indications include:

- **Pro-oestrus** – blood-red discharge.
- **Oestrus** – straw-coloured discharge.
- **Imminent parturition** – dark green discharge.
- **Metritis** – brown/black discharge.
- **Abortion** – foul-smelling, black discharge.
- **Pyometra** – purulent discharge, often green or pale coffee colour.

An accurate history should be obtained to help establish the cause of the discharge to ensure the correct course of action is taken.

Coughing

This may be heard in the hospitalised patient and may vary from a dry, harsh cough to one that is fluid and productive. Coughing may be caused by:

- Congestive heart failure.
- Roundworm infestation in young animals.
- Kennel cough.
- Bronchitis.
- Distemper.
- Inhalation of chemicals or irritant gases.

Any method of restraint that may aggravate the situation should be avoided.

Changes in colour of mucous membranes

The colour of mucous membranes is a good indication of the health of an animal and will sometimes indicate the need for emergency action:

- **Pale mucous membranes** – may indicate haemorrhage, anaemia or circulatory collapse.
- **Blue tinged (cyanosis)** – may indicate respiratory obstruction.
- **Yellow (icterus)** – may indicate liver disease or leptospirosis.

Restlessness

Any animal that appears to be unduly restless should be examined to establish the cause and steps that should be taken if possible to alleviate its distress. Signs of restlessness include:

- Panting.
- Whining.
- Pacing.

- Scratching at bedding.
- Barking.
- Inability to settle.

These signs may be caused by:

- Pain or discomfort.
- Excess heat or cold.
- Need to urinate or defecate.
- Hunger or thirst.
- Loneliness or boredom.
- Dressings too tight.

Temperature, pulse and respiration

These vital signs should be monitored routinely in every hospitalised patient. See Table 2.1.

Temperature

Thermometers

The most common type of clinical thermometer is the veterinary **mercury thermometer**. This consists of a graduated glass tube with a stubby bulb at one end containing mercury. When the temperature rises, the mercury expands causing it to travel along the tube. The thermometer has a kink in the bulb end which prevents the backflow of mercury when it is removed from the animal. This allows an accurate reading of body temperature.

The thermometer may be calibrated in degrees Celsius (°C) or Fahrenheit (°F). Although the veterinary nurse should be familiar with both readings, degrees Celsius is now the standard unit for measurement of temperature. A Fahrenheit reading may be converted to Celsius by use of the formula:

$$°C = (°F - 32) \times 5/9$$

The **electronic thermometer** is now widely used and is designed for rectal or oesophageal use and allows continual monitoring of body temperature. The temperature may be read from a digital readout. The **subclinical thermometer** may be used to record subnormal temperatures and is valuable for anaesthetised patients and those that are critically ill.

Care and storage of the mercury thermometer

The mercury thermometer should be stored in a glass jar with a pad of cotton wool at the bottom. The jar should be filled with antiseptic solution. Both the cotton wool and the antiseptic should be changed daily. The thermometer should be cleaned with cool water and antiseptic. Hot water should not be used as this will cause the mercury to expand and the glass to break.

Thermometers should not be shared between infectious and non-infectious patients.

Great care should be taken when using and storing the mercury thermometer as both broken glass and the mercury can be hazardous.

Table 2.1 Normal range of vital signs in the cat and dog		
	Dog	**Cat**
Temperature	38.3–38.7°C (100.9–101.7°F)	38.0–38.5°C (100.4–101.6°F)
Pulse	60–180 beats per minute (depending on size)	110–180 beats per minute
Respiration	10–30 breaths per minute	20–30 breaths per minute

PROCEDURE FOR TAKING THE TEMPERATURE USING THE MERCURY THERMOMETER

It is usual to take the temperature of an animal via the rectal route.

(1) The patient should restrained by an assistant.
(2) Shake down the thermometer to ensure the mercury returns to the bulb. (To avoid the possibility of breakage, this should never be done near hard surfaces.)
(3) Lubricate the stubby bulb end of the thermometer with Vaseline, K-Y jelly, soap or oil.
(4) Gently insert the thermometer into the rectum with a twisting motion. The anal sphincter of the dog will relax easily but slightly more pressure will be required in the cat to relax its inner sphincter muscle. The thermometer should be directed against the upper surface of the rectum to avoid insertion into a faecal mass.
(5) Hold the thermometer in the rectum for the stated time (30 seconds to 1 minute).
(6) Then gently remove the thermometer and wipe it clean with cotton wool. Avoid touching the bulb.
(7) Hold the thermometer horizontally and rotate it until the mercury level is visible.
(8) Read and record the temperature.
(9) Report any abnormalities to the veterinary surgeon.
(10) Clean thermometer.

Pyrexia (high body temperature) may be caused by:

- Infection.
- Heat stroke.
- Convulsions.
- Pain.
- Excitement.

Low body temperature may be caused by:

- Shock.
- Circulatory collapse.
- Impending parturition.

Fluctuating temperature is known as diphasic and is a symptom of canine distemper.

Pulse

The pulse rate of an animal can be palpated at any point where an artery runs close to the body surface. Each pulsation corresponds with the contraction of the left ventricle of the heart. In the dog and cat, suitable sites include:

- The femoral artery, on the medial aspect of the femur (see Fig. 2.2).
- The digital artery, on the palmar aspect of the carpus.
- The coccygeal artery, on the ventral aspect of the base of the tail.
- The lingual artery, on the underside of the tongue (in anaesthetised patients).

PROCEDURE FOR PULSE-TAKING (Fig. 2.2)

(1) The patient should be restrained by an assistant.
(2) Locate the artery with the fingers.
(3) Count the pulsations for exactly one minute. (With very rapid pulse rates, a shorter period may be all that is possible.)
(4) Record the rate.

Although the rate of pulse is important, the character of the pulse should also be assessed. In a normal patient, the pulse rate increases on inspiration and decreases on expiration, and this variation is known as **sinus arrhythmia**.

A pulse rate that is lower than a corresponding heart rate is known as a **pulse deficit** and is indicative of **dysrhythmia**.

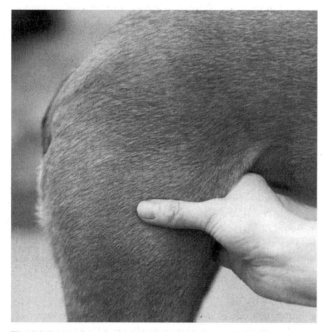

Fig. 2.2 Taking the pulse, using the femoral artery. Photograph courtesy of Roy Hancocks and Rachel Meredith.

POSSIBLE CAUSES OF ABNORMAL PULSE RATES

Raised
- Fever.
- Exercise.
- Hypoxia.
- Pain.
- Fear.

Lowered
- Unconsciousness.
- Anaesthesia.
- Debilitating disease.
- Sleep.

Weak
- Shock.
- Diminished cardiac output.

Strong and jerky ('water hammer' pulse)
- Valvular insufficiency.
- Congenital heart defects such as patent ductus arteriosus.

Respiration

The rhythm and rate of respiration can be assessed by careful observation of the patient or by gently resting the hands on either side of the chest cavity.

POSSIBLE CAUSES OF ABNORMAL RESPIRATION

Tachypnoea (increased respiratory rate)
- Heat.
- Exercise.
- Pain.
- Poisons.

Bradypnoea (decreased respiratory rate)
- Poisons (narcotic or hypnotic).
- Metabolic alkalosis.
- Sleep.

Dyspnoea (difficult breathing)

1. Inspiratory dyspnoea:
   - Obstruction or stenosis of the respiratory tract.
2. Expiratory dyspnoea:
   - Bronchitis and emphysema of the lungs.
   - Pleural adhesions.
3. Mixed dyspnoea:
   - Pneumonia.
   - Pneumothorax.
   - Hydrothorax.
   - Pyothorax.

Cheyne–Stokes respiration often occurs shortly before death and is characterised by alternating periods of deep, rapid and shallow breathing followed by **apnoea** (cessation of breathing).

The respiratory rate should be taken when the patient is at rest but not sleeping or panting. Count either inspirations *or* expirations for exactly 1 minute. Also assess the depth of respiration, which indicates the volume of air inspired with each breath.

General care of the patient

The specific needs of the hospitalised patients will obviously be dependent on their condition. However, all patients have a basic requirement for nutrition, warmth, comfort, hygiene and mental stimulation.

Nutrition

Correct nutrition is of vital importance to the hospitalised patient. A palatable, high-energy diet is required to support the animal during its recovery.

Easily digested foods such as scrambled eggs and chicken may be offered to the inappetent patient. Alternatively, a wide range of commercial diets are available. Strong-smelling foods such as pilchards or meat extract are useful for encouraging animals (especially cats) to eat.

All food should be warmed to blood temperature before feeding. Meals should be fed little and often and any food not eaten after 15 minutes removed.

There are various ways of ensuring that hospitalised patients receive sufficient nutrients. These include:

- Placing food on nose and paws of patient.
- Spoon feeding.
- Syringe feeding.
- Orogastric tubing.
- Nasogastric tubing.
- Pharyngostomy tubing.

Warmth

It is important that all patients are kept warm and free from draughts. The temperature of the hospital ward should be kept constant with adequate ventilation. A temperature of 18–20°C is recommended. Additional warmth may be provided by several means:

Blankets and towels are readily available and often used in the veterinary hospital, but care should be taken that they do not become soaked with urine which could lead to urine scalds in a recumbent or weak patient.

Vetbeds are ideal for use in the ward. They are comfortable, warm and easily washed. Their main advantage is that the base of the vetbed absorbs any fluid, thereby ensuring that the patient remains dry.

Heat lamps should be used with great care. Animals that are unable to move can easily become overheated and possibly burnt if a lamp is used injudiciously. The heat lamp should be no nearer than 61 cm (24 inches) from the patient and constant observation should be maintained.

Hot water bottles are a good source of heat for weak patients, although they do have certain disadvantages. They will require refilling at regular intervals and should always be covered with a towel or blanket. It is possible that the stopper may become loose or that patients may chew the rubber, and scalding may occur as a result. Boiling water should never be used.

Heated pads are useful, but again must be used with care. They should be covered with a towel and the patient checked and turned at regular intervals. Animals with a tendency to chew should not be allowed heated pads as chewing the flex could lead to electrocution.

Incubators are ideal for smaller critical patients and for newborn puppies and kittens. The environment can be automatically maintained at the desired temperature. Newborn animals are **poikilothermic** (body temperature varies with ambient temperature) and therefore a constant temperature of 30–33°C should be maintained for these patients.

Comfort

Patients should be provided with adequate bedding materials. They should be allowed to assume a position that they find comfortable. Fractured limbs, open wounds and dressings should be kept uppermost. Familiar bedding brought in by the owner may provide extra comfort and security.

Recumbent animals should be provided with extra padding, such as foam wedges, to prevent the occurrence of decubitus ulcers. Bony prominences such as the hock, elbow and sternum should be especially protected. The application of a bandage or Vaseline to these areas may be beneficial. The recumbent patient should be turned regularly every 2–4 hours.

Hygiene

A high standard of hygiene must be maintained on the hospital ward. All faeces, urine, vomit and discharge should be removed from the kennel immediately and the patient cleaned thoroughly. Suitable disinfectants, diluted correctly, should be used when cleaning. Protective clothing should be worn to comply with COSHH regulations. Uneaten food should not be left in the kennel as it will be unpleasant for the patient and may attract flies in hot weather.

The mouth, eyes and nose of patients should be kept free of discharge by wiping with damp cotton wool.

Mental stimulation

It is important to maintain the morale of the hospitalised patient. This can be achieved by talking, fussing and stroking with constant use of the animal's name. It should, however, be allowed periods when it can sleep and rest without distraction.

- Regular grooming should be carried out, especially in long-haired breeds. Clipping of hair and bathing may be necessary.
- Long-stay patients may benefit from visits by the owner, although this may not be advisable in all cases as patient and owner alike may become distressed when parting.

- Toys and chews from home may be allowed at the veterinary surgeon's discretion.
- Whenever possible, the patient should be taken outside to enjoy fresh air and a change of environment.

Transport of the patient

Animals should be suitably restrained when they are moved to and from the hospital ward. Dogs that are able to walk should be held on leads and cats confined to a secure basket or carrier.

Anaesthetised or unconscious patients should be supported by stretcher or trolley and observed constantly for struggling, vomiting or respiratory distress. A patent airway must be maintained by extending the head and neck and pulling the tongue forwards. Body temperature of the patient must be maintained during transport and subsequent recovery.

Emesis

Emetics are used to induce vomiting in order to empty the stomach contents. This may be required prior to surgery or more often as a means of eliminating poisonous substances following accidental ingestion. The veterinary nurse may be required to carry out this procedure or she may need to advise clients on how to give an emetic in an emergency. Methods for emesis are given in Chapter 3, p. 33.

> **WARNING**
>
> Emesis is contraindicated in cases of corrosive poisoning or for unconscious or convulsing patients.

Bandaging

The veterinary nurse should be:

- Competent in carrying out routine bandaging procedures.
- Familiar with the more specialised techniques.
- Capable of advising the client on care and protection of the bandage.
- Able to recognise the need for attention or removal of bandaging.

Dressing materials

Various types of dressings are available. They are applied in direct contact with the surface of the skin:

- **Dry dressings** absorb pus or fluid from the wound.
- **Impregnated gauze dressings** may be applied to wounds that need to be kept moist, e.g. burns and scalds.

REASONS FOR BANDAGING

Support
- Fractures or dislocations.
- Sprains or strains.
- Healing wounds.

Protection
- Self-mutilation.
- Infection.
- Environment.

Pressure
- To arrest haemorrhage.
- To prevent or control swelling.

Immobilisation
- To restrict joint movement.
- To restrict movement at fracture site.
- To provide comfort and pain relief.

These dressings are petroleum or Vaseline based and may be impregnated with antibiotic, corticosteroid or chlorhexidine, see Management of wounds, p. 492.

Padding materials

These provide the intermediate layer of many dressings. They cushion and support the wound, and they also provide protection to bony prominences and prevent excoriation. They may be made from natural or man-made fibres, including:

- **Cotton wool**, a natural fibre which is cheap and has good absorptive properties.
- **Softban**, a soft, natural padding material available on rolls of varying width and thickness.
- **Foam**, a useful padding material also available on rolls.

Bandaging materials

These are applied to protect the wound and to hold dressings in place. They include:

- **White open weave**, a natural bandage which is strong and firm, but has the disadvantage of not conforming to the patient's body and a tendency for the cotton fibres to fray.
- **Conforming bandage**, the bandage of choice for most dressings, provides a strong neat bandage that conforms to the patient's body.
- **Cohesive bandage** has self-adhering properties but does not stick to hair or skin. It is strong, flexible and conforming.
- **Tubular bandage**, an elasticated cotton or nylon bandage applied with the use of an applicator, is particularly useful for bandaging limbs or the tail.
- **Crepe bandage**, not frequently used in veterinary practice but it has the advantage of being washable and

therefore may be reused. It conforms to the larger parts of the animal's body and is useful for head and thorax bandaging.

Covering materials

These form the outer layer of the dressing and provide support and protection:

- **Zinc oxide tape**, an adhesive, inelastic, relatively non-conforming material with a tendency to fray. More commonly used as a traction tape.
- **Elastoplast**, an adhesive, elastic material which provides a neat, conforming protective layer.
- **Non-adhesive tape**, a material that will adhere to itself but not to the patient.

Casting materials

- **Fibreglass cast**, a rigid, lightweight material that provides a strong, fast setting cast.
- **Plaster of Paris**, a roll of gauze impregnated with calcium sulphate dihydrate. It is applied by immersing the roll in hot water and winding around the affected part in the manner of a bandage. Once dry, it sets to a hard supportive conforming cast.

Common bandaging techniques

Limb

Limbs are frequently bandaged in veterinary practice to provide protection and support for cuts, torn dew claws and surgical procedures. Various materials may be utilised, including narrow open-weave bandage, conforming bandage or elasticated tubular gauze.

STANDARD PROCEDURE FOR LIMB BANDAGE (Fig. 2.3)

(1) The patient is suitably restrained.
(2) In order to absorb sweat and prevent irritation, cotton wool is placed between the patient's toes, pads and dew claws.
(3) Apply a layer of cotton wool or soft ban around the foot.
(4) Apply the conforming bandage longitudinally to the cranial and caudal surface of the limb and then turn it to wind around the limb in a figure-of-eight pattern. This ensures an even tension throughout the bandage. The bandage is anchored over the hock or carpus.
(5) Apply an external layer of adhesive tape in the same manner.

Ear

One or both ears are often bandaged following trauma, bleeding from ulcerated ear tips or surgical procedures such as aural haematoma or resection.

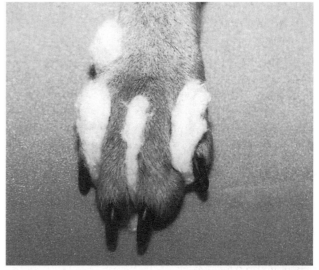

(a)

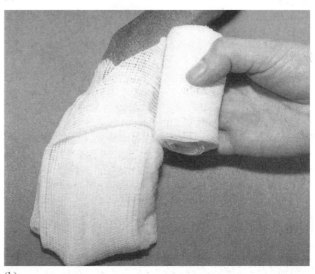

(b)

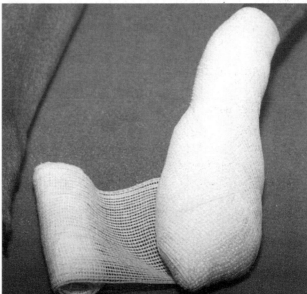

(c)

Fig. 2.3 Procedure for limb bandage: (a) padding between the toes; (b) applying the conforming bandage longitudinally; (c) winding the conforming bandage in a figure-of-eight. Photographs courtesy of Roy Hancocks and Rachel Meredith.

PROCEDURE FOR SINGLE EAR (Fig. 2.4)

(1) Place a pad of cotton wool on the top of the patient's head. Fold the ear back onto the pad.
(2) Apply a dry dressing and place a further pad of cotton wool over the ear.
(3) Apply conforming bandage over the ear and then under the chin; anchor it on either side of the free ear.
(4) The bandage may be covered with adhesive tape.

It is important that the ear bandage is not applied too tightly. The patient should be able to open its mouth normally and its respiration must not be obstructed.

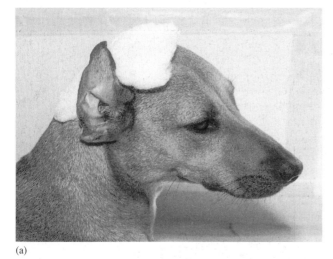

(a)

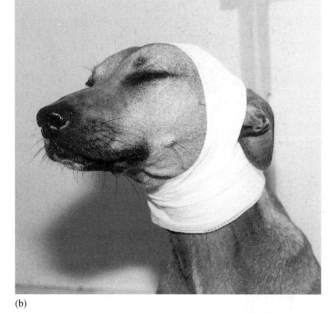

(b)

Fig. 2.4 Procedure for ear bandage: (a) padding the top of the head; (b) the conforming bandage in place. Photographs courtesy of Roy Hancocks and Rachel Meredith.

Abdomen

The abdomen is occasionally bandaged following trauma or surgery. Apply conforming bandage around the abdomen and secure with adhesive tape or tubular gauze. The bandage may have to be extended forwards to the axilla to stop it 'bunching up' later. Care should be taken to prevent the bandage rubbing on the exposed ventral surface of the abdomen – use cotton wool padding or apply Vaseline.

Chest

The procedure for bandaging the abdomen also applies to the chest. The bandage may be anchored between the front legs in figure-of-eight fashion. See Fig. 2.5.

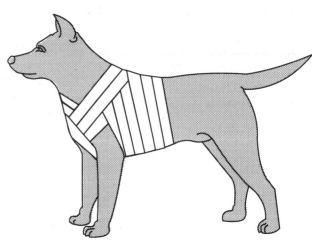

Fig. 2.5 Chest bandage.

Tail

A light bandage may be required following trauma to the tail or amputation of vertebrae. This can be one of the most difficult areas for keeping a bandage in place. See Fig. 2.6.

Specialised bandaging techniques

The three most common special techniques are:

- **Ehmer sling**, to support the hind limb following reduction of hip luxation.
- **Velpeau sling**, to support the shoulder joint following luxation or surgery.
- **Robert Jones bandage**, to provide support and immobilisation to fractured limbs in a first aid situation or following surgery.

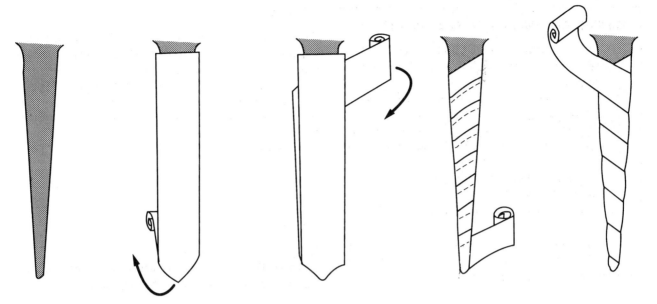

Fig. 2.6 Tail bandage.

PROCEDURE FOR EHMER SLING (Fig. 2.7)

(1) Apply padding material to the metatarsus and stifle.
(2) Flex the leg and rotate the foot inwards. This will force the hip joint into the acetabulum.
(3) Apply conforming bandage to the metatarsus, bringing it medial to the stifle joint.
(4) Continue the bandage over the thigh and back to the metatarsus in a figure-of-eight motion.
(5) Repeat until full support of the hip is achieved.
(6) The bandage is then held in place with adhesive tape.

This dressing is usually kept in place for 4–5 days.

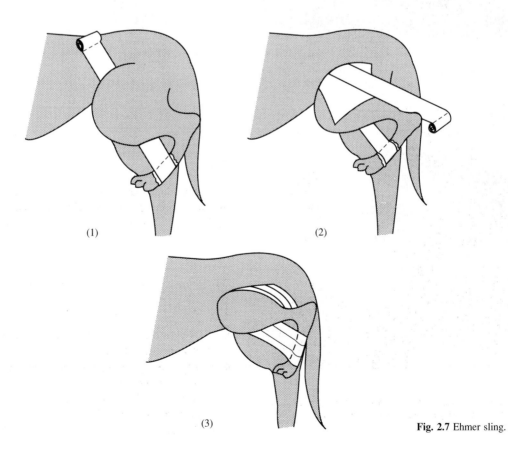

(1)

(2)

(3)

Fig. 2.7 Ehmer sling.

PROCEDURE FOR VELPEAU SLING (Fig. 2.8)

This is applied to support the shoulder joint following luxation or surgery.

(1) Apply a layer of padding material to the foreleg.
(2) Apply conforming bandage to the paw.
(3) Hold the leg in flexion and apply the bandage over the elbow, then over the shoulder and round the chest.
(4) Repeat until full support of the shoulder is achieved.
(5) The dressing is then secured using adhesive tape.

PROCEDURE FOR ROBERT JONES BANDAGE (Fig. 2.9)

(1) Apply zinc oxide traction tapes to the dorsal and ventral surfaces of the foot.
(2) Take cotton wool from the roll and wrap it tightly around the leg and foot. A large quantity should be used to support the limb.
(3) Apply conforming bandage firmly to the padded leg.
(4) Incorporate the traction tapes into the bandage to prevent slipping.
(5) Cover the bandage with adhesive tape for protection and extra support.

On completion, the foot should be visible so that checks may be made for oedema and temperature. This bandage may be kept in place for up to 2 weeks. Occasionally the toes are included in the bandage.

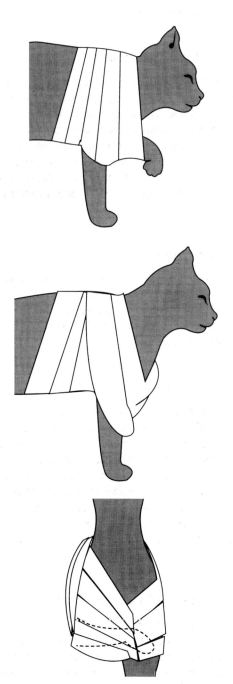

Fig. 2.8 Making a Velpeau sling.

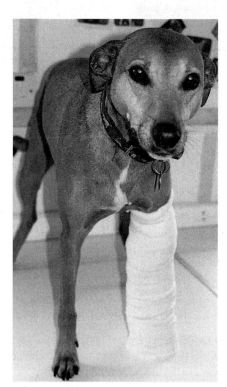

Fig. 2.9 Robert Jones bandage in place. Photograph courtesy of Roy Hancocks and Rachel Meredith.

Care of bandages and dressings

Once the bandage has been applied, constant checks should be maintained until it is removed. Any evidence of odour, oedema, discharge or skin irritation should be reported to the veterinary surgeon. The bandage should be checked to ensure it is not too tight or uncomfortable.

It is important that the dressing does not become soiled or wet. This may be prevented by covering it with a plastic bag when the patient is taken outside.

Constant chewing or licking at the bandage by the patient should be discouraged. If this persists, try one of the following measures:

● Discipline.
● Elizabethan collar (Fig. 2.10).
● Muzzle.
● Application of foul-tasting substance to dressing.
● Sedation.

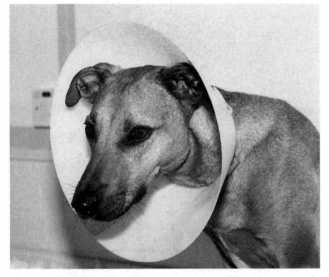

Fig. 2.10 Elizabethan collar. Photograph courtesy of Roy Hancocks and Rachel Meredith.

Local applications of heat and cold

Heat may be provided by applying cotton wool soaked in hot water or by means of a poultice prepared with medicants such as kaolin. The hot application will cause vasodilatation and therefore increased blood supply to the affected area. This will provide white blood cells for wound healing and assist in fluid removal from the area. The application of heat is indicated in cases of:

● Oedema.
● Infected wounds.
● Abscesses.

Cold may be provided by applying gauze soaked in cold water or an ice pack. Burns and scalds should be flushed with cold water from the tap. The cold application will cause vasoconstriction, therefore reducing heat and blood loss. The application of cold is indicated in cases of:

● Pain.
● Haemorrhage.
● Minor burns and scalds.
● Heatstroke.

Administration of medicines

Drug classification, dosage and administration are considered in depth in Chapter 12. The following section is a short introduction to the subject.

Medicines may be administered via various routes:

● **Orally** in the form of tablets, capsules, liquids, pastes or powders.
● **Rectally** in the form of an enema or suppository.
● **Parenterally** by intravenous, subcutaneous or intramuscular injection.
● **Topically** to the skin, eyes, ears, nose or mucous membranes.

Choose the route that is the most appropriate for the patient and for the drug. The following factors should be considered before drugs are administered:

● Pharmacological properties.
● Rate of absorption.
● The patient.
● Convenience for the administrator.

Pharmacological properties

It is essential that the drug to be administered is compatible with the chosen route. Some drugs will not be adequately absorbed from the gastrointestinal tract if given orally, whereas others (e.g. pancreatic enzymes extract) must be given via this route as they act on the digestive system. Some drugs may be dangerous if not administered via the recommended route. If thiopentone sodium is injected subcutaneously, it causes irritation and sloughing of the skin.

Rate of absorption

The requirements for the onset of action of the administered drug should be considered. Generally an intravenous injection will have the fastest action, followed (in descending order) by intramuscular injection, subcutaneous injection and the oral route.

The patient

The condition and temperament of the patient will influence the route of drug administration. It may not be possible to administer drugs to an aggressive patient via the oral, topical or intravenous routes, and therefore an alternative route should be used. Administration of oral drugs to patients with respiratory embarrassment or mouth trauma such as a fractured jaw may cause pain or distress and should be avoided. Continued use of the same injection site may cause soreness and pain and should be minimised if possible.

Convenience of the administrator

Most clients will be able to give drugs orally to their animals and this will allow treatment to be given in the familiar surroundings of home. For the veterinary surgeon or nurse, however, it may be more convenient to administer drugs parenterally.

Routes for the administration of drugs

Systemic routes are those by which the drug affects the body as a whole. They include oral, rectal and parenteral routes.

Oral

Drugs are administered orally in the form of tablets, capsules, powder/granules or liquids. The advantages of oral medicines are:

- Usually the least painful route.
- Easily administered by the client.
- Least risk of introduction of infection, as the skin is not penetrated.

The disadvantages are:

- Possibility of aspiration of medication into respiratory tract, causing choking.
- Variable rate of absorption, depending on metabolic rate, age and condition of patient, motility, and contents of digestive tract.
- May cause irritation or vomiting.
- Patients may not tolerate administration.
- May be difficult to ensure the correct dosage.

Tablets consist of a compressed, moulded mass of drug and may be coated for the following reasons:

- To protect them from moisture.
- To disguise an unpleasant taste.
- To protect the drug (e.g. from hydrochloric acid in the stomach).
- To give a recognisable colour.

Capsules consist of two sections, made of soluble gelatin, fitted together to enclose a powdered drug.

Powders/granules are produced for addition to food or water. They are particularly suitable for the treatment of:

- Young animals.
- Small creatures, such as birds or hamsters.
- Digestive diseases.

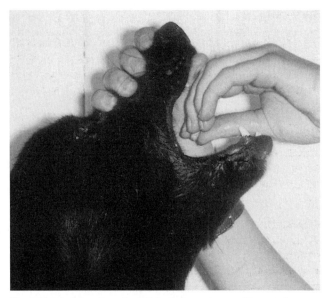

Fig. 2.11 Administration of a tablet via the oral route. Photograph courtesy of Roy Hancocks and Rachel Meredith.

It is important to take precautions when administering cytotoxic drugs as the drug may be inhaled or absorbed through the skin causing irritation or carcinogenic effects.

RECOMMENDATIONS FOR ADMINISTERING CYTOTOXIC DRUGS

(1) Wear gloves, apron and mask.
(2) Do not dispense on surfaces where food is prepared.
(3) Protect work surfaces with disposable absorbent sheets.
(4) Dispose of packaging in a safe manner to comply with COSHH regulations.
(5) Wash hands thoroughly after handling.

Liquid medicines may be in the form of:

- **Solutions** – drugs dissolved in liquid (e.g. glucose solution).
- **Suspensions** – insoluble substance dispensed in liquid (e.g. kaolin and water).
- **Syrup/linctus** – drugs contained in a concentrated sugar solution.
- **Emulsion** – a mixture of two immiscible liquids.

PROCEDURE FOR ORAL ADMINISTRATION OF TABLETS OR CAPSULES (Fig. 2.11)

(1) The patient should be restrained as gently as possible.
(2) The tablet may be lubricated with butter or oil for ease of swallowing.
(3) Open the animal's mouth by placing one hand over the muzzle, while the other hand is used to hold the tablet and also to pull down the lower jaw.
(4) Place the tablet on the base of the patient's tongue.
(5) Close the mouth and stroke the neck to ensure swallowing.

PROCEDURE FOR ORAL ADMINISTRATION OF LIQUID MEDICATION

(1) The liquid should be placed in a syringe for ease of administration.
(2) The patient's head should be tilted back.
(3) Place the syringe into the side of the mouth behind the canine teeth.
(4) Slowly administer the liquid to the back of the throat.
(5) Stroke the neck to ensure swallowing.

Rectal

The rectal route is not commonly used in small animal practice, but drugs such as liquid paraffin or glycerine may be administered in the form of an enema or suppository. Details of enemata are given in Chapter 16 (General Nursing), p. 403.

Parenteral

This term describes the administration of medicines via routes not involving the alimentary canal. This may be achieved using hypodermic injections given via the following routes:

● Subcutaneous.
● Intramuscular.
● Intravenous.
● Intracardiac.
● Intraperitoneal.
● Intrapleural.
● Intra-articular.
● Epidural.

The choice of route should be decided by considering the condition and temperament of the patient, the properties and volume of the drug to be administered, and the desired speed of effect. Hypodermic injections are most commonly administered via the subcutaneous, intramuscular and intravenous routes.

Subcutaneous injections. The loose skin from the back of the neck to the rump is the most common site for the administration of this injection (Fig. 2.12). This area is suitable because of its poor supply of nerves and large blood vessels. Only non-irritant drugs should be administered via

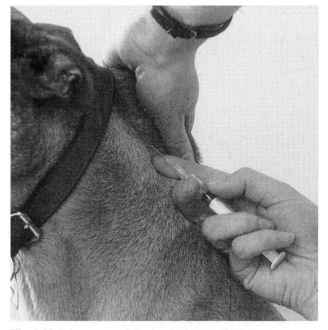

Fig. 2.12 Subcutaneous injection in the scruff. Photograph courtesy of Roy Hancocks and Rachel Meredith.

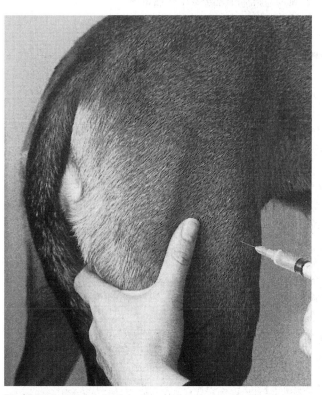

Fig. 2.13 Intramuscular injection in the quadriceps. Photograph courtesy of Roy Hancocks and Rachel Meredith.

this route as there may be irritation or necrosis of tissues. Action following subcutaneous injection will take effect after 30–45 minutes.

Intramuscular injections. The most common site for intramuscular injections is the quadriceps group of muscles in front of the femur (Fig. 2.13). The lumbodorsal muscles and triceps muscles may also be used. The gluteal muscles of the buttocks and the hamstring muscle group should

---

PROCEDURE FOR SUBCUTANEOUS INJECTION (Fig. 2.12)

(1) Prepare the injection by selecting a sterile needle and syringe. Draw up the required volume of drugs.
(2) The patient should be suitably restrained.
(3) Raise a fold of skin from a suitable area.
(4) Moisten the skin with a spirit swab to flatten the hair and remove surface dirt. (Spirit should not be used when injecting a vaccine, as it may inactivate the drug.)
(5) Insert the needle under the skin and withdraw the syringe plunger slightly. If blood appears in the syringe, a blood vessel has been punctured and a new site must be selected.
(6) If no blood appears, the drug may be injected into the patient.
(7) Massage the injection site gently to disperse the drug.
(8) Make detailed records of the medication given.
(9) Dispose of needle and syringe safely

PROCEDURE FOR A CEPHALIC VEIN INJECTION (Fig. 2.14)

(1) The patient, either sitting or in sternal recumbency, should be restrained by an assistant.

(2) The assistant should restrain the patient's head with one hand and use the other hand to extend the leg and 'raise' the vein by applying pressure around the elbow joint with the thumb.

(3) The operator should stabilise the vein and insert the needle through the sterilised and alcohol-cleaned skin into the vein. Blood should flow gently into the syringe.

(4) The assistant should then release the pressure on the vein and the operator may gently introduce the drug into circulation. If large volumes of fluid are to be injected, regular checks should be made to ensure that the needle remains in the vein (by occasionally drawing back a little blood).

(5) Once the injection has been administered, the needle may be removed from the vein and pressure applied to the injection site for a minimum of 30 seconds, to prevent haemorrhage.

be avoided, as there is a danger of bone or sciatic nerve damage.

Because of the density of muscle tissue, large amounts of fluid may be very painful if injected via this route. The maximum administration should be 2 ml in the cat and 5 ml in the dog.

Action following intramuscular injection will take effect after 20–30 minutes.

The technique is similar to that for the subcutaneous route except that the needle should be inserted at right angles into the muscle mass.

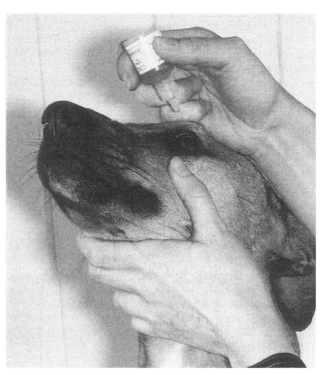

Fig. 2.15 Application of drops to the eye. Photograph courtesy of Roy Hancocks and Rachel Meredith.

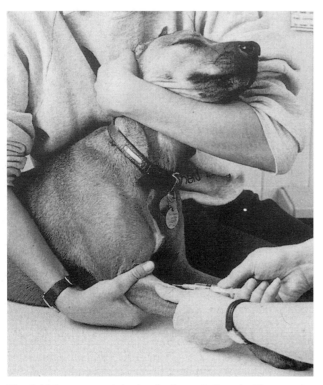

Fig. 2.14 Intravenous injection in the cephalic vein. Photograph courtesy of Roy Hancocks and Rachel Meredith.

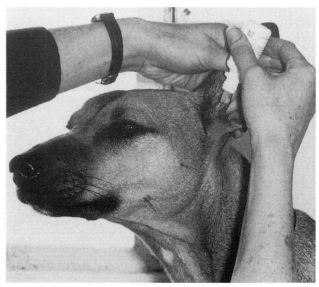

Fig. 2.16 Application of drops to the ear. Photograph courtesy of Roy Hancocks and Rachel Meredith.

Intravenous injections. The common sites for intravenous injection are the cephalic vein in the forelimb, the lateral saphenous vein in the hindlimb and the jugular vein in the neck. The sublingual vein may be used in an anaesthetised or unconscious patient.

Action following intravenous injections will take effect in 0–2 minutes.

Topical

This refers to the application of medication to the external surfaces of the body, e.g. the skin, the eyes and the ears.

The skin. Skin treatment may be applied in the form of:

- **Shampoo** – a solution applied to the whole body by bathing.
- **Ointment** – drugs in a base of wax or jelly acting on the skin surface.
- **Cream** – a semi-solid emulsion which penetrates the skin surface.

The eyes. Eye medication may be applied in the form of drops or ointment. For either medium, the animal's head is tilted back and its eye is held open with the fingers. When applying any substance to the eye, the surface of the cornea should never be touched by the fingers or the nozzle of the applicator.

Drops are applied by dropping liquid on to the centre of the eyeball (Fig. 2.15).

Ointment is applied by gently squeezing a line of the drug on to the inner canthus of the eye, taking care not to touch the surface of the eye with the nozzle or finger. It is often best to approach the patient from the side when using eye ointment, rather than a face-to-face confrontational approach.

After the medication has been applied, the patient should be allowed to blink to disperse the drug evenly over the eye.

The ears. Ear medication may be applied in the form of drops or ointment. The ear should be free from wax and discharge before application. The patient should be restrained and its pinna held firmly. Introduce the nozzle of the applicator into the ear canal and apply the contents gently (Fig. 2.16). Gently massage the external auditory meatus to ensure maximum coverage by the medication.

3

First aid

S. Hiscock

First aid is the immediate treatment of injured animals or those suffering from sudden illness.

Limitations

Under the terms of the Veterinary Surgeons' Act of 1966, no person is allowed to practise veterinary surgery unless registered in the veterinary surgeons' register maintained by the Royal College of Veterinary Surgeons or in the supplementary register to veterinary practitioners. However, amendment to Schedule 3 of that Act in 1991 made special provisions for those whose names are entered in the College's list of veterinary nurses, and their rights and powers are described in more detail in Chapter 7 (The Law and Ethics of Veterinary Nursing).

These changes in the law empower a listed veterinary nurse to do considerably more than a lay person, **but only at the direction of a veterinary surgeon**. In an emergency, when no veterinary surgeon is immediately available to give directions, the veterinary nurse is no different in law from any lay person and, in common with lay persons, has the right to administer first aid treatment to an animal by whatever means are available, **but only as an interim measure, designed to preserve life and alleviate suffering until a veterinary surgeon is able to attend to the animal.**

An example is the passing of a stomach tube in a case of gastric dilatation. This will instantly ease the pain and suffering of the patient and may well be life-saving, and therefore is perfectly permissible. However, any attempts to give medical treatment or gastric lavage through that stomach tube (unless directed to do so by a veterinary surgeon) would exceed the powers given to a veterinary nurse under Schedule 3 as they would not constitute first aid treatments. They are long-term rather than interim measures and do not save the animal's life or lessen its suffering. Wherever possible the veterinary nurse should ask for directions from the veterinary surgeon as soon as possible.

Although in theory veterinary nurses do not have greater powers in law than lay people, in practice they have greater knowledge and training and are obviously far better equipped to assess an emergency case and provide appropriate first aid treatment for the animal until a veterinary surgeon arrives.

Aims and rules of first aid

First aid treatment is based on three aims and four rules. The three aims are:

- To preserve life.
- To prevent suffering.
- To prevent the situation deteriorating.

The four rules are:

- Don't panic!
- Maintain the airway.
- Control the haemorrhage.
- Contact the veterinary surgeon as soon as possible.

If you forget everything else when faced with an emergency case, don't forget these four rules!

Telephone calls

An emergency can be classified as one of three types:

- Life-threatening emergencies, requiring immediate action by the owner at home and the nurse at the surgery.
- Emergencies requiring immediate attention at the surgery but where life is not immediately threatened and there is no action the owner must take at home.
- Minor emergencies where telephone advice enables the owner to alleviate suffering until a veterinary surgeon is able to attend the patient.

Examples of each type are given in Table 3.1.

Immediate classification of an emergency may not be easy over the telephone because owners are often in a panic when they ring the surgery for help. It must be remembered that animals are usually very precious to their owners – emotionally, financially or both. Therefore the owner is rarely able to judge the severity of the illness or injury and may consider that questioning by the veterinary nurse is a waste of valuable time. Bearing these points in mind, the nurse must remain calm but sympathetic and patient (which may not be easy!) and ask specific questions clearly and concisely.

When taking the history, it is always best to speak directly to the owner because 'second-hand' conversations are frustrating and time-consuming and lead to inaccuracies. There are seven basic questions to be asked:

(1) What is the *nature* of the injury (e.g. scalding due to a household accident, haemorrhage from a deep cut, insect sting)? If **poisoning** is suspected, does the owner

Table 3.1 Examples of types of emergencies		
Life-threatening	**Immediate attention**	**Minor**
Unconsciousness	Conscious collapse	Insect stings
Conscious collapse with dyspnoea or cyanosis	Dyspnoea	Minor wounds (where the haemorrhage is easily controlled by bandaging)
Severe haemorrhage	Fractures/dislocations	Minor burns (where there is only slight discomfort)
Severe burns	Haemorrhage	Abscesses
Prolapsed eye	Gaping wounds	Slight lameness (where animal is able to bear some weight on the leg)
Poisoning	Severe dysuria	Haematuria
Snake bites	Dystocia	Aural haematoma

know which poison is involved? (On this subject, further questions during history-taking are suggested in the Poisoning section of this chapter, p. 31.)

(2) What is the *extent* or degree of the injury? Is the animal conscious or unconscious? Is it able to breathe freely? How severe is any haemorrhage? What is the general appearance of the animal?

(3) *When* did the accident happen, or when was the illness first noticed? If the animal is collapsed, was it seen to fall or was it found in the collapsed state? Has the animal's condition improved or deteriorated and how rapidly has any such change occurred?

(4) What age, sex and breed is the patient?

(5) Is it receiving any current veterinary treatment (e.g. insulin injections if a diabetic or NSAIDs if a gastric haemorrhage is reported)?

(6) If injured or taken ill away from home, where exactly is the animal?

(7) What is the owner's name, address and telephone number? (This is very important in case the veterinary surgeon needs more information before deciding on a course of action.)

It is often best to ask these questions in the order set out above because it immediately allows the owner to talk about the problem. It shows that the person receiving the 'phone call is experienced and this in itself gives the owner confidence. There is nothing more frustrating and upsetting for an anguished owner than someone insisting on taking their name and address whilst refusing to listen to details of their pet's illness. Once they have talked to the veterinary nurse and received some reassurance, or been told what to do, they very often calm down and can lucidly give their names, addresses and 'phone numbers. For safety, addresses and 'phone numbers should be repeated back to the caller.

History taking is very important because it enables the nurse to:

● Decide on the type of emergency.
● Give the owner relevant instructions on immediate first aid measures to be carried out in the home (e.g. how to maintain the airway of an unconscious pet).
● Make the necessary preparations to receive the patient at the surgery (e.g. prepare dressings for open wounds).

Handling and transport of the injured animal

Unless life is endangered by falling masonry, fire, poisonous atmosphere, etc., no attempt should be made to move an immobile or collapsed accident victim until it has been given a brief examination. This will ensure that injuries can be adequately protected during handling. The walking wounded may be handled as described later.

General advice on handling and transport is given in Chapter 1 but emergency situations away from the surgery often call for different techniques and a degree of ingenuity.

Approaching the injured animal

An injured animal is usually frightened and shocked which means that it is liable to bite and scratch viciously if cornered or approached too quickly. The gentle approach is usually best but it should not be hesitant. Slow, deliberate movements accompanied by the continuous gentle reassurance of the human voice can do much to calm the anxious patient.

Cats

Shocked and injured cats are not usually aggressive when approached. Observe the animal closely whilst extending the hand to stroke it under its chin. If this is permitted, slide the hand around the cat's face to stroke its neck and then gently grasp its scruff. The animal is now restrained and an examination can be made.

If the animal reacts aggressively when approached, do not attempt to grasp it as this may only provoke an attack or an attempted escape. In these cases an inverted box or basket should be lowered gently over the cat to confine it and a thin piece of hardboard or strong cardboard slid slowly under the inverted box so that the cat comes to lie on it. The whole may then be lifted and made secure for transport to the surgery.

If no box or basket is available, a thick coat or blanket can be thrown gently over the patient but the nurse should be very careful to ensure the head is restrained by grasping the scruff through the material before attempting to lift the animal. Canine teeth can puncture thick material and leather gloves, so this approach must only be used in dire situations.

Dogs

Frightened injured dogs are much more inclined to snap at an approaching human, especially a stranger. Even the dog's owner may be bitten if a normally placid pet is in pain from its injuries. If there is any indication of aggression, form a looped lead as a running 'noose' and try to drop it over the dog's head. Leather leads are better than chain or material ones because the noose tends to hang as an open loop and it is easier to position it around the dog's neck.

Some dogs react to the lead, biting and snapping at the noose as it is lowered towards the head. This makes restraint difficult and, unless there is a 'dog-catcher' available, it is often necessary to ask someone else to stand in front of the dog (at a safe distance), talking to it and **maintaining constant eye contact**. The veterinary nurse can then approach the dog from behind and lower the lead over its head.

Many dogs immediately feel more secure if they are on a lead with a human in control but they still might bite. A muzzle should therefore be tied in place before handling **unless the dog is dyspnoeic or the dog's face is injured**.

Once the animal is under control, a brief but thorough examination should be carried out:

- The **airway** must be checked and cleared if necessary (see Resuscitation, p. 85 and Asphyxia, p. 90).
- **Haemorrhage** must be controlled (see p. 43).
- **Fractures** should be immobilised with splints or dressings if possible (see Fractures, p. 57).
- **Wounds** should be dressed (see Wounds, p. 50).

The patient should then be restrained as gently as possible until it can be transported to the surgery or until a veterinary surgeon can attend the animal. The patient should be allowed to assume the position which it finds most comfortable and most injured animals will lie on the wounded side. This distresses owners but the patient should not be interfered with if it seems to be comfortable. The owner should be asked to stay with the animal to reassure and comfort it.

Transport to the surgery

The aim is to remove the injured animal to the surgery with minimum discomfort to the patient and without disturbing any dressings that have been applied. There are two groups of animals: the ambulatory (able to walk) and the non-ambulatory.

Ambulatory

An ambulatory dog is one that can rise to its feet and is able to walk, even if only to limp slowly. Often these dogs are transported less painfully and with less stress if they are allowed to move themselves rather than submitting to the restrictions of being carried. Gentle encouragement should be used to guide the animal to the transport vehicle, but the patient may need assistance to climb into it.

Non-ambulatory

Lifting in the owner's arms

WARNING

None of the following methods should be used for badly injured animals, e.g. cases of suspected spinal fracture, and the last method must not be used in cases of suspected abdominal or thoracic injury or if the patient is severely dyspnoeic.

Small dogs and cats may be held firmly round the neck with one hand (taking care not to obstruct the breathing) whilst the other hand and arm are slid around the sternum to scoop the body up, supporting the weight along the length of the forearm (Fig. 3.1). The foreleg furthest from the handler's body can then be held firmly in the left hand, to prevent the animal scrabbling to get free, whilst the handler's right hand continues to hold the neck gently in extension, like a wide collar, so that the animal is unable to turn its head round or down to bite the handler.

Medium-sized dogs may be lifted with one arm encircling the front of the sternum, the other around the back of the pelvis to support the hindquarters. The animal is then held against the handler's chest (Fig. 3.2). To prevent injury to the human back, always lift the dog with an almost straight back, using bent knees to provide most of the lifting effort and always ask for help if the dog seems too heavy for one person.

Large heavy dogs should be lifted by two or more people. One person stands at the dog's shoulder with one arm curled around the dog's neck, holding its head against the handler's shoulder to control it, with the other arm under and around its thorax, just behind its forelegs. The second person stands by the hindquarters and places one arm under the abdomen, just in front of the hindlegs, and the other around the pelvis (Fig. 3.3).

Boxes and baskets. These are suitable for cats and small dogs. Types range from wire, wicker or wooden cages to cardboard boxes, laundry baskets, washing baskets and any other containers that might be to hand in an emergency. There are three important criteria:

- The basket should be **escape-proof**. Cardboard boxes, etc., should have a lid firmly secured across the open top.
- **Ventilation** must be adequate. Mesh sides are safer than solid-wall boxes.
- **Constant observation** of the patient must be possible. Wire baskets and plastic laundry baskets are best for this.

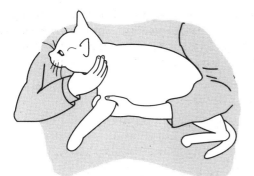

Fig. 3.1 Carrying a small patient.

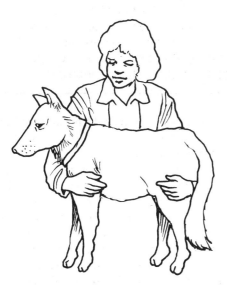

Fig. 3.2 Carrying a medium-sized dog.

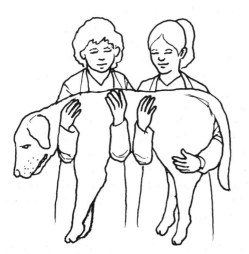

Fig. 3.3 Carrying a large dog.

Lifting badly injured animals. If the animal is collapsed and severe injuries are suspected, it should be lifted with great care to lessen the pain and distress and to prevent further injury.

If the patient is to be transported in a cage or basket, find a sheet of hardboard or thick cardboard which is the same size as the basket or box (or slightly smaller) and slide this gently under the patient. The animal can then be picked up on the support and placed in the container with minimal disturbance.

If no such support is readily to hand, hold the animal's scruff with one hand (to control the head and stop the animal from biting). Slide the other hand, palm up, under the body trunk at the hindquarters and work the hand forwards until the patient's body is laid along the forearm. The animal can then be lifted, using the forearm as a rigid stretcher, and laid gently in the container by reversing the procedure (Fig. 3.4).

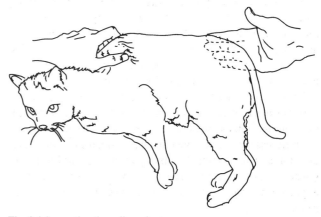

Fig. 3.4 Supporting the collapsed cat.

If the patient is too aggressive to allow either procedure, it may be less distressing and painful if it is lifted up bodily by the scruff in one hand, with minimal gentle support of the hindquarters by the other hand, and placed gently and carefully in the basket, accomplishing the manoeuvre as smoothly and as quickly as possible to minimise the length of painful handling.

Stretchers. Stretchers should always be used to transport the following cases if the animals are too large to fit into boxes or baskets:

- Suspected spinal fractures.
- Collapse with dyspnoea.
- Collapse with thoracic or abdominal injuries.
- Collapse and unconsciousness (these dogs are very difficult to pick up without some support).
- Other severely injured animals, e.g. those with severe lacerations or multiple broken bones, when handling would be too painful for the patient.

The principle is to have a flat, rigid object which is big and strong enough to support the animal in lateral recumbency, yet small enough to fit into the transport vehicle. Stretchers can be improvised from:

- Wood or hardboard sheets (very good for small or medium-sized dogs).
- Wire mesh or plastic-coated fencing wire. (This can only be used if there are two handlers to stretch the wire taut when lifting the animal so that the wire provides a firm support.)
- Sacks or coats mounted on wooden poles. (These are described for human patients in *First Aid, Junior Manual*, British Red Cross Society.)

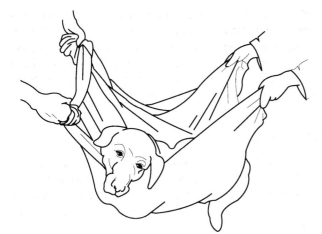

Fig. 3.5 Lifting a large dog with the help of a blanket.

- Blankets. These offer little support for injured spines but may be slid underneath the patient easily (Fig. 3.5) and are usually readily available.

To transfer the patient to the stretcher:

(1) Place the stretcher close to the patient's back as it lies on the ground.
(2) Apply a tape muzzle to a conscious patient if possible, as these animals are often in pain and might bite when handled.
(3) Roll the patient half on to its chest and push the stretcher underneath the animal as far as possible. Then allow the animal to collapse on to its side again and thus on to the stretcher. Several people should help in the transfer and should try to move the animal as a unit, avoiding any twisting of the spine if a spinal injury is suspected (Fig. 3.6a).
(4) Alternatively, grasp the skin along the back at several points – above the scapula, midway along the back and above the pelvis. The patient may now be pulled the short distance on to the stretcher (Fig. 3.6b). This is

(a)

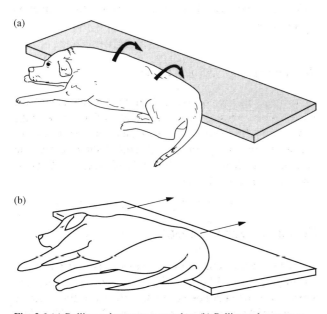

(b)

Fig. 3.6 (a) Rolling a dog on to a stretcher. (b) Pulling a dog on to a stretcher.

particularly useful in cases of spinal damage and fractured limbs as it does not involve twisting the spine, body or limbs. A tape muzzle is strongly advised for this procedure.

Care in transit

Within the vehicle, the patient needs to be observed constantly and restrained to ensure that:

- The condition does not deteriorate.
- Any dressings are not disturbed.
- The animal does not escape from its container (or fall off the seat if it is too large to be contained).
- The animal cannot interfere with the driver of the vehicle.

It is important to have a second person in the vehicle – preferably the owner, who will be able to give a full case history at the surgery and who will want to be with the pet anyway. The owner's presence may also help to calm the patient.

If it is impossible or impractical for a second person to accompany the animal, the ambulatory patient must be restrained on a lead which is securely fastened inside the vehicle. Often the simplest way is to shut the lead in the car door as it is closed, leaving the handle of the lead protruding on the outside of the car. This method has three advantages:

- The dog is securely restrained.
- The animal cannot escape from the vehicle at the last minute as the door is being closed, because the lead is either held by the handler or is jammed in the closed door.
- On arrival at the surgery, the handler can take hold of the lead before opening the door, thus avoiding losing the dog if it makes a bolt for freedom.

Arrival at the surgery

On admission, the animal should be examined, a provisional diagnosis made and treatment given. To avoid errors in treatment when several casualties arrive at the same time, it may be necessary to identify each accident victim individually. Labels can be attached to dogs' collars or identity bands fixed around the front or back leg of each animal.

Examination of the patient

It is necessary to take a full case history and to examine the animal thoroughly in order to make a tentative diagnosis and give the appropriate first aid treatment. Any diagnosis must always be provisional until confirmed by a veterinary surgeon and, if there is any doubt as to the severity of the injury, **the worst should always be assumed** and the patient treated accordingly.

WARNING

Unconscious animals should always take priority and must be examined and treated immediately, as follows:

(1) Check the throat for obstructions and clear the airway as quickly as possible.
(2) Check the heart to see if it is beating. If nothing is detected, start cardiac massage immediately.
(3) Check for respiratory movements. If the animal is not breathing, start artificial respiration. If the patient is trying to breathe, supply oxygen to prevent hypoxia.
(4) Control any severe haemorrhage.
(5) Once the heartbeat is steady, the respiration is maintained (either by the animal on its own or by artificial respiration) and the haemorrhage is controlled, the veterinary nurse may proceed with the more detailed examination.

History taking

A complete and accurate case history can be vitally important in reaching a correct diagnosis. The veterinary nurse will already have a good case history if the owner was able to answer the first six questions outlined previously on pp. 22–23, but further questioning may be needed in cases of suspected poisoning.

It is essential to ask questions about the previous health and treatment (if any) of the animal before the accident or illness because the answers may hold the key to a correct diagnosis. For example, an unconscious bitch may be in a hypoglycaemic coma if she is a known diabetic; or a bitch which has recently had pups may have collapsed because she is hypocalcaemic.

General examination

The first step will have already been completed. The animal has been checked to see that it is alive and that its heart and respiration are functioning adequately. The patient should be observed closely before any attempt is made to touch it, because the general condition and bearing of the patient are important in evaluating the severity of its injuries. The experienced nurse can assess the following three points very quickly whilst taking the case history or even as the patient is carried into the consulting room.

State of consciousness

The unconscious patient must always be treated as a serious case but, in conscious patients, the severity of the injury and risk to life can be more difficult to assess. The animal which follows the movement of human hands with its eyes and responds normally to human voice or touch is less likely to be suffering from potentially fatal injuries. However, the animal which is withdrawn, lies still and seems afraid to move, staring with blank unfocused eyes, is likely to be in serious trouble and severely shocked.

Behaviour

Behaviour is abnormal in some cases. The animal may be excitable, over-reacting to stimuli (**hyperaesthetic**) or, conversely, it may be very depressed and sluggish. Signs of incoordination, muscle tremors or convulsions must be noted.

Respiration

The character and rate of respiration should be observed. Figure 3.28 in the section on Injuries to the respiratory tract illustrates the wide variety of causes which alter the respiratory pattern.

Detailed examination

Ensure that:

● The heart continues to beat steadily.
● Respiration is maintained.
● Severe haemorrhage remains controlled.

Then examine the patient methodically from nose to tail tip, leaving no area of the body unchecked. Table 3.2 sets out the steps for such an examination.

The first aider must be able to appreciate any possible complications which may underlie a seemingly simple wound, e.g. broken bones or penetration of thoracic or abdominal cavities. The mere suspicion that there may be a serious complication can help the nurse to alleviate suffering, preserve life and prevent the situation deteriorating.

Recording the information

Following the examination and first aid treatment of the animal, make notes of the findings and mark the time of the examination. Brain injuries in particular can rapidly deteriorate or improve over short periods and accurate records are an invaluable help in deciding whether the condition is improving or deteriorating.

General nursing care

Accident victims and very ill patients are likely to be severely shocked. Many of the actions taken in first aid nursing are aimed at countering the effects of the shock, a subject which is covered in depth in Chapter 22 (Fluid Therapy and shock).

Table 3.2 Stages of a detailed examination

Nose	Note any haemorrhage (*epistaxis*) and whether it comes from one or both nostrils. Note any swellings which may suggest fracture of the nasal bones

Mouth	• Odours. Carefully open the mouth and smell the breath. Note any unusual smell: e.g. ketones ('pear drops') in cases of untreated diabetics; creosote or phenol in cases of poisoning; urine odour in cases of kidney failure.
	• Haemorrhage. Check for signs of haemorrhage and locate its source, e.g. gums, tongue (dorsal and ventral surfaces), palate, etc. If no injuries are apparent, the blood may have been coughed up from the lungs or issued from wounds in the throat area.
	• Tongue. Check for signs of redness or ulceration, which often occur after licking corrosive poisons.
	• Fractures. Examine the bony structures for signs of fracture: splitting of the hard palate down its centre, jaw fractures.
	• Teeth. Look for any signs of food caked in the crevices. Pesticides are often highly coloured and some evidence may be seen on the teeth if the animal has eaten poisoned bait.
	• Mucosa. Note the colour of the mucosa, which may be:
	
	    (i) normal (pale pink);
	    (ii) congested: brick-red (in toxic or septicaemic animals and heatstroke patients, for example);
	    (iii) pale: may appear white (e.g. in severely shocked patients and those suffering severe haemorrhage);
	    (iv) cyanosed: purple (e.g. patients with severe dyspnoea);
	    (v) jaundiced: orange or yellow (e.g. patients with acute liver damage).
	
	Note whether the mucosa is dry or normally moist, or if the animal is salivating so profusely that it drools. Certain poisons affect the rate of production of saliva.
	If the gums or lips are not darkly pigmented, test the capillary refill by pressing the mucosa to blanch it. In an animal with normal blood pressure, the pink colour returns rapidly within 1–2 seconds of the pressure being removed. In an animal with a low blood pressure, it may take up to 5 seconds before the capillaries refill with blood and the mucosa becomes pink again. This simple test is very helpful in assessing whether the animal has suffered a severe haemorrhage.

Eyes	The eye is a very delicate and sensitive organ and must be treated gently. It is best to examine the animal in a dimly lit or darkened room, where the patient is more likely to open its eye. For detailed examination, an auroscope head or torch may be used to illuminate the eye. • Discharges. Note any discharges of fluid and their appearance and quantity. Clear fluid may indicate that the eyeball has ruptured; purulent discharges could be evidence of a foreign body. • Eyelids. Eyelids can easily be examined for signs of injury and may be opened gently and everted slightly to allow examination of the conjunctiva and nictitating membrane (third eyelid). Check the palpebral reflex and examine the colour of the conjunctival mucosa for an indication of anaemia (pale pink or white), jaundice (yellow) or cyanosis (mauve). • Eyeball. Check for bruising to the sclera or conjunctiva and note any sign of jaundice. Note any injuries to the eyeball, haemorrhage into the anterior chamber, collapsed eyeball, corneal opacity. Note the position of the eyeball in the socket in cases of unconsciousness and any *nystagmus* (involuntary flicking movement of the eyeball from side to side). • Pupils. Note the size of the pupil in each eye and check for response to light. Brain-damaged patients often show a difference in the size of the two pupils; poisoned patients may have very constricted or very dilated pupils which do not respond normally to light.
Skull	Look for signs of depressed fractures, swelling, pain or crepitus. Be very gentle when checking for a suspected fracture of the cranium as heavy handling could depress the bone fragments into the brain cortex and cause enormous damage to the cerebral hemispheres.
Ears	Examine for signs of haemorrhage from the ear canal as this can occur with brain damage.
Limbs	Palpate all limbs, bones and joints, for signs of swelling or pain. In cases of suspected deformity, it is useful to compare the injured leg with its normal partner. If a fracture is suspected, treat it as such pending diagnosis by the veterinary surgeon. Record the way the limb is held and note any obvious *paralysis*: • Flaccid. When the muscles are totally relaxed. • Spastic. When the muscles are contracted to fix the limb rigidly in extension or flexion. Note any loss of feeling, which may be tested by pinching the toes. If the animal is able to feel this stimulus, it will look round at the foot, try to move away or attempt to bite the cause of its discomfort as well as flexing the leg to draw it away from the painful stimulus. This is known as conscious proprioception and should not be confused with the simple withdrawal reflex when the limb is simply flexed to remove it from the pinching stimulus without the animal showing any signs that it is aware of the pain.
Rib cage	Gently palpate for signs of fractured ribs. Listen to any wounds to detect a 'hiss' sound on inspiration which indicates penetration of the pleural cavity.
Abdomen	Palpation of the abdomen is a skilled procedure and can cause considerable harm if attempted by the inexperienced: do not attempt it. Haemorrhage from the penis or bruising or swellings of the abdomen wall should be noted.

Table 3.2 (Continued)

Spine	Note any obvious deformities in the spinal column and gently palpate to detect any gross abnormalities. The spinal column is covered by large muscle trunks and severe spinal fractures are not always obvious. Always assume a fracture is present if there is any doubt. Fractures or dislocations in the cervical region may cause paralysis of all four legs, *quadriplegia*, or, more rarely, paralysis of one side of the body, *hemiplegia*. Fractures or dislocations of the thoracolumbar region may cause paralysis of the hindlegs, *paraplegia*, and many cases show rigid extension of the forelegs and flexion of the hindlegs, with the back arched at the fracture site. It is important to realise that the spinal cord may continue to function normally above and below the fracture site. Thus limb withdrawal reflexes are often unaffected as they are a local reflex arc and do not require input from the brain. However, conscious proprioception may be absent from areas caudal to the spinal injury if nerve impulses are unable to pass to the brain.
Pelvis	Gently palpate the pelvic bones for signs of instability, pain, crepitus and deformity.
Perineal region	The prepuce, vulva and anus should be examined for signs of haemorrhage because signs of blood at these orifices may indicate that internal organs (e.g. the bladder) have been damaged. In cases of paralysis, it is useful to note the presence or absence of the anal ring reflex by watching for anal sphincter contraction when a thermometer is inserted into the anus.
Tail	Observe the signs of voluntary movement, e.g. correct carriage of the tail, wagging, etc.
General body surface	Note any matting of the fur which may indicate an underlying wound. If in doubt as to the severity of the wound, assume the worst and treat accordingly. If foreign bodies are present, removal may be attempted unless they are embedded. Dislodging embedded foreign bodies may provoke more serious injury and must therefore be avoided.

Signs of shock:

- Pallor of mucous membranes (gums, inside lips, conjunctiva).
- Slow capillary refill.
- Increased respiration rate, which may rise markedly if the animal tries to struggle in any way.
- Rapid, feeble pulse. The pulse may be so weak that it cannot be felt.
- Coldness of the inside of the mouth, limbs and tail.
- Dull and depressed attitude – the animal is withdrawn.
- Convulsions and collapse if the brain becomes short of oxygen (**hypoxic**) and ceases to be able to function normally. This is likely to happen in the patient which is haemorrhaging badly (**hypovolaemic shock**) or if the airway is obstructed (**asphyxia**).

Treatment of the shocked patient

The exact treatment given depends on the cause of the shock but the following principles apply to all cases:

(1) **Prevent any further haemorrhage.**
(2) **Do not apply direct heat or give alcohol or other peripheral vasodilator drugs** (e.g. acepromazine). Both actions will cause dilatation of the cutaneous blood vessels, which are a non-essential part of the circulatory system so far as the shocked patient is concerned. The cutaneous blood vessels constrict in shock so that the circulating blood volume is directed towards maintaining sufficient blood supply to vital organs such as the brain, heart and lungs. This is why the extremities (paws and tail) feel cold to the touch and also why the mucosae are pale. If these non-essential blood vessels are encouraged to dilate, the blood pressure will fall as there is more circulatory 'pipework'

to be filled by the circulating blood. Vasodilatation in the skin is also more likely to restart haemorrhage from surface wounds.
(3) **Make the animal comfortable and prevent heat loss** by laying the patient on an insulated surface (such as thick blankets, vetbeds or polystyrene bean-bags) and covering the animal with further insulation (blankets, towels, etc.) to prevent heat loss from the body.
(4) **Set up an intravenous fluid drip**. The drip of choice is warmed Hartmann's solution but normal saline is adequate in an emergency. This measure not only helps to correct the metabolic acidosis of shock but also expands the circulating blood volume quickly and improves the supply of oxygen to all body tissues. It allows the kidneys to function more normally again. If there has been extensive blood loss, a blood transfusion or a plasma expander may be required. In cases of brain damage, some veterinary surgeons use hypertonic solutions to decrease the oedema of the brain tissues (e.g. mannitol solution). These fluids may be warmed, ready for administration if the veterinary surgeon needs them.
(5) **Give fluids by mouth** unless there are contraindications, e.g. vomiting, unconsciousness, severe mouth or throat injuries. Small volumes of fluid (25–100 ml, depending on the size of the animal) should be offered every 30 minutes. Oral Hartmann's solution will help to guard against the effects of shock, but plain water or a prepared solution of half a teaspoonful of salt and half a teaspoonful of bicarbonate of soda, dissolved in 1 litre of water, can be used if no Hartmann's solution is available.
(6) **Check dressings** every 10–15 minutes to ensure that they are comfortable, that the animal is not interfering with them and that any haemorrhage is being controlled.

(7) **Maintain constant observation**. This is essential, especially in cases of brain injury, haemorrhage, dyspnoea and suspected poisoning. The condition of the patient can deteriorate rapidly and the veterinary nurse must always remain on the alert. The state of consciousness, pupillary and palpebral reflexes, mucosal colour, capillary refill, and character and rate of pulse and respiration should be monitored every 10 minutes, or more frequently if the animal seems very distressed. **Make notes of the findings and time of each inspection and record them on the kennel chart.**

(8) **TLC.** All the above measures are aimed at reversing the effects of shock and will therefore make the animal feel more comfortable. However, the emotional needs of the patient should not be overlooked. These animals are often in much pain; they are confused and disorientated because they are alone in a strange and hostile environment (few animals like the surgery!) and they need sensitive and sympathetic handling. It should also be remembered that brain-damaged patients may have lost some faculties (e.g. sight or hearing) in the accident and need even more careful handling.

The nurse can help patients greatly by keeping them in a quiet, warm, darkened room and moving quietly and calmly whilst talking in a soothing manner. It does not matter what you say, rather how you say it. When checks are made, the animal should not be rushed – a gentle approach is much less stressful. Contact with human hands is very important, especially to dogs, and a little fussing is a good idea if time permits, but attention should *never* be forced on the patient. If any apprehension is shown, the animal is best handled as little as possible and it may even be advisable to cover the front of the kennel or basket to allow the patient some privacy between regular check-ups.

As soon as possible, veterinary assistance should be obtained and comprehensive notes should be handed to the veterinary surgeon in charge of the case. Meanwhile, the veterinary nurse may prevent delays by preparing dressings, drips, transfusions, instruments, anaesthetic machines and the operating theatre in readiness for any further treatment which the veterinary surgeon may think necessary once the patient's condition is stabilised. Treatments mentioned later in this chapter may be beyond the scope of veterinary nursing, but have been included to give some idea as to what may be required by the veterinary surgeon. The efficient nurse will save valuable time by having equipment prepared, drugs available, drips warmed, etc., when the veterinary surgeon arrives.

Poisoning

Definitions

● A **poison** or **toxin** or **toxic agent** is a substance which, when it enters the body in sufficient doses, causes harmful effects.
● **Poisoning** is said to have occurred when the poison produces clinical effects in the animal.
● An **antidote** is a substance which specifically counters the action of the poison.

The role of the veterinary nurse

The veterinary nurse should know of the common poisons and their effects in order to be able to act as follows:

(1) **Take a comprehensive case history.** From this the veterinary nurse should be able to recognise that the animal may have been poisoned or be able to reassure the client that the substance is harmless. For example, owners often panic when a puppy eats contraceptive tablets. The hormones contained in these are usually rapidly metabolised and excreted with no harmful effects to the patient!

(2) **Give appropriate first aid advice over the telephone** if the type of poison can be clearly identified from the case history given and the symptoms described by the owner (Fig. 3.7).

(3) **Thoroughly examine the patient and provide the correct supportive treatment** for the animal at the surgery until the veterinary surgeon can attend the case.

(4) **Reserve any vomit, faeces or urine and a sample of the suspected toxic agent** (if it is available) for examination and possible forensic analysis. Even if you are certain that the patient has not been deliberately poisoned, it is always wise to take such samples. Many domestic poisons (e.g. rat and slug baits) are brightly coloured, and the presence of these coloured pellets in the vomit will help the veterinary surgeon in his diagnosis and treatment of the case. The other reason for taking samples is that the owner may require them for analysis at a future date if legal action is taken.

(5) **Label the samples clearly** with:
● The name and address of the owner.
● The animal's name and description (e.g. breed, age, sex).
● The time and date of collection.

(6) **Maintain a diplomatic silence** as regards accusations of malicious poisonings. Unfortunately, there are some owners who are all too keen to assume that poison is the cause for any acute illness and accusations against unfriendly neighbours can flow thick and fast. **It is very important not to agree with any such accusations and it is essential not to make any such suggestion to the owners.** The reasons for this are threefold:
● Cases of malicious poisoning are mercifully rare.
● It is often very difficult to prove exactly which poison is responsible for the illness.
● It is usually impossible to prove in a court of law that the accused person deliberately placed the poison where the patient could reach it in order to harm the animal.

(7) **Ensure that access to a poison information unit is available.** In the UK, the Veterinary Poisons Information Service (VPIS) provides a round-the-clock information service to veterinary surgeons and is able to:
● Supply data on the clinical effects of a great number and range of poisonous compounds.
● Advise on methods of treatment of specific poisons.
● Advise on antidotal therapies (where available).

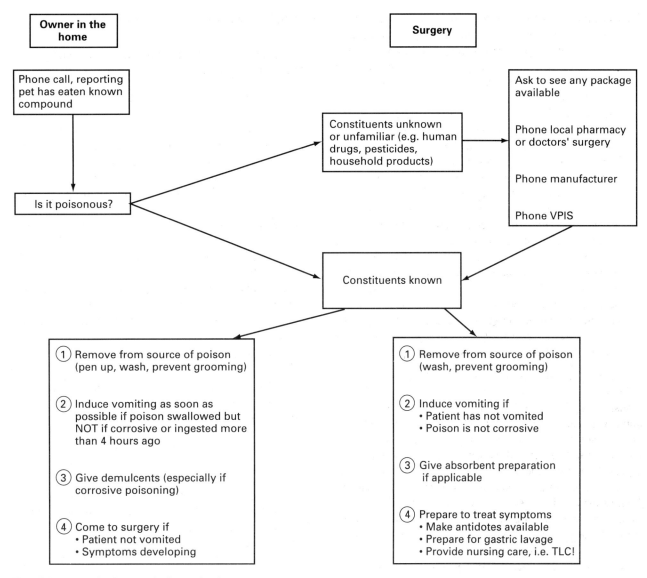

Fig. 3.7 Summary of actions to take for a poisoning case.

In order to enable the staff at the VPIS to give a speedy and rapid response, an accurate case history is needed. This should include as many precise details as possible about the suspected toxic agent (exact trade name, manufacturer, constituents, etc.).

It is very important that the veterinary nurse should only contact the service with the consent of the veterinary surgeon. The VPIS is *not* a public access service and will only accept calls from veterinary practices. It will also make a charge for answering any enquiries, unless the veterinary practice in question already pays an annual subscription to the service, in which case the subscription number should be quoted when the 'phone call is made. To avoid delay, ensure that this number is available.

The VPIS can be contacted on 0171 635 9195 (Fax: 0171 771 5309) or 0113 243 0715 (Fax: 0113 244 5849).

Incidence of poisoning cases

Poisoning is not commonly seen in small animal practice but the veterinary nurse must always bear the possibility

in mind when presented with an acutely ill patient. Sometimes the history offers a clue, e.g. a cat which has been dosed by the owner with paracetamol to ease the pain of an injured leg. At other times, careful questioning is necessary to establish the cause of the problem. Many humans are incurable hoarders and ancient bottles and boxes may be found in many cupboards and garden sheds: strychnine has been banned from use in the UK for a long time but occasional poisonings still occur; some old houses still have linoleum, old lead pipes, lead paint, etc. Table 3.3 suggests possible sources of poisons around the house.

History taking

Many poisons cause common symptoms. This means that, when asking routine questions over the telephone, it can be difficult to decide if an animal has actually been poisoned or has simply had severe gastroenteritis or an epileptic fit. The following points should be considered when trying to come to a conclusion:

Table 3.3 Classification of poisons

Type	Possible sources
Medicines	Sedatives, NSAIDs, etc.
Pesticides	Herbicides, e.g. weedkillers Insecticides, e.g. ant killer Molluscicides, e.g. slug bait
Household chemicals	Rodenticides, e.g. rat poison Garage – engine oils, antifreeze Garden shed – wood preservative Kitchen – disinfectants
Plants	Rare in small animal practice
Reptile bites	Adder bites Exotic species bite if snake, etc., escaped
Insect stings	Wasp and bee stings

(1) **What species is the patient?**
  - **Pups** are indiscriminate chewers of everything from laburnum sticks to old lino, both of which are toxic, and many dogs will eat almost anything, including rat bait.
  - **Cats** are fastidious and cautious about what they consume, but they groom endlessly and are therefore most likely to ingest contact poisons on their coat. They also hunt more and may eat their poisoned prey. The cat also has a poorly developed enzyme system in the liver, which means it is far less able to metabolise and excrete certain poisons. These chemicals therefore build up to toxic levels in the body tissues and poison the animal. The classic example here is paracetamol.
  - **Birds** are more susceptible to inhalation poisoning because of the design of their respiratory system.
(2) **What could be the cause of any poisoning?** Most reported poisonings are due to:
  - **Accidents**, e.g. cats falling into containers of old sump oil or dogs finding slug bait.
  - **Overdosing**, e.g. owners who do not read and follow directions correctly.
  - **Unusual reactions** to normally harmless substances, e.g. allergic (**anaphylactic**) reactions to wasp or bee stings, antibiotics or vaccines (some of these are not poisons but the reaction suggests it).
  - **Carelessness**, when an owner leaves medications where an inquisitive puppy can eat them. This is more of a hazard now that many human medicines are packaged in 'bubble packs'.
  - **Ignorance** of an owner who doses a pet with human preparations. The misuse of ibuprofen and paracetamol are the commonest reported.
  - **Malicious poisoning**, which is in reality extremely rare – it should be considered, but not agreed to without proof.
  The questions the veterinary nurse should ask must therefore concern:
  - The species, age, whereabouts and movements of the patient prior to the onset of illness.
  - The actions of the owner.

Questions about the patient

(1) Has the animal been observed eating anything in the hours preceding the onset of illness? If so, ask the owner to bring a sample of the substance with them or, preferably, to bring the package itself, if it is available. (Most poisons act within hours of ingestion.)
(2) Is there any contaminating substance on the coat, e.g. a smell of creosote, sticky engine oil, greasy paraffin?
(3) What were the patient's movements prior to the illness? For example, was the cat out overnight, or had the dog been shut into a garden shed where slug bait was stored, or is there evidence of chewed tablet packets? Has the animal been anywhere unusual in the last 24 hours – has the dog perhaps been walked in a different area where it may have found something?
(4) How old is the patient? The young are curious and may eat anything. The very young and the elderly are more susceptible to being poisoned since the liver and kidneys may not be functioning efficiently and therefore the poison cannot be detoxified and excreted so quickly. These animals need more rapid treatment and more intensive nursing care.
(5) Are other animals in the household affected (if there is more than one animal)? Simultaneous illness is more likely to be caused by poisoning.

Questions about the home environment

(1) Any medication (human or veterinary) given in the last 24 hours?
(2) Any recent use of toxic products by owner in the house or garden, e.g. pesticides, wood preservative, painting?
(3) Any recent upheavals in the house which may have exposed pesticides or toxic material previously inaccessible, e.g. moving to a renovated house, gutting a kitchen where rat bait has been laid, removing old (lead) pipework, stripping old paintwork where lead-based paints were originally used?
(4) Any recent accident in the home, e.g. overheating of fat or non-stick cooking utensils, accidental spillage of substances onto the animal's coat?

Treatment

Successful first aid treatment depends on four important principles:

- Identify the type of poison.
- Prevent further absorption of the poison.
- Treat the symptoms.
- Give the antidote if a specific one is available.

Identifying the type of poison

Until the nature of the poison is known, correct treatment cannot be given. For example, an animal that has ingested corrosive poisons must not be made to vomit because the poison will cause further damage when it is regurgitated over the already damaged tissues of the oesophagus, pharynx and mouth. Animals poisoned by depressant

Table 3.4 Cleaning solutions for contaminated coats

Non-oily compounds (e.g. disinfectant solutions)	Wash from the coat with copious amounts of water. The immediate use of detergents can actually *increase* the absorption of the toxic material: they make it fat-soluble, which means that it can be absorbed through the skin.
Liquid oily compounds (e.g. sump oil, creosote)	The most efficient way to remove these is to smear the coat liberally with 'Swarfega' (use liquid paraffin or cooking oil if 'Swarfega' is not available) and work it well into the hair. The coat must then be washed clean with three or four baths of detergent in warm water until the smell of the contaminant has completely disappeared.
Solid oily contamination (e.g. tar)	If possible the contaminated fur should be clipped away but often (especially when paws are affected) the tar has become so closely attached to the skin that this is impossible. In these cases, liquid paraffin, vegetable oil or butter can be applied and rubbed well into the area and bandaged to prevent grooming. Solvents such as a mixture of acetone and liquid paraffin are sometimes used.

Warning – It is wise to wear gloves when using these solvents to clean oily contaminants from the coat since regular skin contact with many of these compounds carries a known risk of cancer in humans. If the tar fails to loosen, the area should then be bandaged for 15 minutes, when the heat of the body and the action of the solvent may allow easier removal. If this fails, sedation or anaesthesia may be necessary but the area should be kept bandaged to prevent the animal chewing it. Following successful removal, the area should be well washed with soap and water.

compounds or those likely to cause fits should also not be made to vomit unless the poison has only just been ingested and the patient shows no signs of being affected.

Prevention of further absorption

Some of the following first aid measures can be applied by the owner at home and all may be continued at the surgery as appropriate:

- Remove all animals in the area from the source of the poison by physically restraining them to a known safe area and by washing off any skin contamination.
- Induce vomiting.
- Give gastric lavage.
- Prevent absorption of the poison from the alimentary tract by giving an inert substance by mouth which absorbs the poison and/or giving mild laxatives to speed the rate at which the ingesta passes through the tract.

Removing the animal from the source of the poison

If the poison was eaten or inhaled, the animals must be penned in a *known safe area*. Picking up one pile of rat bait may not be the answer as there could be other similar piles around the house.

If the coat is contaminated, prevent the animal from washing, grooming or preening itself whilst preparing the bath to wash the patient or whilst transporting it to the surgery. Paws and tails may be lightly bandaged. Elizabethan collars can be used or, if the whole body is affected, the animal may be placed in an old pillowcase or bag (with only the head protruding) or wrapped in a towel. Birds should be confined in a darkened box as they are less likely to preen in the dark. The patient must always be kept under constant observation to ensure the dressings are not disturbed.

Cleaning contaminated coats

Suitable cleaning solutions are described in Table 3.4.

Small areas of heavily contaminated coat may be cut away (e.g. tar balls between pads). Bathing the whole animal is a lengthy procedure, requiring as many as three or four repeated washings, especially if oily substances are involved. Thorough bathing is important, particularly for cats which groom continuously.

Towelling the coat dry will help to remove any remaining contamination, but the patient will still be extremely soggy so it will be necessary to use a hair-dryer or heat lamp to complete the process and to ensure that the animal does not succumb to hypothermia. (NB: Anaesthetised or depressed animals must be carefully observed during this process to ensure that they do not become overheated or burnt as the coat is dried because they are unable to move away from the heat source if they become too hot.)

If the patient is too fractious to allow thorough cleansing, a general anaesthetic or some form of sedation will be necessary: cats are particularly difficult to bath as they are well armed with teeth and claws, and hate water. Until the veterinary surgeon arrives to administer the anaesthetic, further ingestion of the poison by grooming must be prevented (see above).

Oiled seabirds require specialist attention as described on p. 35.

Induce vomiting

If the poison has been eaten within the last hour, the patient should be made to vomit as soon as possible except in certain circumstances where corrosive materials have been ingested (see below). Table 3.5 suggests agents which can be used to induce vomiting.

Table 3.5 Agents to induce vomiting

Hydrogen peroxide (1:3 dilution of 10 volume solution)	Give 1–2 tablespoons/10 kg to induce vomiting in 10–15 minutes; if no effect repeat dose after 20 minutes.
Washing soda	One or two pea-sized crystals on the back of the tongue.
Apomorphine	0.1 mg/kg s/c (only available at the surgery and to be given only under the direction of the veterinary surgeon, but very effective).
Xylazine	3.0 mg/kg i/m (subject to the same restrictions as apomorphine).
Mustard	2 teaspoonfuls in a cup of warm water if nothing else is available.

WARNING

- Do *not* suggest that vomiting should be induced if the poison is known or suspected to be corrosive, i.e. petroleum products, disinfectant solutions, strong acids or alkalis.
- Do *not* suggest that vomiting should be induced if the patient is comatose, unconscious or in a fit, or if the poison is of a type likely to make the patient collapse in any way. Collapsed animals can easily inhale the vomit.
- Do *not* suggest that vomiting should be induced if the poison was eaten 2 hours or more previously. Unless a large meal has been consumed, the stomach will have emptied in this time so there will be little point in inducing vomiting as the poison will already be in the small intestine.
- Do *not* suggest the use of salt as an emetic. It is not very effective and the salt swallowed is absorbed and will cause severe electrolyte imbalances, which could be more harmful to the patient than the ingested poison.
- Do *not* encourage the owner to persist in attempting to make the animal sick at home. Most owners find it very difficult to place foul-tasting concoctions on the back of their pets' tongues to make them vomit. If there is no success after 5 minutes, the animal should be brought straight to the surgery as valuable time is being lost.

Gastric lavage

This procedure requires the patient to be unconscious or under a general anaesthetic and should only be performed under the direct supervision of the veterinary surgeon. It is a time-consuming and messy procedure, but can be very rewarding. However, if the poison was ingested over 1 hour ago, the veterinary surgeon may wish to take a plain radiograph of the abdomen to discover if the stomach still contains any ingesta before continuing and the nurse may wish to prepare for this. Warm water or saline at a dose of 5–10 ml/kg is given by stomach tube and then the stomach is drained to wash out the poison. After several flushings, the fluid coming out of the stomach should run clear and then absorbent material (e.g. charcoal, fuller's earth, universal antidote, BCK granules) can be pumped in to absorb any remaining poison.

If poison was known to have been ingested recently (within the last 4 hours) and the patient cannot be made to vomit, the veterinary nurse can prepare the X-ray machine, the anaesthetic machine and warm suitable volumes of saline for gastric lavage whilst awaiting the veterinary surgeon's arrival.

Preventing absorption from the alimentary tract

This may be achieved by:

- The administration of an inert absorptive substance by mouth so that the poison is bound to the ingesta in the gut lumen and is not available for absorption (Table 3.6). In any poisoning, it is advisable to give these preparations as soon as is practicable (e.g. after vomiting has been induced or the stomach lavaged) in order to mop up any toxin which still remains in the alimentary tract. In cases of corrosive poisoning or where treatment has been delayed for 4 hours or more after ingestion, it is the only possible way to prevent more poison being absorbed.
- The use of laxative preparations such as sorbitol to hasten the passage of ingesta so that the poison passes along the tract as quickly as possible. Saline purges are *not* recommended as the salt may be absorbed and upset the electrolyte balance.

Treating the symptoms

In many cases, drugs are needed to control the symptoms of poisonings. These can only be administered by the veterinary surgeon but in the meantime the veterinary nurse can ensure that everything is prepared so that there is no delay caused by searching for the appropriate drugs. However, there are some vital nursing procedures which can be initiated immediately:

- Maintain oxygenation of the depressed patient.
- Give demulcents for gastrointestinal irritation.
- Administer fluids.
- Keep the patient comfortable.
- Prepare drugs to counter symptoms.

Maintaining oxygenation of the depressed patient. If the animal is **dyspnoeic** (struggling to breathe), cyanosed or unconscious, it should be treated as for asphyxiation. Doxapram may be given in the form of drops if breathing ceases.

Giving demulcents for gastrointestinal irritation in cases of irritant or corrosive poisonings. The principle is to coat the alimentary lining with a soothing substance. Mix a beaten raw egg with a little milk and one

Table 3.6 Agents used to bind poisons	
BCK granules	1–3 tablespoonfuls (depending upon the size of the patient) mixed to a slurry with water.
Charcoal	Weigh the patient and allow 1 g activated charcoal/kg bodyweight. Make up to a suspension by adding 5 ml water for every gram of charcoal used.
Kaolin	Generally less effective than charcoal but very useful in cases of paraquat poisoning.

teaspoonful of sugar and give by mouth. The proteins of the egg and milk coagulate, and are deposited on the mucosal surface; the sugar acts to soothe the tissues.

The owner can be advised to give this demulcent at home (especially in cases of corrosive poisoning) to attempt to lessen the damage to the tract and it can also be useful where vomiting and diarrhoea are already evident **but only if the patient is fully conscious and there are no other symptoms** such as excitability or depression. The owner *must* be told that, if other symptoms develop, the animal should be brought to the surgery.

Administration of fluids. As most poisons are metabolised or detoxified by the liver and excreted through the kidneys, it is important to give fluid therapy (Chapter 22) to enable a more rapid flushing of the poison from the body. Many poisons also actively damage the kidney tissue as they are excreted, but this effect can be decreased by ensuring that the urine is as dilute as possible so that the concentration of the poison in the urine is reduced.

Although a conscious animal may be encouraged to drink, it is impossible to ensure adequate fluid intake by mouth and the only effective ways to promote kidney dialysis are as follows:

- **Set up an intravenous drip**. Use lactated Ringer's solution because this will also correct any metabolic acidosis caused by toxic damage to body tissues. As usual, the drip should be warmed unless the poison is one which has caused hyperthermia and the rectal temperature is climbing off the scale. In these cases, it is useful to chill the drip.
- **Make ready a diuretic** to increase the rate of excretion by the kidneys to use on the veterinary surgeon's instructions.

Keeping the patient comfortable. Some poisons (e.g. alphachloralose) depress the body temperature. If the rectal temperature is below normal, the patient should be treated for hypothermia. Conversely, poisons such as dinitro herbicides (2,4-dinitrophenol and dinitro-orthocresol) raise the body temperature so that these patients may suffer from hyperthermia and need to be kept as cool as possible. Treatment for hypothermia and hyperthermia is described in the section on the Unconsciousness (p. 95).

Giving drugs to counter symptoms. The veterinary nurse may not administer prescription-only medicines without the knowledge and consent of a veterinary surgeon but drugs may be prepared so that they are ready for administration as directed by the veterinarian in charge of the case:

- **Barbiturates** (e.g. thiopentone, pentobarbitone) or **diazepam** may be required for convulsing or over-reactive (**hyperaesthetic**) patients.
- **Doxapram** may be given where the depression of the central nervous system is so severe that breathing ceases.

Preparation of specific antidotes

Unfortunately, most poisons do not have specific antidotes or ones that are readily available in veterinary practice. There are a few exceptions, such as warfarin-type rat poisons, where the antidote is vitamin K_1 and organophosphorus compounds, where the antidote is atropine. Again, these are prescription-only medicines and the veterinary nurse may not administer them unless directed to do so by a veterinary surgeon.

Specific poisons

This section is included only to give the veterinary nurse an indication of the relative toxic effects and treatments of the most common poisons encountered in veterinary practice (based on the *Veterinary Poisons Information Service Report, 1996*). When the owner makes the initial telephone call to report an incident involving a *known* substance, the veterinary nurse must be able to give accurate advice immediately or within minutes, but the notes in Table 3.7 are *not* designed to ensure that the veterinary nurse can diagnose which poison has been consumed or absorbed. There are so many toxic compounds encountered in everyday life that it requires a toxicology textbook to describe all the effects, signs and treatments of all toxic agents and the veterinary nurse should consult the publications listed at the end of this chapter for further information.

Treatment of oiled birds

Oiled birds present a real problem, especially wild birds unaccustomed to confinement and close association with human beings.

> **WARNING**
>
> To clean the plumage thoroughly and then maintain the patient whilst the bird's waterproofing oils are revived by natural grooming over a long period requires considerable experience, special facilities and weeks of attention, none of which can be easily provided by busy veterinary nurses in a routine small animal practice. There will also be the problem of returning a wild bird to its natural habitat, and this process of rehabilitation (which is vital to its survival) requires a great deal of knowledge and skill.

The role of the veterinary practice is to admit the bird and then take the following steps:

- Decide if it is well enough to survive. Many oiled birds are in too poor a condition or too badly poisoned and euthanasia is often the kindest treatment.
- Prevent further ingestion of the poison – give superficial cleansing only.

Table 3.7 Toxic agents

Type	Causes	Effects	Treatment
Medicines ACP misuse	Accidental overdosing with tablets in the house. Idiosyncratic reaction to the drug.	Depression or collapse. (Cats may become hyperaesthetic.) Vasodilatation leads to decreased blood pressure and increased susceptibility to heatstroke on warm days. Brachiocephalic dogs are especially likely to suffer. Increased likelihood of fits in epileptic animals.	Induce vomiting if many tablets have been eaten (unlikely, since few surgeries prescribe more than a few tablets for specific occasions). Treat symptoms of collapse/shock, heatstroke and epilepsy as described elsewhere in this chapter.
Abnormal response (anaphylactic reaction)	Allergic-type response to medication, e.g. vaccination, antibiotics.	Depression, occasionally vomiting and diarrhoea, swelling of injection sites. Severe reactions result in collapse, with signs of shock.	Swellings may have cold compresses applied. Treat for shock if collapsed and maintain if unconscious. Prepare corticosteroid injection.
Non-steroidal anti-inflammatory drugs (NSAIDs)	Owners using human preparations on their animals (dosing their pets with so-called pain killers). Dogs 'stealing' owners' medications. *Aspirin* – particularly toxic in cats. *Ibuprofen*, *Flurbiprofen* and *Naproxen* – may be rapidly fatal in some dogs. *Phenylbutazone* – more toxic to cats than dogs	*Aspirin* – Depression. Gastric irritation, leading to vomiting and anorexia. Cats may show some incoordination. *Ibuprofen and Flurbiprofen* – Gastric ulceration and perforation in dogs leads to vomiting and haematemesis, followed by diarrhoea with melaena. Kidney damage may cause acute and fatal renal failure. Dehydration due to fluid losses. *Naproxen* – Gastric inflammation and ulceration leading to vomiting and melaena. Anaemia due to low-grade blood loss. Dehydration.	Stop medication with the drugs. *Before symptoms show*, induce vomiting as soon as possible. *If showing symptoms*, give absorptive preparations and/or demulcents. Dosing with activated charcoal is vital in cases of aspirin poisoning and should be given immediately after vomiting ceases. Prepare intravenous fluids. Prepare **cimetidine** for intravenous injection in cases of naproxen poisoning.
Paracetamol	Owner administered dose or tablet packet chewed.	Dogs tolerate paracetamol well but cats are easily poisoned by as little as half a 500 mg tablet. Poisoning with paracetamol results in haemoglobin being changed to methaemoglobin, which is incapable of transporting oxygen. *Signs* Cyanosis. Depression or excitement. Incoordination due to hypoxia. Facial swelling.	Induce vomiting if no symptoms shown. Give absorptive material by mouth but NOT before consulting veterinary surgeon – if **N-acetyl cysteine** is to be used, the absorptive material may also prevent the absorption of this antidote. Provide oxygen if any sign of cyanosis; ensure that the animal rests as much as possible. Prepare **methionine** or *N*-acetyl cysteine (human preparation 'Parvolex') for oral administration.
Salbutamol	Human preparations that are used to treat asthma and for premature labour.	Stimulation of the sympathetic nervous system, causing peripheral vasodilatation and rapid heart rate (tachycardia). Panting respiration. Muscle weakness.	General first aid treatment but beta blockers may be needed if the heart rate becomes excessively high.
Calcipotriol	Vitamin D derivative contained in psoriasis creams and ointments, chewed by pups.	Similar to vitamin D overdose. Poisoning leads to hypercalcaemia and hyperphosphataemia, causing acute nephritis and damage to gastrointestinal tract. *Signs* Haemorrhagic diarrhoea. Polyuria and polydipsia. Collapse with or without convulsions. Death may occur within 24 hours.	Induce vomiting if ingested within 2–4 hours. Prepare activated charcoal solution. Prepare Hartmann's solution for i/v administration – it is important to flush the calcium and phosphates through the kidneys to minimise renal damage. Prepare frusemide diuretic injection.

Table 3.7 (Continued)

	Causes	Effects	Treatment
Herbicides			
Chlorates	Ingestion of weedkillers or drinking from contaminated puddles – this substance does not degrade readily after use.	Vomiting and diarrhoea with abdominal pain. Cyanosis of mucosa, turning to a muddy brown colour (blood becomes chocolate in colour because poison causes the formation of methaemoglobin – see Paracetamol).	General first aid treatment. Prepare **methylene blue** injection.
Dinitro compounds	Ingestion of 2,4-dinitrophenol (2,4-D) or dinitro-orthocresol (2,4,5-T).	Depression, listlessness, muscle weakness. Rapid respiration and dyspnoea. Hyperthermia with sweating. Urine is almost fluorescent yellow/green.	General first aid treatment. Monitor rectal temperature to detect hyperthermia.
Paraquat	Ingesting weedkiller (though this product is rapidly absorbed onto the soil after application, which renders it harmless). Paraquat has been used in malicious poisonings, but most cases are due to accidents.	Inflammation of the mouth and tongue. Vomiting and diarrhoea, with abdominal pain. Depression and progressive respiratory distress and cyanosis over a period of days, resulting in death.	**Induce vomiting** as soon as ingestion of this chemical is suspected. Even though this is an irritant poison, the effects of the absorbed poison are so severe that treatment is usually hopeless and the only hope is to remove the poison from the alimentary tract as soon as possible. Administering fuller's earth is also helpful because the poison will bind to the fuller's earth and be rendered inactive.
Insecticides			
Borax	Ant killers (e.g. 'Nippon') which are based on honey and therefore very attractive to dogs.	Vomiting and diarrhoea. Collapse, convulsions and possible paralysis. Poisoning may be fatal.	General first aid treatment.
Organophosphates	Overdosing with insecticidal sprays, chewing insecticidal collars, etc.	Vomiting and diarrhoea. Salivation. Constricted pupils. Muscular twitching, excitement, followed by weakness, incoordination. Depression or convulsions.	General first aid treatment. Prepare **atropine sulphate** for injection.
Organochlorines	Woodworm treatments and other insecticides (aldrin, dieldrin, gamma BHC, etc.). Many products are now withdrawn from sale but old stocks still exist.	Involuntary twitching of muscles, especially facial, fore- and hindlimbs and convulsions. Behavioural changes, e.g. aggression, pacing, apprehension, frenzy.	Wash off contamination. Administer absorptive material and/or liquid paraffin to decrease absorption. **Fatty foods and drinks** (including milk) **must not be given** as they may increase absorption of the poison. Prepare **barbiturate** injection to control convulsions.
Molluscicides			
Carbamate	See Organophosphates		
Metaldehyde	Ingestion of slug bait, which some dogs and cats seem to find very palatable.	Incoordination leading to hyperaesthesia and convulsions. Rapid pulse and respiration and possibly cyanosis.	General first aid treatment. Dosing with liquid paraffin may delay absorption of poison as long as it is given before the patient shows any symptoms (do not dose the unconscious patient). Prepare **barbiturate** injection to control convulsions.
Rodenticides			
Alphachloralose	Rat baits and preparations to control pigeon and seabird populations.	Poison acts by lowering the body temperature. Progressive depression, incoordination and coma with hypothermia.	General first aid treatment but warmth is essential.
Calciferol	Ingestion of rat bait.	See Calcipotriol (Medicines).	

Table 3.7 (Continued)

	Causes	Effects	Treatment
Rodenticides (*Continued*)			
Anticoagulant preparations	Rat baits. Several different compounds come under this heading: Warfarin, Coumatetralyl, Chlorophacinone, Difenacoum, Brodifacoum, Bromadiolone.	Interference with clotting mechanism results in haemorrhages in the mucosae, bruising and haematomata, swollen joints, etc.	General first aid treatment. Prepare injections of vitamin K. Large and repeated dosing may be necessary.
Household chemicals			
Alcohol	Ingestion of alcoholic drink or fermenting grain (especially likely with pups).	Hyperaesthesia, incoordination, collapse and even death.	Induce vomiting and provide general first aid treatment.
Chocolate	Ingestion of large amounts of high cocoa content chocolate or cocoa powder. (Not a common poisoning, but causes much public concern.)	Nervous excitement progressing to fits and coma. Tachycardia. Panting.	Induce vomiting (may not be effective if chocolate ingested because of its sticky consistency). Gastric lavage may be required. Prepare activated charcoal solution. Prepare diazepam/phenobarbitone to control fits.
Disinfectants	Household disinfectants, when diluted to correct strength, do not cause a problem but are often used undiluted or incorrectly diluted by over-zealous owners.		
	Phenols – **Cats are particularly susceptible to poisoning by phenols**. Licking paws after walking on wet surfaces recently cleaned with undiluted or incorrectly diluted solutions of disinfectant. Grooming coat after accidental spraying or splashing with strong disinfectant solutions.	**These are corrosive poisons with a strong, distinctive odour**, e.g. pine disinfectants. Convulsions, coma and death in acute poisoning cases. Less acute cases may have inflamed mouths (stomatitis) and occasionally ulcers in the mouth. Animals may also vomit and have diarrhoea and abdominal pain.	**Do not induce vomiting.** General first aid treatment, including thorough washing of contaminated fur.
	Quarternary ammonium compounds – as for phenols.	These are also corrosive poisons but are odourless. Depression and anorexia. Occasionally vomiting. Salivation, stomatitis and mouth ulcers, especially on the tongue tip. Skin ulcerations if compound not washed off quickly.	As for phenols.
Ethylene glycol (antifreeze)	Ingestion of water drained from car radiators (dogs seem particularly prone to drink this).	Incoordination, depression and rapid breathing. Later animal may become uraemic.	General first aid treatment. **Ethanol** is the specific antidote and intravenous injections may be prepared if available at the surgery.
Petroleum products	Usually a problem in cats which have fallen into containers of sump oil, drained from cars. Accidental spillages of petrol, paraffin, etc. Caking of tar in the paws.	These are very corrosive poisons with a distinctive odour. Depression, vomiting, collapse and death if enough ingested. If submersed in the liquid, may also suffer an aspiration pneumonia, which is very severe because of the extremely irritant nature of the inhaled liquid. Inflammation of the in-contact skin and mouth, especially the tongue if the animal has been allowed to groom.	**Do not induce vomiting.** General first aid treatment, including giving olive oil by mouth to decrease the absorption of the toxins.

- Correct hypothermia. Many oiled seabirds are hypothermic because the caked feathers become waterlogged.
- Rehydrate the patient.
- Refer it to the nearest RSPCA treatment centre as soon as possible for proper cleansing and rehabilitation.

Suggested first aid measures are therefore as follows:

- **Prevent ingestion of poison** by carefully wiping as much contamination off the feathers as possible with a clean towel or paper towelling. Take great care not to break the feather shafts and work methodically from the head of the bird to its tail, wiping both topside and underside of each oiled feather. Do not use solvents as this could increase the absorption of the poison.
- **Darkness, warmth and quiet** are the most important requirements. Darkness will calm the stressed bird; it will be less likely to preen and so the danger of absorbing more poison is reduced. Warmth and quiet will counter hypothermia and stress, improving the bird's chances of survival. The worst places for these patients are busy reception areas or noisy kennels. The bird should be placed in a cardboard box of suitable size (such as a cardboard cat carrier for a domestic duck) lined with thick newspaper. Put the box under a heat lamp or next to a radiator or on a hot water-bottle so that the bird is kept in an environment of 17–20°C.
- **Rehydrate by intubating the gullet.** The recommended equipment is a catheter mounted on a syringe. The catheter should be measured against the bird and cut to a length which will pass into the bird's oesophagus and down its neck until well clear of the laryngeal opening (Fig. 3.8). Intubating the gullet is relatively simple: the

larynx can be readily seen attached to the base of the tongue as the bird gapes and so it is easily avoided when passing the catheter down the gullet.

If the bird is bright and alert:

(a) Give warm water to flush the poison from the alimentary system and wait for 20–30 minutes to allow this to work. The volume given will vary according to the size of the patient.

(b) Give Lectade solution diluted in warm water to rehydrate the bird.

(c) Give a slurry mixture of BCK granules and water to prevent absorption of any remaining poison.

(d) If the bird is collapsed, give the Lectade solution every 2 hours to attempt to stabilise the patient's condition.

- **Feeding.** Ideally, a wild bird should not be fed until it has been taken into the care of the RSPCA. In any event, do not feed for at least 30 minutes after giving fluids to ensure that any oil has been flushed out of the intestines. Toxins are more easily absorbed if there is food present. When food is offered, it should be suitable – a mixture of chick pellets, chopped greens and chopped hard boiled eggs is suitable for land birds (a 1:1 mixture of hard-boiled egg and digestive biscuit is a useful substitute in an emergency). Sea birds may be fed small slivers of fresh fish or sprats. Cat food is *not* suitable for birds as it usually causes diarrhoea.
- **Refer to an RSPCA centre as soon as possible** for thorough professional cleaning and rehabilitation. If there is an unavoidable delay, but only with very great care and appropriate handling of the bird, give the feathers a preliminary clean to remove the worst of the oil, paying particular attention to the breast feathers and 'wing pits'. Mild detergents are recommended as these are most readily washed out of the plumage. The bird must be thoroughly rinsed in at least two or three bowls of clean water warmed to around 40–45°C.

Reptile bites

There are two important groups of venomous snakes, *Viperidae* (e.g. vipers, rattlesnakes and adders) and *Elapidae* (e.g. cobras, mambas and coral snakes).

The only indigenous venomous snake in Britain is the adder (*Vipera berus*) but the other exotic reptiles are being kept in ever increasing numbers by the public and should one of these animals escape, it is possible that it might bite the family pet. Although cats are rarely bitten, snake bites can be a problem in dogs because they are more likely to try to attack an escaping snake or to disturb one whilst out walking. The adder has a characteristic dark 'V' or 'X' marking on its head and dark zig-zag markings along the length of its body. It is commonly found basking on warm sunny days on dry, well-maintained heathland. When disturbed, it may strike and bites are therefore usually inflicted on the head, neck or legs of the sniffing dog.

Signs. Following a bite from an adder, the tissues swell rapidly and to such an extent that the two fang marks are rarely visible. The swelling is very painful and oedematous,

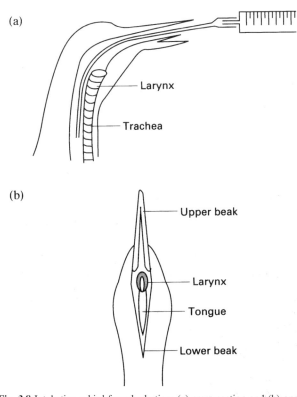

(a)

— Larynx

— Trachea

(b)

— Upper beak

— Larynx

— Tongue

— Lower beak

Fig. 3.8 Intubating a bird for rehydration: (a) cross-section and (b) open beak.

and may be serious if it affects the mouth or throat area, causing narrowing or blockage of the airway. The patient is often dull and depressed but anaphylactic reactions can occur and the animal may rapidly collapse and become comatose.

The effects of bites from other reptiles depends upon the species involved and the owners of the snake should know if that particular species is poisonous. Symptoms can include swelling of regional lymph nodes, bleeding from the gums, hypovolaemic shock, muscular paralysis (which can lead to respiratory failure) as well as possible swelling of the bitten area.

Treatment. If the reptile was a non-poisonous species, the bite wound should be gently washed with 1:4 solution of hydrogen peroxide and then flushed thoroughly with sterile saline. Reptile oral flora is rich in Gram-negative bacteria, which can cause the wound to become badly infected.

If the bite was poisoned, the normal principles apply:

- *Identify the poison involved.* In the case of an exotic reptile, the owner will usually know the species responsible.
- *Prevent further absorption of the poison.* **The animal must be made to rest** so the general circulation is slowed as much as possible. If possible, the bitten limb should be splinted (e.g. using a Robert Jones dressing) to prevent movement. This will also minimise any swelling and therefore decrease the pain. Some elapid snake venoms can cause respiratory paralysis within hours and, if this is suspected, the limb should be bandaged *very* firmly to decrease the venous return (containing venom) from that limb and thus prevent toxins entering the rest of the circulation. Crepe bandage should be used in these cases, applied directly to the leg. Bandaging is started at the toes and continued up the limb as far as is necessary. **Tourniquets must never be used** because, although they prevent all the venous blood from the limb entering the circulation, they also prevent arterial blood from entering the area to keep the damaged tissues alive. If the animal has only been bitten a short while ago (e.g. within 10 minutes), the wounds should be thoroughly flushed with cold sterile saline to wash out as much toxin and infection as possible. However, if the tissues have already begun to swell, this will be an impossible task and should not be attempted. Ice packs may be applied to encourage vasoconstriction and alleviate the pain but it is more important to keep the animal rested and to immobilize the bitten area as described above.
- *Treat the symptoms.* The main symptom will be shock, followed by collapse, unconsciousness and death if sufficient poison is absorbed. General first aid measures should be applied, especially the administration of fluids. Adrenaline, corticosteroids, antihistamines, diuretics, antibiotics, calcium and vitamin D may also be required by the veterinary surgeon and should be made readily available.
- *Antidotes.* Antivenom for adder bites is called **Zagreb** and should be held at all major accident and emergency departments of local hospitals. It may well save valuable

time if the veterinary nurse can telephone the local casualty department, explain the situation and ask if any antivenom is available. Antivenoms for rare and exotic species do exist, but the Veterinary Poisons Information Centre would need to be consulted about availability and supply of these drugs.

Toad poisoning

The common toad secretes toxic venom onto its body surface and, although very few animals will try to pick up toads, it is not unknown for the unwary pup to do so.

Symptoms

Dogs which have picked up toads salivate excessively, pawing at their mouths and may become quite distressed. If part of a toad has been eaten, nervous signs may develop but are not fatal.

Treatment. Little treatment is usually necessary since the dog soon drops the toad and the excessive salivation washes the venom out of the mouth. If the animal is distressed, the mouth may be sponged out or flushed with a hose.

Nervous signs, if shown, may need symptomatic treatment with atropine or corticosteroids.

Insect stings

Wasp and bee stings are very common in the summer and early autumn months, and usually affect the young kitten or puppy as it chases and catches the insect. The areas most affected therefore are the mouth and lips but occasionally the feet may also be stung if the kitten 'bats' the insect with its paws.

Symptoms

Stings in the mouth are rarely severe but may cause considerable swelling, excessive salivation and discomfort. This soon subsides after about an hour.

Stings in the pharynx could cause sufficient swelling to obstruct the airway. The patient will often paw at the mouth and, if the swelling is marked, the breathing may become laboured.

Some animals develop a severe allergic reaction to the sting and may collapse with pale, cold mucous membranes.

Treatment. In event of collapse, the animal must be given first aid for shock and the veterinary surgeon called immediately. Intravenous corticosteroid injections should be prepared.

If the animal has been stung at the back of the mouth, the owners should be advised to keep the patient under close observation for the next hour in case the area swells and obstructs the airway. In the event of airway obstruction, the animal should be brought to the surgery immediately and treated as described under 'Asphyxia' on p. 91.

Wasps rarely leave the sting behind but bees invariably do. The sting shaft of the bee is barbed and the barbs point backwards so that once the stinger has penetrated the skin, the bee cannot withdraw it and the posterior segment of the bee abdomen is torn away as the insect flies off. The muscles in the sting continue to work, forcing the sting deeper into the patient's tissues and emptying the poison sacs at the same time to cause greater and greater inflammation.

In all cases therefore, the area should be examined as soon as possible after the accident to see if a sting remains. Owners should be advised to *scrape* the sting away immediately before it has time to embed itself. A scraping action ensures that the entire sting is removed without disturbing the poison sacs. Grasping the sting with tweezers will simply empty the poison sacs and worsen the pain and inflammation.

If the sting has been present for a few minutes, it will be impossible to scrape it away because it is too embedded. Tweezers have to be used but the sting should be grasped as close to the skin as possible to avoid squeezing the poison sacs.

- **B**ee stings should be bathed with **b**icarbonate solution (one teaspoon of bicarbonate of soda to quarter of a litre of water).
- **W**asp stings should be bathed with **v**inegar (diluted 50:50 with water).

Following swabbing of the area with one of these solutions, ice packs may be used to alleviate the pain and swelling.

If the swelling does not respond to any of these measures, the owner should be told to bring the animal to the surgery. The veterinary nurse should prepare injections of corticosteroids, and make ready the calcium and vitamin D injections used by some veterinary surgeons to stabilize the cell membranes and prevent further swelling and oedema of the area.

Haemorrhage

Haemorrhage is bleeding from any part of the body and is usually caused by injury, but may also occur when blood vessels are affected by disease.

Any haemorrhage must be regarded as serious, for a sudden or severe loss of blood may result in death. Even a slight haemorrhage which continues over a long period may result in loss of blood which jeopardises the life of the patient.

Classification

Haemorrhage classification (Table 3.8) depends on the answers to three questions:

- **What** type of blood vessel is damaged?
- **When** does the haemorrhage occur?
- **Where** did the blood escape to?

Type of blood vessel damaged

- **Arterial haemorrhage.** This is the most serious form of haemorrhage. Blood from an artery is bright red and spurts forcefully from the wound in time with the heart beat. The blood may escape with such force that it sprays walls and floor 2 m away or more, but this depends upon the size of the severed artery. If the wound is large, the blood will be seen to be coming from the side of the wound nearest the heart. Usually a definite bleeding point can be detected.
- **Venous haemorrhage.** This is slightly less serious than an arterial haemorrhage but rapid blood loss will still occur if a large vein is damaged. Venous haemorrhage is usually easier to control, since the blood is under less pressure. Blood from a vein is darker in colour than arterial blood and issues from the wound in a steady stream. When a large vein is damaged, however, the

Table 3.8 Classification of haemorrhage type

Type of blood vessel damaged:

Arterial	Venous	Capillary
Bright red blood	Dark red blood	Bright red blood
Pumps forcefully	No or little spurting from wound	A small volume which oozes slowly from damaged tissues throughout the wound
Issues from side nearest heart	Issues from the side furthest from the heart	
Definite bleeding point	Definite bleeding point	No definite bleeding point

Time at which bleeding occurs:

Primary	Reactionary	Secondary
Immediately	Within 24–48 hours	3–10 days post trauma

Destination of blood loss:

Externally – to body surface and clearly visible	Internally – into body tissues/cavities. Hidden

blood loss may pulsate slightly in time with the heart beat but there is no forceful spurting as is seen in arterial haemorrhage. In large wounds, the blood will issue from the side furthest from the heart and a definite bleeding point is visible.

- **Capillary haemorrhage**. Bleeding from damaged capillaries occurs in all wounds, as the fragile capillary wall is easily damaged. The blood escapes from multiple, pinpoint sources in the tissues and oozes from the wound with very little force. No definite bleeding points are visible.
- **Mixed haemorrhage**. The arteries and veins of the body usually lie very close to one another, so that often all three types of blood vessel are injured simultaneously. When an artery and vein are severed at the same time, the haemorrhage may be so great that the characteristics of arterial haemorrhage are not detectable.

Time of blood loss

- **Primary haemorrhage**. This occurs as an immediate result of damage to the blood vessel wall.
- **Reactionary haemorrhage**. This is haemorrhage which occurs some 24–48 hours after the injury. The primary haemorrhage causes a drop in blood pressure, which may be sufficiently severe to slow the rate at which the blood escapes from the wound. As the blood flow lessens, a blood clot can form around the end of the damaged vessel and seal it so the primary haemorrhage stops. However, if the blood pressure rises again within the next 24 hours (e.g. as the animal recovers from shock or is given intravenous fluid therapy), this clot may be displaced and reactionary haemorrhage will occur.
- **Secondary haemorrhage**. This is haemorrhage that occurs 3–10 days after the injury. The primary haemorrhage stopped because the blood clotted or the vessel was ligated but, if the wound was infected, bacteria invading the blood clot may destroy it and any ligation material.

Destination of blood loss

- **External haemorrhage**. When the blood escapes on to the body surface, it is termed external haemorrhage. It may come from obvious open wounds or escape from regions such as the nose, ear, mouth, stomach linings, intestines, urinary tract or uterus.
- **Internal haemorrhage**. If the blood is lost into the tissues or into a cavity such as the thoracic or abdominal cavity, it cannot be seen and is termed internal haemorrhage. Such haemorrhage occurs:

  (1) if there is severe mucosal bruising;
  (2) if an internal organ is damaged (such as lungs, liver or spleen);
  (3) if there is disease (e.g. a tumour) which erodes blood vessel walls;
  (4) if there is a clotting deficiency (e.g. rat poisoning).

It is very difficult to detect internal haemorrhage although it may cause swelling of the tissues or distension of a body cavity such as the abdomen or joint capsules. In most cases, the only way to detect severe internal haemorrhage is by recognising the general signs of shock which the haemorrhage produces.

Natural arrest of haemorrhage

Four factors tend to stop initial bleeding:

- Retraction of the cut ends of the blood vessels.
- Falling blood pressure.
- Back pressure.
- Blood clotting.

Retraction of cut ends

Retraction of cut ends of arteries, arterioles and large veins is due to the elastic nature of their walls. When the cut ends recoil, the elastic tissues contract and bunch up at the end of the vessel. This closes or reduces the size of the aperture through which blood is flowing. Tearing of the blood vessel produces a better recoil as the vessel is stretched before it breaks. Therefore a lacerated wound bleeds less than an incised wound. (Compare the amount of mess caused by a cut pad with that caused by a lacerated foot wound following a road accident. Although there may be much more tissue damage, the lacerated wound bleeds far less.) A lessening of blood flow allows more rapid clot formation to seal the blood vessel completely.

Fall in blood pressure

Loss of blood will result in lowered blood pressure so that less blood reaches the affected vessel and there is less pressure to force it out of the cut end of the vessel.

Back pressure

Internal haemorrhage will eventually fill the cavity (e.g. abdomen) or distend the surrounding tissues (**bruising**) until the lowered blood pressure *in* the severed vessel is equal to the pressure of the fluid *surrounding* the severed end of the vessel. When the pressures are equal, no further blood can escape from the damaged blood vessel.

Blood clotting

Clotting takes place in the wound, both within and around the cut end of the vessel. This clot acts as a plug, sealing the severed vessel and preventing further blood loss. (This mechanism cannot work in cases of warfarin poisoning.)

Repair of blood vessels

When haemorrhage has been arrested, the body will repair the damaged vessel. If this is not possible (e.g. in complete severance of a vessel, where the two ends have recoiled away from each other) the vessel will become permanently sealed. The flow of blood will be redirected via other vessels, which enlarge to cope with the increased flow. New vessels will develop to re-establish the natural circulation. This bypass system works well unless all arteries supplying a part of the body are severed. The circulation cannot then be re-established in time to prevent the tissues dying, as is often seen in crushing injuries to the tail and digits.

First aid treatments of haemorrhage

A number of methods can be used to stop bleeding:

- Direct digital pressure.
- Use of artery forceps.
- Pad and pressure bandage.
- Pressure points.
- Tourniquet.

The risks, advantages and disadvantages of each method are described in Table 3.9, p. 44.

Direct digital pressure

Haemorrhage is controlled by applying pressure to the wound with *clean* hands. It is best to apply the fingers to the *intact* skin on either side of the wound and to pinch the wound edges together gently to avoid further bacterial contamination of the wound itself. The finger pressure will collapse the walls of the severed blood vessels, so preventing blood loss from the cut ends (Fig. 3.9).

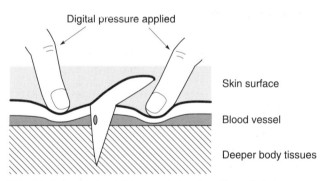

Fig. 3.9 Cross-section of a wound showing direct digital pressure to stop bleeding.

If the wound is too large to apply effective pressure along its entire margin, clean hands or a piece of clean, non-fluffy material (e.g. a tea-towel) should be placed in the wound and direct pressure applied to the bleeding points in the wound itself.

Use of artery forceps

In cases of severe arterial haemorrhage, it is acceptable for a skilled nurse to use a pair of artery forceps to occlude the offending vessel and then ligate it with catgut. **This procedure must only be considered when the cut end of the artery can be clearly seen.** It may usefully be used as a follow-up procedure to direct digital pressure, use of pressure points or the use of a tourniquet.

Pad and pressure bandage

A pad of gauze swabs or gauze overlaid by a thick pad of cotton wool is applied to the wound and bandaged very firmly into position. If the wound is high up on a limb, the whole leg may need to be bandaged because otherwise the tissues below the bandaged area will swell.

If the bleeding continues, a second pad may be bandaged over the first; it is best not to remove the first dressing as the blood clots will be disturbed and the bleeding will start again. Deep wounds may need to be packed with sterile gauze before the pressure pad is applied.

If internal bleeding is suspected, a crepe bandage may be firmly applied to the area, effectively increasing the back pressure in the affected tissues. Blood loss is quickly controlled and there should be minimal swelling and bruising of the tissues.

Pressure points

A pressure point is a site in the body where it is possible to press an artery against a bone. This prevents arterial flow along the vessel and stops arterial bleeding from the wound further down the leg or tail. The method is limited to three points in the dog or cat:

- **The brachial artery** as it runs down the medial shaft of the humerus and swings cranially behind the fleshy biceps muscle (Fig. 3.12). The pulse can clearly be felt in the distal third of the humerus. Pressure applied to this vessel will arrest serious arterial haemorrhage from below the elbow. (Note that this pressure point is not easily found and so it is a good idea to practise feeling the pulse here on a healthy animal.)
- **The femoral artery** as is passes obliquely over the proximal third of the femur on the medial aspect of the thigh. It lies just in front of the small taut pectineus muscle and pressure applied to this vessel will arrest arterial haemorrhage from below the stifle.
- **The coccygeal artery** as it passes backwards along the underside of the tail (Fig. 3.13). Pressure at the root of the tail (where the pulse can easily be felt ventral to the coccygeal vertebrae) will arrest arterial haemorrhage from the rest of the tail.

Tourniquet

A tourniquet stops bleeding by constricting all the arteries supplying blood to a wound on a limb or a tail. Correct application is essential and the tourniquet should only be used in cases where there is severe haemorrhage that cannot be controlled by other methods.

Many forms of tourniquet are available, but in an emergency the tail/leg can be held very tightly by the human hand whilst a more permanent tourniquet is found. The usual tourniquet is one consisting of a flat elastic bandage with a fastening clip but a length of strong bandage, a piece of material, a piece of rubber tubing, a thick elastic band or a narrow belt can be effectively applied. String and rope are not good materials as they dig in and cause severe tissue damage at the point of application.

Table 3.9 Methods of stopping bleeding: risks, advantages and disadvantages

	Risks	Advantages	Disadvantages
Direct digital pressure	If a foreign body is suspected in the wound, care must be taken not to push it deeper. Similarly, in the case of underlying fractures, care must be taken not to displace fracture fragments.	(i) Direct pressure on a wound, particularly when applied to a bleeding point, is both quick and effective and stops blood loss immediately. (ii) It needs no equipment other than a clean finger and thumb – instruments which are always available. (iii) This method alone may be sufficient to control venous haemorrhage because constant digital pressure for five minutes stops the flow for a sufficient time to allow a clot to form and this clot may well seal the blood vessel. However, a constant pressure must be maintained for this time because lessening the pressure even for a few seconds allows the haemorrhage to start again, destroying any clot structure which may have begun to form in the blood vessel. It is a wise precaution to apply a pressure bandage to the wound in any case, even if the haemorrhage has completely stopped, because the blood vessels may also start to haemorrhage again as the animal moves and the blood pressure rises. (iv) If there is a protruding foreign body, direct digital pressure can be applied without disturbing the foreign body as pressure can be applied to the wound edges rather than into the wound itself.	This is a temporary emergency measure and is not suitable for the longer term control of haemorrhage.
Use of artery forceps	Arteries and nerves commonly lie close together and fishing blindly in a wound with artery forceps may crush these nerves to functionless pulp. The artery forceps should never be used as a clamp across the edges of a bleeding wound.	This method permanently controls haemorrhage.	(i) It can be difficult to identify the cut end of an artery when blood is pumping out of the wound. To clear the field, it is often necessary to apply direct digital pressure or a tourniquet to stop the haemorrhage temporarily so that the wound can be examined and the end of the cut vessel identified, clamped and ligated. If the vessel cannot be identified (and these vessels may be surprisingly small), the digital pressure or tourniquet should be released gradually whilst the wound is examined carefully to detect the first sign of bleeding which will mark the location of the offending blood vessel. (ii) This method requires specialised equipment (artery forceps and ligation material). In an emergency, household tweezers and cotton thread may have to be substituted to save the animal's life.

Table 3.9 (*Continued*)

	Risks	Advantages	Disadvantages
Pad and pressure bandage	Where there is an embedded protruding foreign body or shallow underlying fracture, a ring pad should be used so that the foreign body is not driven deeper into the tissues and the fracture is not complicated or displaced. The ring pad may be fashioned from material (Fig. 3.10) or several thick rolls of bandage can be arranged as a ring around the wound and bandaged in position to create the same effect. If the foreign body is large and protrudes a long way, it may also be necessary to carefully cut off the protruding end so that the ring can be effective. The principle behind ring pads is that they should only prevent overlying pressure bandages from applying direct pressure to the protected area (Fig. 3.11). However, since the pressure bandage will still apply pressure to the ring pad, it forces the pad down and, in so doing, effectively creates a ring of direct digital pressure around the wound. This will prevent haemorrhage from superficial blood vessels but does not affect the haemorrhage which wells up from the deep tissues around a fracture site. The deep haemorrhage is controlled by back pressure as the area in the centre of the ring fills with blood until the pressures equalise. (Penetrating foreign bodies usually act as a plug in the wound they have created and so deep external haemorrhage is rarely a problem in these cases.)	(i) Pressure bandages are easy to apply and comfortable for the animal. (ii) The bandage can be left in place until the veterinary surgeon attends the case, and needs little attention from the veterinary nurse except continued observation to ensure that the dressing is not disturbed and that blood is not seeping through the bandage. (iii) Most forms of haemorrhage respond well to this method of control and this is the commonest form of first aid for haemorrhage used in practice.	(i) This method requires first aid equipment and a certain degree of co-operation from the patient. (ii) Some areas of the body can be difficult to bandage effectively, e.g. the shoulder and upper thigh regions.
Pressure points	Only major arterial haemorrhage is controlled using this method so blood loss will continue from other vessels. As the tissues of the lower limb which are supplied by the artery will also be deprived of an arterial blood supply, this method can only be used for a limited period (see Tourniquet).	(i) Equipment (i.e. fingers) is always available. (ii) Arterial haemorrhage is quickly controlled, allowing identification of bleeding points and ligation of severed vessels. (iii) In cases where the damaged tissues are macerated beyond recognition (e.g. loss of limbs or severe injuries following road accidents), these pressure points allow haemorrhage control at a site far removed from the injured area, which lessens the pain for the animal.	(i) Pressure points can be difficult to find. Plenty of practice in detecting the pulse of normal animals in these sites is essential in order to be confident of finding the correct location in an emergency case, where the blood pressure may be very low. (ii) This procedure does not immediately cause all bleeding to cease, because venous bleeding is unaffected and will continue. (iii) As with direct digital pressure, this is only a temporary measure and some other form of control such as ligating the artery must be applied to contain the haemorrhage if veterinary help is delayed for any length of time.
Tourniquet	A tourniquet should be used for as short a time as possible because it cuts the circulation to all the tissues of the limb or tail so that they will start to die from the moment the tourniquet is applied. Therefore, a tourniquet should never be left in place for more than 15 minutes before being released for at least 1 minute to allow blood to circulate and revive these tissues.	(i) Tourniquets are quick and easy to apply. (ii) No special equipment is necessary. If nothing is available, the limb or tail may be held as tightly as possible by hand. This usually controls the haemorrhage sufficiently until a tourniquet can be found or the haemorrhage is controlled by some other means.	(i) All the blood supply to the limb or tail is cut off. (ii) Tissues are damaged at the point of application because of the pressure exerted by the tourniquet. (iii) Constant observation of the patient is essential.

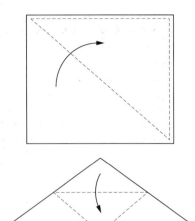

Step 1
Take a clean tea-towel,
headscarf, or any material
3 foot square or oblong.
Fold diagonally.

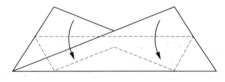

Step 2
Fold point down on to
diagonal fold.

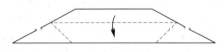

If cloth is oblong, fold
both points down.

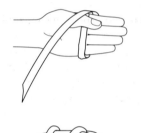

Step 3
Fold in half again to
create a narrow band.

Step 4
Hold one end of the band
between ball of thumb and
palm of hand. Make loop
around the fingers.

Step 5
Remove the loop from the
fingers and wind the long
free end tightly around the
loop. Tuck in the end to
make a compact ring.

Fig. 3.10 Ring-pad dressing.

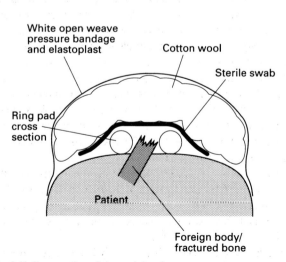

Fig. 3.11 Cross-section of ring-pad dressing.

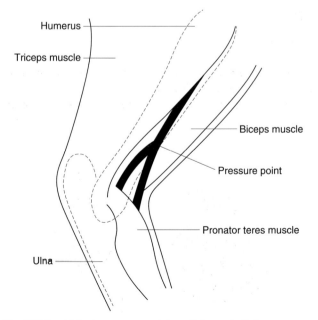

Fig. 3.12 Brachial artery pressure point, medial aspect of elbow.

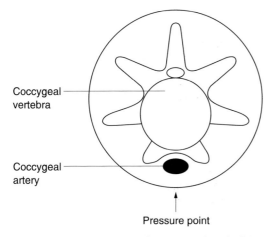

Fig. 3.13 Coccygeal artery pressure point, cross-section of tail base.

Table 3.10 Classification of wounds

Open	Closed
Incised	Contusion
Lacerated	Haematoma
Puncture	Haemorrhage into body cavity
Abrasion	e.g. cranial cavity
	epidural space
	chambers of the eye
	thorax
	pericardium
	abdomen
	joint spaces

The tourniquet is fixed firmly round the limb or tail, at a point a few inches above the wound. It should be adjusted so that the pressure is just sufficient to stop the haemorrhage. This is achieved by adjusting the clip of the conventional tourniquet. With other tourniquets, a half-hitch is tied firmly against the skin and then a stick or rod (e.g. ballpoint pen) is tied over the half-hitch. Twisting this stick will twist and gradually tighten the tourniquet until the haemorrhage is just controlled (Fig. 3.14).

Some other method of control should be attempted as soon as the tourniquet has controlled the bleeding, e.g. ligating the large blood vessels or applying a pressure bandage. Then the tourniquet should be slackened off slowly and the wound or dressings observed for signs of further haemorrhage. If bleeding starts again and it is necessary to replace the tourniquet, it should be applied a little closer to the wound to allow the tissues at the original site to recover from the effects of the constriction. **At no time should a tourniquet be covered with a dressing and no animal should be returned to a kennel with a tourniquet in place.**

Wounds

Definitions

A **wound** is an injury in which there is a forcible break in the continuity of the soft tissues.

An **open wound** is one where the injury causes a break in the covering of the body surface, i.e. skin or mucous membranes. These wounds can be seen and blood loss evaluated.

A **closed wound** is one where the injury does *not* cause a break in the body covering. This category contains everything from minor bruising to serious damage to internal organs, e.g. rupture of the spleen. The wounds cannot be seen and blood loss is difficult to evaluate.

An **abrasion** is a wound where the epidermis has been eroded to expose the underlying dermis, i.e. the injury does not penetrate the entire skin thickness.

An **avulsed** wound is any wound in which a flap of skin has been forcibly plucked off or torn away from the underlying tissues and yet still remains attached at some point (Fig. 3.15b, d and f).

A **contused** wound is any wound in which there is bruising.

The classification of wounds is set out in Table 3.10.

Open wounds

Table 3.11 and Fig. 3.15 illustrate and describe the characteristics of open wounds.

Incised wounds

Incised wounds may be caused by sharp cutting instruments such as surgical scalpel blades, knives, broken glass or cats' claws. Barbed wire tears may also be incised wounds.

The edges are clean cut and clearly defined and usually gape, especially on movement. Avulsed incised wounds are often V-shaped and are commonly seen on the legs and feet. The top layer of a foot pad may be almost sliced away if the animal stood on a piece of broken glass. Simple small incised wounds (say 1 cm in length) may seal together very rapidly and remain closed, which can make them difficult to find.

Incised wounds usually bleed freely as there is little elastic recoil from the cut ends of the blood vessels to allow natural arrest of haemorrhage. Such wounds often penetrate deeply and there is often damage to underlying structures such as nerves and tendons.

Incised wounds tend to heal quickly if the edges are held together, leaving little scar formation.

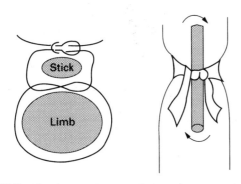

Fig. 3.14 Tourniquet.

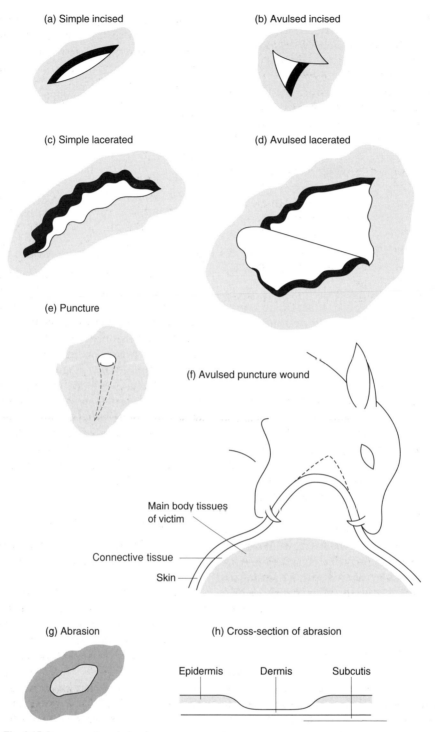

Fig. 3.15 Open wounds and abrasions.

Table 3.11 Characteristics of open wounds and abrasions

Incised	Lacerated	Puncture	Abrasion
Any size	Any size	Small	Any size
Usually deep	May be deep	Deep wound	Superficial
Haemorrhage freely	Little haemorrhage	Little haemorrhage	Little haemorrhage
Gapes unless small	Gapes	Closes very quickly	No gaping skin edges
Rarely grossly contaminated	Often grossly contaminated	Often contaminated	Often contaminated
Heals rapidly by first intention	Heals slowly by granulation	Rapid healing if infection controlled	Rapid healing
May be avulsed	May be avulsed	Rarely avulsed	Cannot be avulsed
Rarely contused	Often contused	Often contused	May be contused
Little pain	Painful	Little pain unless infected	Painful

Lacerated wounds

These are the most common type of wound encountered in small animals and are usually caused by road accidents, dog fights, tearing by barbed wire, etc. The wounds are irregular in shape, with jagged uneven edges. Areas of skin may literally be worn away, especially following road accidents when the animal has been dragged along the road. The edges of any lacerated wound always gape because the skin has been torn apart.

The severity of these wounds depends on how deeply the wound penetrates, but often underlying muscle, tendons, ligaments and even bones may be affected. Haemorrhage, even from large wounds is often surprisingly little as the ragged tearing of the blood vessels causes good elastic recoil and natural control of haemorrhage. There is, however, considerable risk of infection from ingrained dirt, saliva and bacterial contamination.

Healing is often slow and there is usually considerable risk of extensive scar formation.

Puncture wounds

These are produced by blows from sharp pointed instruments such as nails, stakes, thorns or fish hooks, and also from the canine teeth in bite wounds. Airgun pellets and bullets also cause puncture wounds.

The actual skin wound may be quite small but this will often lead to a long narrow track which penetrates deeply into the underlying tissues. Puncture wounds commonly become infected because bacteria may be carried deep into the tissues at the time of injury. The small skin wound usually heals rapidly, trapping infection in the tissues, and an abscess will form. Bleeding from puncture wounds is often small and **such wounds are liable to be overlooked.** The only sign of such a wound may be a small tuft of matted, bloodstained fur over the site of the injury. Cat bite wounds may carry such a small tuft that it is more easily felt than seen in the depths of the fur.

In some staking injuries, the cause of the wound may be seen projecting from the surface. In other cases, the damaging foreign body may be hidden below the surface. Airgun slugs and shotgun pellets usually remain in the depths of the puncture wound but a bullet can penetrate right through the body, leaving wounds at the points of both entrance and exit and a trail of devastation in its path through the body, e.g. broken bone, damaged muscle and haemorrhaging internal organs.

Occasionally avulsion wounds can occur (Fig. 3.15f) and are most often seen in the scruff following dog-fight injuries if the injured dog has been picked up or shaken by its opponent. The area of skin grasped by the teeth is pulled away from the patient's body, creating a cavern underneath the skin where the connective tissue holding the skin to the underlying body is torn apart. Little is seen on the outside except two or four puncture wounds at either side of the cavern, which were created by the canine teeth of the attacker, but the space will readily fill with pus if the wound becomes infected. Since bite wounds are always contaminated, this is a very common occurrence.

Successful healing of a puncture wound can only occur if the wound granulates from the bottom up, i.e. the skin wound remains open until the underlying tissues have healed so that any infection can drain out as the wound heals. Once the infection is controlled, healing is rapid because the wound edges do not gape as the wound is so small.

Abrasion

This is the name given to a graze or scrub wound. Such wounds do not penetrate the entire skin thickness (Fig. 3.15g and h) and therefore are not true open wounds, but they do affect the body surface and have been included here for completeness. They are usually caused by a glancing blow or road accident where the animal is dragged along the ground. Occasionally, some dogs (especially labradors and retrievers) suffer 'hot spots', when the dog scratches and rubs the side of the face/neck so intensely that it becomes red raw and bleeding within hours.

The wound is superficial and the haemorrhage consists of capillary bleeding, so that these wounds, though often contaminated, are rarely serious. They are, however, very painful, often more so than any of the other wounds because the epidermis may be worn away to expose large areas of the sensitive dermis with its multiple nerve endings. In open wounds, which penetrate through the total skin thickness, the dermal nerve endings are only exposed at the edges of the wound, which is a relatively small area when compared with an extensive graze.

Healing of open wounds

Wounds heal by one of two methods: **first intention** healing or **granulation** (Table 3.12). See Chapter 19, p.491.

First intention healing. The edges of the wounds are not widely separated and are held together by blood clots. New blood vessels grow into these clots from the sides of the wound, carrying with them the healing components that will produce the fibrous scar tissue to tie the wound edges together permanently. Epithelial cells quickly spread across the narrow scar and start producing a new skin layer over the scar tissue (Fig. 3.16). Provided that there is no sepsis to interfere with the process, healing will be complete in 7–10 days.

Table 3.12 Healing of open wounds

First intention	Granulation
Usual for incised wounds and simple puncture wounds	Usual for lacerated and infected puncture wounds
Edges of wounds remain close together	Wound edges are widely separated
Healing complete in 7–10 days	Healing can take weeks or months
No infection present	Wound often contaminated and may become infected
Minimal scarring	Scarring is extensive

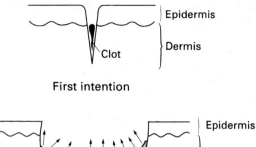

Fig. 3.16 Healing of wounds.

First intention healing can only take place in incised wounds where the edges remain close together. This may be achieved by stitching or bandaging whilst the healing takes place.

Granulation. Granulation tissue usually heals lacerated, avulsed and infected wounds and the repair process may take several weeks, as the wound edges are widely separated (Fig. 3.16). Clusters of cells are produced on the exposed tissue of the wound and they multiply rapidly to form areas of granulation tissue which gradually expand to cover the entire wound area. The tissue is moist and bright red, with a bubbly, uneven surface. It is easily damaged and bleeds if disturbed, as it has a very rich blood supply. It grows up towards the skin surface level, filling the gap between the wound edges. When it is level with the surface, new epithelial cells can spread across the top to complete the healing process but as there is a far larger area to be covered (compared with a case of first intention healing), this process can take weeks to complete. The new epithelial tissue first shows as a thin, smooth, white-blue line around the edge of the wound. It gradually spreads inwards towards the centre of the granulating area – the reversal of ripples on a pond.

Factors delaying wound healing

Movement. If the wound edges move against each other, the delicate healing tissues are continually destroyed and need to reform. Injuries over joints will take longer to heal than injuries where skin movement is minimal.

Infection. Most wounds are contaminated because they have been inflicted by unsterile objects which leave bacteria in the body tissues. For example, lacerated wounds caused by road traffic accidents are usually grossly contaminated by dirt, grit and hair, all of which are covered with bacteria that may be harmful to living tissues. If the wound is not treated correctly or the body defence mechanisms are poor, the bacteria will multiply and invade the body tissues, killing them. The healing tissues are destroyed and wound healing is seriously delayed. Infected wounds show all the signs of inflammation and may discharge pus.

Disturbance in circulation. Heavily contused wounds may take longer to heal as the local circulation to the wounds is impaired. The skin at the edge of the wound dies and the wound edges cannot heal until this dead tissue has been removed.

Avulsed wounds also may result in areas of skin which have lost their blood supply and die. The dead skin becomes hard, leathery and dry and will eventually separate from the healthy tissues. The wound created by this loss of skin then has to heal by granulation.

Self-trauma. Continual licking will cause movement of the wound, introduce infection and damage the healing tissues.

Treatment of open wounds and abrasions

The aims of treatment are:

- To arrest haemorrhage.
- To treat shock.
- To prevent sepsis.

The first two are the most important and it is sometimes preferable to delay the treatment against infection until the general condition of the patient has improved.

There are certain pitfalls to be avoided when presented with the patient and it is best to follow a set course of action:

(1) Treat for shock.
(2) Remove any dressings applied by the owner.
(3) Control any severe haemorrhage.
(4) Remove the cause of the injury.
(5) Clip the hair around the wound.
(6) Remove any contaminating foreign bodies.
(7) Cleanse the wound.
(8) Dress the wound.

Treating for shock. See earlier, p. 29. If the animal is collapsed, fluid therapy should be commenced at an early stage.

Removing dressings applied by the owner. This allows the veterinary nurse to inspect the injuries sustained but must be done with care as it will probably be painful for the patient. If the animal becomes too distressed, it may be better to leave these in place so long as the patient is comfortable and its condition is stable. Incautious or rough removal of bandages may also tear away blood clots and restart haemorrhage.

Controlling haemorrhage. Immediate steps must be taken to control any severe haemorrhage. All instruments used in treating the wound should be sterilised if possible and hands should always be washed (preferably in surgical scrub) to prevent further contamination of the wound. **Blood that has clotted should never be removed by the person applying first aid** as this will invariably restart the haemorrhage.

Removing the cause of the injury. The cause should be removed where this is possible, particularly if it is likely to cause further damage or continuing pain. Superficial items such as traps, snares or fish hooks may be removed, but deeply penetrating foreign bodies should be left alone: glass fragments can be triangular, with only the tip showing above the skin so that attempts to remove them will cause the animal pain and may only drive the glass deeper into the tissues; stakes penetrating the chest wall or abdomen may have entered the thoracic cavity or ruptured a large blood vessel, and the attempted removal of these foreign bodies may cause a pneumothorax or may disturb clots formed around the blood vessel, restarting a serious haemorrhage.

Large penetrating foreign bodies which protrude from the body should be cut off so that they only just protrude above the skin surface. A ring-pad dressing can then be applied over the whole wound (see Figures 3.10 and 3.11 on p. 46).

Clipping the hair. The hair around the wound should be clipped carefully to avoid contaminating the wound with multiple individual hairs. If the hair is matted with blood, it can be clipped away quite cleanly, but normal fur should be smeared with aqueous cream (which can be easily removed before surgery) or at least dampened with saline so that it sticks together in clumps and can be removed more efficiently.

Contaminating foreign bodies. Grit and dirt usually contaminate road accident wounds. Hair is commonly found deeply buried in gunshot wounds and bite injuries. Such foreign bodies should be removed if possible by the careful use of dressing forceps or similar instruments.

Cleansing the wound. The aim at this stage is to flush the wound mechanically, irrigating the damaged tissues with a soothing, non-toxic solution which will wash away the superficial contaminating dirt and bacteria. Isotonic sterile saline, syringed with gentle force into the wound, will achieve all of these objectives (this is a good use for half-used sterile intravenous drips). If no sterile saline is available, a saline solution may be made up from half a teaspoonful of salt to one litre of cooled, boiled water. Failing all else, warm tap water may be used. In general, *antiseptic solutions should not be used* to cleanse wounds: although they hinder the growth of micro-organisms, they can also have harmful effects on the raw body tissues, especially if not made up to the precise strength recommended by the manufacturer.

Puncture wounds caused by canine, feline or reptile bites are the exception to this rule and should be gently but thoroughly flushed with a solution of hydrogen peroxide, diluted 1:4 with warm water, or a *correctly diluted* solution of povidone-iodine could be used. These bites are usually heavily contaminated with pathogenic bacteria, many of which are anaerobes.

The cleansing procedure should be gentle but thorough. Make sure that the irrigating fluid penetrates into the depths of the wound, but **take care that the clots in the wound are not disturbed** and that the wound is not further contaminated by dirt derived from the skin.

Dressing the wound. A suitable dressing should now be applied. The aims are:

- To prevent further contamination of the wound.
- To prevent further damage to the tissues, e.g. by the patient licking the wound or the exposed tissues drying out.
- To prevent blood clots being disturbed.

Firstly, to protect any exposed areas of raw tissue, a protective gel (e.g. Intrasite Gel) should be applied. This step is usually only necessary with lacerated wounds since incised wounds and puncture wounds do not gape open or may be bandaged so that the skin edges come together, protecting the underlying tissues.

A sterile, non-adhesive wound dressing is then placed on the wound, covered by cotton wool and a bandage. (Bandaging techniques are described in Chapter 2, p. 13.) If a non-adhesive dressing is not available, a sterile gauze swab may be used, but these tend to stick to the wound and may cause further damage to the tissues when removed at surgery. *Cotton wool should never be applied directly to the wound* because it will stick to the wound and the wisps will contaminate the wound.

If it is not possible to dress the wound (the animal may have a suspected broken spine and a large lacerated chest wound that cannot be bandaged without moving the patient and causing intense pain), it is important to keep the tissues moist and viable by applying a protective gel and covering the area with 'cling film' to stop the moisture evaporating.

NB: It is better to use protective gel on exposed tissues than to apply antiseptic preparations. If antiseptics are used, choose a water-soluble cream, not an oily ointment, which will be difficult to remove at subsequent surgery.

Closed wounds

There are three types of closed wound: contusions, haematomas and injuries to internal organs.

Contusions

A contusion (bruise) is produced by a blow with a blunt instrument which causes rupture of blood vessels in the skin and in the soft tissues beneath. The escaping blood seeps into the surrounding damaged tissues and will eventually clot. As the damaged tissues heal, the red blood cells in the clot are broken down and the breakdown products of the haemoglobin pigment account for the yellow/green discoloration of the skin.

The signs of a contusion are **heat, pain** and **swelling**. White-skinned animals show **discoloration** of the skin, which is first red (immediately after the blow), then purple (within a few hours) and finally yellow/green (after several days). Deep bruising of muscles will cause a swelling which often increases in size as it heals. This severe bruising remains painful for a period of weeks until healing is complete.

Treatment of contusions

- **Cold compresses** should be applied immediately to cause vasoconstriction in the damaged area. Constriction of the blood vessel walls will decrease the amount of blood entering the area and thus limit the volume of blood lost and help to prevent swelling of the tissues. The cold will also help to alleviate pain.
- **Firm bandaging** will increase the back pressure, control haemorrhage and limit swelling.
- If several hours have elapsed since the injury and the area is already swollen, **hot fomentations** should be used: they will speed recovery by causing vasodilatation to *increase* the blood supply to the damaged tissue so that the injury can be repaired more rapidly.

Haematomas

These injuries most commonly affect the earflaps of dogs and cats. Occasionally, a small blood vessel may spontaneously rupture or the animal may scratch hard at the earflap or shake its head violently. The escaping blood from these damaged veins fills a pocket of connective tissue under the skin, ballooning it out until back pressure results in a natural arrest of haemorrhage.

Haematomas may also be seen following intravenous injections or blood sampling if pressure is not applied to the vein as the needle is withdrawn. Accidental puncture wounds which damage large blood vessels may also create haematomas.

Unlike a contusion or an abscess, the swelling of a haematoma is soft, usually painless and cool to the touch. In time, the blood will clot, and the clots contract over a period of weeks to become hard and knobbly.

Treatment of haematomas. The only first aid treatment of value is to bandage the affected area firmly, as soon as possible, or apply firm pressure with a cold compress if bandaging is impractical. Once the area is swollen, surgical intervention may be necessary to drain the haematoma of the earflap.

Damage to internal organs

Crushing injuries of the body may result in damage to internal organs. Details of first aid are given later in this chapter, in sections relevant to various body systems.

Burns and scalds

Definitions

A **burn** is an injury to the body caused by:

- Dry heat (house fires, contact with hot surfaces, etc.).
- Excessive cold (frostbite, cryosurgery).
- Corrosive chemicals (strong acids, petroleum products).
- Electric currents or radiation (after a major disaster, e.g. a nuclear disaster).

A **scald** is an injury caused by the effect of moist heat (such as boiling water, tar or oil).

The distinction between burns and scalds is not of practical interest, for the signs and principles of treatment are the same in each case. It is far more important to identify the cause of the injury so that the correct first aid is given. For example:

- **Heat burns** must be cooled immediately.
- **Chemical burns** must be cleaned with a suitable solvent.

Classification

Classification depends upon the depth of the injury and the size of the area affected.

Depth of injury

This classification used to be divided into six degrees but the modern classification recognises only two types of burns or scalds:

- **Superficial**, penetrating no deeper than the skin surface (1st and 2nd degree burns).
- **Deep**, penetrating through the skin thickness into the tissues beneath (3rd, 4th, 5th and 6th degree burns).

Percentage of the total body surface affected

This is simply a rough estimation based on examining the patient (e.g. a burn which affects the whole of one side of an animal would be estimated to be a 40% burn). Evaluation of the skin area affected is useful because it gives some idea of the degree of pain suffered by the animal and the rate of loss of body fluids. Extensive burns can cause dehydration as appreciable volumes of body fluids evaporate from a large area of exposed flesh.

Clinical signs

The clinical signs of all burns and scalds are very similar but appear at different times depending on the cause of the injury. Heat and electrical burns produce symptoms immediately, but with chemical, cold and radiation burns it may take several hours or even days before the signs appear. The signs are also more severe in young animals, which have more delicate skin.

The signs may be summarised as follows:

- **Redness and heat.** The blood vessels of the skin dilate as the area becomes inflamed. Redness is most easily seen in white unpigmented skin.
- **Swelling**. The tissues swell and the surface becomes *moist* as the inflammatory changes allow tissue fluid to escape from the capillaries into the damaged tissues and on to the surface of the wound. Blisters are rarely seen in animals.
- **Pain**. Pain is variable but, as a rule, deep burns are less painful than large superficial ones. This is because the deep burn destroys the sensory nerve endings in the dermis, so the central area of the burn becomes relatively

insensitive. However, the edges of the wound which are superficially burnt will be painful because the sensory nerve endings are still intact.

- **Loss of fur**. The fur will fall out after a few days (if it was not burnt away by dry heat at the time of the accident) because the hair follicles in the dermis are damaged so the hair shaft is shed.
- **Skin surface becomes leathery.** Surface tissues are destroyed in deep burns and dry out to become leathery and totally insensitive in the days following the injury. The dead tissues will peel away from the surrounding healthy, healing tissues and the open wound created will heal by granulation.

Specific injuries: treatment and complications

Table 3.13 sets out the likely causes and clinical signs of heat burns, scalds, electrical burns and chemical burns.

Extensive heat burns and scalds

Burns and scalds from, for example, domestic fires can be extremely painful and animals resent interference. All cases of extensive burns or scalds should be treated by a veterinary surgeon as soon as possible. First aid measures involve:

- Cooling the damaged areas as quickly as possible.
- Keeping the patient warm once the initial cooling treatment is complete.
- Dressing the wound.
- Splinting to limit movement if necessary.
- Preparing intravenous drips.

Cooling the damaged areas. Cold water should be gently hosed on to the burnt areas as soon as the animal is removed from the fire. This will rapidly decrease the heat in the tissues so that fewer cells die and tissue damage and pain are kept to a minimum. It will also guard against the risk of hyperthermia.

A gentle, continuous stream of water is better than an ice pack because larger areas can be treated and it avoids putting any pressure on the extremely painful, damaged tissues. This treatment must be discontinued if it causes the animal pain or if the animal shows signs of becoming chilled, which can happen within a few minutes if large areas of the body are affected. The rectal temperature should be monitored as in cases of hyperthermia (see Hyperthermia in the section on Collapse, p. 96).

Keeping the patient warm. This is difficult because, although the body needs to be kept warm, any heating of the burnt areas will cause the animal considerable pain. **Heat lamps and other forms of direct heat must never be used in these cases.** It is best to conserve the body heat by wrapping the unaffected parts of the body in warm, dry blankets and shielding the animal from draughts. The injuries may be kept cool by covering the dressed wound (see below) with a cold, wet towel or ice packs.

Dressing the wound. Burns and scalds are sterile wounds as the initial heat destroys the bacteria on the skin surface. Dressing the wound is useful because:

- It prevents body fluid loss from the exposed tissue.
- It protects the damaged tissues from further damage.
- It prevents the animal contaminating the wound by licking at it.

Table 3.13 Burns and scalds: causes and signs

	Causes	Clinical signs
Heat burns and scalds	House fires Kitchen accidents Burns to the feet as the result of walking on hot surfaces (e.g. unwary cats walking on hot ceramic hobs).	Clinical signs immediate in both cases. *Burns* Any area of the body may be affected. Singed or burnt hair indicates damaged area. Wounds may be very deep or superficial, depending on the cause. *Scalds* Usually occur on the head, neck or dorsum because hot liquids drop on animal from a height. Splashing with hot liquids results in 'inverted pear-shaped' wound (bulk of liquid lands on animal and then drains down the skin in an increasingly narrowing stream). Hair may be matted with liquid if fatty/high sugar content. Usually superficial wounds.
Electrical burns	Burns are seen in pups that chew through electrical cables and also in cases of electrocuted animals.	Clinical signs immediate. Burns seen where current enters and leaves the body: Pups often have red areas on lips, tongue and gums if chewed cable. Electrocution victims show burns to nose (if sniffing), sternum (if lying down), feet (where current usually exits the body) or neck (if wearing metal collar). Wounds are usually superficial.
Chemical burns	Splashing by strong acids or alkalis (e.g. quicklime) or accidental immersion in containers or corrosive or irritant substances (e.g. battery acid, sump oil).	Clinical signs take hours to develop. Burns may occur anywhere on the body but feet and hindquarters are particularly prone to injury (animals walking on contaminated ground or falling into containers of sump oil, etc.). Wounds usually superficial.

However, remember that these wounds are extremely painful and thorough cleansing and conventional bandaging will probably only be possible under general anaesthetic when strict aseptic precautions can be observed.

The wound should be gently cleaned with cool sterile saline to remove any loose or charred remnants of hair before a dressing is applied. Protective wound gel and sterile non-stick dressings or paraffin tulle covered by a **minimal** amount of sterile absorbent dressing should be applied and bandaged in place. The absorbent dressing should be kept as light as possible because:

- Thick layers prevent heat loss from the inflamed, overheated area and the cooler the area is kept, the less the pain.
- This layer will absorb fluid from the wound surface, causing more damage to the surface tissues by drying them further.

Polythene bags wrapped around the completed dressing will prevent evaporation of moisture.

If no dressings are available at the site of the accident or if the wound is too large or painful to be dressed using conventional bandaging, a *clean* sheet of polythene or 'cling film' may be laid directly over the injured area and a cold, wet towel laid on top to keep it in place and cool the burnt area.

Splinting. Splinting can be used to limit movement if there are severe burns to the limbs, but must be applied in such a way that there is no pressure on the damaged area. In practice, this is very difficult to achieve with the shocked, conscious patient which is in considerable pain. However, bandaging of a limb will limit movement to some extent.

Preparing for the veterinary surgeon. Intravenous drips will be needed to replace the fluid lost by evaporation in extensive burns and to combat the shock. Dextrose saline or normal saline are both suitable.

Pain-killing drugs should be to hand and it may be necessary to anaesthetise the patient so that the wounds may be properly dressed.

Less extensive heat burns or scalds

The treatment of minor scalds from kitchen accidents is similar:

- Cool the affected area as soon as possible to limit tissue damage and alleviate the pain.
- Clean the area, as for extensive burns. (In long-haired animals, the fur covering a scalded area should be clipped away if possible to allow the skin to cool before it is dressed.)
- Apply dressings, as for extensive burns.

Cooling the affected area. This needs to be done immediately by the owners at home. It may be necessary to first cut the soaked fur away in long-coated animals because this will remove the source of the heat and expose the underlying skin for easier washing and cooling. It will be too painful for the patient if an attempt is made to shave the area, but even if a 'crew cut' style is achieved, it will allow the cooling water to reach the skin instead of running off over the surface of the coat.

Scalds caused by water-soluble fluid (e.g. milk, boiling water) and burn injuries can be flushed *immediately* with cold, running water. It may be necessary for the owner to put the animal under the shower in the bath or to hose off the patient outside.

Scalds caused by fat or oil must be cleaned quickly before the fat congeals in the coat and seals in the heat. Paper towel should be used to soak up as much fat as possible (taking care not to scald the hands of the owner or nurse) and then a warm detergent solution should be poured on to the area and **gently** worked into the coat for a few seconds to help to remove the fat. Finally, the scalded area must be washed well with cold water to remove the detergent and cool the tissues.

Ice packs are very useful to continue cooling the injured area after washing and can be made from polythene bags filled with crushed ice, frozen peas or anything else readily to hand in the household freezer. As only a relatively small area of the body is to be treated, there is no risk of causing hypothermia and the ice pack may be gently bandaged over the wound and left in place for 10 minutes, after which it can be renewed or removed if necessary.

Owners who are unable to give this treatment at home should be advised to hold an ice pack onto the injured area or cover the area with a cold, wet towel and bring the animal to the surgery immediately so that the veterinary nurse can proceed with the treatment.

Complications of heat burns and scalds

Shock. The degree of shock is very severe in cases of extensive burning and is caused by:

- Pain.
- Tissue damage and inflammation.
- Loss of body fluids from the damaged areas.
- Infection in the days following the injury.

Tissue death and wound infection release toxins which, when absorbed into the bloodstream, may cause toxaemia or septicaemia. This, in combination with the shock of fluid loss, may be severe enough to cause the death of the patient.

Dyspnoea or asphyxia. Animals rescued from house fires may suffer from pulmonary oedema (fluid on the lungs) as the irritant smoke inhaled in the fire can cause severe inflammation of the respiratory tract. These patients often develop bronchitis or pneumonia 2–3 days after the accident (see Asphyxia, p. 90).

Infection. The moist tissues on the surface of the burn easily become infected and this will delay wound healing.

Scar formation. These wounds heal by second intention and scar formation may be extensive in a large wound. This will cause problems if the wound overlies a joint because the healthy, elastic skin is replaced by inelastic scar tissue which is unable to stretch freely as the joint is flexed and extended. Thus the range of movement of the joint may be restricted.

Electrical burns

> ### WARNING
> Do not touch an electrocuted animal until the electricity supply has been disconnected (see Electrocution, p. 95).

Wounds should be treated and dressed in the manner described for heat burns.

The most serious complication associated with electrical burns is that of electrocution. Longer term problems could include the complications mentioned for heat burns and scalds. However, electrical burns are rarely extensive and so local infection of the wound is the most likely problem – if the animal survives the initial accident.

Chemical burns

It is advisable for the handler to wear gloves to prevent any human skin burns before attempting to deal with the situation. Copious volumes of water should be used to wash the worst of the chemical contamination off the skin and then the coat should be washed with a mild detergent to ensure complete removal of the chemical. If the chemical is a known alkali (e.g. caustic soda or quicklime), prepare an acid solution by mixing equal quantities of household vinegar and water and use it to wash away the chemical. If the burn is caused by a known acid, use a concentrated solution of bicarbonate of soda or washing soda. However, the secret of successful treatment is the rapid washing away of the chemical and the prompt use of a hosepipe is usually sufficient.

Chemical burns are rarely deep but may be very extensive and very irritating to the animal. The major complication in these cases is that of poisoning as the patient tries to clean the corrosive chemical from its coat. It is a wise precaution to tell the owner to give demulcents and absorptives at home to prevent any poisoning. (See Poisoning p. 30.)

Fractures

Definitions

A **fracture** is a forcible break in the continuity of bony tissue, i.e. the bone is broken.

Fragments are the pieces of bone that are formed as the result of a fracture.

There are varying degrees of injury, but any damage to the bony cortex which is caused by force is still technically a fracture. Some fractures are as slight as a hairline crack (*incomplete fractures*), i.e. the bone cortex is broken on one side only but the bone itself is not broken into pieces (see Fig. 3.17) but other cases may have *complete fractures* where the bone is completely broken into two or more fragments (Fig. 3.18).

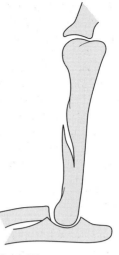

Fig. 3.17

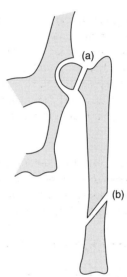

Fig. 3.18

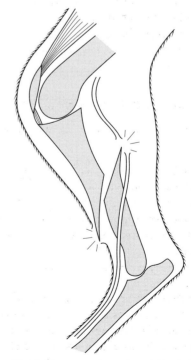

Fig. 3.19

The fragments are usually sharp and jagged and are thus likely to cause further damage, especially when they are displaced by muscular spasms and spear into surrounding tissues (Fig. 3.19).

Fractures are also described according to the damage done: see Fracture classification, p. 499.

- A **simple** fracture is one where the bone is broken cleanly into two pieces.
- A **compound** fracture is one where there is a wound communicating between the skin or mucous membranes and the fracture site. There is a real risk that infection can occur in these fractures.
- A **complicated** fracture is one where important structures or organs around the fracture site are damaged, e.g. blood vessels, nerves, the spinal cord, the lungs or the heart. (Fig. 3.19).
- A **multiple** fracture is one where the bone is fractured in two or more places, but where there is an appreciable distance between the sites of the fractures (Fig. 3.18). NB: A multiple fracture is *not* one where there are lots of fragments at the fracture site. This is known as a comminuted fracture.

A fracture may be described using several of the above terms. Figure 3.19 illustrates a simple compound complicated fracture of the tibia. It is a *simple* fracture because the bone is broken into two pieces but it is also *compound* because the sharp proximal fragment has penetrated the skin and it is *complicated* because the saphenous nerve has been damaged by the sharp distal fragment.

Signs of fracture

- Pain at or near the site of the fracture.
- Swelling.
- Loss of function.
- Deformity.
- Unnatural mobility.
- Crepitus.

The last three signs are not often detected in incomplete fractures and it must not be expected that all of the above signs will be found in every case. If there is any reason to suspect a fracture, the injury should be treated as such pending diagnosis by a veterinary surgeon.

Pain on or near the site of the fracture

It must be remembered that pain increases shock and gentle handling is essential to avoid increasing the pain. The severity of the pain depends upon:

- **The amount of movement** which can occur between the bone fragments and how much the fragments rub against each other. Incomplete fractures are less painful than complete fractures, as the fragments scarcely move. Overriding fractures (e.g. Fig. 3.19) tend to be less painful because the broken ends do not grate on each other.

- **The damage to other tissues involved.** In cases of vertebral fractures, the pain is usually intense because of the pressure exerted on the spinal cord by the displaced bones and fragments.

Swelling

Swelling occurs soon after the accident due to haemorrhage from the bruised muscles and inflammation of the soft tissues surrounding the fracture site. The swelling will be made worse if the sharp fracture fragments are allowed to move freely following the accident and cause more soft tissue damage.

Loss of function

This may be partial or complete. There is always some limitation of use after a bone has been fractured and the animal is usually 90–100% lame.

Deformity

Fractures of limb long bones are often obvious because the fracture fragments can be severely displaced and the limb is markedly deformed. Fracture deformities of other bones (e.g. the pelvic bones or the vertebrae) may be more difficult to detect because the bones are covered by large muscle masses.

Unnatural mobility

This is usually noted in fractures of the limb long bones the bone will bend where it should not bend, e.g. the lower leg may swing from side to side after a femoral fracture. Unnatural movement may be noticed at the fracture site as the animal moves or as the limb is gently examined.

Crepitus

A grating sound may be heard or felt when the broken ends move against one another. This, and unnatural mobility, should not be tested for by the person giving first aid, but gives positive evidence of the presence of a fracture if noticed during the course of an examination.

First aid treatment

The principle of first aid treatment for a fracture is to minimise the movement of the fracture fragments. This alleviates pain and stops the situation deteriorating because the sharp fracture fragments are not allowed to jar against each other nor can they cut into the surrounding soft tissues every time the animal moves. The following treatment route is recommended:

- Handle the broken bone as little as possible.
- Control haemorrhage in a compound fracture.
- Support the fracture.

Handling

> **WARNING**
>
> **Under no circumstances should resetting of the limb or reduction of the fracture be attempted.** If a vertebral fracture is suspected, the patient must be moved with extreme care, keeping the whole of the spinal column supported *at all times* and avoiding any twisting movements of the spine. This means that the animal should not be turned over unless absolutely necessary (e.g. to examine wounds on its underside). If the patient does have to be moved, seek the assistance of several people to turn the animal.

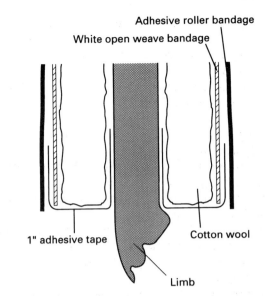

Fig. 3.20 Robert Jones dressing (cross-section).

Haemorrhage

Haemorrhage in a compound fracture should be controlled by applying a dressing if possible. Digital pressure must only be used with care as this could displace the fragments and cause complications. A ring-pad dressing is very useful here. The wound may be cleansed as described earlier.

Support

It is really only practical to support limb fractures.

Support for the fracture should be applied as soon as possible to limit movement and prevent further damage. However, splinting should be abandoned if it is impossible without a struggle – provoking the animal to thrash around will do it more harm than the splint will do good. Such animals are best kept still, warm and comfortable until professional help is available or until the animal has calmed down and will allow a splint to be applied without a struggle.

Support dressing for fractured bones

Robert Jones dressing

This is used for fractures of the elbow and stifle joints and bones below, and is one of the most useful limb dressings which may be applied in veterinary practice. It consists of layers of cotton wool, which are then bound tightly with a roller bandage until the cotton wool is compressed and becomes almost rigid. It is thus a soft dressing, which conforms perfectly to the contours of the limb and is difficult to apply too tightly. It also controls soft tissue swelling superbly and, most important of all, is very well tolerated by the patient.

Application of a Robert Jones dressing

● Cut two strips of 1 inch (25 mm) adhesive plaster, long enough to cover the length of the metacarpal/metatarsal region of the foot, plus a couple of inches. Apply these strips longitudinally to the anterior and posterior aspects of the metacarpals/metatarsals (Fig. 3.20).

● Using a roll of cotton wool as a roller bandage, cover the entire length of the leg with four to five layers of cotton wool (a 500 g roll should be sufficient for an Irish wolfhound). If orthopaedic bandaging is used (e.g. 'Softban'), as many as 12–15 rolls will be needed.

● Bandage the cotton wool firmly in place using white open-weave bandage. This is better than conforming bandage because it will not contract once applied. Conforming bandages can increase the pressure in the dressing to such an extent that the blood supply to the limb is cut off. White open-weave bandage relaxes slightly after application and so it is difficult to apply it too tightly and the blood circulation can function normally (for signs of an overtight bandage, see Application of splints, p. 58).

● To test if sufficient tension has been used to compact the cotton wool, 'flick' the completed dressing with a finger. It should make a resonant sound similar to that heard when testing a ripe melon.

● Reflect the longitudinal strips of adhesive bandage upwards over the bandage and stretch them as tight as possible. These prevent the dressing slipping down the leg.

● Bandage these strips in place, using 2–3 inch (8 cm) wide adhesive roller bandage wrapped around the layer of white open-weave bandage. The bandage now consists of the layers shown in Fig. 3.20. The toes may be left exposed for observation (see Chapter 2, p. 16).

Bandaging

The affected part of the body is bandaged firmly to unaffected parts of the body, so that the healthy body is used as a splint. This technique is used for the *scapula*, which can be bound against the rib cage, or for single fractured *metacarpals, metatarsals* or *digits* which may be bound to adjoining unaffected bones of the same foot by bandaging the foot. Such support will also decrease the amount of swelling following the fracture and thus minimise the pain.

Splinting

A splint is an appliance which restricts the movement of an injured part. Splints are of limited value:

- They can only be applied successfully to the bones and joints below the elbow and stifle joints. Above these joints, the bones are surrounded by large muscle masses and it is impossible to immobilise the fracture fragments by applying a simple external splint.
- They are time-consuming to apply and can cause the patient pain as they are fitted.

Therefore, the use of splints is restricted to those cases where professional help may be delayed for some time (e.g. the patient has to travel a long way to the surgery) or where the animal must be manhandled (e.g. the large, collapsed dog with a fractured tibia which has to be lifted into a car).

Criteria for a successful splint. The splint used should be:

- Long enough to immobilise the joints above and below the fractured bone.
- Rigid, so that it will not bend and allow movement of the injured part.
- Smooth, so that there are no projections which can dig into the patient's underlying tissues.
- Conforming, so that it holds the injured part firmly in position, does not allow movement and is comfortable for the patient.

Materials used for splints. Many materials can be used, depending on the initiative of the person at the scene of the accident and the size of the patient. Broom handles, rolled-up newspapers and magazines, ice-lolly sticks and wire coat-hangers have all played a part. More conventional splinting materials are as follows:

- **Wooden splints** – straight pieces of wood of appropriate length.
- **Preformed metal splints** made of tin or aluminium. Zimmer splints (malleable aluminium splinting of different widths, backed by foam) are very useful and can easily be bent to conform to the shape of the leg.
- **Plastic gutter splints** of varying diameters, lined with foam, may be snapped off at the desired length.
- **Plaster or resin.** Roller bandages made of coarse material and impregnated with plaster of Paris or resin are commonly used in fracture treatment. The bandage should *not* encase the limb – this is beyond the scope of first aid – but may be used as a slab to form a gutter splint on one side of the leg only. (Plaster of Paris splinting should not be used on a compound fracture because any wound dressings will become saturated with water and the wound could become contaminated by the plaster of Paris. Resin materials hold hardly any water and will not contaminate the injury, and so these splints may be used over a dressed wound.)
- **Inflatable airbags** could be used around a limb of a suitable size to immobilise a broken leg. (There is a range of such appliances for human first aid.) There may be a risk of obstructing the circulation if the bags are too tightly inflated.

Application of splints. **If the splint itself is not padded, the limb should always be covered with two layers of orthopaedic bandaging** (e.g. 'soft ban') or a thin layer of cotton wool before the splint is applied. This layer should be thick enough to prevent the hard splint from pressing on the skin and causing damage or discomfort, but thin enough to allow the splint to be placed as close to the fractured bone as possible to immobilize the fracture efficiently.

Wooden, metal and plastic splints. If wooden splints are used, the leg must be bandaged first as described above. Metal and plastic splints are usually already padded.

The splints may be attached by strips of 1 inch adhesive tape, bound firmly but not tightly around the leg (Fig. 3.21). Where possible, these strips should not encircle the limb at the actual fracture site for fear of causing complications. The whole leg is then bandaged with a support dressing such as a thick layer of cotton wool firmly bandaged in place with white open weave or conforming bandage. This support dressing will also prevent swelling in tissues *not* bound by the adhesive strips.

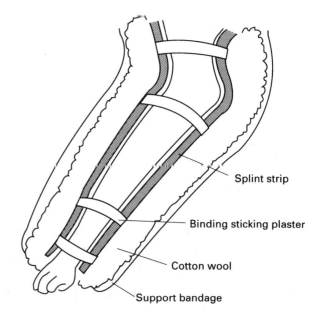

Fig. 3.21 Applying metal splints.

Splint strip

Binding sticking plaster

Cotton wool

Support bandage

Resin or plaster splints. The leg must first be bandaged with orthopaedic bandage – cotton wool is not suitable as it will absorb too much water if plaster of Paris is used.

The splint should be fashioned as follows:

- Cut a suitable length of **resin cast** material from a roll and soften as appropriate before applying to the limb. Note that only *one* layer of resin casting material is needed, except when very large dogs are being treated (when it may be necessary to use two layers). This material is very strong, so that if several layers are used it may be impossible for the veterinary surgeon to remove the splint easily and give further treatment.
- A **plaster of Paris** bandage (Fig. 3.22) needs to be soaked in water, wrung out, unrolled on a smooth surface and folded on itself 3–4 times to form a slab of the desired length. It is then moulded upon the affected limb

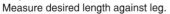

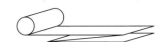

Step 1
Measure desired length against leg.

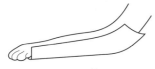

Step 2
Create a slab of wet or dry bandage (plaster of Paris only).

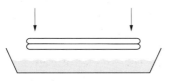

Step 3
Soak bandage and squeeze if necessary. (Hold in both hands for plaster of Paris. Use scissors etc. to immerse resin bandage in hot water).

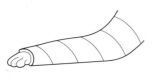

Step 4
Mould on to limb to form a gutter.

Step 5
Bandage in place and allow to set.

Fig. 3.22 Making a plaster splint.

and secured in position by an ordinary roller bandage, used wet. (It may be easier to unroll the bandage and make a slab of the desired length *before* wetting the bandage – it is very difficult to wet an entire roll and also difficult to find the end of the bandage when it is wet. The ends of the dry slab should be held in either hand whilst immersing the bandage in the water so that the slab can easily be straightened out and applied to the limb after the excess water has been squeezed out of the dressing.)

The cast should be strapped firmly in place using crepe bandages and movement restricted until the casting material hardens.

Support dressing. In all cases where a support dressing is used, the toes should not be completely covered by the final dressing if possible, so that they can be examined frequently to ensure that the circulation is not hindered by too tight a splint. The tissues at the fracture site may continue to swell for a short time after the splint is applied so that the tension under the dressing rises and the bandaging becomes overtight. Overtight bandaging will obstruct the venous return up the leg and the toes will swell.

> **WARNING**
> If both arterial and venous flows are obstructed, the toes may become swollen and cold. If any swelling should occur, **the dressings must be removed immediately** and replaced by looser bandaging.

Observation. Finally, once any dressings are in place, patients should be observed constantly for signs of discomfort – usually indicated by biting at the splint. If this occurs, the dressings should be checked and, if the animal persists, the dressings should be removed and replaced.

The state of consciousness (in cases of trauma to the head and spine), the breathing (in cases of rib fractures) and the passage of urine and faeces (in cases of pelvic fractures) must also be closely monitored.

Dislocations, sprains, strains and ruptured tendons

Definitions

A **dislocation** or **luxation** is a persistent displacement of the articular surfaces of the bones which form a joint (Fig. 3.23).

A **sprain** is an injury which occurs when a synovial joint has been violently forced to move too far in one direction, stretching and damaging the synovial membrane, ligaments and other soft tissues in the process but where the anatomy of the joint remains normal (unlike dislocations).

A **strain** is the stretching or tearing of a muscle or tendon.

A **ruptured tendon** is a form of severe strain or injury in which the tendon is either partially or completely torn as a result of sudden violence. Wounds to the distal limbs should always be checked to find out if the tendons are damaged. Tendons may also rupture due to indirect violence, e.g. twisting the leg awkwardly can rupture the Achilles tendon.

Common sites, clinical signs and treatment of these conditions are given in Table 3.14.

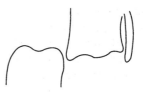

Luxation

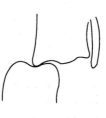

Subluxation

Fig. 3.23 Luxation and subluxation of a joint.

Table 3.14 Dislocations, strains, sprains and ruptured tendons

	Common sites	Clinical signs	Treatment
Dislocations	*Carpus and tarsus* (especially in association with deep lacerated wounds following road accidents where the ligaments have been destroyed). *Hip joint.* *Patella* (but these are usually long-standing injuries).	*Pain* on manipulation of the joint (much less in the chronic case). *Swelling* of the joint. *Loss of function* of limb, resulting in 90–100% lameness. *Deformity.* Usually obvious in cases of complete dislocation (the leg may be abnormally angled or obviously shorter than its partner). Subluxations are more difficult to detect because there is less deformity. *Limited movement* of the joint. *Crepitus* may be noticed but much less obvious than with fractures.	*Do not attempt to reduce the dislocation.* *Cold compresses* to limit swelling and ease pain. *Bandage* with suport dressing (e.g. Robert Jones dressing). Analgesics may be given by the veterinary surgeon.
Sprains	*Shoulder.* *Stifle* (usually resulting in the rupture of one or both cruciate ligaments). *Carpus and tarsus.*	*Pain* which is more severe if the joint is moved in the direction with stretched damaged tissues but much less intense than in cases of fracture or dislocation and *tenderness* on palpation of the actual joint. *Swelling* of the joint capsule, which develops shortly after the injury and is due to inflammation of the synovial membrane and bleeding from the damaged tissues. *Loss of use*: 50–70% lameness. *No gross deformity* of the limb.	These injuries are minor emergencies (Table 3.1). *Rest.* *Cold compresses* do not prevent swelling but will help to alleviate pain. *Bandaging.* A support crepe bandage may be applied at home by the owner to minimise the swelling. If preferred, a cold compress could be incorporated into the dressing to ease the pain.
Strains	*Muscles of the legs*, usually as the result of a sudden wrench. Racing and high-performance dogs are particularly prone to these injuries.	*Sudden loss of use* whilst exercising. The animal pulls up to 30–70% lame and further exercise is impossible. *Tenderness and swelling* over the affected muscles. *No deformity* of the limb.	*Rest* must be enforced. If necessary, the limb may be splinted. *Cold compresses and support bandages* to limit the swelling immediately after the accident. *Hot fomentations or electric heating pads* for longer term use to alleviate the pain and speed recovery.
Ruptured tendons	*Distal tendons of legs and feet.* Lacerated wounds (e.g. road accident injuries of carpus and hock downwards). Incised wounds of palmar and plantar surfaces of feet (e.g. the deeply cut pad/posterior surface of metacarpals and metatarsals). Spontaneous rupture (e.g. injuries in racing dogs). *Gastrocnemius tendon.*	*Visibly damaged tendons* in the depths of the wound if this is the cause of the injury. The torn ends of the gastrocnemius tendon are often palpable through the intact skin, although there may be a gap of several centimetres between the ends. *Unusual foot/leg conformation* In cases of flexor tendon foot injuries, the claw of the affected toe(s) sticks upwards rather than curving neatly to the ground (Fig. 3.24) – the so-called 'knocked-up toe'. In cases of gastrocnemius tendon injury, the hock sinks downwards, especially if there is any weight bearing. As the animal puts its foot to the ground, the tarsus sinks to the floor and the patient walks with the metatarsus on the ground like a kangaroo (Fig. 3.25). *Lameness.* The tendon injury itself is not very painful as tendons have a very limited blood supply and there is little bruising after the injury. Lameness occurs because: The joints of the limb have lost normal support and are abnormally stretched as weight is borne. Any lacerated wounds associated with injury are painful.	*Bandaging.* Cut ends of damaged tendons recoil up the leg and can be very difficult to find at subsequent surgery. If possible, the leg should be splinted in such a way as to keep the ruptured ends together: Flexor tendon injuries of the foot bandaged so the toes are flexed. Extensor tendon injuries bandaged in the normal foot position. Gastrocnemius tendon injuries bandaged with the hock in extension. *Wounds* should be cleansed and dressed as described earlier.

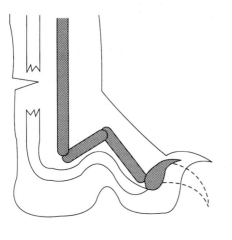

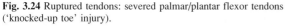

Normal position of claw

Fig. 3.24 Ruptured tendons: severed palmar/plantar flexor tendons ('knocked-up toe' injury).

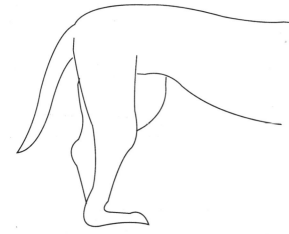

Fig. 3.25 Ruptured Achilles tendon, 'kangaroo' stance.

Injuries to the respiratory tract

WARNING

Injuries to any part of the respiratory tract may be fatal because the respiratory tract is the only source of the body's oxygen supply. Therefore, all patients showing dyspnoea should be very carefully and continuously observed. (See Table 3.15 for causes of dyspnoea.)

Nose

Causes

- **Trauma** – haemorrhage from the nose (**epistaxis**) most commonly occurs following a direct blow to the nasal bones, which rarely causes any problems, but occasionally it may be associated with severe skull fractures.

- **Tumours** of the nasal cavity may haemorrhage from time to time.
- **Foreign bodies.** Grass seeds, grass blades and occasionally splinters may become lodged in the nasal chambers of the dog and cat. It is not uncommon to find that a blade of grass works its way forwards down the cat's nose from the pharynx (Fig. 3.26).

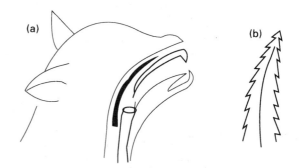

Fig. 3.26 (a) Grass in the nasopharynx. (b) A magnification of a grass blade showing barbed edges which prevent grass being swallowed and enable it to work forwards into the nasal passages.

Table 3.15 Causes of dyspnoea	
Laboured breathing	
Obstructed upper airway	Nasal passages, e.g. by blood, exudates, etc.
	Pharynx, e.g. large foreign body, swallowed tongue, swollen pharyngeal walls, etc.
	Larynx, trachea, e.g. strangulation injuries, collapsed trachea.
Fluid in the alveolar spaces (See *Asphyxia*, p. 90)	Drowning accidents. Congestive cardiac failure. Haemorrhage into the lungs. Irritant smoke inhalation (e.g. after house fires).
Collapsed lungs	Pneumothorax. Haemothorax. Pyothorax. Diaphragmatic ruptures.
Decreased oxygenation of the blood	Alveolar wall thickens (gaseous exchange is prevented, e.g. as in paraquat poisoning). Oxygen uptake by haemoglobin prevented by: Formation of methaemoglobin (as in paracetamol, chlorate poisonings – see p. 91). Formation of carboxyhaemoglobin (in carbon monoxide poisoning – see p. 91). Severe blood loss (decreased number of RBCs available to transport oxygen leads to hypoxia).
Rapid shallow breathing	
Shock	
Interference with respiratory movement	Paralysis of respiratory muscles (e.g. strychnine poisoning).
Pain	Gastric dilatation or torsion (compresses the thorax and is painful). Thoracic wall injuries.

Signs

- **Sneezing/head shaking.** The linings of the nasal passages are irritated by a foreign body, blood clots or the presence of a tumour. The bouts of sneezing are often violent and prolonged, accompanied by head shaking and pawing at the face as the animal attempts to reach the cause of the problem.
- **Haemorrhage. Epistaxis** or bleeding from the nose usually arises from the vascular turbinate mucosa and is not in itself a serious haemorrhage. The blood loss varies in each case and it is important to note whether the blood escapes from one or both nostrils.
  - *Trauma* – blows to the head usually result in haemorrhage from both nostrils, which is free-flowing immediately after the accident, but congeals within minutes, blocking both nostrils. In the following days, the patient usually sneezes a watery blood-stained discharge as the clots in the nose organise and contract. The haemorrhage rarely restarts.
  - *Tumours* bleed from time to time. The bouts of haemorrhage are therefore recurrent and are usually associated with sneezing and often only one nostril is affected.
  - *Foreign bodies* – severe sneezing will cause haemorrhage, usually from only one nostril (as above).
- **Purulent discharge** is usually unilateral (from one nostril) and occurs with foreign bodies and occasionally in cases where there is a tumour present.
- **Mouth-breathing** or **noisy nasal breathing** occurs as the nostrils and airways are completely or partially blocked.
- **Swelling of the nasal or frontal sinus area** can be caused by trauma or tumours.
- **Crepitus, deformity** or evidence of **depressed fractures** at the point of impact of a blow.

Complications

- **Concussion.** If the blow to the head was sufficiently serious, the cranium may be fractured and the fracture fragments displaced into the cranial cavity. The pressure this produces on the brain can cause collapse, unconsciousness and possibly death. (See Direct trauma, p. 89.)
- **Dyspnoea.** The patient may find it difficult to breathe because the nasal passages are blocked. In cases of head trauma, the nasal bones may be fractured and collapse, distorting and narrowing the nasal airways.
- **Vomiting.** Any blood lost is usually swallowed, either because it drains to the back of the nose or because the animal licks away discharge from the nostrils. If much blood in ingested, it may cause the animal to vomit.
- **Infection** is the greatest problem in foreign body cases and will not be controlled until the foreign body is removed from the nasal passages.

Treatment

If the animal is dyspnoeic or facial bone fractures are suspected, the nose must *not* be taped to restrain the animal. Patients with blocked nasal passages *must* be

Table 3.16 Treating dyspnoea	
Rest	Decreases the body's demand for oxygen. Confine the patient to a small basket or kennel in which it can lie down comfortably but has little space to move around.
Gentle handling	To avoid distressing the patient and provoking a struggle.
Oxygen	To ensure that the reduced volume of gas reaching the alveoli is rich in oxygen and thus hopefully supplies enough for the body's needs. (See *Treatment and resuscitation* for methods of giving oxygen, p. 85.)
Close observation	The patient's condition may deteriorate very rapidly.

allowed to mouth-breathe and taping may displace fractured bones.

- **Dyspnoea** should be treated (Table 3.16).
- **Cold compresses** applied externally to the nose will help to control the haemorrhage, reduce soft tissue swelling and alleviate pain, but in some cases adrenaline swabs inserted into the nostril opening may be needed to treat the condition. This should not be attempted without the consent of the veterinary surgeon: it is usually impossible to position the swab effectively in a conscious animal and incorrect insertion will do more harm than good.
- **Constant observation** is needed so that delayed concussion, if it occurs, can be detected at the earliest opportunity. If the patient already shows signs of concussion, it should be monitored.
- **Foreign bodies** visible at the nostrils may be carefully removed. If nothing is visible except a purulent discharge, the advice of the veterinary surgeon must be sought.

Pharynx and oesophagus

Causes **Foreign bodies** may lodge in the pharynx:

- The partly swallowed ball which lodges just behind the tongue on top of the larynx, being just too large to pass down the oesophagus, can asphyxiate the animal (Fig. 3.27).
- Cats eating grass may get a blade of grass stuck in the pharynx as they try to swallow it (Fig. 3.26).
- Sewing needles and fish hooks are occasionally found embedded in the walls of the pharynx or come to lie across the pharynx of young animals.
- Bones may also become lodged. The worst culprits are either fish bones (which usually lodge across the pharynx as a needle might) or rough irregular bones such as chop bones or chicken bones, which have projections which prevent them from being swallowed down or retched up.

Inflammation of the pharynx as a result of trauma, stings, etc. can cause severe problems if the walls of the pharynx become swollen.

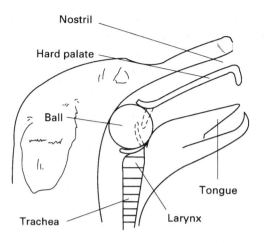

----- Normal positions of soft palate and epiglottis

Fig. 3.27 Pharyngeal foreign body: ball lodged in pharynx.

Signs

- **Altered behaviour.** Cats are usually subdued and are reluctant to groom normally because the actions of the tongue move the foreign body in the pharynx and may cause severe discomfort. Dogs are often restless and may paw at the mouth to try to remove the foreign body.
- **Gagging, retching and gulping** when swallowing or when the pharynx is gently palpated externally. If the foreign body is sharp, handling this area will cause intense pain and may drive the object deeper into the pharyngeal tissues. Great care is needed when handling these animals.
- **Salivation.** If swallowing is too painful, the patient may drool; this is usually seen when sharp objects are lodged.
- **Dysphagia.**
- **Dyspnoea** varying from heavy breathing to asphyxia, depending upon the degree of pharyngeal obstruction. If the walls of the pharynx are simply inflamed and slightly swollen, the breathing may be slightly harsher than normal. If the pharynx is completely blocked by a foreign body, the patient will very soon suffocate (Fig. 3.27).

Complications. Asphyxia has already been mentioned. Another complication might be **nasal discharge** in cats with grass pharyngeal foreign bodies. If the grass is not or cannot be removed, it will usually start to track forwards into the nasal passages over a period of days or weeks (see Injuries to the respiratory tract, p. 61).

Treatment

- **Treat asphyxia** (see Resuscitation, p. 85).
- **Remove the foreign body.** With the animal held firmly, the mouth should be opened as far as possible to inspect the throat. Pharyngeal foreign bodies are rarely removable without an anaesthetic, as they are often lodged beyond reach, but it may be possible to attempt careful removal of a foreign body with fingers or forceps if it can be seen clearly and is not embedded in the walls of the pharynx. *Never* attempt to remove a **fish hook** because of the barbed point (see Injuries to the alimentary tract, p. 66).

- A **thread** should not be pulled, but traced to find out if it is attached to a needle or fishhook (but often no foreign body can be seen as it has been swallowed). If the foreign body cannot be seen or removed, the two ends of the thread should be tied together to prevent it becoming unthreaded. The veterinary surgeon will then be able to use the thread to trace the needle/fishhook at subsequent surgery.
- **Dyspnoeic patients** should be kept under constant observation. Intubation may be necessary in cases of obstructing foreign bodies or if the swelling of the pharyngeal tissues gets steadily worse, as may happen in cases of allergic reactions to insect stings (see Asphyxia, p. 90). Prepare a suitable endotracheal tube in case the animal loses consciousness. Also prepare the site for a tracheotomy by clipping up the midline ventral neck and giving it a preliminary scrub.
- The Heimlich manoeuvre may be attempted to remove smooth foreign bodies but **only if the patient has asphyxiated and is unconscious.** (See later section on Asphyxia, p. 90.)

Larynx

Causes

- **Bite wounds.** Dog bite injuries occasionally result in severe wounds to the ventral neck area as the dog attacks its victim's most vulnerable part.
- **Laceration wounds to the neck**, e.g. a dog injured by running into a strand of barbed wire hidden in the grass. These wounds are also occasionally seen following road accidents. Incised wounds may occur if the animal falls through glass.
- **Strangulation injuries** usually occur because the animal's collar is caught on some projection as it falls or jumps from a height.

Signs

- **Swelling and pain.** The tissues of the neck may be swollen and painful because of extensive bruising and inflammation. **Subcutaneous emphysema** may develop around the injuries if the larynx has been punctured. The air in the larynx escapes into the tissues around the injury, creating a unique type of swelling: the swollen tissues 'crackle' under the fingertips when palpated as the tiny pockets of air in the tissues are popped.
- **Harsh, noisy breathing and dyspnoea.** The laryngeal cartilages may be distorted or collapsed and the lining of the larynx is inflamed and swollen, narrowing the air passageway.
- **Hissing and ballooning.** Any wound penetrating the larynx allows air to be sucked in and blown out of the wound during respiration, so that a 'hissing' sound may be heard on each inspiration as the air is sucked in through the tissues. On expiration, the tissues frequently balloon out as the air is forced into then.
- **Frothy haemorrhage.** Haemorrhage from these wounds is likely to be frothy as the blood is mixed with air.

Complications

- **Asphyxia.** If the trauma is severe and the lining of the larynx is very swollen or the laryngeal cartilages collapse, the patient will asphyxiate. If the wound penetrates the larynx, blood may be sucked into the respiratory tract as the patient inhales. Large volumes of blood will severely compromise the breathing as the clotting blood blocks the airways and fills the alveolar spaces.
- **Contamination of the airways.** Hair, dirt and bacteria may be sucked into the respiratory airways if an open wound penetrates the larynx.

Treatment

- **Asphyxia** should be treated as described on p. 91 (Unconsciousness). Dyspnoeic patients should be treated as outlined in Table 3.16. A suitable endotracheal tube must be immediately to hand in case the animal loses consciousness so that the airway may be maintained. The veterinary surgeon may have to perform a tracheotomy (e.g. in cases of severe laryngeal injury where a tracheal tube cannot be passed in the normal manner) and the site can be prepared by clipping up the midline ventral neck and giving it a preliminary scrub.
- **Haemorrhage** should be controlled quickly to prevent any inhalation of blood and to save the patient's life. The haemorrhage may be fatal if branches of the jugular vein and carotid artery are also damaged in the accident.
- **Wounds** should be treated as described elsewhere but *great care must be taken when cleansing the wound that no fluid is allowed to enter the air passages* (use well wrung-out swabs). Dressings may be applied, but only with great care because any pressure may further collapse the airway and make the situation worse.

Trachea

Causes, signs, complications and treatment are as described above for the larynx.

Lungs

Causes

- **Trauma.** Indirect violence such as a blow to the chest causes multiple minor haemorrhages into the lung tissues. Direct violence such as a displaced fractured rib, penetrating gunshot wounds or staking injuries can tear the delicate tissue.
- **Paraquat poisoning** causes irreversible changes to the lung tissue (see section on Poisoning, p. 30, for signs and treatment).
- **Fluid in the alveolar spaces** occurs as a result of drowning accidents, acute congestive heart failure, etc.
- **Lung collapse** may follow damage to the chest wall.

Signs

- **Trauma.** External wounds and haemorrhage may or may not be present in both cases, but animals are usually shocked and breathing is often rapid and shallow because of the painful chest wall. Bleeding from the lungs (**haemoptysis**) may be present, in which case bright red, frothy blood is coughed up. The haemorrhage is not severe and usually clears within a few hours.
- **Fluid in the alveolar spaces** causes the patient to cough continuously in an attempt to clear the lungs. Dyspnoea and cyanosis may be evident if there is much fluid in the lung spaces (see Asphyxia, p. 91).

Complications

- **Infection of the pleural cavity** will occur in cases of open wounds.
- **Haemothorax and/or pneumothorax** may be present in trauma cases. If the injury also damaged a major blood vessel in the chest cavity or tore the lungs so badly that a large volume of air escapes from the bronchioles, the lungs would collapse (see Chest wall injuries, below).
- **Cyanosis, air hunger and death** if oxygenation of the blood is prevented, e.g. by fluid in the alveolar spaces.

Treatment. Lung injuries must always be regarded as serious because the complications may be so serious. **Rest is essential** and the animal should be allowed to assume the position which it finds most comfortable. Wounds, haemorrhage and shock should be treated as discussed elsewhere and additional oxygen supplied (see Resuscitation, p. 87).

Chest wall

Causes

- **Road accidents,** when the chest has been crushed by the vehicle.
- **Severe bites,** especially those inflicted to the chest walls of toy dogs which have been grabbed from above by larger dogs, picked up and shaken.
- **Staking accidents, gunshot wounds,** etc.

Signs

- **Abnormal breathing patterns.** Breathing is painful for the patient and so animals with these injuries tend to have rapid, shallow respiratory patterns which cause minimal movement of the chest wall. However, if the lungs are collapsed, the need for oxygen overcomes the pain and the animal starts to gasp, trying to draw the air into the lungs. If the situation deteriorates, the patient will show increasing signs of 'air hunger' (see Asphyxiation and Unconsciousness, p. 91).
- **Thoracic wounds causing an open pneumothorax,** often 'hiss' on inspiration as the air is drawn in through the wound (Fig. 3.28a and b), but there are few external signs in cases of closed pneumothorax. Fractured ribs tend to stay in position because they are effectively splinted to those ribs on either side which are not damaged.
- **Subcutaneous emphysema** may be present in any case of pneumothorax (Fig. 3.28a and b) but it is usually more marked in a closed pneumothorax.

(a)

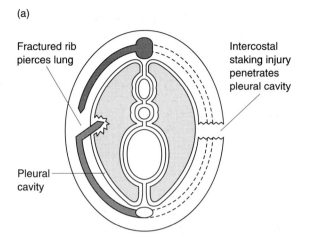

Fractured rib pierces lung

Intercostal staking injury penetrates pleural cavity

Pleural cavity

(b) Lungs collapse as pneumothorax develops

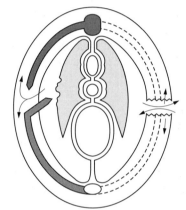

→ Direction of air flow during respiration movements.
Note subcutaneous emphysema developing under the skin of both injuries.

Fig. 3.28 Chest wall injuries.

(c) Haemothorax

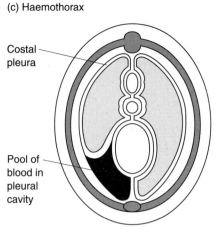

Costal pleura

Pool of blood in pleural cavity

(d) Diaphragm rupture

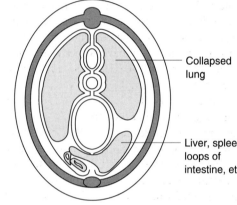

Collapsed lung

Liver, spleen, loops of intestine, etc.

Complications. **Lung collapse.** There are four possible reasons why the lungs may collapse following injury to the chest wall:

● **Open pneumothorax** occurs when a wound penetrates into the pleural cavity. Air is sucked into the pleural cavity each time the animal inhales and the negative pressure in the pleural cavity is therefore destroyed so that the lungs will gradually collapse.
● **Closed pneumothorax** occurs when there is no wound leading from the body surface to the pleural cavity. This can happen if the lung is torn during a crushing injury to the thorax or if the lung is pierced by a sharp fragment of fractured rib. In these cases, the air escapes from the damaged lung tissue and fills the pleural cavity.
● **Haemothorax** occurs if a blood vessel is damaged in the thorax and a large volume of blood collects in the pleural cavity. The lungs float up to the top of the thoracic cavity but are unable to expand properly because of the fluid beneath them (Fig. 3.28c).
● **Diaphragmatic rupture** may occur if the chest wall is distorted (see Rupture of the diaphragm as in (d) above).

The other complications which may arise are **infection and contamination of the pleural cavity**, which may occur in cases of penetrating open wounds. **Anaemia and shock** will follow extensive haemorrhage into the thoracic cavity.

Treatment

> **WARNING**
>
> Any wound of the thoracic wall should be treated with caution since it may not be obvious how deeply it penetrates. These animals should be handled with care because these injuries are very painful and fractured ribs may be displaced, causing further damage. The nose should *not* be muzzled unless absolutely necessary as these patients may need to mouth-breathe in order to satisfy their demand for oxygen.

The wounds should be cleaned carefully, taking care that no fluid is drawn into the pleural cavity. **Do not remove**

penetrating foreign bodies, as this may lead to sudden lung collapse and death. Instead, the protruding portion should be cut off close to the skin and a ring-pad dressing used to protect the remaining portion from being pushed deeper into the wound. The torn tissues may be folded back over the injury to seal the hole and a moist lint or gauze pad placed over the wound and bound to the thorax to keep the tissues in position. If the 'hissing' noise can still be heard after the tissues are folded down, a sheet of *clean* 'cling film' or polythene may be placed over the raw tissues to seal the hole before the tissues are folded down, so that the air-tight film is trapped in the depths of the wound.

In larger wounds, it may also be necessary to place a smooth, flat, rigid object (e.g. a credit card) over the folded tissues before bandaging the chest firmly. The rigid object will compress the tissues of the wound without allowing them to be forced into the chest cavity by the pressure of the dressing. It will also prevent the dressing pressing any fractured rib fragments into the chest cavity because it can be placed across the wound like a bridge, supported at either end on sound, undamaged ribs.

After the dressing is in place, the animal should be rested and oxygen given if necessary. Radiography will probably be needed to assess the extent of the damage and chest drains required when the injury is surgically repaired. These can be prepared whilst awaiting the veterinary surgeon's arrival.

Rupture of the diaphragm

Causes. This injury is seen more commonly in cats than dogs and is usually the result of a road accident or falling from a considerable height. The thin muscular diaphragm tears when the abdomen is crushed or the rib cage is distorted in the accident.

Signs. Diaphragmatic rupture alone causes no problem. It is only when the abdominal organs migrate through the diaphragm and cause lung collapse that any symptoms are seen. Very small tears may cause no problems immediately after the accident because the hole in the diaphragm is initially too small to allow large abdominal organs to enter the chest. Signs may occur later on as the omentum finds its way through and the hole gradually enlarges (Fig. 3.29).

Complications. The complications of this condition are **cardiac compression** and **lung collapse** (Figs 3.28d and 3.29). Animals with large diaphragmatic tears, where the omentum and a liver lobe or two have entered the pleural cavity, may show only slightly laboured breathing at rest. The lungs are collapsed to some degree but still able to expand sufficiently to cope with the low oxygen demands of the resting animal. However, the animal may become quite distressed and dyspnoeic on exercise (e.g. if it struggles whilst being examined) because the lungs cannot expand sufficiently to cope with an increased oxygen demand.

Patients with extensive diaphragmatic tears may suffer partial asphyxia at rest because the omentum, liver, intestines and even the stomach and spleen have entered the

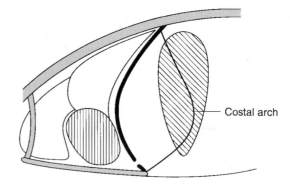

(a) Ruptured diaphragm

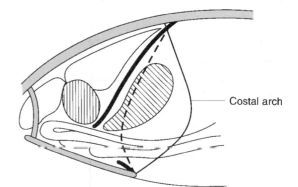

(b) Ruptured diaphragm with displaced viscera

Key: ☐ Lung   ⑪ Heart
      ☒ Stomach   ▬ Diaphragm
      ▩ Vertebral column,   – – Normal position
        1st rib, sternum   of diaphragm

Fig. 3.29

pleural cavity and the lungs are collapsed. The abdomen of these animals often appears thin and sunken because many of the bulky abdominal viscera are in the chest cavity.

Treatment. Asphyxia should be treated as described in the section on Resuscitation on p. 87. Otherwise, there is no specific first aid treatment for these patients except to encourage the animal to rest on a slope, with the head higher than the hindquarters. This should allow the abdominal viscera to fall back into the abdomen, or at least to the back of the pleural cavity so that pressure is taken off the heart and apical lung lobes, enabling them to inflate more efficiently. The patient should be kept under constant observation.

Injuries to the alimentary tract

The mouth

Causes

- Curious cats and dogs may get their **head or noses wedged** into plastic containers, discarded food tins, etc.
- **Lips.** *Insect stings* commonly affect the lips. *Fish-hooks* can also become embedded.

- **Bone structures**. *Compound fractures* of the hard palate and mandible are commonly seen following road accidents or in animals which have fallen from a great height (so-called 'tenement disease' after cats which fall from top floors in blocks of flats).
- **Teeth**. *Foreign bodies* such as pieces of stick or bone sometimes become wedged transversely across the roof of the mouth between the molar teeth (Fig. 3.30) or portions of soft bone may become wedged on or between the teeth. In older animals, *teeth may become so loosened in the sockets that they only remain attached at the gum margin*, which can be acutely painful for the animal.
- **Tongue**. *Foreign bodies* such as needles and fishhooks are occasionally found embedded in the tongue. Corrosive and irritant substances contaminating the coat will cause *tongue-tip ulceration*, especially in cats, as the corrosive chemical comes into contact with the tongue when the animal grooms itself. *Open wounds* are seen after an animal has licked out a sharp-edged can or bitten through its tongue after a major trauma (e.g. a road accident). Dogs playing with sticks occasionally 'run on to' the stick, which can cause extensive lacerations, especially to the underside of the tongue and pharynx. *Loops of string*, fishing line or thread may catch round the base of the tongue when a bundle of twine, etc. is swallowed. The loop embeds deeply into the frenulum on the underside of the tongue and the two ends of the loop disappear into the oesophagus (Fig. 3.31).

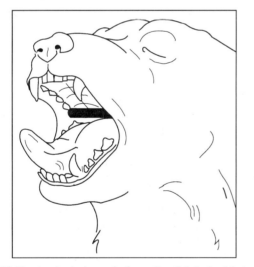

Fig. 3.30 Foreign body in roof of mouth: stick lodged between carnassial teeth.

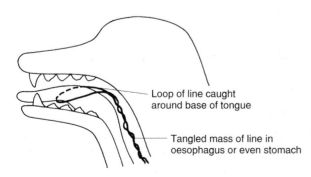

Fig. 3.31

Signs of oral pain

No matter what the cause, the signs of pain in the mouth are common to all:

- Profuse salivation and drooling.
- Pawing at the face or rubbing the face on the ground.
- Dysphagia (difficulty in swallowing) – the animal is interested in food and may go to the bowl and sniff the food, but then turns away because it is too painful to feed.

Signs of specific injuries

Inflammatory conditions (e.g. stings, ulcerations) induce signs of acute pain. The swollen tissues around the area of the sting or the denuded, red raw tongue ulcers are usually easily spotted when the mouth is opened.

The pain associated with **foreign bodies** is usually less severe but the patient is more likely to paw at its face and may also continuously 'mouth' with its tongue and jaw as it tries to dislodge the problem. However, the animal with a penetrating foreign body (e.g. a needle) may remain very quiet and apprehensive, reluctant to move its tongue or swallow because of the pain that this causes.

Fractures in the mouth are usually easily recognised, if not easily seen:

- **Hard-palate fracture** presents as a thin reddened crack running longitudinally in the midline of the roof of the mouth.
- **Mandible fracture** results in one or both sides of the jaw being totally unstable. The most common site of such fractures is at the mandibular symphysis, when the two halves of the mandible can be freely moved against one another.

Wounds are also easily seen, except in those affecting the underside of the tongue. Dogs which have 'run on to' sticks may show few signs at the time of the accident. The owner often reports that the dog yelped as it reached the stick, rushed back to the owner for reassurance and has been subdued ever since. There is usually surprisingly little haemorrhage from even quite deep and extensive cuts. If the injury is relatively long-standing (e.g. a foreign body that has been embedded for 2 3 days), there may well be halitosis because these wounds soon become infected.

Complications

- **Inability to eat or drink**. Some patients have such severe damage to the structures of the mouth that it is impossible for them to eat or drink. Such animals need to be supported with intravenous therapy and may need to have a pharyngostomy or nasopharyngeal tube implanted.
- **Unconsciousness**. Fracture of the hard palate may occasionally be associated with other cranial fractures which cause brain damage and unconsciousness.
- **Infection** follows any injury, because the mouth is not a sterile environment.
- **Damage to pharyngeal tissues** and **deeply embedded foreign bodies** following the 'running on to a stick' injury. Many of these lacerations are very deep, often

extending 15 cm from the root of the tongue into the pharyngeal tissue. It is not uncommon for a small fragment of stick to break off and remain buried deep in the wound, where it festers and may abscessate on to the skin of the neck many weeks after the initial injury.

Treatment. For **insect stings** and **tongue ulceration**, refer to the Poisons section, p. 30.

There is no specific first aid treatment for **fractures** unless the mandibular injuries are so severe that the lower jaw hangs down because both rami are fractured. In these cases, the fracture can be stabilised by gently bandaging the jaws together so that the upper jaw acts as a splint for the lower jaw. **This must not be attempted if the animal is dyspnoeic.**

Removal of **foreign bodies** (including loose teeth) should be attempted cautiously, as the animal will often resent handling of the mouth, and general anaesthesia may be required.

Sticks and bones lodged across the roof of the mouth are often easily levered out if a pair of closed artery forceps or dental forceps is gently slipped between the foreign body and the roof of the mouth. A small pair of forceps must be used as these objects are usually jammed tightly against the soft tissues. If the foreign body does not dislodge easily, do not apply excessive force: the object might have penetrated the tissues more deeply than it appears to have done.

String caught around the tongue should be left in place as the bulk of the string cannot be seen – it may be just down the oesophagus or it may have passed all the way into the animal's stomach. It will also be painful for the patient when the embedded loop is pulled free of the tongue tissues. A general anaesthetic is usually needed to treat these cases.

WARNING

No attempt should be made to pull out a fish-hook. Because of its barbed end, the shaft should be pushed still further into the tissues until the barb comes out through the skin (Fig. 3.32). This is not easy to do as fish-hooks are often rusty and blunt. Spraying the buccal mucosa with local anaesthetic can help to deaden the pain whilst this procedure is carried out, but it may be impossible to do with the animal conscious. Once the barb is pushed free of the mucosa, the shaft of the hook is cut through and the two halves are removed independently.

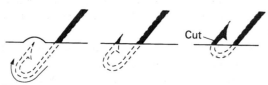

Direction to
push to expose
barb

Fig. 3.32 Removing a fish-hook.

Wounds in the mouth are not easily cleansed without a general anaesthetic. Extensive wounds may also require suturing, so theatre should be prepared.

Pharynx

See Injuries to the respiratory tract, p. 61.

Oesophagus

Causes. **Foreign bodies.** The oesophagus is very distensible, with strong muscular walls, so that most smooth foreign bodies (e.g. balls) pass through uneventfully and enter the stomach. **Rough, irregular objects** such as chop bones might lodge in the oesophagus when the projections stick into the oesophageal wall. There are three sites where a bone or any other obstructing foreign body might lodge in the oesophagus:

- The thoracic outlet at the base of the neck.
- Over the base of the heart.
- At the cardia of the stomach.

Wounds to the oesophagus may occur in severe neck injuries (e.g. dog bite lacerations) but this is uncommon as the oesophagus is a tough, elastic structure, buried under layers of muscle and it tends to stretch rather than tear.

Signs. Signs of **foreign bodies** include:

- **Vague discomfort** – the patient is usually slightly subdued and withdrawn.
- **Regurgitation.** Food, if taken, is regurgitated almost immediately and is unchanged, i.e. there is no stomach acid present and no acidic smell to the vomit. Fluids often pass through unhindered because the obstruction is usually incomplete.
- **Dyspnoea.** Large foreign bodies which lodge at the base of the heart may press on the tracheal bifurcation, narrowing the airway.
- **Traumatic damage** to the oesophagus is usually only detected at surgery, when the wound is being sutured. Occasionally, swallowed saliva may be detected leaking from a neck wound.

Complications. Obstructing irregular or sharp foreign bodies may penetrate through the walls of the oesophagus, especially if they have been lodged there for some days because the owner does not realise the severity of the situation. If this occurs in the chest, the infected material surrounding the foreign body can leak out of the oesophagus and enter the pleural cavity, causing pleurisy or even a pyothorax if the condition is left untreated.

Treatment. There is no specific first aid treatment. Dyspnoea should be treated as described in Table 3.16. In cases of suspected foreign bodies, the patient should be prepared for endoscopy and/or radiography and a barium or other contrast medium swallow. Surgery will probably be necessary in long-standing cases.

Stomach

Causes

- **Foreign bodies**. Many objects may be swallowed and lodge in the stomach, e.g. stones, bones and assorted household objects. Young, inexperienced and curious animals are the most at risk. Dogs tend to suffer more than cats because they do not mind what they eat and the greedy dog is the worst of all.
- **Infections or disease** causing persistent vomiting, e.g. parvovirus, renal failure.
- **Poisoning** by corrosive substances.
- **External trauma**, e.g. a blow to the abdomen sustained during a road accident.
- **Gastric dilatation and torsion** (as described later).

Foreign bodies

Signs

- **Vomiting**. Patients harbouring a foreign body are bright, alert and normally healthy for most of the time, but suffer bouts of acute vomiting if the foreign body jams in the pylorus and obstructs the emptying of the stomach. If the object then falls back into the stomach, the symptoms disappear again.
- **Pain**. The stomach is a roomy organ and it is rare that any foreign body causes much discomfort unless it lodges in the entrance or exit of the stomach.

Complications. Occasionally, a large foreign body may irritate the gastric lining, which leads to **haematemesis** (vomiting blood), but this is rare.

If the foreign body should squeeze through the pylorus into the small intestine, it may well obstruct and cause problems (see Intestine, p. 70).

Treatment. Food and water should be withheld until the veterinary surgeon has been consulted. Radiographs and barium meals may be necessary to diagnose the problem and a laparotomy may have to be performed if a foreign body is present.

Inflammation (i.e. infection, poisoning, trauma)

Signs

- **Vomiting**. Inflammatory conditions of the stomach result in more consistent, prolonged periods of vomiting, especially after food or water is ingested.
- **Haematemesis**. The vomit may contain blood, which haemorrhages from the sore and possibly ulcerated stomach lining. (Note that animals will vomit back ingested blood which they have swallowed, e.g. after licking wounds, and so haematemesis is not always a sign of gastric irritation/ulceration.) Fresh blood appears bright red or gives a pinkish tinge to the vomit. Blood which has remained in the stomach for any length of time is brown in colour and resembles coffee grounds as it is partially digested.

- **Pain**. The stomach lining is sore and becomes rapidly more inflamed as the vomiting persists. The animal is often depressed and obviously ill and may show abdominal guarding, a tucked-up abdomen or it may assume a 'praying position' (see Fig. 3.36).

Complications. Dehydration and electrolyte imbalance (loss of chloride ions) occur due to prolonged vomiting. Other complications arise because of the underlying conditions (see sections on Poisoning, p. 61; Infectious diseases, p. 30; Renal failure, p. 452, etc.).

Treatment

- **Withhold all fluids and food**. In some cases, great thirst may be exhibited, but no food or fluid should be given by mouth. A piece of ice placed on a flannel in a dish (so that the water formed as the ice melts is absorbed and cannot be taken) may be given to the animal to lick.
- Prepare intravenous fluids. Normal saline will replace the chloride ions lost. In cases of kidney failure, Hartmann's solution should be used.
- **Treat for shock**.
- **Reserve samples** of vomit and/or diarrhoea in cases of suspected poisoning.

Gastric dilatation and torsion

Cause. The cause of this syndrome is not known, but it is an extremely serious condition. The stomach fills with gas and swells to enormous proportions (gastric dilatation). Very often, the gas is unable to escape because the whole stomach has twisted around in the abdomen, effectively knotting the cardia and the pylorus together and occluding both entrance and exit (gastric torsion). As the gas pressure continues to build, the condition becomes more and more serious and will be fatal within hours unless the first aider is prepared to take certain emergency measures.

The condition is almost always seen in large, deep-chested dogs, usually 2–3 hours after they have eaten a large meal. Dilatations also occasionally occur in elderly small dogs.

Signs

- **Restlessness** and signs of discomfort are the first signs as the stomach begins to swell. Nothing else is usually noticed at this stage. The dog is unable to settle and may eat grass and try to vomit without success. In some cases, gas may be belched up.
- **Swelling** of the anterior abdomen follows as the pressure builds, distending the stomach so much that the posterior rib cage is pushed out. Gentle tapping on the abdominal wall with finger-tips produces a hollow, drum-like sound.
- **Breathing becomes laboured** as the swelling enlarges and the condition becomes more painful. The diaphragm is pushed forwards by the hugely distended stomach, which makes breathing more difficult and painful. The stomach of a weimaraner-sized dog may be as big as a large washing-up bowl at this stage.

● **Collapse**. The dog collapses gradually into lateral recumbency, when the gas-filled, bloated stomach can be clearly seen to bulge on the left side, just behind the rib cage. The blood circulation has also been upset by this stage as the enormous stomach presses on the posterior vena cava and portal veins, slowing the return of blood to the heart from the posterior abdomen. The patient is now severely shocked and close to death.

Complications. Gastric rupture and death. If untreated, the dog will become unconscious, the stomach will rupture and the animal will soon die.

Treatment

● **Veterinary assistance must be sought immediately.**
● **Relieve the pressure in the stomach.** If the dog is collapsed and unconscious and veterinary help is delayed, the pressure must be eased or the dog will die. There are two possible courses of action: passing a stomach tube or, if that is unsuccessful, piercing the abdominal wall.
● **Treat for shock.**
● In all cases, **emergency surgery** will be necessary and the nurse should prepare the patient and the theatre accordingly.

Stomach tube. Some cooperative animals will swallow a stomach tube when fully conscious. A roll of bandage, placed between the molar teeth, can be used as an improvised gag. Unconscious animals should be intubated first with a cuffed endotracheal tube to maintain the airway before the stomach tube is passed.

Procedure. The distance from the mouth to the costal arch is first measured against the outside of the patient: lay the stomach tube on the dog, bending it so that it follows the course of the oesophagus down the neck and through the thorax. Make a mark on the tube where it lies level with the canine tooth (Fig. 3.33). This precaution ensures that the operator knows how far to pass the tube in order to position one end inside the stomach.

Lubricate the blunted end of the stomach tube and pass it down the oesophagus.

When the cardiac sphincter of the stomach is reached, there will be some resistance, but gentle pressure may overcome this. If not, **do not persist** in the attempt to enter the stomach. The stomach may have twisted on itself and force will only rupture the oesophagus.

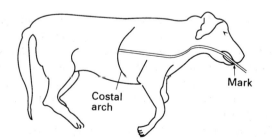

Fig. 3.33 Measuring the stomach tube (gastric torsion).

Emergency deflation by piercing the abdominal wall

> **WARNING**
>
> **This procedure must only be performed with the knowledge and consent of the veterinary surgeon.** It must only be attempted as an emergency measure to save the dog's life, i.e. if the patient has become unconscious and is cyanosed.

If stomach tubing is unsuccessful, the gas may be allowed to escape by using a wide-bore (16 G) intravenous needle/catheter to pierce the **left** abdominal wall at the point of maximum distension.

● The skin is quickly clipped and prepared for surgery.
● The large-bore needle is **inserted at right angles to the skin at the point of maximum distension.**
● As soon as the stomach is entered, a gust of gas or frothy fluid will escape and the pressure will reduce. If a catheter is used, the stylet should now be withdrawn. The needle hub must be held in position, pressed against the skin at right angles as the stomach slowly deflates.
● The release of gas may be slowed by placing a finger tip over the needle hub. If the stomach deflates too rapidly, the blood trapped in the posterior vena cava is suddenly released and floods into the heart, overloading it and causing cardiac failure.

Intestine

Causes

● **Obstruction**. The small intestine can become blocked by:
  (a) Foreign bodies similar to those found in the stomach. Various examples have been quoted, but often an object can be in the stomach for months before it finally moves into the small intestine and causes a problem.
  (b) Portions of intestine which 'telescope' into one another (**intussusception**).
  (c) Strangulation of hernias/ruptures of the abdominal wall.
● **Infection**. Organisms such as *Clostridium perfringens*, canine parvovirus, *Giardia* and feline enteritis can cause sudden and acute sickness and diarrhoea, involving severe inflammation of the intestine.
● **Poisonings**. Several poisons damage the intestines.

Foreign bodies

Signs

● **Vomiting** which, if the obstruction is complete, is often brown, foul-smelling faecal vomit. The patient may be sick every hour, day and night, as the normal bowel secretions are unable to pass down the intestine and have to be vomited back.

- **Pain** varies, depending on how much the intestinal wall is damaged. If the object is large or too rough, with irregular, sharp projections (e.g. bones), the animal may suffer acute abdominal pain, shown by restlessness, adopting the 'praying position' and tucking up the abdomen (see Fig. 3.36). Some animals may suffer conscious collapse. Smooth objects do not cause the same discomfort and the animal may remain quite bright, despite regular bouts of vomiting.
- **Lack of faeces.** As nothing is passed through the intestine, faecal production gradually ceases or very few faeces are passed. When the temperature is taken, the rectum feels sticky and dry as the thermometer is inserted.

Complications. Rupture of the intestines and subsequent peritonitis – a sharp projection from a foreign body may erode the intestinal wall and rupture the intestine. In cases of intussusception, the wall may rupture as the telescoped tissues lose their blood supply and die.

Dehydration occurs due to the fluids lost by the continual vomiting.

Treatment

- Keep the patient comfortable and give nothing by mouth.
- Radiographs and contrast studies may be needed to help diagnose the problem.
- Intravenous fluids will be required to correct the electrolyte loss (chloride ions) and dehydration.

Infections and poisonings

Signs

- **Vomiting.** Acute intestinal infections and certain poisons may cause bouts of prolonged vomiting. The vomit may be clear, bile stained or tinged with blood, which may be fresh or partially digested. It is rarely faecal vomit.
- **Diarrhoea** is often observed in these cases as the whole of the intestines are irritated and inflamed. In these acute cases, it is usually bloody and foul smelling.
- **Collapse and shock.** These patients are acutely ill and rapidly dehydrate. The mucosa is pale and the pulse is thin and rapid.

Complications. Other animals may be infected by these patients. They should be isolated as soon as possible.

Dehydration is a real problem and needs to be corrected rapidly. In cases of poisonings, other body systems may also be affected, e.g. kidneys, central nervous system.

Treatment. Drugs may be needed to control the vomiting (e.g. metoclopramide) and the patient should be treated for shock. Intravenous Hartmann's solution is the drip of choice as the diarrhoea leads to loss of bicarbonate ions.

Rectum and anus

Prolapse of the rectum

Cause. This condition involves a protrusion of the rectum through the anal opening. The rectum is literally pushed out

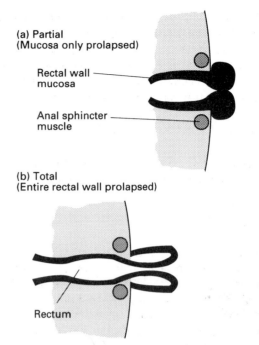

(a) Partial
(Mucosa only prolapsed)

Rectal wall mucosa

Anal sphincter muscle

(b) Total
(Entire rectal wall prolapsed)

Rectum

Fig. 3.34 Rectal prolapses.

of the anus and, not surprisingly, these prolapses are usually associated with conditions producing diarrhoea and/or **tenesmus** (straining to pass faeces).

Signs. Rectal prolapses are usually seen in young puppies or kittens but can also occur in hamsters of any age. They range in severity from partial prolapses (where only the mucosal rectal lining is prolapsed, Fig. 3.34a) to total prolapses (where the entire thickness of the rectal wall prolapses, Fig. 3.34b).

A **partial prolapse** appears as a pinky-red rosette centred on the anal opening. As the prolapse is small, it frequently disappears (i.e. reduces spontaneously) between bouts of straining and thus the mucosa usually remains moist and may not ulcerate.

Total prolapses present as red, oedematous, tubular structures protruding from the anus. The prolapsed mucosa is often coated with thick mucus and is frequently congested; it may dry out and ulcerate if not replaced promptly. The length of the prolapse varies, depending on how much rectal wall is involved, but can be surprisingly large – particularly in hamsters, where 2 cm prolapses are not unknown. In the female it is sometimes difficult to distinguish this mass from a prolapse of the vagina.

Complications

- **Swelling.** The venous return and lymphatic drainage are often partially blocked by the pressure on the tissues at the anal ring (comparable with overtight bandages on limbs which cause the toes to swell). Thus the prolapse swells and becomes congested, which makes the patient strain even harder and makes it more difficult to replace the prolapse.
- **Drying of mucosa.** Dry mucosa is very fragile and easily damaged and so ulcers and haemorrhage are common.

The tacky mucosa is also easily contaminated by cat litter, bedding, etc., and it can be very difficult to bathe these foreign bodies away without further damaging the mucosa.

● **Self-trauma**. As the animal automatically tries to clean the area, its rough tongue inflicts much damage. It is not unknown for patients (particularly hamsters) to groom so obsessively that they severely mutilate or even chew off the prolapsed tissues.

Treatment

● **Moisten and lubricate** the prolapsed tissue. Warm saline (0.9% solution) should first be used to rehydrate the mucosa, followed by liquid paraffin to lubricate the tissues and prevent them from drying out again. Several applications of liquid paraffin may be required if the prolapse cannot be reduced to ensure that the surface stays moist until veterinary help arrives.
● **Attempt to replace the prolapse**. Gentle pressure should be used – a finger-and-thumb 'pinching' movement on the end of the protrusion is usually the most successful, encouraging the tip of the prolapse to turn back in on itself. Once the exposed tip has been persuaded to invert again, the rest of the tissues usually follow – but not invariably. If the prolapsed mucosa starts to bleed, the attempt should be abandoned. Many cases require surgical treatment to reduce them successfully.
● **Prevent further straining**. An analgesic suppository may be inserted to prevent further straining or, if this is unavailable or impractical to use (e.g. the patient is too small or the tissues are too fragile to handle), the prolapse can be sprayed with local anaesthetic.
● **Prevent self-trauma**. The patient should be fitted with an Elizabethan collar and kept under constant observation.
● **Prepare the patient for surgery**. Even if the prolapse can be reduced, most cases readily recur and it is usually necessary to place a purse-string suture around the anal ring to keep the prolapsed tissues in place.

Anal foreign bodies

Cause. Sharp bone fragments or small pieces of bone impacted into a mass may become lodged in the posterior rectum and anus. This is a particular problem of the middle-aged or elderly dog which has been given cooked bones to eat. As dogs age, they become less able to digest such 'treats' and the bone passes through the system virtually unchanged, gathering together in the colon to form a concreted mass of bony spicules.

Pins, safety pins, needles, sharp bits of plastic, etc., may lodge transversely across the rectum or anus, or penetrate their walls. This condition is seen more frequently in the young animal, which is more inclined to chew things up and swallow foreign bodies.

Signs. The animal is restless and unable to sit comfortably; it may show persistent irritation by continually licking the anus.

Constant straining which either produces only a mucoid discharge from the anus or may result in small, hard, blood-stained faecal pellets being passed.

Pain when straining – non-penetrating foreign bodies cause some discomfort but the foreign body lodged across the rectum causes the animal to cry out as it strains to pass faeces.

Haemorrhage may be seen if the obstruction penetrates the rectal wall.

Vomiting is not uncommon in cases of constipation, possibly related to the continual strong abdominal straining.

Complications. Rectal prolapse due to the excessive straining (see above); wounding and inflammation of the rectal mucosa.

Treatment

● **Attempt to remove the foreign body**. The area should be lubricated with liquid paraffin and the bone may then be removed very carefully with fingers or forceps if it is not too firmly lodged. If a thread is found to be hanging from the anus, a search should be made to discover the other free end and the two ends tied together. Gentle pulling may remove the needle, but no force must be applied. If the foreign body cannot be removed easily, the animal should be referred to a veterinary surgeon.
● **Attempt to remove the impacted mass**. A gentle 'milking' action, as used when emptying anal glands, may cause the impacted mass to pop out of the anus. Liquid paraffin should again be used to lubricate the area before this is attempted.

Impacted anal sacs

Cause. Blockage of the ducts of the anal sacs and subsequent impaction may lead to abscess formation. Such an abscess will usually burst just below and to one side of the anus.

Signs. The animal shows initial irritation of the area but, as the abscess forms, the area is swollen and the skin becomes reddened, shiny and very painful. The patient becomes depressed and febrile, with a full, bounding pulse. The abscess soon bursts and the patient then recovers dramatically!

Treatment. Hot fomentations may speed the 'pointing' of the abscess and alleviate the pain in the earlier stages. A pad of cotton wool moistened with hot water can be held against the perineum.

When the abscess has burst, the matted hair should be clipped away from the area and the wound washed as described earlier. Antibiotics are usually needed to control the infection.

Perineum

Deep wounds in this area may also involve injury to the urogenital tract (see later).

Fly strike

This is not a life-threatening condition, but is particularly distressing to owners and causes several emergency calls during the summer months.

Rabbits are usually affected, but old, debilitated, incontinent dogs and cats can also suffer if allowed to lie outside on a fine day.

Cause. Blow flies (e.g. 'greenbottles' and 'bluebottles') will lay clutches of eggs on heavily soiled fur. If the animal is too fat, old or ill to be able to groom, the perineal region becomes smelly and attracts the flies. The patient is unable to chase the flies away and the eggs laid in the fur can hatch within hours, releasing hundreds of tiny maggots. These burrow into the depths of the coat and begin to feed voraciously on the skin and underlying tissues. The fur falls away and large areas of raw tissues are exposed.

Signs. The areas commonly affected in rabbits are the recesses on either side of the rectum and the folds of skin at the tail base, where the tail curls upwards. Owners frequently find the problem in the evening, when they go to clean/feed the pet and notice a nasty smell. When the animal is turned over, the cause of this smell is obvious.

The wounds resemble superficial burns – the exposed tissues look clean and moist but the edges of the denuded area are soiled with a purulent discharge which mats the fur. It is here that the maggots are most often found.

Treatment. The maggots must be prevented from causing further damage and this is most effectively achieved by spraying the fur at the edges of the wound with an insecticidal spray, which will rapidly kill them. However, **care must be taken not to spray the raw tissues** as the insecticide could be absorbed into the bloodstream and the propellant may cause severe tissue irritation. Therefore, before the spray is applied, the raw area should be covered by a barrier, e.g. a water-based cream or damp swab. Bigger, more mature maggots can be picked off using tweezers, but this is impossible if there are large numbers and if they are in the depths of the fur.

All soiled fur should be clipped away close to the skin (using electric clippers) and the clipping continued until a border of 2 cm of healthy skin has been exposed all around the affected area. This may not be possible in the conscious animal as the wounds will be painful and an anaesthetic may be required. It may also be necessary to suture large or deep wounds in certain cases so theatre should be prepared.

It should be remembered that these patients, like those suffering large superficial burns, will be losing water through the exposed tissues and may be ill for other reasons (e.g. the open pyometra case). Fluid therapy may be necessary.

Injuries to the abdominal wall

Definitions

Evisceration occurs when an organ or organs escape from a body cavity.

A **rupture** is said to have occurred when abdominal viscera escape through a *traumatic tear* in the muscles bounding the abdominal cavity, i.e. the muscular abdominal wall and diaphragm.

A **hernia** is said to have occurred when abdominal viscera escape through a *natural body opening* in the muscular abdominal wall, i.e. the inguinal canals and umbilicus.

A **reducible** hernia or rupture is one where the viscera can be pushed back into the body cavity through the original defect in the wall (Fig. 3.35a).

An **irreducible** hernia or rupture is one where the viscera cannot be replaced into the body cavity without enlarging the original defect in the wall (Fig. 3.35b).

A **strangulated** hernia or rupture is one where the arterial supply to the escaped viscera has been cut off because the tissues have swollen so much or become twisted, etc. (see also Chapter 19, p. 518).

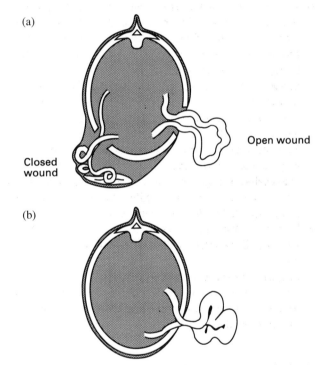

Fig. 3.35 Abdominal wall injuries.

Causes. **Ruptures** may be caused by:

- Road accidents, when the wheels of vehicles may roll over the abdomen causing severe crushing injuries.
- Staking injuries, when the animal becomes impaled on sharp object.
- Severe bites.
- Gunshot wounds.
- Surgical procedures.

Hernias occur when the natural openings in the body wall (i.e. the umbilicus and the inguinal canals) are larger than normal but it may be years before any abdominal contents find their way through the enlarged openings and come to lie just under the skin. If these organs then become trapped and strangulate, the animal will become acutely ill and may present as an emergency.

Signs of rupture

As with the thoracic injury, abdominal wounds must be treated cautiously as it can be difficult to appreciate the depth of the wound.

Open wounds. If the muscles making up the body wall have been ruptured, part of the abdominal contents (particularly the lacy fat of the omentum) can escape and protrude through the rupture (Fig. 3.35). Fatty tags on the surface of the wound may therefore indicate that the wound penetrates deeply into the abdominal cavity and is much more serious than it appears to be.

Closed wounds. Occasionally, no external wound is apparent and yet the muscles of the abdominal wall have still been ruptured, allowing the abdominal organs to escape from the peritoneal cavity. In these cases, there is little to see except the skin discoloration produced by the bruising and an abnormal swelling under the skin. This swelling may not be obvious because the surrounding tissues are bruised and swollen themselves so that the edges of the swelling are not clearly defined.

The most serious of this type of injury is the **diaphragmatic rupture** (see Injuries to the respiratory tract, p. 61). Other serious injuries commonly occur in the inguinal region of cats involved in road accidents.

Signs of hernia

Hernias only present as emergencies if they involve viscera other than omentum and strangulate. The owner may report a soft, painless swelling in the umbilical or inguinal region which has suddenly become hard and painful as the hernia becomes irreducible and then strangulates. The skin over the swelling becomes inflamed and the swelling itself is very painful. The patient may vomit because loops of intestine are obstructed.

Complications. **Evisceration**. The most common organs to escape from the abdominal cavity are the omentum and loops of small intestine.

Open wounds.

- *Reducible ruptures*. Omentum tissue looks like small fatty tags in the depths of the open wound and can be difficult to distinguish from torn subcutaneous fatty tissue. Loops of intestine are unmistakable. Usually several loops of intestine protrude from the wound and will dry out when exposed to the air. The surface becomes tacky and is therefore often heavily contaminated by dirt, grit, etc. The intestine is inflamed and bright red in colour but the walls remain soft and pliable (c.f. irreducible hernias and ruptures, below).
- *Irreducible ruptures*. Any organs trapped outside the peritoneal cavity may gradually swell if the venous blood return from the organs is cut off or reduced. The organs then become very painful, swollen and inflamed and cannot be replaced into the abdomen. Loops of intestine involved in irreducible ruptures appear dark red in colour, with turgid, stiffened walls. Small tears are often seen in the serosa. If the loops are parted, it is usually possible to see the bounding arterial pulse in the mesentery.

- *Strangulated rupture*. The arterial blood supply to the eviscerated organs is reduced and the tissues start to die. As the irreducible condition becomes strangulated, the viscera take on a blackened appearance and the arterial pulse becomes thin and weak before ceasing completely.

Closed wounds. If the wound is closed and no viscera can be seen, evisceration should always be suspected if there is a large swelling under a bruised area of skin (in the case of traumatic rupture) or in the umbilical or inguinal areas (in cases of herniation). **Gentle** palpation of the swelling may replace the eviscerated organs back into the abdomen and then the edges of the rupture/hernia can sometimes be felt.

If the hernia or rupture becomes irreducible or strangulated, the swelling becomes very painful and the skin overlying the area is often reddened and inflamed. The tense and painful nature of the swelling and its position (if a hernia) should lead the veterinary nurse to suspect the cause of the problem.

Ruptures and hernias also become irreducible when a distensible organ such as a bladder is involved. An empty bladder which slips through a defect in the abdominal wall and fills with urine over a period of hours becomes impossible to replace into the abdomen. The bladder is too large to empty at this stage and the pressure within the bladder rises, causing the patient excruciating pain. This can be a serious complication of a perineal rupture. Owners of an elderly entire male dog may notice a large, tense, painful swelling to one side of the anus because the bladder has slipped through torn muscle at the posterior end of the abdominal cavity.

Shock. Animals with evisceration injuries are frequently toxic and collapsed. If a loop of intestine is involved, they will also vomit because the bowel is obstructed as it passes into and out of the hernia or rupture.

Self-trauma. Animals with open eviscerated wounds are liable to damage the viscera when licking the wound. Sometimes, as with rectal prolapses, they may actually eat away the exposed organs in their desperation to clean the wound.

Trauma. Abdominal organs may have been damaged in the accident which injured the abdominal wall. This can lead to peritonitis (if the bowel or bladder is perforated) or severe or even fatal haemorrhage (if the liver, kidney, spleen, etc., are damaged). Eviscerated organs may be so damaged that they need to be surgically removed in order to save the life of the patient.

Collapsed lungs. In cases of diaphragmatic rupture, the lungs may be collapsed (see Injuries to the respiratory tract, p. 61).

Infection. As with any open wound, abdominal wounds are prone to infection, but the consequences are more severe if the abdominal cavity has been entered as peritonitis can develop.

Treatment

- **Clean the wound**. In cases where abdominal viscera protrude through an open wound, the hair should be clipped away in the normal manner, but antiseptics must *never* be used in case irritant chemicals penetrate the peritoneal cavity. The protruding viscera should be washed with warmed sterile saline to remove any grit or dirt.
- **Attempt to replace viscera into the abdominal cavity**. No force should be applied and it is easier to restrain the animal in such a position that the wounded side of the abdomen lies uppermost so that gravity assists the replacement. However, if there is any difficulty in breathing, the animal should not be forced to lie on its side or back as this could prove fatal.
- **Prevent damage to exposed viscera**. If it is impossible to replace the viscera, they must be kept warm, moist and undamaged by a covering of sterile swabs soaked in sterile saline and bandaged firmly but gently in place, using a crepe bandage which encircles the abdomen, or a many-tailed bandage. Cling film or clean polythene may be laid over the swabs before bandaging to prevent the swabs drying out. *This is an important first aid measure that the owner should take at home to keep the exposed tissues viable during transport to the surgery.* Sterile saline solutions, such as used in the care of contact lenses, are ideal to moisten the dressings, but cooled, boiled water may be used if no such solution is available. The viscera should be inspected every 15 minutes to renew the dampened swabs and check that the bandaging has not interfered with the circulation of the protruding viscera.
- **Observation and treatment for shock**. The animal must be constantly observed to prevent it tampering with the dressings and damaging the protruding viscera. All patients should be confined, made comfortable and treated for shock.
- **Prepare the theatre**. Veterinary assistance must be sought as soon as possible because irreducible ruptures or hernias may progress to strangulated conditions and these injuries, unless rapidly reduced, cause irreversible damage. Surgical interference is invariably necessary and the veterinary nurse should prepare the theatre accordingly.

Injuries to abdominal organs: liver, spleen, pancreas

Signs of abdominal pain

Injury to any abdominal organ can cause acute abdominal pain. The symptoms displayed are the same, regardless of the cause or organ affected:

- **Body posture**. The animal stands with its back arched and its abdomen tightly 'tucked up' (Fig. 3.36a) or it may adopt the 'praying position', lying down on its sternum but with its hind legs still standing (Fig. 3.36b).
- **Abdominal boarding**. The slightest touch on the abdominal wall usually results in the abdominal muscles

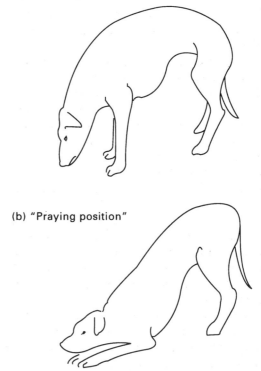

(a) Tucked-up abdomen

(b) "Praying position"

Fig. 3.36 Abdominal pain stance.

stiffening to become as hard as a board. This is also termed **guarding** of the abdomen.
- **Depression**. The patient is usually very ill and may even be collapsed. These animals are also commonly pyrexic.

Liver

Causes

- Trauma to the liver may occur in road accidents.
- Infectious canine hepatitis and *Leptospira icterohaemorrhagia* can both severely injure the liver of the dog.
- Poisons (e.g. antifreeze) may cause acute liver damage in the dog and cat.

Signs

- **Pain**. Acute liver damage is usually accompanied by acute abdominal pain.
- **Vomiting**. Patients with liver problems are usually vomiting and there may be diarrhoea in cases of infection.
- **Jaundice**. Depending on the type, severity and duration of the injury, the patient's mucous membranes may also be jaundiced. Infections and poisons act directly to damage the liver tissues and so the signs are observed within days.

Complications

- **Haemorrhage**. The liver is a very vascular organ and trauma may result in severe internal haemorrhage.
- **Diaphragmatic rupture**. Injuries which crush the anterior abdomen and damage the liver may also tear the diaphragm (see Injuries to the respiratory tract).

Treatment. No specific first aid treatment is possible, but the veterinary nurse should remain alert to the possibility of infectious conditions in the unvaccinated animal and isolate the patient.

WARNING

It is also important to ensure that rigorous hygiene precautions are enforced because leptospirosis is a zoonosis which can be fatal in humans.

Pending the attention of the veterinary surgeon, all patients should be made comfortable and treated for shock. It is generally not advisable to give fluids by mouth as this may provoke an attack of vomiting. If the animal does vomit, a sample should be kept in case the animal may have been poisoned.

Intravenous fluids may be required (e.g. Hartmann's solution) and plasma expanders (e.g. Haemaccel) or blood transfusions may be necessary in cases of internal haemorrhage. The veterinary nurse may also prepare for X-ray because it may be necessary to check for a ruptured diaphragm.

Spleen

Causes

- **Tumours**. Some dogs suffer from malignant tumours of the spleen, which can cause collapse from a very sudden major internal haemorrhage if they erode through the splenic capsule.
- **Trauma**. The spleen may be ruptured following a crushing injury to the abdomen.
- **Torsion**. Very occasionally, the spleen rotates in the abdomen, twisting the loose gastrosplenic mesentery into a tight cord-like structure. This results in serious venous congestion of the spleen as the thin-walled veins collapse in the tightening gastrosplenic mesentery and the spleen can swell to enormous size.

Signs. Haemorrhage from the spleen, whether caused by an invading cancer or by external injury, is often severe and can be fatal. The animal is collapsed; it breathes rapidly and has a thin, rapid pulse and extremely pale mucous membranes. Tumour cases often suffer periodic haemorrhages, which worsen with time. Therefore, there may be a history of a previous partial collapse with pale mucosa, from which the dog recovered (because of a natural arrest of haemorrhage).

Splenic torsions cause acute abdominal pain and it is sometimes possible to see the engorged spleen distending the anterior abdominal wall.

Complications. Severe internal haemorrhage and death.

Treatment. No specific first aid treatment is possible, though the abdomen may be firmly bandaged in cases of internal haemorrhage to attempt to increase the back pressure and control the haemorrhage. The animal should be made as comfortable as possible and **treated for shock**. Surgical intervention may be necessary and plasma expanders or blood transfusions can be prepared for intravenous administration.

Pancreas

Cause

Acute pancreatitis can cause sudden death or acute illness in dogs. The problem arises because certain changes allow the trypsin in the pancreas to set off a chain reaction, which results in the digestion of the tissues in the pancreas, i.e. the animal starts to digest its own body. This digestion releases even more trypsin, which causes even more autodigestion. Once the process has started, it can rapidly escalate and bring about severe shock and the death of the patient, often in great pain.

Signs. The animal is extremely ill; it shows signs of acute abdominal pain and may vomit.

Treatment. There is little that can be done except to give parenteral fluids to correct the acid–base balance, give antibiotic cover and provide relief from pain by administering pain-killing drugs. The veterinary nurse should therefore treat the animal for shock and make it as comfortable as possible until the veterinary surgeon can give the necessary treatment. Hartmann's solution may be warmed in readiness for intravenous administration and corticosteroid injections may be prepared for intravenous use. *Give nothing by mouth unless instructed to do so by a veterinary surgeon.*

Injuries to the urogenital system

Definitions

Anuria is the complete absence of passage of urine.

Oliguria occurs when the animal only passes a very small volume of urine over a period of time.

Tachyuria is the passing of very small amounts of urine at very frequent intervals. A normal volume of urine is passed over a period of time, but as little-and-often dribbles rather than normal streams.

Dysuria occurs when the patient has difficulty passing urine. This may be because it is too painful (as in cases of cystitis) or because the outlet is obstructed (as in cases of urethral obstruction).

Haematuria is the passing of blood in the urine.

WARNING

Care must be taken when examining a bitch to ensure that the normal bleeding of the oestrous cycle is not confused with haematuria.

Cystitis is the term given to inflammation of the bladder.

Kidney

Causes

- **Trauma**. Crushing or staking injuries of the abdomen which rupture the kidney result in instant death due to internal haemorrhage. Less severe trauma may bruise the kidney tissue and result in haematuria.
- **Back pressure damage**. If the outflow of urine is obstructed at any point along the tract (e.g. by stones blocking the urethra), back pressure will build up in the kidney tissues as the urine continues to be produced but cannot drain away from the renal tubules. This pressure will eventually destroy the delicate filtration beds in the kidney.
- **Infection** with *Leptospira canicola* causes inflammation and destruction of the kidney tissues.
- **Ingestion of certain poisons** (e.g. antifreeze, chlorate herbicides, mercury compounds) can also cause acute kidney damage.

Signs

- **Abdominal pain**. Patients with acute kidney damage are frequently in severe pain and may stand with an arched back and be 'tucked up' in the abdomen or show signs of abdominal guarding when the abdomen is touched (Fig. 3.36a).
- **Elevated temperature** in cases of infection.
- **Oliguria and haematuria**. The amount of urine which is produced by the kidney is reduced and often bloodstained.

Complications. Acute renal failure is always a risk following sudden damage to the renal tissues by poisons, infection and back pressure. The signs include vomiting, oliguria, dehydration, collapse and death.

Hypovolaemic shock and/or death may follow trauma to the kidney. The blood supply to the kidneys is extremely good and the effect of crushing the kidney is nearly as dramatic as severing the abdominal aorta.

Treatment. There are no specific first aid measures but the veterinary nurse should always be alert to the possibility of kidney damage if the abdomen has been crushed or poisons consumed. The volume and appearance of any urine passed should be recorded and the presence and severity of haematuria noted. **Samples should be kept for the veterinary surgeon to examine and for analysis in cases of suspected poisoning/infection.**

These animals rapidly become uraemic/acidotic and may collapse, and intravenous fluid therapy, using Hartmann's solution will greatly increase the chances of survival. The only contraindication for this treatment is an obstruction of the urinary tract, in which case it is best if the back pressure is first relieved (e.g. by catheterizing the bladder) before fluids are given.

Bladder

Causes

- **Trauma**. Rupture of the bladder may occur following crushing injuries to the abdomen if the bladder was full of urine. If the trauma is less severe, the bladder wall may simply be bruised and become inflamed. This is a common complication of pelvic fractures.
- **Irreducible hernias and ruptures**. If the bladder escapes from the abdominal cavity and then becomes trapped outside the body wall, the urethra may become obstructed. If this is not corrected, the bladder will become distended and may rupture.
- **Bladder stones**. The presence of bladder stones inflames the mucosal lining of the bladder and causes cystitis. If the urethra becomes obstructed, the bladder will distend and may rupture.
- **Infection**. Female patients are particularly prone to infection of the bladder, which can cause sudden and dramatic cystitis.

Signs of inflammation of the bladder (cystitis). If the bladder is simply bruised or inflamed, the animal shows dysuria, tachyuria and haematuria in many cases. These patients are not severely ill and may continue to eat normally, but are very restless and may cry continually, especially when straining to pass urine.

Signs of bladder distension. If the urethra is blocked, the animal will constantly strain to pass urine but only a few bloodstained drops or small teaspoonfuls may be produced. The patient is obviously unwell, loses its appetite and becomes withdrawn. As the bladder distension increases, the animal becomes more and more depressed and will collapse. A hard, painful ball-shaped mass is sometimes noticed in the ventral abdomen as the animal is handled. The bladder may be so distended that it can be seen as a bulge distorting the abdominal wall as the animal lies on its side. **No attempt must be made to palpate the abdomen and the veterinary surgeon must be informed of this finding as soon as possible** as bladder rupture is imminent.

Signs of rupture of the bladder. Animals with ruptured bladders are pale and shocked and often collapsed. Occasionally a small drop of bloodstained urine is seen at the vulva or prepuce. **No urine is passed** subsequently because the urine draining from the kidneys simply floods out through the ruptured wall of the bladder and collects in the abdominal cavity.

Complications. Bladder stones causing cystitis may pass into the urethra and cause obstructions in male animals.

Severe bladder distension and bladder rupture result in uraemia and peritonitis as the urine cannot drain from the body.

Treatment. No specific first aid measures are possible but the veterinary nurse must observe whether or not urine is passed and must also note its appearance, smell and quantity.

If a rupture is suspected, the veterinary nurse should prepare catheters and X-ray plates so that a pneumocystogram can be performed to ascertain how severely the bladder is damaged. Emergency surgery will be necessary to repair the damaged wall. Catheters will also be required in cases of blockage of the urethra (see Urethra, below). Intravenous Hartmann's solution drips should be prepared.

Urethra
Causes

- **Trauma**. Fragments from pelvic fractures may pierce or bruise the urethra as it runs over the pubic symphysis. Occasionally the urethra may also be damaged in male animals if there are wounds to the perineum or penis.
- **Calculi**. The urethra of the male may become blocked by small stones which have been washed out of the bladder and may lodge firmly in the narrow part of the urethra as it passes through the os penis in the dog or just proximal to the tip of the penis in the cat. As this problem recurs in certain individuals, a good case history can be invaluable in reaching a correct diagnosis.

Signs of obstruction. If the urethra is simply inflamed following trauma, urine will be passed normally but there may be some haematuria and dysuria, especially if the tissues swell so severely that they block the passage of urine and the animal really has to strain to pass anything at all. Bladder stones cause severe dysuria and the patient may be anuric. These patients usually progress to show signs of severe bladder distension (see Injuries to the urogenital system, p. 77).

Signs of rupture. Some urine will be passed through the penile opening, but some may also leak out of the wound. Haemorrhage may be quite severe if the erectile tissue surrounding the urethra is damaged.

Complications

- Haemorrhage if the wound damages the erectile tissues of the vascular penis.
- Distension/rupture of the bladder.
- Acute renal failure following damage to the kidneys due to back pressure.

Treatment. There is no specific first aid treatment for either of the above conditions except if there are complications. Haemorrhage from erectile tissue is best controlled by digital pressure, pinching the tissues together. There is little force behind this haemorrhage and so constant pressure applied for 5 minutes should suffice to control it if the animal can be made to rest and does not interfere with the wound.

The animal should be made as comfortable as possible and treated for shock, pending the arrival of the veterinary surgeon. Fluid therapy (Hartmann's solution), catheterisation and surgical intervention are usually necessary and the theatre should be prepared accordingly.

Prostate gland

Causes. Acute prostatitis in the dog is the only prostate condition which may present as an emergency. Any mature, entire dog can suffer from this problem, but it is more often seen in the hypersexed animal. The cause is usually a bacterial infection.

Signs

- **Dysuria and possible haematuria**. The patient will strain to pass urine because the enlarged, inflamed prostate gland presses down on the urethra and partially occludes it.
- **Preputial discharge**. The fluids from the infected gland drain into the urethra and out of the penis.
- **Vomiting** occurs in many cases, possibly because of endotoxaemia.
- **Pyrexia**. The temperature is usually markedly raised (104°F/40°C). Care must be taken when inserting the thermometer in small dogs because this procedure can be very painful if the thermometer should press into the gland (the prostate lies just ventral to the rectum and often bulges up, narrowing the rectum).
- **Abdominal pain** (Fig. 3.36a). Typically, the patient is in acute pain and stands still, with the back arched high, refusing to walk. Any pressure on the abdominal wall results in groaning or the animal will turn and snap at the handler.
- **Depression**, followed by collapse in severe cases.

Treatment. There is no specific first aid treatment for this condition except general nursing care. Treatment usually consists of dosing with antibiotics and delmadinone acetate injections.

Penis
Causes

- **Trauma**. The tough fibrous coat of the penis may be damaged by self-inflicted injury in the oversexed dog, exposing the cavernous tissues beneath.
- **Swelling**. The erect penis may become too engorged with blood to slide back into the prepuce and remains protruding. This is termed **paraphimosis**.
- **Foreign bodies**. Grass seeds, etc., occasionally work their way up inside the prepuce.

Signs. Trauma to the fibrous coat of the penis results in bouts of dramatic and copious haemorrhage every time the dog starts to get an erection. This is when the cavernous tissues fill up with blood and, in cases of penile damage, the blood can flood out though the damaged fibrous coat.

In cases of paraphimosis, the penis is very swollen and reddened and the preputial opening appears to cut into the engorged tissues. The normally moist surface of the penis will dry out after a while, which makes replacing the protruding penis much more difficult.

Foreign bodies inside the prepuce cause a heavy purulent discharge (which may be bloodstained) and irritation. The animal licks continually at the preputial opening and is very restless, unable to settle comfortably. Palpation of the prepuce can be extremely painful. (Note that many hypersexed dogs normally have a thick green/yellow preputial discharge but there is no pain or discomfort associated with the condition.)

Complications. The only complication to note is that of haemorrhage if the penis is traumatised.

Treatment for trauma cases. Veterinary assistance should be sought immediately in cases of penile injury but first aid can be given in the meantime. Cold compresses and ice packs will markedly decrease the blood flow to the penis and **pinching the skin just in front of the scrotum** further reduces the blood supply. These measures will help to control haemorrhage from the damaged penis.

The wound may be gently cleansed but great care should be taken to avoid disturbing the clots in the wound. Surgical repair is usually necessary.

Treatment for paraphimosis. Cold compresses and pinching the skin just in front of the scrotum will also decrease the size of the engorged penis sufficiently to allow it to slide back into the prepuce in many cases. However, if the tissues of the penis have become dry and tacky, liquid paraffin or K-Y jelly should be used to lubricate the tissues and aid reduction of the paraphimosis.

If these measures are not successful, the penis should be kept moist and **veterinary assistance must be sought** as it may be necessary to enlarge the preputial opening surgically. Set out surgical instruments and prepare the theatre.

Treatment for foreign bodies. Foreign bodies can be removed if seen, but a general anaesthetic is often needed so that the penis can be fully extruded and the whole of the inside of the prepuce examined to ensure that all foreign bodies are removed and there is no other injury.

Vagina and vulva

Causes. Most first aid situations in this area are associated with parturition (Chapter 18). Other conditions are:

- **Pyometra.** Owners may report that the bitch is 'bleeding' from the vulva, but this discharge usually turns out to be a reddish-brown purulent discharge from an open pyometra.
- **Vaginal polyps** and vaginal **prolapses** may occasionally be presented as an emergency.
- **Vaginal foreign bodies** do occasionally occur.
- **Trauma.** In some instances (e.g. road accidents), injuries to the peritoneum can affect the vulva.

Signs of open pyometra. Open pyometra cases are usually fairly bright and alert but there is much soiling of the fur around the vulva and the discharge is often unpleasantly smelly. The condition is classically seen in middle-aged animals (6–8 years old) and most bitches are midway between seasons, though these infections can occur immediately after a season. The patient is usually polydipsic.

Signs of polyps and prolapse. Vaginal polyps and prolapses are usually observed at the time of the oestrus and appear as red, round, glistening masses which suddenly protrude from the vulva or are seen sitting between the lips of the vulva. The animal is well in herself and usually unconcerned about the prolapse, though she may strain occasionally, but the suddenness of the appearance of the prolapse worries the owner. Occasionally protruding masses may become ulcerated and bleed but the haemorrhage is usually capillary in nature and, though messy, is not severe.

Signs of foreign bodies. Any foreign body in the vagina causes intense irritation, licking of the vulva and a purulent vaginal discharge if present for any length of time. The discharge is not as great as in the case of many open pyometras and can occur in any bitch, whether spayed or not.

Signs of wounds. Wounds to the vulva are usually lacerations or abrasions when the animal has been hit with force from the rear. There is usually much bruising.

Complications. Trauma to the perineum may also involve a fracture of the pelvis and damage to the urethra.

Treatment. Surgical intervention will usually be necessary in cases of open **pyometra** but rarely is emergency surgery necessary.

Vaginal polyps or **prolapses** which protrude from the vulva should be replaced as soon as possible to prevent the surface from drying out and becoming damaged when the bitch sits down or licks the prolapsed tissues. Gentle pressure applied to the **prolapse** is usually sufficient to replace it. If the surface has already become dry and sticky, it may also be necessary to lubricate the tissue with liquid paraffin or K-Y jelly. Where large **polyps** protrude, try to ease the lips of the vulva gently around the mass at the same time as applying pressure to the polyp to replace it into the vagina.

Irreplaceable prolapses and polyps should be kept moist until the veterinary surgeon can attend the case. The patient should be kept under observation to ensure that she does not cause any damage to the prolapse and an Elizabethan collar can be fitted to prevent self-trauma.

Foreign bodies may be removed if they can be seen easily but no undue force should be applied in case the foreign body is embedded in the wall of the vagina. A general anaesthetic is usually required. Any materials removed should be retained in case of possible litigation.

Wounds may be treated as described elsewhere in the text.

Injuries to the eye

General signs of painful injury to the eye

Whatever the cause of pain in the eye, the clinical signs are similar:

- The eyelids are screwed up against the light (**blepharospasm**) and the patient may hide away in dark corners to avoid bright light (**photophobia** = hatred of light).
- Tear production is increased and may overflow the eyelids (**epiphora**).
- The sclera and conjunctiva are often reddened and inflamed.
- Self-trauma: the animal may rub the eye with a forepaw, or rub its head against furniture, etc.

Examination

The eye is a delicate and sensitive structure and should only be examined as described in Table 3.2. It is especially important to avoid touching the surface of the cornea with the finger because this may cause corneal ulceration.

Eyelid
Causes

- **Wounds** to the eyelid are seen following road accidents, fights, etc., or may be the result of self-trauma.
- **Inflammatory reactions** occur as the result of allergic reactions, insect stings, etc., and may produce severe oedema of the eyelid and conjunctiva.
- **Foreign bodies** (e.g. grass seeds) may become lodged under the eyelids or beneath the nictitating membrane. This is often a problem in rabbits and guinea pigs which are bedded on straw.

Signs of injury. Injuries to the eyelids are usually the most painless of all three conditions. There is rarely much swelling or bleeding and it can be quite difficult to see simple wounds because the wound edges rarely gape.

The cornea should always be carefully examined in any case of lid injury to check for signs of corneal damage which may have occurred at the same time as the eyelid injury.

Signs of inflammation. Inflammatory reactions may result in severe head-rubbing until the entire skin of the eyelids and adjoining area is severely abraded, red raw and swollen. The conjunctiva is often so oedematous that it bulges up over the eyelid margin like a pink cushion (**chemosis**). If both upper and lower eyelids are affected, it may be difficult to see the eye itself because both upper and lower palpebral conjunctivae are so swollen (Fig. 3.37).

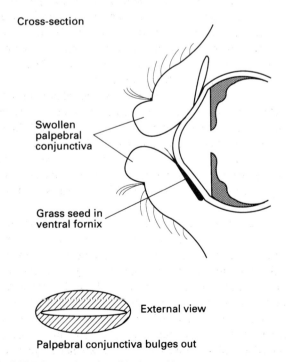

Cross-section

Swollen
palpebral
conjunctiva

Grass seed in
ventral fornix

External view

Palpebral conjunctiva bulges out

Fig. 3.37 Inflammation of eyelid (chemosis).

Signs of foreign bodies. The presence of foreign bodies is the most painful condition of all and it can be impossible even to examine the eye because the patient keeps it tightly shut. There may also be **corneal damage**, caused by the sharp foreign body scraping on the cornea every time the animal moves its eyeball.

If the object has been lodged in the eye for any length of time, it will cause a **purulent ocular discharge**.

Occasionally, foreign bodies lie deep in the ventral or dorsal fornix (the pocket where the palpebral conjunctiva turns inwards to become the bulbar conjunctiva, Fig. 3.37) or become lodged behind the third eyelid so that they can easily be missed. Only the tip of the foreign body may protrude and the eye must be examined very thoroughly and carefully before deciding that there is no foreign body present.

Treatment. Any wounds should be cleansed with care to ensure that contamination (dirt, hair, etc.) is not washed into the eye. Antiseptic solutions should not be used near the eye of the conscious animal.

The pain associated with inflammation, however caused, may be alleviated by the use of ice packs, applied gently to the area. The veterinary nurse may also apply two or three drops of an ophthalmic local anaesthetic preparation to the eye if these are available.

Non-penetrating foreign bodies should be removed wherever possible. It is best if local anaesthetic is administered as described above before the removal is attempted, as this is usually an acutely painful procedure and if the patient wriggles uncontrollably at the crucial moment, further damage may be done when implements accidentally jab into the eye.

Large foreign bodies (e.g. grass seeds) may be grasped manually and removed. No undue force must be used because part of the seed may break off and be left in the eye.

Smaller foreign bodies (e.g. grit) should be flushed into the corner of the eye using warmed sterile saline solution. Once lying on the sclera or lid conjunctiva, the culprit can be removed more easily and safely as the tissues are far less sensitive than the cornea, and more robust. A piece of moistened lint, a cotton bud or fine paintbrush is used to lift the foreign body from the eye surface.

If the foreign body does not move when saline is flushed across the eye, it must be assumed to have penetrated the eyeball and should not be disturbed. Veterinary advice must be sought immediately.

Eyeball
Causes

- **Fractured skull**. The eyeball is well protected by the bony orbit and the eyelids. However, the force which fractures the orbital bones can produce severe bruising of the eye.
- **Blows to the eye**. Direct trauma to the eye can cause haemorrhage within the eye, despite the protective eyelids.

- In short-nosed breeds which have a very shallow bony orbit and protuberant eyes, injury to the orbital area (e.g. resulting from a road accident or a fight) can **prolapse** the eye.

Signs with skull fracture

- The eyeball often protrudes slightly from the socket because of a **retrobulbar haemorrhage** (bleeding into the soft tissues behind the eye in the orbit) and the eye may even prolapse.
- There is usually **bruising of the bulbar conjunctiva** (seen as a bright red blood blister on the white sclera).
- The **pupillary reflexes** may be decreased or absent and the pupil may be constricted if the nerve supply to the iris is damaged.
- The animal may also be **concussed** and the signs of pain are variable, depending on the state of consciousness.

Signs of injury to the eyeball. Affected animals show signs of ocular pain but often the pain is duller and less acute than in cases of eyelid inflammation or foreign bodies. Bruising of the conjunctiva is commonly seen and the anterior chamber of the eye may look clouded with a red mist because the delicate iris haemorrhages and the blood swirls round in the aqueous humour.

Prolapse of the eyeball. The entire eyeball sits exposed on the side of the patient's face. It becomes inflamed and congested within minutes as the eyelids close behind it and the cornea rapidly dries. Because the eyeball is now totally unprotected, other damage can occur.

Treatment. If any injury to the eyeball results in a protruding eye and loss of pupillary reflexes, the patient must be observed carefully in case this partial prolapse becomes a total prolapse.

The prolapsed eyeball is the only condition where specific first aid measures may be applied. **The eyeball must be replaced as soon as possible** because the dry cornea will soon ulcerate and the optic nerve may suffer permanent damage.

Liquid paraffin, olive oil or preferably 'false tears' (e.g. methyl cellulose preparations) should be used to lubricate the eyeball, and a gentle attempt made to draw the lids out and over the eyeball. **The eyeball itself must never be pushed back in.** No force should be used and, if the attempt is unsuccessful, the cornea should be kept well moistened with a sterile saline or 'false tears' until a veterinary surgeon can attend the case.

If owners ring up and report that a pet's eye has prolapsed, they **must be advised to keep the eyeball lubricated** as described above so that the tissues do not dry out before the animal reaches the surgery. Contact lens saline is an ideal solution which may be available in the home; failing this, owners can make their own sterile saline by dissolving half a teaspoonful of salt in 1 litre of cool, boiled water. The use of these solutions is much kinder to the traumatised tissues of the eye than pure water, but cold boiled water is better than nothing if owners are unable to prepare saline solutions.

The animal must be closely observed at all times to ensure that it does not cause further damage to the eye. It must also be treated for shock and made as comfortable as possible.

Cornea

Causes. Non-penetrating wounds (ulcers) may be caused by foreign bodies in the eye, or sharp objects such as cats' claws or thorns. The surface of the cornea may also be damaged by splashes from scalding fluids, paint, acid or alkali.

Penetrating wounds occur as the result of more serious injury received in fights, road accidents, etc., and may be complicated by injury to, or prolapse of, the internal structures of the eye, particularly the vascular iris.

Signs of ulceration. The cornea is extremely sensitive and any injury causes pain. There is often a bluish or white tinge to the cornea at the site of the injury but otherwise the cornea looks normal.

Signs of penetrating wounds. Penetrating wounds result in a loss of pressure in the anterior chamber of the eye as the aqueous humour escapes through the wound. The cornea often appears wrinkled like the skin of a raisin instead of being smooth and rounded. Any pressure on the eyeball (as may be applied when parting the lids to examine the eye, for example) results in a gush of clear or bloodstained watery fluid as aqueous humour escapes from the eye.

Treatment. **An eye splashed by chemicals or detergents should immediately be treated by repeated flushing of the eye surface.** Sterile saline or contact lens solutions should be used, but tap water can be used in an emergency in the home. Bicarbonate solutions may be applied to neutralise acid splashes and vinegar solutions used for alkali damage. Cold liquid paraffin may be used in the case of hot fat splashes to prevent the fat from congealing on the cornea but these measures are mainly academic – **thorough flushing of the eye** is what really counts.

After the initial 'panic' flushing, a saline solution must be used (as in cases of eyeball injury) as this is more comfortable for the animal and will remove any residual chemical. At the surgery, the cornea should be flushed with sterile saline and a sterile gauze pad fixed loosely in position over the eye with adhesive plaster (if the patient permits this) but the eye must always be checked by a veterinary surgeon to assess and treat any corneal damage.

Penetrating wounds of the eyeball should be disturbed as little as possible to avoid loss of aqueous humour. Sometimes thorns may transfix the cornea but should be left for the veterinary surgeon to remove. Surgery may be necessary to repair penetrating wounds and theatre should be prepared.

Following the first aid measures above, the animal should be confined in a darkened room or kennel to alleviate discomfort, but steps must be taken (e.g. by fitting an Elizabethan collar) to ensure that the wounded eye is not disturbed.

Injuries to the ear

Injuries to the ear flap

Causes

- **Trauma**. The ears may be a site of injury following road accidents, or more often from fights and bites. Dogs exercised in dense undergrowth may catch the ear flaps on thorns or barbed wire.
- **Insect stings and snake bites** can also affect the ear flap.
- **Aural haematomas** occur as a result of self-trauma or head shaking.

Signs. Open wounds of the ear bleed freely and may cause shaking of the head and irritation. Scratching at the ear will increase the haemorrhage and may enlarge the wound.

Closed wounds result in swelling. If there is inflammation present (e.g. sting and snake bite injuries), this swelling is hot, hard and painful. Aural haematomas do not inflame and the swelling is cool and soft.

Treatment. Wounds to the ear flap should be treated by normal methods, but care must be taken when clipping the fur that the ear flap itself is not cut. Haemorrhage from ear flaps is not life-threatening but it is very messy. The haemorrhage constantly restarts as the animal shakes its head and blood will be splattered widely. It is usually necessary to bandage the ear flap by folding it back to lie over the top of the head and fixing it with a wide bandage which encircles the head tightly. Large wounds may require surgical treatment later.

Stings and snake bites should be treated as described in the section on poisoning.

Aural haematomas should be treated as described in the wounds section (haematomas; p. 52).

Foreign bodies in the ear

Signs. Grass seeds commonly gain access to the ear canal and travel downwards to lie in the horizontal ear canal, up against the ear drum. The animal will show intense irritation and pain, holding the head to one side, shaking its head violently and rubbing the ear with a forepaw, or along the ground. If the base of the vertical ear canal is palpated externally, the patient will often cry in pain.

Treatment. The foreign body, if visible, should be gently removed with forceps. If this is not possible, warmed olive oil or liquid paraffin may be poured into the ear to alleviate the discomfort. No attempt should be made to probe the ear, but veterinary attention should be sought. No food must be given because a general anaesthetic will usually be needed before any foreign body can be removed from the depths of the ear canal.

Vestibular syndrome (including 'strokes')

Causes. This condition does not appear to be caused in the same way as human strokes, but the symptoms are so similar that it is often labelled as a stroke for convenience.

(A true stroke is the result of a circulating embolus.) The symptoms result from injury to the vestibular system (balance organ) in the inner ear but the cause of injury is often unknown, although inflammation of the inner ear or inflammation of brain tissue itself (encephalitis) are responsible in certain cases.

Signs. The patient is usually an older dog but cats and rabbits with severe ear infections also suffer, as do the cage pets, hamsters, gerbils, rats and mice. The onset of the problem is sudden and the symptoms vary, but all patients will have marked head tilt and loss of balance. The affected dog almost always has some degree of nystagmus.

Severe cases are unable to lie in sternal recumbency and stay collapsed on their sides. There may be reduced pain sensation in the feet of the affected side and pedal reflexes may be slowed but eye reflexes are usually unaffected. The patient may be depressed, but this is largely due to the animal being unable to understand what is happening rather than true depression due to brain dysfunction. Many of these animals want to eat if they can get the food into their mouths.

Patients which are less affected are able to stand but show incoordination and a stumbling gait. They may walk in circles and fall over on the affected side. The animal is usually bright and appetite is unaffected if coordination permits prehension of food – it can be difficult to eat if the head is twisted on one side.

Treatment. There is little that a veterinary nurse can offer as first aid except to reassure the owner and patient. Owners are always fearful that a fatal 'stroke' may follow these symptoms and the patient may panic because it cannot coordinate its movements. Confine the animal to a small kennel or basket to restrict movement and to force it to rest. Once it stops falling over, it will feel more secure and settle down calmly.

Propentofylline is a very useful drug to try in these cases. Injections of diuretics and corticosteroids may also be required, but complete recovery is rare and most patients are left with a varying degree of head tilt.

Death, unconsciousness and collapse

The first fact to establish when presented with an immobile, collapsed animal is whether the patient is alive or dead. Table 3.17 gives the comparisons between unconscious collapse and death.

Signs of death

Signs of death include:

- Absence of heartbeat.
- Absence of respiratory movement.
- Dilatation of the pupil and loss of light reflex.
- Loss of the corneal reflex.
- Glazing of the cornea.
- Body cooling and rigor mortis.

Table 3.17 Comparison between death and unconsciousness

Sign	Death	Unconscious collapse
Heartbeat	Absent for more than 3 minutes	Regular, though slowed
Respiratory pattern	Absent, although occasionally Cheyne–Stokes respiration is observed	Varies according to the depth of CNS depression (mimics anaesthesia)
Eyeball position	Central	Turned down or central, according to the depth of CNS depression
Cornea	Glazed	Normally moist
Corneal reflex	Absent	Present (unless eyelids paralysed)
Pupil size	Fully dilated	May vary in size, but are rarely fully dilated
Pupillary light reflex	Absent	Usually present unless iris paralysed
Movement	Absent, except Cheyne–Stokes respiration. Rigor mortis in a few hours	May be roused in stupor. Pedal reflexes present in mild cases of unconsciousness
Body temperature	Cools within 15 minutes	Remains constant

Absence of a heartbeat

Absence of the heartbeat for 3 minutes is detected by palpation of the chest for the apex beat and listening to the chest with a stethoscope.

The heartbeat may be felt by placing one hand on either side of the chest wall so that the fingertips come to rest on the costal cartilages of ribs 5–6, i.e. at the bottom of the rib cage just behind the elbow. (The area would lie just under the elbow of the standing dog; in the collapsed patient it appears to be behind the elbow as the forelegs are usually extended when the animal lies on its side.) Apply *gentle* pressure with the fingertips, pressing the costal cartilages inwards until the pulsations of the ventricles can be felt through the chest wall. (No pressure is needed in cats or dogs with deep, narrow chests.) In barrel-chested breeds such as bulldogs, it may be impossible to feel an apex beat so a stethoscope must be used.

The veterinary nurse should take every opportunity to practise feeling this apical heartbeat in healthy, unconscious animals. Many opportunities arise when observing anaesthetized animals admitted for routine surgery and familiarity with techniques leads to confidence in an emergency.

If no heartbeat is immediately obvious, a stethoscope must be used to detect *any* cardiac activity. The cardiac muscle contractions may be too slight or weak or the conformation of the chest may be too broad. The head of the stethoscope should be placed in the area of intercostal space 7–8. Again, the veterinary nurse should practise auscultating the heart of normal, unconscious animals to be confident of placing the stethoscope in the correct position for this emergency.

Absence of respiratory movement

The nurse should be familiar with shallow breathing and should watch closely for any breaths. Fogging of a cold mirror or movement of a fine tuft of hair held at the nostrils will detect the slightest expiration.

Dilatation of the pupil and loss of light reflex

This is tested using a pen torch or auroscope head light source in a darkened room.

Loss of the corneal reflex

The cornea is easily damaged and so this reflex should only be tested by touching a wisp of moist cotton wool on to the cornea. This will be sufficient to make the eyelids blink.

Glazing of the cornea

The surface of the eyeball lacks its usual lustre.

Body cooling and rigor mortis

After the muscles have relaxed, they gradually stiffen due to chemical changes in the muscle cells. Rigor mortis usually takes about 12 hours to set in throughout the body, but the rate is variable depending on the room temperature, cause of death and physical condition of the animal. The cooling of the body also takes several hours, again depending on the room temperature.

Rigor mortis will pass off after several days as decay sets in.

Unconsciousness

Definition

Loss of consciousness occurs when the brain is affected so that the animal is unable to respond normally to external stimuli.

In most cases, the brain is depressed and the patient becomes totally relaxed and comatose, but in other cases (e.g. epilepsy) the brain is overactive and the body muscles contract convulsively.

Signs of unconsciousness

Many of the signs of flaccid unconscious collapse mimic those seen in anaesthetised animals because general anaesthesia is, after all, a state of flaccid unconscious collapse. Therefore, the veterinary nurse may apply the knowledge and experience gained in theatre to assess the degree of depression of the patient and the seriousness of the situation.

Heart and pulse rates. The heartbeat in the flaccid unconscious patient is usually regular but slowed. As the situation deteriorates, the rate slows further until cardiac arrest occurs.

Respiratory movements. Deep, regular breathing may quicken as the animal regains consciousness or it may progress to rapid, shallow gasps as the brain becomes more and more depressed. **Cheyne–Stokes** respiration (deep, convulsive gasps for breath at infrequent intervals) heralds the onset of death.

Position of the eyeball in the socket. In cases of epileptiform convulsions, the eyeball may stay in its usual position but remains in a fixed, unfocused stare. The eyes do not turn to follow movements or towards the owner in recognition.

In cases of flaccid unconsciousness, the eye position will often indicate the depth of unconsciousness **unless the muscles of the eyeball are paralysed**. Evidence of **nystagmus** (rapid involuntary side-to-side or up and down movement of the eyeball) or **strabismus** (squint) should be noted.

Palpebral reflex. This should *not* be tested in the convulsing animal as the stimulus may worsen the convulsions. In the flaccid animal, the presence or absence of this reflex is another indication of the severity of brain depression. If the palpebral reflex is absent, the **corneal reflex** may be tested as described earlier (see Signs of death, p. 82). The cornea is so sensitive that this is one of the last reflexes to be lost as the animal loses its fight for life. However, it should be remembered that, in some cases of head trauma where the motor nerves of the eyelid muscles are damaged, the animal will be unable to respond and may not necessarily be dying.

Pupil size. Compare the pupil size of each eye. Asymmetry of pupil size (**anisocoria**) can indicate unilateral brain damage.

Pupillary light reflex. This reflex should be tested in a darkened room, using a torch or auroscope head as a source of bright light. Both pupils should constrict equally as the light shines into the eye. Failure to do so indicates brain damage but, if the nerves to the pupil are damaged (e.g. by trauma as occurs in a prolapsed eyeball), the reflex may be absent in that eye because the reflex is unable to work. The unaffected eye should react normally.

Again, this test should not be carried out on the convulsing animal as it may make the situation worse.

Depth of consciousness. This is assessed by the various eye reflexes described above. The pedal reflexes are also a useful indication as to the depth of unconsciousness, since they are the first reflexes to be lost as brain activity becomes depressed and the last to return as the condition improves.

There are two terms used to describe the depth of unconsciousness:

- In **stupor**, the animal can be roused with difficulty and the pedal withdrawal reflex is still present, though the toes may need to be pinched quite hard. Pupillary and palpebral reflexes are also still present.
- In **coma**, the animal cannot be roused, the pedal reflexes are absent and the eye reflexes indicate a plane of surgical anaesthesia or deeper. The pupils become dilated as the condition deteriorates and death approaches.

Convulsions. Convulsions are violent, irregular involuntary movements of the body. The time of onset and duration should be noted.

Incontinence. Urine or faeces may be passed by the unconscious animal either passively (a gradual seepage because the sphincter muscles relax) or actively (e.g. a pool of urine passed during an epileptiform fit).

Collapse

Definition

Collapse is said to have occurred when a conscious animal is unable or unwilling to stand up.

'Collapse' is the most common emergency reported by owners and covers a multitude of situations from an arthritic dog which is reluctant to get up and go for a walk, to a deceased pet. The cause and severity of the 'collapse' must therefore first be discovered so that the correct first aid procedure may be carried out.

Signs of collapse

The difference between collapse and unconsciousness is whether the animal is still conscious or not. **The conscious patient responds normally to sound, sight and touch.** A dog will turn its eyes, if not its head, when its name is called. The conscious animal has all the normal eye reflexes and can focus on objects and follow movements with its eyes. The patient will respond to handling: either the animal will become calm or affectionate following gentle stroking, or it may be aggressive to any handling. Beware: the response of the collapsed aggressive patient is coordinated and deliberate, so that the animal is able to bite, even if it is unable to get up. If a patient has all these normal responses and yet is unwilling or unable to get up, it may be said to have collapsed.

The collapsed animal should always be treated with care because its condition may not be stable. In some cases, the patient may lapse into unconsciousness and die. In other cases, there may be a rapid improvement to normal health. As with cases of unconsciousness, a collapsed patient must be constantly observed and its reflexes assessed to ensure that the situation is not deteriorating.

Causes of collapse and unconsciousness

The causes of collapse and unconsciousness are listed in Table 3.18, but this is often not a clear-cut situation. It must be remembered that all the causes of unconsciousness may also cause the animal to collapse if the brain is only mildly depressed. Conversely, most causes of collapse may progress to unconsciousness if the situation deteriorates. Therefore, the categories listed in Table 3.18 (i.e. whether a condition causes collapse or unconsciousness) simply reflect the most likely presenting symptom seen in day-to-day practice.

Some conditions are placed in both categories. This is because that condition may be so acute in some accidents that the patient becomes unconscious almost immediately and the conscious collapse phase is scarcely noticeable. In other accidents, the situation may not be so severe and the patient is simply collapsed when presented. For example, hyperthermia (heatstroke) can present as either case, depending on the vigilance of the owner. If an animal is confined to a car on a hot, humid day and left, it will be unconscious within an hour. If the same animal is left for 20 minutes in the same conditions, it will probably be collapsed but still conscious.

Treatment and resuscitation procedures

When an unconscious animal is first presented, the veterinary nurse should follow the **ABC (airway, breathing, circulation)** treatment regime laid out in the first section of this chapter under 'Arrival at the surgery' (see box on p. 27). In practice, if presented with a dying patient, the veterinary nurse needs to give cardiac massage and artificial respiration simultaneously – the one is pointless without the other. However, this is impossible to portray in a textbook because the procedures must be separated in order to describe the methods but the treatments have been arranged in the following order to indicate their priority in an emergency.

Maintaining the airway

The first action when presented with a collapsed unconscious patient is to clear an airway. Tight collars should be removed and the mouth examined as swiftly as possible to ensure that there is no obstruction at the back of the throat, e.g. blood, mucus, etc. Fluids should be swabbed away and any foreign body should be removed or pushed to one side (see Asphyxia, p. 90). The trachea should be intubated if

Table 3.18 Causes of collapse and unconsciousness

Body system	Cause	C	U
CNS	Epilepsy	–	+
	Brain trauma, e.g. blow to head	+	+
	Vestibular syndrome	+	–
	Disc protrusion	+	–
	Atlanto-axial subluxation	+	–
	Spinal fractures	+	–
Respiratory	Obstruction of the airway	+	+
	Fluid in the alveolar spaces	+	+
	Collapsed lungs	+	–
	Interference with respiratory movements	+	–
	Interference with oxygenation of the blood	+	–
Circulatory	Cardiac failure	+	+
	Hypovolaemic shock – acute haemorrhage	+	+
	– severe fluid loss	+	–
	Traumatic shock, e.g. RTAs	+	–
	Anaemia (long-term blood loss)	+	–
	Thrombosis – brachial or iliac	+	–
Abdominal catastrophe	Gastric torsion, bowel rupture	+	–
	Bladder rupture	+	–
	Urethral obstruction	+	–
	Acute prostatitis	+	–
	Acute hepatitis	+	–
	Splenic torsion	+	–
	Acute pancreatitis	+	–
Locomotor conditions	Dislocations and fractures of the limbs	+	–
	Arthritis, muscle wasting	+	–
Metabolic disturbances	Hyper/hypoglycaemia	+	+
	Hypocalcaemia	+	+
	Uraemic fits	+	+
	Toxaemia, e.g. pyometra	+	–
Physical causes	Electrocution	–	+
	Hypothermia	+	+
	Hyperthermia	+	+
Drugs and poisons	Any compound causing CNS depression	+	+

Key: C = Conscious collapse; U = Unconscious collapse; RTA = Road Traffic Accident; CNS = Central Nervous System, i.e. the brain and spinal cord.

possible and the cuff inflated to avoid inhalation of fluids. NB: The patient must be observed closely as many of these cases regain consciousness rapidly and the endotracheal tube may need to be removed in a hurry.

If no endotracheal tubes are available or the trachea cannot be intubated, the patient should be laid in the veterinary recovery position (see Non-intubated patients, below).

Cardiac massage

Cardiac massage must be started immediately if there is no pulse and no heartbeat can felt or heard when using a stethoscope.

The heart may be stimulated by rhythmical compression of the lower rib cage over ribs 3–6. Cats' chests are easily compressed by placing the fingertips of both hands on either side of the thorax and applying gentle, firm pressure. Large dogs need to be laid on their side in the recovery position (Fig. 3.38) and punched with a closed fist to stimulate the heart effectively.

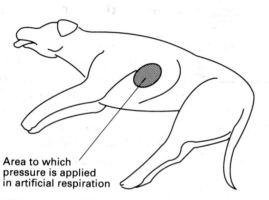

Area to which pressure is applied in artificial respiration

Fig. 3.38 Recovery position.

Pressure should be applied at half-second intervals in the case of small animals. In larger patients, compressions at one-second intervals are sufficient.

Artificial respiration must be maintained at the same time as the cardiac massage is given and therefore it is best if two people cooperate in resuscitating the patient. If alone, the veterinary nurse should apply cardiac massage for 5 seconds then inflate the chest 3 times, then cardiac massage, then chest inflation, etc. In this way, there is oxygen available in the lungs as soon as the circulation restarts, but the cardiac massage is continued almost uninterrupted.

If the heart does not restart after 3 minutes of cardiac massage, the patient may be declared to be dead.

Artificial respiration

If respiratory movements have ceased, respiratory stimulant drugs may be used (e.g. doxapram hydrochloride) but, until the animal starts to breathe on its own, **the lungs must be mechanically inflated** if the patient is to continue to live.

It is *always* preferable to intubate these patients because:

● The tube ensures the airway remains patent.
● The inflated cuff avoids any inhalation of fluids.

● It is much more hygienic to give artificial respiration by giving gases or blowing down a clean tube than attempting mouth-to-nose resuscitation.

Intubated patients. Intubated patients should be connected to an oxygen supply from a closed-circuit anaesthetic machine and **the re-breathing bag used to inflate the lungs**. Only very gentle pressure may be needed at frequent intervals to mimic panting respiration, i.e. approximately 120 breaths per minute, two breaths a second. Massive inflation of the lungs (equivalent to drawing a deep breath) can overinflate them, causing damage to the lung alveoli and possibly driving the lungs against sharp fragments of broken ribs. This panting form of artificial respiration can be so effective that it is possible to 'rest' the respiration for 5 seconds in every 15 seconds to see if the breathing has restarted. However, if there is any sign of cyanosis, the respiration should be maintained continuously.

If no anaesthetic machine is immediately available, the animal should be intubated and the lungs inflated by gently blowing down the tube at 1 second intervals. **Do not overinflate the lungs** – use gentle puffs which just cause the rib cage to lift a little. Carbon dioxide in the nurse's exhaled breath may stimulate the animal to breathe.

Artificial respiration is continued until the animal starts to breathe on its own (which may take up to an hour or more) or until death has intervened.

Non-intubated patients. Non-intubated patients should be placed in the recovery position (Fig. 3.38):

● The animal is laid on its right side.
● The head and neck are extended.
● The tongue is pulled out to clear the airway.
● The front legs are pulled forwards so the upper leg does not rest on the chest, weighing it down and making inspiration more of an effort.
● Lay the palm of the hand in the middle of the chest wall, just behind the mass of the triceps muscle of the foreleg.
● Apply firm steady pressure and then release so that the elastic rib cage springs back, drawing air into the lungs. **Reapply the pressure at 0.5–1 second intervals** depending upon the size of the animal.

This procedure must *not* be used in cases where any damage to the thoracic wall is suspected, as fractured ribs could easily be displaced and pierce the lungs or heart during compression of the thorax. In such cases **mouth-to-nose resuscitation** should be used if no intubation facilities are to hand:

● The patient's tongue is first pulled forwards to ensure an unobstructed airway.
● Then the nose is grasped firmly but gently in the left hand so that the thumb and fingers curl round the snout to hold down the upper lip-folds and create an airtight seal. This is important because, if the mouth is not sealed, air blown into the nose escapes through the mouth instead of being forced into the lungs.
● The right hand is placed under the lower jaw to support the weight of the animal's head (Fig. 3.39).

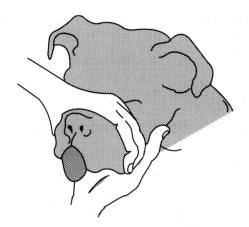

Fig. 3.39 Mouth-to-nose resuscitation: holding the nose.

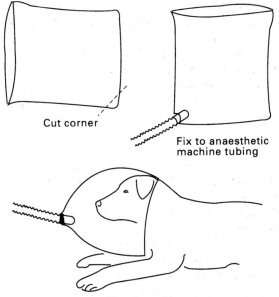

Fig. 3.40 Using a plastic bag as a face mask.

- If the patient is a large dog, with lip margins too long for the left hand to cover so that the lips cannot be sealed effectively, the right hand should also be used to seal the part of the lips which the left hand cannot reach.
- **Always wear a face mask when attempting this procedure** because of the risk to human health. Try to blow air away from your mouth and do not inhale saliva or air from the patient. Inhale through your nostrils not your mouth.
- Care must also be taken not to overinflate the lungs or the delicate lung tissue may be damaged. Use gentle puffs as when the patient is intubated.

Prevention of hypoxia

Hypoxia occurs when the blood does not contain as much oxygen as normal.

Intubated unconscious patients can be connected to the oxygen supply of an anaesthetic machine.

If the animal is dyspnoeic but conscious, **it is most important that it is made to rest as much as possible**. Attempts to examine the mouth for obstructions should be abandoned if they cause distress. Struggling will only increase the body's demand for oxygen, so that the hypoxia becomes more severe and the patient's condition deteriorates.

The animal should be encouraged to breathe oxygen or oxygen-enriched air to correct the hypoxia. Small dogs and cats can be placed in wire baskets, which in turn are placed in large plastic bags which may be inflated with oxygen to create a small oxygen tent. 'Gas out' boxes (used in some veterinary surgeries for anaesthetising recalcitrant cats) can be used as oxygen tents if connected to an oxygen-only anaesthetic machine.

Larger dogs must be encouraged to lie still while a stream of oxygen is directed at the nostrils. Forcing a dog's head into a mask will only distress the animal and worsen the problem. However, a plastic bag may be used to create a light, flexible mask that funnels oxygen to the face. The bag should be large enough to fit comfortably over the entire head of the animal. Cut off one of the bottom corners and push the tube from the oxygen-only anaesthetic machine through the resulting hole. Adhesive tape may be used to attach the bag to the end of the tube. Gently draw the open end of the bag over the animal's face. Because the polyethylene is lightweight and transparent, the animal does not feel trapped and restricted and will often tolerate the arrangement very well (Fig. 3.40). The bag must hang freely ventrally to allow water vapour and expired air to escape. If the bag fits the face too tightly, a hot and humid atmosphere develops in the bag and distresses the patient.

Some animals may allow a nasal catheter to be inserted into the nostrils, especially if they are only semi-conscious.

Control of severe haemorrhage

This has already been described (see p. 42).

Conservation of heat

These animals are in a state of shock and should not be allowed to lose heat. The exception to this is, of course, the collapsed heatstroke patient.

Administration of fluids

Fluids should never be given by mouth to an unconscious animal unless the trachea is intubated with an inflated cuffed tube and a stomach tube is passed. The only indication for such measures is the hypoglycaemic diabetic patient, when glucose solution should be given via the stomach tube.

Constant observation

When the patient has been stabilised and made comfortable, it is most important to **maintain constant, keen observation.** Every 10–15 minutes, the eye reflexes, breathing pattern and pulse rate of the unconscious patient should also be checked and the findings and time of testing recorded on a chart. Such charts enable the veterinary nurse to monitor the progress of the patient and are essential for the veterinary surgeon to estimate the rate of deterioration or improvement in the animal's condition. Evidence of rapid worsening of the situation may prompt surgical intervention in cases of head trauma or may mean that further drugs must be given in other cases. The charts also enable the veterinary surgeon to give a more accurate prognosis.

Specific causes and treatment of unconsciousness

The causes of unconsciousness are shown in Tables 3.18, 3.19 and 3.20.

Primary causes are those causing unconsciousness as an immediate result of injury or dysfunction of the nervous system itself.

Secondary causes are those causing unconsciousness because of another system failure or metabolic dysfunction.

Table 3.19 Classification of causes of unconsciousness

Primary causes	(a) Epilepsy (b) Direct trauma to the brain (c) Chemical causes – poisons

Secondary causes	(a) Asphyxia
	(b) Metabolic disturbances
	    ketoacidosis
	    hypoglycaemia in diabetics
	    hypocalcaemia in eclampsia
	    uraemia in kidney failure
	(c) Circulatory disturbances
	    cardiac failure
	    hypovolaemic shock
	(d) Physical causes
	    electrocution
	    hyperthermia (heatstroke)
	    hypothermia

Table 3.20 Classification of types of unconsciousness

Spastic (rigid)
unconsciousness
	Primary epileptic convulsions
	Metabolic dysfunction, e.g. uraemic fits,
	    eclampsia
	Physical causes – electrocution
	Chemical poisonings, e.g. strychnine,
	    slug bait

Flaccid (relaxed)
unconsciousness
	Oxygen deprivation – asphyxia
	Metabolic dysfunction, e.g. diabetes
	    mellitus
	Circulatory dysfunction, e.g. cardiac
	    failure, severe haemorrhage
	Central nervous system injury, e.g.
	    trauma following road accidents, etc.
	Chemical poisoning
	Physical causes, e.g. heatstroke

Death	

Epileptiform fits

Cause. The condition is more common in dogs than in cats and is usually seen in animals 1–3 years old, especially if inclined to nervousness or over-excitability (**primary fits**). Older animals may suffer **secondary fits** which occur following brain damage by diseases (such as distemper), trauma (such as a blow to the head) or toxaemia (as seen in uraemic patients and poisoning cases).

Signs. Fits vary in severity and are described as *petit mal* (when the patient does not collapse) or *grand mal* when the patient does collapse and becomes unconscious).

Grand mal fits often occur as the animal is waking up from sleep, but may also happen when it is fully conscious. In the latter case, the animal often becomes restless just before the fit commences and may be unusually affectionate, continually seeking reassurance from the owner. Occasionally the dog becomes hysterical, barking and rushing madly around before succumbing to the fit. The fit itself usually happens suddenly.

The animal having a fit collapses on to its side and goes into violent convulsions in what is known as the **ictal phase**. Its legs are extended, its head pulled back and neck extended; there is involuntary champing of the jaws, which churns saliva into a foaming froth around the lips. Its eyes are open and stare fixedly. The respiratory rate is much increased and defecation and urination are common during severe fits. Most convulsions subside after 5–10 minutes but occasionally the dog will remain in a fit for hours, relaxing from one attack only to start shaking with the next fit.

Following an attack, the dog usually rises and wanders about aimlessly and unsteadily, looking dazed and confused. Soon it recognises its owner and, although very tired, will be back to normal.

The 'petit mal' fit is often less dramatic: the animal simply wanders around, staring fixedly, unresponsive to the owner and unable to settle.

Complications. The possibility of **rabies** must always be considered in cases of unusual nervous signs in the dog and cat, although the likelihood of this lethal disease manifesting itself in the household pet in the UK is still at present remote. In first aid history taking, the owners should be asked how long they have owned the pet and whether the animal has been abroad, especially within the past 6 months.

In the case of **secondary fits**, the underlying cause may make treatment impossible (see uraemia). Samples of urine, faeces and vomit should be saved in cases of suspected poisoning.

Fits are not fatal in most cases but, very rarely, the animal may have a **swallowed tongue** (see Fig 3.42) and chokes. The patient's breathing becomes extremely laboured but soundless as no air can be inhaled. The mucosae are purple because of the cyanosis. The convulsions subside as the animal becomes hypoxic and the patient will soon die.

Treatment. Whatever the cause of the attack, the first aid treatment remains the same. These attacks represent gross overactivity of the central nervous system 'circuits' and any extra stimulus usually only worsens the situation and prolongs the fit.

- Owners should be advised to contain the dog in a darkened (no visual stimulus), quiet (no auditory stimulus) room.
- They should remain in the room with the dog but should **not touch it** (minimal tactile stimulus) unless the dog threatens to injure itself.
- Above all, **the owners must remain calm** and any member of the family who threatens to become hysterical should not be allowed to stay with the dog.
- As the fits are often of short duration, it is best to leave the dog in the house to avoid stimulating it any further.
- Should the fit persist, or should the owner be unable to cope with the situation, the patient may be brought to the surgery.

At the surgery, the animal should be confined to a dark, quiet kennel for observation until the veterinary surgeon can attend to it. Injections of barbiturate or diazepam should be prepared because it may be necessary to anaesthetise or sedate the patient to control the fit.

When the dog is recovering from the fit and pacing around, reassurance may be given **if the dog seeks it** (i.e. if the dog approaches the owner), but no attempt should be made to prevent the restlessness as this may simply spark off another fit. Similar advice should be given in the case of the very mild epileptic dog. See Chapter 17, Fits pp. 454–5.

Should the patient show signs of **cyanosis**, it must be carefully observed because the tongue may be obstructing the pharynx. If the breathing becomes soundless (see above), the animal may be picked up and suspended by the hind legs in the hope that this will ease the obstruction.

WARNING

Under no circumstances should the owner or veterinary nurse attempt to put a hand into the animal's mouth until the convulsions subside. Such attempts are fruitless and can lead to severe bites being inflicted if the patient's jaws are still champing.

If the convulsions have stopped (the patient may be nearly dead), the mouth should be opened and the tongue can be unrolled with difficulty (a finger inserted into the fold and pulled forwards is usually the best way – see Fig. 3.42). Resuscitation should then be carried out as described earlier.

Direct trauma (concussion)

Causes. Any blow to the head, as sustained in a road accident or following a kick from a horse, etc., may result in unconsciousness because pressure is exerted on the delicate cerebral hemispheres. Depressed fractures of the cranium will obviously cause such pressure and damage, but concussion is frequently seen without any fracture being

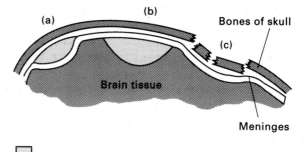

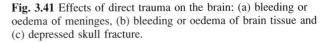

Tissues swollen by haemorrhage or inflammation

Fig. 3.41 Effects of direct trauma on the brain: (a) bleeding or oedema of meninges, (b) bleeding or oedema of brain tissue and (c) depressed skull fracture.

present. In these cases it is due to intracranial haemorrhage or oedematous swelling in the meninges overlying the hemispheres, or in the nervous tissue itself. As the entire cranium is formed by bone, any swelling must press inwards on the brain itself (Fig. 3.41).

Signs. The signs of concussion are very variable, ranging from a slightly dazed animal to the comatose patient, depending on the degree of injury. The following signs may be seen:

- Shock.
- Haemorrhage from the nose, mouth or ears.
- Fracture of the cranium or hard palate also indicate trauma to the head. (Note that any palpation of the cranium must be carried out very gently for fear of depressing the fracture even deeper into the brain tissues.)
- The pupils may be unequally dilated and vary in their reactions to light, indicating that one side of the brain is more affected than the other. The eyes may also show nystagmus or strabismus. In severe cases, the palpebral and corneal reflexes may be absent and the pupils dilated, but the veterinary nurse should test both eyes. It may be that the reflexes are absent because the sensory or motor nerve involved in the tested reflex is damaged, not because the animal is profoundly unconsciousness. For example, paralysis of the facial nerve on one side of the face will mean that the eyelid cannot blink as the palpebral reflex is tested but the other side of the face may be totally unaffected and react normally.
- Respiration is usually slow and shallow and the heart rate is depressed in severe cases.
- Movement in the conscious patient is often uncoordinated. The unconscious patient is flaccidly collapsed but occasionally there may be spasmodic muscular shivering.
- Conscious patients may vomit.
- In other cases, damage to certain areas of the brain leads to paralysis. Symptoms can be very variable depending upon the part of the brain injured and the extent of the injury.

Treatment. The most important first aid measures are to maintain the airway and to **constantly assess the eye reflexes and degree of depression of the nervous system.** Constant monitoring of these patients is an essential part of the veterinary nurse's duties. The reflexes should be checked every 10 minutes, noting the time and observations fully on the kennel chart. Otherwise, there is no specific treatment except to conserve heat and minimise the shock by confining the animal to a quiet, warm, darkened kennel.

Spinal injury

Spinal injuries themselves do not cause unconsciousness but may be the cause of acute, conscious collapse and are therefore included here.

Cause. The causes of acute spinal injury fall into three categories:

- **Disc protrusion**, a problem seen in dogs, which usually affects the cervical region (e.g. poodle, spaniel) or the thoracolumbar region (e.g. dachshund, Pekinese).
- **Spinal dislocation**, seen less commonly as an acute problem but which can cause sudden collapse in toy breeds with malformed atlantoaxial joints because the odontoid peg slips upwards to hit the spinal cord.
- **Spinal fractures**, which can occur in any animal following severe trauma. Rabbits suffer spontaneous spinal fractures if their powerful hind legs kick out in panic whilst the shoulders are firmly held (either by a human or because the animal is wedged in the corner of the hutch/run). Sufficient force may be generated to fracture the lumbar vertebrae.

Signs of spinal injury depend upon the place and degree of injury.

Cervical injury. These patients are usually in intense pain and lie still, reluctant to move, screaming whenever the spine twists. In severe cases, all four legs are paralysed (quadriplegia or tetraplegia) and the patient is incontinent. There may be withdrawal reflexes when the foot is pinched (a local reflex), but proprioception (i.e. conscious realisation of pain) is reduced or absent because the nerve impulses cannot pass easily up to the brain as the pathways are damaged at the site of the trauma (see Table 3.2).

If the injury is less severe, the patient may appear uncoordinated, scuffing its toes as it walks, or it may appear lame in one leg if the injury affects one side of the spinal cord more than the other. It is reluctant to turn its head and may yelp every time it does so.

Thoracolumbar injury. The patient shows pain and may cry out if the back is made to move suddenly. Intense trauma (usually seen as the result of a spinal fracture) may result in a collapsed patient with front legs rigidly extended and hind legs tightly flexed. Other severe injuries show paralysis of the hind legs (paraplegia) and incontinence. The animal may try to move around, walking normally with its front legs whilst the hind legs trail out behind. Withdrawal reflexes in the affected legs are normal but proprioception is reduced or absent for reasons explained above.

Patients able to stand do so with the back arched but will cry out if any force is applied to the midline of the back which pushes the arch downwards. The hind legs are often uncoordinated if the animal tries to walk around. In many cases, the owner will report that the dog cried out in pain when trying to jump up, e.g. into a car, going upstairs, etc.

Treatment. There is no specific first aid treatment for these cases. If spinal injury is suspected, the most important advice to owners over the telephone is:

- Move the animal as little as possible.
- Lift the animal as a unit so that the spine is *never* twisted.

Methods for transporting these animals are described at the beginning of the chapter. Upon arrival at the surgery and following a thorough examination, the patient should be confined to a kennel so that it moves as little as possible.

Radiographic examination will be necessary and the relevant preparations should be made.

Poisons

Poisoning should be considered in the case of unconscious animals if no other cause is apparent.

Asphyxia (suffocation)

Asphyxia or suffocation results from any failure to oxygenate the blood. **Partial asphyxia** occurs when small supplies of oxygen manage to reach the lungs, but the blood is only partially oxygenated and hypoxia results. **Hypoxia** occurs when there is an abnormally low level of oxygen in the tissues.

Causes (see Table 3.15)

(1) **Partial or total airway obstruction**:
   - Pharyngeal foreign bodies (Fig. 3.27).
   - Swallowed tongue (Fig. 3.42).
   - Swelling of the pharyngeal walls.
   - Collapsed trachea as seen in cases of strangulation, choke chain injuries, etc.
(2) **Interference with respiratory movements**:
   - Paralysis of the respiratory muscles by poisons (such as strychnine or scoline) or nerve damage.
   - Crushing injuries preventing normal respiratory movement.
(3) **Interference with oxygenation of the blood**.
   - Fluid in the alveolar spaces prevents the air entering these structures where the blood can be oxygenated. Drowning accidents, bleeding from the lungs, congestive heart failure and irritant smoke inhalation may all cause asphyxiation because of the effects they have on the alveolar spaces.
   - Inhalation of noxious fumes from house fires may result in oxygen starvation because there is little oxygen contained in the gases inhaled (most of the oxygen has been 'used up' by the flames) and the gases may be irritant which provokes inflammation of the respiratory tract and fluid release into the alveolar spaces. Animals that survive house fires but

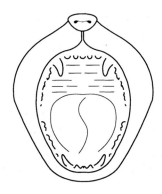

View of open mouth

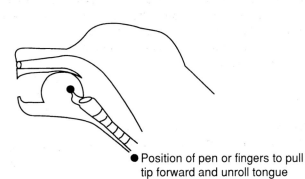

● Position of pen or fingers to pull
tip forward and unroll tongue

Cross-section through dog's head

Fig. 3.42 The 'swallowed' tongue.

have inhaled smoke or fumes may be expected to develop bronchitis 48 hours after the incident. The nurse should anticipate this complication and advise the owner to bring the animal to the surgery for treatment, even if it seems fine at the time of the accident.

● Paracetamol and chlorate poisoning interferes with the oxygenation of red blood cells because these compounds convert oxygen-carrying haemoglobin into methaemoglobin, which cannot combine with oxygen.

● Carbon monoxide poisoning from car exhaust fumes interferes with oxygenation of red blood cells because the haemoglobin combines with the carbon monoxide in preference to oxygen, so that the oxygen content of the blood is severely reduced. Carbon monoxide poisoning in the home is often the result of badly ventilated gas heaters and closed fire-stoves.

(4) **Pleural cavity problems**:

● Pneumothorax, haemothorax and diaphragmatic hernia will all cause lung collapse (see Injuries to the respiratory tract, p. 61).

● Fluid pleurisy (**pyothorax**) is quite common in the cat and may produce lung collapse and asphyxia.

Signs. Signs include air hunger and cyanosis.

Air hunger: the animal will often lie in sternal recumbency with its neck extended and often mouth-breathing. Respiratory movements are strenuous and exaggerated, the animal literally gasping for breath, and the respiratory rate is increased (**tachypnoea**). These patients are always hypoxic and often in great distress, especially if they struggle or try to move around too much. As the blood's oxygen levels fall still further, the animal becomes **hyperaesthetic** (excitable), reacting with abnormal violence to any stimulus and throwing itself around in an uncontrollable manner until unconsciousness intervenes. Death will soon follow.

Cyanosis occurs rapidly in cases of airway obstruction, but more slowly with other causes of asphyxiation. The mucosa changes from pink to mauve and the animal will die unless rapid action is taken. Carbon monoxide poisoning is the exception to the cyanosis rule: the blood remains a brilliant cherry red despite the fact that there is very little oxygen in the bloodstream. This is because the blood corpuscles carrying the carbon monoxide are the same colour as the corpuscles carrying oxygen.

General treatment. **These animals must be handled as gently and quietly as possible and must not be hurried.** They need much reassurance because they are fighting for their lives and will panic and lash out if they become distressed.

The mouth should be opened and the pharynx inspected for signs of obstruction, but only if this can be done without upsetting the patient. If the animal is unconscious, the airway must be cleared and the patient resuscitated as described earlier (see p. 86).

Oxygenation is vital in all these cases and providing pure oxygen for the animal to breathe means that the small volume of gas reaching the alveolar spaces is at least pure life-giving oxygen instead of the mere 20% present in inhaled air. If nothing else can be done for the patient until the veterinary surgeon arrives, the nurse should administer oxygen by face mask or other suitable method (see Resuscitation, p. 86).

Rest is also vital so that the body's demand for oxygen is kept to a minimum.

Specific treatments for obstruction by foreign bodies. Foreign bodies which obstruct the airway will kill animals very quickly and **must be removed or held to one side to allow air to pass** down the trachea.

Beware – removal of a smooth pharyngeal foreign body, such as a ball, looks possible but is usually impossible as the ball is tightly jammed in the pharynx and coated copiously with slippery saliva. **Do not persist with fruitless efforts –** it is more important to maintain the airway.

If the patient is conscious, trying to open its mouth to examine the pharynx could provoke a struggle which will worsen the patient's condition and risk injury to the nurse's hands. **Do not persist** but keep the animal under constant, close observation and provide oxygen until the veterinary surgeon arrives.

If the patient is unconscious, the following procedures may be tried:

● Smooth, round-ended instruments may be used to hold the obstruction to one side. Whelping forceps are ideal, but teaspoons, dessertspoons or fingers can be used in an emergency. **Great care is needed because these patients regain consciousness very rapidly** and objects in the mouth could get badly chewed. This is no more than a temporary measure.

● A small endotracheal tube may be passed down the trachea beside the foreign body to maintain the airway in the asphyxiated unconscious patient. The animal must be very carefully observed for returning consciousness because the tube may need to be removed quickly to avoid complicating the situation with a chewed-off, inhaled endotracheal tube. Should unconsciousness return, the patient must be intubated again with all speed.

● Suspending the animal by its hind legs encourages the foreign body to fall forwards in the pharynx, taking the pressure off the laryngeal opening and allowing air to pass through the nasal passages and into the trachea. If the animal coughs, the object may even dislodge and fall out of the mouth. If this is not successful, the Heimlich manoeuvre as applied to animals can be a life-saving procedure.

The Heimlich manoeuvre. The principle is to administer a sharp punch to the abdominal wall just above the xiphisternum, angled downwards towards the diaphragm (Fig. 3.43) so that the animal coughs and the smooth foreign body is dislodged. In order to get the object to fall out of the mouth, the procedure should be carried out with the patient suspended upside-down by the hind legs. A large dog may have to be suspended from a table edge or a wooden fence if out of doors. First aid workers also refer to this Heimlich manoeuvre as the 'abdominal thrust', which suggests the technique used in removing a foreign body.

The problem is that, once the animal is suspended in this way, it can be difficult to deliver an effective punch in narrow-chested patients because the weight of the body draws the costal arches even closer together at the xiphisternum and the abdominal muscles are stretched tight. If attempts prove useless, try placing the hands on either side of the suspended patient's chest wall (Fig. 3.43b) and delivering a sharp punch-like compression of the thorax. This usually has the desired effect. If a dog is too large to be suspended by its rear legs, its hindquarters should be raised as high as possible and its head allowed to hang down before the blow is administered. The procedure may be repeated up to 4 times, but further attempts should be discontinued for fear of causing internal injury and the theatre should be prepared for an emergency tracheotomy. The ventral throat area should be clipped and scrubbed to save time. The patient should be kept alive using any of the other methods already described until the veterinary surgeon arrives.

Interference with respiratory movements. If the muscles are paralysed, the veterinary nurse should carry out artificial respiration, giving oxygen if possible (see Resuscitation, p. 86).

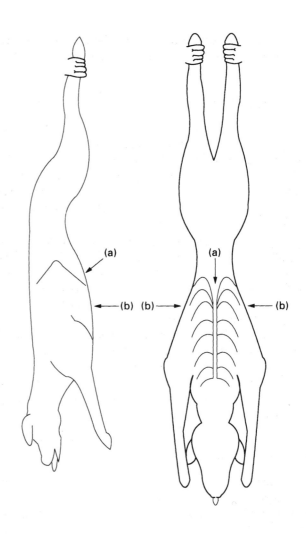

⟶ **Direction and point of impact of blow.**

Fig. 3.43 The Heimlich manoeuvre: (a) standard Heimlich manoeuvre and (b) modified version.

If respiration is painful because of chest wall trauma, the only useful first aid treatment is to give the animal oxygen to breathe through a loose-fitting face mask.

Fluid in the alveolar space. Where this is as the result of a drowning accident, the fluid must be drained out immediately. Any weed, etc., in the mouth should be removed and the animal held up by its hind legs if possible and swung round in a circle or arc so that the centrifugal force encourages the fluid to drain out of the lungs. (This applies the same principle as used to revive puppies, only on a large scale.) If the animal is too big for this method, it must be laid on as steep a slope as possible and artificial respiration applied to encourage oxygenation and drainage of the chest. Once the animal has been resuscitated, it should be dried and kept warm. Direct heat may be applied in these circumstances because these patients are often hypothermic.

Suspending the animal on a slope may also be necessary in other cases where there is much fluid in the alveolar spaces (e.g. congestive heart failure). If the animal arrives at the surgery, cyanosed and blowing frothy mucus from its mouth and nose, the fluid must be drained off as quickly as possible and gravity is a great help.

Treatment for pleural cavity problems. This is described in the section about injuries to the respiratory tract (see p. 64).

Cardiac failure

Causes. Cardiac failure is usually seen in the older animal, often as a result of thickened heart valves which cannot close properly. These leaking valves decrease the efficiency of the heart as a pump and the rate at which the blood circulates around the body is slowed. If the right side of the heart is affected, the lung circulation is poor and the blood will not be oxygenated so efficiently. If the left side of the heart is affected, fluid may build up in the lungs because the left side of the heart cannot pump efficiently enough to move the venous blood from the lungs and around the systemic circulation. Inefficiency of the bicuspid valve may also lead to fainting fits as the heart is unable to pump sufficient oxygenated blood to the brain.

Acute heart failure can also occur in young animals if there is a heart defect which only becomes apparent as the animal matures and becomes more active.

Giant breeds of dog are prone to **cardiomyopathies**, which result in damaged heart muscle. These dogs may suffer acute cardiac failure.

Signs. This condition is more often seen in dogs than in cats. The signs are as follows:

- Reluctance to exercise, which has gradually increased over a period of months in most cases.
- Coughing on exercise or exertion. The coughing fits become more prolonged and severe as the condition advances.
- Cyanosis as fluid builds up in the lungs and interferes with the oxygenation of blood. Patients collapse on exercise, showing signs of air hunger (see Asphyxia, p. 90).
- Sudden collapse in acute heart failure or when the left side of the heart is affected. The animal may have suffered fainting fits in the past but these were so brief (with the patient completely recovering after a few seconds) that the owner was not unduly worried. However, in acute heart failure, the animal does not revive spontaneously and there may be no heartbeat when it is presented at the surgery.

Dogs usually show all the above signs as they are inclined to try to carry on as normal despite coughing bouts and fainting fits. However, cats rarely show signs of cardiac failure until the condition is serious because they will rest sensibly if feeling short of breath. The owner may report that the cat has become lazier over a period of months, but rarely reports that the animal has been coughing. Therefore, the onset of signs may seem very acute and the animal is presented with a chest full of fluid, gasping for breath and going gently blue on the slightest exertion.

Treatment. If there is no heartbeat, cardiac massage should be applied as soon as possible. These cases rarely respond unless they are presented to the surgery within minutes of collapse.

If the heart is still beating, the animal should be treated as for hypoxia (see Resuscitation, p. 86) and must be made to rest.

Shock

Causes

- Acute haemorrhage.
- Severe fluid loss as in prolonged or severe bouts of vomiting and diarrhoea. There will also be dehydration in cases of renal failure, or in cases of water deprivation (e.g. a cat that has been trapped for days without access to water).
- Traumatic shock. The body's response to severe trauma is to shut down the non-essential circulation.

Signs and treatment

Signs and treatment for shock are given in an earlier section, General nursing care (see p. 29).

Anaemia

Causes

- Flea infestation. Young, underweight kittens that have been rescued may be found to be collapsed because poor nourishment and flea burden have caused severe anaemia.
- Feline infectious anaemia. This usually occurs in older cats and the onset is more gradual so that the animal is rarely presented as an emergency.
- Any other cause of blood loss or bone marrow depression.

Signs

- Stupor.
- Extreme pallor of mucous membranes.
- Thin, very rapid pulse.
- Rapid shallow breathing.
- Depressed rectal temperature.

Treatment. Insulate to conserve body heat, but do not warm the body because as much blood as possible must be kept flowing to the brain. Supply oxygen-enriched air to breathe so the little circulating blood available is rapidly oxygenated in the lungs. De-flea, preferably using a non-toxic preparation, e.g. 'Frontline'.

These cases usually carry a very poor prognosis.

Thromboses

Causes. The cause of this condition is a circulating clot (**embolus**) which lodges in the arteries supplying the hind- or forelimbs so that the artery becomes blocked, depriving the limb of its oxygenated blood supply. One or both back legs may be affected because the clot may lodge where the arteries branch from the aorta and cause both to be blocked. In the front leg, the blockage occurs at some distance from the aorta and only one limb is affected.

Signs. This condition is more commonly seen in cats than in dogs. The animal is presented in extreme and acute pain, collapsed and howling. It frequently tries to drag itself around as if trying to escape from its own rear end. The distinctive signs are:

- Absence of pulse in the affected limb. No femoral or brachial pulse can be detected.
- Coldness of the limb. As no warm blood is flowing into the leg, the tissues of the leg cool rapidly and the foot feels ice-cold and clammy.
- Spastic contraction of the muscles. This tends to hold the leg in extension. Because of the lack of oxygen in the muscle tissue, changes occur in the muscle cells which are similar to those occurring in rigor mortis.
- Decreased withdrawal reflexes. The leg has not lost its reflexes but the animal finds it difficult to move because of the spastic contractions. The motivation to withdraw the foot is also not great because the animal is in such intense pain that a nip on the toe is insignificant.

Treatment. These animals are very shocked and in great pain. They need to be handled carefully.

Warm the limb, using a heat lamp, heated pads, etc. Vasodilatation is to be encouraged in these cases as it may enlarge the diameter of the affected artery at the site of the blockage so that the blood can once again flow past the obstruction.

Massage the limb. This may also help to dilate the blood vessel and stimulate the circulation down the leg. In practice this treatment is usually impossible because the patient is very likely to resent handling of its leg because of the pain.

The animal should be encouraged to rest as much as possible because there is often an underlying heart condition. Cyanosis may develop and oxygen should be available.

Hypoglycaemic coma

Cause. Hypoglycaemia occurs in the diagnosed diabetic animal when there is an imbalance between the insulin given and the glucose available. Too much insulin removes the soluble circulating glucose and converts it to insoluble glycogen in the liver. The animal becomes hypoglycaemic (low levels of blood glucose) and the metabolism slows down. The causes of this condition are explained in Chapter 17 (Medical Disorders and their Nursing).

Signs. The time of onset depends upon the type of insulin used but usually the following signs occur about 10 hours post injection:

- Dullness and lethargy.
- Ataxic (uncoordinated) movements.
- The mouth and body feel cold to the touch.
- Collapse – as the situation becomes more grave, the animal may start to twitch uncontrollably and may go into convulsions.
- Coma and death soon follow.

Treatment in the home. **Glucose solution** should be administered immediately the first signs are seen. One or more tablespoons should be given by mouth. If glucose is not available, honey should be used instead. If neither of these is available, sugar water can be given, but this has the disadvantage that the disaccharide of sugar must be digested first to release the glucose molecule and this may not happen quickly enough to arrest the onset of the diabetic coma.

Treatment at the surgery. If the patient is unconscious, the owners should bring the animal to the surgery immediately for an intravenous injection of glucose. The injection should be prepared ready for administration by the veterinary surgeon and a glucose solution may also be prepared for oral administration by stomach tube.

Hypocalcaemia (eclampsia)

Cause. Lack of circulating calcium ions causes malfunctions of nervous and muscular tissue. The problem of eclampsia is usually seen in lactating bitches with large litters soon after birth when the pups are 2–3 or 5 weeks old. It has also been seen in cats nursing kittens. The demand for milk by the rapidly growing offspring is enormous and drains the calcium from the mother's body. To meet this demand, she must either take in calcium from the diet or reabsorb calcium from her bones. The latter is a slow process so that, unless enough calcium is given in the diet to cope with the demand, the mother will soon become deficient in circulating calcium ions and show signs of eclampsia. Rabbits may also develop eclampsia.

Signs

- Restlessness and inability to settle to feed the litter.
- Panting respiration.
- Muscular tremors – the muscular tissue becomes unable to function normally as the calcium levels fall.
- Collapse and hyperaesthesia – the slightest sound now causes convulsive twitching.
- Unconsciousness. As the brain becomes more affected, the twitching lessens and ceases. Death will soon follow.

Treatment. Calcium given by mouth is not effective as it is poorly absorbed. Intravenous calcium must be injected and syringes should be prepared (usually with 10% calcium solution) ready for injecting when the veterinary surgeon can attend the case.

The pups should be removed as further feeding will drain yet more calcium from the system.

Uraemia

Cause. Uraemic fits are usually seen in old dogs with chronic kidney failure and are due to a build-up of toxic substances (especially phosphates) in the bloodstream which would normally be excreted by the kidneys.

Signs. In most cases there is a long-standing history of polydipsia and weight loss, culminating in vomiting, anorexia and lethargy and, in the last stages, epileptiform convulsions. The breath may smell of urine. Occasionally, the onset of the uraemia is rapid (e.g. antifreeze poisoning) but the clinical signs are similar, e.g. vomiting, anorexia, lethargy.

Treatment. Euthanasia is usually necessary and the animal should be made comfortable and treated as an epileptic pending diagnosis by the veterinary surgeon. Fluid therapy (Hartmann's solution) may be required if the animal is to be treated.

Electrocution

Cause. Electrocution occurs when a high voltage passes through the animal's body. If the line of conduction passes through the animal's heart, the result is instantaneous cardiac arrest.

Most cases occur because of electrical faults in everyday equipment and the most extraordinary things can happen. In one case the wire mesh of a kennel's exercise run became 'live' following an electrical fault and all the dogs in that block were electrocuted. In another case, a dog urinated on a lamppost and electrocuted himself because the lamppost was 'live'. (Water in any form is a marvellous conductor of electricity.)

Signs. The animal is found collapsed by the source of the problem, but it may not be obvious exactly what has happened.

If the animal is still alive, the entire body is stiff and twitching. The muscles of the face may be spastically contracted so the animal appears to grin or snarl. The ears are very sharply pricked and the fur over the entire body surface stands on end. Breathing is sharp and short and the animal may scream with every exhalation.

Treatment

> **WARNING**
>
> **SWITCH OFF THE ELECTRICITY SUPPLY**
> before touching the animal – the animal may well be electrically 'live' though clinically dead.
>
> If the mains switch cannot be located quickly, **stand on a dry insulated surface** (e.g. a dry wooden board) and **use a dry wooden pole** (remember that water and metal both conduct electricity) to push the animal well away from any object which may be electrically active.

The animal should be given cardiac massage if no heartbeat can be felt and the airway of an unconscious animal must be maintained, but these cases are usually rapidly dead or rapidly recovered. However, non-fatalities should be checked for signs of electrical burns and may need treatment for meningeal oedema, so they should be brought to the surgery.

Heatstroke

Cause. The cause is usually overexposure to heat, classically seen in short-nosed breeds left in a closed car in the full sun, but it is also seen in hairy dogs that have undergone considerable exercise or have become very excited when the weather is warm and humid. Elderly animals with thick coats may occasionally suffer heatstroke with no history of recent exercise.

Signs. Initially, the animal is distressed, panting excessively and restless. As the situation worsens and the body temperature increases, the animal starts to become cyanosed, drools saliva copiously and becomes unsteady on its feet. If the body temperature continues to climb, the animal will collapse; it becomes comatose and soon dies. The body feels burning hot and the rectal temperature is off the scale.

Treatment. Maintain oxygenation. Swab saliva away from the unconscious patient and intubate. Give oxygen at the first sign of cyanosis in the conscious patient.

Cool the animal immediately using cold water baths, soaking the animal by running water from a hosepipe on it, covering the body with blankets and towels soaked in cold water, applying ice packs, etc. Dogs with dense hairy coats are difficult to cool as the water runs straight off the coat and the coat insulates the body from ice packs, etc. The only solution is total body immersion in a bath/pond or to run a hosepipe over the body, pushing the end into the depths of the fur and moving from one part of the body to another in an attempt to keep the whole skin wet. These measures will have limited use as the sudden cooling will cause vasoconstriction in the skin, so that the blood arriving at the surface of the body to be cooled will be much reduced, but it is a valuable first step which may be done at home.

As the blood is the body's transport system, cooling the blood is the most efficient way to cool the whole body and chilled intravenous drips may be set up as soon as possible. If no chilled drip is available, lay the giving set tube in a bed of crushed ice so that the intravenous fluid is chilled as it runs through the drip tubing.

Confine the patient to a cool, airy kennel, preferably one with a concrete floor to encourage further heat loss by conduction. Lay a wet blanket over the animal to keep the coat wet and decrease its insulative properties.

Check the rectal temperature every 15 minutes to avoid overdoing the cooling of the body. As soon as the temperature has fallen to 102°F (39°C), the animal should be dried off and placed in a cool kennel with access to cold drinking water. The temperature must then be checked every 30 minutes to ensure that it is not allowed to rise again.

Hypothermia

Cause. Hypothermia is a common problem of the very small and the very young and in victims of drowning accidents. Small mammals and birds readily suffer hypothermia; young puppies and kittens, with little or no temperature regulation, are helpless if warmth is not given.

Signs. The animal becomes sleepy and lethargic and does not bother to feed. Its movements become weaker and the patient becomes comatose. Its body feels cold to the touch and the rectal temperature is subnormal (around 98°F (38°C)).

Treatment. Massage with warm, rough towels to stimulate young neonates and to open up the cutaneous circulation so that the body is able to pick up radiant heat more efficiently. Towels also dry the fur of a patient suffering from exposure so that it regains its insulating cover.

Conserve heat by laying the animal on thick bedding (e.g. Vetbed). Light coverings may be laid over the patient, but thick blankets should be avoided as they will prevent the animal from absorbing direct warmth.

Apply heat by:

- Warmed intravenous drips (the most efficient method).
- Heat pads, hot water-bottles and avian hospitalisation cages (these are controlled forms of heating that are unlikely to overheat the patient).
- Heat lamps for the mature animal, which can move away from the heat source when it becomes too hot.
- Space blanket (reflective foil).
- Hair drier (use on low heat setting).

Check the rectal temperature every 15 minutes – or every 10 minutes with the young patient since these animals absorb the heat more quickly than the larger, adult animal. Recovery is usually rapid in the young and signs of returning consciousness and movement can also be used as a guide.

Maintain the temperature by confining the patient to a warm box or kennel. (See Chapter 19, p. 498.)

Further reading

Andrews, A. H. and Humphries, D. J. (1982) *Poisoning in Veterinary Practice*, 2nd edn, National Office of Animal Health.

Campbell, A. and Chapman, M. J. (1999) Handbook of Poisoning in Small Animal Practice, Blackwell Science.

Gfeller, R. W. and Messonier, S. P. (1997) *Handbook of Small Animal Toxicology and Poisonings*, Mosby, St Louis.

Humphries, D. J. (1988) *Veterinary Toxicology,* 3rd edn, Baillière Tindall, London.

Marsden, A. K., Moffat, Sir C. and Scott, R. (1992) *First Aid Manual of the St. John's Ambulance, St. Andrew's Ambulance Association and British Red Cross*, 6th edn, Dorling Kindersley, London.

South West Oiled Seabird Group (1993) *First Aid for Oiled Seabirds*, RSPCA, Horsham.

Taylor, D. T. (1992) *BVA Guide to Dog Care*, 2nd edn, Dorling Kindersley, London.

4

Occupational hazards

R. Butcher

The laws relating to occupational health

The very nature of veterinary practice means that staff, clients and visitors can be exposed to potential hazards and the work situation is such that accidents are possible. The Health and Safety legislation attempts to make the workplace as safe an environment as possible, by ensuring that practices examine their working procedures to reduce to a minimum the risk of exposure to hazardous materials or circumstances in which accidents can occur. Even so, accidents will happen and practices should draw up contingency plans to deal with them. The legislation also makes provision for the recording and reporting of diseases and injuries that occur in the workplace.

It is important that veterinary nurses are familiar with this legislation, not only because they have specific obligations as employees but also because they may become involved in formulating the practice policy or ensuring that other staff adhere to it. The most important Health and Safety legislation relating to veterinary practice include:

- The Health and Safety at Work Act (1974).
- The Control of Substances Hazardous to Health (COSHH) Regulations (1998).
- The Ionising Radiation Regulations (1985).
- The Control of Pollution Act (1974).
- Controlled Waste Regulations (1992).
- Environmental Protection Act (1990).
- Reporting of Diseases and Dangerous Occurrences Regulations (RIDDOR) (1995).
- Manual Handling Operations Regulations (1992).
- Health and Safety (Display Screen Equipment) Regulations (1992).
- The Management of Health and Safety at Work Regulations (1992).

In addition to these major regulations, a number of others have relevance to the practice of Health and Safety and some of these are considered in Chapter 7 (The Law and Ethics of Veterinary Nursing).

The Health and Safety at Work Act (1974)

This Act applies to all businesses, however small, and relates to all persons in the workplace, whether employers, employees or visitors. It sets out the specific duties of both employers and employees, and indicates that the ultimate responsibility rests with the senior partner of the practice.

The general provisions of the Act dictate that every *employer* should ensure that:

(1) Proper provision is made to establish safe systems of work. These should be written down as '**Local Rules**' and be displayed on Health and Safety notice boards at the appropriate work stations.
(2) All equipment is adequately maintained to the manufacturer's specification.
(3) The premises (including vehicles) should be kept in a good state of repair and adequate attention given to providing safe access or exit in times of emergency.
(4) All articles and substances used within the practice should be handled, stored and transported in a safe manner.
(5) Information, instruction and supervision of employees should be carried out regularly.
(6) All appropriate protective clothing is provided free of charge.
(7) A satisfactory working environment is maintained with adequate facilities and arrangements for employees' welfare at work. This should include adequate washing and toilet facilities as well as a separate hygienic area for rest and refreshment.
(8) Appropriate first aid facilities are available. In addition all accidents should be recorded, and the more serious ones reported to the Health and Safety Executive (see below).

In addition, an employer with five or more employees must prepare, and when necessary revise, a written **Health and Safety Policy Statement**. This must outline the general policy of the practice, as well as listing the general duties of all members of the practice. It may be necessary to appoint (in writing) individual members of staff to jobs with special responsibilities (e.g. practice safety officer, fire officer, first aid officer, etc.), providing written job specifications for these posts. It is essential that this statement, and any revision, is brought to the attention of all employees.

The Act also highlights the responsibilities of all *employees*, who must:

- Take reasonable care for the health and safety of themselves and of other persons who may be affected by their acts or omissions.
- Co-operate with the employer so far as it is necessary to enable any duty or requirement under the Act to be performed or complied with.
- Not interfere, recklessly or intentionally, with anything provided in the interests of health, safety and welfare.

These broad guidelines to the Act are highlighted on a poster and leaflet produced by the Health and Safety Executive (HSE) entitled *Health and Safety Law – What You Should Know*. The poster should be displayed on the practice notice board and the leaflets should be provided to all staff.

The Control of Substances Hazardous to Health (COSHH) Regulations (1998)

These Regulations were introduced to cover areas that were not dealt with adequately by the more general Health and Safety at Work Act. They require that all practices should make an assessment of all the potential hazards that are in the work place (**COSHH Assessment** – see below). This will involve the development of written **Standard Operating Procedures (SOPs)**. In reality, there is often much overlap between these and the 'Local Rules' as required by the Health and Safety at Work Act, so that it may be preferable to write a single document, combining:

● Local Rules.
● SOPs.
● COSHH Assessment.
● Health and Safety Policy Statement (if applicable).

Hazards and risks

A **hazard** is defined as something with the potential to cause harm. A **risk**, however, is something that is likely to cause harm. The essence of the COSHH Regulations is to identify all the hazards to which the staff are exposed and then to develop work protocols that reduce the risks from these hazards to a minimum.

The range of potential hazards within a veterinary practice is vast, but can usefully be classified into:

● Pharmaceutical products.
● Laboratory reagents.
● Cleaning materials.
● Miscellaneous (non-laboratory) solvents.
● Explosive/flammable agents.
● Laboratory micro-organisms.
● Zoonotic infectious agents.
● Hypersensitivity to animal tissues.
● Unidentified allergens.
● Sharps.
● Inhalation of fumes.
● Radiation.
● Direct injury inflicted by animals.
● Injury from faulty equipment.
● Manual lifting procedures.
● Display screen equipment.

Warning labels. All hazardous chemicals have clear warnings on the bottle and are classified as:

● Toxic.
● Highly flammable.
● Corrosive.
● Harmful.
● Irritant.

Examples of warning labels are shown in Fig. 4.1.

A more complex numerical code system employed for the purposes of the classification and labelling of hazardous chemicals was introduced as a result of the **Chemicals (Hazard Information and Packaging for Supply) Amendment Regulations (1996) (CHIP 96)**. This classification includes data relating to the potential risks and safety precautions required for these chemicals. Although much is of little relevance to veterinary practice, the veterinary nurse should be aware of its existence.

Maximum Exposure Limit (MEL). The MEL of a hazardous substance is assessed in relation to a specific reference period when calculated by a method approved by the Health and Safety Commission. Exposure should not exceed this level.

Occupational Exposure Standard (OES). Where an OES has been approved for an inhalation agent, control can still be regarded as adequate if the level is exceeded and yet the employer identifies the reasons and takes the appropriate action to remedy the situation as soon as is reasonably practical.

The COSHH Assessment

A detailed discussion of how to perform a COSHH Assessment is beyond the scope of this chapter (see Further Reading). Very broadly, the assessment can be approached in three stages:

(1) Consideration of the individual hazards.
(2) The production of SOPs.
(3) An overall assessment of the safety within each work station, in the light of (1) and (2).

Individual hazards. The veterinary nurse should consider each hazard in relation to:

● **The nature of the hazard**. What symptoms are seen if exposure occurs? Is there a published MEL or OES?
● **Route of exposure**. Remember that there may be more than one for each substance, and that accidents may result in unexpected routes of exposure (e.g. injectable drugs could enter the body by accidental self-injection, but also via the skin or eyes if the bottle is broken).

Fig. 4.1 Hazard warning labels.

- **First aid**. Are there any specific first aid measures if accidental exposure occurs?
- **Preventative measures**. Does this particular substance need to be used or is a safer alternative available? Will strict SOPs, possibly involving the use of protective clothing, greatly reduce the risk?
- **High-risk staff**. Are there any members of staff who may be at a greater risk (e.g. those with known allergies or at risk during pregnancy)? In this regard it is important that staff feel able to notify the practice safety officer or senior partner in confidence if they consider there is any chance of being pregnant, or if they have any disease or condition that might increase the risks when working in a particular environment.
- **Recording of exposure**. Are there any monitoring schemes available to record exposure? This would include dosimetry for X-ray radiation exposure and any monitoring for halothane and nitrous oxide in the operating theatre.

Many of the individual hazardous substances can be grouped together since the hazards are similar. Further subdivisions can then be made within the major groupings (e.g. pharmaceutical drugs can be split into smaller groups such as: injectable antibiotics, topical steroid creams, cytotoxic drugs, organophosphate insecticides, etc.). Much of the technical data can be gleaned from the *COSHH Hazard Data Sheets* that should be available for each product from the manufacturers. (Note that these are not the same as the standard Product Data Sheets.)

Standard Operating Procedures (SOPs). Written SOPs should be produced to cover the range of all work performed at the surgery. They must above all be clear and concise, and be tailored to the work protocols of each individual practice. Copies should be posted at the appropriate work stations, so that the group of SOPs in that area forms the basis of the Local Rules as required by the general Health and Safety legislation. A pictorial component would give more impact to SOPs posted on notice boards. Specimen SOPs are available as part of the BSAVA Members' Information Service.

The actual SOPs required by each practice may vary, but suggested topics (some of which are discussed in greater detail in relevant chapters of this book) include:

- Radiation protection.
- Accidents and first aid.
- Health surveillance.
- Laboratory procedures.
- Postage of laboratory specimens.
- Safe prescribing and handling of medicines.
- Injections.
- Restraint of animals.
- Spillages.
- The dental scaler.
- Waste disposal.
- Disinfectants and floor cleaning.
- Kennel management.
- Anaesthetic gases – scavenging and monitoring.
- Fire precautions.

- Mortuary/post-mortems.
- X-ray processing.
- Sterilisers.
- Manual handling/lifting.
- Display screens.
- The practice vehicle.
- On the farm/stable.

Overall assessment of each practice work area. This builds on the information collated above and is basically a critical look at the safety of each work station within the practice. The format discussed below is that suggested in *COSHH: BVA Guide to the Initial Assessment in Veterinary Practices*.

At each work station (or room or department) the assessment involves methodical listing:

(1) Hazardous substances/pathogens that may be encountered in that area. For each one the practice must assess the degree of risk and allot a hazard code (H = high; M = moderate; L = low; N = negligible). If the substance has a known MEL or OES, this too should be recorded.
(2) All the members of staff present in this area. This should include their sex, official job title and a brief summary of their involvement in this area.
(3) All the practice SOPs that may be of relevance in this area.
(4) The control measures in use in the area. This may simply require reference to specific SOPs.
(5) Safety clothing provided and used.

Having completed this stage of the assessment, it is important to record a comment that represents an overview of the exposure and actual risks in that area. It is possible that various deficiencies are highlighted. These should be listed and a note made when they have been corrected.

An important part of the assessment is to ascertain where further staff training or instruction is required. This too should be planned and a note made when completed.

Finally, the date of the next assessment should be set (at least annually). The COSHH Assessment is therefore an ongoing process promoting continual improvements to the practice's safety standards.

Ionising Radiation Regulations (1985)

These apply specifically to the hazards associated with radiography and are dealt with fully in Chapter 24 (Radiography).

Clinical Waste Regulations

The principal regulations relating to this subject are:

- Control of Pollution Act (1974).
- Controlled Waste Regulations (1992).
- Environmental Protection Act (1990).

Together they regulate the correct segregation, storage, transfer and eventual destruction of waste products produced at the surgery. The waste produced at veterinary practices must be classified by the veterinary nurse (clinical waste, 'sharps', special waste, cadavers and industrial waste) and disposed of correctly see p. 128.

Clinical waste includes all waste that consists wholly or partly of animal tissues, blood or other body fluids, excretions, drugs or pharmaceutical products likely to be hazardous to health. It should be collected and stored in approved colour-coded plastic sacks (yellow with the words 'Clinical waste' clearly printed on the outside).

'Sharps' is a special category of clinical waste that includes used needles, scalpel blades or other sharp instruments. These should be discarded *immediately* after use, into special yellow plastic tubs that can be sealed once full.

Special waste, a further category of clinical waste, includes bottles and vials contaminated with pharmaceutical products. These too are stored in specific plastic bins.

Cadavers are technically clinical waste. Strict interpretation of the law would cause problems for owners who wish to bury their pets in their garden. The Department of Environment Management Paper No. 25 states:

> Pets deceased at a veterinary practice remain the property of the owner and may be disposed of by the owner within the curtilage of their dwelling in their capacity as a private individual without breach of duty of care. Where the pet suffered from an infectious disease or for other reasons may be significantly hazardous, then it should be dealt with by the veterinary surgeon as clinical waste. Low hazard deceased pets should be classed as non-clinical commercial waste where the owner requests disposal by the veterinary surgeon, who will be subject to the duty of care.

This is of importance to the owner who wishes to bury their own pet in their garden.

The remainder of the practice waste is regarded as **industrial waste**. This is non-hazardous and can be removed by the local authority or other registered carrier (an appropriate charge may be levied for the service).

Segregation and storage within the practice

The practice must have a strict policy on the segregation of waste. To be practical this must allow for the immediate disposal of material after use and hence there must be sufficient receptacles to allow for segregation at each work station. This should also apply to practice vehicles. Prior to collection, clinical waste should be stored in a secure place within the practice.

Transport and disposal

Clinical waste is collected by a registered carrier in a 'dedicated' vehicle, licensed specifically for the transport of clinical waste. It is transferred to a licensed plant where final disposal is achieved, preferably by high temperature incineration. Each collection (or batch of collections) should be accompanied by the appropriate certification, copies of which should be kept by the practice.

The regulations place a duty of care on the producers of clinical waste to ensure that, from production to ultimate disposal, the waste is dealt with according to the law. The practice itself is responsible for checking that both the carrier and incineration plant have the appropriate licences (ideally keeping photocopies for its own records).

General maintenance and care

It is important that all buildings are kept in a good state of repair, especially with regard to electrical or gas installations and fittings.

All equipment (X-ray machines, anaesthetic machines, autoclaves, etc.) should be regularly serviced according to the manufacturer's recommendations and service records should be kept.

Fire precautions

Adequate precautions should be taken to avoid or combat fires. This is covered by the Fire Precautions Act 1971 and may involve:

- The provision of adequate fire-fighting equipment. Advice needs to be taken on the correct extinguishers for different work stations, and these should be checked regularly.
- An alarm system, regularly maintained.
- Well signposted emergency exits.
- Emergency lighting.
- Clear local rules stating what to do in case of fire. These should be posted in strategic places, and reinforced by regular fire practices.
- Care in the storage of inflammable and explosive material.
- The provision of fire doors where appropriate.

The practice should appoint a fire officer to oversee these precautions. Very valuable advice can be obtained from the local Fire Prevention Officer.

Protection of the person against physical attack

Unfortunately, veterinary practices are not immune from the attentions of criminals. Nurses or veterinary surgeons 'on call' at night and weekends are especially vulnerable and it might be worth incorporating personal 'panic buttons' into the practice alarm system. The local Crime Prevention Officer may give useful advice on this matter. Staff should always state where they have been called out to and obtain phone numbers.

First aid and reporting accidents

First aid

Despite every precaution, accidents will occur. The practice must keep an approved first aid box, the size and contents of which reflect the number of staff. The practice's first aid officer should ensure that this is regularly checked and re-stocked as necessary. It would be valuable to train one or more members of staff in basic first aid techniques, perhaps by the attendance at courses run by the Red Cross or St Johns Ambulance groups.

It is worth considering (in relation to the COSHH Regulations) that the blood from another member of staff, or a client, is potentially hazardous and so adequate precautions (disposable gloves, etc.) should be taken by those administering first aid.

Recording accidents

It is the duty of the practice to record all accidents and injuries that occur. An accident book approved by HSE (Form B1 510) is available from HMSO. The information that is to be recorded includes:

(1) The full name, address and occupation of the person who had the accident.
(2) The signature (with date) of the person filling in the book. This must also include the address and occupation if the person is different from (1).
(3) When and where the accident happened.
(4) Details about the cause of the accident. Record details of any personal injury.
(5) Indicate whether the injury needs to be reported under RIDDOR.

Reporting accidents

Under the provisions of RIDDOR 1995, the practice is obliged to report certain serious events direct to the HSE. These can be broadly divided into three categories:

● Major or fatal accidents.
● 'Three-day' accidents.
● Dangerous occurrences and near misses.

Major or fatal accidents must be reported as soon as possible by telephone, followed by written confirmation within seven days on Form 2508. Major accidents are defined as:

● A fracture of the skull, spine or pelvis.
● A fracture of a long bone of the limb.
● Amputation of a hand or foot.
● Loss of sight of an eye.
● Any other accident which results in an injured person being admitted into hospital as an in-patient for more than 24 hours, unless only detained for observation.

Fatal accidents include those instances where a fatality occurs within 1 year as a result of an original accident at work.

'Three-day' accidents relate to absences from work for a minimum of 3 days as a result of an accident at work. The DHSS will notify the HSE, who in turn will require a written report from the practice.

There is a list of **dangerous occurrences** that should be reported to the HSE (Form F2508) whether or not an injury occurs. These include:

● Explosion from a gas cylinder or steriliser.
● Uncontrolled release of substance (including gases, vapours and X-rays) liable to be hazardous to health.
● Any escape of substances that might result in problems due to inhalation or lack of oxygen.
● Any cases of acute ill health that could have resulted from exposure to pathogens in infected material.
● Any unintentional ignition or explosion.

See also Chapter 13, p. 342.

Manual handling procedures

More than a quarter of the accidents reported each year to the enforcing authorities are associated with manual handling, i.e. the transporting or supporting of loads by hand or body force. Indeed, statistics published by the HSE indicate that this may be as high as 55% for those working in medical, veterinary and other health services. Sprains and strains arise from the incorrect application and/or prolongation of bodily force. Poor posture and excessive repetition of movement can be important factors in their onset. Many manual handling injuries are cumulative rather than being truly attributable to any single handling incident.

The Manual Handling Operations Regulations (1992) expand on the general provisions of the Health and Safety at Work Act (1974) in this regard. The HSE booklet *Manual Handling – Guidance on Regulations* clearly outlines the requirements and application of these regulations.

The general provisions highlight a hierarchy of measures:

● Avoid hazardous manual handling operations so far as is reasonably practicable.
● Assess any hazardous manual handling operations that cannot be avoided.
● Reduce the risk of injury so far as is reasonably practical.

The assessment

Though the HSE Guidelines give some practical help, the regulations set no specific requirements such as weight limits. The importance of an ergonomic approach to the assessment of each procedure is stressed – giving consideration to the **task**, the **load**, the **working environment**, the **individual's capability** and the relationship between them. The intention is to fit the operation to the individual rather than the other way around.

Factors to be considered in making an assessment are fully explained in the HSE Guidelines and specific references to some problems in veterinary practice are made. When carrying animals, for example, the load lacks rigidity, there is a concern on the part of the handler to avoid damaging the load and sudden movements of the load add an element of unpredictability. All these factors serve to increase the likelihood of injury compared to handling an inanimate load of similar weight and shape.

It should be realised that an individual's physical capability varies with age, the risk of injury being higher in the teens or above the age of 50 years. Pregnancy also has significant implications for the risk of manual handling injuries. Hormonal changes can affect the ligaments, increasing the susceptibility to injury; and postural problems may increase as pregnancy progresses. Particular care should also be taken for women who may handle loads during the 3 months following a return to work after childbirth.

Display screen equipment work

Possible hazards associated with the use of display screens are those leading to musculo-skeletal problems, visual fatigue and stress. The likelihood of experiencing these is related mainly to the frequency, duration, intensity and pace of spells of continuous use on the display screen equipment.

The HSE booklet entitled *Display Screen Equipment Work – Guidance on Regulations* clearly outlines the provisions and requirements of the regulations (e.g. the provision of appropriate eye and eyesight tests for designated '*operators*' and '*users*').

In general it is very unlikely that many staff working in a veterinary practice would be classified as '*operators*' or '*users*' under the provisions of the regulations, since most of the display screen work is intermittent. However, the guidelines do give some useful points to consider in relation to the physical layout of the work station (e.g. lighting, correct posture, layout of screen and keyboard, etc.). Such considerations would be part of the normal Health and Safety assessment irrespective of whether the specific Display Screen Equipment Regulations apply.

Practical health and safety in the practice environment

The following section indicates the veterinary nurse's responsibility for looking at some of the areas that should be of concern when formulating the practice's Health and Safety policy statement and COSHH Assessment. These can only act as hints, as each practice will have its own particular hazards and work practices.

General points

Many items covered by the SOPs will be common to all parts of the practice (e.g. first aid, fire precautions, floor cleaning and disinfectants, etc.) and will not be mentioned below.

In all work areas where hands are likely to become contaminated, it is worth considering the use of elbow taps on sinks and disposable towels.

Waiting room/reception

Probably the major potential hazard in this area is injury from unrestrained animals. Clients should be made aware (ideally by a sign outside the building) that all animals must be suitably restrained. Leads and cat baskets should be available in reception for clients who arrive without them.

Recently washed floors must be dried well or 'wet floor' warning notices displayed.

The consulting room

A special consideration here is the potential hazard of children becoming injured by contact with sharps or pharmaceutical products. Ideally drugs should be stored outside the consulting room. Where this is not practical, they must be kept well out of reach of children.

Clinical waste, including sharps, should be disposed of in the appropriate manner immediately after use.

The dispensary

The correct storage and dispensing of drugs (as recommended by the RCVS), including special provisions for controlled drugs, is an important factor and is discussed fully in Chapter 12 (Medicine, Pharmacology, Therapeutics and Dispensing).

Care must be taken when dispensing drugs that can be absorbed through the skin (e.g. cytotoxic drugs). Some individuals show skin hypersensitivity to antibiotics and so disposable gloves should be considered when handling tablets. The use of automatic tablet counters avoids direct handling altogether. Care must also be taken when dispensing small quantities of powdered material that could be a hazard if inhaled. Face masks should be worn. Similarly, precautions may be needed if dispensing small volumes of liquid from a larger stock solution.

Stores

In most practices space is at a premium and so storage often involves high shelving. Full consideration of the provisions of the Manual Handling Regulations should be made. Avoid putting heavy material on the highest shelf and provide non-slip stools in each store room where they may be required. Where heavy items need to be transported within the practice (e.g. trays of petfood or anaesthetised dogs), a trolley should be available to avoid back injury. It is important to keep corridors free from stored material as this could impede rapid exit in the case of fire.

The practice laboratory

There are many potential hazards in the practice laboratory and strict attention to SOPs is required. This is considered in more detail in Chapter 13 (Diagnostic Aids).

In practices without a laboratory, it is important to adhere to the regulations for the postage of pathological specimens.

The X-ray room

The problems associated with radiation hazards are discussed fully in Chapter 24 (Radiography). It is worth considering here the problems of disposing of spent developer and fixer solutions. The appropriate protective clothing should be worn when dealing with these chemicals and good ventilation is essential to avoid inhalation of fumes. Consideration should also be given to the extraction of silver from spent fixer before this is discharged into the normal waste water supply. See Chapter 24, p. 659.

The preparation area

The problems related to anaesthetic gas scavenging and monitoring are of significance in this area. In addition, the amount of animal hair should be reduced to a minimum, not only to improve general hygiene but also to reduce the risk of hypersensitivity reactions in some individuals.

Dental scalers are often used in this area, and an SOP should be formulated to cover the use of masks and eye protection. It is also recommended that chlorhexidine is added to the coolant water.

In practices using oscillating saws to remove plaster casts, thought should be given to the control of the amount of dust, which could be hazardous if inhaled.

The operating area

There are no specific problems here not already dealt with elsewhere but it is worth considering the transport of animals to and from the theatre using trolleys and providing hydraulic tables to avoid excessive heavy lifting of animals.

The level of waste anaesthetic gases in the recovery area is likely to be high as the animals exhale it on recovery. Good ventilation is therefore essential in this area.

Hospital kennels and catteries

Thought should be given to hygienic kennel protocols that reduce the risk of infection from zoonotic agents. The practice might consider the provision of isolation facilities (see Chapter 5) in cases where there is a known risk of zoonoses.

There should also be clear instructions to staff relating to the handling of animals and their transport within the building to avoid physical injury from bites and scratches, as well as from manual lifting procedures.

Mortuary

Correct protective clothing and disinfection regimes are essential in this area. Special thought should also be given to precautions taken if post-mortems are performed on parrots, since there is the additional risk of the inhalation of the agent causing psittacosis from feather debris.

Staff rest room

Adequate rest room facilities should be provided to allow refreshments to be enjoyed away from the working areas. A sink should be provided specifically for the supply of drinking water and for washing up crockery.

Office

There are guidelines relating to the minimum temperatures and lighting conditions for the workplace. The use of display screen equipment is referred to earlier.

Car park/entrance

The Health and Safety legislation extends to the limit of the practice boundaries. Ensure adequate lighting at night and consider providing bins for the disposal of dog faeces.

Practice vehicles

Within vehicles, ensure that all drugs are stored safely and securely. Also make provision for the immediate disposal of clinical waste and sharps. The habit of bringing trays of used syringes and needles back to the surgery for others to dispose of greatly increases the risk of accidental self-injection (especially important in relation to drugs like prostaglandins).

On the farm

The same principles of Health and Safety apply when working on the farm. Many potential hazards relate to zoonotic infections and the BVA guidelines are very useful in this regard. Farmers also have responsibilities under the Health and Safety at Work Act and the COSHH Regulations, and the veterinary surgeon's advice is very important in helping farmers to formulate their own SOPs with regard to zoonotic infections.

Further reading

BSAVA Members' Information Service (1993) *Guides to Local Health and Safety Rules.*
BVA (revised 1989) *Health and Safety at Work Act – A Guide for Veterinary Practices.*
BVA (1991) *COSHH: BVA Guide to the Initial Assessment in Veterinary Practices.*
HSE (1992) *Display Screen Equipment Work – Guidance on Regulations.*
HSE (1992) *Management of Health and Safety at Work – Approved Code of Practice.*
HSE (1992) *Manual Handling – Guidance on Regulations*
HSE (1992) *Personal Protective Equipment at Work – Guidance on Regulations.*
HSE (1992) *Work Equipment – Guidance on Regulations.*
NOAH (1990) *The Safe Storage and Handling of Animal Medicines.*
RCVS Guidelines (1988) *Dispatch of Pathological Specimens by Post* (reprinted by BSAVA Members' Information Service).

5

Management of kennels and catteries

C. A. van der Heiden

It is essential that those persons who are responsible for animals should have a good basic knowledge of the needs, care and welfare of the normal healthy domestic animal, whether it is in a one-pet household or in a large kennel or cattery. This knowledge can then be built upon so that the many and varied requirements of patients that are entrusted to the care of the veterinary nurse can be taken into account.

Although this chapter is relevant to accommodation for pets and is therefore likely to assist the nurse in advising pet owners, it deals mainly with the care of groups of dogs and cats in kennels or catteries. Veterinary nurses are often responsible for running the hospital kennels, and it is important to understand fully the construction and efficient management of such establishments and their effects on the health and well-being of the animals.

Basic requirements for a kennel or cattery

The design and construction of a kennel or cattery will depend upon its main use. Kennels and catteries range from those owned by private individuals (for housing their pets, breeding and show animals or working dogs) to large boarding, quarantine or dog training establishments, as well as the specialist hospital accommodation provided within veterinary practices. The requirements for the housing of all dogs and cats are basically the same, with some variations for different use of accommodation.

Construction requirements

Essential requirements

Above all, kennels should be designed and managed to meet the needs of the animal to be housed in comfort. This first and most important consideration for the housing of any animal should not be prejudiced by other requirements such as ease of management, as this could result in housing to suit the human operators rather than the animals.

> **BASIC NEEDS**
>
> The animals' basic needs are:
>
> - Warmth, comfort and security.
> - Companionship, mental stimulation and opportunities for expression of normal behaviour.
> - Exercise as appropriate to the animal.
> - Protection from disease and injury.
> - Protection from fear and distress.
> - Provision for appropriate feeding.
> - Opportunities for defecation and urination away from the sleeping area.

Warmth, comfort and security

For the normal healthy dog, a relatively cool environmental temperature is quite acceptable (though it should not drop below 7°C (44°F)) as long as the accommodation is dry and draught free and with suitable and sufficient bedding material. The working party report 'Model Licence Conditions and Guidance for Dog Boarding Establishments' recommends that there must be some part of the dog's sleeping area where the dog is able to enjoy a temperature of at least 10°C (50°F). A higher temperature is required by very young, elderly or ill animals and by some specialist breeds. Under normal circumstances a maximum temperature of 26°C (80°F) should not be exceeded as this becomes uncomfortable for dogs (see Table 5.8).

Dogs are generally more relaxed when they feel comfortable and secure. The design of the sleeping area will aid this: they tend to seek out darker areas where they can lie behind or underneath something, or in a corner. All dogs should be given the opportunity to sleep in a conventional sleeping area, which they will usually prefer once settled into kennel life, but they often initially have the desire to create their own sleeping area by moving the bedding material. Some individuals pull the bedding out to the centre of the kennel or into the run if they can. This is a form of nesting behaviour and the dog will often be much more relaxed if it has been able to achieve this, though at times there seems to be quite a frantic period of activity before the dog finally settles.

Cats require a comfortable ambient air temperature of at least 10°C (50°F) in the sleeping area (recommended maximum temperatures as for dogs). The sleeping area should be sited and designed to encourage cats to feel secure and comfortable. A bed should be provided with adequate protective sides. Many shy cats take to the 'igloo' style of bed, which has its own roof. Even a simple upturned cardboard box can give a greater feeling of security in an unfamiliar environment.

Companionship, mental stimulation and opportunities for expression of normal behaviour

Dogs are pack animals by nature and prefer companionship. Domesticated dogs need the attention and physical presence of humans as well as other dogs. Association with the latter can (or, in quarantine, must) be achieved without actual physical contact (see Quarantine and Isolation, p. 139).

Kennelled dogs and cats need stimulation – by sight, sound, smell and touch, as found in their normal environment – to avoid boredom and, ultimately, the stereotyped behaviour patterns that boredom would produce. This can be a particular problem in long-stay establishments and in institutional or 'rescue' kennels. Opportunities to look out at distant views may be preferable to face-to-face kennels that encourage dogs to bark at each other.

Exercise

To understand the dog's natural exercise behaviour, it is necessary to look at the domestic animal's wild cousins. These dogs would exercise at a trot over many miles per day, with short bursts at full speed when hunting or at play, interspersed with rest periods (particularly after feeding). This behaviour is modified in the domestic dog, though it is still seen in some working dogs.

Age and health affect exercise requirements, e.g. young adult dogs require more than the middle-aged, elderly or very young. The breed of dog also has an enormous influence on the amount of exercise required. All dogs require daily exercise, though the requirement of gun dogs, herding dogs and sight hounds, for example, is much higher than for toy breeds. Dogs are more contented and relaxed when exercised on a regular daily basis, and so kennel design and practices must take the need for exercise into account.

Cats in a domestic environment exercise themselves by playing hunting games where stalking, pouncing and killing are practised on small inanimate objects. Cats at liberty act in contrast to dogs: they usually walk and then stalk, with jumping and running over short distances only. They jump much higher than dogs and they have the ability to climb. Cats that have outdoor access sometimes range a considerable distance when hunting. They are territorial and identify their territory by scent marking, guarding the area against intruding cats. Intruders have the choice of standing and fighting or running away when challenged.

The normal exercise requirements for cats differ from those of dogs and this should be borne in mind when keeping cats indoors or in a cattery. The cat should be provided with suitable 'toys' to stalk and chase, some of which can be suspended to simulate airborne prey. Opportunity should be provided for cats to climb and jump by providing ledges or similar at different heights. In a cattery, window-sills or similar vantage points are provided within the run.

Protection from disease and injury

This is one of the major contributions made by humans to the well-being of the domestic dog and cat. Many factors contribute to this and in a kennel or cattery environment they are as follows:

- Safe housing: no sharp edges; escape-proof accommodation and secure run fencing; no areas to get caught or fall into; use of non-toxic and non-combustible materials; prevention of access to dangerous areas or materials.
- Hygiene and cleanliness of the living areas, and surrounding environment: specialist kennels for sick dogs (e.g. hospital for non-infectious, isolation for infectious cases).
- Health care: vaccination and antiparasitic control programmes; grooming and checking for abnormalities; prompt recognition of any signs of ill health, presentation to the veterinarian and subsequent application of prescribed treatments.

Protection from fear and distress

It is important to take into account that if kennelled animals have been parted from their owners and are accustomed to living in a domestic situation, when put into kennels or a cattery for the first time they may be distressed until they become accustomed to the new routine. They should be handled with consideration and care, taking into account their temperature and mental state (recognised by body posture and behaviour). Time should be taken to reassure distressed animals, particularly recent admissions.

Provision of appropriate feeding

Dogs and cats must receive adequate nutrition appropriate to their specific requirements and must have access to clean, fresh drinking-water at all times (unless contraindicated by a specific condition). Automatic drinking-water systems can be incorporated into the design of the kennel. Nutrition requirements are dealt with in Chapter 8.

Opportunities for defaecation and urination

Dogs are instinctively reluctant to foul their sleeping area. During early training this instinct is extended to human living areas via house-training. It is therefore necessary to provide frequent opportunities for urination or defaecation in designated areas to avoid the breakdown of this training.

Dogs prefer to relieve themselves on a similar surface to the area they used as puppies, which is often grass. This behaviour will probably have to be modified during a stay in the kennels, as grass is not practical for kennel 'relief areas' due to reasons of hygiene. However the preference should be borne in mind if a particular dog is very reluctant to relieve itself in the designated concrete area.

Exercise is the time used by many owners to give their dogs the opportunities for urination and defecation, but elimination behaviour should be separated from free exercise where possible. Many local authorities have laws on the fouling of public areas by dogs and so owners are encouraged to 'relieve' their dogs on command in their own gardens before exercising. Alternatively they should clean up after their dogs; this is easier if the command is given just before exercise so that the faeces are easily found and removed.

When dogs are in kennels, therefore, it is important that opportunities for urination and defecation are regular and are separate from exercise periods, so that training habits are not disrupted.

Cats are also instinctively reluctant to foul their sleeping area and they usually have the desire to bury their excreta. This assists greatly in normal domestic house-training as loose, readily dug materials considered suitable by the cat can be provided by the owner in a 'litter' tray. Sometimes cats will deposit faeces that remain uncovered for marking their territory.

Cats which do not have free access to areas that they would naturally find suitable (e.g. loose soil) should be provided with sanitary trays containing material that they find acceptable. The trays should be regularly cleaned and replenished.

Design factors for kennels and catteries

They should be built for the purpose for which the animals are housed (Table 5.1).

They should meet all local authority licensing, building, planning requirements and regulations.

Table 5.1 Examples of kennels and uses

Private owner unlicensed
  pet dogs
  gun dogs/herding dogs
  small-scale breeding (one or two bitches)
  show dogs
Private owner licensed breeding (two breeding bitches or more)[a]
Boarding kennels/cattery[a]
Training kennels
  Police, customs, security, defence
  Guide dogs for the blind, hearing dogs for the deaf, dogs for the disabled, etc.
Charity rescue kennels
  e.g. Wood Green Animal Shelters, RSPCA, NCDL, etc.
Quarantine kennels
Veterinary practices with hospital kennels

[a] Need to be licensed. Requirements are available from the licensing body as regards building materials and accommodation sizes.

They should be designed with the factors set out in Table 5.2 in mind, as well as those essential requirements already discussed.

The sizes and construction materials depend upon the proposed use of the kennels. Many kennel owners refer to recommended boarding kennel sizes and construction details when building private kennelling, and this is increasingly made easier by the availability of ready-made sectional kennelling (Table 5.3). Medium-sized to large establishments tend to build traditional permanent buildings, built to a specific design using suitable permanent materials such as brick or breeze-block structures.

The walls have impervious coverings and are built on to foundations. Internal concrete flooring is laid with a minimum fall of 1 in 80 running towards built-in drains, or guttering and drains. The floor is then either painted, tiled, or covered with asphalt, vinyl or similar internal flooring material in such a way as to prevent ponding of liquids. Particularly useful are materials that can be moulded up at the edges and secured to create a watertight seal with the walls. Any material for kennel or cattery flooring must be impervious and capable of being regularly hosed and disinfected, in addition to being non-slip (even when wet) for the safety of both animals and kennel personnel.

Sound-proofing

All kennels have a potential noise problem caused by the barking of the dogs and every effort should be made to prevent barking becoming a problem. The effective handling and control of the dogs is of great importance. All staff should be aware of dog behaviour, including why dogs bark and how to reduce the noise. Where a dog is barking from excitement, it should be handled calmly and firmly – and without shouting, as this can in itself contribute to further excitement and noise.

Staff cannot be in the kennel 24 hours a day and spontaneous barking will usually occur if the dogs are disturbed by external noises. Efficient sound-proofing will reduce the likelihood of such disturbance as well as assist in reducing the noise of barking reaching outside the kennels. Sound-proofing is achieved by either absorbing the sound, deadening it with suitable materials rather than reflecting it from hard surfaces, or preventing the free passage and escape of the sound from the buildings and perimeters (Table 5.4).

Purpose-built kennel blocks

Individual kennels designed and arranged together in a group under one roof are generally referred to as a kennel block. There are many different designs for differing requirements, each with certain advantages and disadvantages. The main features of the more common designs (run-access, corridor kennels, circular 'parasol' and 'H'-block kennels) are given in Table 5.5 and illustrated in Fig. 5.1.

Table 5.2 Factors in kennel and cattery design

Accessibility	Cleaning and disinfection. Safe handling of the animal (for animal and staff). Maintenance work. Rapid access in emergency situation.
Efficiency	Animal housing close to service area (food preparation areas, store rooms, etc.). Service fittings appropriately positioned, e.g. handles, switches and service controls within easy reach; work surfaces at the correct height and situation; storage space suitable for equipment and stocks. Construction materials should be easy to clean and dry, with drains to remove water when cleaning (via a fall in the floor towards the drain); non-permeable surface materials should be used.
Adequate care facilities	Grooming and bathing areas for dogs. Food storage and preparation areas. (If both dogs and cats are kept, separate areas should be allocated for the foods.) Treatment room (surgery). Hospital and isolation facilities. Whelping or puppy facilities (where appropriate to the purpose of the kennels).
Health, safety and fire prevention	The accommodation should be designed to meet all the health and safety and fire regulations. Adequate fire precautions should be in operation with all staff aware of procedures. Safe construction materials should be used. Kennels and catteries should be designed to avoid hazards, e.g. no deep drains or unsafe steps, no high shelves that may be difficult for the staff to reach. Safe working practices should be observed. Electric power-points should be covered with approved coverings when water is used nearby.
Designed for the purpose	Designed to be appropriate for the purpose that the animals are housed for, e.g. quarantine kennels where high security from escape and contact between animals is of vital importance.
Licensing and planning regulations	Designed to meet all licensing, building and planning requirements and regulations.
Cost and maintenance	Construction materials and installations should be of a reasonable cost but able to withstand constant use. Balance between expensive and durable fittings and economy in construction. Materials used and basic design should contribute to maintenance required, being as low as possible; metal fitments may become corroded by urine and chemicals used for disinfection; wooden window frames should be avoided, due to the need for frequent painting.

Kennel construction and siting	It is usual to site a kennel/cattery in a reasonably isolated position but close to a large area of population, particularly if the purpose is boarding animals.
	Factors taken into account when choosing a site for commercial kennelling include:
	    Site suitable for building, e.g. not sloping excessively, not liable to subsidence, etc.
	    Sufficient space for the proposed kennels and ancillary buildings. (The space required depends upon the number of dogs to be housed and the type of kennel design to be built.)
	    Good road access for clients. Access for goods delivery, etc.
	    Adequate space for parking of clients/delivery vehicles, etc.
	    Whether a licence and planning permission is likely to be granted.
	    Noise control. If not totally isolated or there is any possibility of future planning permission being granted for building within the area surrounding the kennel site (this cannot be totally ruled out), then sufficient space must be available to erect noise control structures (earth banks) around the kennels.
	
	Availability of local services:
	Sewage water (mains or septic tank) where suitable for proposed use. Availability of electricity, gas, etc.
	Refuse collection or the possibilities of running an incinerator for kennel waste.
	
	Cattery siting
	As for dog kennels but noise control is not a major consideration.
	The Feline Advisory Bureau recommends that dogs are not housed in close proximity. It also recommends that $\frac{1}{3}$ to $\frac{1}{2}$ of an acre is sufficient for building accommodation for 45–50 cats and that cat cabins are built with the runs to face south or south-west. This is recommended for the following reasons:
	
	    It reduces the possibility of overheating the sleeping compartments in the summer.
	    It assists the drying out of runs after cleaning.
	    Cats can sit in the sun.
	
	It is also recommended that the runs are built giving the cats maximum visibility of the surrounding area, to provide mental stimulation.
	Dog kennels can also be built facing south or south-west for similar reasons, if they are designed with the runs all facing the same way. Other factors, such as allowing maximum visibility, may lead to excessive barking, therefore a balance must be made to ensure sufficient mental stimulation to combat boredom but a low noise level.

Table 5.3 Sectional prefabricated kennels

Concrete kennel bases with drainage	Where any type of demountable kennelling such as sectional kennels (or catteries) are erected, first lay a concrete base and drainage system. This base usually forms the kennel floor (if a floor is not incorporated in the kennel design) and the kennel run. The base is laid on hard-core with a damp-proof membrane. The concrete is laid a minimum of 4 inches thick with a fall towards drains and/or drainage guttering. Precast concrete gutter units can be set into the concrete to assist water drainage towards the kennel and run drains. Drains are either connected to the mains effluent disposal system or other systems approved by the Water Authority.
Wooden kennelling	Generally wooden kennels are not recommended (unless covered by an impervious material) due to (a) the risk of escape by chewing out and (b) being impossible to disinfect properly. However, many private owners do use wooden kennels, as cross-infection is not such a common problem when only the owner's own dogs are being accommodated. These kennels are relatively inexpensive and are easily erected and dismantled. Many designs are available.
Fibreglass and other modern materials	Twin insulated fibreglass and other easily cleaned modern materials are likely to phase out the use of wood; they are as convenient and have many advantages, such as the ease of cleaning and disinfection. Many new types of kennelling are appearing on the market aimed at all types of user, from the pet owner to the commercial kennel/cattery.

Table 5.4 Sound-proofing

Absorbing the sound	Use of acoustic tiles or materials with similar properties on upper walls and roof (hard surfaces are preferable for hygienic reasons lower down). Tiles must be out of dogs' reach (easily damaged if chewed or scratched). Some acoustic tiles cannot be cleaned/disinfected easily – carefully use spray disinfectants for those that should not be wetted. Washable tiles are now available but can still be damaged with rough use.
Preventing the free passage and escape of sound	Construct the building to prevent free passage of sound down corridors: use double doors offset to one another. Double glazing throughout the kennels. Perimeter structures such as earth mounds or 'buns' surrounding the kennels – require additional space and are expensive but can be very effective. To be fully effective: ● They must be at least as high as the kennel roof. ● There must be no near neighbours with buildings higher than the mounds. Other effective structures that take up less space: ● 'Green' or 'willow' walls of woven willow fencing and earth. Shrubs that are planted in these 'walls' to stabilise and create attractive appearance. ● Tree belts. Require large area for maximum effect with bushy non-deciduous trees/shrubs. Not effective until trees are well grown and even then not as effective as solid structures such as earth mounds.

Table 5.5 Main kennel types – advantages and disadvantages

Run-access kennels	These are the type most commonly used by private owners and breeders as they are very convenient, relatively inexpensive and widely available as sectional units. Some of the more modern designs are used by small boarding establishments or as additional overflow/emergency kennelling. Any number of individual kennels can be erected side by side or back to back. The main drawback: this type is essentially basic outdoor kennelling – services are not usually installed such as active ventilation, central heating or internal kennel lighting. Therefore it is difficult to control the living environment of the dogs. Other drawbacks are: They are more time consuming for staff to run. They are not particularly suitable for dealing with aggressive dogs as staff cannot reduce contact with the dog by having access to the kennel without entering through the run and confronting the dog. The dogs when confined to the kennel cannot usually see out and cannot easily be seen by staff. With this type of kennel it is usual to allow the dog free access from kennel to run during the day. This can lead to noise problems of persistent barking occurring. Heating the kennels is also inefficient.
Corridor kennels	This design has been commonly used where a number of individual kennels are required to be incorporated into one compact block and as such is suitable for medium to large establishments. Large establishments may have a number of these blocks. These can be sectional buildings or traditionally built. Entry to the kennels is via a central corridor with individual kennels along the corridor at each side. The runs are connected to the individual kennels by either an external door which can be opened by staff walking through the kennel to let the dogs into the run or a hatch operated via a pulley system that can be operated without entry into the kennel. The dogs can be allowed either free access to the runs or limited access depending upon the weather, policy of the kennel or the control requirements for individual dogs.

Table 5.5 Continued

	This kennelling usually has food preparation and grooming areas situated at the end of the corridor of kennels. This enables staff to work near the dogs and supervise them, which will help to reduce the noise and other problems. Any animals requiring close supervision should be kennelled near to the staff working area to assist staff having prompt access to deal with them. As the individual kennels face one another, all dogs can see another animal. This can help dogs to settle as it fills the need for companionship even if they have no physical contact. Where this design is used for large establishments many blocks require to be built. It is more time-consuming for staff to run more than one block of kennels where they are separated this way. The dogs will also be supervised less if one staff member runs more than one block. However, where large numbers of dogs are housed, the risk of spread of disease is higher. The construction of several separate blocks of kennels is therefore an advantage for disease control, provided the dogs have no external contact with others, and the kennel blocks are spaced to prevent contact via kennel runs. It is then possible to prevent infectious conditions such as kennel cough running through entire kennels. Drawbacks to this design, besides staff time, etc., are that firstly the bed has to be along the side wall or in a corner. Therefore the type of bed that can be used is limited as the kennel shape is usually long but narrow. Secondly, if transparent external doors are used from the kennel to run, although it is light in the kennel and the dogs can see interesting things outside during the day time, during the night this is a disadvantage and can lead to restlessness, leading to noise problems when the kennels are unattended overnight.
Circular 'parasol' kennels	This more recent design is used for medium to large establishments. It has been notably successful when used for animals requiring a great deal of supervision and observation such as those housed in quarantine and animal rescue kennels. Although it has some advantages, it has been more expensive to build as it is circular. The individual kennels are built in a circle with a large circular central area instead of a corridor. The runs are attached to each kennel via an external door or hatch which can be operated in a similar method to the corridor kennel-run doors, i.e. staff opened or a pulley system. The main advantage of this design is an improved ability to supervise the dogs. A staff member in the central kennel area can see all the dogs in the block from one position. Equally important the dogs can see both the staff member and more of the other resident dogs than with any other kennel design. This is particularly important for long-stay animals as it assists in fulfilling the need for companionship and mental stimulation: 'confinement without the solitude'. This also applies to the dog runs, as the dogs have a wide area of vision due to the area radiating outwards, ending with a relatively wide terminal fence. As with the corridor kennels, a grooming area and food preparation area are usually incorporated in the design at the entrance to the block or in the central area that may otherwise be wasted space. For large establishments, rather than increase the size of the circular kennel it is usual to have either several individual units (as with the corridor kennels with similar advantages regarding disease control) or two or three units joined. In the latter case, the normally separate auxiliary buildings can be incorporated resulting in the entire kennel buildings being under one roof and therefore more convenient and less time-consuming for staff. Some of the drawbacks to this design (apart from the cost of building by traditional methods) are: ● The kennels use a larger amount of ground space per animal housed than in some more compact designs. ● The size of each block is limited, as the larger the block becomes the larger the central space becomes, which unless utilised may be wasted floor space. ● The kennels may be difficult to fit with some types of beds due to the shape of the individual kennels. ● The size of the runs may be limited depending upon the number of kennels in the block and ground space available.
'H'-block kennels	The true 'H'-block kennel has four main kennel blocks arranged together in the form of an 'H' with the service areas forming the cross bar of the 'H'. There is a corridor between the individual kennels and the runs therefore, allowing no free access option for running the dogs. This arrangement is used for training establishments such as those of the Guide Dogs for the Blind Association where a large number of dogs are to be housed with the best possible use of ground space. All the normal auxiliary buildings and a hospital and other special need kennels (except the isolation block) are under one roof, and the space between the four wings of the 'H' is fully utilised. The major advantage to this design is that it is compact and therefore easy to manage. Staff time can be used very efficiently as all the major auxiliary service areas are close to hand, without having to leave the dogs unsupervised for long periods (thus aiding noise control). All four kennel blocks are quickly accessible from the central area. Staff do not get cold and wet during the winter when moving from block to block, or to and from the main service areas. Another advantage is that centralised systems can be installed to control heating, air conditioning, etc., in all areas under the one roof. The drawback of this type of kennelling is that it is too large and therefore expensive for all but those establishments requiring to house a relatively large dog population of say 80 or more dogs. Additionally, with a large number of dogs under one roof, a strict disease control regime is essential, with an efficient active ventilation system being particularly important in the control of airborne diseases. The presence of a corridor between the individual kennels and runs requires staff to take each dog out of its kennel individually to the run. This is therefore not a suitable design where aggressive dogs are likely to be housed. The other disadvantage to the one-side layout and corridor is that the dogs have restricted vision while in the kennel – they cannot see outside (but this is an advantage regarding noise control). They cannot see other dogs either and unless more than one dog is housed in one kennel the dog may lack companionship and mental stimulation.

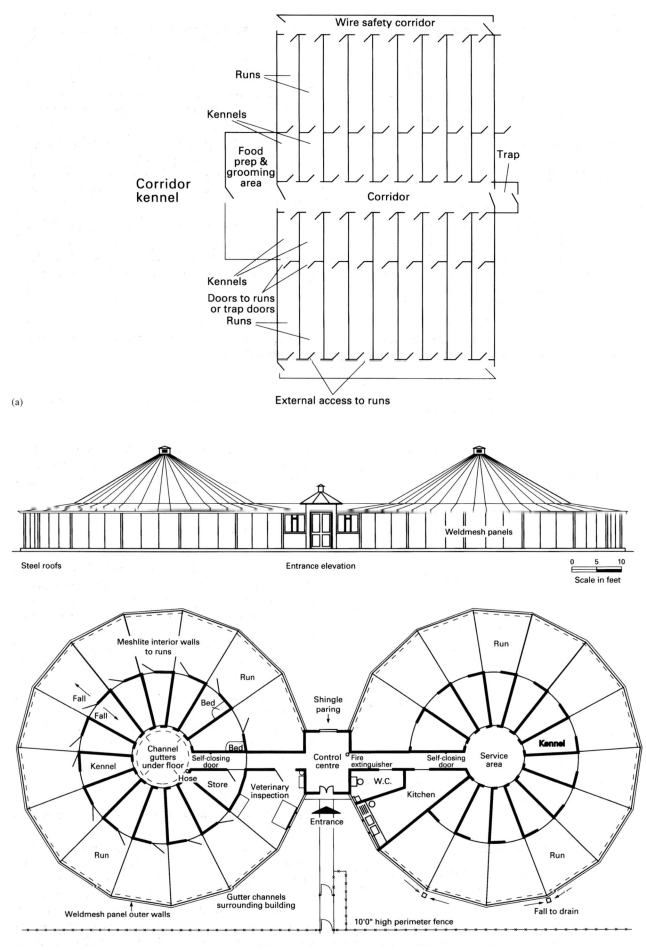

(a)

Corridor kennel

Wire safety corridor

Runs

Kennels

Food prep & grooming area

Trap

Corridor

Kennels

Doors to runs or trap doors

Runs

External access to runs

Steel roofs

Entrance elevation

Weldmesh panels

0   5   10
Scale in feet

Meshlite interior walls to runs

Fall

Fall

Run

Bed

Bed

Run

Channel gutters under floor

Self-closing door

Shingle paring

Control centre

Fire extinguisher

Self-closing door

Service area

Kennel

Kennel

Hose

Store

Veterinary inspection

W.C.

Kitchen

Run

Entrance

Run

Weldmesh panel outer walls

Gutter channels surrounding building

10'0" high perimeter fence

Fall to drain

(b)   **Circular 'parasol' kennel**

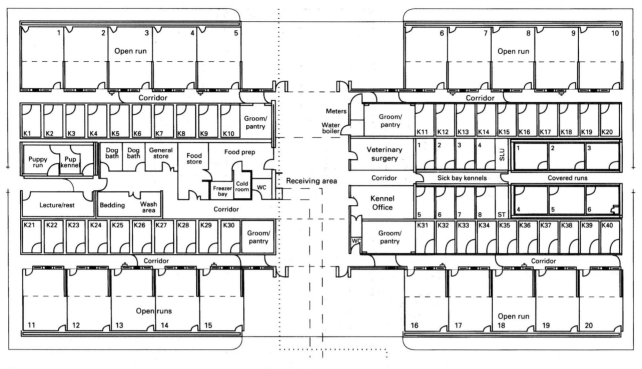

(c)   **H-block kennel**

Fig. 5.1 Main kennel types. (The design of the 'H'-block kennel is credited to the Guide Dogs for the Blind Association and architects Abbey Hanson Rowe Partnership. The circular kennel plan is courtesy of the Animal Inn, Deal, Kent.)

Contents of kennel accommodation

Whatever the design, each individual kennel should contain:

- A plinth for the bedding or a removable bed.
- Some form of heating, e.g. an infrared dull emitter (if not centrally heated).
- A bulkhead electric light or similar (unless corridor lighting is sufficient to light the kennel).
- A water bowl or automatic drinking-water system.
- Some form of ventilation, e.g. controllable vents, if there is no centralised active ventilation system.

The kennel block should contain:

- Electricity points, protected or removed from possible contact with water.
- Water points or taps conveniently situated for hose connection.
- A sink and water-heating system.
- Work tops, shelves, cupboard, etc.
- Dustbins and other waste disposal receptacles.
- Various items such as brushes, buckets, shovels and other cleaning equipment; grooming equipment; feed and water bowls, etc.

Cattery design and construction

The essential requirements in cattery design are similar to those for the housing of dogs but two further factors must be taken into account:

- The cat's agility in climbing to escape.
- The greater risk of infectious respiratory disease among cats, which means that segregation is more important.

The two common types of cattery (the 'outdoor' and the 'indoor') can both be built using traditional methods but modern sectional catteries are increasingly becoming available.

Outdoor catteries

These are similar to the run-access kennels for dogs, with entrance to the cat accommodation through the outdoor run. Major differences are that the run is totally roofed (part of which must be translucent) and that the run access is via a safety passage covered with mesh to prevent any likelihood of escape.

The cat accommodation units are side by side, with full height 'sneeze barriers' and/or gaps of 0.6–1.2 m (2–4 ft) minimum between the runs (Fig. 5.2).

Correctly positioned and managed, outdoor catteries provide the least risk for cross-infection between cats. This advantage can be lost if two of the blocks are positioned with their runs facing into the same safety passage from opposite sides.

Indoor catteries

Indoor catteries are similar in layout to corridor kennels for dogs (Fig. 5.1), with access to each cat housing unit via a central passage. The major disadvantage is the risk of cross-infection due to air exchange between the units via the central passage. The exterior doors from the units on both sides of the block open into totally enclosed runs. Each unit is completely enclosed, to prevent escape, with roofing of runs as for outdoor catteries. Within the cattery building, the doors and internal partitions should be solidly constructed to prevent air circulation between the units. Due to the

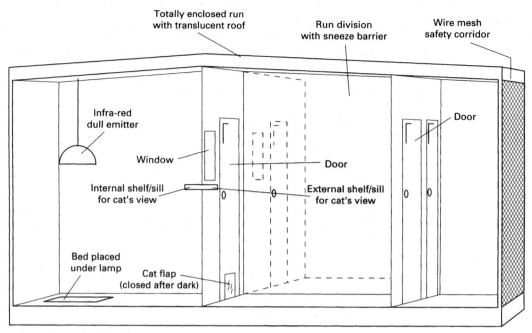

Fig. 5.2 Outdoor cattery design.

increased risk of cross-infection good ventilation is of major importance in an indoor cattery. (Ventilation is discussed later in this chapter.) The solid doors between the units and central corridor must have viewing panels incorporated in all new catteries to allow the inspection of the whole area.

Cattery windows

It is recommended in the 'Model Licence Conditions and Guidance for Cat Boarding Establishments' that each sleeping compartment should have its own window, with a shelf beneath it to allow natural daylight into the unit and to permit the cat to look out. Due to the agility of cats, windows may pose a security risk and therefore must be escape proof at all times. It is therefore recommended that windows are either protected by welded mesh, or be made of reinforced glass, polycarbonate or other impact-resistant material.

CATTERY UNIT SIZES

Recommended in 'Model Licence Conditions and Guidance for Cat Boarding Establishments'.

Sleeping areas can be at ground level or raised (penthouses).

No. of cats	Sleeping area size (min) sq m (sq ft)	Exercise area size (min) sq m (sq ft)
1 cat	0.85 (9)	1.70 (18)
2 cats	1.50 (16)	2.23 (24)
4 cats (max)	1.85 (20)	2.79 (30)

Height of sleeping area at least 91 cm (3 ft).

Raised sleeping areas must be a minimum of 91 cm (3 ft) above floor level with a maximum depth of 106 cm (3 ft 6 inches).

Minimum internal height of unit 1.8 m (6 ft).

Contents of cat accommodation

Each cat accommodation unit should contain:

- A cat bed, possibly on a shelf or plinth.
- Heating, such as an infrared dull emitter or a heated bed.
- Lighting and ventilation systems.
- Dustpan and brush (for exclusive use in a single unit).
- Two each of water bowls, feed bowls and litter trays (for exclusive use of one cat).
- Scratching post.
- Toys (possibly suspended) to encourage play.
- A shelf or window-sill in the run to allow the cat a view.

The cattery block should contain:

- Electricity points (for heating and lighting) situated away from any water sources.
- Water points, external stand pipes/taps (one over a sink), with a drain for litter trays and one tap for a hose connection.

Auxiliary buildings and facilities

Kennels and catteries require some auxiliary facilities, the size, contents and type of which depend upon the type of kennels. Three facilities are essential to all establishments:

- Reception office (attached to the block or separate).
- Small kitchen (Table 5.6).
- Isolation unit (described in depth later in this chapter).

Other facilities (Table 5.6) might include:

- Stores for equipment, cleaning materials, bedding, etc.
- Grooming and bathing room.
- Surgery or veterinary examination room.
- Secure area for storage of medicines and disinfectants.

Table 5.6 Other facilities in a kennel or cattery

Kitchen with food stores	It is advisable to have the kitchen separate from the kennel blocks, particularly if it is to service more than one block. Where it is separate each kennel block should have a small utility area with worktops and sink, for final mixing of feeds, washing of dishes, etc. The main dog and cat kitchen should be easy to clean and disinfect and be equipped as follows: At least one sink with hot and cold water. At least one refrigerator. A deep freeze (size dependent on the kennel use of frozen foods). A small cooker and/or microwave oven. Work surfaces, shelves and cupboards. Vermin-proof bins for in-use sacks of food. A cool, dry and vermin-proof store room where sacks of food can be stored, raised off the floor. Various cutlery scoops, tin openers, etc. Scales for accurate weighing of feeds.
Stores for equipment, disinfectants, cat litter, bedding, etc.	The size of the stores will depend upon the size of the kennels and the types of materials used. Relatively large storage areas may be required if it is possible to bulk-buy items.
Grooming and bathing room	The size of the grooming area, type of bath and equipment held depend on the use. Some kennels run animal grooming services where owners bring the animals in for the day; they therefore require a large fully kitted grooming and bathing room with small holding kennels. Where the grooming facilities are for boarding/hospitalised animals a small area in each kennel block may be used for grooming individuals. A small central bath room/area can then be used if bathing of animals is fairly infrequent.
Surgery or veterinary consulting room	This room, built as a separate facility for non-veterinary practice kennels, is usually only necessary for large establishments. Separate facilities are particularly useful where the animals are long-stay and the population is relatively static. It is more usual for the animal to be examined and treated either in its own housing or in a hospital ward where suitable examination facilities are made available.

Specialised animal housing

Specialised housing is used for animals that have specific needs regarding their environment and care. Specialised housing includes:

● Hospital kennelling.
● Whelping kennelling.
● Puppy kennelling.
● Isolation kennelling.

The same type of kennelling can be used for veterinary practice kennels or private kennelling, as the principles are the same. The precise requirements depend upon the category of animal.

Hospital kennelling

Hospital kennels or cages are designed and constructed for animals that are undergoing treatment or for post-operative convalescence. These short-stay animals require a high degree of supervision and the kennelling is deliberately restrictive in size (Table 5.7). In many cases strict rest is required, particularly for post-operative animals that may dislodge sutures, etc.

It should be remembered that these units are designed for a short stay. Where animals do not specifically require confinement and their stay is likely to be medium to long term, they should be housed in a larger kennel.

Hospital kennelling can be either of the 'walk-in' type or the more restricting 'locker' type. It is usual to have a

Table 5.7 Hospital kennel sizes (locker type): some size ranges in common use

Type/size of animal	Width		Height		Depth	
	cm	(inches)	cm	(inches)	cm	(inches)
Cats	45.72	(18)	45.72–60.96	(18–24)	72.39	(28.25 or slightly less)
Dogs						
Small breeds	60.96–76.20	(24–30)	45.72–76.20	(18–30)	72.39	(28.25 or slightly less)
Medium breeds	76.20–91.44	(30–36)	76.20–91.44	(30–36)	72.39	(28.25 or slightly more)
Large breeds	121.92	(48)	76.20–91.44	(30–36)	72.39–100	(28.25)–(39.4)
Giant breeds	152.40–182.88	(60–70)	91.44	(36)	72.39–100	(28.25)–(39.4)
Walk-in kennels	approx 140 cm		180		100	

With the smaller sized kennels where space is limited and for top rows the depth can be reduced from 72.39 cm (28.25 inches) to 60.96 cm (24 inches) or a minimum of 45.72 cm (18 inches).

choice of both types in a hospital ward to allow selection of the most suitable housing for each animal, depending upon the animal's size and temperament and the degree of confinement required.

Metabolic kennels. Metabolic monitoring kennels, available in some veterinary hospitals, are usually smaller and therefore even more confining than standard hospital kennels. Animals are only housed in them for the short duration of any tests before being rehoused in standard hospital kennelling.

Intensive care kennels. Some form of intensive care kennelling is available in many hospitals. It is usually in the form of an airtight kennel with the supply of oxygen to the interior. The front of the kennel is transparent to allow constant observation of critically ill animals.

Whelping kennelling

A whelping kennel and its run should be large enough to accommodate a whelping bitch and her litter up to at least 6 weeks of age. The whelping box should be designed to allow the use of an additional heating unit (such as an infrared dull emitter) and to give the bitch privacy, with an observation panel that enables staff to observe her unnoticed. Kennelling must be escape-proof; a bitch should never leave the confines of the whelping area, because of the high risk of introducing disease to her pups from contact with other dogs. The whelping kennels should be situated away from other dog housing and be managed in a similar manner to the isolation unit detailed later in this chapter, to achieve 'protective isolation' for the vulnerable pups.

In a hospital, it is highly unlikely that the bitch and pups will be housed longer than the duration of the whelping itself. It is therefore only necessary to have a kennel large enough to hold the whelping bed but it should be the quietest site available. The bitch and pups should still be subject to protective isolation procedures within the hospital environment.

Puppy kennelling

Breeding kennels and others that commonly house very young animals for a short time usually require safe housing for these vulnerable animals. Puppy kennels should be situated away from adult dogs and managed so as to reduce the risk of unvaccinated youngsters coming into contact with disease. A puppy kennel should be able to house an additional heating unit, with any possible contact with electric wiring totally eliminated.

There must be no gaps between the dividing partitions and the floor for kennelling and runs as puppies can squeeze through very small spaces, including those used for drainage in the kennels of adult dogs.

Where litters of puppies are to be housed, a divided 'stable door' is invaluable: when its top half is opened, attending staff can step over the closed bottom half which confines the pups. When a standard kennel door is opened, it can be very difficult to stop a number of pups escaping or, worse, getting trapped by the door.

Kennel services

Lighting

It is necessary for the kennels to be well lit so that all procedures can be carried out effectively and safely, from cleaning the kennels to safe handling and effective observation of the boarders.

Lighting and its effects on dogs

Dogs require mental stimulation for their general well-being, and in this the use of sight plays its part. It is therefore important for the welfare of the dog that adequate lighting is provided during the active hours of daylight. This may seem obvious but, in kennels that have no natural light through windows, the dogs can be left in total darkness when staff switch off the lights. The dog should be able to observe other dogs and staff, creating an interesting environment preventing boredom.

It is preferable to allow as much natural light as possible but to bear in mind the likelihood of overheating the kennels in mid-summer.

Lighting and restfulness

While it is necessary to have good lighting to create an interesting environment during the active daylight hours, it is also necessary to have reduced lighting in sleeping areas to encourage rest.

During daylight periods of inactivity, dogs take short periods of rest. To sleep, they often seek out darker areas. This should be taken into account when designing kennel sleeping areas, e.g. a 'skylight' over the sleeping bench should be avoided. Where a great deal of natural light is provided (via windows and glass doors) it is useful to be able to reduce this overnight so that the dogs are more restful and less likely to bark. In winter, the long hours of darkness achieve this naturally but in summer months the dogs become restless at dawn and start to bark, which can cause problems with neighbours.

Artificial lighting

It is usually necessary to supplement natural light with some form of artificial lighting in a kennel block. The most commonly used is fluorescent strip lighting with a diffuser, which provides few shadows and is therefore helpful when cleaning.

The lighting is usually situated in the corridor, or in the central area of circular kennel blocks. If this does not provide sufficient visibility for cleaning, bulkhead lights can be positioned in the kennels. These are securely attached, to either the ceiling or the upper wall, and are completed covered. Hanging light-bulbs are not recommended: some dogs may try to grab them if they dangle low, and there is also a danger of kennel staff knocking the bulbs while scrubbing out the kennels.

All wiring and switches should be inaccessible to the dogs and all electrical fittings should be protected from contact with water. One method is to use waterproof switch units and screw-on covers for power points when not in use.

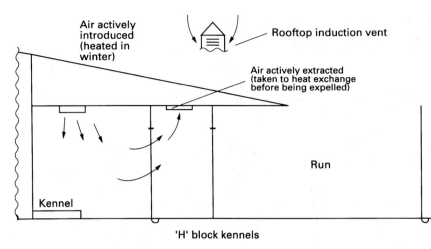

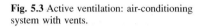

Fig. 5.3 Active ventilation: air-conditioning system with vents.

Ventilation

Ventilation must be provided in kennels and catteries to:

- Provide transmission of clean air for the animals and staff by removing any foul air containing fumes, obnoxious gases and smells, e.g. stale air (CO_2 from exhalation), ammonia, methane and unpleasant odours from animal soiling.
- Reduce to a minimum the concentration of possible airborne infective agents that may cause disease.

The two types of ventilation commonly used in kennels are known as active and passive.

Active ventilation

Active ventilation mechanically pulls air into or out of the kennels, usually by means of extractor fans or an air-conditioning system. In the case of air-conditioning, a heat exchange system to prevent loss of heat from the unit can be incorporated with a heating system, providing a dual-purpose ventilation and heating system.

In some specialised kennels much thought is given to the ventilation system and attempts are made to reduce the potential transmission of airborne infection. The aim is to introduce clean air into each kennel, and extract the 'used' air from the kennel, in such a way as to reduce the likelihood that the air exhaled by one animal is inhaled by another. There are two common systems: either air-conditioning with induction vent or extractor fan with vent.

Air-conditioning system with induction vent. In this system there is an induction vent in each kennel unit, actively pushing air into the kennel from an external 'clean' source such as the central area of the kennel roof. The air is actively extracted by another vent immediately outside the individual kennel in the corridor (Fig. 5.3).

Air-conditioning units are usually installed to suit the conditions within the unit when closed, which means that leaving doors and windows open can affect their efficiency. Always seek advice from the manufacturers or installation engineers to ensure effective management and operation.

Active ventilation enables control over the number of air changes per hour, usually set at 6 for kennels, with the ability to increase up to 12 changes (or to decrease the rate in some circumstances), depending on weather conditions, number of kennel occupants, etc.

Extractor fan and vent. Vents to introduce air are placed in the kennels and are themselves passive, the air being drawn through them by the activity of the extractor fan. The success of the system depends upon the correct placing of the vents in relation to the extractor fan. Figure 5.4 demonstrates the system in use in a circular 'parasol' kennel. The system is also suitable for the smaller indoor catteries and small-scale hospital accommodation.

This system can be used in reverse, with air drawn in through the central fan rather than being extracted by it. This creates positive pressure so that the air is forced out through the passive vents.

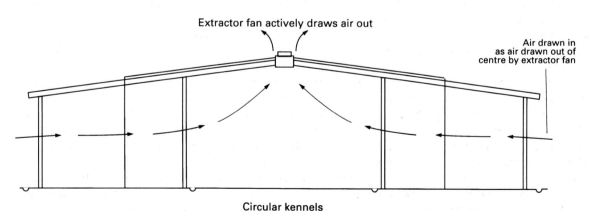

Fig. 5.4 Active ventilation: extraction fan and vents.

Even though a ventilation system is designed to reduce airborne infection in a working kennel, it should be remembered that it is not infallible. There is a strong possibility of the transmission of airborne infection if the dogs are passing along the corridor to grooming or relief areas or for exercise, or if they are allowed to exercise in adjoining runs with free airflow between them. For disease control, in addition to a scientific ventilation system:

- The kennels should be managed in such a way as to reduce likely contact, particularly at high risk times (e.g. when kennel cough is known to be affecting dogs in the area, or the kennels are full). All staff should be aware of the risk of airborne disease and be able to quickly identify suspect cases.
- Animals infected or suspected of being infected should be placed in an isolation unit immediately and their living area disinfected immediately.

Passive ventilation

Passive ventilation is achieved by opening and closing vents, windows and doors. Although widely used in many kennels and found to be satisfactory for situations where only a few animals are kept, there are some disadvantages:

- No control over air changes.
- Draughts may be caused.
- Loss of heat may be a problem.

Insulation and heating

Insulation and heating are provided for several reasons:

- For the warmth and comfort of the dogs.
- To enable rapid drying of kennels and service areas after cleaning and disinfection (heating combined with through airflow provides the most rapid drying).
- For the maintenance of buildings and contents (without heating, some deterioration or damage may occur – such as the freezing and fracturing of insufficiently insulated water pipes). A good heating system, combined with proper ventilation, also controls condensation, the dampness of which leads to mould and other problems.
- To a lesser extent, for the comfort and health of staff working in the kennel area: they will also benefit from dry, well-ventilated and warm environments.

Temperature control

It is advisable to check the temperature at different sites within the kennel building, particularly within the kennels themselves. The use of a 'maximum/minimum' environmental thermometer can be helpful in assessing the variations in temperatures throughout the day and night. The range may be significant enough to warrant changes to the system. During the day the general opening and closing of doors associated with the normal running of kennels may have a noticeable effect. During the night, when there is no movement, the temperature range and air quality may be

Table 5.8 Environmental temperatures for housing dogs	
Adult dogs	Should not drop below 7°C (44°F). Boarding/private kennels in sleeping area at least 10°C (50°F).
Whelping and puppy accommodation	18–21°C (65–70°F), with the temperature in the whelping bed for pups in the nest at 26–29°C (80–85°F) during their first week, 21–26°C (70–80°F) in their second week, then 20°C (68°F) thereafter until weaning. The pups require a higher temperature than the bitch. The bitch can leave the bed if she becomes too hot without the pups becoming chilled.
Hospital and isolation kennels	Usually 18–21°C (65–70°F). Should not fall below 15.5°C (60°F).

significantly different from that in the daytime. Table 5.8 gives recommended environmental temperatures for housing dogs.

Types of heating

Heating for kennelling and catteries should be:

- Economical to install and run.
- Easy to control, operate and maintain.
- Safe, i.e. not easily knocked over, with no naked flames and free from fumes.

Various options are available for heating kennels but they generally fall into two groups: environmental or 'central' heating of the whole kennel space and local heating for individual animals.

Central heating is controlled by a thermostat. Local heating is more economical to run: it provides additional heat for individuals with special needs, enabling the overall environmental temperature of the block to be lower so that it is more comfortable for individuals not requiring such a high degree of warmth. This allows animals with different needs to be housed in the same block. Table 5.9 sets out the advantages and disadvantages of typical systems used for both central and local heating.

Insulation and draught-proofing

Whatever type of heating is installed, it will not be efficient or economical if heat can easily be dissipated due to poor insulation or draughts.

Automatic door closers may be found helpful. If doors and windows are unnecessarily left open when the heating is operating, this will obviously also reduce the effectiveness of the heating systems.

In cat accommodation, cat flaps are required in the door from the sleeping area to permit access for the cat to the run. As this is a potential source of draughts, positioning and design of the flaps should be taken into account when constructing catteries.

Table 5.9 Types of heating: advantages and disadvantages

Type	Advantages	Disadvantages
Central heating **Gas, oil or electricity powered boilers.** These heat water-filled radiators, usually placed outside individual kennels in the corridor.	Easy to operate and maintain, commonly available.	The corridor is often warmer than the kennels (a thermostat or thermometer should be used to ensure individual kennels are at the correct temperature, not only the corridor). Requires suitable wall space for fitting. Likely to be difficult to keep clean and disinfect as many pipes/corners in the apparatus.
Electrical underfloor heating. Usually situated under the individual kennel flooring.	Floors dry very quickly, dogs have local heating when in closer contact with the floor when resting.	If insulation is poor the floors can become uncomfortably hot as the system attempts to increase the air temperature. Animal faeces dry hard to the floor, making removal difficult. System faults may be difficult and expensive to repair if the fault is under the floor. Electrical 'leaks' may eventually require the excavation of the whole floor.
Electric fan-assisted warm air heating. This form of heating is more often used to provide supplementary heating but can be installed in some cases as a central heating system.	The main advantage of this form of heating is its ability to provide rapid heat by circulating heated air.	As the air is very hot when it leaves the heater, great care should be taken not to place a heater too close to a patient's kennel as overheating of the patient could occur. This type of heating is fairly noisy and relatively expensive to run if used for more than as a supplementary heating option.
Total air conditioning/heating system. This system is usually installed when the building is purpose-built and is centrally operated. It is only suitable for large establishments where many kennels or kennel blocks are under one roof.	Heat and clean air can be fed directly into individual kennels and extracted in the corridor, ensuring the kennels themselves are at the correct temperature and air is pushed/pulled out of the kennels. This reduces the air flow from kennel to kennel, which is advantageous in reducing the distribution of airborne infection.	Expensive to install and not suitable for many types of kennel design with low roofs. Running costs may be high in winter.
Local heating **Infra-red dull emitter.** Widely used in all types of kennels, the unit is suspended from the roof by a chain or other strong adjustable material over the sleeping area. This is assessed before the animal is housed by placing a thermometer on an object such as a box, at the height of the sleeping animal's back. Once the optimum temperature has been reached by raising and lowering the unit and leaving for a few minutes each time, the unit can then be fixed in position and a mark or strip of tape can be permanently put on the wall indicating the height and temperature expected.	Easy to install. Correct heat can be directed into the animal's sleeping area. Produces heat without light, thus aiding restfulness. The height of the unit can be adjusted to regulate the heat reaching the animal.	Requires a power point either in each kennel or the means to direct an electric lead safely into the kennel. Unless correctly positioned the animal may be either too hot or cold. (The FAB recommend the use of individually thermostatically controlled infra-red dull emitters in cat accommodation to reduce the risk of over- or under-heating.) Some animals may be able to tamper with it with disastrous results if hung too low and not firmly fixed to the ceiling (by a chain or similar). Fires can occur if: – The animal pulls it down and it is in contact with bedding. – It is hung too low scorching the bedding. – Water is splashed onto the bulb which then bursts.
Heated bed/pad. This type of supplementary heating is widely used and enjoyed by many animals, healthy or ailing in kennel or hospital situations. It is essential that this type of heating is only used to supplement the environmental heating system as only the bed is warmed.	The animal can be directly heated by contact with a low constant heat being emitted from directly below.	Frequently damaged by chewing (even when metal casing used for wires) leading to a risk of electrocution of animal. These should be used with a circuit breaker to minimise the risk. Increased risk of contamination as directly in contact with the animal and may prove difficult to disinfect thoroughly. Some users feel that continual contact with a heated surface can lead to hair loss.

Table 5.9 (Continued)

Type	Advantages	Disadvantages
Hot water-bottles Hot water-bottles are often used as temporary heaters for very young puppies (with the water at normal body temperature).	Cheaply available for providing rapid direct warmth to the animal. They are suitable for sending home with tiny puppies or kittens after a Caesarean operation.	There is a danger of using water too hot and burning the animal. There is also a risk of bursting and wetting and/or scalding the animal, particularly as the animal may bite or claw the hot water-bottle. The water cools rapidly and therefore hot water-bottles are only used for short-term emergency use where an animal can be supervised.
Portable radiant heaters.	Widely available and provide rapid heat. Good for emergency use, heaters can be hired.	They should never be used when they cannot be supervised as if in contact with any combustible material can cause fires. They should never be used in a busy ward where they can be knocked over or have anything dropped on them, as fires can start very rapidly.
Electric fan heaters	Can be used to boost the heat rapidly in cold weather or act as a temporary rapid emergency heating in the case of the main heating system malfunctioning.	As for electric fan-assisted warm air heating.
Electrically heated oil-filled radiators. Widely available and provide heat without light.	Mobile and relatively safe as there is no single concentrated heat source.	Can take much longer to heat an area than some of the other forms of supplementary heating. They therefore may not benefit the animals for a long time after switching on.

Beds and bedding

Beds are used to contain the animal while resting or sleeping. They should provide a sanctuary where the animal may retire to feel safe and secure. The bed will represent its own territory in the kennels.

For these reasons all dogs and cats, whether housed in human accommodation or in any type of kennelling, should have a bed. The basic requirements for most types of bed are that they should:

- Be raised to some extent from the floor.
- Give easy access for the animal (particularly the old and very young).
- Have sides and back (and front where used) high enough to prevent draughts, to promote the animal's feeling of security and to contain the bedding material.

Types of bed

Many types of bed are available for purchase (Table 5.10). The majority are designed with the domestic pet owner in mind, rather than for kennel use, although some are suitable for both. Most require the addition of bedding material but some have this incorporated in the bed.

Bedding

Bedding is used:

- To provide warmth by insulation of the animal's body heat.

- To provide comfort, by allowing padding between the animal and hard surfaces.
- To avoid injury from constant contact between skin over bony areas and hard surfaces that cause pressure or 'bed' sores.

Properties of suitable bedding material:

- It should be a good insulator.
- It should be soft and flat with some give, and large enough to accommodate a stretched-out animal (it is important that older animals should not be forced to sleep curled up), but it can be arranged by the animal when curling up to sleep.
- It should permit drainage of body fluids. This is essential in keeping ill or incontinent animals dry.
- It should not contain anything that is harmful if ingested or is irritant, for example, to skin or eyes.
- It should be easy to physically manage.
- It should be easily cleaned, disinfected or disposed of.
- It should be easy to store.
- It should not soil or damage the animal's coat.
- It should be economical to use – inexpensive if disposable – durable, long-lasting and not easily chewed or destroyed if reusable.

The materials that are commonly used for bedding are either disposable or non-disposable (Table. 5.11).

Non-disposable bedding. Non-disposable materials are laundered, disinfected and reused; they are used mainly in

Table 5.10 Types of bed for domestic animals

Type of bed	Use	Qualities	Additional bedding type
Wicker basket	Domestic	Popular with owners, flexible, attractive, traditional. Liable to chewing by some dogs, difficult to clean/disinfect, can harbour flea eggs.	Blanket or similar.
Bean bag	Domestic	Liked by many dogs and can be 'arranged' by dog. Warm polystyrene beads insulate. Beads mould to body shape assisting comfort. Outer cover is washed/disinfected, remainder difficult to wash. Not suitable for incontinent animals. Not suitable for chewers as small holes allow the polystyrene beads to escape.	None
Foam and fabric (traditionally shaped)	Domestic	Are popular with more designs becoming available. Are available for cats and small dogs with a 'roof', igloo style. Flexible, small beds are machine washable.	Foam pad. (Additional blankets can be used.)
Metal frame	Domestic	Collapsible dog bed raises animal well off floor, liked by many dogs. Removable covers or blankets used to allow washing. Some elderly animals may have difficulty in getting in.	Blankets or similar for some types.
Radiator cat beds	Domestic	Radiator fixed cat beds, a fixed radiator is required. The bed hooks over the top of the radiator. A removable washable cover is used. Popular with some owners and many cats. The bed protrudes and cannot always be conveniently placed. Elderly/very young or infirm cats may not be able to get in and out. Cats will seek warmth while radiator is on, but will be less comfortable when the heating is off, e.g. at night.	
Plastic moulded	Domestic/kennels	Widely available in many sizes. Used with removable bedding. They can be washed and adequately chemically disinfected. Can be chewed by some dogs resulting in quite sharp edges being formed. Occasionally animals have been found to have allergic reactions to prolonged contact with some types of plastic, especially if the dog's nose rests on the plastic.	Covered foam pad, blankets, etc.
Sleeping benches	Kennels	(A) *Fixed (built-in plinth)*. This is an area of kennel that is raised. It is either a low, slightly raised floor in one area, or a structure projecting from a wall with supports at each end. Bedding material must be used. It may have difficult corners to clean/disinfect dependent on design.	Blankets or similar, or disposable bedding such as shredded paper can be used, if retaining board used.
		(B) *Removable*. Slide/lift out. Fold down. Wood laminated (aluminium reinforced edges). These have the advantage over the fixed plinth in that they are removable, and have some degree of 'give' or flexibility and usually are slightly better at insulating body heat. Bedding material used should be either of the disposable or non-disposable type. It may be chewed by some dogs if any unreinforced edges are accessible to the dog.	Bedding as above.

longer-stay kennels. They can be expensive to purchase and require suitable facilities for laundering and disinfection. The size of storage area for this type of bedding is far less than for the disposable type as less stock is required. Non-disposable bedding includes blankets, acrylic bedding and covered foam pads.

Disposable bedding. Disposable materials are relatively inexpensive and are discarded once soiled. A large stock of materials will be required and needs a suitable storage area situated as near to the kennel accommodation as possible.

Provision must also be made for disposal according to current regulations. Commonly used disposable materials include newspaper, shredded paper and woodwool. Less frequently used (and not advised for regular use) are straw, straw bags, peat, woodshavings and sawdust.

General principles of kennel and cattery management

Kennel and cattery management consists of ensuring a planned and methodical approach, by designing and

Table 5.11 Types of bedding

Non-disposable	Disposable
Blankets Unless donated or old blankets are used they can be an expensive form of bedding, particularly as they may be chewed and torn up by some destructive dogs. Dogs with allergies to dust mites may not be suited to this type of bedding if it is not laundered regularly using very hot washing water. Blankets are, however, a traditional warm bedding and are often used in domestic circumstances, and owners like to see them used in kennels. They are not suitable for hospital kennels or housing infectious disorders as they are difficult to sterilise. **Acrylic bedding** This type of bedding is widely used both domestically and in kennels. It is very expensive to purchase but more resistant to chewing than blankets. This type of bedding is easier to launder than blankets as it is resistant to organic material, even dried-on debris can usually be removed by soaking. The properties that make it particularly suitable for hospital use are that it allows body fluids through thus keeping an animal relatively comfortable and dry and it is sufficiently supportive as to reduce the occurrence of pressure sores in elderly and recumbent animals. **Covered foam pads** These are generally used in conjunction with a traditionally shaped foam-and-fabric or plastic-moulded bed. They can also be chewed and once damaged should be repaired or removed as soon as possible as chunks of foam can be more easily torn off by a dog once the pad has been initially damaged. This bedding is fairly easily laundered and warm and comfortable. It is sufficiently supportive as to reduce the occurrence of pressure sores. In some cases thick foam pads covered with waterproof material are found useful in a hospital situation where very large breeds are recumbent. The additional thickness assists in the support of these very heavy animals. Due to the thickness and size of these pads they are very difficult to launder. The waterproof covering can, however, be cleaned/disinfected by using chemical disinfectant and a cloth to wipe over.	**Newspaper** Newspaper is widely used by kennels and hospitals as it is freely available and absorbent. Many kennels line the bed area with newspaper and place a blanket or similar on top. It is rarely used on its own as a bedding as it is not warm or comfortable enough for the animal. A disadvantage of newspaper is that the newsprint will stain, particularly when wet. Dogs with light coloured coats and light coloured kennelling are likely to stain. **Shredded paper** This has the advantage over newspaper in that it is bulky and therefore warmer. If shredded newspaper is used the staining previously mentioned can be a problem. It can be messy to deal with in kennels, as are all materials with similar properties unless retained in the sleeping area by some method. It will stick to an animal's coat if damp and is not suitable for use with animals that have discharging wounds as it is liable to attach itself to such areas. Healthy dogs in a kennel situation find this form of bedding very comfortable and appear to enjoy arranging it and burying their toys in it. Some animals may eat it and small amounts usually cause little harm. **Woodwool** Woodwool is used in some kennels as it is warm and liked by the dogs though it is more recently being replaced by the use of shredded paper. Woodwool is expensive and can on occasion cause allergic reactions. Small pieces may occasionally get into an animal's eyes. It is less absorbent than paper but this can be an advantage if body fluids are required to drain through a bedding rather than being absorbed. (It is thought that pine oil may repel ectoparasites where wood-origin materials are used.)

executing efficient routines and procedures for the care and welfare of the animals. Such management will ensure that:

- All tasks are carried out in a logical order, with the needs of the animals high in priority.
- The best possible use is made of labour and materials.
- Health and safety requirements are met.
- All staff are fully instructed about how to carry out their tasks.
- All staff are aware of set standards and can recognise when they have been achieved.
- Consistency of standards is maintained by supervision and by checking procedures.
- Morale of staff is kept high by making them fully aware of what is expected and the reasons for carrying out their tasks.
- Confidence generated by the staff and management conveys to clients that their animals are being well cared for.

Daily work routine within the kennel block

The daily work routine is an amalgamation of tasks that must be carried out to a strict timetable, e.g. animals receiving medications at specific times of day and other tasks that are more flexible. Experienced staff will fit into these routines as appropriate. All new and inexperienced staff should carry out tasks as instructed by their supervisor.

The five main factors to consider when planning daily work are as follows:

- *External influences*. These can be almost anything that will affect the working day, from the weather (e.g. ice and snow hampering the cleaning of external exercise runs and requiring more time to complete the task) to several owners being due to collect their dogs on a particular day, or perhaps an unusual number of long telephone calls.
- *Weekly or non-routine tasks*. The relevant documentation (usually a diary) should be checked for weekly or

non-routine tasks due to be carried out on a particular day.

- *Time allowed for completion of tasks.* Because many and varied tasks have to be included, it is important that all work is started promptly and that the time taken for each task is assessed appropriately.
- *Adaptability.* Adaptability is essential when working with animals, as sudden changes will require the rescheduling of tasks. Animals may become ill or there may be unexpected requests to collect animals, e.g. when an elderly owner has been admitted into hospital as an emergency.
- *Communication.* As in any business where more than one person is working, it is important to communicate effectively with all other personnel likely to be affected by any decision or action. In addition to verbal communication, it is advisable to use some form of written instructions. Typical systems are kennel diaries, check-lists that can be ticked-off, and clearly written lists of the routine daily tasks. Table 5.12 gives practical examples of daily kennel and cattery routines.

Kennel management procedures

The kennel manager should design and introduce set procedures within the kennel to ensure smooth running and minimise error. These should be supported by some form of documentation for record and checking purposes. Set procedures should include admission (intake of animals), discharge (animals leaving the kennels) and others as appropriate to the type of kennels.

Documentation

All documentation must be:

- Legible and accurate.
- Up-to-date and relevant.
- Able to record action taken.
- In the correct terminology.

All documentation must be easy to read and accurate in order to avoid mistakes being made (e.g. special feeding requirements or medication) and to ensure that all legal requirements are covered. Information should be recorded promptly (to ensure that records and instructions are up to date) and should be concise and brief. When instructions have been followed, the action taken must be recorded (this can be simply a tick column, or initials and date where two or more members of staff are responsible for the duties). The correct terminology should be used, and any abbreviations must be those that are understood and commonly used by all staff.

Table 5.13 gives examples of admission and discharge procedures.

Kennel cleaning and disinfection

All animals require a hygienic environment in order to remain healthy. Where animals are housed in large numbers

---

Table 5.12 Daily routines in kennels and catteries

Example of daily kennel routine

7 a.m. start. Open kennels: check all dogs (walk through kennel block).
Gather equipment.
When initial excitement subsides, take dogs quietly to the runs.
Clean kennels and replace or change bedding.
Check that each dog has urinated and defecated (record) and return dogs to kennel.
Remove faeces from runs and rinse away urine patches.
Check water supply, water bowls and buckets.
Carry out any early morning treatments or medications.
Breakfast. Break for staff.
Make up feeds: feed dogs; wash dishes (if water bowls/buckets are used, wash and renew water supply).
Take dogs quietly to runs and see to any soiled kennels.
Record any urination and defecation; return dogs to kennels.
Remove faeces from runs and hose-clean entire run area.
Carry out kennel tasks (e.g. washing blankets/cleaning dog kitchen, checking feed/disinfectant/bedding supplies).
Exercise dogs according to type, age, condition, etc.
Remove any faeces from exercise runs.
Commence grooming and checking long-haired dogs (if time).
Lunch. Break for staff.
Take dogs to runs, etc.
Continue checking and grooming all dogs (long-haired dogs first).
Bath/groom any dogs being discharged and prepare belongings for return to owners.
Feed any dogs receiving p.m. feeds; wash dishes.
Take dogs to runs, etc.
Disinfect and thoroughly rinse and dry all runs.
Reception/discharge of dogs (there may be two reception/discharge times during the day, one in the morning, one in afternoon).
Settle in new dogs, feed, take to runs, etc.
Supper. Break for staff.
Any uncompleted documentation, paperwork; discussions, planning.
Break for staff; then in late evening:
Take all dogs to runs, etc., opportunities for urination and defecation.
Check all dogs.
Lock up kennels. Set any security devices.

Example of daily cattery routine

Starting 7–8 a.m. Check all cats.
Remove feed and water bowls.
Adust heating if necessary.
Wash water bowls.
Feed cats and supply water (with milk as appropriate).
Clean kennels (cat units). Sweep cat housing unit and tidy bed (using the unit's individual dustpan and brush).
Wash down any soiled surface (with disinfectant/detergent solution).
Litter trays emptied, disinfected, cleaned and refilled (records of urination/defecation kept).
Thoroughly sweep clean.
Sweep safety passage. Soiled litter/waste bags removed and prepared for disposal. Clean and disinfect any vacated units.
Treatments carried out. Grooming carried out.
Feed list for afternoon feeds made up and dated as necessary. Second feed given (8 hours after a.m. feed).
Attend to litter trays (check at intervals and attend to trays as necessary during the day).
Prepare any documentation for any admissions or discharges the following day.
Dusk:
Secure cats in housing units.
Late evening:
Check each cat, adjust heating if necessary.
Lock up all buildings. Set fire and other security alarm systems.

or the population is constantly changing, as in most kennels and catteries, an effective cleaning and disinfection routine should be in place and strictly followed. When setting up such a routine it is important to maintain a balance: constant washing creates damp kennels and a humid atmosphere in which micro-organisms thrive and, in any case, dogs and cats are more comfortable in dry accommodation.

Daily cleaning

Whilst animals are resident, one thorough daily cleansing (and disinfection where conditions dictate) using the method described on p. 124 should be sufficient and is better than, say, three half-hearted floor wipes with a cloth or mop and bucket. When animals accidentally soil their accommodation, this should be dealt with on a local area basis and must be attended to at once.

Tidying kennels

For removal of dust and hair from the kennel during the day, consider the use of a vacuum cleaner. It is more effective and less time-consuming than a broom or dustpan and brush and it reduces the amount of water used in the kennels. (Take care to use a quiet machine and be aware that some animals may object to the noise.) At this point the bedding is usually tidied and shaken out.

Cleaning and disinfection on departure

On an animal's departure from the kennels, its accommodation and fittings must be thoroughly cleaned and disinfected, and preferably left empty for a few days. All bedding is removed and either disposed of or disinfected.

If disinfecting bedding some types of detergent/disinfectant may be used in washing machines, e.g. halogenated tertiary amines (that are a mix of special detergents and disinfecting agents). However, strongly acidic oxidising or bleaching agents should not be used (always check the manufacturers' recommendations before use).

All toys belonging to the kennels (rather than to the individual) should be disinfected, or discarded if this is not possible.

Post-operative kennelling

The highest possible standards of disinfection are essential in veterinary hospital kennels, especially where a risk of infection is likely, as in post-operative kennelling.

Principles and methods of cleaning and disinfecting kennels

The cleaning and disinfection of kennels is achieved by physical and chemical actions. The action of all chemical disinfectants is dependent upon being in direct contact with the target micro-organisms. This means that all traces of organic material such as dirt, grease, faeces, urine, blood and vomit must be physically removed from the surface prior to disinfection, as it will prevent such contact. Begin

by removing the bulk of the material with a shovel and scraper (or similar). Tackle the remainder by hosing out the kennel liberally with water; then use a detergent and energetically scrub with a suitable brush.

Precautions and use of chemical disinfectants

When using any chemicals, including disinfectants and cleaning materials, care should be taken to ensure their correct handling:

- Store in the original containers with the lids fully secured.
- Keep away from animals and children.
- Wear protective clothing when recommended and take care to avoid contact with skin.
- Wash hands thoroughly after use, particularly before eating and drinking.
- Only use disinfectants for the purpose recommended by the manufacturer.
- Use the correct concentration.
- Wear gloves.

Manufacturers of disinfectants give recommended dilution rates. There is usually more than one rate, depending upon where the chemical will be used and the type of organisms to be killed or inactivated. To simplify use, most manufacturers do not provide a list of micro-organisms and a recommended strength for each, but they give a recommended strength for routine or general use and (usually) a stronger solution for certain specific disease-causing organisms.

In some kennels the recommended 'routine' strength is used for the normal daily cleaning and disinfection of kennels where no specific problems exist. A recommended higher concentration is often used in disinfecting a kennel after its occupant has been discharged and before admitting another animal into it. Some general rules can be applied to the use of disinfectants:

- Too weak a solution will be ineffective, whereas a solution that is stronger than the recommendation is not only wasteful but also may, with some types of disinfectant, lead to problems with the animals' feet, eyes and other sensitive areas. Inadequate rinsing may lead to similar problems.
- A disinfectant should have no substances other than water added to it. It is potentially dangerous to mix disinfectants together or disinfectants with detergents, unless recommended by the manufacturer, as combinations of chemicals can negate the effect of the active ingredient in both products as well as producing noxious gases or cause corrosive action. This problem can occur accidentally if adequate safeguards are not in place – always be cautious of the chemicals and always use and store as recommended.
- Use at the chemicals' optimum temperature for action. Many disinfectants are more effective when used with hot water than with cold, although with others there is no advantage. It is advisable to check this feature.
- Using very hot water can be hazardous. If it spills on the operator or the animal, injury will occur. Safety should

Table 5.13 Admission and discharge procedures

Admission	The date/time of admission should have been previously written in the diary/day book. A kennel should be available/prepared for the animal.
On arrival	*Vaccination certificates must be checked BEFORE the animal is admitted to ensure animal is properly vaccinated and up to date.* Record details of admission – card or forms are usually designed to fulfil the individual kennel needs. However, generally the information is: owner details: owner name, address and telephone number (plus a contact address/number if the owner is working or on holiday); animal details: name, species, breed, age, sex (and if neutered); animal's normal behaviour, characteristics or peculiarities; details of food/normal feeding time/normal relief pattern and surface used (urination and defecation)/normal amount of exercise given. List items admitted with the animal and label them: collar, lead, toys, carrying box, etc. (Try to avoid admitting many personal items as even if labelled they can still be lost causing embarrassment to the kennels or veterinary practice.) Details of stay: arrival time and date; reason for stay, e.g. boarding, hospitalisation. Time and date of the animal's discharge: other details/policies. Consent forms may be required to be filled in, or if the kennels are not attached to a veterinary practice details of the client's veterinary surgeon should be recorded. It MAY also be policy in some kennels to: (a) Ask the owner how they will be paying. (b) Inform the owner if they are expected to settle all debts upon collection. (c) State the cost of the service. This is usually done in a predetermined way as part of the normal administration procedure so that it does not offend or embarrass the owner. It does however save embarrassment or misunderstanding when the account is to be settled on collection as the owner knows what to expect. Any other kennel policy may need to be stated and the owner may be asked to sign a form in some cases agreeing to abide by the policy. If it is possible, check the animal over in the presence of the owner and identify to the owner any abnormalities found. It is sometimes possible that they are aware of, say, a small swelling for example, but have forgotten to inform you of it, and which later may develop into a large hernia. It is helpful to carry out this check with the owner present to avoid any disagreement regarding whether an animal sustained an injury while in your care or was injured prior to admission. Check at this stage for signs of parasites and if present deal with them with the consent and knowledge of the owner.
Weigh the animal	If the animal is likely to stay in kennels for a prolonged period it should be weighed on entry and thereafter at weekly intervals. This should be part of the condition monitoring of all long-stay animals.
Admit the animal	Firmly but pleasantly take the animal from the owner. Always remember that the separation may in some cases be distressing for both animal and owner. Make sure the animal cannot escape from you if it should struggle. It is best to use a kennel slip lead for dogs but with cats, due to their agility when determined to escape, strict precautions should be imposed to prevent possible escape. The cat should be presented in an escape-proof container (basket, carrying box, cage) and the owner should accompany the member of staff to the cage.
Kennel the animal securely	All animals should be transferred to their housing using an escape-proof technique, as when first admitting an animal is the time when the risk of potential escape is very high. The animal should be offered water and food if appropriate. The animal should be closely observed and reassured as it settles into the kennel routine.
Discharge	The date and time of the animal's discharge should be written in the diary or day book. The day prior to departure, any preparations that are required for the animal's departure should be carried out. These may be: the preparation of any written materials such as reports/special care instructions for the owner to continue, or the preparation of any prescription. The account should be prepared and checked.
Feeding	Animals travelling a distance or not used to car journeys should not normally be fed less than four hours before their departure. This will help to reduce the likelihood of the animal vomiting and if it does vomit there will be less solid vomit for the animal to soil itself or the owner's car.
Grooming	The animal should be checked and groomed before departure. This may fit in with the animal's normal daily grooming depending on the departure time. If not, the grooming will require to be rescheduled to be carried out earlier in the day to ensure that the animal is groomed before collection.
Items admitted with the animal	Check that all the items admitted with the animal are ready for collection and are clean and undamaged.
Report on the animal's stay	If the animal has been hospitalised, a written or verbal report may be required. Where an animal has been boarding, a verbal report will be required by the owner. This should never come as a surprise and efforts should be made to report as fully as possible on the animal. This inspires confidence in the establishment as the owner is satisfied that the staff have taken an interest in the animal that is naturally regarded as special to them. This should ensure future custom from them and enhance the reputation of the kennels when they relay to others the high standard of care and attention that they feel was given to their pet. The account or method of payment must be resolved. If it is policy for the account to be settled on collection of the animal, the itemised bill should be ready. The owner, having been previously made aware of the kennel policy, will be expecting it to be ready for payment.

be of paramount importance, as with all actions in kennels.

● The contact time should be taken into account when planning a disinfection routine. All disinfectants require time to kill or inactivate micro-organisms and are ineffective if rinsed off immediately after application. The required contact time varies considerably, depending on the type of disinfectant and the organisms to be killed. Take note of the manufacturers' recommended contact times when selecting a disinfectant: it may be able to kill certain organisms but may take up to 24 hours' contact time to do its work.

● Use freshly made-up solutions to ensure effectiveness. Some disinfectants begin to deteriorate when made into solution with water.

● Equipment and receptacles used with disinfectants should be thoroughly cleaned and rinsed before use. Any organic material present may reduce the effectiveness of the disinfectant.

It should also be noted that the efficiency of some disinfectants may be hindered by 'hard' water, some plastics and certain other materials. Read all the literature relating to the chemicals before use.

● All disinfectants should be thoroughly rinsed off once the contact time is completed, unless otherwise recommended.

● Always adhere to recommendations on product COSHH sheets. Specific use and precautions to be taken when using chemical disinfectants are stated on the COSHH sheet provided by the manufacturer.

It is essential that veterinary nurses understand the COSHH (Control of Substances Hazardous to Health) regulations 1998 and adhere to standard procedures (see Chapter 4).

Cleaning and disinfection of kennel equipment

Equipment such as shovels, buckets, mops, dustpans and brushes, kitchen utensils, feed bowls, beds and bedding must all be cleaned and disinfected regularly. Wash them first in detergent and water to remove any organic material. To disinfect, soak the equipment in a solution of disinfectant appropriate to the material at the manufacturer's recommended strength and for the recommended contact time. Then thoroughly rinse and dry the equipment before storing it.

Special care must be taken that the disinfectant is in fact 'appropriate to the material' as some items can be corroded by certain chemicals. Particular care should be taken with the disinfection of items made of plastic (including thermoplastic floor tiles), rubber and mild steel; the soaking of these materials in an oxidising disinfectant should be avoided unless the manufacturer states otherwise (if so, the stated contact times should not be exceeded, with items being thoroughly rinsed and dried). If bedding is disinfected by soaking it can be laundered in the normal way afterwards.

SUMMARY OF ROUTINE PROCEDURE FOR CLEANING AND DISINFECTION OF KENNELS

(1) Remove animal from kennel into a run or other secure holding area (not another dog's kennel).
(2) Remove bed, bedding, toys and any other portable objects.
(3) Remove any gross soiling with shovel and scraper or similar equipment.
(4) Hose out hair and any debris. Pressure hoses or steam cleaners are used in some establishments.
(5) Scrub out with detergent.*
(6) Rinse with water.*
(7) Apply disinfectant* (or scrub out with detergent/disinfectant).
(8) Time contact.
(9) Rinse thoroughly.
(10) Dry (remove excess water with a 'squeegee' drier).
(11) Leave to air dry.
(12) Return/replace bedding as necessary.
(13) Return animal to kennel.

* Many of the more recently developed kennel disinfectants are a combination of specialist detergents and disinfectant agents. These specialist detergent/disinfectants are mixed by manufacturers as part of the active ingredient formulation. This principle potentiates the activity of the disinfectant and accelerates the microbiocidal process.

When using these products follow actions 1–4 (using the correct dilution), cut out steps 5 and 6 and proceed with step 7, second option.

These products are often used in low-risk areas for routine cleaning/disinfection where no disease problems exist.

Antiseptics and disinfectants

The terms 'antiseptic' and 'disinfectant' are often used loosely when referring to chemical agents but they actually describe the chemicals' action against micro-organisms.

Selecting disinfectants and antiseptics

The choice of product depends upon many factors but some of the main considerations are:

● The intended use of the product.
  – environmental (kennels, runs, equipment)
  – on living tissue (skin, wounds, body cavities, etc).
● The product's activity against specific micro-organisms.

- **Antiseptics** are chemicals that cause the destruction or inhibition of micro-organisms, preventing their growth or multiplication, without damaging an animal's cells. Antiseptics applied topically have many uses, such as the cleansing of wounds or the skin.

- **Disinfection**. This term describes a process that is used to reduce the number of micro-organisms (not usually including bacterial spores) to a level which is not harmful to health. This term applies to the treatment of inanimate objects and materials and may also be applied to the treatment of skin, mucous membranes and other body tissues and cavities. Methods of achieving disinfection include the use of chemicals and some physical processes such as boiling.

- **Skin disinfectants** are antiseptic preparations designed either for pre-operative skin cleansing or for use on inanimate objects.

- **Environmental disinfectants** are designed for use on inanimate objects only; many of them require the user to wear protective clothing and they should *never* be used on the skin.

- **Sterilant** is a term used to describe some types of chemical disinfectant which can under certain conditions destroy bacterial spores, viruses and vegetative organisms. Physical methods of sterilisation are superior to chemical sterilants in their effectiveness, e.g. steam sterilisation.

- **Sterilisation** is the term applied when an inanimate object is rendered free from all micro-organisms, including bacterial spores, by their removal or destruction. This procedure must be used when the efficient destruction of all micro-organisms is vital, such as in the preparation of instruments for surgery. When selecting methods for destroying micro-organisms on inanimate objects, it is important to remember that a method producing sterilisation is far more satisfactory than one that produces disinfection.

- **Decontamination** refers to rendering an item safe by the destruction or removal of microbial contamination. This is usually achieved by cleaning, disinfection or sterilisation.

SUFFICES

- **-cide** indicates that a chemical kills a particular type of micro-organism. For example, a bactericide kills bacteria; a fungicide kills fungi.

- **-stat** describes the action of a chemical that prevents or inhibits the growth of a particular type of micro-organism, for example, a bacteriostat inhibits the growth of bacteria. Some antiseptics have this characteristic, although it is preferable to select a chemical with the ability to kill the micro-organism rather than one that merely prevents or inhibits its growth.

- The contact time required.
- Known local conditions (e.g. water hardness).
- Safety of staff and animals – ideally the product should be non-irritant, non-toxic and non-corrosive – check manufacturer's COSHH sheets for details of any hazards and for recommended suitable protective clothing for the user.
- Stability of the product in storage.
- Odour of product. Ideally products should be either odourless or have a pleasant aroma that is agreeable to staff and animals.
- Ease of use – it should disperse easily in water if dilution is required.
- Economy of use, assessed by cost per litre of ready-to-use solution.

It should be noted, for example, that:

- Some products which are very effective for kennel disinfection will stain bedding and other porous materials.
- The presence of even relatively small amounts of organic material in water may affect some products.
- Some animal species are sensitive to some types of disinfectant (e.g. cats are sensitive to phenol; and vapours given off by some chemicals such as glutaraldehyde will cause irritation to the eyes of many animals).
- Strong odours or perfumes are offensive to some animals, promoting sneezing and irritation to the ocular mucous membranes.

Effectiveness. The product should have been tested for action against specific significant organisms, for example, parvovirus. The results of these tests should be available so that the user knows what strength/dilution and contact time are effective. Early tests, such as the Rideal–Walker and Chick–Martin tests, only give accurate results for phenolic-based disinfectants; more modern techniques such as the Kelsey–Sykes test are suitable for the assessment of most disinfectants.

The bacteria-killing capability of a disinfectant varies as some forms of bacteria are more resistant than others. The Gram-positive group are the most easily destroyed; the Gram-negative group, acid-fast group and bacterial spores are progressively more difficult to destroy. The literature for many disinfectants now available for use in kennels and catteries states that they are effective against specific important viral diseases of the dog and cat.

Types of disinfectants and antiseptics

There are a number of different products available on the market, with new products appearing frequently. Most chemical disinfectants available will fit broadly into the main groups, some of the recognised general characteristics of these chemicals being listed below. However, it should be recognised that advances in manufacturing and blending of chemicals may mean that certain disinfectants may perform slightly differently. It is therefore advisable when selecting products to refer to the manufacturers' performance data.

The main groups of disinfectants

Phenolics

The phenolic disinfectants have a wide range of bactericidal activity but variable activity against viruses (usually poor against non-enveloped viruses such as parvovirus). The activity against bacterial spores is poor.

Black, white and clear phenolics. These disinfectants are inexpensive and not as susceptible to inactivation by organic materials as some other chemicals. They are toxic and irritant to varying degrees and should not come into contact with the skin. These types of disinfectant can be absorbed by rubber and plastics. They are also strong smelling and black fluids can leave sticky residue on some materials.

Chloroxylenols (synthetic phenol/chlorinated phenol). Chloroxylenol is less irritant than other types of phenolic but can be inactivated by hard water and organic material. Active against Gram-positive bacteria but poor activity against Gram-negative bacteria (though improved by the addition of EDTA in some products).

Hexachlorophane. This type of chemical is more active against Gram-positive than Gram-negative bacteria, but has little other activity. Hexachlorophane has been used in soap and detergent preparations, for skin disinfection, as it has a good residual effect. Recently there have been concerns regarding its possible cumulative toxicity (with human neonates). This has restricted its use in some areas.

Triclosan (cloxifenol) has similar characteristics to hexachlorophane but no concerns regarding toxicity. It is now used in a similar manner to a skin disinfectant.

Halogens

Hypochlorites (bleach). These disinfectants are generally inexpensive and are effective against bacteria, fungi, viruses and spores when used correctly. However, there are some disadvantages: chlorine is a strong oxidising agent which is corrosive to metals and bleaching of some materials occurs. Chlorine gas may be liberated if in contact with acids, therefore, it should not be used in the presence of urine. It should be noted that these chemicals can gradually lose strength in storage and that the presence of organic matter can affect the disinfectant activity.

Halogenated tertiary amines (HTA)

This is a new group of compounds developed in the UK and used now worldwide. The term 'halogenated' provides association with the chlorine derivative which is reacted in combination with other complex chemistries. Tertiary means 'third level' and in this case is used to specify a particular molecular structure of substances reacted with a chloride salt and where there are two other compounds. Generally these new compounds contain one or more highly sophisticated **quarternary ammonium compounds** (QACs) which work with very specific amine salts. These products with their specialist detergents have wide-ranging activities. These include action against Gram-negative and Gram-positive bacteria. There is also good action against viruses, including enveloped and non-enveloped types. These disinfectants also act against spores and fungi. These compounds are more resistant to inactivation by organic materials than some other types of disinfectant. Although they are thought to be irritant at concentrate level (the use of gloves is recommended), they are generally of low toxicity and low corrosion potential.

Dichloroisocyanurates

Sodium dichloroisocyanurate is a chlorine-releasing agent available in tablet/powder or granule form. Advantages are that they have similar disinfectant activities to hypochlorite but less of a corrosive tendency. They are also generally more resistant to inactivation by organic materials and although unstable when made up into solution they are very stable when stored correctly as powder, granules or tablets.

Iodine/iodophors

This group of disinfectants has a wide range of activity including some activity against bacterial spores. Iodine has been used for well over one hundred years in the treatment of wounds. The properties of iodine and iodophors ('iodine carriers') are similar in many ways to the hypochlorites but are most often used on the skin rather than environmentally. It should be noted, however, that some people may be allergic to iodine. Staining can also be a problem with iodine products. Iodophors have an added substance (often a non-ionic surfactant) these products are less irritant and do not stain in the same way as iodine. Povidone-iodine products (water-soluble complex of iodine and polyvinylpyrrolidone) are used in veterinary practice.

Peroxides

Peroxygen compounds (peracetic acid, hydrogen peroxide, potassium monopersulphate, peroxygenated chlorine compounds). Hydrogen peroxide and peracetic acid are oxidising agents that have a wide range of bactericidal, virucidal and fungicidal activity when used appropriately. There is, however, variable sporicidal activity with hydrogen peroxide, but good activity for peracetic acid. The activity is greatly reduced in the presence of organic matter and there can be corrosion of some metals. Hydrogen peroxide has low irritancy and toxicity but peracetic acid is highly toxic and irritant. The characteristics of other peroxygen compounds are similar to those of peracetic acid and hydrogen peroxide but some can be highly corrosive to many metals and break down plasticisers in rubber and plastic products. Manufacturers' approval must be obtained for use of their products with equipment that may be prone to corrosion or degradation.

Biguanides

This group contains chlorhexidine preparations which have low toxicity and irritancy, and are therefore frequently used in skin cleansing agents and surgical scrubs. Biguanides are more active against Gram-positive than Gram-negative bacteria but have no activity against bacterial spores. There is good fungicidal activity but limited activity against viruses. They can be inactivated by organic matter, soap and other anionic detergents.

Alcohols

Alcohols are very effective against many organisms with the notable exception of spores and some viruses (but only if organic material has first been removed). Ethanol (70%) and isopropanol (70%) are used for clean areas such as trolley tops. Hand rubs containing alcohol and other chemicals such as chlorhexidine and glycerine are often used for disinfection of hands between clean tasks. Alcohols are flammable and care should be taken when using and with storage.

Aldehydes

Glutaraldehyde. This chemical has a wide range of bactericidal activity and is known to be active against many bacterial spores and some viruses. Glutaraldehyde is relatively slow acting but organic matter has less effect on its activity than some other disinfectants. Some products containing glutaraldehyde may also have QAC combined. This type of disinfectant is useful for disinfecting some types of equipment that cannot be heat sterilised. Disadvantages include high irritancy and toxicity; it is irritant to the skin, eyes and respiratory mucosa. Glutaraldehyde can also cause sensitisation, leading to further health problems with continued exposure. It is therefore only used where the recommended necessary precautions for user protection can be applied. The Health Service Safety Council recommends that disinfectants employing this substance should not be used as general 'wash down' disinfectants.

Formaldehyde. Formaldehyde is active against many microbes but is considered too irritant to be used as a disinfectant.

Surfactants

Chemical compounds that lower the surface tension of an aqueous solution. Commonly used as wetting agents, detergents and emulsifiers.

The types of surfactant are:

- Anionic.
- Cationic.
- Amphoteric (ampholytic).
- Non-ionic.

Anionic surfactants. These types are generally referred to as soaps. The most important action is the physical emulsification of lipoidal secretions of the skin which contain bacteria; the bacteria are thus suspended in the lather and are rinsed away. The inclusion of certain antiseptics has increased the antibacterial action of anionic surfactants.

Cationic surfactants. The most important example of this type of surfactant is the QACs. QACs have low toxicity and some detergent properties. These disinfectants are more active against Gram-positive than Gram-negative bacteria, have good fungicidal activity, but have variable activity against viruses. They are not active against bacterial spores. They are widely used in the cleansing of food preparation areas. They can be inactivated by many materials including soaps and organic matter. These surfactants are frequently used in products in combination with other chemicals to increase the disinfectant activity. Benzalkonium chloride is one type of QAC used in veterinary practice.

Amphoteric (ampholytic) surfactants. These agents have similar characteristics to the anionic and cationic surfactants in that they have good detergent and bactericidal properties. The food industry uses compounds based on dodecyldi(aminoethyl)glycine.

Non-ionic. The non-ionic surfactants are considered to have no antimicrobial properties; however, polysorbates are believed to weaken some bacteria making them more sensitive to other agents. For example, they are frequently used in iodophor preparations.

Table 5.14 lists some disinfectants that are available, their main active ingredients and recommended uses (for detailed information regarding each product's suitability in veterinary practice, the manufacturer's data sheets should be read).

Disposal of waste

All establishments, whether domestic or industrial, have to dispose of waste materials. Veterinary practices and commercial kennels are classed as industrial users for this purpose.

Since April 1992 the Environmental Protection Act 1990 imposed a 'duty of care' on the disposal of waste classed as Controlled Waste, of which there are three types; household, industrial and commercial. Of particular importance to the veterinary practice is the fact that some of the items in the

Table 5.14 Antiseptics and disinfectants – some examples of types available

Active ingredients	Examples of products	Presentation and recommended use
Phenol compound (black fluids)	Jeyes fluid	Liquid concentrate – environmental use.
Phenol compound (white fluids)	Izal	Liquid concentrate – environmental use.
Phenol compound (clear soluble)	Clearsol	Liquid concentrate – environmental use.
Chloroxylenol (chlorinated phenol)	Dettol	Liquid concentrate – environmental use and skin disinfectant.
Chloroxylenol (chlorinated phenol)	Ibcol	Liquid concentrate – environmental use and skin disinfectant.
Hypochlorites (bleaches)	Chloros	Liquid concentrate – environmental use.
Hypochlorites (bleaches)	Domestos	Liquid concentrate – environmental use.
Halogenated tertiary amine	Trigene	Liquid concentrate – disinfectant cleaner. Environmental use
Sodium tosychloramide	Halamid	Powder concentrate – environmental use.
Sodium dichlorisocyanurate	Vetaclean Parvo	Tablet – environmental use.
Povidone-iodine	Pevidine Antiseptic Soln	Solution – topical application – burns, wounds, etc.
Peroxyacetic acid Acetic acid Hydrogen peroxide surfactants	Vetcide 2000	Liquid concentrate. Environmental use.
Peroxygen compound Inorganic salts, organic acid, anionic detergent	Vircon (concentrate)	Powder. Environmental use.
Chlorhexidine gluconate 4%	Dinex Scrub	Liquid concentrate – pre-op. skin disinfectant.
Chlorhexidine gluconate	Hibiscrub Vet	Rapid bactericidal skin cleanser/surgical scrub.
Chlorhexidine acetate 0.1%	Nolvadent	Solution and spray – oral cleanser.
Chlorhexidine acetate	Nolvasan Surgical Scrub	Solution – skin and wound cleanser.
Chlorhexidine gluconate cetrimide	Savlon Vet Concentrate	Solution – wounds (dilute). Pre-op. instruments.
Glutaraldehyde	Cidex	Liquid concentrate – environmental use.
Glutaraldehyde	Formula H routine spray	Spray – environmental use.
Glutaraldehyde	Formula H concentrated disinfectant	Liquid concentrate – environmental use.
Cetrimide (quaternary ammonium compounds)	Cetavlon	Liquid concentrate – environmental use and skin disinfectant
Ampholytic surfactants	Tego	Liquid concentrate – environmental use.
Quaternary ammonium compound Non-ionic surfactant	Vetaclean	Liquid concentrate – surface disinfectant, sanitising feeding utensils, etc.
Octyl decyl dimethyl ammonium chloride	Quinticare	Liquid concentrate.
Dioctyle dimethyl ammonium Alkyl dimethyl benzyl ammonium chloride	(Quinticide)	Environmental use – especially stainless steel.
Benzalkonium chloride	Roccal	Liquid concentrate – environmental use and skin disinfectant.
Benzalkonium chloride	Marinol Blue	10 or 50% solution. Pre-op. Topical (diluted) or environmental.

Table 5.15 Clinical waste and its disposal

Sharps. Needles, syringes, broken glass, scalpel blades, etc.	Waste containing blood, body fluids, excretions, drugs. Swabs and dressings, blood/body fluids.	Non-agricultural animal carcasses and animal tissue. Non-domestic kennel excreta and bedding.

Unless rendered safe is clinical waste.

Pre-disposal handling

Sharps. Approved sharps container (sealed).	Swabs and soiled disposable bedding. Kennel excrement. Approved yellow containers or bags identifiable (with name and source of waste) prior to collection.	Cadavers. May be deep frozen for storage prior to collection.

Collection by local authority or licensed contractors.
All clinical waste is destroyed by high temperature incinerator, licensed for this use.

Industrial class are further classified as Clinical Waste and it is essential that the veterinary nurse should be aware of items in this category, with particular regard to methods of disposal and how they should be handled and stored prior to disposal. Table 5.15 identifies items classed as clinical waste and their ultimate disposal.

Handling clinical waste

For the health and safety of staff and to comply with the regulations, clinical waste must be handled, segregated and disposed of with great care. See Clinical waste, p. 100. It must be placed in yellow polythene bags marked 'For Incineration Only', with the name and origin of the waste. The specification is in 'The Safe Disposal of Clinical Waste' published by HMSO.

Disposal of clinical waste

All items classed as clinical waste must be disposed of by incineration in a licensed high-temperature incinerator. These incinerators must conform to the regulations regarding clean discharge into the atmosphere.

As clinical waste is classed as Industrial Waste, the duty to arrange for it to be collected and correctly disposed of is with the person who controls it – the veterinary practice is responsible, not the local authority. Some local authorities do offer a service for the disposal of clinical waste but licensed contractors must be used where this service does not exist. The collection and disposal of clinical waste incurs a charge if collected by either local authority or licensed contractors.

In the veterinary context, clinical waste includes carcasses. The veterinary profession has the 'duty of care' for the disposal of dead dogs and cats. The advice of the Department of Environment is that pets which die on veterinary premises remain the property of the owner and may then be disposed of by the owner within the 'curtilage' of their own dwelling in their capacity of a private individual without breach of the veterinarians 'duty of care'.

Bereaved owners may wish to take bodies home with them for disposal (see Chapter 26). If an animal has suffered from an infectious disease, however, or for any other reason may be significantly hazardous, then it should be dealt with by the veterinarian as clinical waste and disposed of by licensed incineration.

Non-clinical practice waste

Non-clinical waste is classed as domestic waste. This includes empty food cans, outer packaging and office waste. (All confidential records should be shredded prior to disposal.) Domestic waste continues to be collected regularly by the local authority. Normal 'day-to-day' deposits of pet owners' dog faeces are also classed as refuse rather than clinical waste. Black plastic bags are commonly used for the refuse that is not classified as clinical waste.

Animal care

Daily care of hospitalised animals

The specific requirements in the care of hospitalised animals depend to some degree on the conditions under treatment. Table 5.16 suggests a care routine.

Defecation and urination

Dogs. The opportunity to defecate and urinate is sometimes referred to as 'relief' and sometimes as 'exercise'. Most hospitalised dogs require restricted exercise but frequent opportunities to relieve themselves. It is therefore less confusing to refer to 'opportunity for relief' rather than 'exercise' in this context.

All dogs should be taken to a run and given frequent opportunities for relief, unless they are not mobile or movement is contraindicated by their condition. It is important not to leave a dog so long that it is forced to urinate

Table 5.16 Care routine for hospitalised animals

Check	Care routine
General check	All animals are inspected briefly by touring the kennels/cages. This is to establish that there are no urgent problems that require immediate attention.
Individual checks	Each individual should be looked at for some time, noting the behaviour of the animal compared with its normal, e.g. whether it is lively, aggressive, unresponsive. Its posture should be noted – whether it is standing, lying down or in an abnormal position.
Observe respiration	This should be done before the animal is disturbed.
Pulse and temperature	The animal's pulse and temperature may be taken (before exercise).
Soiling, etc.	Check for soiling of kennel, and record details of quantity and type of eliminations. If the animal has urinated or defecated, note if it is normal. If the animal has vomited, note the appearance or amount, assess what has been eaten and record the observation before removing it. It is not usual practice to leave food in with dogs overnight except in the case of difficult or shy feeders. It is more frequently necessary to leave food in with cats, as overnight is often the only time that some hospitalised cats will eat.
Check the water bowl	Note how much has been taken and if any spilling has occurred (if there is spilling the assessment of intake will be inaccurate).
Physical check on patient	Any abnormalities should be noted and recorded. Wounds may be inspected. Any discharges should be gently removed.

or defecate in its kennel, which would cause considerable distress to normally clean house-trained dogs.

When the dog is taken to a run, its gait and general body stance should be noted. When it passes urine and faeces, any difficulty should be noted along with the appearance and the amount passed.

Reluctance to urinate or defecate in kennel runs. A reluctant dog should not be returned to its kennel until every effort has been made to encourage it to urinate and defecate. This is particularly important if the dog has been confined for a long period (such as overnight) and has not soiled its kennel.

Some dogs are reluctant to relieve themselves with the handler in close proximity. If so, retire a suitable distance to observe. If the dog is still reluctant, it may be unused to defecating on a hard surface such as concrete or slabs (as described in the discussion on kennel design earlier in this chapter). These dogs may be used to relieving on grass or soil surfaces, and it may need a little ingenuity to encourage them. Initial effort will ensure less stress to the dog and will save time for the handler on future occasions as the dog should relieve itself without delay once it understands the routine.

Put some sawdust or peat on a small area at the end of a run and then praise the dog when it urinates or defecates there, so that it understands that this is the right place. The sawdust or peat can be lifted along with any urine or faeces and the run cleaned as normal.

If this ploy fails, it may be necessary to walk the dog for some distance and then 'leash relieve' it on grass. However, this is not generally recommended as it is unhygienic: grass cannot be disinfected. (Dogs with suspected infectious disease should never be relieved on an area that cannot be adequately disinfected.)

Cats. All hospitalised cats should be provided with a litter tray unless their condition contraindicates. Clean the tray regularly and record the presence and characteristics of the faeces and urine produced. If the tray is not cleaned frequently enough, some cats are so fastidious that they will not reuse the tray but will soil elsewhere in the kennel.

Some cats prefer privacy, which can be provided by covering the litter tray with an upturned box with an entrance hole cut into it.

Feeding

All animals should be observed when feeding to check that they are eating normally and without difficulty.

Each animal should have the same feed and water bowls throughout its stay to reduce the possibility of cross-infection. The bowls can be labelled or numbered to identify them with the kennel or animal.

Medication

Adhere strictly to any specific medication times, as instructed by the veterinary surgeon. Keep up-to-date records of all medications given.

Where medication has been given with food, check that the food has been consumed.

Weighing

All dogs should be weighed on entry to the hospital and weekly thereafter. This is important with long-stay animals to ensure that the feeding and exercise regime maintains the dog's condition and that any loss of weight due to illness is monitored and reported.

Grooming of hospitalised animals

Every effort should be made to keep hospitalised animals in a hygienic and comfortable condition. The grooming of hospitalised dogs should be carried out as part of their general nursing care, unless their condition contraindicates it (e.g. an animal admitted for warfarin poisoning should not be handled vigorously – see Chapter 3).

Grooming as part of normal animal care

There are various reasons why grooming is beneficial and all of them can be placed broadly under five headings:

- **C**leanliness.
- **H**ealth.
- **A**ppearance.
- **I**nspection.
- **R**elationship.

The initial letters of these headings form a useful memory aid: CHAIR.

Cleanliness

Keeping the animal clean by the removal of dirt and discharge and assisting in the casting of hair contributes towards the animal's health and well-being. At home, the regular grooming of dogs and cats reduces the amount of hair deposited on furniture and carpets.

It is important that animals with dense or long coats are groomed regularly, as their coats rapidly become tangled, matted and soiled.

Health

By keeping the animal's coat clean, grooming assists the condition of the skin and hair and thus contributes to the animal's health:

- Grooming stimulates anagen (the hair growth stage) by the removal of dead, shedding hairs.
- The removal of discharge and prevention of matting prevents skin irritation.
- The close inspection of the animal during grooming assists in early problem recognition.
- During grooming, daily care and attention to any bony prominences, skin folds, feet and claws, eyes and ears, mouth and teeth, anus, vulva and prepuce contribute to the health of the animal.

Appearance

Owners usually give this as the first reason for grooming, though it is the least important for the animal itself. Many owners take a pride in the appearance of their animals – and this becomes very apparent when a post-operative animal with large areas of denuded skin is returned to an owner who was not forewarned. Owners of pedigree dogs often want their pets to look like the breed as seen at championship dog shows and this means that many dogs are trimmed and clipped by professional groomers, a practice that also assists the owner's daily grooming of the dog. The appearance of the true show dog is of major concern to its owner and show preparation often involves hours of careful grooming and trimming or clipping.

The veterinary nurse needs to appreciate this emphasis on appearance: many owners, rightly or wrongly, judge the standard of care at the practice or kennels by the appearance of the animal when it is returned to them.

Inspection

The daily inspection of an animal during the grooming routine contributes to its health by giving an opportunity for early recognition of problems. For example, flea excreta will only be discovered on close examination of the coat. It is recommended that inspection is carried out in a logical daily sequence so that any problems found can be attended to before further damage or discomfort is caused to the animal during the actual grooming.

Relationship and contact

This may seem a strange reason for grooming, but for the dog in the wild state grooming is part of pack socialisation activities. Dogs lower in the pack order submit to grooming by a more dominant member, while dominant dogs make it clear whether or not they consent to being groomed by other members of the pack. When dogs are groomed by their handlers, the activity strengthens the bond between them and confirms to the dog its place in the hierarchy: the handler is the 'pack leader'. The act of grooming, therefore, should assist in the handling and training of the dog.

Grooming can also assist in teaching a dog to sit or stand still whilst the procedure is carried out, which will be of great assistance for veterinary examinations. If a dog resents grooming for no physical reason, it is likely to prove generally difficult to handle.

Introducing an animal to grooming

Ideally the process of grooming should be introduced (to all domesticated species) at a very young age as part of socialisation and habituation. Even short-haired puppies and kittens should be handled each day and introduced gently to brushes and combs. The experience should be made pleasant for the animal, with praise given for good behaviour but a firm tone if the animal struggles.

Table 5.17 Factors affecting hair growth and type

Factors	The average rate of hair growth in the dog is 0.5 mm per day. An average smooth-coat type takes about 6 months to regrow completely. Fine, silky long-haired coats take up to 18 months; a similar growth rate can be expected in cats.
Environmental temperature and time of year	Dogs kept in housing with constantly high environmental temperatures (usually centrally heated) will often shed hair almost continuously throughout the year but with noticeable increases in spring and autumn. Shedding in dogs kennelled out of doors or with less environmental heating tends to be more obviously seasonal – shedding is very noticeable in spring and autumn. This seasonal coat change is a natural process triggered by increasing day length in spring and decreasing day length in autumn.

	Spring = increasing day length
	      Production of summer coat triggered
	      Increased hair shedding (of winter coat)
	      Coarser coat with reduced density
	plus
	      Increased sebaceous gland activity
	
	                = Summer coat
	
	      Allowing increased air circulation through coat

	Autumn = decreasing day length
	      Production of winter coat triggered
	      Increased hair shedding (of summer coat)
	plus
	      New coat growth and reduced sebaceous gland activity
	
	                = Winter coat
	
	Increased coat density = Insulation against the cold.

Health and reproductive status	Condition can often be assessed by observing the coat and noting any unseasonal loss or thinning of hair. Thinning during periods of ill health is due to interruption of the growth cycle: fewer individual hairs are in the growth stage. An animal suffering from ill health may also have a dull and harsh coat. The reproductive status of an animal can have an effect on the coat growth and this can be quite obvious during pregnancy and lactation and occasionally after neutering. These and other so-called hormonal alopecias usually involve thinning of hair on certain areas of the body.
Feeding and nutrition	Diet affects hair growth, as it does all other functions. Nutrients essential for good health of skin and hair include amino acids, essential fatty acids, zinc, iodine, etc. (see Chapter 8).

Table 5.18 Coat types

Coat	Type	Example
Most coat types can be divided into five broad groups for the purpose of grooming:		
1. **Smooth coat**	Short fine	Boxer, Dachshund, Chihuahua.
	Intermediate or coarse	German shepherd dog, Pembroke corgi. Wild dogs and wolves have
	Dense	this coat type and it is therefore sometimes referred to as a normal coat.
2. **Wire coat**		Wire-haired terriers.
3. **Double coat**		Rough collie, long-haired German shepherd dog.
4. **Silky coat**	Medium	Most spaniels, setters and some retrievers.
	Long fine	Afghan hounds, Bearded collies.
5. **Woolly coat**		Poodle, Bedlington terrier, Curly-coated retriever, Irish water spaniel.

There are some more unusual or specialised coat types, such as corded coats. Where animals with such coats are under the nurse's care, a professional groomer or the individual breed society should be contacted for specific advice if the owner is unable to provide details on coat maintenance.

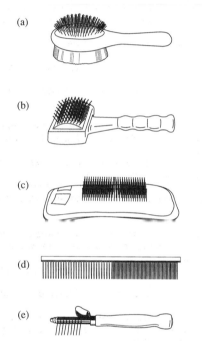

Fig. 5.5 Grooming equipment: (a) double-sided grooming brush (pins and bristles), (b) slicker brush, (c) hound glove, (d) metal grooming comb, (e) de-matting comb.

As with all training, grooming should be carried out for a few minutes at a time at first and gradually built up as the animal becomes accustomed to it. Each session should end on a successful note with the animal being praised for compliance.

Owners of long-haired animals should in particular be advised that time spent in the early stages of ownership will ensure that the animal is easier to groom in later years and is less likely to be presented at the practice for de-matting when an owner is unable to groom the pet because it objects, struggles or even attempts to bite.

Routine grooming

Routine grooming is part of the daily care of a normal healthy animal but the veterinary nurse can be faced with

quite a problem as there are so many different types of coat. In addition, various factors have a direct effect on the coat and it is necessary to have a broad understanding of them so that the coat can be correctly maintained while the animal is in the nurse's care and so that owners' queries regarding grooming at home can be answered. It can be seen from Table 5.17 that the major factors affecting hair growth include:

- Environmental temperature and time of year.
- Health.
- Endocrine and reproductive status.
- Feeding and nutrition.

The type of coat is governed by combinations of individual hair types that make up the coat. These are the rigid primary or 'guard' hairs and the soft, thinner secondary or 'lanugo' hairs. The various proportions, lengths and weights of these hair types account for the many and varied types of coat seen in dogs and cats (Table 5.18).

Grooming equipment and methods

A fairly wide range of attention and equipment is required to deal with the various types of coat. For the routine maintenance grooming of patients and boarders, it is advisable to stock a range of basic grooming equipment (Table 5.19 and Fig. 5.5).

Although different coats require different attention, a logical general sequence can be adopted for all common breeds to ensure that nothing is missed out during the grooming session:

- Assess the animal's temperament.
- Carry out a physical inspection of the animal (Table 5.20).
- Loosen dead hair.
- Comb, brush and finish (Table 5.21).

De-matting

Sometimes the coat of a long-haired animal has been so grossly neglected and become so matted that it would be unkind to try to de-mat it while the animal is conscious. The

Table 5.19 Grooming and trimming equipment

	Types	Features and use
Brushes	Pin brush	Metal pins with rounded ends, mounted on a rubber back cushion. If used correctly, cannot break or pull out hair. The straight pins are able to be used more effectively than bristle with silky coats. Used for general grooming-out of silky and double coats and on feathering. Used to separate hairs and smooth and lay the coat. The action assists in promoting a smooth shine by distributing natural oils. Not so useful for tangled coats (a comb should be used first).
	Bristle brush	Often wooden or plastic with natural or synthetic bristles, with or without a handle. Denser than pin brushes and less able to brush through thick coats to achieve hair separation. Used for removal of dirt and debris. As the bristles are flexible, can be used with more pressure: flicks dirt deep in the coat on to the surface and then removes it with the following brush action. To remove dirt and debris from most types of coat, is most commonly used for routine grooming of short-coated breeds. For short coats it can be used fairly vigorously on the animal's back, sides, hindquarters and shoulders.
	Slicker brush	One-way hooked pins on a rubber pad. Stiff and softer pinned varieties are available. The hooks assist in pulling out dead hair. The action can be quite fierce and care should be taken with its use. Pressure should not be used as the hooks easily damage the dog's skin. Usually designed for one-way use only, towards the handle; the operator pulls the brush through the coat. Very useful for removing dead hair clogging coats and can be used to break up some coat tangles. Commonly used in the grooming of dogs with silky coats (especially feathering), wire, woolly and double coats.
	Hound glove	Designed to fit over the hand; flexible, with either short wire or plastic bristles, small plastic projections or a velvet surface or similar type of material. Often double sided with short bristles one side and velvet on the opposite side. As the glove is flexible it allows palm pressure and vigorous use (heavy pressure and vigorous use should be avoided with wire bristle types). Can be used to assist moulting by removing dead hair, with the smooth velvet side being used to promote a shine. Commonly used for the routine grooming of short-coated breeds.
Combs	Metal combs	Two types of comb commonly used for dog grooming: handle and non-handle comb. Both are ridged combs with metal rounded teeth, available in various tooth widths depending on density of coats being groomed. Handle comb has one size of teeth at one end and handle at the other. Easier to use for a longer period than a non-handle comb. Advantage of a non-handle comb is that it usually has two widths of teeth on the one comb. The combs are used only with the lay of the hair, at approximately 45° angle. Used for removing dead hair and the selective grooming of longer hair behind ears in silky coats etc. Also used for de-tangling and breaking up small mats.
	Rake	Ridged metal teeth with rounded ends set perpendicular to the handle. Designed to achieve a greater pull through dense coats. Great care should be used with the rake as damage can easily be inflicted on the dog's skin. Commonly used with dense coats for removal of dead undercoat and breaking up and removal of some small mats (with great care).
	De-matting comb	Specialised teeth, rounded and blunt on one side with sharp blades on the opposite side of each tooth. Substantial handle and thumb grip. Only used to cut out mats; it is a much safer way to remove mats than by the use of scissors. Used by placing blunt side towards the animal's skin and drawing the sharp edge against the mat, thus cutting and breaking up the mat for removal. Allows the maximum amount of coat to be preserved once the mat is removed.
Scissors	Trimming scissors	Long very sharp blades tapering to a point. Different sizes available. Used to trim neatly around the edges of ears, etc.
	Toe scissors	Short blades with blunt ends. Used to trim delicate areas between toes, etc.
	Thinning scissors	Specialised blades cut small amounts of hair and leave an equal amount uncut at intervals with easy use. The hair is thinned by this action without leaving 'steps' in the coat. Used anywhere the coat requires thinning to enhance features, e.g. the shoulders, sides of chest.

Table 5.20 Physical inspection routine before grooming

Aims	Method
Assess the state of the animal's coat and therefore the need for the use of non-routine equipment such as the de-matting comb.	The inspection should be carried out in a logical sequence, checking the dog from head to tail, checking closely both visually and by running the hands carefully over the animal. Areas requiring special attention, particularly with elderly or hospitalised animals, include:
Assess the state of the animal's health. This is very important as it ensures close observation of the animal so that lesions normally obscured by the coat are found prior to the use of any equipment that may cause injury to the animal. (It is too late to find a wart once you have stuck the comb in it causing it to bleed!)	Mouth, teeth, gums and lip folds. Eyes and ears – discharges wiped away with clean damp cotton wool. In some breeds the long hair on the ears (and face) may gather food whilst the animal is eating. This should be removed by washing. Either trim the hair carefully to prevent recurrence; or, for a pedigree breed where this long hair is a feature, make a note to use a 'snood' when feeding the dog (these hold the long hair and ears back during feeding and are often used for Afghan hounds) or a narrow but deep feeding bowl that allows the long hair and ears to fall on each side of the bowl and not in the food. Hocks and elbows – any pressure sores noted and attended to (improve bedding and apply white petroleum jelly if there is hard skin but no sign of breaks in the skin). Foot pads – may be cracking, or in dogs that pace about continually in hard-surfaced runs they may be reddened and thin due to the abrasive action. Claws – these should be checked for injury and condition (e.g. they may be overgrown when a dog has restricted exercise or is walked on grass). Some dogs that have a long-term abnormal gait may wear their claws unevenly, resulting in the need to trim some of the claws on a regular basis. Body orifices – anus, vulva and prepuce may require the regular removal of discharges/soiling. With long-haired animals it may be necessary to trim or clip away some of the surrounding hair to allow easier cleaning of these areas. Any treatment or attention to any abnormalities found should be dealt with at this stage.

neglect may have arisen because the animal has been so difficult to groom when conscious anyway.

In such cases the veterinary surgeon might sedate or anaesthetise the animal and request the veterinary nurse to 'de-mat' it. This should be carried out with great care: it is very easy to cut the skin and scissors should not be used by unskilled nurses. Cats are especially at risk when hair lumps are cut away.

Clipping and trimming

Under normal circumstances a nurse is unlikely to be involved in the long-term maintenance of a coat that requires clipping or trimming. However, it is essential that all those who care for hospitalised animals should know how to look after a variety of coat types.

The routine clipping or trimming of some areas in long-haired dogs will assist in maintaining cleanliness but care should be taken not to take the scissors to an animal without its owner's consent – it may be a pedigree show dog, which needs experienced clipping and trimming.

The clipping, hand stripping and trimming of specific breeds is generally within the realms of the professional dog groomer and showing kennel. Interested veterinary nurses can attend special courses on this art but in general practice it is more usual for a nurse to clip or trim a pet dog at its owner's request because the animal is difficult or impossible to groom. This may be due to the animal's temperament, or because the dog is elderly or infirm with perhaps an elderly owner. In the latter case, trimming and clipping may be carried out as part of a geriatric care policy (for the dog, that is). Where temperament is the problem, it is

usually necessary to sedate the dog or, in extreme cases, to anaesthetise it as already discussed for de-matting.

In general practice, then, the veterinary nurse needs to know how to use common equipment for trimming or clipping a dog neatly and tidily. The regular trimming of some types of coat assists grooming and general hygiene, while clipping can assist in grooming by keeping the coat short enough to be managed easily.

Trimming is carried out with special scissors. Areas that are commonly trimmed to assist in grooming are those prone to matting or collection of soiling in breeds such as some spaniels and setters. This includes the ears, to avoid the collection of food when eating, and the matting of the long silky hair just behind the ears. Feet are trimmed particularly between the toes, where mud can collect and dry on the hair so that it causes discomfort by rubbing and by pushing the toes apart. In bitches, it may be necessary to trim soiled areas post-whelping if soiling and staining from whelping fluid cannot be removed easily any other way.

If a dog soils itself or mats easily, grooming will be simplified if hair is judiciously trimmed from the anal area and hindleg feathering – but do not be scissor-happy. Strike a balance between the need to keep the dog hygienic and the owner's need for the dog's appearance to be acceptable.

Clipping is by means of special clippers. There are set styles of clip designed to enhance breed features, e.g. some of the hair of terrier breeds is removed or thinned out by professional hand-stripping. Non-showing owners of breeds with long, heavy coats such as the Old English sheep dog will have their animals clipped out for the summer. Dogs such as poodles do not moult normally and it is essential to clip the coat regularly, otherwise it would become

Table 5.21 Grooming procedures	
Procedure	**Aim**
Loosening the dead hair	Most coats will benefit from the groomer pulling the fingertips along the skin through the coat against the lay of the hair. This will help to loosen the dead hair and therefore stimulate normal hair growth. Dogs tend to find this procedure pleasant and some will get excited and see it as a game, so firm but friendly handling is required to insist that the dog stays fairly still.
Combing	Using a traditional comb, any tangles can be eased out gently and any loose hair removed from the coat at this stage. The comb is used with the lay of the hair at an angle usually about 45°.
	Particular attention should be paid to areas on the longer haired breeds that have a tendency to tangle and mat such as behind the ears and feathering between and on the backs of the hindlegs. As the comb is more accurate than a brush and is usually smaller it can be used with care on areas that are difficult to assess, ensuring that no areas are missed or tangles remain underneath a superficially groomed coat. If mats are found during combing and they are not able to be removed or teased out gently during a traditional comb, then a specialised de-matting comb can be used where appropriate to remove the mat, followed by a combing out of the remaining hair gently with the traditional comb. Where a mat has been removed it is important to check the skin underneath it for damage as the area may be reddened or even suppurating. If the mat has caused irritation to the skin, this should be dealt with, depending on the severity.
Brushing	This is carried out with a brush type depending upon the coat; the action of brushing depends on the brush. Exercise great care when grooming with pin or slicker brushes, as it is possible to damage the skin with some types if used too vigorously. It is not generally advisable to use this type of brush against the lay of the hair.
	For a smooth coat of the intermediate type the following brushing technique could be adopted:
	Once the combing is complete a bristly brush can be used.
	Firstly it is used on the hair covering the trunk. The brush is used against the lay of the hair in short straight strokes. This is begun at the base of the tail and thighs and moves gradually forward as each area is brushed.
	The brushing against the lay stops at the back of the head and at the base of the skull, leaving the head untouched at this stage.
	The brush is then used gently on the head with the lay of the hair and thereafter working downwards and backwards with short straight strokes, until the entire body and legs have been brushed.
	Taking hold of the tail, gently but firmly brush carefully from base to tip. Care is required when grooming tails as many dogs are quite sensitive about their tails being groomed and some may react sharply to all but the most gentle brushing.
	During the brushing phase the brush should be periodically cleaned to remove any build-up of hair. This can be done by drawing a traditional comb through the bristles.
Finishing	After combing and brushing, a smooth or silky medium type of coat can be finished off by using a damp cloth or smooth hound glove (or a piece of velvet or damp synthetic chamois cloth).
	The face is gently wiped over followed by the remainder of the body, working from front to back.
	This action smooths down the coat and removes stray hair and dust from the coat surface, giving a sleek shine to a healthy coat. This is not done generally with coats that are of the woolly or wire coat type, as these are usually required to stand up and are brushed into shape and left.

unmanageable for the owner and would cause discomfort and distress to the dog.

Clippers should only be used according to the manufacturer's instructions as they are easily damaged by misuse. For example, the hair must be completely dry, as wet hair quickly blunts the blades. The blades should not be forced through a thick coat or matting as they may be clogged by the hair and stop the machine, possibly causing damage to the equipment. If the clippers become hot during use, they should be allowed to cool down before continuing.

Clipping machines should be regularly serviced and maintained. They need to be thoroughly cleaned and oiled after each use and then stored in a dry environment. A variety of blades should be available, with spares of those used most commonly to enable a rotation for regular sharpening.

Bathing

Bathing is carried out for three main reasons:

- To eradicate and control ectoparasites.
- To treat skin conditions and apply topical medication.
- To cleanse and condition the coat.

Cleansing may be required for various reasons, such as:

- The coat is soiled with a substance that cannot be removed by normal grooming.
- To remove odours (e.g. when a dog has rolled in excreta).
- To assist in the removal and masking of the scent from a bitch just out of season who is still receiving the attention of male dogs.
- To improve the appearance of the coat before a show.

Shampoo

There are many products for shampooing dogs. Some are generally available; others (for specialised medical or antiparasitic use) are only available by prescription. The preparations fall into three categories:

- Insecticidal (to eradicate and control parasites, most commonly fleas, lice and ticks).
- Medicated (containing some form of antiseptic or other active ingredient and prescribed for dogs with minor skin problems).
- Cleansing (general purpose or also for conditioning).

The latter category includes those most widely used – shampoos for general coat cleansing. A conditioning agent is often added to improve the hair texture by lubrication, so that the coat is more manageable for brushing out when dry.

Specialised shampoos are available from the pet trade for different types of coat. The two most notable are the 'mild' shampoo for puppies and dogs with sensitive skins, and 'colour enhancing' shampoos for particular coats, such as products containing optical whiteners for white coats.

Note that if the shampoo is in a glass bottle the amount required should be decanted into a plastic cup or a similar small, unbreakable receptacle before bathing commences. A small amount of water may be added to the shampoo at this stage so that it is easier to distribute when applied to the dog's coat.

Dog baths

The ideal dog bath should:

- Allow the handler to get the dog in and out of the bath easily but also to contain the dog safely, deterring escape.
- Allow access to all parts of the dog being bathed without the handler having to bend or reach excessively.
- Have a non-slip area for the animal to stand on, with the surrounding area also non-slip for the safety of the handler.
- Have a flexible shower hose with a spray head.
- Have easily adjustable water and heat controls.
- Have an easily cleaned surface allowing access for cleaning all parts of the bath.

Many specially designed dog baths are available from the pet trade but in some small establishments, where the bathing of dogs is not carried out regularly, it is possible to modify other installations, e.g. non-slip mats can be added to a shower cubicle in which the floor has been raised and the shower-hose and controls lowered, or the mats can be added to a bath designed for a disabled person and fitted with a shower-hose.

The domestic bath. Clients who bath their dogs in a domestic bath should always be advised to use a non-slip mat and that they should not put the plug in the bath. An inexpensive mixer shower-hose can be fitted to the bath taps. Clients should be warned that some modern domestic baths scratch easily and can be damaged by the claws of a scrambling dog.

Drying the dog. Several towels are needed to dry a dog after it has been bathed. It is always advisable to put out at least two extra ones, to save having to search for more towels while a half-dry dog shakes itself and distributes water all around the bathing area.

The number of towels needed can be reduced by first using a synthetic chamois cloth to remove excess water. This can be wrung out several times and reused before towels finish the drying off.

Dogs that are bathed regularly may be familiar with hair-driers but these can frighten a dog that is new to the experience. Never blow the drier towards the dog's face.

Instead, blow towards the hind end from the front, moving towards the rear and directing the hot air along the hair shaft, not directly at the skin. Continuously test the heat by keeping a hand in front of the air jet at the approximate distance of the dog's skin. The same hand can assist the drying process by lifting the dog's hair, running the fingers through to ruffle the coat.

The dog should be sitting comfortably. Panting or shivering would indicate distress or discomfort.

Protective clothing

It should be standard practice for the handler to wear protective clothing when bathing a dog. It not only keeps the handler's clothes dry but may also be required for safety. The usual clothing is:

- Waterproof overall or apron.
- Water-resistant boots or shoes with non-slip soles.
- Protective gloves where suggested by a shampoo manufacturer. (Those who have sensitive skin may prefer to wear protective gloves anyway.)

Handling and restraint for bathing

All dogs must be adequately restrained during bathing. A large wet dog leaping out of a bath can injure both itself and handler, and back injuries are not uncommon. A collar and lead, or nylon slip-lead, should be looped over the handler's arm so that it is readily accessible if restraint is required. With a large or boisterous dog, it is advisable to have a second person to steady or restrain it.

WARNINGS

- A dog should never be encouraged or allowed to jump in or out of the bath at any time, as it may easily slip on a wet surface and injure itself.
- A dog should never be left unattended in a bath, as it may try to jump out, injuring itself if it slips.
- A dog should never be tied up in the bath as it could leap over the side and strangle itself in a few seconds while the handler reaches away.

Where there are no steps for the dog to be encouraged to walk into the bath, it will require to be lifted. With large dogs, this should be carried out by two people for safety.

Bathing procedure

The procedure for bathing dogs depends to some extent on the reason for the bath. The following is a general procedure for coat cleansing:

(1) Know why the dog is being bathed.
(2) Assess the dog's temperament and arrange assistance if necessary.

(3) Assemble all the equipment and prepare the bathing area.

(4) Put on protective clothing.

(5) Bring the dog into the bathing area and encourage it up steps into the bath, or lift it in (with help if needed).

(6) Reassure the dog and start water flow away from the dog, running the water over a hand until a constant acceptable temperature is maintained.

(7) Carefully apply the water, soaking the dog well but taking care not to alarm it. Protect the dog's eyes with a hand and do not spray water directly on to its face.

(8) Apply shampoo sparingly to the entire coat but avoid sensitive areas such as the face, or into the vulva or sheath. (If the head requires particular attention due to a medical condition, protect the eyes by applying a bland eye ointment or smearing the lids with petroleum jelly.)

(9) Massage shampoo into the coat, or use as directed (e.g. leave it on for the recommended time before rinsing).

(10) Rinse thoroughly, starting at the upper front and moving in a downwards and backwards sequence so that every part is thoroughly rinsed.

(11) Squeeze out excess water; then remove as much water as possible with a synthetic chamois leather cloth, squeezing it out as necessary and reapplying.

(12) Remove the dog from the bath, either by encouraging it to step out or by lifting it carefully.

(13) Towel-dry.

(14) Use hair-drier if it is safe to do so (keep electric driers away from risk of contact with water) and if the dog's temperament permits.

(15) Return the dog to a warm kennel to avoid chilling.

(16) Record that the bath has been carried out, stating what shampoo has been used.

Dental care (oral hygiene)

Dental disease is one of the most common problems seen in veterinary practice and the veterinary nurse is increasingly involved with client education in this respect. Many owners of show animals have been carrying out some form of teeth-cleaning for cosmetic reasons for some years but the routine brushing of pets' teeth as part of the daily grooming procedure has been overlooked by most pet owners until quite recently. Changes in the consistency of petfood have led to a greater need for routine teeth-cleaning, which is now recognised as necessary for dental health and therefore referred to correctly as 'oral maintenance'. For optimum results, all teeth should be cleaned daily.

Toothbrushes and toothpaste

Animal toothbrushes have bristles that are designed to enable the operator to reach and clean under the gumline, and the small spaces that surround each tooth where plaque readily accumulates. Other cleaning methods can be used to accustom the animal to the cleaning routine such as the use of pads and swabs; these can only remove the plaque above

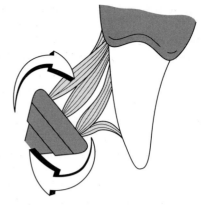

Fig. 5.6 The most effective way of tooth-brushing. Reproduced by kind permission of the St Jon VRx Products Ltd.

the gumline, therefore brushing is by far superior. The selection of the correct toothbrush is very important. Initially a finger brush can be used for dogs to accustom them to the feel of bristles before progression on to a toothbrush. There are now available brushes, specifically designed for dogs, with a long handle and dual-ends for easy access to all areas. Cats also require a specially designed toothbrush as they have very little room between the back teeth and inside of their cheeks.

Toothpaste specifically designed for dogs and cats should be used as the toothpaste designed for humans can lead to problems such as fluoride toxicity and excessive sodium intake when used with dogs and cats. Additionally the flavours of human toothpastes are less than appealing to dogs and cats.

Introducing an animal to the oral hygiene procedure

Advice regarding the method of cleaning teeth and the introduction of an animal to the procedure is offered by the manufacturers of the various products that are now widely available. Some general considerations are as follows:

- Before attempting oral maintenance, always assess the temperament of the animal and handle accordingly, but always proceed with caution.
- As with all training it is better (where possible) to begin by simulating the procedure while the animal is still very young, so that it become accustomed to being handled in this way.
- The experience should be as pleasant as possible for the animal.
- Always reward good behaviour but be firm if the animal struggles or misbehaves.
- Exercise patience and do not try to proceed too quickly. Initially, do not expect the animal to tolerate the brushing for more than a few minutes at a time.
- Incorporate short rest breaks into the routine to avoid the animal becoming uncomfortable and restless.

Practical application. Begin by gently handling the animal's mouth daily and praising good behaviour. Increase the handling time to 5 minutes or so after a few days.

Once the animal tolerates the handling, hold its mouth closed with one hand, opening the mouth on one side and gently rub the teeth with a finger of the other hand. When this stage is tolerated, use a toothbrush on a few teeth and increase the number brushed as the animal becomes accustomed to the experience.

When the animal has accepted brushing of the outside of its teeth, gently pull its top jaw upwards to open its mouth. Gently introduce the brush into the mouth to clean the inner surfaces of the teeth, again increasing the number brushed as the animal becomes accustomed to the procedure. Finger-stall toothbrushes are useful for cleaning the inside of dogs' teeth. The most effective way of brushing is to point the bristles upwards while brushing the upper teeth and downwards for brushing the lower teeth. This angling allows cleaning of the small space that surrounds each tooth where the gum meets it. See Fig. 5.6.

Clipping claws

The average healthy animal does not usually require attention to its claws which, under normal circumstances, wear naturally with everyday use – with the notable exception of the 'dew claw' (though this claw tends to be slow growing). Dogs that have dew claws should be checked regularly for signs of abnormal length or the claw curling into the skin.

Where disease, injury or any type of immobility occurs, the claws may overgrow. This can lead to further immobility if the claws have grown to such as extent that they prevent or restrict the animal's normal gait. In extreme cases the claws may be so long that they curl around and begin to grow in towards the foot pad, causing the animal discomfort or even pain if the skin is penetrated.

Where animals do require some attention, the problem usually arises in one of the following categories:

- Animals that are only exercised on soft ground. (Dogs exercised on grass only, particularly very lightweight ones, are more likely to require claw-clipping than those that do a lot of road work or use concrete or similar runs daily.)
- Animals whose normal behaviour or exercise is restricted by their housing and management. (This includes most small mammals kept as pets – the problems of rabbits and budgerigars, for example, are discussed in Chapter 10.)
- Elderly animals that are unable to exercise normally. (Dogs that are stiff or generally less active due to old age are more likely to require regular attention to their claws.)
- Dogs with immobilised fractured limbs. (The nails will not wear on the injured limb and therefore need to be trimmed while the leg is immobile.)
- Animals with injury or disease conditions of the foot or nail. (The claws of a foot affected by disease need to be trimmed. A nail that is partly broken off will need to be trimmed.)
- Previous injury to the foot or leg causing abnormal gait. (Previous injuries such as fractures or damaged tendons may cause a change in the normal gait, leading to uneven wearing of some of the claws.)

- Puppies in the nest. (The claws of nursing pups are very sharp and grow rapidly, and the bitch's glands can become very sore from their scratches. To prevent or reduce damage to the lactating bitch, clip the puppies' claws weekly.)
- Animals causing damage to owners' property. (Cat owners often request claw-clipping when a pet damages their furniture. Waterbeds are especially at risk. However, clipping of cat claws is a controversial issue and only of very short-term usefulness in this situation. Instead owners should be encouraged to provide scratching-posts.)

Equipment

Essential equipment for claws includes clippers suitable for the size and thickness of the claw. There are various types available. They should be kept sharp and in good working order and should always be used as recommended by the manufacturer.

In case bleeding occurs due to inadvertent cutting of the quick, have cotton wool to hand and a silver nitrate pencil (to be applied with care).

Procedure for claw-clipping

(1) The animal should be suitably restrained and reassured throughout the procedure.
(2) Take the foot firmly, using thumb or fingers to push up each toe in turn and fully expose the nail.
(3) Inspect each nail in turn for damage and length of quick (if it can be seen – if the nail is black the quick will not be seen). A very bright light is helpful.

(a)

(b)

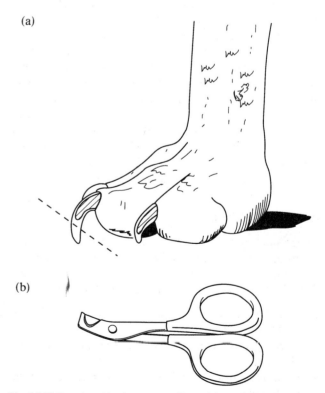

Fig. 5.7 Nail-cutting: (a) where to cut, (b) special cat claw scissors for precise trimming.

(4) If the quick is visible, place the clippers below the quick and cut the nail at an angle (Fig. 5.7). Do this with a rapid action before the animal detects pressure and attempts to withdraw its foot.

(5) Take great care not to cut into the quick – it causes pain. An animal that has been caused pain during claw-clipping is likely to be very uncooperative and distressed on all future occasions.

(6) If the quick is not visible, estimate where it should be. Apply slight pressure with the clippers and note the animal's reaction. If necessary, revise the estimated position and cut well below it. Err on the side of caution: it is better to make one or two safe small trial cuts than to make one large cut that causes pain and bleeding.

(7) If the animal reacts strongly, watch for bleeding. If bleeding does occur it may be stemmed by pressure from a pad of cotton wool. If bleeding persists, traditional styptics such as friar's balsam can be applied with a cotton bud but a silver nitrate pencil, applied with great care, is more effective.

(8) Once each foot is completed, move to the next. Check each time for the presence of a dew claw, which can easily be hidden in long-haired dogs.

(9) Once the procedure is over, always praise the animal for compliance. A food reward may be offered at the end.

Quarantine and isolation

The terms 'quarantine' and 'isolation' both refer to the separation and segregation of animals to protect and prevent the transfer of infectious disease. This usually means that an animal which is infected, or is suspected of being infected, is housed in such a way as to prevent other animals coming into contact with the disease-causing organisms.

In the UK, 'quarantine' usually refers to a period of detention of animals entering the country from overseas to avoid introducing infections, especially the virus disease, rabies. 'Isolation' is a situation of reduced contact with infectious disease, e.g. in an isolation kennel at a veterinary hospital or boarding kennels. In the case of 'protective isolation', an uninfected but susceptible animal – a very young one, perhaps, or an animal with a lowered resistance (e.g. a post-surgical case) – is itself housed in such a way as to prevent its contact with disease-causing organisms.

Methods of isolation

The methods used for isolation or quarantine depend upon the mode of transmission of the disease and the species of animal involved. Four factors are essential to the transmission of infectious disease from one animal to another:

- A micro-organism capable of causing disease and capable of transmission.
- An environment favourable to the growth of a particular micro-organism.
- A mechanism by which the micro-organism can be transferred.
- A susceptible host.

Micro-organisms capable of causing disease are always present under normal conditions in most environments where animals are housed. A favourable environment for the spread of many micro-organisms usually exists where several animals are housed together, such as in kennels or hospitals. Animals that are likely to be more susceptible as hosts to disease are generally more common in a hospital situation (e.g. post-operative cases are more susceptible than the average healthy adult animal) and hospital accommodation is therefore designed and managed to reduce this risk by means of high standards of hygiene. Unfortunately, even with the best standards of kennel design and hygiene, risks can never be totally removed, particularly where there is a potential mechanism by which micro-organisms can be transferred.

Thus it becomes apparent that three out of the four factors in the above list can never be wholly removed. It is therefore important to concentrate on the other factor – the essential link of the transfer mechanism by which a micro-organism is transferred from one animal to another. The prevention of this mechanism is achieved by 'barrier nursing' or 'isolation nursing' of the infected animal.

To achieve effective isolation of an infected animal, the particular transfer mechanism of the specific disease must first be understood (see Chapter 17).

Admission of infected animals

As general kennel or practice policy, ideally no animal should be admitted that has (or is suspected of having) an infectious disease which poses a potential risk to other animals housed. An infected animal should never be admitted into a hospital or kennels where no separate, specific isolation facilities exist.

The usual reason for providing isolation facilities in kennels and catteries is to enable the isolation of animals that have developed suspicious symptoms after they have been admitted. By then, this will be the only course of action to protect the other animals housed. Where this occurs, the correct care and housing depends upon the nature of the disease and the type of infection risk.

Isolation kennelling

The size of isolation facilities is dependent on the numbers of animals housed. The recommended rate for dog isolation is at least one isolation kennel for up to 50 kennels (licensed for 50 dogs) and pro rata above that number.

The recommended rate for cat isolation is at least one isolation unit for up to 30 units (licensed for 30 cats).

When isolation kennelling is being designed, all possible disease transmission factors should be taken into account. The kennelling should comprise a totally self-contained unit so that all procedures can be carried out within the unit itself.

Isolation kennels must be separate from the main kennels and are usually physically separated by at least 5 m (15 ft) (this distance is based upon the distance that a dog sneeze travels). In existing catteries there must be a minimum of 3 m (10 ft) physical separation from the main cat accommodation units.

Where new kennels or catteries are being built it is recommended that isolation facilities are built 10 m (30 ft) from the main accommodation units. However, intervening buildings and other constructional details such as the positioning of doors, windows and exercise runs, when taken into account, may allow for variation of the distance.

All equipment should be kept and used in the isolation unit only and the unit should be equipped to enable the intensive care of acutely ill patients.

Isolation and infectious disease

Certain disease management methods are used routinely when managing a case in isolation:

- If possible, one or two staff members should be allocated to deal only with the infected animal and they should not handle any other animals. If this is not practical, they should be restricted to handling animals that have a low risk of contracting the disease. On no account should they also care for high-risk animals such as the very young.
- A foot-bath should be used at the entrance of the isolation unit and should contain a freshly prepared disinfectant solution. The disinfectant type depends upon the disease.
- All hygiene procedures should be carried out using disinfectants known to be effective against the disease concerned.
- A change of protective clothing should be available in a suitable area at the entrance to the isolation unit. The type of clothing depends upon the disease but may be:
  – a boiler suit or other coverall;
  – wellington boots;
  – disposable gloves and apron;
  – surgical mask;
  – hat (particularly for staff with long hair).
- There should be facilities for washing and disinfection and for safely discarding disposable items at the exit from the isolation unit.
- The infected animal should be nursed and treated as is appropriate to the disease.

Where purpose-built isolation facilities are not available, a measure of isolation can be achieved in less than ideal situations by strict nursing techniques (see Chapter 17).

Quarantine in the UK

The British Isles have been fortunate in being separated by sea from the continent of Europe. This separation has provided a natural barrier to diseases that spread through wild or domestic animals where free passage across borders is otherwise difficult to prevent. Pet animals require human assistance to cross the sea and it is therefore relatively easy to control and restrict the entry of animals, despite the constant movement of humans and even when a tunnel link with Europe is now available.

Britain has been free from the disease of rabies for many years and the continued prevention of its entry is of major concern. The principal control measure has been the quarantine of all animals susceptible to transmitting the disease, i.e. dogs, cats, etc., entering the country but in recent years there has been much debate with the other European Community member states regarding the freer movement of animals. The argument put forward is that effective vaccination is now possible and so is thought to reduce the likelihood of rabies entering the UK. Although the use of quarantine still stands as the principal method of preventing the entry of rabies, Britain has now agreed to certain new arrangements regarding the movement of animals, but only in cases where the conditions provide controls at least as stringent as quarantine. The Ministry of Agriculture, Fisheries and Food (MAFF) announced that changes relating solely to commercially traded breeding animals came into force in July 1994. These new arrangements are known as the 'Balai' arrangements and at the time of writing the present quarantine regulations are under review by an independent team 'the advisory group on quarantine'. However until such time as quarantine from Europe ceases the existing arrangements will continue to be fully and rigorously enforced.

The 'Balai' arrangements – exception from quarantine

(1) Under tightly controlled conditions, commercial traders in dogs and cats for breeding may use an alternative to quarantine. Movements between registered premises will depend on residency, vaccination at least 6 months prior to the intended movement, blood test, identification and certification requirements involving checks at origin, notification of a consignment, controlled movement and checks at destination. These arrangements take into account the most recent scientific advice and the need for arrangements to be fully enforceable. Any trader who fails to observe the rules will lose this possibility and their animals would be subject to quarantine, as will pet dogs and cats which do not meet these very strict conditions.

(2) The second change refers to the fact that other categories of captive bred rabies susceptible animals present no real risk of bringing rabies into the British Isles, e.g rabbits, rats and guinea pigs. From 1 January 1994 there was no requirement to quarantine such animals, provided that they have been born and reared on the holding of origin without coming into contact with any other rabies susceptible animal. (Domestic farm livestock and horses have never been included in the rabies quarantine arrangements as they are not considered a risk on import.)

MAFF will only agree to further these changes provided that the British quarantine arrangements for pet animals are replaced only with alternative measures which provide for at least the same level of protection.

Animals still subject to quarantine are:

- Primates.
- Carnivores.
- Wild mammals not born and kept in captivity.

In view of further changes to the rules, it is strongly recommended that those who wish to import or export dogs and cats into or from the UK should contact the MAFF for the most recent information regarding relevant regulations and the specific requirements for each country of destination. At present the quarantine period for dogs and cats entering the UK is six calendar months, the only exceptions being those previously mentioned.

The requirements of quarantine kennelling

The principles of quarantine kennelling for the prevention of rabies entering Britain are that the animal should be confined humanely for a period of 6 months in a secure establishment. The animal must have no possibility of contact with other animals (either internally or external to the kennels) that may risk being infected by rabies. To meet these principles:

● No physical contact of any kind is allowed between animals.
● No animal may have contact with the body fluids of another animal (e.g. urine must not seep through or be directed from one run to another through fences, and screens must protect cats from spitting at one another).
● No animal may have contact with any item used by another animal prior to disinfection (e.g. dog beds and non-disposable bedding materials).
● There must be no possibility of escape from the kennel or compound.

The only exception to the above is where animals from the same household share a kennel, in which case both animals are isolated from others as if they were one animal.

The standard sizes and other factors regarding quarantine accommodation for dogs and cats are set out in Table 5.22.

Licensing of quarantine kennels

Kennels and catteries used for the quarantine of animals in the UK are authorised by MAFF. The primary concern is that the kennels should be secure and meet standard requirements necessary to achieve all the principles previously mentioned in relation to the design, construction, operation and management.

If a lay person owns the kennels they must employ a veterinary surgeon who is appointed as veterinary superintendent and who must visit the premises daily from Monday to Saturday, and on Sunday when necessary.

General safety procedures in quarantine establishments

● All staff must be instructed on the dangers of rabies.
● Quarantine kennels must be run separately from all other units on the same site.
● Security and fire precautions and procedures must comply with current regulations.

Table 5.22 Quarantine facilities

	Sleeping area (not less than)	Adjoining exercise area (run) (not less than)	Other comments
Small dogs (less than 12 kg (26 lb))	1.1 m² (12 sq ft) Width and length: 0.9 m (3 ft)	3.7 m² (40 sq ft) Width: 0.9 m (3 ft)	*Height of dog compartments*: not to be less than 1.8 m (6 ft). Walls of sleeping area must be floor to roof or with all walls measuring at least 1.8 m (6 ft) and any gap above partitioned with escape-proof weld mesh. Wire diameter must not be less than 2 mm (14 swg), with mesh size not exceeding 50 mm (2 inches).
Medium sized dogs (12–30 kg (26–66 lb))	1.4 m² (16 sq ft) Width and length: 1.2 m (4 ft)	5.5 m² (60 sq ft) Width: 1.2 m (4 ft)	Runs should be constructed to allow dogs to see beyond the confines of the unit wherever possible.
Large dogs (more than 30 kg (66 lb))	1.4 m² (16 sq ft) Width and length: 1.2 m (4 ft)	7.4 m² (80 sq ft) Width: 1.2 m (4 ft)	They must be constructed to allow no nose or paw contact and no passage of urine from one run to another. *Dividing partitions between runs*: At least 1.8 m (6 ft) high. An impervious material with a smooth hard finish is used for the first part of the dividing partition, to a height of 0.4 m (18 inches) for small to medium sized dogs and 0.6 m (2 ft) for large dogs. The upper part of the dividing partition must be constructed of a see-through material that is nose and paw proof. *Run fencing*: Minimum height of 3 m (10 ft) with a weld mesh guard of 0.6 m (2 ft) set at an inward 45° angle; or Runs roofed over completely.
Cats	Total floor area (sleeping compartment and run) not less than 1.4 m² (15 sq ft). Width and length: 0.9 m (3 ft) Height not less than 1.8 m (6 ft).		Quarantine accommodation for cats should be of the 'walk-in' type. It must be securely roofed with all partitions solid to prevent cats spitting at one another.

- All animals must be transported to the kennels by an authorised carrying agent from the airport or ship's dock, and in a special vehicle and container.
- A high-security area must be used for the transfer of animals from the transporting vehicle to the kennel accommodation units.
- Rabies vaccination should be carried out on arrival or within 24 hours (regardless of current vaccination status).
- An animal must be kept in one accommodation unit for the duration of its stay.
- Animals housed in each accommodation unit should be clearly identified.
- Strict hygiene procedures should be observed at all times, using approved disinfectants.
- Animals in quarantine have restricted access by owners or any other person. Special authorisation is required if owners visit before 14 days of the arrival in quarantine.
- Strict recording procedures must be carried out regarding any movements of the animal, visits by the owner and all health records.

See Chapter 17 Rabies, p. 438.

The welfare of dogs and cats in quarantine premises

A voluntary code of practice regarding the welfare of dogs and cats held in quarantine premises has been produced. These standards were compiled by MAFF in consultation with the owners of quarantine premises and animal welfare organisations.

The standards include:

- Identification of who is responsible for the welfare of the animals.
- Transport to and moves within the premises.
- Minimum standards for sizes of units housing dogs and cats.
- General standards including hygiene, non-slip and other construction hazards, visual stimulation and ventilation, sleeping compartment, and heating recommendations.
- Feeding and management standards include, weighing, feeding and supervision, provision of water, diet, and condition and frequency of feeds.
- Recommended animal checking intervals.
- General conduct including reporting structure, supervision and training of staff.

Copies of the booklet are available on request.

Procedure if a rabies case is suspected

Where the suspected case is held in quarantine

If an animal in quarantine displays unexplained nervous signs, it should immediately be confined and the MAFF should be informed that a case of rabies is suspected.

If the suspect case dies or is euthanased, the animal is removed by the Ministry veterinary officer. Its head will be removed and taken to the MAFF diagnostic laboratory where the brain is removed under very strict conditions for tests to determine if the animal was infected by rabies.

Where a suspected case occurs in general practice

> The veterinary nurse should always have emergency plans prepared for various events, including natural disasters such as fire and flood. Rabies should be considered as a potential 'disaster' and requires a plan of action by the head nurse to keep the veterinary practice prepared.

It is possible that an animal brought into the practice for consultation with a veterinary surgeon displays clinical signs and a case history which raise the suspicion that it may be a case of rabies. Even a sick bat brought in might have to be viewed with suspicion. The veterinary surgeon will take into account all the symptoms and the history in making a decision to report the case as suspected rabies.

Where an animal is a suspected case but with insufficient grounds to report. In these circumstances a second opinion may be requested.

The MAFF Duty Veterinary Officer at the local Animal Health Divisional Office (AHDO) should be contacted to arrange for a veterinary officer to visit and examine the animal in consultation with the veterinary surgeon. The animal will be isolated and the veterinary surgeon will remain with the suspect animal until the veterinary officer arrives.

Where the veterinary surgeon makes a decision to report a suspected case. There is a statutory requirement that any suspicion of a case of rabies must be reported to:

- A MAFF inspector (Veterinary Officer).
- The local authority animal health inspector.
- A police constable.

Where a case is suspected in general practice, it is likely that the first contact will be with the Duty Veterinary Officer at the AHDO, by telephone.

The owner or person in charge of the animal should be advised by the veterinary surgeon:

- That rabies is suspected.
- That the animal must be detained and isolated.
- That it will be necessary for an official enquiry to be carried out by the Ministry veterinary officer who is being called to attend the case.

Isolation of the suspected case. The suspect animal must be isolated in escape-proof accommodation in order to prevent any further contact with animals or humans. It must remain on the premises on which it has been examined by the veterinary surgeon until the Ministry veterinary officer's enquiries are completed.

Identification of all contact animals. The names and addresses of the owners or person in charge of all animals that may have come into direct contact with the suspect case, along with descriptions of those animals, should be recorded. Reception records for the day will be needed for verification.

Any animal that has been bitten, scratched or come into contact with the saliva of the suspect animal should be detained at the premises until the Ministry veterinary officer's enquiries are completed.

The officer will advise if any further action is necessary with regard to contact animals.

Human contacts. Once the animal has been detained and isolated, all persons who have handled it should carry out a thorough personal disinfection:

- Hands should first be washed with soap or detergent and hot water.
- Clothing or overalls, if contaminated with discharges from the suspected animal, should be removed and sterilised before reuse.
- Equipment used on the animal should be removed and sterilised before reuse.

All cases of human contact with the suspected animal must be referred to the Medical Officer or the Environmental Health Office for further action and advice immediately.

WARNING

It is of paramount importance that anyone bitten or scratched by the suspected animal should have the wound treated immediately.

(1) Wash and flush the wound with soap or detergent and water.
(2) Flush repeatedly with running water alone – this is imperative.
(3) Apply either:
   - 40–70% alcohol; or
   - tincture of aqueous solutions of iodine; or
   - 0.1% quaternary ammonium compounds (NB: soap neutralises quaternary ammonium compounds, therefore all traces of soap must be removed before application).

General routine of admission of dogs and cats into the UK

The routine of admission at the time of writing is as follows. For information on imports, contact MAFF.

Government ban on certain breeds of dog

The Government has, under the Dangerous Dogs Act 1991 (as amended 1997) placed a ban on the ownership of certain breeds of dog. The dogs affected by the ban are certain breeds bred for fighting and cross-breeds of these types.

The following are affected by the ban:

- Pit Bull Terrier.
- Japanese Tosa.
- Dogo Argentino.
- Fila Braziliero.

The UK police and local authorities may seize any dog that **appears** to belong to one of these breeds. The owner will then be prosecuted.

If convicted the owner will face a fine or imprisonment and the dog may be destroyed on the order of the court.

Import licence

No pet dog or cat may be imported unless an import licence has been granted by or on behalf of MAFF (or the Secretary of State for Scotland, Northern Ireland or Jersey or the Welsh Office Agriculture Department if appropriate). Commercial trade in dogs or cats may be allowed under the 'Balai' arrangements provided that all of the conditions can be met.

A condition of the licence is that the animal will be held in quarantine for six calendar months from the date of its landing in the UK.

Application for import licences must be made in good time. As it is essential that the licence is issued on time, it is necessary for applications to be made at least 8 weeks in advance of the proposed date of importation.

Licences will not be granted unless the Ministry or relevant Department of Agriculture is satisfied that the necessary arrangements have been made, i.e. that the quarantine kennels and carrying agent have given notice of the booking.

Quarantine kennels. Accommodation must be reserved at approved quarantine premises well in advance of the proposed date of importation. A list of approved premises is available from MAFF or the relevant Department of Agriculture.

Authorised carrying agent. The services of an authorised carrying agent must be reserved to meet the animal at the port or airport and be responsible for its safe custody to the quarantine premises (some quarantine premises are also authorised carrying agents).

The port of entry. Animals may only be landed at certain ports and airports. A list is available from the Ministry or relevant Department of Agriculture.

Granting of the licence. The Ministry or relevant Department of Agriculture will confirm the booking with the quarantine premises and carrying agent. They will then:

- Send the import licence to the carrying agent. (The carrying agent is responsible for clearing the animal through customs.)
- Send a boarding document to the applicant (usually owner of the animal) or a named representative. (The boarding document will confirm the licence number and act as written evidence that a licence has been granted. This document will be shown to the shipper or airline before the animal will be allowed to leave for the UK.)

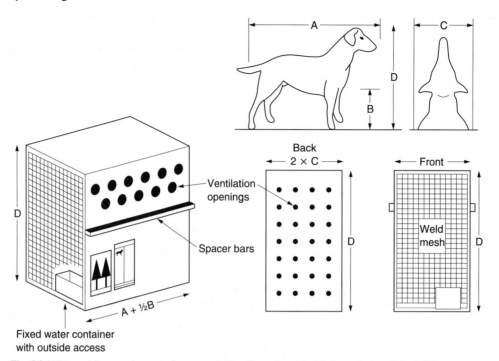

Fig. 5.8 IATA container requirements for cats and dogs. Reproduced by kind permission of the IATA.

● Send a red label to the applicant or named representative if the animal is to be transported by air. The red label is to be completed and affixed to the crate prior to embarkation.

Container or crate. If the animal is to travel by air, the container or crate must conform to IATA standards, i.e. it must be large enough for the animal to stand and lie in a natural position and turn around (Fig. 5.8).

The animal will travel to the UK as manifest cargo in the freight compartment.

Procedure for exporting dogs and cats from the UK

The factors governing the requirements for the export of dogs and cats from the UK are determined by the country to which the animal is being exported. No British laws are in force which govern the export of animals – the only laws presently in force govern imports.

The regulations relating to the export of dogs and cats to other countries vary considerably and may change depending upon the circumstances within the individual country at the time.

It is recommended that the export section of MAFF be contacted for the up-to-date requirements for each country.

Breeds: the recognised groups of dogs and cats

Pedigree dog breeds

The Kennel Club

The Kennel Club has been in existence since 1873 and its main aim is 'To promote in every way the general improvement of dogs'. The kennel club is the governing body for all official shows, trials and competitions held in the UK. All dogs exhibited in the UK at official shows must be of a breed recognised by the Kennel Club and must be registered through a system by which each has a registered name, usually combined with its breeder's registered prefix. Any change of ownership is also registered with the Kennel Club. The breeds recognised by the Kennel Club are broadly classified as 'sporting' and 'non-sporting', subdivided into 'groups' as follows:

● *Sporting*
  Hound group
  Gundog group
  Terrier group
● *Non-sporting*
  Utility group
  Pastoral group
  Working group
  Toy group

Within these groups there are at present 188 different breeds eligible for registration; each of these breeds has a 'breed standard'. The breed standard is a description of how the ideal dog of each breed should look, behave and move. The breed names are not necessarily a guide to the breed's group. For example, not all dogs with the word 'terrier' in their name are classed as terriers. The Australian silky terrier, English toy terrier and Yorkshire terrier are in the Toy group, while the Boston and Tibetan terriers are in the Utility group. Most but not all spaniels are in the Gundog group but the Tibetan spaniel is in the Utility group and the King Charles and Cavalier King Charles spaniels are in the Toy group.

Tables 5.23 and 5.24 give maximum/minimum or ideal height and weight where stated in the breed standard.

Table 5.23 Sporting breeds

Breed name	Height at withers (top of shoulder) Ranges	Weight
Hound Group		
Afghan Hound	Dogs 68–74 cm (27–29 in)	
	Bitches 63–69 cm (25–27 in)	
Basenji	Dogs 43 cm (17 in)	11 kg (24 lb)
	Bitches 40 cm (16 in)	9.5 kg (21 lb)
Basset Fauve de Bretagne (Interim)	32–38 cm (12.5–15 in)	
Basset Griffon Vendeen Grand (Interim)	39–43 cm (15.5–17 in)	
Basset Hound	33–38 cm (13–15 in)	
Beagle	33–40 cm (13–16 in)	
Bloodhound	Dogs 63–69 cm (25–27 in)	41–50 kg (90–110 lb)
	Bitches 58–63 cm (23–25 in)	36–45 kg (80–100 lb)
Borzoi	Dogs 74 cm (29 in) minimum	
	Bitches 68 cm (27 in) minimum	
Dachshunds	Standards	9–12 kg (20–26 lb)
	Miniatures	4.5–5.0 kg (10–11 lb)
Deerhound	Dogs 76 cm (30 in) minimum	45.5 kg (100 lb)
	Bitches 71 cm (28 in) minimum	36.5 kg (80 lb)
Elkhound	Dogs 52 cm (20.5 in)	23 kg (50 lb)
	Bitches 49 cm (19.5 in)	20 kg (43 lb)
Finnish Spitz	Dogs 43–50 cm (17–20 in)	14–16 kg (31–35 lb)
	Bitches 39–45 cm (15.5–18 in)	
Foxhound (Interim)	58–64 cm (23–25 in)	
Grand Bleu De Gascoigne (Interim)	Dogs 63.5–70 cm (25–27.5 in)	
	Bitches 60–65 cm (23.5–25.5 in)	
Greyhound	Dogs 71–76 cm (28–30 in)	
	Bitches 68–71 cm (27–28 in)	
Hamiltonstovare	Dogs 50–60 cm (19.5–23.5 in)	
	Bitches 46–57 cm (18–22.5 in)	
Ibizan Hound	56–74 cm (22–29 in)	
Irish Wolfhound	Dogs 79 cm (31 in) minimum	54.5 kg (120 lb)
	Bitches 71 cm (28 in) minimum	40.9 kg (90 lb)
Norwegian Lundehund	Dogs 35–38 cm (14–15 in)	7 kg (15.8 lb)
	Bitches 32–35 cm (12.5–14 in)	6 kg (13 lb)
Otterhound	Dogs 67 cm (27 in)	
	Bitches 60 cm (24 in)	
Petit Basset Griffon Vendeen	33–38 cm (13–15 in)	
Pharaoh Hound	Dogs 56–63 cm (22–25 in)	
	Bitches 53–61 cm (21–24 in)	
Rhodesian Ridgeback	Dogs 63–67 cm (25–27 in)	
	Bitches 61–66 cm (24–26 in)	
Saluki	Dogs 58.4–71.1 cm (23–28 in)	
Segugio Italiano (Interim)	Dogs 52–59 cm (20.5–23 in)	
	Bitches 48–56 cm (19–22 in)	
Sloughi (Interim)	60–70 cm (23.5–27.5 in)	
Whippet	Dogs 47–51 cm (18.5–20 in)	
	Bitches 44–47 cm (17–18.5 in)	
Gundog Group		
Bracco Italiono (Interim)	55–67 cm (22–27 in)	
Brittany	Dogs 48–50 cm (19–20 in)	
	Bitches 47–49 cm (18–19 in)	
English Setter	Dogs 65–68 cm (25.5–27 in)	
	Bitches 61–65 cm (24–25.5 in)	
German Short-Haired Pointer	Dogs 58–64 cm (23–25 in)	
	Bitches 53–59 cm (21–23 in)	
German Wire-Haired Pointer	Dogs 60–67 cm (24–26 in)	25–34 kg (55–75 lb)
	Bitches 56–62 cm (22–24 in)	20.5–29 kg (45–64 lb)
Gordon Setter	Dogs 66 cm (26 in)	29.5 kg (65 lb)
	Bitches 62 cm (24.5 in)	25.5 kg (56 lb)
Hungarian Vizsla	Dogs 57–64 cm (22.5–25 in)	20–30 kg (44–66 lb)
	Bitches 53–60 cm (21–23.5 in)	
Hungarian Wire-Haired Vizsla (Interim)	Dogs 57–64 cm (22.5–25 in)	
	Bitches 53–60 cm (21–23.5 in)	
Irish Red and White Setter		
Irish Setter		
Italian Spinone	Dogs 60–70 cm (23.5–27.5 in)	34–39 kg (75–86 lb)
	Bitches 59–65 cm (23–25.5 in)	29–34 kg (62–75 lb)
Kooikerhondje (Interim)	35–40 cm (14–16 in)	
Large Munsterlander	Dogs 60–65 cm (23.5–25.5 in)	25–29 kg (55–65 lb)
	Bitches 58–63 cm (23–25 in)	25 kg (55 lb)
Nova Scotia Duck Tolling Retriever (Interim)	Dogs 48–51 cm (19–20 in)	
	Bitches 45–48 cm (18–19 in)	

Table 5.23 (Continued)

Breed name	Height at withers (top of shoulder) Ranges	Weight
Pointer	Dogs 63–69 cm (25–27 in) Bitches 61–66 cm (24–26 in)	
Retriever		
– Chesapeake Bay	Dogs 58.5–66 cm (23–26 in) Bitches 53.5–60.9 cm (21–24 in)	
– Curly Coated	Dogs 67.5 cm (27 in) Bitches 62.5 cm (25 in)	
– Flat Coated	Dogs 59–61.5 cm (23–24 in) Bitches 56.5–59 cm (22–23 in)	27–36 kg (60–80 lb) 25–32 kg (55–70 lb)
– Golden	Dogs 56–61 cm (22–24 in) Bitches 51–56 cm (20–22 in)	
– Labrador	Dogs 56–57 cm (22–22.5 in) Bitches 54–56 cm (21.5–22 in)	
Spaniel		
– American Cocker	Dogs 36.25–38.75 cm (14.5–15.5 in) Bitches 33.75–36.25 cm (13.5–14.5 in)	
– Clumber	Dogs Bitches	36 kg (80 lb) 29.5 kg (65 lb)
– Cocker	Dogs 39–41 cm (15.5–16 in) Bitches 38–39 cm (15–15.5 in)	12.75–14.5 kg (28–32 lb)
– English Springer	51 cm (20 in) approx.	
– Field	45.7 cm (18 in) approx.	18–25 kg (40–55 lb)
– Irish Water	Dogs 53–58 cm (21–23 in) Bitches 51–56 cm (20–22 in)	
– Sussex	38–41 cm (15–16 in)	23 kg (50 lb)
– Welsh Springer	Dogs 48 cm (19 in) approx. Bitches 46 cm (18 in) approx.	
Weimaraner	Dogs 61–69 cm (24–27 in) Bitches 56–64 cm (22–25 in)	
Terrier Group		
Airedale Terrier	Dogs 58–61 cm (23–24 in) Bitches 56–59 cm (22–23 in)	
Australian Terrier	25.5 cm (10 in)	6.34 kg (14 lb)
Bedlington Terrier	41 cm (16 in)	8.2–10.4 kg (18–23 lb)
Border Terrier	Dogs Bitches	5.9–7.1 kg (13–15.5 lb) 5.1–6.4 kg (11.5–14 lb)
Bull Terrier	(no height/weight limits)	
Bull Terrier (Miniature)	35.5 cm (14 in) maximum	
Cairn Terrier	28–31 cm (11–12 in)	6–7.5 kg (14–16 lb)
Cesky Terrier (Interim)	Dogs 28–35.5 cm (11–14 in) Bitches 28–35.5 cm (11–14 in)	8 kg (17.5 lb) 7 kg (15.5 lb)
Dandie Dinmont Terrier	20–28 cm (8–11 in)	8–11 kg (18–24 lb)
Smooth Fox Terrier	Dogs Bitches	7.3–8.2 kg (16–18 lb) 6.8–7.7 kg (15–17 lb)
Wire Fox Terrier	Dogs 39 cm (15.5 in) maximum Bitches slightly less than above	8.25 kg (18 lb)
Glen of Imaal Terrier (Interim)	35–36 cm (14 in) maximum	
Irish Terrier	Dogs 48 cm (19 in) Bitches 46 cm (18 in)	
Kerry Blue Terrier	Dogs 46–48 cm (18–19 in) Bitches slightly less than above	15–16.8 kg (33–37 lb) 15.9 kg (35 lb)
Lakeland Terrier	Dogs 37 cm (14.5 in) Bitches 37 cm (14.5 in)	7.7 kg (17 lb) 6.8 kg (15 lb)
Manchester Terrier	Dogs 40–41 cm (16 in) Bitches 38 cm (15 in)	
Norfolk Terrier	25–26 cm (10 in)	
Norwich Terrier	25–26 cm (10 in)	
Parson Jack Russell Terrier	Dogs 33–35 cm (13–14 in) Bitches 30–33 cm (12–13 in)	
Scottish Terrier	25.4–28 cm (10–11 in)	8.6–10.4 kg (19–23 lb)
Sealyham Terrier	Dogs 31 cm (12 in) maximum Bitches 31 cm (12 in) maximum	9 kg (20 lb) 8.2 kg (18 lb)
Skye Terrier	Dogs 25–26 cm (10 in) Bitches slightly less than above	Bitches somewhat less
Soft Coated Wheaten Terrier	Dogs 46–49 cm (18–19.5 in) Bitches slightly less than above	16–20.5 kg (35–45 lb)
Staffordshire Bull Terrier	Dogs 35.5–40.5 cm (14–16 in) Bitches	12.7–17 kg (28–38 lb) 11–15.4 kg (24–34 lb)
Welsh Terrier	39 cm (15.5 in) maximum	9–9.5 kg (20–21 lb)
West Highland White Terrier	28 cm (11 in)	

Table 5.24 Non-sporting breeds

Breed name	Height at withers (top of shoulder) Ranges	Weight
Utility Group		
Boston Terrier		Not exceeding 11.4 kg (25 lb)
	Lightweight	Under 6.8 kg (15 lb)
	Middleweight	6.8–9.1 kg (15–20 lb)
	Heavyweight	9.1–11.4 kg (20–25 lb)
Bulldog	Dogs	25 kg (55 lb)
	Bitches	22.7 kg (50 lb)
Canaan Dog (Interim)	50–60 cm (20–24 in)	18–25 kg (40–55 lb)
Chow Chow	Dogs 48–56 cm (19–22 in)	
	Bitches 46–51 cm (18–20 in)	
Dalmatian	Dogs 58.4–61 cm (23–24 in)	
	Bitches 55.9–58.4 cm (22–23 in)	
French Bulldog	Dogs	12.7 kg (28 lb)
	Bitches	10.9 kg (24 lb)
German Spitz	Klein 23–29 cm (9–11.5 in)	
	Mittel 30–38 cm (12–15 in)	
Japanese Akita	Dogs 66–71 cm (26–28 in)	
	Bitches 61–66 cm (24–26 in)	
Japanese Shiba Inu	Dogs 39.5 cm (15.5 in)	
	Bitches 36.5 cm (14.5 in)	
Japanese Spitz	Dogs 30–36 cm (12–14 in)	
	Bitches slightly smaller	
Keeshond	Dogs 45.7 cm (18 in)	
	Bitches 43.2 cm (17 in)	
Leonberger (Interim)	Dogs 72–80 cm (28.75–32 in)	
	Bitches 65–75 cm (26–30 in)	
Lhasa Apso	Dogs 25.4 cm (10 in)	
	Bitches slightly smaller	
Miniature Schnauzer	Dogs 35.6 cm (14 in)	
	Bitches 33 cm (13 in)	
Poodles	Standard – over 38 cm (15 in)	
	Miniature – 28–38 cm (11–15 in)	
	Toy – under 28 cm (11 in)	
Schipperke		5.4–7.3 kg (12–16 lb)
Schnauzer	Dogs 48.3 cm (19 in)	
	Bitches 45.7 cm (18 in)	
Shar Pei	46–51 cm (18–20 in)	
Shih Tzu	26.7 cm (10.5 in) maximum	4.5–8.1 kg (10–18 lb)
Tibetan Spaniel	25.4 cm (10 in)	4.1–6.8 kg (9–15 lb)
Tibetan Terrier	Dogs 35.6–40.6 cm (14–16 in)	
	Bitches slightly smaller	
Pastoral Group		
Anatolian Shepherd Dog	Dogs 74–81 cm (29–32 in)	50–64 kg (110–141 lb)
	Bitches 71–79 cm (28–31 in)	41–59 kg (90.5–130 lb)
Australian Cattle Dog (Interim)	Dogs 46–51 cm (18–20 in)	
	Bitches 43–48 cm (17–19 in)	
Australian Shepherd (Interim)	Dogs 51–58 cm (20–23 in)	
	Bitches 46–53 cm (18–21 in)	
Bearded Collie	Dogs 53–56 cm (21–22 in)	
	Bitches 51–53 cm (20–21 in)	
Belgian Shepherd Dog	Dogs 61–66 cm (24–26 in)	
	Bitches 56–61 cm (22–24 in)	
Bergamasco (Interim)	Dogs 58–62 cm (23–25 in)	32–38 kg (70–84 lb)
	Bitches 54–58 cm (21–23 in)	26–32 kg (56–70 lb)
Border Collie	Dogs 53 cm (21 in)	
	Bitches slightly less	
Briard	Dogs 62–68 cm (24–27 in)	
	Bitches 56–64 cm (23–25.5 in)	
Rough Collie	Dogs 56–61 cm (22–24 in)	
	Bitches 51–56 cm (20–22 in)	
Smooth Collie	Dogs 56–61 cm (22–24 in)	20.5–29.5 kg (45–65 lb)
	Bitches 51–56 cm (20–22 in)	18–25 kg (40–55 lb)
Estrela Mountain Dog (Interim)	Dogs 65–72 cm (25.5–28.5 in)	
	Bitches 62–68 cm (24.5–27 in)	
	(A tolerance of 4 cm (1.5 in) above allowed)	
Finnish Lapphund (Interim)	Dogs 46–52 cm (18–20.5 in)	
	Bitches 41–47 cm (16–18.5 in)	
German Shepherd Dog (Alsatian)	Dogs 63.5 cm (25 in)	
	Bitches 57.5 cm (23 in)	
	(2.5 cm (1 in) above/below permissible)	
Hungarian Kuvasz (Interim)	Dogs 71–75 cm (28–29 in)	40–52 kg (88–114 lb)
	Bitches 66–70 cm (26–27.5 in)	30–42 kg (66–92 lb)

Table 5.24 (Continued)

Breed name	Height at withers (top of shoulder) Ranges	Weight
Hungarian Puli	Dogs 40–44 cm (16–17.5 in) Bitches 37–41 cm (14.5–16 in)	13–15 kg (28.5–33 lb) 10–13 kg (22–28.5 lb)
Komondor (Interim)	Dogs – Average 80 cm (31.5 in) Bitches – Average 70 cm (27.5 in)	50–61 kg (110–135 lb) 36–50 kg (80–110 lb)
Lancashire Heeler (Interim)	Dogs 30 cm (12 in) Bitches 25 cm (10 in)	
Maremma Sheepdog	Dogs 65–73 cm (25.5–28.5 in) Bitches 60–68 cm (23.5–26.5 in)	35–45 kg (77–99 lb) 30–40 kg (66–88 lb)
Norwegian Buhund	Dogs 45 cm (17.5 in) Bitches somewhat less	
Old English Sheepdog	Dogs 61 cm (24 in) Bitches 56 cm (22 in)	
Polish Lowland Sheepdog	Dogs 43–52 cm (17–20 in) Bitches 40–46 cm (16–18.5 in)	
Pyrenean Mountain Dog	Dogs 70 cm (28 in) minimum Bitches 65 cm (26 in) minimum	50 kg (110 lb) minimum 40 kg (90 lb) minimum
Pyrenean Sheepdog (Interim)	Dogs 40–48 cm (16–19 in) Bitches 38–46 cm (15–18 in)	
Samoyed	Dogs 51–56 cm (20–22 in) Bitches 46–51 cm (18–20 in)	
Shetland Sheepdog	Dogs 37 cm (14.5 in) Bitches 35.5 cm (14 in)	
Swedish Lapphund (Interim)	Dogs 45–51 cm (18–20 in) Bitches 40–46 cm (16–18.5 in)	
Swedish Vallhund	Dogs 33–35 cm (13–13.75 in) Bitches 31–33 cm (12–13 in)	11.4–15.9 kg (25–35 lb)
Welsh Corgi – Cardigan – Pembroke	 30 cm (12 in) 25.5–30.5 cm (10–12 in)	 Dogs 10–12 kg (22–26 lb) Bitches 9–11 kg (20–24 lb)
Working Group Alaskan Malamute	 Dogs 64–71 cm (25–28 in) Bitches 58–66 cm (23–26 in)	 38–56 kg (85–125 lb)
Beauceron (Interim)	Dogs 65–70 cm (25.5–27.5 in) Bitches 63–68 cm (24.75–26.75 in)	
Bernese Mountain Dog	Dogs 64–70 cm (25–27.5 in) Bitches 58–66 cm (23–26 in)	
Bouvier Des Flandres	Dogs 62–68 cm (25–27 in) Bitches 59–65 cm (23–25.5 in)	35–40 kg (77–88 lb) 27–35 kg (59–77 lb)
Boxer	Dogs 57–63 cm (22.5–25 in) Bitches 53–59 cm (21–23 in)	30–32 kg (66–70 lb) 25–27 kg (55–60 lb)
Bullmastiff	Dogs 63.5–68.5 cm (25–27 in) Bitches 61–66 cm (24–26 in)	50–59 kg (110–130 lb) 41–50 kg (90–110 lb)
Dobermann	Dogs 69 cm (27 in) Bitches 65 cm (25.5 in)	
Dogue de Bordeaux (Interim) Eskimo Dog	 Dogs 58–68 cm (23–27 in) Bitches 51–61 cm (20–24 in)	 34–47.6 kg (75–105 lb) 27–41 kg (60–90 lb)
Giant Schnauzer	Dogs 65–70 cm (25.5–27.5 in) Bitches 60–65 cm (23.5–25.5 in)	
Great Dane	Dogs 76 cm (30 in) minimum Bitches 71 cm (28 in) minimum	54 kg (120 lb) minimum 46 kg (100 lb) minimum
Hovawart (Interim)	Dogs 63–70 cm (25–27.5 in) Bitches 58–65 cm (23–25.5 in)	30–40 kg (66–68 lb) 25–35 kg (55–77 lb)
Leonberger Mastiff Neopolitan Mastiff (Interim)	 Dogs 65–75 cm (26–29.5 in) Bitches somewhat less	 50–70 kg (110–154 lb)
Newfoundland	Dogs 71 cm (28 in) Bitches 66 cm (26 in)	64–69 kg (140–150 lb) 50–54.5 kg (110–120 lb)
Pinscher (Interim)	43–48 cm (17–19 in)	
Portuguese Water Dog (Interim)	Dogs 50–57 cm (19.5–22.5 in) Bitches 43–52 cm (17–20.5 in)	19–25 kg (42–55 lb) 16–22 kg (35–48 lb)
Rottweiler	Dogs 63–69 cm (25–27 in) Bitches 58–63.5 cm (23–25 in)	
St Bernard	Taller the better	
Siberian Husky	Dogs 53–60 cm (21–23.5 in) Bitches 51–56 cm (20–22 in)	20–27 kg (45–60 lb) 16–23 kg (35–50 lb)
Tibetan Mastiff (Interim)	Dogs 66 cm (26 in) Bitches 61 cm (24 in)	

Table 5.24 (Continued)

Breed name	Height at withers (top of shoulder) Ranges	Weight
Toy Group		
Affenpinscher	24–28 cm (9.5–11 in)	3–4 kg (6.5–9 lb)
Australian Silky Terrier	23 cm (9 in)	4 kg (8–10 lb)
Bichon Frise	23–28 cm (9–11 in)	
Bolognese (Interim)	Dogs 27–30.5 cm (10.5–12 in)	
	Bitches 22.5–28 cm (10–11 in)	
Cavalier King Charles Spaniel		5.4–8 kg (12–18 lb)
Chihuahua		
– Long coat		1–2.7 kg (2–6 lb)
– Smooth coat		1–2.7 kg (2–6 lb)
Chinese Crested Dog	Dogs 28–33 cm (11–13 in)	5.5 kg (12 lb) maximum
	Bitches 23–30 cm (9–12 in)	
English Toy Terrier (Black & Tan)	25–30 cm (10–12 in)	2.7–3.6 kg (6–8 lb)
Griffon Bruxellois		2.2–4.9 kg (5–11 lb)
Havanese (Interim)	23–28 cm (9–11 in)	
Italian Greyhound	32–38 cm (13–15 in)	3.6–4.5 kg (8–10 lb)
Japanese Chin		1.8–3.2 kg (4–7 lb)
King Charles Spaniel		3.6–6.3 kg (8–14 lb)
Lowchen (Little Lion Dog)	25–33 cm (10–13 in)	
Maltese	25.5 cm (10 in) maximum	
Miniature Pinscher	25.5–30 cm (10–12 in)	
Papillon	20–28 cm (8–11 in)	
Pekingese	Dogs	5 kg (11 lb) maximum
	Bitches	5.5 kg (12 lb) maximum
Pomeranian	Dogs	1.8–2 kg (4–4.5 lb)
	Bitches	2–2.5 kg (4.5–5.5 lb)
Pug		6.3–8.1 kg (14–18 lb)
Yorkshire Terrier		3.1 kg (7 lb) maximum

Table 5.25 Pedigree cat breeds/colours as classified by the GCCF

Long-hair	Bicolour LH – inc. Van (coat pattern)
	Black LH
	Blue LH
	Blue cream LH
	Cameo – Cream/Blue-cream/Red/Tortie LH
	Chinchilla
	Chocolate LH
	Colourpoint – Blue/Seal/Tabby/Tortie/Self Colourpoint AOC
	Cream LH
	Exotic short-hair (short coated Persian type)
	Golden Persian
	Lilac LH
	Pewter LH
	Red Self LH
	Smoke LH Black/Blue/Blue-Cream/Chocolate/Chocolate Tortie/Cream/Lilac/Lilac Cream/Red
	Tabby LH – Brown/Silver/Red
	Tortoiseshell LH
	Tortie/Chocolate Tortie and White LH inc. Van
	Blue/Lilac Tortoiseshell and White LH inc. Van
	White LH – Blue eyed/Orange eyed/Odd eyed
Provisional breed status long-hair	Chocolate tortie LH
	Lilac cream LH
	Tabby AOC LH
Assessment classes	Shaded silver
	Tabby AC-, Bi- or Tri-Colour
Semi-long-hair	Birman – Blue point/Seal point
	Birman – Chocolate point/Lilac point/Red point/Tabby point/Tortie Group point/Tortie tabby point
	Turkish van – (Auburn and Cream)
	Somali – Usual/Silver/Sorrel/AOC (ex silver)
	Maine Coon
	Norwegian Forest Cat

Table 5.25 (Continued)

Provisional breed status semi-long-hair	Bicolour Ragdoll AC Colourpointed Ragdoll AC Mitted Ragdoll AC
British Short-hair	Bicolour BSH Black BSH Blue BSH Blue Cream BSH Blue Tortie and White BSH Colourpointed inc. Smoke and Silver BSH Cream BSH Manx Smoke BSH Spotted BSH – Brown/Red/Silver/Silver spotted AOC/Spotted AOC Tabby BSH – Cream/Blue/Brown/Red/Silver/AOC Silver/Tortie Tipped BSH Tortie BSH – Black/Chocolate/Lilac Tortie and White BSH – Black/Chocolate/Lilac White BSH – Blue eyed/Orange eyed/Odd eyed
Provisional breed status British short-hair	Lilac BSH
Preliminary breed status (assessment) British short-hairs	Tabby Chocolate/Red/ChocolateTabby BSH Tabby – Lilac BSH Tipped – Golden BSH
Foreign	Abyssinian – Blue/Sorrel/Usual/AC Silver (exc. sex-linked colours) Asian Smoke/Burmilla Asian Tabby (Spotted, Classic, Mackerel or Ticked) Korat Rex – Cornish/Devon Russian Blue
Provisional breed status foreign	Abyssinian Fawn Asian Self/Tortie inc. Bombay
Preliminary breed status (assessment) foreign	Abyssinian Asian-Tiffanie Bengal Ocicat Russian – White/black Singapura Tonkinese
Burmese	Blue Burmese Brown Burmese Chocolate Burmese Cream Burmese Lilac Burmese Red Burmese Tortoiseshell – Brown/Tortie Burmese AOC
Orientals	Foreign White Havana Oriental – Black/Blue/Cinnamon/Red Oriental shaded inc. Apricot Oriental Tabby – Classic/Mackerel inc. Apricot/Spotted inc. Apricot/Ticked inc. Apricot Oriental Tortoiseshell
Provisional breed status Orientals	Angora Oriental – Apricot/Cream Oriental – Smoke inc. Apricot
Preliminary breed status (assessment) Orientals	Oriental – Caramel/fawn
Siamese and Balinese	Balinese AC (inc. Caramel series) Siamese – Seal point/Blue point/Chocolate point/Lilac point/Tabby point/Red point/Tortie point/Cream point
Preliminary breed status (assessment) Siamese and Balinese	Siamese – Cinnamon/Caramel/Fawn – Tortie points/Tabbie points/Tortie tabby points

Key to abbreviations: AC, Any Colour; exc., excluding; inc, including; AOC Any Other Colour; LH, Long-hair; BSH, British short-hair; SH, short-hair; ex, except.

Cats

There are more than 5 million non-pedigree cats in Britain. All types are seen due to the free-range nature of the breeding of cats in this country and resulting mix of genes. Both long- and short-hair types occur naturally in the present population. All colours are found but the most common is tabby, of which there are two types: those with 'mackerel' stripes (narrow bands of colour similar to the coat of the Scottish wildcat) and those with the more common blotched tabby markings. The tabby colouring is followed in frequency by black and white colouring. More unusual colours like chocolate, colour point and chinchilla suggest that a pedigree cat has been involved in an individual ancestry.

Pedigree cat breeds are recognized and classified in the UK by the Governing Council of the Cat Fancy (GCCF), which is similar to the Kennel Club in that it:

- Classifies breeds and issues breed standards by which cats may be judged.
- Licenses cat shows and appoints judges.
- Prepares and publishes the rules to control these functions.
- Protects the welfare of cats and improves cat breeding.
- Protects the interests of cat owners.
- Exercises disciplinary powers.

In 1992 there was a major change in the GCCF's classification and grouping of cats with the introduction of a new section, the 'semi-long-hairs'. The major groups are now:

- Long-hairs.
- Semi-long-hairs.
- British short-hairs.
- Foreign.
- Burmese.
- Orientals.
- Siamese and Balinese.

The GCCF has a breed numbering system first adopted in 1910, which has evolved into a master series of numbers and letters. Each cat breed is individually numbered according to the major group, breed type, coat pattern and colour.

Table 5.25 lists the cat breeds that are catered for at GCCF championship shows, with coat patterns and colour variations recognized for each breed. Please note, that for ease of identification this list is in alphabetical order not by breed number. Also note that some breeds are comparatively new to Britain and have only provisional or preliminary status.

References and further reading

Kennel and cattery construction

Hamilton-Moore, S. and Cruickshank, C. (1988) *Boarding Cattery Construction and Management*, Feline Advisory Bureau Boarding Cattery Information Service.
Heginbotham, G. and S. (1984) *Boarding Kennels and Catteries (Their Design and Management)*, 2nd edn, The Kennels Agency and Hurst Publications, Reading.
Working Party Report (1995) *Model Licence Conditions and Guidance for Dog Boarding Establishments*, Chartered Institute of Environmental Health, London.
Working Party Report (1995) *Model Licence Conditions and Guidance for Cat Boarding Establishments*, Chartered Institute of Environmental Health, London.
Zabawa, S. (1988) *Running Your Own Boarding Kennels*, Kogan Page Ltd, London

Antiseptics and disinfectants

Ayliffe, G. A. J., Coates, D. and Hoffman, P. N. (1993) *Chemical Disinfection in Hospitals*, 2nd edn, PHLS, London.
Rutala, W. A. (1990) APIC guideline for selection and use of disinfectants. *American Journal of Infection Control*, vol. 18, no. 2, pp. 99–117.
Stucke, V. A. (1993) *Microbiology for Nurses*, 7th edn, Baillière Tindall, London.

Management and hygiene

Officers of the BVA (1993) The veterinary surgeon's duty of care in handling and disposing of clinical waste. *The Veterinary Record*, January 9, pp. 25, 43, 44, 45.
Price, C. J. (1991) *Practical Veterinary Nursing (Nursing of In-patients)*, 2nd edn, BSAVA, Cheltenham.
Taylor, R. (1992) An introduction to dog grooming (parts 1 and 2). *BVNA Journal*, vol. 7, nos 5/6, pp. 158–164.
Watson, D. (1992) The skin, mother nature's barometer of health. *Veterinary Practice Nurse*, vol. 4, no. 2, pp. 9–11.

Quarantine, isolation and quarantine kennels

Evans, J. (ed.) (1989/90) *Rabies – Guidance Notes, Henston Vade mecum (small animal)*.
Simpson, G. (ed.) (1994) *Practical Veterinary Nursing*, 3rd edn, Chandler, S., pp. 182–183, Isolation, BSAVA Cheltenham.
MAFF Rabies information literature inc. *Rabies – Guidance Notes for Practising Veterinary Surgeons*, provided by MAFF Tolworth, Surbiton.
MAFF (1995) *The Welfare of Dogs and Cats in Quarantine Premises, Voluntary Code of Practice*, MAFF Publications, London.

Dog and cat breeds

Governing Council of the Cat Fancy (March 1998) *List of Breeds to be Catered for at GCCF Championship Shows*, GCCF.
Spall, J. (ed.) *Showing Cats (the GCCF Guide to Shows and Show Cats)*, GCCF/Pedigree Petfoods.
The Kennel Club (1998) *The Kennel Club's Illustrated Breed Standards*, Ebury Press. London.

6

Basic organisation and management

Sue Morrissey

We will in this chapter consider why a practice needs to be 'managed' at all, how we know if that management is succeeding, and, in more detail, those non-clinical aspects of practice management in which support staff, primarily nurses and receptionists are involved.

No one decides on a career in veterinary care because it is an easy way to make money. Indeed, when entering the profession it is not uncommon for individuals to think that it is somehow wrong for a practice to seek to be profitable.

Why profit?

A veterinary practice is an expensive business to run. From the fees paid by clients must be met the cost of drugs, salaries of staff and all the other overheads associated – rent, business rates, vehicle running costs, etc. It is imperative that a fee structure is in place which will not only cover these costs but also leave a surplus (profit) which can be used both to develop the practice and also reward the owners for their investment.

Planning for success

The successful practice is one which achieves its objectives. Objectives should always include profitability. Success does not just happen – plans must be made, systems set up and monitored, and changes made to meet changing circumstances.

It is of fundamental importance that the aims and objectives of the practice are defined and known, understood and accepted by all members of the practice. These aims are most usually set out in two documents:

The **Mission Statement**. This is a written statement of the practice's purpose and ethos. It is usually brief and may cover such items as

- The geographical area served by the practice, e.g. '10 mile radius of Anytown'.
- The type of work undertaken by the practice, e.g. 'companion and farm animal work'.
- Whether the practice is for first opinion or referral cases.
- The standard of patient care to which the practice aspires.
- How clients may expect to be treated when they visit the practice.
- Pricing policy.

The Mission Statement is displayed in public areas of the practice for clients to see and may even be incorporated into literature produced by the practice such as the practice brochure.

The **Business Plan**. This again is a written statement. It sets out in precise terms what the practice aims to achieve over a given period (3–5 years), and how it will achieve those objectives. It is a living document which is constantly being updated to take account of changes in circumstances.

Before formulating its Mission Statement or Business Plan, the practice must first analyse its current position, performing what has come to be known as a 'SWOT' analysis.

- **S** – *Strengths*. What are the strengths of the practice? Excellent location? Longstanding reputation for good service? Highly trained and committed staff?
- **W** – *Weaknesses*. What are the weaknesses of the practice? Poor premises? Lack of equipment? Inadequately trained staff?
- **O** – *Opportunities*. What opportunities are open to the practice? Neighbouring practice closing down? Growth in local population bringing potential new clients?
- **T** – *Threats*. What is the potential threat to the practice? Pet superstore opening locally? Declining population?

The whole practice should be involved in the SWOT analysis, initially often most successfully undertaken as a 'brainstorming' session. The SWOT analysis should be performed on an annual basis and changes reflected in the Business Plan.

Armed with the self-knowledge derived from the SWOT analysis and Mission Statement, the practice can then set about the task of writing a Business Plan.

To be successful it is essential that the Business Plan is:

- *Achievable*. Planning to have 100% of the cat-owning population of an area as clients within 12 months is unrealistic, as is seeking to convert an inner city small animal practice into a profitable farm business.
- *Resourced*. The Business Plan must take account of financial and human resources required and available.
- *Targeted*. The Business Plan should set very specific goals.
- *Measurable*. To assess whether a target has been achieved, that target must be measurable and the method of measurement laid down.

Either as part of the Business Plan, or as a series of associated documents, detailed Action Plans for all the tasks necessary for achievement of the plan will be made.

An example

To illustrate this process, let us follow through a simple example. The Anywhere Veterinary Practice conducted a SWOT analysis. Amongst the results of this were:

- Strengths – a highly trained nursing team.
- Weaknesses – included the lack of any programmes designed to encourage client loyalty and market practice services, and poor morale in the practice.
- Opportunities – included an increased number of potential clients from a newly completed housing estate.
- Threats – thought to exist from the planning consent which had been granted for another practice to open in the same locality.

The practice discussed these SWOT results at some length and decided that it was not happy with the situation, wishing instead to be perceived as a practice which was interested in maintaining the health of pets rather than one where the only contact between client and surgery was when an animal was sick. In addition, it was agreed that practice members would be happier and more fulfilled if they had the opportunity to use more of their skills. When the Mission Statement was written, it included 'This practice seeks to work with clients to keep pets as happy and healthy family members'.

Through a series of meetings, practice members were encouraged to put forward ideas for ways in which the aspirations expressed in the Mission Statement could be fulfilled and the positive and negative points arising from the SWOT analysis tackled. Amongst other ideas, the nurses said that they would like to set up puppy parties, as this was a service requested by clients and an area in which they felt they could use skills which were currently redundant. It was agreed that puppy parties could be a positive development of practice services and that they should be incorporated in the Business Plan.

The entry in the Business Plan read 'Puppy parties will commence on 1st March 1999. The programme of material to be included at the parties, and a suggested marketing scheme for them, will be drawn up by the Head Nurse and submitted for Partners' approval by 1st November 1998. Initially the parties will be held once a month. No charge will be made for the parties. Annual costs, including promotional material and overtime payments, are estimated to be c£1000 per annum'.

No practice will achieve the goals set out in the Mission Statement and Business Plan unless practice members accept responsibility for and understand their personal role in fulfilling those goals. Plans which are formulated by practice owners without the involvement of the rest of the practice and issued simply as sets of instructions are less likely to succeed than those which have involved staff and sought input from everyone in the practice from their inception.

The purpose of management is to achieve the objectives of the practice, using resources effectively and efficiently. It is the responsibility of every member of the practice to contribute to this, often outside what may be considered the narrow confines of their professional discipline. **This is probably more true for veterinary nurses than for any other group of staff.**

We will now consider in more detail those areas of practice activity, outside clinical work, where the veterinary nurse can, quite literally, 'make or break' a practice.

Client contact: interpersonal skills

A veterinary nurse, whether officially designated 'receptionist' by the practice or not, will often be the first point of contact between the client and the practice. Poor interpersonal skills at this stage may lead to clients taking their pets elsewhere with consequential loss of fee-earning potential to the practice. Brusque treatment of a client who has come to purchase wormers for their puppy does not result simply in the loss of that £5 sale for the practice, it means that the practice has lost the capacity to earn hundreds of pounds over the lifetime of the dog in vaccination and neutering fees alone, without even considering any fees resulting from treatment for illness. *An even more damaging consequence of poor client service is that the client concerned will undoubtedly tell friends and family of their dissatisfaction, harming the reputation of the practice and possibly causing other clients to go elsewhere.*

The receptionist is usually the first person with whom a client or the general public have contact when they telephone or come into the practice. The image that the receptionist portrays at that point of contact will be what the person remembers and perceives as the image of the practice as a whole. It is essential that this first impression, be it by telephone, direct contact or letter, is the one the practice wishes to portray. Reception is often the hub of internal and external communication within the practice.

Those working in reception must understand the policies and procedures of the practice for greeting visitors and clients and for security, safety and emergencies, as well as policy relating to routine work such as neutering, vaccination, worming and dealing with second opinion or referral cases. All these protocols should be incorporated into a staff handbook which forms the basis for induction training.

The reception area must be kept clean and tidy. With the use of plants, attractive and well-maintained posters or pictures, up-to-date reading material and comfortable seats, the area can project a warm, pleasant feeling which will encourage client confidence.

The personal appearance and hygiene of all members of staff are often perceived as representing the cleanliness and quality of the entire practice. Therefore it is important that a professional image is given. Clients like to know to whom they are talking and many practices now provide name badges.

Clients are like paying guests and they should be greeted as soon as they arrive. Ascertain the purpose of the visit and obtain all relevant details. Listen carefully and interpret the information that is given. Also look at the person who is communicating with you: non-verbal communication (body language) may tell you more than you are hearing.

Client contact: answering the telephone

The telephone should be answered promptly, confidently and efficiently, saying 'Good morning' (or afternoon or evening) and giving the name of the practice. Speak clearly and remember that your greeting will create a favourable or unfavourable impression of the practice as a whole.

Some practices may require that you then state your name and ask, 'How may I help you?'; however this will vary. Always ask who is calling. If you are unable to deal with the enquiry yourself, obtain as much information as possible and notify the caller that you are placing them 'on-hold' while you see if someone else is able to assist.

Pre-empt any queries or lapses of memory by surgery staff about the waiting caller by giving them the relevant information before putting the call through. This will also create a favourable impression with the client. In the meantime, keep going back to the caller 'on-hold' to apologise for the delay. They may be required to call back at a more appropriate time or you may need to obtain details from them so that the call can be returned. All telephone messages should be recorded in writing.

The practice should have a clear policy about the information that may be given over the telephone to clients and non-clients. All staff must be aware of these policies and then the relevant information can be given out in a clear and informed manner. If there is any doubt, the veterinary surgeon should be consulted and the client asked to bring the animal into the practice for examination.

A client may require telephone advice on animal first aid procedures. This should be given in a clear, calm manner by someone who has received training or instruction in the aims and procedures of animal first aid. You may need to advise the owner on how best to transport the animal to the practice or alternatively arrange a visit depending on the situation.

Client contact: rules for good communication

A few basic rules should ensure an accurate and effective system of internal and external communication:

- All forms of communication must be polite, clear and unambiguous.
- Information must be easily understood by both parties.
- Do not forget that the style and tone of a message or conversation can affect the response given.
- One of the most important aspects of communication is to be able to listen to others, to understand their viewpoint or requirements and to try to fulfil their expectations.

There will be occasions when communication fails, leading to a complaint from the client. In the case of complaints made at the reception desk, try to take the client to a private area where the problem can be discussed, and hopefully resolved, without interruption. At all times the client must be treated with courtesy.

Client contact: accuracy and efficiency

Appointments for consultation

Ensure that all those booking appointments know who is consulting and what length of consultation they require for certain procedures. Primary kitten vaccination consultations are sure to take longer than a post-operative check on a dog castration.

Nothing annoys clients more than surgeries that always run late. Try to ensure that surgeries start on time and that time is allotted for possible unexpected cases or emergencies.

Appointments for surgery

Ensure that all those clients booking animals in for operative or medical procedures are aware of the practice protocol for such cases. All animals should have been examined recently by the veterinary surgeon or be booked in for an appointment on the day of admission. Full details about the animal in question should be obtained from the owner plus a detailed list of procedures required to be undertaken whilst admitted into the practice.

Clients should be given accurate and detailed instructions on the preparation of the animal prior to admission.

Appointments for second opinions

When clients indicate to a veterinary surgeon that they are seeking referral for a second opinion from another veterinary surgeon, the original veterinary surgeon should make all the arrangements for such a consultation, including providing a full case history to the second veterinary surgeon.

Clients often telephone the practice themselves to arrange for a second opinion and it is essential that all staff dealing with such calls know what procedures should be followed to avoid the unethical situation of supersession. The original veterinary surgeon should be contacted by the practice and notified of the client's wish, so that both veterinary surgeons can discuss the case.

If the owner subsequently decides not to use the services of the original veterinary surgeon, the latter should be notified as soon as possible.

The following relevant definitions are given in the RCVS's *Guide to Professional Conduct*:

- **Second opinion** – when the original veterinarian or the client requests a second opinion from another veterinarian on diagnosis or on treatment, the intention being that the continued responsibility for treatment of the case should remain with the original veterinarian.
- **Referral** – when at the request of a veterinarian or client a case is referred to a second veterinarian or to another therapist for further diagnosis and treatment with the objective of return to the responsibility of the referring veterinarian at a mutually agreed time.
- **Supersession** – when a second veterinary surgeon assumes responsibility for diagnosis and treatment of the case without reference to the first veterinary surgeon or against the latter's wishes.

House calls

Ensure that the client's full name, address and telephone number are obtained when arranging a house call. It is helpful if the client gives suitable directions on how to reach the house. It is essential to obtain as full a description of the animal's condition as soon as possible to ensure that the veterinary surgeon takes not only the correct equipment and drugs but also support staff if necessary. Staff should be aware that the personal security of a veterinary surgeon going out on a visit may require that a nurse is taken along for safety in numbers. The time of the visit should therefore be arranged according to the urgency of the visit and the availability of staff.

Admission of animals

The admission of animals is best carried out by appointment in a separate room, allowing the owner time to discuss the case with the veterinary surgeon or nurse. This is usually done the evening prior to surgery, or at least 2 hours prior to surgery, thus giving time for the animal to settle and any preoperative procedures to take place.

Owners are frequently concerned about leaving a pet and often need the reassurance of a talk with a neatly dressed, friendly and knowledgeable person. There should be clear practice policies on who admits animals (if not the veterinary surgeon) and when an animal's preoperative check should take place. Owners often wish to see the premises where their animal will be hospitalised and there should be a clear practice policy on this matter also.

On admitting an animal, the nurse should write down routine details and ask relevant questions about the condition of the animal. These should include checking the owner's details and contact telephone number, the animal's details and an up-to-date weight. Ask the following questions:

- Have there been any changes since the veterinary surgeon last saw the animal?
- When did the animal last eat any food?
- When did the animal last take fluids?
- When did the animal last have any medication, particularly if on a current course prescribed by the veterinary surgeon?
- To the owner's knowledge, does the animal have any allergies or adverse reactions to particular foods or drugs?
- When was the last bowel movement/urine passed?
- If the animal is female and entire, when was she last 'in season'?
- Vaccination status?
- Temperament?
- Have any abnormalities been noticed?

Also take the following action:

- Make a note of all objects brought in with the animal, to ensure that they are returned with the animal when it is discharged.

- All cats should be brought into the surgery in some form of carrier – if not they should be placed in one immediately. For security, cats should always be carried in a carrier, even from one room to another.
- To ensure that dogs do not escape by slipping collars and leads provided by the owner, place practice slip-leads on all dogs when transferring them to and from the kennels.
- It will depend on practice policy whether owners accompany their pets to the kennels. If not, it is best to ask the owner to leave the room before the dog is taken through.
- Any animal booked in for a procedure requiring the administration of a general or local anaesthetic should normally be admitted only after the owner or agent has read, understood and signed a fully completed anaesthetic consent form. Only someone over the age of 18 years may sign this form.
- It is often practice policy that all operative and investigative procedures are paid for on collection of the animal. The veterinary surgeon admitting the animal should be able to give the owner some idea of the cost, but this can always be confirmed when the owner arranges an appointment on the date of collection.

Kennels

Kennels and cages must be labelled clearly and a system used to ensure that animals are not mixed up. It is possible to obtain identification collars for dogs and cats similar to the wrist bands placed on people when in hospital.

There must also be some method of correctly linking an animal in a kennel or cage with its full records, wherever these are kept. They might be on the front of the cage, or on clip-boards kept in a place corresponding to the appropriate kennel. If a computerised system is used, there must be a proper reference on the kennel which can be used to access with certainty the right patient's data on the computer.

Think about the allocation of cages according to the species and the disease:

- Cats are best separated from dogs.
- Small animals need to be put in an appropriate place and type of cage.
- Birds and nocturnal animals prefer a secluded, dimmed area.
- Infectious animals must be isolated and their cages labelled with relevant information so that staff may handle and care for them accordingly.

The stress for a hospitalised animal can be reduced to a minimum with gentle, caring nursing and a little thought. Animals often settle very well if regularly visited by the owner, who may bring in a well-loved blanket or toy (as long as the animal is unlikely to eat it). Feeding an animal from its own bowls may also reduce stress. If this does not work, early discharge may need to be considered in the interest of the animal's wellbeing.

Discharging of animals

This process must be undertaken by someone who will be able to answer the owner's routine questions about the case.

No animal should be allowed to go home if the owner feels unable to care for it properly, be it wound management, stabilisation of an animal's fluid balance, digitalisation or diabetic stabilisation. Some animals are bright and well enough to go home but it is more convenient if the practice keeps the animal hospitalised, e.g. when a dog has a discharging Penrose drain in a wound that needs flushing four times daily. A sleepy Pomeranian is easy enough to care for post-operatively, but this may not be the case with a Great Dane. Each case should be considered individually and discharged at an appropriate time that is convenient for the owner, but in the best interest of the animal.

Before discharging the animal:

- The owner should be given full details on the procedures undertaken and any results of investigative procedures carried out on the animal.
- Detailed information on immediate post-operative/investigative care with regard to wound care, diet, exercise and medication should be given.
- If the animal is present whilst this information is being given, the owner is likely to take in very little – it is better to give the information before the animal is brought through. Many owners benefit from being given these instructions in writing as well. They should always be reassured that they can contact the surgery staff if they have any queries.
- If any medication is being dispensed, owners are often very glad to be given a practical demonstration on how best to administer it, particularly if they have no previous experience.
- All drugs should be suitably packaged and labelled.
- Remember to return the animal's belongings and always ensure that they are clean before going out.
- Despite the animal's state on arrival for admission, every effort should be made to ensure that it goes out clean and well groomed. With certain animals the coat is in such a bad state on admission that it would require more than a good brush to remove the dirt and mats. Permission must be sought to go ahead with such a procedure.
- Finally, make an appointment for a return visit if required and deal with payment of the account according to the practice policy.

Client contact: keeping records

Computers

The use of computers is growing rapidly and they are playing an increasingly important role in the day-to-day running of veterinary practices. They can be extremely useful in a number of areas, including:

- Client record keeping.
- Sales and purchase controls.
- Stock control.
- Costing and budgetary control.
- Personnel records.
- Wages/salary systems.
- Market research.
- Cash-flow analysis.
- Word processing.
- Desktop publishing.

All users of computers must be aware of the Data Protection Act 1984, which is supervised by the Data Protection Registrar. All employers holding computerised data including personnel records need to register as 'data users' and must state the following before registering:

- The types of data held.
- Why the data is held.
- From whom and how the information is obtained.
- To whom the information will be disclosed.

Employees and clients have a statutory right to access all computerised information held about themselves. Reference to any manual records from the computer system are not covered by this Act provided that any such manual records contain purely factual information.

Eight principles within the Act govern the processing of computerised personal data:

- Data must be obtained fairly and lawfully.
- Users are required to register the personal data held with the Data Protection Registrar and it must be held only for specified and lawful purposes.
- Data must only be disclosed and used for the purpose registered.
- Data must be relevant, adequate but not excessive for its requirement.
- Data must be accurate and up to date.
- Data must not be held any longer than necessary.
- Individuals have a right to be granted access to their own personal data at reasonable intervals without undue expense and must be provided with a copy of it, in an understandable form. Data must be amended or removed where appropriate.
- Necessary precautions must be taken by data users to ensure security in order to prevent unauthorised access, disclosure, alteration or removal of personal data and accidental loss of data.

Computer hardware

The physical parts of a computer are described as hardware:

- **Terminal** – a visual display unit (VDU) and keyboard linked to a computer, in effect the point of use for the operator.
- **Peripheral device** – any input or output device that is used to communicate with the computer; a typical set includes keyboard, mouse, VDU and printer.
- **Central processing unit (CPU)** – controls the operation of the computer.
- **Keyboard**, through which the operator enters data into the computer.

- **Visual display unit (VDU)** – displays data on a screen.
- **Mouse** – portable input device on a rolling ball; it is used to move a pointer on the screen, the position of which is activated when the mouse button is 'clicked'.
- **Printer** – data printed out on paper by the printer is described as **hard copy**. The wide choice of printers currently falls into two main categories: character printers, which print one character, i.e. letter or number, at a time (e.g. dot matrix or inkjet), and page printers, which print a complete page at a time (e.g. laser).

Computer disks

Hard disks, normally of metal, might be:

- Fixed (Winchester) type – fixed inside a micro-computer and able to store from 20 to more than 1000 megabytes of data.
- Exchangeable type – in stacks of up to six disks enclosed in a plastic case (generally used only by large organisations).

Floppy disks are of thin, flexible plastic protected by a hard or soft plastic cover, usually 3.5 inches in size (though some 5.25 inch disks are still available for old machines). The size and the density of the disk determines the volume of data that can be stored on it. A 3.5 inch disk holds more information than a 5.25 inch disk; high-density (HD) disks hold more than single-density (SD) or double-density (DD) disks. The choice of size and density is dictated to some degree by the CPU.

Floppy disks are placed into the appropriate **disk drive** mounted on the computer. They can be used as a method of filing computer data but for large volumes (as in a veterinary practice system) it is more usual to store the information on hard disk and perhaps use a tape back-up system. Different types or sources of data can be stored on separate disks but these must be clearly labelled and stored safely in a disk box.

Computer tapes are used for back-up storage where quick access is not required.

Optical disks include computer disk (CD) Read Only Memory (ROM) disks that look like compact disks and are designed as bulk storage systems for information that does not require changing. They are usually produced commercially and hold data such as textbook information – they have a role in teaching.

Computer systems

Single-user systems include personal computers (PCs), i.e. one VDU, one keyboard and one CPU, and usually with one person accessing the information. Some of these are 'dedicated' as word processors.

Network systems are groups of single-user PCs linked (by cable) to a terminal so that data and expensive resources such as printers can be shared.

Multi-user PCs, using special software, allow a number of terminals to operate a single computer (one CPU and a number of 'dumb' terminals). This is the system most commonly used in large, fully computerised veterinary practices.

Software

The program that dictates what the hardware does is described as the **software**. The process of switching on the computer and loading the software into its memory is described as **booting up**.

Software application packages are written for particular functions. For example:

- Games.
- Drawing or painting.
- Design drawings.
- Management information systems (appointment system/ meetings).
- Database (sales/purchases/wages systems).
- Word processing.
- Spreadsheets (calculations and accounts).

Database programs are designed to manage and store large quantities of data. They are often custom-written and a veterinary practice's database program might include information on vaccinations, species, coat colours, etc. The program allows the creation, amendment and deletion of records so that client and animal information is kept up to date.

Spreadsheets are powerful calculating tools used in managing numerical information quickly and efficiently. For example:

- Plotting graphically the values of monthly vaccination sales.
- Calculating the costs of an operation by inputting figures, e.g. if you enter the number of hours an animal is under an anaesthetic, the flow rate of the gases and the unit cost of the gases, the computer will calculate how much it costs to provide the gases for that particular operation.
- Calculating averages and standard deviations, e.g. calculating the average transaction fee. If the practice price list is stored on a spreadsheet it is very simple and quick to increase prices by the rate of inflation without having to calculate and change each price individually.
- Accounts and VAT records can also be kept.

Desktop publishing is a facility for preparing documents containing both text and graphics of a quality adequate for use in publications – incorporating pictures with the text, laying out pages with multiple columns, etc., as required for a practice newsletter.

Word processing

A variety of documents can be produced using a word-processing applications program on a PC or stand-alone (dedicated) word processor (WP). The screen displays typed input or text, either with codes that control its design and layout or as straight text on the basis of WYSIWYG ('what you see is what you get').

There are many word-processing applications:

- Processing articles, letters, reports, minutes, etc.
- Amending and updating documents without retyping all of the information (e.g. drug lists, mailing lists, price lists, telephone numbers).
- 'Merge-printing' standard letters with a mailing list so that each letter is individually addressed and detailed (e.g. booster reminders).

More sophisticated WP programs have extended capabilities such as database, spreadsheet and desktop publishing facilities.

Computer communication

It is possible to create high-speed links between computer systems at different locations and these are increasingly being used both by practices with more than one site as a means of transferring or viewing information and also by practices as a means of placing orders with drug wholesalers. The most common types of linkages are made using telephone lines, and include modem, ISDN and kilostream. All have significant costs for installation and usage but can repay these costs to the practice through increased efficiency.

Data safety

Floppy disks are prone to damage which can corrupt the information stored on them unless they are handled and stored correctly:

- Do not handle the exposed parts of a floppy disk.
- File disks in a dust-free box when not in use.
- Do not drop them.
- Keep coffee and other liquids well away from disks (and keyboards).

Information held on the computer in a veterinary practice is irreplaceable. It is essential to have a **back-up routine** that will minimise the loss of information in most eventualities. Each practice should devise a regular back-up routine and should ensure that the routine is followed rigorously. The essence of backing up is to copy data on to a separate disk or tape, stored separately from the originals.

- Back-up daily (or more frequently in a very busy practice). Daily back-ups are often performed automatically overnight.
- In addition, back-up weekly to ensure that data is saved in case corruption of information goes unnoticed for a number of days.
- For added insurance, back-up on a monthly basis as well. (This is a 'belt-and-braces' system – many practices follow only a daily back-up routine.)

Intelligent tills

Intelligent tills incorporate some of the elements of a computer. They may be able to read item prices, using a bar-code reader or have dedicated buttons for items and services sold. Some also have the capacity to check stock levels and create automatic orders. Certain intelligent tills can be used to update vaccination reminder information. If a practice uses a manual medical record-card system, an intelligent till provides a cheap and effective way of automating certain routines such as stock control and vaccination reminders.

The future of electronic technology

Increasingly, computers are replacing manual filing systems. Digital data may be stored (filed) 'on-line' in a computer, or 'off-line' on disks or other magnetic media. Advances in technology have resulted in significant changes in the way that data is generated, stored and utilised, particularly in the fast-moving world of veterinary medicine. It is now possible to use the following in the day-to-day running of many practices:

- Storage of ECGs on computer.
- Interpretation of ECGs by computer.
- Storage of radiographs on computer.
- Scanning of radiographs by computer.
- Digital cameras linked to the computer to take and store information such as skin conditions.
- Electronic drug-ordering – the order to the wholesaler is transmitted direct from the computer.
- Laboratory reports transmitted electronically from the laboratory directly to the practice computer.

The management of information may be in the form of one or a combination of the following increasingly sophisticated systems:

- Card system and an ordinary till.
- Card system and an intelligent till capable of stock control.
- Card system and an intelligent till capable of stock control and producing vaccination reminders.
- Word processor and intelligent till holding clinical data as well as controlling stock and producing vaccination reminders.
- Multi-user system.
- Computer system at the main surgery linked to the branch surgeries by dedicated lines, ensuring access of information gathered at all sites.

Clinical information held on a card system at a practice that runs more than one site can be difficult to access when, say, an animal normally seen at a branch is brought into the main surgery out of normal working hours. Practices that encounter this problem will probably favour the computer-link system described above.

Filing systems

Filing is often an unpopular job but it is a vital one. A poorly managed system will produce hours of extra work spent looking for misfiled or lost material. If the filing of records is carried out regularly and accurately, a fast efficient system for the retrieval of information can be developed.

The storage system must be suitable for the information being stored and accessibility required. The storage of radiographs in labelled envelopes or cardboard sleeves placed in suspension filing cabinets is more appropriate than stacking them all on top of one another in a box.

The ideal filing system should incorporate the following features:

- Guaranteed fast retrieval of information.
- Easy identification of misfiled material.
- Easy identification of active material and archive material.
- Allowance for expansion of the system.
- Determination of the period of retention of documents.
- Consideration of security and safety.
- Identification of file users by a system of tracer cards or 'out' guides showing users' names and date borrowed, placed in position of file removed.
- Suitable system of indexing.
- Index and cross-references if necessary.
- Colour coding for awareness of misfiling and for ease of identification.

Commonly used indexing systems include:

- Alphabetical.
- Numerical.
- Alpha-numerical.
- By subject.
- Geographical.

The alphabetical system is most commonly used in practice for client files.

Storage of documents

Due to the nature of the work carried out in a veterinary practice, a variety and large volume of documents and correspondence need to be stored. Each practice should draw up an appropriate retention and disposal policy to ensure that essential, irreplaceable information is protected and non-essential documents and records are disposed of at appropriate intervals. Depending on the subject matter and legal obligations, certain correspondence and documents must be kept for certain periods:

- Accident records: 3 years.
- VAT records: 6 years.
- PAYE records: at least 3 years after the income tax year to which the earnings relate.

There is no statutory obligation to keep the following records but the Veterinary Defence Society recommends that they are kept for a minimum of 2 years; if there is any possibility of dispute about a case, keep them for longer:

- Anaesthetic consent forms.
- Medical/hospital records.
- Laboratory reports.
- Radiographs.
- ECG/EEC traces.

The Royal College of Veterinary Surgeons recommends that records are kept for a minimum of 6 years. In disputed cases that are taken to the Veterinary Defence Society, the Society is advised to keep papers and documents with reference to the case, for court purposes, for 6 years and 364 days.

Many practices keep documents and records for longer than is legally required. These are termed 'dead files' and it is important to ensure that the storage system is both cost-effective and easily accessible.

Financial control

Every successful practice has a written budget which includes targets for fees earned and estimates of overheads, etc. It is formulated annually, based on the Business Plan. During the year, financial management reports are produced regularly for the practice owners so that they can assess progress against budgets, identifying and taking action to correct any problems quickly.

Methods of payment

Strict procedures must be in place for the handling of payments made by clients, and accuracy of recording is vital.

Each method of payment has advantages and disadvantages:

- **Cash**. This has the benefit of being instant but it is easy to make mistakes, e.g. in counting change, when working under pressure. The security of cash in the practice and when being taken to the bank also has to be considered, as well as the possibility of theft within the practice.
- **Cheques**. A more secure form of payment in that it is less subject to dishonesty or mistakes than cash, but it has disadvantages in that there is a delay in the cheque clearing through the banking system. Banks usually charge the practice for processing cheques and unless the cheque is covered by a guarantee card, a bank may refuse to honour it.
- **Credit/debit cards**. These are increasingly being used by clients and should be accepted by all practices. Electronic terminals give instant authorisation and same-day credit of the amount paid directly into the practice account. The practice is charged a percentage of each transaction by their service provider for credit card transactions and a flat fee for debit card transactions.

All monies received from clients must immediately be accounted for, either through the computerised or manual cash book.

At the end of each day, or when a change of shift occurs, cash/cheques/credit and debit card slips in the till must be reconciled against the cash book and any discrepancies immediately investigated. It is just as serious to be 'over' in the till as 'under', as it means that payments have not been attributed to a client's records and a non-existent debt chased by the practice, to the annoyance of the client concerned.

Debt control

Constant vigilance is required to ensure that all fees earned by the practice are collected. All practices have a policy for collection of fees and this procedure must be followed at all times. Small animal practices usually operate on the basis of payment at the time work is done (though there may be a few exceptions, e.g. breeders may be allowed account facilities with settlement on a monthly basis) whereas large animal practices usually bill their clients at regular intervals. The practice's terms of business must be made known to clients before the provision of services, though care must be taken with the tone of any communication to avoid the impression that the practice's primary concern is financial rather than clinical.

Debt must be dealt with assertively and promptly. Many practices use the services of solicitors, debt collecting agencies or the County Court to collect debt.

Security

Security in a veterinary practice covers many areas and all members of staff should be aware of the implications of a lax system with reference to theft, damage and personal safety.

Premises

Burglaries are not uncommon and it is wise to ask the local Crime Prevention Officer for advice on how best to secure the premises. All doors, windows, skylights and shutters should be locked and checked before the building is left unattended.

Personal safety

It is unwise for anyone on their own at the practice to open the surgery door to a caller who may appear to be the owner of an animal in distress. A telephone intercom may be fitted so that you may speak directly to the person without opening the door. Then contact the veterinary surgeon on call before proceeding any further. A good source of light should make it easier to see and identify the caller and their vehicle (write down its colour, make and number).

To minimise the risk of personal danger of a nurse, arrangements can be made with known clients to call at the surgery at a specified time. They should have given a description of themselves, their vehicle and the animal. Ensure that all staff are aware of practice policy on this matter and that they all **think** before putting themselves in potentially dangerous situations. The fitting of 'panic buttons' in strategic places within the practice can make staff feel more secure.

Tills

Never leave an open, unlocked till unattended, even if you are staying in the same room. Never place the money tendered by the client into the till until you have counted out and given them their change and receipt.

It is very easy to accept into the till a £10 note for a small transaction only to be told, on giving the person their change, that they had given you a £20 note. Unless there is a detailed list of what was in the till, it is very difficult to prove that they did not in fact pass over £20.

Dangerous drugs cupboard

Only veterinary surgeons and nominated staff should hold keys to the dangerous drugs cupboard and these should never be left lying around or lent to unauthorised staff. Nor should the cupboard be left unlocked.

Staff-only areas should be well signposted and clients should never be left unattended in areas that contain anything other than GSL drugs.

Prescription pads and headed paper should not be left lying around. Stolen pads have sometimes been used by drug users trying to obtain prescription-only medicines or controlled drugs.

Animals

Always ensure the security of the animals in your charge and lock cages if necessary to prevent escape.

Measuring practice success

In order to assess progress in achievement both of the specific objectives of the practice as set out in the Business Plan and also its general health as a profit-making organisation, regular measurements must be taken. Most practices use broadly similar measurements, adding parameters to suit their particular circumstances. All practices produce annual Profit and Loss Accounts. Additional commonly used methods of assessing practice performance are:

- *Average transaction value (ATV).* The total value of turnover in a period, divided by the number of invoices raised in that period. For example, if in a month the practice has achieved a turnover of £60 000 and during that time 3000 invoices have been raised, then the average transaction value would be £20. ATV should be regularly monitored and changes investigated.
- *Annual health check and booster appointments.* Responses to reminder letters should be monitored each month and compared with previous months. The practice should aim to achieve as near 100% compliance from clients as possible.
- *Active and bonded clients.* An active client is one who has used the practice within a given period – often taken as the preceding 2 years. Definitions of 'bonded' vary but commonly a bonded client is said to be one whose pets' vaccinations are kept up to date. Practices seek both to increase the number of active clients and ensure that these clients are bonded. The practice should target these clients for marketing of services available.
- *Practice activity.* The number of procedures and appointments in a given period, compared with past months or years.

- *Team member's activity.* The income achieved by each member of the practice. Care should be taken in interpreting the results of this analysis as almost inevitably not all individuals will have the same opportunities to contribute directly to the income of the practice.
- *Overheads.* These are the costs associated with running the practice and must be constantly monitored, with any variations against budget investigated promptly.

Particular care should be taken following any increase in the price of services. Some areas of practice activity are likely to be more 'sensitive' to an increase in prices than others. These 'sensitive' areas are generally those where the service is elective and it is apparently straightforward to the client to compare prices between practices, e.g. neutering and vaccination.

Further reading

Blaney, D. *Information Technology,* Institute of Administration Management.

Bower J., Gripper, J. and Dixon-Gunn *Veterinary Practice Management,* 2nd edn, Butterworth-Heinemann, Oxford.

Corsan and MacKay *The Veterinary Receptionist,* Butterworth-Heinemann, Oxford.

Denyer, J. C. *Office Management,* Pitman.

Graham, H. T. *Human Resources Management,* M & E Handbooks.

Lysons, K. *Manpower Administration,* Institute of Administration Management.

Osuch, D. *Administration in the Office,* Institute of Administration Management.

Sheridan, J. and McCafferty, E. *The Business of Veterinary Practice,* Butterworth-Heinemann, Oxford.

7

The law and ethics of veterinary nursing*

A. R. W. Porter

Origins

Although veterinary surgeons have relied on the help of lay assistants of various kinds since time immemorial (and we are told that a Canine Nurses Institute was established in London at the beginning of the century), it was not until 1961 that the present veterinary nurse training scheme was set up by the Royal College of Veterinary Surgeons (RCVS).

At that time, legislation designed to limit the title 'nurse' to those who were already trained and qualified to nurse human patients prevented its use in the veterinary field – even with the use of the word 'animal' as a prefix. Accordingly persons who qualified under the new RCVS scheme (and only a handful of men sought the qualification) had to be content with the rather clumsy title of Registered Animal Nursing Auxiliary. They very soon became known as RANAs.

In the course of time the statutory position changed and it became possible for the title 'nurse' to be applied to those engaged in nursing animals, provided the particular nature of their work was made plain. Accordingly on 1 November 1984, the title of RANA passed into history and the new title of **Veterinary Nurse** came into being.

With effect from January 1999, veterinary nurse training has become part of the National Vocational Qualifications (NVQ) system. Those candidates who are enrolled with an Approved Training and Assessment Centre (ATAC), fulfil the prescribed training requirements and pass the 'independent assessment' which was formerly known as the Part I examination, will now be awarded a NVQ at level 2. Candidates who then go on to fulfil the further requirements and pass the next 'independent assessment' (formerly Part II examination) will be awarded an NVQ at level 3 and, on completing 24 months' full-time training at an ATAC, will be entitled to have their names entered on the list of veterinary nurses maintained by the RCVS and, of course, to describe themselves as veterinary nurses (VNs).

Career prospects

The scope of the work open to veterinary nurses can be quite wide but the majority are still employed in small animal practice. This reflects the fact that the main employment area is in companion animal work. At present, the syllabus for training relates to small animals and does not yet relate either to the horse or to farm animals.

---

* The law contained in this chapter is the law in operation at 31 December 1998.
† See Appendix in volume 2 for *Guide to Professional Conduct for Veterinary Nurses.*

Nevertheless, nurses now work in mixed or equine practices where they have been extensively involved with these larger animals, and the extension of veterinary nurse training to include horses is expected to come about in the relatively near future.

Companion animals are treated and nursed, not only in private veterinary practices but also in other centres such as the university veterinary schools and animal welfare society clinics and kennels and so veterinary nurses will be found working there.

Other career opportunities are available as practice managers, with pharmaceutical companies, in teaching and in other establishments where animals must be well cared for, such as zoos. Many holders of the veterinary nurse qualification have found that it is highly regarded overseas and have therefore gone to work permanently or for a time in other countries. Graduate veterinary nurses are expected to have wider opportunities in many of these fields.

The law relating to veterinary nursing†

The Veterinary Surgeons Act 1966

The Veterinary Surgeons Act 1966 is the written law or 'statute' which governs the practice of veterinary surgery in the UK. It provides that (with certain specified exceptions) no one may practise veterinary surgery unless he or she is registered with the RCVS. The title of **veterinary surgeon** is reserved by law to those whose names appear in the Register of Veterinary Surgeons maintained by the RCVS. Persons so registered are members of the RCVS and use the letters MRCVS or FRCVS if they are qualified as Fellows. Veterinary surgeons may also be colloquially referred to as **veterinarians**, a title that was one of the earliest names used and it is one widely recognised in North America and continental Europe. **Veterinary practitioner** is a title which the members of the Supplementary Veterinary Register may use. This small group of persons do not have formal qualifications in veterinary medicine and no further names may be added to this Register.

Veterinary surgery is defined in the Act as meaning:

...the art and science of veterinary surgery and medicine and without prejudice to the generality of the foregoing, shall be taken to include:

(a) the diagnosis of diseases in, and injuries to animals, including tests performed on animals for diagnostic purposes;
(b) the giving of advice based on such diagnosis;
(c) the medical or surgical treatment of animals; and
(d) the performance of surgical operations upon animals.

The exceptions referred to give certain limited powers of treatment – under specified conditions – to doctors, dentists and animal owners, and, under Statutory Orders, make provision for lay persons to carry out certain minor procedures which are applicable to farm animals.

Schedule 3 to the Veterinary Surgeons Act 1966

Veterinary nurses, like other non-veterinarians, may take advantage of those provisions in Schedule 3 to the Act which permit lay persons over the age of 18 to amputate the dew-claws of a puppy before its eyes open and allow anyone to render **first aid** in an emergency for the purpose of saving life or relieving pain or suffering.

The question is sometimes asked as to the extent of the treatment which may be considered permissible under the term 'first aid'. Precise definition is impossible, but the RCVS has advised that first aid should be restricted to what is necessary to save an animal's life, or to stop pain or suffering as an interim measure until a veterinary surgeon's services can be obtained.

Since 1991, Schedule 3 has also included very special provisions which extend the rights and powers of veterinary nurses to do things which other non-veterinarians cannot do, and these provisions are dealt with below.

Schedule 3 provisions relating to veterinary nurses

The heading to Schedule 3 to the Veterinary Surgeons Act is 'Exemptions from restrictions on practice of veterinary surgery'. Part 1 of the Schedule is entitled 'Treatment and Operations which may be given or carried out by unqualified persons'. In this context, 'unqualified persons' are people who are not qualified as veterinarians, and if it were not for the special provisions written into the Schedule in 1991 to cover veterinary nurses, they would be in the same position as any non-veterinarians.

Those special provisions referred to consist of the following additions to Part 1 which makes lawful:

Any medical treatment or minor surgery (not involving entry into a body cavity) to a companion animal by a veterinary nurse if the following conditions are complied with, that is to say:

(a) the companion animal is, for the time being, under the care of a registered veterinary surgeon or veterinary practitioner and the medical treatment or minor surgery is carried out by the veterinary nurse at his direction; and

(b) the registered veterinary surgeon or veterinary practitioner is the employer or is acting on behalf of the employer of the veterinary nurse.

In this paragraph, 'companion animal' means an animal kept as a pet or for companionship, not being a horse, pony, ass, mule, nor an animal used in agriculture, as defined by the Agriculture Act 1947. 'Veterinary nurse' means a nurse whose name is entered in the list of veterinary nurses maintained by the RCVS.

Interpretation of the provisions

It should be noted that these provisions do *not* permit:

- The making of a diagnosis.
- The carrying out of any procedure which is neither medical treatment nor surgery.
- Entry into a body cavity (e.g. a laparotomy). (The RCVS has advised that, in law, this prohibition applies also to cat castrations.)
- Any medical or surgical treatment carried out on any animal that does not meet the definition of a companion animal.

Further, from 1 July 1993, by virtue of an amendment to Schedule 3, dogs' tails may no longer be docked by unqualified persons. The only persons now permitted by law to dock dogs' tails are veterinary surgeons.

However, how should one interpret the positive aspects of these provisions? One can do no better than to summarise the advice given by the RCVS itself:

The amendment to Schedule 3 does not attempt to define what constitutes 'medical treatment or minor surgery' (which is a term used elsewhere in Schedule 3) but leaves it to the directing veterinary surgeon to interpret the phrase with common sense, allied to professional judgement. There should be less difficulty in construing the term 'medical treatment' than the term 'minor surgery', since it may be a matter of opinion as to what is minor or not. It may, however be helpful to note that Stedman's *Medical Dictionary* defines a minor operation as a 'surgical procedure of relatively slight extent and not in itself hazardous to life'.

The Royal College Council gave very careful consideration (when the proposed amendment to Schedule 3 was being discussed with the Ministry of Agriculture) to the possibility of producing a list of procedures which veterinary nurses might carry out, and rejected this idea in favour of a more flexible system whereby each veterinary surgeon would decide not only what he or she considered could reasonably be described as 'minor surgery', but whether or not the experience and expertise of the veterinary nurse to whom it was proposed to entrust the minor surgery, justified such a decision.

The advice of the Royal College is therefore that veterinary surgeons, rather than seeking guidance as to what procedure should or should not be entrusted to veterinary nurses, should make an individual assessment of whether or not each qualified nurse whose name is on the list maintained by the RCVS ought to be directed to carry out medical treatment or minor surgery. The following considerations should therefore be taken into account by the directing veterinary surgeon:

(1) How difficult is it to carry out the procedure in question competently and successfully and bearing in mind the risks inherent in the procedure?

(2) Have the veterinary nurses who are to be asked to carry out a procedure been given training and gained experience in the performance of the procedure, been made aware of the risks associated with the procedure and are they competent to carry it out?

(3) Do the veterinary nurses feel confident that they can competently and successfully carry out the procedure in question – or are they anxious that they may be asked to undertake tasks beyond their capabilities?

(4) Do they have not only the expertise and general competence to carry out the procedure, but also the experience and good

sense which will enable the nurse to react appropriately in the event of any problem arising?

(5) If necessary, will a veterinary surgeon be available to respond sufficiently quickly to a request for assistance?

The RCVS stresses that the directing veterinary surgeon is always responsible for the actions of the veterinary nurse. Consequently in deciding whether or not a veterinary nurse should be permitted to carry out a particular procedure within the guidelines set out above, directing veterinary surgeons must be confident that their decision would withstand any action for negligence that might arise.

Administration of anaesthesia

The process of inducing and maintaining anaesthesia does not fall within the meaning of the term 'minor surgery or medical treatment' contained in Schedule 3 and cannot, therefore, be entrusted to a veterinary nurse by virtue of the provisions of that Schedule. Accordingly, the question of the part that a veterinary nurse may legally play in the anaesthetising of an animal has to be approached by reference to the Veterinary Surgeons Act itself, and the RCVS has offered the guidance set out below, in relation to the anaesthetisation of companion animals as defined in Schedule 3:

Induction and maintenance of anaesthesia and the management to full recovery of consciousness involve a number of separate steps which are integrated:

(1) A clinical examination is required to assess the fitness of the patient to undergo anaesthesia.

(2) Evaluation of clinical signs may be followed by further examination and, when necessary, additional diagnostic tests.

(3) The anaesthetic regime has to be planned accordingly and a suitable technique has to be selected which is suitable for that animal and the type of procedure that is to be performed.

(4) It is necessary to select the appropriate sedative, analgesic and other agents which may have to be administered as premedication.

Only a veterinary surgeon should be responsible for these initial procedures, and for the selection of the anaesthetic technique, the doses of premedicant, anaesthetic agents and the selection of the route by which they are to be administered. Furthermore only a veterinary surgeon should administer and monitor the anaesthesia where the induction dose is either incremental or to effect i.e. intravenous or inhalation.

Provided the veterinary surgeon is physically present during anaesthesia and immediately available for consultation, it would be in order for a veterinary nurse, whose name is on the list maintained by the RCVS (and subject to the guidance set out above as to the basis on which procedures should be entrusted to veterinary nurses), to provide assistance by:

(1) Administering the selected pre- and post-operative sedative, analgesic or other agent.

(2) Administering prescribed non-incremental anaesthetic agents on the instruction of the directing veterinary surgeon.

(3) Monitoring clinical signs and maintaining an anaesthetic record.

(4) Maintaining anaesthetic by administering supplementary incremental doses of intravenous anaesthetic agents or adjusting the delivered concentration of anaesthetic agent under the direct instructions of the supervising veterinary surgeon.

The meaning of the word 'direction'

The amendment to Schedule 3 provides that a veterinary nurse may carry out medical treatment or minor surgery 'at the direction' of the employing veterinary surgeon. That means that it is sufficient for the veterinary surgeon to instruct the veterinary nurse to carry out the procedure in question. There is no requirement in law for the veterinary surgeon to be present and/or supervise the veterinary nurse.

The veterinary nurse in training

It must be clearly understood that Schedule 3 provisions as set out and explained above do not apply to student veterinary nurses. They apply only to veterinary nurses whose names appear on the RCVS's list of veterinary nurses. While in training, and not yet qualified, student nurses cannot take advantage of the special status conferred on qualified and listed veterinary nurses, and cannot lawfully be directed by an employing veterinary surgeon to carry out any of the procedures covered by the amendment to Schedule 3.

They can, however, still administer first aid in an emergency and also amputate dew-claws of a puppy before its eyes open provided they have reached the age of 18. These are rights granted to all lay persons.

They can also carry out nursing duties and assist veterinary surgeons in any way which does not involve an act of veterinary surgery

Procedures that are not 'acts of veterinary surgery'

Some years ago the solicitors to the RCVS advised that there were certain common procedures which did not constitute even minor acts of veterinary surgery and therefore could be carried out by veterinary nurses, nurses in training or other non-veterinarians.

These procedures included the removal of sutures, the replacement of dressings, the cutting of nails and beaks (unless performed for the treatment of a pathological condition), and the scaling of teeth carried out for prophylactic or cosmetic reasons. The RCVS was further advised that there were a number of 'borderline' procedures which might or might not be considered to be acts of veterinary surgery. These included the giving of enemata, oral and anal hygiene measures, and the administration of medical products (other than controlled drugs and biological products) by the subcutaneous, intramuscular, intravenous and intraperitoneal routes, following specific instructions from the veterinarian as to dosage.

The RCVS's solicitors advised even at that time (prior to the amendment of Schedule 3) that it would be unlikely that a veterinary nurse would be prosecuted for carrying out any such procedures if she did so at the direction of a veterinary surgeon. The advice would also apply to a student veterinary nurse although the veterinarian would wish to be particularly sure of her competence before directing her to carry out such a procedure.

A qualified veterinary nurse should now be on firm legal ground, since the carrying out of the procedure mentioned, on companion animals at the direction of an employing veterinary surgeon (or veterinarian acting on behalf of the nurse's employer), would be covered by the amendment to Schedule 3.

Insurance cover for nursing duties

The employing veterinary surgeon carries the responsibilities for the incompetent or negligent actions of the veterinary nurse. Although a client who wished to bring an action in the courts could also sue the veterinary nurse, it is likely that the employer would be the plaintiff's target as being better able to meet any damages awarded.

All veterinary practices insured with the Veterinary Defence Society Ltd are covered for acts and omissions not only of themselves, but also their nursing and other lay staff. The RCVS has advised its members insured with other companies to make certain that their policies provide equivalent cover.

Professional ethics for nurses

All veterinarians on the Register of Veterinary Surgeons or the Supplementary Veterinary Register of veterinary practitioners (both maintained in terms of the Veterinary Surgeons Act by the RCVS) are subject to the investigative jurisdiction of the College's Preliminary Investigation Committee and the judgements of its Disciplinary Committee – both statutory committees. As an aid to the better understanding of the veterinary profession's ethical obligations, the RCVS publishes (and revises triennially) its Guide to Professional Conduct, and any veterinarian whose ethical conduct is found by the Disciplinary Committee to be so seriously flawed as to amount to conduct disgraceful in a professional respect is in danger of having his or her name removed (or suspended for a stated time) from the Register.

The RCVS has no such powers in relation to veterinary nurses and neither the British Veterinary Nursing Association nor any other body has powers of this kind either. Nevertheless, veterinary nurses must be aware that ethical misbehaviour on their part could be held to be the responsibility of the veterinarian for whom they work – particularly if it were to be considered that the misbehaviour was permitted, condoned or due to lack of adequate instruction or supervision. All veterinary nurses should

therefore be aware of the main provisions of the RCVS's Guide to Professional Conduct in order that they may avoid acting in a way which might call their employing veterinarian's conduct into question.

Some of the most important obligations which veterinary nurses should bear in mind are as follows:*

(1) Never to carry out any act of veterinary surgery other than one which they are permitted to perform in terms of Schedule 3 to the Veterinary Surgeons Act or any other exemption order under the Act in terms of which they hold an individual qualification (e.g. the Veterinary Surgery (Blood Sampling) Orders).
(2) To respect client confidentiality in exactly the same way as a veterinarian must do in the terms of the RCVS's Guide to Professional Conduct.
(3) At all times (again like veterinarians) to do all in their power to ensure the welfare of animals entrusted to their care.
(4) Not to make any adverse comment to a client or other member of the public regarding the treatment administered to an animal by a veterinary surgeon, whether a member of their own practice or organisation or any other.
(5) Not to participate in, or allow themselves or their qualifications to be used in relation to the promotion of veterinary medicinal products, animal foods, or any other products directly associated with veterinary practice or animals.

All these obligations apply equally to veterinary nurses and to student nurses.

In regard to confidentiality (item 2 in the above list) there are a few specific exceptions which are clearly set out in the appropriate sections of the RCVS Guide to Professional Conduct, and all veterinary nurses must familiarise themselves with these parts (paragraphs 2.46 and 5.3) of the Guide. These exemptions apart, the ability of clients to consult professional advisers, secure in the knowledge that their discussions and any information passing between them will remain totally confidential, is the hallmark of the profession. If there is no certainty of complete confidentiality, information relevant to the well-being and treatment of the animal in question may be withheld – to the disadvantage of the animal.

Second opinions, referrals and specialists

The Guide to Professional Conduct lays down for all veterinarians the procedures that need to be followed when a case is being referred to another veterinarian for a second opinion or on a referral basis. As the veterinary nurse is often the first person to be contacted by animal owners, she must familiarise herself with the correct procedures and see that, in so far as any referral needs to be arranged by her, the correct procedures are followed.

---

* For the full provisions of the *Guide to Professional Conduct for Veterinary Nurses*, see the Appendix to volume 2.

Veterinary nurses must be aware that the description '**specialist**' may only be applied to those veterinarians specifically authorised by the RCVS to use this designation and listed in the appropriate sections of the RCVS's Register of Veterinary Surgeons. They should not, therefore, whether orally or in writing, refer to any member of the veterinary profession as a 'specialist' if that person is not recognised as such by the RCVS. Veterinarians who provide services of a particular nature or for a particular species simply have a special interest or particular skills: they are not 'specialists' until and unless those skills, allied to their qualifications and experience, have enabled the RCVS to endow them with specialist status.

Care must also be taken in referring to a veterinary surgeon as a **consultant**. He or she may be providing consultancy services in a practice, as a person with experience or expertise in a particular field, but should not be referred to in such a way (e.g. 'consultant in veterinary dermatology') as would suggest that he or she is authorised to use the title 'specialist' if that is not the case.

The Health and Safety at Work Act 1974

The Act applies to all persons at work (other than domestic servants) and covers every business (such as veterinary practice) and the self-employed. It has relevance to both employers and employees, and also to the health and safety of members of the general public who may come into contact with the business or work in question.

The objective of the Act is to ensure that all employers and self-employed persons carry on their businesses in such a way as to ensure that no one is exposed to risks to their health or safety. Employees, who will include veterinary nurses, must:

● Take reasonable care for the health and safety of himself or herself and of other persons who may be affected by his or her omissions at work.
● Co-operate with the employer (or other persons) so far as is necessary to enable any duty or requirement under the Act to be performed or complied with.
● Not interfere, recklessly or intentionally, with anything provided in the interests of health, safety and welfare.

The Health and Safety Executive, which has responsibility for enforcing and advising on the Act, has shown interest in health and safety in veterinary practice. Of particular relevance in this area are the regulations that have been in force since October 1989 on the control of substances hazardous to health (COSHH 1998). These regulations require employers and the self-employed to assess and then prevent or control the exposure to hazardous substances of all their employees and others who might be affected by exposure to hazardous substances at work. This includes microbiological agents, dusts of any kind in substantial quantities and all chemicals hazardous to health. Lead, asbestos and ionising radiation are covered by separate sets of regulations.

The British Veterinary Association's journal *In Practice* has published at regular intervals helpful articles on Health and Safety requirements in general and COSHH in particular, and these are deserving of study.

Chapters 4 (Occupational Hazards) and 12 (Medicines: Pharmacology, Therapeutics and Dispensing) look at the Health and Safety at Work Act and the COSHH regulations in greater detail.

Environmental protection law

The Environmental Protection Act 1990 has a relevance to the work of veterinary nurses, especially in the handling of clinical waste. The Act imposed a duty of care upon all producers of clinical waste to ensure that waste is handled and stored safely on their premises, and also disposed of safely and legally by the producers and others to whom the waste is passed on for this purpose. This very complex matter is considered in more depth in Chapters 4 (Occupational Hazards) and 20 (Theatre Practice). For a clear explanation of the provisions of the legislation, the article which appeared in the *Veterinary Record* (9 January 1993, pp. 43–45) under the title 'The veterinary surgeon's duty of care in handling and disposing of clinical waste' is essential reading.

In that article, the view was expressed that since the legislation allows waste producers to hand over waste for subsequent disposal only to an authorised person, pets which were put down or died at a veterinary surgery (and thereby became clinical waste) could not be returned to owners for burial or other disposal at home. Although that would appear technically correct, the British Veterinary Association was subsequently advised by the Environment Minister that the Act need not be interpreted so strictly. The pet owner retained ownership of the body in law and therefore had a right to have it returned (*Veterinary Record*, 30 January 1993, pp. 99–100). This interpretation seems to have been strengthened by virtue of the provisions of the Waste Management Licensing Regulations 1994.

The Environmental Protection Act 1990 is also the legislation which made it obligatory for all councils to provide a Dog Warden service from April 1992 and an offence for dogs to 'stray' on the public highway.

Other relevant legislation

Although the Veterinary Surgeons Act 1966 is the statute of principal relevance to veterinary practice and therefore to the work of veterinary surgeons and veterinary nurses alike, there are a number of other Acts of Parliament of which both must be aware. Within the compass of this chapter it is not possible to provide more than a very brief account of each Act: for a fuller understanding of the provisions of each it may be necessary to consult the statutes themselves. The following are the principal statutes with relevance to companion animal practice, with which veterinary nurses should be familiar.

The Medicines Act 1968

This Act controls the manufacture, importation, sale and supply of medicinal products in the United Kingdom, for both human and veterinary use. Its purpose is to secure the safety, quality and efficacy of all such products.

Medicinal products are substances or articles manufactured, sold, supplied, imported or exported for use, wholly or mainly for administration to humans or animals for a medicinal purpose. A **medicinal purpose** is defined in the Act so as to include diagnosis, treatment, or prevention of disease, contraception, inducing anaesthesia, and preventing or interfering with the normal operation of a physiological function.

Medicinal products are divided into three main categories:

- **GSL** products (on a general sales list).
- **POM** products (on prescription only).
- **P** products (pharmacy only medicines).

There is also a fourth category of veterinary medicinal products, which is commonly referred to as the Merchant's List and indicated as **PML**. These are mainly for sale to farmers and horse keepers. Chapter 12 (Medicines: Pharmacology, Therapeutics and Dispensing) deals with this Act in more detail.

Misuse of Drugs Act 1971

Chapter 12 (Medicines: Pharmacology, Therapeutics and Dispensing) also considers this Act which, with its subsidiary legislation, controls the possession, supply and use of what used to be known as 'dangerous drugs'. In terms of the Act, these are now known as 'Controlled Drugs'.

The Act allows veterinarians to possess, use, supply and prescribe most controlled drugs, but for veterinary use only. It is important to note that all controlled drugs are also prescription-only medicines in terms of the Medicines Act (see above).

The Protection of Animals Acts

There is a group of statutes, beginning with the Protection of Animals Act 1911 and known collectively as the Protection of Animals Acts 1911–1988, which seeks to prevent cruelty to animals and alleviate suffering.

The Act of 1911 provides that the following actions constitute cruelty, punishable by a fine or imprisonment:

(a) Cruelly to beat, kick, ill-treat, over-drive, over-load, torture, infuriate or terrify an animal.
(b) To cause suffering by doing or omitting to do any act.
(c) To convey or carry any animal in such a manner as to cause it unnecessary suffering.
(d) To perform any operation without due care and humanity (in relation to which the provisions of the Anaesthetics Acts are relevant).
(e) The fighting or baiting of any animal or the use of premises for such a purpose.
(f) The administering of any poison or injurious drug or substance to any animal.

It should be noted that the legislation is not concerned with whether or not the cruelty was intended. It is the result of the relevant act or omission which is important. When an owner of an animal is convicted of cruelty, the courts may order:

- The destruction of the animal(s) either with agreement or on the evidence of a veterinary surgeon.
- The disqualification from having custody of a particular kind of animal or any animal at all.

The Protection of Animals (Amendment) Act 1988 has made it an offence either to be present, without reasonable excuse, when animals are placed together for the purpose of fighting, or to publish, or to cause to be published, an advertisement for a fight between animals.

The Anaesthetics Acts

The Protection of Animals (Anaesthetics) Acts 1954 and 1964 are intended to prevent the infliction of unnecessary suffering on an animal during an operation. It provides that the carrying out of any operation with or without the use of instruments, involving interference with the sensitive tissues or the bone structure or an animal, shall constitute an offence unless an anaesthetic is used in such a way as to prevent any pain to the animal during the operation. An operation of this kind, performed without or with inadequate anaesthetic, is said to be performed 'without due care and humanity' – see subparagraph (d) of the previous section. Exceptions to this general rule (which may be relevant to companion animal practice) are as follows:

(1) The making of injections or extractions by means of a hollow needle.
(2) Experiments authorised under the Animals (Scientific Procedures) Act 1986.
(3) The rendering of emergency first aid for the purpose of saving life or relieving pain.
(4) The docking of the tail of a dog or the amputation of the dew-claws of a dog before its eyes open.
(5) Any minor operation performed by a veterinarian which, by reason of its quickness or painlessness, is customarily so performed without an anaesthetic.
(6) Any minor operation whether performed by a veterinarian or by some other person, being an operation which is not customarily performed only by a veterinarian.

The Animals (Scientific Procedures) Act 1986

This Act prohibits the carrying out of experiments on animals except under licence from the Home Office. This is a very specialised piece of legislation and for those wishing to study its provisions in depth, reference to the Home Office and its publications available through HMSO is advised. Nevertheless, the veterinary nurse in companion animal practice should be aware of the following three points:

- All establishments breeding and supplying the most commonly used laboratory animals are required to obtain a certificate of approval from the appropriate Secretary of State.

- The Act prohibits the use of cats and dogs unless they are obtained direct from the designated establishment where they were bred. The use of stray or stolen pets will not be allowed in any circumstances.
- Demonstrations using live animals will be permitted where absolutely necessary for professional training but the Act prohibits their use in the education of school children or others at the same level.

Legislation covering animals kept commercially

There are four statutes which are designed to control the premises on which companion animals are kept for commercial purposes, and ensure the welfare of such animals. These are:

- The Pet Animals Act 1951.
- The Animal Boarding Establishments Act 1963.
- The Breeding of Dogs Act 1973.
- The Riding Establishments Acts 1964 and 1970.

The responsibility of enforcement of these Acts rests with the local authority, from whom licences to operate such premises must be obtained, but inspections are normally carried out on behalf of the authorities by veterinary surgeons. Environmental Health Officers and Dog Wardens may also be involved in the inspection of premises.

The Pet Animals Act relates to the keeping of pet shops and prohibits the selling of animals as pets in any street or public place. It also prohibits the sale of pets to children under 12 years of age.

The Animal Boarding Establishments Act relates only to establishments which board dogs and cats, and not to the boarding of other animals. It should be noted that the fact that a boarding establishment is kept and is run by a veterinary surgeon (as distinct from having cages for his patients) does not exempt him or her from the need to obtain a licence.

The Breeding of Dogs Act requires the licensing of any premises (including a private dwelling) where more than two bitches are kept for the purpose of breeding for sale.

The Riding Establishments Acts deal with ponies and horses used in riding schools for hire and riding tuition. Each of these Acts is concerned with making sure that the animals are properly accommodated, watered, bedded, exercised, and protected against disease and fire. The Acts relate to the inspection by approved veterinary surgeons of horses let out for hire or where money is exchanged for riding lessons on a horse or pony not belonging to the rider. Pony trekking centres are also involved in inspections but both riding clubs and livery yards are exempt if no tuition is involved using hired horses.

The British Veterinary Association has published guidelines for the inspection of each type of establishment.

The Dangerous Dogs Act 1991

This Act, together with subsidiary legislation, is designed to stop people keeping dogs which are bred for fighting. The dogs currently specified as falling within this category are the **Pit Bull Terrier**, the **Japanese Tosa**, the **Dogo Argentino**, and the **Fila Braziliero**, but other types may be added by statutory order.

The Act prohibits the breeding, sale, exchange or gift of dogs of the specified types. The only such dogs which anyone may now lawfully possess are those which, by the appropriate date (now past), had been reported to the police by the owners and which the owners had ensured were neutered, permanently identified and made the subject of third-party insurance. Even then such a dog may be allowed in a public place, only if it is muzzled and on a lead, securely held by someone of not less than 16 years of age. To abandon such a dog or allow it to stray is an offence. In the case of convictions for offences under the Act, the court has the power to order the destruction of the dog in question, but, since the passing of the Dangerous Dogs (Amendment) Act 1997, has a wider discretion than before.

The Act also creates the separate offence of owning or being in charge of a dog of any type which is dangerously out of control in a public place.

Some other Acts of importance

Under the **Abandonment of Animals Act 1960** it is an offence for the owner or possessor of an animal to abandon it without good reason (whether permanently or not) in circumstances likely to cause unnecessary suffering. The **Animals (Cruel Poisons) Act 1962** prohibits the killing of any mammal by any cruel poison, which is specified as including red squill, strychnine and yellow phosphorus. The **Dangerous Wild Animals Act 1976** provides that no one shall keep a dangerous wild animal without a licence from the local authority. The question often arises as to whether an animal is dangerous and wild in terms of legislation. All animals covered by the Act are set out in a Schedule to the Act.

Regulations on the import and export of cats, dogs and birds

In general terms, dogs and cats may not be **imported** into the UK without spending 6 months in quarantine in terms of the **Rabies (Importation of Dogs, Cats and other Mammals) Order 1974**. See Chapter 5, p. 140. Any queries in regard to importation and this order should be addressed to the Rabies Branch of the Ministry of Agriculture, Fisheries and Food. From time to time a veterinary practice may be presented with a dog or cat that has been imported but has not met the quarantine requirements. Although the practice may consider there is a dilemma between reporting this serious breach of the law and the ethical requirements of preserving client confidentiality, the RCVS has resolved the problem by stating in its Guide to Professional Conduct that the exceptions to the confidentiality rule include this very situation. Accordingly, the veterinary surgeon should at once report such a breach of the quarantine regulations to the Rabies Branch of MAFF or to the Divisional Veterinary Officer.

Special provisions have been made for the importing of cats and dogs from other Member States of the European Community with effect from July 1994 *provided that they are being imported for commercial purposes only*. Such animals may be imported without quarantine provided they are accompanied by the necessary certificates testifying to the facts that they are at least 8 months old, were born and have remained in a single rabies-free establishment since birth, and are identified by microchip, have been vaccinated against rabies and blood tested to confirm immunity.

The import of any live poultry, or other birds or hatching eggs, is prohibited, except under licence, in terms of the **Importation of Birds, Poultry and Hatching Eggs Order 1979**; however, the Ministry of Agriculture, Fisheries and Food publish a leaflet (IM98A: rev. 4/96) entitled 'Information about importing family pet birds into Great Britain'. With regard to the **export** of birds, cats and dogs to other countries, the veterinary certificates, vaccinations and other requirements will vary from one country to another. (It should be borne in mind that the formalities are not so much designed for the export from the UK as for the import into another country.) If information is required regarding the importation of a dog, cat or bird into another country, enquiries should be made of the Export Branch of the Ministry of Agriculture, Fisheries and Food as far in advance of the proposed date as possible.

8

Nutrition

Sandra McCune

Proper nutrition is essential for the maintenance of optimum health and activity in all living creatures. Wild animals can obtain all the nutrients they need through a combination of hunting, scavenging and foraging, but the opportunity for companion animals to access their natural diet has been limited by the process of domestication. It is the responsibility of the owner, therefore, to ensure that the diet they provide meets all the nutritional and behavioural needs of their pet, and professional advice in this area is frequently sought.

Failure to provide a nutritionally adequate diet can result in disease or sub-optimal performance, but nutritional factors may impact on the health of animals in a number of other ways. Many medical conditions will respond to modification of some aspect of the diet and nutritional support is particularly important at times of illness or other forms of stress. See Fig. 8.1.

Nutrients and nutrient requirements

Food may be defined as any solid or liquid which, when ingested, can supply any or all of the following:

- Energy-giving materials from which the body can produce movement, heat or other forms of energy.
- Materials for growth, repair or reproduction.
- Substances necessary to initiate or regulate the processes involved in the first two categories.

The components of food which have these functions are called **nutrients** and the foods or food mixtures which are actually eaten are referred to as the **diet**. Any nutrient which is required by the animal and cannot be synthesised in the body is called an **essential nutrient** and a dietary source

must be provided. If any essential nutrient is lacking or present in insufficient quantity in the diet, then the diet, as a whole, must be considered inadequate.

Energy

In addition to providing specific nutrients, food also supplies energy. Energy is a fundamental requirement of all living species and provides the power for cells to function. The energy content of the diet is derived from carbohydrates, fats and protein, and the amounts of each of these nutrients in a food will determine its energy content. Dietary fat supplies twice as much energy as protein or carbohydrate per gram and is therefore a more efficient fuel for metabolism. Water has no energy value, so the energy density of food varies inversely with its moisture content.

Energy intake must be carefully regulated and maintained at a level close to requirements. When maintained over long periods, energy intake in excess of energy expenditure can be detrimental and leads to obesity or, in some young dogs, growth abnormalities. An inadequate energy intake results in poor growth in young animals and weight loss in adults. Although most animals are efficient self-regulators of their energy intake, this ability may be overridden by a number of factors, particularly in dogs.

No animal is able to utilise all the energy from its food. Energy intake is therefore considered at three different levels: gross energy (GE), digestible energy (DE) and metabolisable energy (ME).

- **Gross energy** of ingested food is the maximum amount of energy that can be released by a food and is assessed by bomb calorimetry. Although a substance may have a high GE content, it is of no use unless the animal is able to digest and absorb it.
- **Digestible energy** is the energy available from a food when it has been absorbed into the body after digestion in the digestive tract and is calculated as GE minus faecal losses.
- **Metabolisable energy** is the energy which is ultimately utilised by the tissues and is calculated as DE minus urinary losses.

The DE and ME contents of foods depend both upon their composition and upon the species which consumes them. The digestive systems of animals differ markedly between species and even two fairly similar animals, such as the dog and the cat, show differences in digestibility values when fed the same food. In addition to these species differences there will be variations between individual animals in their own metabolic efficiency.

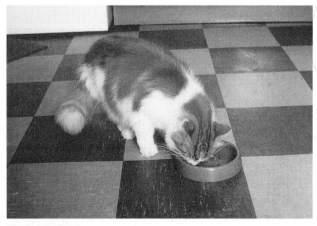

Fig. 8.1 Cat feeding.

Table 8.1 Calculation of metabolisable energy in cat and dog foods (kcal/100 g food[a]) (after Wills, 1996)

Species	Food type and ME equation
Cat	Canned $(P \times 3.9 + F \times 7.7 + C \times 3.0) - 5$
	Dry $(P \times 5.65 + F \times 9.4 + C \times 4.15)\, 0.99 - 126$
	Semi-moist $(P \times 3.7 + F \times 8.8 + C \times 3.3$
Dog	All $(P \times 3.5 + F \times 8.5 + C \times 3.5$

P = protein g/100 g of food, F = fat (acid ether extract) g/100 g of food.
C = carbohydrate (calculated by difference) g/100 g of food.
[a] For result in kJ/100 g food, multiply by 4.18.

Table 8.2 Estimated energy requirements of healthy dogs in various physiological states

Physiological state	Energy requirement
Work 1 hour light work	MER $\times$ 1.1
1 full day light work	MER $\times$ 1.5
1 full day heavy work (sledge dog)	MER $\times$ 2–4
Gestation (<42 days)	MER $\times$ 1
(>42 days)	MER $\times$ 1.1–1.3
Peak lactation (21–42 days)	MER $\times$ (1 + [0.25 $\times$ no. in litter])
Growth birth to 3 months	MER $\times$ 2
3 months to 6 months	MER $\times$ 1.6
6 months to 12 months	MER $\times$ 1.2
Cold wind chill factor of 8.5°C	MER $\times$ 1.25
wind chill factor of <0°C	MER $\times$ 1.75
Heat – tropical climates	MER $\times$ 2.5
Inactivity	RER $\times$ 1.3

RER = resting energy requirement (kcal) = $70 \times BW^{0.75}$ [kg].
RER (kJ) = $4.184 \times 70 \times BW^{0.75}$ [kg].
MER = maintenance energy requirement = RER $\times$ 2.

Table 8.3 Estimated energy requirements for healthy cats in various physiological states

Age	Physiological state	MER[a] (kcal [kJ]/kg BW)
10 weeks	Growth	250 [1046]
20 weeks	Growth	130 [544]
30 weeks	Growth	100 [418]
40 weeks	Growth	80 [355]
Adult	Inactive	70 [293]
Adult	Active	80 [335]
Adult	Gestation	80 [335] $\times$ 1.1–1.3
Adult	Lactation	80 [335] $\times$ (1 + (0.25 $\times$ no. in litter))

[a] Maintenance energy requirement.

Simple formulae have been developed which give reasonable approximations of the ME in a food from its carbohydrate, fat and protein contents, allowing for the losses in absorption and efficiency (Table 8.1).

Within the body, energy is used to perform muscular work, basic processes such as breathing and physical activity to maintain body temperature. There are two components of energy expenditure, basal metabolic rate and thermogenesis:

- **Basal metabolic rate (BMR)** keeps the body 'ticking over', and includes processes such as respiration, circulation and kidney function. It may be affected by many factors including bodyweight and composition, age and hormonal status.
- **Thermogenesis** is simply an increase in metabolic rate over the basal level and includes the cost of digesting, absorbing and utilising nutrients (the 'thermic effect of food'); of muscular work or exercise; of stress; or of maintenance of body temperature in a cold environment. Unlike BMR, the degree of thermogenesis can vary widely and may cause large variations in daily output.

Energy requirements of individual animals are based on the weight of actively metabolising tissue and may be influenced by bodyweight, body surface area, body composition and hair type. Dogs are a unique species in that there is such a wide variation in normal adult bodyweights, and estimations of energy needs are calculated from an allometric equation which relates energy requirements to the animal's metabolic bodyweight, BW $(kg)^{0.75}$ (see p. 193). For other species, including cats, with a relatively narrow range of bodyweights, a linear equation which links energy requirements directly to bodyweight is appropriate in most situations (see p. 193). These basic energy requirements may then be modified according to the animal's physiological status (including life stage and state of health or disease), level of activity and environmental conditions (Tables 8.2 and 8.3).

The energy density of the diet must be high enough to enable the dog or cat to obtain sufficient calories to maintain energy balance. This is the principal factor determining the quantity of food eaten each day and thus the amount of each nutrient ingested by the animal. Nutrient requirements are usually expressed in terms of the ME concentration so that the values are applicable to any type of food or diet regardless of its water content, nutrient content or overall energy value.

Macronutrients

Protein

Proteins are large complex molecules which are composed of long chains of amino acids linked together by peptide bonds. There are only about 20 amino acids, but these may be arranged in any combination to give an almost infinite variety of naturally occurring proteins, each with its own characteristic properties. Proteins are essential components of all living cells where they have several important functions including regulation of metabolism (as enzymes and some hormones) and a structural role in cell walls and muscle fibre. They are thus an important requirement for tissue growth and repair. Proteins are also a source of energy in the diet.

Animals need a dietary source of protein to provide the specific amino acids that their tissues cannot synthesise at a rate sufficient for optimum performance. Amino acids may be classified as either essential (indispensable) or non-essential (dispensable). **Essential** amino acids cannot be synthesised by the body in sufficient amounts and must, therefore, be provided in the diet (Table 8.4). **Non-essential** amino acids are equally important as components of body proteins, but they can be synthesised from excesses of certain other dietary amino acids or other sources of dietary nitrogen.

Protein is required during normal maintenance to replace protein lost during the natural turnover of epithelial surfaces, hair and other body tissues, and in secretions. Additional protein is needed during periods of growth, pregnancy, lactation and for repair of damaged tissue. It is during these critical stages that protein quality (the amino acid composition of the protein) and digestibility are most important. Animal proteins generally have a more balanced amino acid profile, with a greater proportion of essential amino acids and better digestibility than plant proteins. The biological value of a food protein is the proportion which can be utilised for synthesising body tissues and compounds and is not excreted in urine or faeces. Good-quality animal proteins have a higher biological value than plant-based proteins.

Protein deficiency can result from either insufficient dietary protein or from a shortage of particular amino acids. Signs of protein deficiency include poor growth or weight loss, rough and dull hair coat, anorexia, increased susceptibility to disease, muscle wasting and emaciation, oedema and finally death. Deficiency of a single essential amino acid results in anorexia and subsequent negative nitrogen balance.

Cats exhibit a number of nutritional peculiarities, many of which are reflected in their protein and amino acid requirements. Not only do they have a higher maintenance protein requirement than many other mammals, but they are also particularly sensitive to an arginine-deficient diet and they have a specific dietary need for the amino-sulphonic acid, taurine. Taurine is vital to the functioning of a wide range of mammalian organ systems but unlike other animals, cats are unable to synthesise sufficient quantities to meet their exceptionally high requirements. A deficiency of taurine in cats results in **feline central retinal degeneration**, and has also been linked to **dilated cardiomyopathy**, reproductive failure in queens, developmental abnormalities in kittens and impaired immune function.

Dietary protein in excess of the body's requirements is not laid down as muscle but is, instead, converted to fat and stored as adipose tissue.

Fat

Dietary fats consist mainly of mixtures of triglycerides, where each triglyceride is a combination of three fatty acids joined by a unit of glycerol. The character of each fat is determined largely by the different fatty acids in each. Fatty acids may be described as **saturated**, where there are no double bonds between carbon atoms, or **unsaturated**, where one or more double bonds are present. Those containing more than one double bond are referred to as **polyunsaturated.** Most fats contain all of these types but in widely varying proportions.

Dietary fat has several roles. It serves as the most concentrated source of energy in the diet and it lends palatability and an acceptable texture to food. However, its most important functions are as a provider of **essential fatty acids (EFA)** and as a carrier for the fat-soluble vitamins A, D, E and K. There are currently three recognised EFA, all of which are polyunsaturated; linoleic, α linoleic and arachidonic acids. Linoleic and α-linoleic acids are the parent compounds from which the more complex, longer chain compounds (derived EFA) can be made. The cat is unusual in that it is unable to convert the parent EFA into longer chain derivatives and therefore requires a dietary source of arachidonic acid, which in practical terms means a requirement for EFA of *animal* origin.

The EFA are involved in many aspects of health, including kidney function and reproduction. They are essential components of cell membranes and they are necessary for the synthesis of prostaglandins. Signs associated with EFA deficiency in dogs and cats include dull, scurfy coat, hair loss, fatty liver, anaemia and impaired fertility.

It should be noted that diets high in polyunsaturated fatty acids may become rancid through oxidation, which can lead to the destruction of other nutrients, particularly vitamin E.

Carbohydrate

Carbohydrates provide the body with energy and may be converted to body fat. This group includes the simple sugars (such as glucose) and the complex sugars (such as starch) which consist of chains of the simpler sugars. All animals have a metabolic requirement for glucose, but provided the diet contains sufficient glucose precursors (amino acids and glycerol), most animals can synthesise enough to meet their metabolic needs without a dietary source of carbohydrate.

Table 8.4 Essential amino acids for dogs and cats

Amino acid	Dog	Cat
Arginine	✓	✓
Histidine	✓	✓
Isoleucine	✓	✓
Lysine	✓	✓
Methionine	✓	✓
Cystine	✓	✓
Phenylalanine	✓	✓
Tyrosine	✓	✓
Threonine	✓	✓
Tryptophan	✓	✓
Valine	✓	✓
Taurine	✗	✓

✓ = essential; ✗ = non-essential.

Sugars and **cooked** starches are economical and easily digested sources of energy, whereas uncooked starches are less readily digested. Some species (e.g. some dogs) may find sugars palatable, but others, such as the cat do not respond to the taste of sugars. The value of disaccharides such as sucrose or lactose is limited in most animals by the activity of the intestinal disaccharidases, such as sucrase and lactase. In particular, the activity of lactase declines with age and an excessive consumption of lactose-containing (dairy) products can lead to the production of diarrhoea.

Dietary fibre

Dietary fibre, or roughage, is the term applied to the group of indigestible polysaccharides such as cellulose, pectin and lignin. They are usually associated with plant material and typically constitute the cell walls of plants. These materials generally escape digestion and pass through the digestive tract relatively unchanged. The role of dietary fibre in the animal depends to a large extent on the physiology of the animal's digestive tract, but in most species, a limited amount of dietary fibre may provide bulk to the faeces, regularising bowel movements and thus helping to prevent constipation or diarrhoea. Soluble and insoluble sources of dietary fibre are used to improve glycaemic control in dogs with diabetes mellitus and in the dietary management of a number of other 'fibre-responsive' diseases.

Micronutrients

Minerals

Minerals are inorganic nutrients, which are sometimes referred to collectively as 'ash'. They may be divided into macro minerals (which are required in relatively large amounts) and trace elements or micro minerals (which are required in relatively small or trace amounts). Electrolytes are minerals in their salt form as found in the body tissues. Table 8.5 lists the function of the main minerals and Table 8.6 the dietary requirements.

Macro minerals

Calcium (Ca) and phosphorus (P). Calcium and phosphorus are closely interrelated nutritionally and will therefore be discussed together. They are the major minerals involved in maintaining the structural rigidity of bones and teeth and approximately 99% of body calcium and 80% of body phosphorus are stored in the skeletal tissues. Calcium and phosphorus requirements are increased during growth, late pregnancy and lactation. The metabolism of calcium and phosphorus is closely linked with vitamin D.

Calcium is also essential for normal blood clotting and for nerve and muscle function. The level of calcium in the blood plasma is crucial to these functions and is very carefully regulated.

Phosphorus also has many other functions (more than any other mineral) and a complete discussion would require coverage of nearly all the metabolic processes of the body. Phosphorus is involved in many enzyme systems and is also

Table 8.5 Established functions of minerals in the dog and cat

Element	Function
Macrominerals	
Calcium	Bone and teeth development. Required for blood clotting, nerve and muscle function.
Chloride	Maintains osmotic pressure, acid–base and water balance.
Magnesium	Bone and teeth development. Energy metabolism.
Phosphorus	Bone and teeth development. Required for energy utilisation and various enzyme systems.
Potassium & Sodium	Maintain osmotic pressure, acid–base and water balance. Required for nerve and muscle function.
Microminerals	
Arsenic	Required for growth and red blood cell formation.
Chromium	Required for carbohydrate metabolism.
Cobalt	Component of vitamin B_{12}.
Copper	Required for haemoglobin synthesis, structure of bones and blood vessels, melanin production and various enzyme systems.
Fluoride	Bone and teeth development.
Iodine	Thyroid hormone production.
Iron	Component of haemoglobin and myoglobin. Needed for the utilisation of oxygen.
Manganese	Required for chondroitin sulphate and cholesterol synthesis. Various enzyme systems associated with carbohydrate and fat metabolism.
Molybdenum	Various enzyme systems.
Nickel	Function of membranes and nucleic acid metabolism.
Selenium	Component of glutathione peroxidase.
Silicon	Bone and connective tissue development.
Vanadium	Growth, reproduction and fat metabolism.
Zinc	Various enzyme systems including alkaline phosphatase, carbonic anhydrase and digestive enzymes. Maintenance of epidermal integrity and immunological homeostasis.

a component of the so-called 'high energy' organic phosphate compounds. These are mainly responsible for the storage and transfer of energy in the body.

Although the absolute concentrations of these minerals in the diet are of paramount importance, the ratio of calcium to phosphorus is also of great significance. The minimum calcium:phosphorus ratio for growth is generally considered to be about 1:1. For adult animals it is somewhat less critical. Imbalance in this ratio, where calcium is much less than phosphorus, leads to a marked deficiency of calcium in relation to bone formation.

Table 8.6 Dietary requirements: minerals

Mineral	Cat		Dog	
Calcium	Growth:	110–173 mg/kg BW/day or approximately 160–250 mg/100 kcal (418 kJ) ME.	Growth:	320 mg/kg BW/day or approximately 275 mg/100 kcal (418 kJ) ME.
	Maintenance:	87–156 mg/kg BW/day or approximately 125–200 mg/100 kcal (418 kJ) ME.	Maintenance:	119 mg/kg BW/day or approximately 130–160 mg/100 kcal (418 kJ) ME.
Phosphorus	Growth:	90–150 mg/kg BW/day or approximately 120–200 mg/100 kcal (418 kJ) ME.	Growth:	240 mg/kg BW/day or approximately 200–225 mg/100 kcal (418 kJ) ME.
	Maintenance:	90 mg/kg BW/day or approximately 120 mg/100 kcal (418 kJ) ME.	Maintenance:	89 mg/kg BW/day or approximately 120–160 mg/100 kcal (418 kJ) ME.
Copper	Growth:	100–160 µg/kg BW/day or approximately 300–460 µg/100 kcal (418 kJ) ME.	Growth:	160–500 µg/kg BW/day or approximately 150–440 µg/100 kcal (418 kJ) ME.
	Maintenance:	75 µg/kg BW/day or approximately 100 µg/100 kcal (418 kJ) ME.	Maintenance:	80 µ/kg BW/day or approximately 150 µg/100 kcal (418 kJ) ME.
Iodine	Growth:	20–30 µg/kg BW/day or approximately 27–33 µg/100 kcal (418 kJ) ME.	Growth:	30–50 µg/kg BW/day or approximately 16–25 µg/100 kcal (418 kJ) ME.
	Maintenance:	7–15 µg/kg BW/day or approximately 10–20 µg/100 kcal (418 kJ) ME.	Maintenance:	12 µg/kg BW/day or approximately 16–24 µg/100 kcal (418 kJ) ME.
Iron	Growth:	4–4.5 mg/kg BW/day or approximately 12–18 mg/100 kcal (418 kJ) ME.	Growth:	1.74–2.3 mg/kg BW/day or approximately 1–2 mg/100 kcal (418 kJ) ME.
	Maintenance:	1.2 mg/kg BW/day or approximately 1.6 mg/100 kcal (418 kJ) ME.	Maintenance:	0.65 mg/kg BW/day or approximately 100–130 mg/100 kcal (418 kJ) ME.
Magnesium	Growth:	7.5–9.4 mg/kg BW/day or approximately 10–12.5 mg/100 kcal (418 kJ) ME.	Growth:	22 mg/kg BW/day or approximately 25 mg/100 kcal (418 kJ) ME.
	Maintenance:	6 mg/kg BW/day or approximately 8 mg/100 kcal (418 kJ) ME.	Maintenance:	5.5–8.2 mg/kg BW/day or approximately 11 mg/100 kcal (418 kJ) ME.
Manganese	Growth and Maintenance:	80–250 µg/kg BW/day or approximately 100–250 µg/100 kcal (418 kJ) ME.	Growth:	280–1000 µg/kg BW/day or approximately 200–600 µg/100 kcal (418 kJ) ME.
			Maintenance:	100 µg/kg BW/day or approximately 140–200 µg/100 kcal (418 kJ) ME.
Selenium	Growth:	5–13 µg/kg BW/day or approximately 2–5 µg/100 kcal (418 kJ) ME.	Growth:	6–13 µg/kg BW/day or approximately 3–8 µg/100 kcal (418 kJ) ME.
	Maintenance:	5 µg/kg BW/day or approximately 6 µg/100 kcal (418 kJ) ME.	Maintenance:	6 µg/kg BW/day or approximately 7 µg/100 kcal (418 kJ) ME.
Sodium	Growth:	15–30 mg/kg BW/day or approximately 20–40 mg/100 kcal (418 kJ) ME.	Growth:	30 mg/kg BW/day or approximately 20–25 mg/100 kcal (418 kJ) ME.
	Maintenance:	14 mg/kg BW/day or approximately 18 mg/100 kcal (418 kJ) ME.	Maintenance:	14 mg/kg BW/day or approximately 18 mg/100 kcal (418 kJ) ME.
Chloride	Growth and Maintenance:	29 mg/kg BW/day or approximately 38 mg/100 kcal (418 kJ) ME.	Growth:	46 mg/kg BW/day or approximately 40 mg/100 kcal (418 kJ) ME.
			Maintenance:	17 mg/kg BW/day or approximately 21–30 mg/100 kcal (418 kJ) ME.
Potassium	Growth and Maintenance:	100–125 mg/100 kcal (418 kJ) ME.	Growth and Maintenance:	100–125 mg/100 kcal (418 kJ) ME.
Zinc	Growth and Maintenance:	2.5–3.9 mg/kg BW/day or approximately 1–2 mg/100 kcal (418 kJ) ME.	Growth:	1.9–3.3 mg/kg BW/day or approximately 0.97–2 mg/100 kcal (418 kJ) ME.
			Maintenance:	0.72 mg/kg BW/day or approximately 0.92–1.200 mg/100 kcal (418 kJ) ME.

Calcium deficiency (absolute or relative) results in **nutritional secondary hyperparathyroidism** in which there is increased bone resorption to restore circulating calcium levels. This results in skeletal deformities and lameness in the growing animal. Calcium–phosphorus imbalance may also occur in association with deficiency of vitamin D. This gives rise to **rickets** in the growing animal or **osteomalacia** in the adult. Hypocalcaemia in lactating bitches (particularly of the toy breeds) causes **eclampsia**, with nervous disturbances. This occurs where there is an inability of the calcium regulatory mechanism to compensate for the loss of calcium in milk.

There is evidence that very high levels of calcium and phosphorus or a very high ratio are also harmful. Conditions such as **hip dysplasia, osteochondrosis syndrome, enostosis** and **wobbler syndrome** have been related to excessive calcium intake in the growing dog.

Magnesium (Mg). In association with calcium and phosphorus, magnesium is required for healthy bones and teeth. About 60% of body magnesium is found in skeletal tissue, but it is also to be found in the soft tissues of the body. Heart and skeletal muscle and nervous tissue depend on a proper balance between calcium and magnesium for normal function. Magnesium is also important in sodium and potassium metabolism and plays a key role in many essential enzyme reactions, particularly those concerned with energy metabolism.

A deficiency of magnesium is characterised by muscular weakness and in severe cases, convulsions. Nevertheless, a dietary deficiency of magnesium is very unlikely. In contrast, very high intakes of magnesium have been associated with an increased incidence of **feline lower urinary tract disease**.

Potassium (K). Potassium is found in high concentrations within cells and is required for acid–base balance and osmoregulation of the body fluids. It is also important for nerve and muscle function and energy metabolism. Potassium is widely distributed in foods and naturally occurring deficiencies are rare. However, requirement is linked to protein intake so care may be needed in ensuring that high protein diets contain adequate potassium.

A potassium deficiency causes muscular weakness, poor growth and lesions of the heart and kidney. In cats, the use of diets containing urinary acidifiers with a marginal potassium content has recently been associated with hypokalaemia.

Sodium (Na) and Chloride (Cl). Together, sodium and chloride represent the major electrolytes of the body water and are required for acid–base balance and osmoregulation of the body fluids. Chloride is also an essential component of bile and hydrochloric acid (which is present in gastric juice).

Common salt (NaCl) is the most usual form in which these two minerals are added to food, so the dietary recommendation is often expressed in terms of sodium chloride. As with potassium, salt is widely distributed in normal diets, so deficiencies are rare.

Signs of deficiency may include fatigue, exhaustion, inability to maintain water balance, decreased water intake, retarded growth, dry skin and hair loss. Excess will cause greater than normal fluid intake and it has been suggested that some dogs with hypertension may benefit from a lower sodium diet.

Trace minerals

Iron (Fe). Iron is an essential component of the oxygen-carrying pigments, haemoglobin (in blood) and myoglobin (in muscle). It is also an essential part of many enzymes which are involved in respiration at the cellular level.

A deficiency causes anaemia with the typical clinical picture of weakness and fatigue. Conversely iron, like most trace elements, is toxic if ingested in excessive amounts and is associated with anorexia and weight loss.

Copper (Cu). Copper is required for the formation and activity of red blood cells, as a co-factor in many enzyme systems, and for the normal pigmentation of skin and hair.

Copper deficiency impairs the absorption and transport of iron and decreases haemoglobin synthesis. Thus a lack of copper in the diet can cause anaemia even when the intake of iron is normal. Bone disorders can also occur as a result of copper deficiency and in this case the cause is thought to be a reduction in the activity of a copper-containing enzyme, leading to diminished stability and strength of bone collagen.

Ironically, *excess* dietary copper may also cause anaemia which is thought to result from competition between copper and iron for absorption sites in the intestine. Bedlington Terriers are known to display an unusual defect which results in hepatitis and cirrhosis and appears to be inherited. It has also been identified in other breeds including West Highland White Terriers and Dobermann Pinschers. For these particular breeds, foods with a high copper content and copper-containing mineral supplements should be avoided.

Zinc (Zn). Zinc is an essential component of many enzyme systems, including those related to protein and carbohydrate metabolism, and is essential for maintaining healthy coat and skin. Zinc is required by all animals, but the zinc requirement is particularly affected by the other components of the diet. For example, a high dietary calcium content or a vegetable protein-based diet can dramatically increase the zinc requirement and this latter effect may be related to that reported for iron absorption.

Zinc deficiency is characterised by poor growth, anorexia, testicular atrophy, emaciation and skin lesions. Although all nutrients are important, the link between zinc and skin and coat condition makes this trace element particularly crucial for the companion animal. This is because a marginal deficiency may occur where an animal is not obviously unwell but its skin or coat condition is sub-optimal and significantly detracts from its appearance.

Zinc is relatively non-toxic, but high levels may interfere with the absorption and utilisation of iron and copper.

Iodine (I). Iodine an essential component of thyroid hormones, which regulate basal metabolism in the body, and this is its only recognised function. Goitre (enlargement of the thyroid gland) is the principal sign of iodine deficiency but other factors may also produce goitre.

Hypothyroidism has been reported in dogs and iodine deficiency has also been observed in zoo felids, domestic cats, birds and horses. Clinical signs include skin and hair abnormalities, dullness, apathy and drowsiness. There can also be abnormal calcium metabolism and reproductive failure with foetal resorption.

Excessive iodine intakes can be toxic, producing acute effects similar to those of a deficiency. The high doses in some way impair thyroid hormone synthesis and can produce so-called iodine myxoedema or toxic goitre. Anorexia, fever and weight loss may occur in cats.

Selenium (Se). Selenium is closely interrelated with vitamin E, such that the presence of one nutrient can 'spare' a deficiency of the other, and together they protect against damage to cell membranes. Nevertheless, it has been shown that selenium cannot be completely replaced by vitamin E and has a discrete, unique function. Selenium is an obligatory component of glutathione peroxidase, the enzyme which protects cell membranes against damage by oxidising substances. Selenium may also have other roles including protection against lead, cadmium and mercury poisoning and has been implicated as an anti-cancer agent.

Selenium deficiency has many effects but one described in dogs is degeneration of skeletal and cardiac muscles. Effects of deficiency in other species include reproductive disorders and oedema.

Selenium is highly toxic in large doses and the difference between the recommended allowance and the toxic dose may be quite small. Injudicious supplementation of foods is therefore particularly dangerous in this respect.

Manganese (Mn). Manganese is involved in many enzyme-catalysed reactions and is required for carbohydrate and lipid metabolism and cartilage formation. A deficiency is characterised by defective growth, reproduction and disturbances in lipid metabolism.

Cobalt (Co). Cobalt is an integral part of the vitamin B_{12} molecule and a deficiency is unlikely to occur if adequate vitamin B_{12} is present in the diet.

Other trace elements. A number of trace elements have been demonstrated as necessary for normal health in mammals, although specific requirements have not been established for companion animals. These elements are listed in Table 8.7 with a brief summary of their functions. It appears that the amounts required in the diet are very low and the likelihood of a deficiency of any of these nutrients in a normal diet is consequently almost non-existent.

Conversely, as with the majority of the trace elements these substances are all toxic if fed in large quantities, although the amounts which can be tolerated vary from one element to another. Arsenic, vanadium, fluorine and molybdenum are the most toxic, whereas relatively large amounts of nickel and chromium can be ingested without adverse effects.

Vitamins

Vitamins are organic compounds which help to regulate the body processes. Most vitamins cannot be synthesised in the body and must, therefore, be present in the diet. They may be classified as **fat-soluble** (vitamins A, D, E and K) or **water-soluble** (B-complex vitamins and vitamin C). A

Table 8.7 Functions of additional trace elements (after Wills, 1996)

Element	Function
Chromium	Carbohydrate metabolism, closely linked with insulin function
Fluoride	Teeth and bone development, possibly some involvement in reproduction
Nickel	Membrane function, possibly involved in metabolism of the nucleic acid RNA
Molybdenum	Constituent of several enzymes, one of which is involved in uric acid metabolism
Silicon	Skeletal development, growth and maintenance of connective tissue
Vanadium	Growth, reproduction and fat metabolism
Arsenic	Growth, also some effect on blood formation, possibly haemoglobin production

Table 8.8 Essential features of the major vitamins

Vitamin	Features
A	Fat soluble. Essential in diet. Found in liver, fats, oils, egg yolks and cereal grain germ. Exists as a pro-vitamin in vegetable sources. Stored in the body. Deficiencies affect vision, hearing, respiratory tract lining, skin and bones. Excesses are toxic.
B group	Comprises thiamine (B_1), riboflavin (B_2), niacin, pyridoxine (B_6), pantothenic acid, folic acid, biotin and cobalamin (B_{12}). Water soluble. Many are produced by intestinal bacteria. Found in liver, egg yolks, yeast and whole cereal grains. Exists as the active form in vegetables. Not sorted in the body, except vitamin B_{12}. Deficiencies affect appetite and metabolism. Excesses are not usually toxic.
C	Water soluble. No dietary requirement in healthy dogs and cats. Found in fresh fruit and vegetables. Found as the active form in vegetables. Not stored in the body. Deficiencies affect wound healing and capillary integrity. Excesses are not toxic.
D	Fat soluble. Essential in diet. Found in liver, fats, oils, egg yolks and cereal grain germ. Exists as a pro-vitamin in vegetable sources. Stored in the body. Deficiencies affect bone, teeth and calcium/phosphorus absorption/utilisation. Excesses are toxic.
E	Fat soluble. Essential in diet. Found in liver, fats, oils, egg yolks and cereal grain germ. Found as active form in vegetables. Stored in the body. Deficiencies affect muscle, fat and reproductive ability.
K	Fat soluble. Minimal requirement in diet as it is manufactured by intestinal bacteria. Found in liver, fats, oils, egg yolks and cereal grain germ. Exists as a pro-vitamin in vegetable sources. Not stored in the body. Deficiencies cause a coagulopathy.

frequent intake of water-soluble vitamins is necessary since they are poorly stored in the body, with excesses being lost via the urine. The fat-soluble vitamins are stored to a much greater extent and, consequently, a daily intake is less critical. However, because they are stored, the risk of toxicity arising through excessive intake is far greater with the fat-soluble vitamins. Tables 8.8 and 8.9 list the essential features of vitamins and the cat's and dog's dietary requirement.

Fat-soluble vitamins

Vitamin A. In nature, vitamin A (retinol) is found to a large extent in the form of its precursors, the carotenoids, which are the yellow and orange pigments of most fruits and vegetables. Of these, β-carotene is the most important. Vitamin A is a component of the visual pigments (which transmit light) in the eye and is important for proper vision. It is also concerned with cell differentiation and main- tenance of normal cell structure, so is important for sustaining healthy skin, coat, all mucous membranes and for normal bone and teeth development.

A deficiency of vitamin A may be associated with anorexia, weakness, ataxia, weight loss and abnormalities of the squamous epithelium which are usually manifest as seborrhoeic coat conditions; xerophthalmia, which will ultimately lead to corneal opacity and ulceration; increased susceptibility to microbial infections; crusting lesions of the external nares and accompanying nasal discharge; and epithelial degeneration of the seminiferous tubules and endometrium, leading to infertility.

Deficiencies of vitamin A are not common and dogs are able to synthesise vitamin A from plant-derived β-carotene. Cats, however, are unable to perform this conversion and their diet must therefore include a source of pre-formed vitamin A, which may only be found in animal fat.

Excesses of vitamin A are stored in the liver and a toxicity can lead to liver damage. Clinically, the most recognisable signs of hypervitaminosis A are those of a crippling bone disease which results in the formation of bony exostoses and ankylosis of joints, particularly in the cervical vertebrae and the long bones of the forelimb. Cats are particularly susceptible to hypervitaminosis A and the problem usually arises following prolonged oversupplementation of the diet

Table 8.9 Dietary requirements: vitamins

Vitamins		Cat per kg BW/day	Cat per 100 kcal (418 kJ)		Dog per kg BW/day	Dog per 100 kcal (418 kJ)
Vitamin B						
Choline	Growth:	120–130 mg	48 mg	Growth	50 mg	34 mg
	Maintenance:	120–130 mg	48 mg	Maintenance	25 mg	34 mg
Biotin	Growth:	1.5–3 μg	1.4–3.2 μg	Growth:	20 μg	12.5 μg
	Maintenance:	1.5 μg	1.4 μg	Maintenance:	20 μg	12.5 μg
Cobalamin	Growth:	1 μg	0.4–1.25 μg	Growth:	1 μg	0.7 μg
	Maintenance:	0.32 μg	0.4–0.5 μg	Maintenance:	0.5 μg	0.7 μg
Folate	Growth:	25–40 μg	16–25 μg	Growth:	8 μg	5.4 μg
	Maintenance:	16–20 μg	27 μg	Maintenance:	4 μg	5.4 μg
Niacin	Growth:	1.8 mg	1.8–2.4 mg	Growth:	0.45 mg	0.3 mg
	Maintenance:	0.9 mg	1.8 mg	Maintenance:	0.225 mg	0.3–0.45 mg
Pantothenic acid	Growth:	75–180 μg	100–250 μg	Growth:	400 μg	270–330 μg
	Maintenance:	75–180 μg	100–250 μg	Maintenance:	200 μg	270–400 μg
Pyridoxine	Growth:	0.128–0.2 mg	0.08–0.16 mg	Growth:	0.06 mg	0.03 mg
	Maintenance:	0.07 mg	0.08–0.1 mg	Maintenance:	0.022 mg	0.03 mg
Riboflavin	Growth:	150–320 μg	130–280 μg	Growth:	100 μg	68–80 μg
	Maintenance:	90 μg	120 μg	Maintenance:	50 μg	68 μg
Thiamine	Growth:	100–250 μg	0.125–0.16 mg	Growth:	54 μg	27–40 μg
	Maintenance:	80 μg	0.1 mg	Maintenance:	20 μg	27 μg
Vitamin A	Growth:	64–75 U	80–100 U/kg	Growth:	202 U	100–170 U
	Maintenance:	64–75 U	80–100 U/kg	Maintenance:	75 U	100–150 U
	Reproduction:	90–100 U	120–140 U/kg			
Vitamin D	Growth:	18–22 U	15–25 U	Growth:	22 U	11–18 U
	Maintenance:	8 U	10 U	Maintenance:	8 U	11–15 U
Vitamin E	Growth:	1–1.5 U	0.9–1 U	Growth:	1.4 U	1.25 U
	Maintenance:	0.45 U	0.6 U	Maintenance:	0.5 U	0.6–1 U
Vitamin K	Growth:	16–60 μg	2–20 μg	Growth:	16–60 μg	2–20 μg
	Maintenance:	16–60 μg	2–20 μg	Maintenance:	16–60 μg	2–20 μg

One international unit (1 U) of Vitamin D is equivalent to 0.025 mg.
One international unit (1 U) of α-tocopherol is equivalent to 1 mg.

with vitamin A (in cod liver oil, for example) or by feeding large quantities of liver.

Vitamin D. Metabolites of vitamin D stimulate calcium absorption in the intestine and, in conjunction with parathyroid hormone, stimulate resorption of calcium from bone. The requirements for vitamin D are closely linked to the dietary concentrations of calcium and phosphorus.

Most mammals are able to synthesise vitamin D_3 from lipid compounds in the skin provided they have exposure to sunlight and are otherwise well nourished.

A deficiency of vitamin D is extremely rare but is frequently confounded by a simultaneous calcium and phosphorus imbalance, causes **rickets** in the young animal and **osteomalacia** in the adult, characterised by a failure of mineralisation of newly formed osteoid. In the young animal, endochondral ossification of the growth plates is disturbed, giving rise to the typically enlarged metaphyses, particularly of the radius/ulna and ribs.

Toxic effects of excess vitamin D cause adverse effects and are generally related to hypercalcaemia which, if prolonged, results in extensive calcification of the soft tissues, lungs, kidneys, and stomach. Deformations of the teeth and jaws can also occur and death can result if the intake is particularly high.

Vitamin E. Acting with selenium, vitamin E protects cell membranes against oxidative damage. The requirement for vitamin E is increased when dietary levels of polyunsaturated fatty acids (PUFA), which are easily oxidised, are high.

In cats, vitamin E deficiency can be induced by feeding diets of oily fish (especially red tuna) which are rich in polyunsaturated fatty acids or with feeding rancid, oxidised fat. This causes a painful inflammatory condition of body fat (especially subcutaneous fat) known as **pansteatitis (yellow fat disease).** Vitamin E deficiency in dogs has been associated with skeletal muscle dystrophy, reproductive failure and impairment of the immune response.

In practice, vitamin E toxicity is unlikely to occur and relatively high doses may be tolerated.

Vitamin K. Vitamin K regulates the formation of several blood-clotting factors (factors VII, IX, X and XII). In normal, healthy animals the requirement for vitamin K is met by bacterial synthesis in the intestine and a simple deficiency is unlikely to occur. Hypoprothombinaemia and haemorrhage may occur in some animals when bacterial synthesis is suppressed, or there are vitamin K antagonists (such as warfarin or other coumarin compounds) in the diet.

Excess vitamin K has low toxicity but very large intakes may produce anaemia and other blood abnormalities in young animals.

Water-soluble vitamins

B-complex. The B-complex vitamins are used to form co-enzymes (co-factors) which are involved with normal metabolic function, especially energy metabolism and synthetic pathways. They are now usually referred to by their chemical names rather than by a letter/number combination.

Thiamine (Aneurin, Vitamin B_1). Thiamine is involved in carbohydrate metabolism and the requirement for this vitamin is dependent on the carbohydrate content of the diet. Thiamine deficiency can occur in cats as a result of feeding large amounts of certain types of *raw* fish which contain the enzyme thiaminase. In addition, the vitamin is progressively destroyed by high temperatures and under certain conditions of processing. Most pet food manufacturers supplement their products to compensate for possible losses, but some home-prepared diets may require additional thiamine.

Thiamine deficiency is expressed clinically as anorexia, neurological disorders (especially of the postural mechanisms) followed ultimately by weakness, heart failure and death. Like other water-soluble vitamins, thiamine is of low toxicity.

Riboflavin (B_2). Riboflavin is a constituent of two co-enzymes which are essential in a number of oxidative enzyme systems. Cellular growth cannot take place in the absence of riboflavin.

Riboflavin deficiency is associated with eye lesions, skin disorders and testicular hypoplasia. Toxicity of this vitamin has not been reported.

Pantothenic acid. Pantothenic acid is a constituent of co-enzyme A which is essential for carbohydrate, fat and amino acid metabolism. This vitamin is widespread in animal and plant tissues and a deficiency is unlikely to occur in normal circumstances.

Signs of experimentally induced deficiency include depressed growth, fatty liver, gastrointestinal disturbances (including ulcers), convulsions, coma and death. Toxicity has not been reported.

Niacin (nicotinamide and nicotinic acid). Niacin is a component of two important co-enzymes, the nicotinamide adenine dinucleotides, which are required for oxidation–reduction reactions necessary for the utilisation of all the major nutrients. In mammalian species, the requirement for niacin is influenced by the dietary level of the amino acid tryptophan, which can be converted to the vitamin. In cats, however, this conversion does not occur because an alternative pathway in the metabolism of tryptophan is favoured, so the dietary requirement for niacin is greater.

A deficiency of niacin causes a condition known as pellagra in humans and blacktongue in dogs and cats, which is characterised by inflammation and ulceration of the oral cavity with thick, blood-stained saliva and foul breath. Neither form of niacin is considered toxic.

Pyridoxine (vitamin B_6). This vitamin is involved in a wide range of enzyme systems associated with nitrogen and amino acid metabolism and consequently, increased levels are required as the protein content of the diet increases.

A deficiency of pyridoxine results in anorexia, weight loss and anaemia. In cats, irreversible kidney damage can occur. Pyridoxine and its derivatives are not considered toxic.

Biotin. Biotin is required for a variety of reactions involving the metabolism of fats and amino acids. The vitamin is important in maintaining the integrity of keratinised structures, such as the skin and hair.

Deficiencies of biotin are unlikely to occur since the daily requirement is normally met by intestinal bacterial synthesis. However, a deficiency may develop following the prolonged use of oral antibiotics which suppress microbial synthesis or the feeding of large amounts of raw egg white containing avidin, a protein which binds biotin. Eggs should, therefore, be cooked if they are to form a significant proportion of the diet.

Signs of biotin deficiency include dry, scaly skin with dull, brittle hair, hyperkeratosis, pruritus and skin ulcers.

Folic acid (pteroylglutamic acid, folacin). The folates are important for a number of reactions including the synthesis of thymidine, an essential component of DNA. It is essential for normal maturation of red blood cells in bone marrow and the typical signs of folic acid deficiency are anaemia and leucopenia. However, deficiencies are unlikely to occur since it is likely that most, if not all of the daily requirement can be met by intestinal bacterial synthesis.

Vitamin B_{12} (cyanocobalamin). The function of vitamin B_{12} is closely linked to that of folic acid. It is also involved in fat and carbohydrate metabolism and in the synthesis of myelin. A deficiency results in pernicious anaemia and neurological signs.

Choline. Choline is a constituent of phospholipids which are essential components of cell membranes and it is also the precursor of acetylcholine, a neurotransmitter chemical. A dietary deficiency of choline is unlikely to occur, but experimentally it causes fatty infiltration of the liver.

Ascorbic acid (vitamin C). Vitamin C is required for many intracellular reactions and protein synthesis, but most mammals are able to synthesise it from glucose. The main exceptions are man and other primates and the guinea pig. Although there is no dietary requirement for vitamin C in normal, healthy companion animals, some researchers believe that a dietary source may be beneficial under certain circumstances (such as stress or high activity levels) or in certain individuals.

Water

An animal's requirement for water is at least as important as that for any other nutrient; life may continue for weeks in the absence of food but only for a few days, or even hours, when water is not available. Water performs many vital functions within the body and the body water content is regulated within quite narrow limits. A daily intake is necessary to replace obligatory water losses from the body which occur mainly via the urine, faeces, skin and lungs and in productive secretions such as milk.

Water is taken into the body in several forms: as fluid drunk, as a component of food or as metabolic water (that released during the breakdown of protein, fat and carbohydrate). The daily water intake of any individual will depend on a number of factors including the moisture content of the food, environmental temperature, level of activity and physiological state. A plentiful supply of fresh drinking water should, therefore, always be available.

A balanced diet

A diet which is balanced will supply all the key nutrients and energy needed to meet the daily needs of the animal at its particular life stage. Nutrient and energy content are therefore important considerations but other related factors include digestibility and palatability of the food. Animals eat to satisfy their requirement for energy, so if all key nutrients are balanced to the energy content of the diet, then providing the correct quantity of energy also ensures an appropriate intake of essential nutrients. The need of animals requiring a higher plane of nutrition (as in gestation or lactation) will inevitably receive a higher intake of all key nutrients when they increase the amount of food consumed to meet their energy demands.

Nutrient balance

Nutrient requirements are bounded by a minimum and, in some cases, a maximum value. In other words, the amount of nutrient needed in the diet must lie on a 'plateau' between deficiency on the one hand and toxicity on the other (Fig. 8.2). The main criteria for what constitutes a complete diet can therefore be summarised as:

- The content of each nutrient must be on the plateau.
- Each nutrient must be present in the correct ratio to the energy content of the diet.
- Each nutrient must be at the correct ratio to other nutrients (where appropriate).
- Each nutrient must be in a form that is usable by the animal for which the diet is made.

Nutrient interactions

Deficiencies of a specific nutrient may occur as a result of interactions with other components of the diet, which reduce their bioavailability. For example, excessive amounts of phytate (as is found in cereal-based diets) will interfere with the intestinal absorption of zinc and high levels of calcium will reduce the absorption of both copper and zinc. The absorption of iron is known to be influenced by a number of factors.

Digestibility

The digestibility of a food is a measure of the biological availability of its constituent nutrients to the animal. Although analysis of a particular food may give an

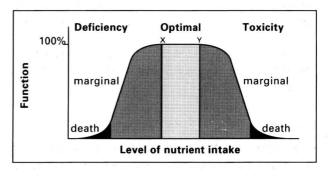

Fig. 8.2 Relationship of nutrient intake to health.

indication of its total nutrient content, it is only the portion of nutrients which are actually absorbed from the gut that have any true nutritional value. Factors which affect the digestibility of a substance include chemical composition of the food, its state of subdivision and its method of preparation or processing.

Palatability

The palatability of food is a complex subject, including a knowledge of the factors affecting appetite and behaviour, as well as an understanding of taste, smell and texture of food and their interrelationships. The importance of palatability cannot be overemphasised since a food which is left uneaten, whatever its nutrient content, is of no nutritive value to the animal.

First impressions of a food are always important and food must always be presented in a manner which is appropriate to the size of the animal. Cats and small dogs prefer food in small pieces which are not too sticky, whereas larger dogs are able to eat foods with a much broader spectrum of shape and size.

Smell and taste are necessary sensory components of any meal and animals with poor appetites can often be tempted to eat by providing strong-smelling foods, particularly if the food is warmed to about 35°C. Cats can distinguish between sweet and bitter tastes but do not respond to the addition of glucose in their food. In general, meat is very palatable to dogs and cats, and its acceptance can often be further enhanced by the addition of fat, especially animal fat.

Most animals enjoy variety in their diet, although they may be initially suspicious of a food which differs markedly from their previous diet. Above all, it is important to recognise that, like humans, all animals are individuals with their own dietary likes and dislikes.

Foods and food types

Prepared pet foods

In the developed countries, the vast majority of dogs and cats are fed commercially prepared pet foods. The enormous range of manufactured pet foods available offer the pet owner a convenient method of feeding their pet; the preparation time involved is minimised, and the animal can be provided with a variety of flavours and textures in its diet. All these diets are nutritionally balanced when fed according to the instructions on the label and are all prepared to the same exacting standards.

Prepared diets for pets are either complete or complementary and this information should be stated on the product label. A **complete** diet will provide a balanced diet when fed alone, although the specific lifestage (such as growth, reproduction or adult maintenance) for which it is designed must be specified. A **complementary** diet is designed to be fed in combination with an additional, specified food source, such as canned meat and biscuit mixer.

There are three main forms in which prepared pet foods are usually presented:

- **Dry foods**, which have a moisture content of 10–14%, include both complete diets and biscuits. The complete diets are usually a mixture of dry, flaked or crushed cereals and vegetables, and many include a meat-based dry protein concentrate. They may be fed dry or the owner may add gravy or water before feeding. Biscuits are generally made from wheaten flour and may be fed whole or broken and used as a mixer with moist foods.
- **Moist foods** are the most popular means of feeding pet dogs and cats. Their moisture content is 60–85% and they may be packed in cans, plastic or semi-rigid aluminium. They tend to have a higher meat content and are filled with gravy or set in jelly, both of which provide important vitamins and minerals and improve the palatability of the product. Canned meat products tend to be the most palatable.
- **Semi-moist foods** have a moisture content of 25–40%, and are composed of a meat and cereal mixture which is cooked to a paste and extruded into small, shaped pieces. The main advantage of this type of diet is its convenience.

The product packaging provides useful data, some of which is legally required, that should help the pet owner to make important decisions about how to feed the product. In addition to information which identifies the product and the

---

Table 8.10 Some ingredients used in commercial pet foods

Dry foods	Canned foods	Semi-moist
Ground cereals (corn, oats, wheat, sorghum)	Ground cereals (corn, oats, wheat, sorghum)	Ground cereals (corn, oats, wheat, sorghum)
Meat and bone meal	Meat and bone meal	Sucrose
Whey	Meat	Meat and bone meal
Soyabean meal	Meat by-products	Wheat bran
Animal fat	Liver	Meat
Iodised salt	Lung	Meat by-products
Vitamin/mineral mix	Corn flour	Tallow
	Heart	Milk
	Lard	Soy flour
	Blood	Propylene glycol
	Vitamin/mineral mix	Iodised salt
		Vitamin/mineral mix

species for which the food is intended, the pet food label should state:

- The ingredients in descending order of predominance by weight (Table 8.10).
- The typical (or guaranteed) analysis giving the concentrations of protein, oil, fibre, ash and moisture (if over 14%) in the product.
- Whether the food is complete or complementary in respect of the particular lifestage for which it is designed.
- The manufacturer's directions for use, including feeding recommendations or guidelines.

EC regulations do not currently permit the declaration of energy content on pet food labels, but this may be roughly estimated from its carbohydrate, fat and protein contents (Table 8.1). This reinforces the importance of reliable feeding recommendations, but these should always be regarded as guidelines only. Observation of the health, condition and bodyweight of the animal will help to determine whether adjustments are necessary in the amounts fed. Where supplementary foods are provided, as snacks, treats or table scraps, their nutritive value must be taken into account when determining the daily food allowance.

Home-prepared diets

For a variety of reasons, many dog and cat owners prefer to feed their pets on fresh foods prepared at home. However, formulation of a balanced diet for any animal requires a detailed knowledge of its specific nutritional needs; of the nutritive value of different foodstuffs from which the diet is to be prepared; of dietary interactions; and of methods of preparation and storage which may affect the availability of individual nutrients (Tables 8.11 and 8.12). Considerable time, effort and expertise are therefore required to be able to offer the animal a consistent and nutritionally adequate diet.

The following foods are common ingredients of home-prepared diets for dogs and cats:

- *Meat.* Lean muscle meat is a poor source of calcium and the feeding of an 'all-meat' diet is the most common cause of **nutritional secondary hyperparathyroidism**.
- *Offals.* These do not constitute a balanced diet and should not be fed exclusively. In particular, cats may become 'addicted' to liver and risk the development of **hypervitaminosis** A.
- *Fish.* Care should be taken when feeding raw fish as some types contain thiaminase, leading to thiamine deficiency with prolonged feeding. Large amounts of oily fish, especially red tuna, can precipitate **pansteatitis (yellow fat disease)** due to vitamin E deficiency.
- *Eggs.* These are a valuable source of good-quality protein but should be fed cooked to destroy avidin (which binds biotin)
- *Milk, cheese and other dairy products.* These are a good source of protein, fat, calcium and phosphorus but some individuals may be intolerant of lactose.

Table 8.11 Selected common protein sources and quantities required to supply 10 g of protein in home-made diets

Type of food	Approximate amount (g) required to supply 10 g protein[a]	Ca	P	Na	Cu	Fi	Fa	BV
Chicken meat	50	L	M	L	L	L	L	H
Chicken skin	62	L	M	L	M	L	H	M
Giblets	47	L	M	L	M	L	L	H
Cod	57	L	M	L	M	L	L	H
Haddock	53	L	M	L	L	L	L	H
Halibut	48	L	M	L	M	L	L	H
Shrimp	55	L	M	H	M	L	L	H
Tuna canned in oil	41	L	M	H	M	L	H	H
Tuna canned in water	36	L	M	L	M	L	L	H
Beef lean meat	48	L	M	L	H	L	M	M
Beef normal meat	56	L	M	L	H	L	H	M
Beef heart	59	L	M	M	–	L	L	M
Beef kidney	65	L	M	H	–	L	M	M
Beef liver	50	L	M	H	–	L	L	M
Lamb meat	65	L	M	M	–	L	H	M
Cottage cheese creamed	74	L	M	H	L	L	L	M
Cottage cheese non-creamed	59	L	M	H	L	L	L	M
Cheddar cheese	40	M	M	H	L	L	H	M
Egg whole	78	L	L	M	L	L	L	H
Egg white	92	L	L	M	L	L	L	H
Egg yolk	63	L	L	L	L	L	L	H

[a] The amounts required will vary between products. The amount required to supply 10 g protein can be calculated in the following way: amount required in g = (100 ÷ protein content per 100 g of the food) × 10.
Ca, calcium; P, phosphorus; Na, sodium; Cu, copper; Fi, fibre; Fa, fat; BV, protein biological value.
L = low levels (provides <50% of daily requirements on an ME basis).
M = medium levels (provides >50–150% of daily requirements on an ME basis).
H = high levels (provides >150% of daily requirements on an ME basis).
– = unknown or variable levels.
The sodium levels are assuming food is cooked in unsalted water.

Table 8.12 Selected common protein sources and quantities required to supply 100 kcal (418 kJ) in home-made diets

Food	Approximate amount (g) required to supply 100 kcal (418 kJ) energy[a]	Ca	P	Na	Cu	Fi	Fa	BV
Bread white	37	L	L	H	M	H	L	L
Bread whole wheat	41	L	L	H	M	H	L	L
Corn flour	27	L	L	L	–	M	L	L
Corn meal	27	L	L	L	–	M	L	L
Corn flakes (breakfast cereal)	26	L	L	H	M	M	L	L
Macaroni, cooked	75	L	L	L	L	M	L	L
Oatmeal, cooked	181	L	L	L	–	M	L	L
Potato, cooked	133	L	L	L	–	M	L	L
Rice long grain, cooked	80	L	L	L	L	M	L	L
Soybean flour high fat	26	L	M	L	–	–	L	L
Soybean flour low fat	28	L	M	L	–	–	L	L
Spaghetti (quick cook), cooked	77	L	L	L	L	M	L	L
Spaghetti (ordinary), cooked	91	L	L	L	L	M	L	L
Wheat dry	27	L	L	L	–	M	L	L
Wheat cooked	240	L	L	L	–	M	L	L
Wheat flour	30	L	L	L	–	M	L	L
Fat, trimmed from beef	14	L	L	L	L	L	H	0
Lard	11	L	L	L	L	L	H	0
Margarine	14	L	L	H	L	L	H	L
Oils – salad/cooking	12	L	L	L	L	L	H	0

[a] The amounts required will vary between products. The amount required to supply 100 kcal can be calculated in the following way: amount required in g to supply 100 kcal = 100 ÷ energy density kcal/g; amount required to supply 418 kJ = 418 ÷ energy density kJ/g.
Ca, calcium; P, phosphorus; Na, sodium; Cu, copper; Fi, fibre; Fa, fat; BV, protein biological value.
L = low levels (provides <50% of daily requirements on an ME basis).
M = medium levels (provides >50–150% of daily requirements on an ME basis).
H = high levels (provides >150% of daily requirements on an ME basis).
– = unknown or variable levels.
0 = does not apply to these ingredients.
The sodium levels are assuming food is cooked in unsalted water.

- *Cereals and vegetables.* These should be cooked to improve digestibility. High levels of phytate in cereals may reduce the availability of some minerals, especially zinc. Palatability may be low for some dogs and cats and, being obligate carnivores, cats cannot be maintained on an exclusively plant-based diet.

Cooking is advisable for most foods, especially meats, since this will kill most bacteria and parasites and will improve the digestibility of some materials. Overcooking should be avoided, however, since this will destroy vitamins and reduce the food value of proteins. A minimal amount of cooking water should be used and, if possible, fed with the meal in order to conserve vitamins and minerals. Home-prepared diets will almost certainly require careful vitamin and mineral supplementation.

Dietary supplementation

Contrary to many advertisements and popular beliefs, young animals and lactating females do not require large quantities of minerals and vitamins. Provided they are fed a balanced diet appropriate to their lifestage, their needs will be met as their food intake increases to meet their energy requirements. There is no advantage to be gained by overdosing.

Supplementation should be undertaken with care as this may unbalance an otherwise balanced diet, and many nutrient interactions can result in a reduced availability of specific nutrients. This can lead to the possibility of toxicities occurring, as may readily occur with vitamins A and D, for example. Dietary supplementation can be expensive and is unlikely to be of benefit in non-deficient animals. Table 8.13 lists the deficiencies of foods commonly used in home-prepared diets.

However, the value of vitamin/mineral supplements used in moderate amounts should not be dismissed. They can act as an insurance for those individual animals who may experience difficulties in either absorption or utilisation of specific nutrients. Although they are unnecessary when a commercially prepared pet food is fed, supplements are likely to be required in order to produce nutritional balance in home-prepared diets. In addition, they have a psychological benefit for people who need to give what they see as extra care. Nevertheless, in cases of diet-related nutrient deficiencies, it is considered preferable to correct the deficient diet itself rather than to rely on blanket supplementation.

Feeding healthy dogs and cats

Pet owners tend to treat their dogs and cats as individuals and will develop their own feeding practices which must take account of the particular circumstances, likes and dislikes of the animal and their own view of convenience, cost, variety and suitability of foods. They must identify the particular needs of their animal and find a combination of foods to meet them.

Table 8.13 Nutrient imbalances of selected foods

Food	Deficiencies	Excesses
Meat	Calcium, phosphorus, sodium, iron, copper, iodine, vitamins A, D, E	Protein
Fish (bones removed)	Calcium, phosphorus, iodine, vitamins A, D, E	
Fish (including bones)[a]	Iron, vitamins A, D, E	Calcium, phosphorus
Fats and oils		Energy, vitamin D (fish oils)
Eggs	Calcium, phosphorus	Fat, avidin
Milk		Lactose
Cheese, cottage cheese	Calcium, phosphorus	
Liver	Calcium	Vitamin A
Vegetables	Calcium, phosphorus, protein, fat	
Cereals	Calcium, phosphorus	

[a] Cooked and finely ground fish.

The feeding recommendations in the following sections are intended only as **guides** for the average dog or cat in the usual range of environments found in European households. These guides can be used as a starting point to obtain an approximate estimate of a pet's needs, then by observation of the animal to decide whether to feed more or less, and by substitution of one food for another, the owner will arrive at a suitable regime.

Maintenance

Nutritionally speaking, the stage of adult maintenance is considered to be the period of basal requirements. An adult animal is said to be **in maintenance** when it is not subjected to the additional physiological stresses of growth; pregnancy or lactation; regular work or high levels of activity; or extremes of environmental temperature. During this period, the diet must provide the correct amount, balance and availability of energy and nutrients required to maintain optimal health and activity and promote peak condition in the animal. Since animals eat to satisfy their requirement for energy, all essential nutrients must be present in the correct amounts relative to the energy content of the diet.

Dogs

Dogs are represented by a wide diversity of breeds of different body types, with adult bodyweights which range over 100-fold from 1 to 115 kg. Energy expenditure is directly related to the weight of actively metabolising tissue, so for animals with such widely differing bodyweights, energy requirements are more closely related to the animal's **metabolic bodyweight** than to bodyweight itself. For moderately active pet dogs, maintenance energy requirements may be calculated using the equation:

$$ME \text{ (kcal/day)} = 110W^{0.75}$$

where W is the dog's bodyweight in kg. For more active dogs, the allowance can be increased to $125W^{0.75}$. However, variations in body composition, shape and coat type are complicating factors in determining energy requirements, particularly for the larger breeds. For example, Newfound-lands tend to need less than the predicted amounts, whereas Great Danes need more, despite these two breeds being of comparable bodyweight.

The amount of food needed to meet these requirements may then be calculated from a knowledge of the energy values of foods. Feeding recommendations are only ever given as guidelines and are subject to individual variability between dogs and to differences in activity level and environmental conditions. If extra snacks, treats or table scraps are added to the diet their energy content must be taken into account when calculating the daily food allowance. In addition, spaying may reduce the resting energy requirement of bitches by up to 10%. Regular weighing of the animal allows the owner to monitor the adequacy of the feeding regime on a quantitative basis.

Most adult dogs in maintenance are able to eat all they require in a single meal and it is perfectly acceptable to adopt a once-a-day feeding regime. It is usually best to avoid late evening meals since dogs may need to excrete faeces or urine within a few hours of feeding and this can be inconvenient in the middle of the night. There is no disadvantage in feeding more frequently, provided that the total daily intake is limited to the dog's daily needs, and feeding 2–3 times a day to coincide with family meals is a common practice. Whatever the frequency of feeding, a routine should be established and adhered to as far as possible. See Table 8.14.

Cats

Domestic cats show a relatively narrow range of adult bodyweights (from 2.5 to 6.5 kg) and their energy requirements may be calculated from a linear relationship. In normal circumstances, an adult cat requires 70–90 kcal/kg bodyweight/day, depending on its level of activity. However, large, overweight individuals and very inactive or caged cats (such as those in a hospital environment) have lower maintenance energy requirements and allowances should be based on 50–70 kcal/kg bodyweight/day.

Cats have the ability to regulate their energy intake from day to day and unless they are fed an exceptionally palatable diet or lead a particularly sedentary life, they will normally adjust the amount of food they eat to achieve the correct balance.

Table 8.14 Recommended nutrient requirements for the dog, according to physiological status

Status	Minimum ME density (kcal (kJ)/g)	Digestibility (%)	Protein (%ME)[a]	Fat (%ME)[a]	Fibre (%DM)[b]	Ca	PO₄ (mg/100 kcal (418 kJ))	Na
Maintenance	3.5 (14.6)	>75	16–20	30–50	5	130–160	110–160	15
Growth Gestation Lactation	3.9 (16.3)	>80	22–28	30–50	5	280	200–250	23
Geriatric	3.75 (15.7)	>80	14–18	30–50	4	130–150	110–140	15
Stress: Environmental Psychological Physical	4.2 (17.6)	>82	20–25	30–50	4 max	150–250	130–230	23

[a] The proportion of metabolisable energy supplied by that nutrient.
[b] g/100 g dry matter.

The cat exhibits a number of nutritional peculiarities which distinguish it from the dog and reflect its naturally predatory lifestyle. Several aspects of feline metabolism have evolved in adaptation to a strictly carnivorous diet which is typically high in protein and low in carbohydrate. In addition, the cat has a dietary requirement for a number of nutrients which are only found naturally in significant quantities in animal tissues. Specific nutritional differences of the cat may be summarised as follows:

- A limited ability to regulate amino acid catabolism resulting in a higher dietary requirement for protein than dogs and an inability to adapt to extremely low protein diets.
- A high dietary requirement for taurine partly because of an inability to conjugate bile acids with glycine instead of taurine.
- A particular sensitivity to arginine deficiency.
- A limited ability to synthesise niacin.
- An inability to convert β-carotene to retinol (vitamin A), resulting in a dietary requirement for preformed vitamin A.
- A limited ability to convert linoleic acid to arachidonic acid.
- A limited ability to metabolise carbohydrate, resulting in an intolerance of high carbohydrate diets.

Cats may be considered as **obligate carnivores** since taurine, preformed vitamin A and arachidonic acid are only found in significant quantities in animal tissues. It is thus essential that the cat is supplied with at least some animal-derived materials in its diet. In view of these nutritional specialities, it should be noted that long-term feeding of dog foods to cats is unacceptable since these diets may not meet the specific nutritional requirements of the cat.

When allowed continuous access to food, cats tend to adopt a pattern of small, frequent (usually eight to 16) meals throughout the whole 24-hour period. However, cats readily adapt to different feeding schedules imposed by their owners and are commonly fed two meals per day. Nevertheless, if feeding time is restricted then sufficient food must be provided to satisfy their daily nutrient and energy requirements.

Environmental factors are also known to affect the volume of food a particular animal will eat. Most cats do not relish cold food straight from the refrigerator and prefer to eat food that is close to their own body temperature and that of freshly killed prey. This response may reflect a behavioural strategy in the wild which ensures that only the freshest prey is eaten.

Cats do seek variety in their diet, as long as the new food is not *too* different from the familiar one, or the palatability too low. However, during times of stress, such as when hospitalised, a familiar diet is preferred. Repeated exposure to fresh supplies of a new food which is not initially acceptable to the cat may encourage the cat to overcome its reticence. Furthermore, cats can often detect and may reject diets that are deficient in certain nutrients, so it is important that any diet offered is nutritionally complete. See Table 8.15.

Table 8.15 Recommended nutrient requirements for the cat, according to physiological status

Status	Minimum ME density (kcal (kJ)/g)	Digestibility (%)	Protein (%ME)[a]	Fat (%ME)[a]	Fibre (%DM)[b]	Ca	PO₄ (mg/100 kcal (418 kJ))	Mg	Na
Maintenance	>3.7 (15.7)	>75	24–26	>25	5	130–200	120	80	15
Growth Gestation Lactation	3.9 (16.3)	>80	30–35	>40	5	160–250	120–200	150	30
Geriatric	3.75 (15.7)	>80	24–26	>34	5	130–150	120	80	15

[a] The proportion of metabolisable energy supplied by that nutrient.
[b] g/100 g dry matter.

Reproduction

The reproductive lifestage is a nutritionally demanding time for the bitch or queen. During this period, her intake of energy and nutrients must be adequate not only to meet her own maintenance requirements but also to support normal growth and development of her offspring during pregnancy and, through milk production, during lactation. At peak lactation her energy and nutrient requirements may rise to up to 3–4 times the level required for maintenance. This may involve eating large volumes of food and, at times of high demand, achieving a sufficient intake can be a problem. This may be offset to some extent by feeding a diet which is:

- Concentrated with respect to energy and nutrient density.
- Palatable to encourage feeding.
- Highly digestible to reduce bulk.

The additional requirements imposed by pregnancy are relatively small and can usually be met by simply increasing the amount of the animal's normal food, provided that this is well balanced. In late pregnancy and particularly if the litter is large, the space occupied by the gravid uterus may be so great that the physical capacity for food intake is limited. In this case, feeding a concentrated diet can help to ensure an adequate intake and offering smaller, more frequent meals can also be beneficial. To meet the high demands of lactation a palatable, highly digestible, concentrated diet should be fed. Milk production is affected by protein quantity and quality in the diet and it is important that the extra food supplied is of good quality. It is not appropriate to simply increase the dietary energy content by adding fat or carbohydrate sources. Diets formulated for growth or specifically for gestation and lactation are suitable for feeding at this time.

During pregnancy and lactation, the content and balance of nutrients in the diet are critical and must be carefully regulated. Provided that a balanced diet is fed, the increased requirement for nutrients is met when food intake is increased to meet the energy needs of the bitch or queen. Further supplementation with vitamins or minerals is *not* required and could actually be harmful by causing an imbalance in the diet.

Dogs

The average duration of pregnancy in the bitch is 63 days, but her energy requirements do not increase appreciably until the last third of gestation when most foetal weight gain occurs. It is important, therefore, to avoid overfeeding in early pregnancy since this will lead to the deposition of unwanted fat and may predispose the bitch to problems at whelping. A gradual increase in food allowance over the second half of gestation is all that is required and a satisfactory regime would be to increase the amount of food by 15% of the bitch's maintenance ration each week from the fifth week onwards. During the week before whelping, the bitch should, therefore, be eating 60% more than when she was mated. Appetite may be reduced in the later stages of pregnancy, particularly with large litters, and it is sensible to divide the daily allowance into several small meals.

Lactation represents the most nutritionally demanding lifestage for the bitch. During the first 4 weeks post whelping, she must eat enough to support both herself and her rapidly growing puppies which may double their weight within a matter of days. The extra energy and nutrients needed over and above her normal intake depends on the size and age of the litter but at peak lactation (3–4 weeks after whelping), she may need to eat anything up to 4 times her normal maintenance allowance. Failure of the diet to meet these demands means that the bitch will nurse her young at the expense of her own body reserves, with a resultant loss of weight and condition.

The food allowance should be increased steadily throughout the first 4 weeks of lactation in accordance with the bitch's needs. A highly palatable, digestible and concentrated food should be offered in several small meals or *ad libitum* and food should be made available throughout the night. An unlimited supply of drinking water should also be provided to cater for the large volumes that may be involved in milk production.

Weaning of the litter should be accomplished gradually in order to prevent mastitis in the bitch and growth check in the puppies. Most puppies begin to take an interest in solid foods from about 3–4 weeks and once they are eating well, the bitch may be separated from the puppies for progressively longer periods to allow her milk supply to diminish. Weaning may be completed between 6 and 8 weeks of age and it may be advisable to cut the bitch's ration down to half her maintenance level immediately following total separation. Her food allowance may be gradually increased over a period of days and if she has lost condition during lactation, extra food may be introduced as soon as her milk supply has dried up.

If the litter is large and particularly if the bitch's milk supply seems inadequate, supplementary feeding of the puppies should be encouraged from about 3 weeks. **Eclampsia (post-puerperal hypocalcaemia)** is a condition which can affect lactating bitches, especially of small breeds, with larger litters. Lowered blood calcium concentrations lead to signs which range from restlessness and ataxia to muscle tremors and collapse with tetanic convulsions. Treatment involves the oral or intravenous administration of calcium, depending on the severity of signs, and puppies should be removed immediately from affected bitches and hand-reared. Although some owners give calcium and vitamin D supplements to bitches in late pregnancy and lactation as an 'insurance policy', these do *not* prevent eclampsia and may, in fact, increase the risk of eclampsia or calcinosis in the bitch and produce developmental abnormalities in the puppies.

Cats

Gestation length for cats is similar to that of dogs and is in the region of 64 days. However, unlike dogs and most other mammals, pregnant queens start to eat more and gain weight within a week of conception. By the end of the third week of gestation, the pregnant queen will have gained almost 20% of the extra weight she will carry at term. Following parturition, only about 40% of this extra weight is lost (compared with almost 100% in the bitch) and the remaining 60% is lost during the course of lactation.

This unusual pattern of bodyweight gain in early pregnancy is thought to be due to the extra-uterine deposition of fat and protein reserves which may be mobilised in late pregnancy and lactation, when dietary intake of the queen may be insufficient to meet her greatly increased nutritional demands.

Throughout pregnancy, food intake of the queen rises continuously to fuel her extra weight gain and peaks at around 7–8 weeks of gestation. The food allowance may be gradually increased from 1 week of a successful mating and since cats rarely overeat, an *ad libitum* feeding regimen is perfectly acceptable. Voluntary intake may drop slightly just before and immediately after parturition, after which food consumption rises progressively to meet the increased demands of lactation. As with the bitch, energy require- ments of the lactating queen vary with litter size and age and at peak lactation may be anything up to 4 times her maintenance level. Again, a highly palatable, digestible and concentrated diet should be fed as frequent small meals and *ad libitum* feeding is preferred to allow the queen to successfully control her energy intake. Food should be available throughout the night and an unlimited supply of fresh drinking water must be accessible at all times.

It is normal for the queen to lose weight during lactation as her body reserves are used up, but she should achieve her pre-mating weight by the time the kittens are weaned at 6–8 weeks. Although kittens begin to take solid food from about 3–4 weeks of age and demand less of the queen, her energy requirements remain elevated to allow for restoration of her depleted body reserves. After weaning, the additional food allowance can be gradually cut back until the queen is eating her normal amount or adjusted to compensate for any observed weight loss or gain.

Growth

In relation to bodyweight, growing animals require a much higher plane of nutrition than their adult counterparts. For young animals, the diet must not only supply all the nutrients required for maintenance but also those required to fuel rapid growth and development and to support their active lifestyle. In particular, they have higher demands for energy, protein (which must be digestible and have an amino acid profile appropriate for growth), vitamin E and certain bone-forming minerals, such as calcium and phos- phorus. Both the *amount* and *balance* of nutrients provided are critical for the growing puppy or kitten and dietary errors at this stage can have damaging effects, particularly on skeletal development, which may be long lasting and potentially irreversible.

To meet these high demands, young animals must eat large amounts of food relative to their size, but their physical capacity to do so is limited by their small stomach volume. The daily food allowance should therefore be divided into several small meals to compensate for this and

the diet itself should meet certain criteria. A suitable diet for growth is formulated to ensure an adequate intake of energy and nutrients in a relatively small volume of food and should be

- Concentrated.
- Nutritionally balanced.
- Highly palatable.
- Highly digestible.

For the first few weeks of life, all the nutritional needs of the puppy or kitten are met by their mother's milk and no supplementary feeding is necessary, unless the milk supply is inadequate. As their interest in solid food gradually increases, finely chopped soft foods or dry kibble moistened with milk or gravy may be provided in shallow bowls. The food may be the same as that offered to the mother or may be one designed specifically for growth.

Contrary to popular belief, milk is not essential in the diet of weaned puppies or kittens. After weaning, their ability to digest lactose becomes progressively less efficient and feeding large quantities of milk can result in diarrhoea. Nevertheless, milk remains a useful source of nutrients for individuals that can tolerate it, if fed in restricted amounts.

Puppies

Most owners are aware that correct nutrition is fundamental to achieving normal growth and development in the growing dog, but there is a common tendency to overfeed (to produce rapid growth rates) or to oversupplement the diet (to prevent classic deficiency syndromes). Excessive energy intake, however, is likely to cause obesity in the small breeds, and rapid growth rates in the large and giant breeds, which may be detrimental to the animal. The aim should be to allow the puppy to grow sufficiently quickly to enable it to fulfil its genetic potential while the bones are still capable of growth. A more rapid increase in body weight can place undue stresses on the juvenile skeleton, particularly in the fast-growing large and giant breeds, and may predispose to a variety of disorders which are characterised by abnormalities of bone growth and develop- ment. Examples of these include **osteochondrosis syn- drome**, **hip dysplasia**, **wobbler syndrome** and **enostosis (panosteitis)**. In some cases, excessive dietary calcium intake may also play a major contributory role. It is therefore unwise to overfeed growing dogs in an attempt to obtain the maximum possible rate of growth and a more advantageous approach is to moderately restrict their intake and allow them to take slightly longer to reach their adult weight. See Fig. 8.3.

Oversupplementation with fat-soluble vitamins A and D may also result in skeletal and other abnormalities, and care should always be exercised with supplements such as cod liver oil, which is a rich source of both these vitamins. A properly balanced diet which is formulated for growth does not need any form of supplementation and careless use of additives can result in serious dietary imbalances with deleterious consequences. This is true even of the large breeds since their extra needs are catered for by their increased food intake to meet their energy requirements.

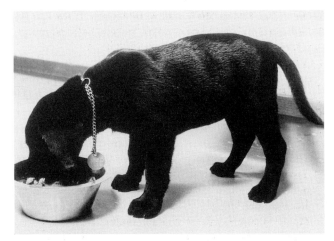

Fig. 8.3 Young animals should be fed diets specifically designed for their growing needs.

All puppies grow very rapidly in the early stages and by 5–6 months of age most breeds will have reached about half their adult weight. However, because of the wide variation in adult bodyweight, different breeds continue to mature at different relative rates and, in general, the larger breeds take longer to mature than the smaller breeds. Small and toy breeds may reach their adult weight at 6–9 months of age. Larger breeds will still be growing at this age and take longer to mature. Labrador Retriever or Newfoundland puppies, for example, may not reach their adult weight until 16 months or 2 years, respectively.

At weaning (between 6 and 8 weeks of age), the puppy's energy requirements are about double those of an adult of the same breed, per unit of bodyweight. As the puppy grows, this requirement declines progressively and by the time it has reached 40% of its mature weight, the energy requirement is only 1.6 times that for adult maintenance. At 80% of its mature weight, the puppy needs only 1.2 times as much energy as an adult per unit of bodyweight.

High levels of high-quality protein are also required for growth. Although it is often thought that large amounts of additional protein in the puppy diet will aid the development of good condition and muscle, this is not the case. Instead, protein eaten in excess of requirements is metabolised to produce energy or stored as fat

Most puppies can be weaned onto a varied diet or a single, complete food between 6 and 8 weeks of age. At this stage, it is better to feed them four small meals a day than to allow continuous access to food. Commercial diets designed specifically for growth are ideal and it is recommended that a growth formulation is fed until the puppy attains at least 75% of its adult weight. Although such diets require no further supplementation, some owners may like to offer alternative foods from time to time. Meat, offal, cheese, eggs and bread are often fed to dogs but only a few different food sources should be introduced gradually at any one time, to allow the digestive system to adapt. Nevertheless, if alternative foods are to form the major part of a home-prepared diet, food composition tables should be consulted and careful supplementation with vitamins and minerals will almost certainly be required.

Puppies should have their food allowance divided into four or five meals a day until about 10 weeks of age and then three meals a day until they have reached approximately 50% of their expected adult body weight. At this stage (5–6 months), the frequency of feeding can be reduced to twice daily. As the puppy approaches its adult weight, the daily food allowance can be gradually incorporated into a single meal, as in the adult. *Ad libitum* feeding is not recommended for growing dogs since they tend to overeat and this can lead to obesity or skeletal developmental abnormalities. As a guide, feeding at a level of 85% of *ad libitum* feeding has been shown to result in optimal growth and body composition in dogs. Precise recommendations on the amounts to feed are difficult to give because of huge variations in individual requirements and in the caloric densities of the foods themselves. It is important, therefore, that the health and condition of growing dogs is regularly assessed 'by hand and eye' to monitor their progress and allow any necessary dietary adjustments to be made.

Kittens

Kittens weigh between 85 and 120 g at birth and may gain up to 100 g per week in the early stages of growth, so that at weaning they should weigh between 600 and 1000 g. Males grow at a faster rate than females and by 6 weeks of age they are already significantly heavier. At 1 year, male cats can be up to 45% heavier than females from the same litter.

At weaning, the energy requirements of kittens per unit of bodyweight are between 3 and 4 times that of an adult and reach a peak at about 10 weeks of age. Unlike puppies, kittens do not tend to overeat and are not prone to the same problems of obesity and skeletal developmental abnormalities as growing dogs. It is usual, therefore, to allow kittens unrestricted access to food during the rapid growth phase, although multiple small feeds throughout the day (at least 4–5 per day at weaning) may also be offered. Moist food which is left uneaten should be discarded at least twice daily.

Concentrated diets designed for kitten growth are ideal at this stage to ensure an optimal intake of energy, protein, taurine and calcium, in particular. Growing kittens tend to have acidic urine due to the liberation of hydrogen ions during bone growth and it is important that urine-acidifying diets designed for the management of struvite-associated lower urinary tract diseases are avoided in young cats.

Although male kittens take slightly longer to mature than females, most kittens will have attained 75% of their ultimate adult bodyweight by 6 months of age. Further weight gains after this are attributable to developmental changes rather than skeletal growth, and at this stage the growth diet may be changed to an adult formulation. If desired, the frequency of feeding may be reduced to twice daily but many people continue to offer multiple feeds throughout the day, even to adult cats. This pattern of feeding fits in well with the cat's natural preference to snack feed during both day and night rather than eat a small number of large meals. Total food intakes continue to rise between 6 and 12 months to coincide with continued slow growth, but tend to stabilise at an adult level towards the end of the first year.

Feeding orphaned puppies and kittens

Hand-rearing of puppies and kittens may be necessary if the mother has an inadequate supply of milk, if she is sick or if the litter is orphaned (see Chapter 18, p. 487). The ideal alternative is to cross-foster the young on to a lactating bitch or queen whose young are old enough to be weaned, but this is not always a practical option. Motherless puppies and kittens have vital requirements in two main areas, that is, provision of a suitable environment and nutrition. Important husbandry aspects of orphaned puppies and kittens may be summarised as follows:

- Ideally, the environment should be controlled by an incubator. Alternatively, a heating pad with adequate insulation of the pen can be used.
- After they have been fed, the mother would normally provoke reflex defecation and urination in the puppies and kittens by licking the anogenital area.
- This action can be simulated by applying a piece of damp cotton wool at the anogenital area or simply by running a dampened forefinger along the abdominal wall.
- Between 16 and 21 days, puppies and kittens no longer require stimulation to urinate and defecate and from 28 days, when they completely control their body temperature, they begin to explore their surroundings and become more independent.

The food supplied must be a concentrated source of nutrients based on the composition of normal bitch or queen's milk. Table 8.16 shows the average composition of milk from bitches, cows, goats and queens. It is clear that cow's and goat's milks are inadequate as a substitute for rearing puppies and kittens since the protein and fat levels are too low. Calcium levels are also considerably lower than that of bitch's milk. Many commercially available milk substitutes are now available for dogs and cats. They are usually based on cow's milk which has been modified to resemble bitch or queen's milk more closely. They can be administered by means of a small syringe or a puppy or kitten feeding bottle.

Dried milk feeds should be reconstituted daily and fed warm (38°C). Food must be given slowly and must not be forced into the animal. Frequent, small feeds (at least four) should be offered throughout the day. When feeding from a miniature bottle, the hole in the teat may need to be enlarged so that the flow is improved and the puppy or kitten does not suck in air. When they begin to explore their surroundings (at 3–4 weeks), a high-quality puppy or kitten food can be introduced. This can be mixed with a milk substitute to begin with and then offered separately. See p. 487 for examples of commercially available milks.

Senior animals

As a general guideline, dogs and cats may be considered to be geriatric once they have reached the final third of their anticipated lifespan. The aim of feeding elderly but otherwise healthy animals is to slow or prevent the progression of metabolic changes associated with ageing and thus to increase longevity and preserve the quality of life. Old age is often, however, accompanied by clinical disease for which dietary management may constitute an important component of therapy. Chronic renal failure is a particular problem of middle-aged and old cats, whereas old dogs tend to be more susceptible to heart disease. There is a tendency towards obesity in older animals, especially dogs, and oral hygiene measures have particular significance in old age. Free access to a clean supply of water is essential to prevent dehydration.

Dogs

Most senior dogs have an energy requirement which is approximately 20% less than that of a younger adult of equivalent bodyweight. This decline in energy requirement appears to be linked to both a reduction in physical activity and a reduction in lean body tissue, which has a lower basal metabolic rate. To reduce the risk of obesity, therefore, older

Table 8.16 Nutrient content of milk from different sources

| Nutrient | % Nutrient as fed (g/100 kcal (418 kJ) ME) | | | | |
	Bitch's milk	Cow's milk	Queen's milk	Goat's milk	Evaporated milk + water[a]
Water	77 (0)	88 (0)	81.5 (0)	87 (0)	80 (0)
Protein	8.2 (6.6)	3.2 (5.4)	7.4 (8.4)	3.5 (5.5)	5.3 (5.5)
Fat	9.8 (7.8)	3.7 (6.3)	5.2 (5.9)	4.2 (6.6)	6.1 (6.3)
Lactose	3.6 (2.9)	4.6 (7.8)	5.0 (5.7)	4.5 (7)	7.6 (7.8)
Calcium	0.28 (0.22)	0.12 (0.2)	0.035 (0.04)	0.13 (0.2)	0.19 (0.2)
Phosphorus	0.22 (0.18)	0.1 (0.17)	0.07 (0.08)	0.11 (0.17)	0.15 (0.16)
ME					
kcal/100 g[b]	125	59	88	64	97
kJ/100 g[b]	522	246	360	267	406

[a] 3 parts whole evaporated milk diluted with 1 part water.
[b] ME content as-fed was estimated using nutrient energy densities of 3.5 kcal (14.6 kJ)/g for protein and lactose, and 8.5 kcal (35.6 kJ)/g for fat.

dogs should be fed to a lower energy requirement than younger dogs without restricting the intake of other essential nutrients. Nevertheless, some individuals have a reduced appetite and may be underweight if intake does not meet their energy requirements. This may be exacerbated by a tendency towards reduced digestive efficiency in the older animal.

Although protein digestibility may be slightly reduced in older animals leading to higher dietary requirements, high levels of dietary protein may increase the renal workload when kidney function may already be impaired to some extent. Conversely, very low protein diets may be associated with a risk of protein malnutrition and tend to be unpalatable. In general, healthy older dogs should have diets based on their individual needs which will be related to bodyweight, condition and physical activity. Early clinical and biochemical signs of chronic renal failure would support the introduction of a diet with a low phosphorus and moderately reduced protein content. As a rule, protein sources for older dogs should be highly digestible and of high biological value.

Although restriction of dietary sodium or phosphorus may be indicated in old dogs with cardiac or renal diseases, respectively, there is no evidence that healthy individuals have altered requirements for these or other minerals. Similarly, vitamin requirements of healthy senior dogs are not thought to differ markedly from those of younger adults and although the importance of vitamin E is often cited, no benefits of an increased intake have been demonstrated in older dogs.

Cats

As with dogs, the energy requirements of cats decline with increasing age. However, obesity is not considered a significant problem in old cats and there is a greater tendency for geriatric cats to be underweight. Cats show a significant decline in digestive function with age, resulting in a significant decrease in the digestibilities of protein, fat and, hence, energy. Most healthy cats are able to compensate for this effect by increasing their food intake to maintain bodyweight but in some cases, provision of a more energy-dense food may be appropriate.

In view of the high protein requirements of the cat and reduced digestive efficiency in old age, restriction of dietary protein is not recommended in healthy individuals because of the associated risk of protein malnutrition. However, moderate restriction of dietary protein to alleviate clinical signs of uraemia may be implemented, together with dietary phosphorus restriction, in cats with evidence of chronic renal failure. Again, highly digestible protein sources of high biological value should be employed for all older cats.

Careful monitoring of food intake is important in the senior cat and may help to identify conditions associated with altered food intake. For example, hyperthyroidism is characterised by weight loss despite an increased appetite, and prolonged inappetence may predispose an obese cat to hepatic lipidosis.

Table 8.17 summarises the age-related changes in dogs and cats and their effect on nutritional status.

Table 8.17 Ageing changes in dogs and cats and their effect on nutritional status

Ageing change	Effect on nutritional status
Metabolism	
Reduced sensitivity to thirst	Dehydration
Reduced thermoregulation	Increased energy expenditure with extremes of heat
Reduced immunological competence	Increased susceptibility to infection
Decreased activity and metabolic rate (possibly due to decreased thyroid function)	Decreased energy needs predisposes towards obesity
Increased body fat	Predisposes towards obesity
Special senses	
Decreased olfaction	Reduced food intake which
Decreased ability to taste	may lead to a loss of
Decreased visual acuity	weight and condition
Oral cavity	
Dental calculus	
Periodontal disease	Reduced food intake which
Loss of teeth	may lead to a loss of
Decreased saliva production	weight and condition
Gingival hyperplasia	
Urinary system	
Decreased renal function	
Decreased renal blood flow	Decreased protein
Decreased glomerular filtration rate	requirement
Skeletal system	
Osteoarthritis	Decreased mobility reduces energy requirements
Reduced muscle mass	Decreased protein reserves
Cardiovascular system	
Congestive cardiac failure	Decreased salt intake

Working dogs

Working dogs perform at a wide range of activity levels and in a variety of environmental conditions, from acting as guide dogs for the blind to pulling sledges in polar regions. The diet and feeding regime employed in each case varies widely according to the role the dog is asked to perform and its individual work and training schedule. Any increase in physical activity requires extra energy to sustain the increase in muscular work but a further allowance must be made for the element of stress that is associated with strenuous activity. Both physiological and psychological stresses further increase the demand for energy and certain nutrients in hard-working dogs.

The main fuels for muscular exercise in the working dog are fats and carbohydrates. Sprinting dogs, such as the racing greyhound, require short but very intense bursts of energy. In these circumstances, the muscle fibres contract very rapidly and rely mainly on readily available glucose as an energy source. Muscle glycogen stores supply approximately 70–80% of the energy required for this type of exercise, with fats providing the rest. For these working dogs, a diet which provides a relatively large quantity of carbohydrate may be appropriate since this helps to maximise muscle glycogen reserves. Useful sources of carbohydrate include corn, oat flakes, rice and potatoes.

However, high carbohydrate diets are not suitable for most other working dogs and may actually reduce performance. They may exacerbate the accumulation of lactic acid in muscles during prolonged exercise, leading to muscle damage and exhaustion. For working dogs which are active for long periods (endurance performers), energy for sustained muscle activity is produced through aerobic fatty acid oxidation with fat providing 70–90% of the energy and carbohydrates providing the rest. Dogs which perform this type of work may benefit from training on a high fat diet. This also applies to dogs which operate in a hostile environment (such as sledge dogs or avalanche rescue dogs) where extra energy is required to maintain body temperature as well as for increased muscular activity. For most other working dogs, the optimal dietary ratio of fat:carbohydrate falls somewhere between these two extremes.

The protein requirements of hard-working dogs may be slightly increased over maintenance levels but there is no evidence to suggest that a high protein diet will promote superior muscle development. Exercise stress may increase the demand for specific amino acids and has been associated with anaemia, so a good-quality protein source is essential for dogs in work. Suitable protein sources include meats, fishmeal, powdered whole egg and casein.

Little is known about the requirements of hard-working dogs for vitamins and minerals, but there may be a higher requirement for iron because of its involvement in haemoglobin production and oxygen transport. Similarly, vitamin E and selenium requirements may be increased since they act as antioxidants and protect cell membranes, including red blood cells, from damage. If the diet is nutritionally balanced, however, these increased demands will be met when the dog consumes more to satisfy its energy requirements.

The amount of extra energy required by working dogs depends on environmental conditions, the amount of exercise and the nature of the work. A dog which travels long distances in the course of its work may need as much as 2–3 times the normal adult maintenance ration. Despite this, food intake may be reduced in some dogs due to fatigue and to offset this, the diet should be concentrated, palatable and highly digestible. This type of diet is also lower in bulk, which is a significant advantage to the working dog. As well as being an ideal energy source for most working dogs, fat is an excellent means of increasing the energy density of the diet and both fat and protein may be used to enhance palatability.

Where the type of work performed is not overly strenuous, the additional needs may be met by simply feeding more of the dog's nutritionally balanced maintenance diet. At higher levels of performance, a more concentrated source of energy and nutrients is recommended and complete diets formulated for active dogs are ideal. Alternatively, supplementary foods, such as fish or meat, may be added to the maintenance ration but this strategy will require suitable vitamin and mineral supplementation. On rest or training days, the dietary requirements will differ and the amounts fed must be adjusted accordingly. A smaller allowance of the same meal is most appropriate.

Working dogs should receive only a small concentrated meal before working, as a full stomach limits performance and increases the risk of bloat. If the working period is prolonged, a further small meal may be given during the rest period. The main meal should provide two-thirds of the daily ration and should be reserved until after work. A rest period of about an hour should be allowed before feeding if the work is strenuous. To prevent dehydration, working dogs should be given free access to water.

Clinical nutrition

Nutritional factors may affect the health of any animal in a number of ways. The provision of a nutritionally adequate diet is clearly important in the prevention of disease associated with deficiencies of imbalances of specific nutrients. Nutritional diseases are now rare in companion animals, thanks to the widespread feeding of nutritionally balanced commercial diets, but problems do occasionally arise when

- The animal's intake is reduced.
- The diet is poorly formulated or stored.
- An otherwise balanced diet is carelessly over-supplemented.
- The animal is unable to digest, absorb or utilise the nutrient as a result of disease or genetic factors.

Nutritional support at times of stress, disease or injury is a second area in which nutrition may impact on disease. Failure to consider this aspect of disease management may have a detrimental effect on the animal's recovery. Finally, dietary modification may form an integral part of the management of a variety of clinical conditions.

Nutritional support

The nutritional requirements of the stressed or traumatised patient differ markedly from those of the healthy animal and, coupled with this, there is often a reduced desire or physical ability to eat. Failure to address these altered needs can result in malnutrition of the critical care patient and will have an adverse effect on the animal's recovery. Conversely, the therapeutic benefits of appropriate nutritional support for these animals are well established and include:

- Increased survival rates.
- Improved tolerance to invasive procedures.
- Shorter hospitalisation periods.
- Decreased risk of infection.
- Earlier return to mobility.
- More rapid wound healing.

Altered nutritional needs of the stressed patient

In the healthy animal, short-term fasting results in a series of adaptive mechanisms which are designed to maintain blood glucose concentrations, preserve lean body tissue and promote survival. Because there is little or no intake of food, the body mobilises its own tissue reserves to provide essential nutrients and lowers its metabolic rate to reduce energy expenditure.

Most cells adapt to using fatty acids, instead of glucose, as an energy source and within a few days, fat becomes the major source of fuel in the fasting animal. However, the cells of some tissues, such as the brain, kidney and red blood cells, still require a constant supply of glucose for energy. To meet this demand, tissue proteins are broken down to provide amino acids which can then be converted to glucose. In starvation, therefore, fat reserves are used to supply energy but even in the healthy animal there is inevitably some loss of tissue protein. When feeding is resumed, amino acid mobilisation decreases and metabolism returns to normal within 24 hours.

In conditions of stress or trauma, however, these adaptive mechanisms to food deprivation are overridden. An initial 'ebb' or 'shock' phase lasts for a few hours up to 2 days, during which intravascular fluids are redistributed (**hypovolaemia**) to maintain tissue perfusion. Treatment during this phase is aimed at life-saving procedures. Metabolism *may* be lowered (**hypometabolism**) during this phase.

This phase is quickly followed by a 'flow' period of accelerated metabolism which is designed to support the healing of wounds and resistance to infection. This stage can last from days to several weeks, depending on the severity of the injury. During this period of **hypermetabolism**, energy requirements increase in accordance with the severity of the injury and are particularly high in cases of head trauma (because the brain has a particularly high energy requirement), septicaemia, extensive burns or following radical surgery. Even healthy animals undergoing minor elective surgery may experience a transient increase in energy requirements of up to 10% above normal.

In stressed animals, glycogen reserves are rapidly depleted and fat becomes the major and preferred energy source. In addition, healing tissues and some tumours require glucose as an energy source and the breakdown of tissue proteins increases markedly in order to maintain blood glucose levels to meet this demand. Nevertheless, high levels of dietary carbohydrate are contraindicated in hypermetabolic patients since they commonly exhibit a peripheral insulin resistance and are unable to utilise glucose efficiently. An excessive intake of carbohydrate during this period can result in respiratory acidosis and other complications. Unlike in the healthy animal, these metabolic changes are not immediately reversed when feeding is resumed.

Protein–energy malnutrition (PEM)

The cumulative drain on tissues may continue for weeks and, if not corrected, can result in PEM. During this time, nutritional support becomes a crucial part of the treatment. PEM can have a number of adverse effects which, in combination, can delay recovery and increase the patient's susceptibility to infection and shock. The most obvious effects of PEM are muscle wasting and weakness, but other side effects include reduced immune function, increased risk of infection and delayed wound healing. Impaired digestive function exacerbates the problem. In extreme cases, death can occur due to sepsis and failure of the heart, lungs and other organs.

Patient assessment

Some form of nutritional support is required for any animal that is unable or unwilling to eat voluntarily, but a thorough veterinary examination is necessary to assess the individual requirements of the patient and the most appropriate method of administering support.

Specific nutritional support is indicated if:

- Oral intake is reduced for 3–5 days or if it is anticipated to be interrupted for this length of time as a result of surgical or other in-hospital procedures.
- There is an acute weight loss of more than 5–10% of body weight (excluding fluid losses).
- Actual weight is 15% or more below ideal body weight.
- Body condition, as scored on a scale of 1 (cachectic) to 5 (obese), is below the optimal score of 3.
- Physical changes are accompanied by hypoalbuminaemia.
- Recent trauma, surgery or sepsis is accompanied by anorexia.

Patients which have recently undergone major surgery or trauma, especially when this is associated with head injuries, blood loss, sepsis, severe burns or open wounds, are prime candidates for nutritional support. Another group of patients are those which are physically unable to eat (e.g. with jaw fractures) and those with chronic wasting diseases, such as cancer.

Once an initial assessment has been made, the degree and duration of nutritional support can be estimated and a nutritional plan formulated on an individual basis for each patient. For surgical patients, preoperative assessment is particularly important so that invasive tube placement can be performed at the time of the initial surgery. See Table 8.18.

Table 8.18 Practices that may adversely affect the nutritional status of sick animals

Failure to record daily weight.
Failure to observe, measure and record the amount of food consumed.
Delay of nutritional support until the patient is in an irreversible state of depletion.
Withholding food for diagnosis procedures.
Failure to recognise and treat increased nutritional needs brought about by injury or illness.
Failure to appreciate the role of nutrition in the prevention of and recovery from infection: unwarranted reliance on drugs.
Prolonged administration of glucose and electrolyte solutions.
Rotation of staff at frequent intervals and confusion of responsibility for patient care.
Inadequate post-operative nutritional support.
Limited availability of laboratory tests to assess nutritional status.

Techniques for nutritional support

Nutritional support for small animals may be provided by either the enteral or the parenteral route. See also Chapter 16, p. 398. Total parenteral nutrition is the provision of nutrients by the intravenous route, but this technique is expensive with inherent technical problems and is usually reserved for a small number of patients with gastrointestinal failure.

Where there is a functional gastrointestinal tract, enteral nutrition is a more economical and physiologically sound option. Prolonged lack of enteral nutrition can result in intestinal mucosal atrophy, with an associated reduction in functional capacity and risk of intestinal bacterial translocation into the portal blood. A number of techniques are available for enteral feeding, the choice of which depends on various factors including type of injury, medical condition or surgical procedure and should be based on individual patient assessment. .

If voluntary intake is adequate, nutritional support may simply take the form of providing a more concentrated source of energy and nutrients. Other patients may be encouraged to feed by hand feeding, providing aromatic foods or heating the food offered to stimulate the appetite. Inappetent cats may respond to the intravenous administration of diazepam but this method of appetite stimulation should not be continued for longer than 3 days.

Where the patient's needs cannot be met through voluntary intake, some form of involuntary tube feeding must be considered. Force feeding by syringe, by daily orogastric intubation or by rolling the food into small balls and 'pilling' the animal are short-term options, but these methods can be stressful for the patient and may not satisfy the animal's nutritional needs.

Surgical placement of a **pharyngostomy tube** has been used successfully for feeding patients with prolonged anorexia and an inability to pick up or chew food. However, the popularity of this method of tube feeding has recently declined in favour of nasal feeding or gastrostomy tubes.

Naso-oesophageal or nasogastric intubation requires no sedation and is well tolerated by most cats and dogs. The tube may be left in place for several weeks, but since the tube size is limited, this method can only be used for feeding larger animals. It can, however, be used for long-term administration of fluids to any size of animal. Nasal feeding is recommended as an adjunct to voluntary feeding or where sedation or anaesthesia of the patient poses too great a risk for surgical placement of a gastrostomy tube (Fig. 8.4).

Gastrostomy tube feeding is indicated where long-term involuntary nutritional support is anticipated and the presence of pharyngeal or oesophageal lesions precludes the use of pharyngostomy tubes (Fig. 8.5). The use of gastrostomy tubes is increasing in small animal medicine thanks to the development of a technique for percutaneous tube placement without the need for laparotomy. Percutaneous endoscopic gastrostomy (PEG) is a simple and well-tolerated procedure, but requires the use of a flexible endoscope. Alternatively, a large-bore Foley catheter can be placed into the stomach at laparotomy and secured to the abdominal musculature. Complications associated with this method include peritonitis and tube displacement or blockage. Gastrostomy tubes are wide bore and so will accommodate most types of diet. The tube may be left in place for weeks to months and tube feeding by this method can be continued by most owners at home.

Feeding directly into the small intestine by **enterostomy catheter** may be required when serious conditions of the upper gastrointestinal tract, such as pancreatitis or major gastric or small bowel surgery, are present. Animals fed in this way require liquid elemental diets that require little digestion and are readily absorbed from the jejunum and ileum. Parenteral nutrition would be an alternative if small bowel function was not satisfactory.

Energy and nutrient requirements

Daily energy requirements of the hospitalised patient are based on basal energy requirements (BER) or cage-rest maintenance energy requirements (MER) multiplied by an arbitrary factor, the size of which varies according to the severity and nature of the illness. In some cases, energy requirements may be below normal because the animal is

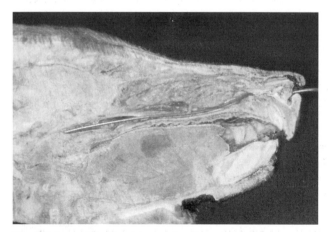

Fig. 8.4 A nasal feeding tube passing through the ventral meatus.

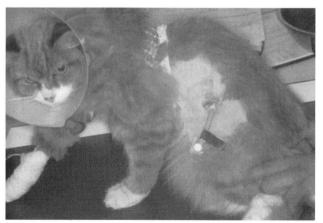

Fig. 8.5 Gastrostomy tube placed to provide nutrition to a cat with empyema.

hypometabolic or because it is physically inactive as a result of the injury.

Maintenance energy requirements (MER) are calculated using the formula:

MER (kcal/day) = $110 \times BW^{0.75}$ (dog)
MER (kcal/day) = $70 \times BW$ (cat)

where BW is the animal's bodyweight (kg).

The volume of food required is calculated by dividing the total daily energy requirement (kcal) by the energy density of the diet (kcal/ml) as recorded on the product label. The total volume required is divided into four to six feeds per day, depending on previous oral intake and individual animal tolerance. The normal stomach capacity is no more than 90 ml/kg in dogs and 50 ml/kg in cats. All dietary transitions should be made slowly and in the initial stages of nutritional support, the calculated amount of nutrients should be approached over a period of 48 hours to avoid vomiting, abdominal discomfort and diarrhoea. For animals that have been inappetent for prolonged periods, slow rates of administration (over 10 minutes) are recommended.

Weight and body condition score should be recorded on a daily basis to enable accurate calculation of the patient's energy requirements and to monitor its progress. Adjustments in food allowance can then be made on an individual basis according to observed changes in the animal's body weight and body condition.

Stressed, hypermetabolic patients use fat, rather than carbohydrate, as their main source of energy and most cells become progressively less able to use glucose efficiently. High levels of carbohydrate in the diet during this period can, in fact, give rise to serious metabolic disturbances which may lead to respiratory or cardiac failure. High fat diets are therefore recommended and tend to be more palatable, digestible and calorie-dense, which are advantages for feeding potentially anorexic patients. Protein requirements of the stressed animal are higher than normal to maintain wound healing and immunity and to compensate for the higher rate protein breakdown. However, some restriction of dietary protein may be indicated in certain specific conditions, such as chronic kidney or liver disease.

Supplementation of the diet with certain amino acids, including **glutamine** and **arginine**, may be beneficial in the nutritional management of critical care patients. There may also be an increased requirement for water-soluble **B-complex vitamins**, and **zinc** may have an important role in wound healing.

Suitable diets

In selecting a diet for enteral administration, it is important to consider the most appropriate dietary formulation, the caloric density of the diet and, where appropriate, the diameter of the feeding tube. Commercial liquid enteral diets or liquidised canned diets may be used for most purposes. Elemental diets containing amino acids or glucose

may be useful if gastrointestinal function is compromised or to supplement other diets.

Ideally, diets for the critical patient should be highly palatable, highly digestible and nutrient dense in order to ensure an adequate intake of nutrients in a reduced volume of food. Although healthy dogs (but not cats) can be maintained on a plant-based diet, such diets are unsuitable for the metabolically stressed animal and should be replaced by a meat-based diet for the duration of the dog's illness and convalescence. Following injury, the metabolism of the dog tends to revert to its more carnivorous origins and is more closely aligned with that of the cat. Thus, protein and fat utilisation is increased and carbohydrate is used with decreasing efficiency. In addition, plant-based diets are less digestible than meat-based diets and can cause digestive upsets in the stressed patient.

Complications of nutritional support

Following a period of food deprivation, all dietary transitions should be made slowly to avoid complications including the development of potentially serious metabolic derangements (Table 8.19). In the initial stages of refeeding, vomiting may occur due to gastrointestinal hypomotility and diarrhoea may result from reduced intestinal surface area, decreased enzyme activity and hypoalbuminaemia. Normal digestive function is usually restored within a few days of appropriate enteral feeding.

Calorie intake has an important effect on convalescence. An insufficient intake can result in PEM, but overfeeding can be equally detrimental, particularly when the carbohydrate intake is excessive. In starved, hypometabolic patients, excessive carbohydrate can lead to insulin-induced transport of phosphorus and potassium into cells and, subsequently, hypophosphataemia and hypokalaemia. The resultant respiratory and cardiovascular failure could prove fatal in some cases.

Other complications of nutritional support include mechanical problems or infections related to the feeding tube. Tube obstructions can be minimised by using liquid diets with fine-bore tubes, by sieving liquidised canned diets prior to administration via pharyngostomy or gastrostomy tubes, and by flushing with water after each feed. Occasionally, naso-oesphageal tubes may be regurgitated and pharyngostomy tubes can cause gagging, airway obstruction and related problems.

Table 8.19 Food reintroduction schedule for animals recovering from vomiting, diarrhoea or pancreatitis

Day	Percent of normal daily food quantity
1	33
2	66
3	100

Feed small, frequent meals (4–6 day) of a highly digestible, low fat (<15% DM; <30% ME), low fibre (<2% DDM; 0.5 g/100 kcal (418 kJ) ME) diet.

Dietary sensitivity

The term 'dietary sensitivity' describes any clinically abnormal response to a particular food item and may be further classified as either **food intolerance** or true **food allergy (hypersensitivity)**. True dietary hypersensitivity is an immune-mediated phenomenon whereas food intolerance denotes any other clinically abnormal response to a dietary component. Food intolerance can result from an impaired ability to digest the food (often because a specific enzyme is lacking) or from pharmacological, metabolic or toxic reactions. With the exception of certain specific conditions, the clinical signs associated with hypersensitivity reactions are often indistinguishable from those produced by food intolerance and management protocols are identical for both.

In the dog and cat, dietary sensitivity usually manifests as skin or gastrointestinal disease and a number of cases will present with signs involving both systems. Pruritus is the most frequently observed presenting sign, which is accompanied by a gradation of clinical signs associated with self-inflicted trauma. Dietary sensitivity has also been implicated in some cases of **otitis externa** in dogs and of **miliary dermatitis** and **eosinophilic plaque** in cats. Certain forms of food intolerance, notably **lactose intolerance** and **gluten-sensitive enteropathy of Irish setters**, usually manifest as diarrhoea. In addition, a number of chronic conditions of the gastrointestinal tract have been reported in which dietary hypersensitivity may play a role, including **inflammatory bowel disease** in cats and canine **idiopathic chronic colitis**.

Food sensitivity may be associated with any dietary ingredient, including additives, but most reactions are caused by dietary proteins. In cats, reactions to cow's milk, beef and fish account for more than half the reported cases whereas reactions to cow's milk, beef and cereal (alone or in combination) are more common in dogs. The successful management of dietary sensitivity involves identification of the offending ingredient and its elimination from the diet. By examining the animal's detailed dietary history, it may be possible to identify foods which the animal has never eaten (or at least within the previous month) and these can be used to form the basis of an elimination diet which is 'hypoallergenic' for that individual. Such restricted diets should contain a minimum number of protein sources which, preferably, are not commonly associated with sensitivity reactions. Elimination diets that have been used successfully in dogs and cats include chicken, lamb, rabbit, venison and a variety of fish species which are typically fed with rice or potatoes. Traditionally, these ingredients have not been used widely in commercially prepared pet foods and the animals is less likely to have had previous exposure to these foods.

The elimination diet should be fed for a minimum of 3 weeks although a trial period of up to 60 days may be necessary in animals that do not respond initially. Failure to respond within this time suggests that either dietary sensitivity is not involved, other factors may be contributing to the clinical disease or the animal is sensitive to the protein in the elimination diet. During the diagnostic period, there should be **no access to any other source of nutrients**, including treats, chews or nutritional supplements. A small number of animals will react to commercially prepared elimination diets but not to home-prepared diets using the same ingredients and it may be preferable to use a home-prepared diet in the initial diagnostic stages.

If clinical improvement occurs, a diagnosis of dietary sensitivity may be confirmed by challenging with the original diet and demonstrating an exacerbation of clinical signs within 1–14 days. Reintroduction of the elimination diet should result in an improvement in signs and, at this stage, it may be possible to introduce a commercially prepared diet with the same ingredients. Individual protein sources can then be introduced at weekly intervals to identify specific dietary allergens that should be avoided. Once a diagnosis has been established, it is usually possible to manage cases of dietary sensitivity using commercial diets with novel, restricted protein sources of high digestibility.

Alternatively, it may be possible to identify a range of standard products that the animal is able to tolerate.

Obesity management

Obesity is the most common form of malnutrition seen in companion animal practice, with an estimated incidence of 25–33% in dogs and 6–25% in cats. Although cats tend to be more efficient regulators of their energy intake, this ability may be overridden and recent trends towards the free-choice feeding of palatable dry cat foods together with a more sedentary, indoor lifestyle may have increased the frequency with which feline obesity is observed in some parts of the world. Obesity may not only reduce the animal's enjoyment of life but a number of serious clinical problems have now been linked to the condition, including:

- **Osteoarthritis**.
- Respiratory distress and reduced exercise tolerance.
- **Diabetes mellitus**.
- Circulatory problems.
- Lowered resistance to infections.
- Liver disease, including **idiopathic hepatic lipidosis** in cats.
- Dermatological problems which, in cats, may be linked to difficulties in self-grooming.
- Increased risk of **feline lower urinary tract disease**.
- Increased surgical and anaesthetic risk.

Obesity is a consequence of energy intake exceeding requirement at some stage in the animal's life. During this phase, excessive energy intake results in the deposition of fat in adipose tissue and is associated with an increase in fat cell size (**hypertrophy**) in the adult, or fat cell numbers (**hyperplasia**) in the growing animal. Once fat cell hyperplasia has occurred, the animal retains a lifelong predisposition for excessive weight gain and it is important that food intake of growing dogs, in particular, is controlled to avoid obesity in the adult. The initial dynamic phase of fat deposition is followed by a static phase in which the animal remains fat but its bodyweight is fairly stable.

Appetite may be normal or even reduced and this apparent anomaly may be confusing for the owners.

An animal is considered obese if its bodyweight is 15% or more above the ideal. Breed standards may provide useful guidelines for determining the ideal weight of purebred dogs, but are of little value in crossbred dogs and cats. Practical assessment of the degree of obesity involves subjective evaluation of the animal's appearance and palpation of the subcutaneous fat deposits. In normal animals, the ribs should be palpable but covered with a moderately thin layer of fat and there should be a definite indentation, or waistline, behind the rib cage when viewed from above. Dogs also tend to accumulate fat around the tail head and obese cats may develop an 'apron' of fat in the groin. Accumulation of fat in the abdominal cavity must be differentiated from abdominal enlargement due to other causes, such as ascites, gas, pregnancy or abdominal organ enlargement.

Dietary therapy of obesity is aimed at moderate, controlled energy restriction. Rapid weight loss should not be attempted in obese cats since this can lead to the development of **hepatic lipidosis**, which is potentially fatal. In general, it is recommended that an initial target weight is set which represents a 15% reduction in bodyweight. Further reductions can then be planned once this target weight has been reached. For dogs, this degree of weight loss can be achieved within 12 weeks by feeding 40–50% of the animal's energy requirement for maintenance at its target weight. In cats, a 15% reduction in weight can be safely achieved over 18 weeks by feeding 60% of the animal's target energy requirements.

Simply feeding less of the normal diet is not recommended since prepared pet foods are balanced to a normal energy intake and by restricting energy intake, essential nutrients may also be restricted. This can produce deficiency states that may be dangerous or even lethal. In additional, this technique rarely forms part of a structured weight loss programme and success rates tend to be low. A more effective strategy is to feed a prepared low-calorie diet which has been specifically formulated to achieve weight loss and ensures an adequate intake of essential nutrients. This is particularly important when the diet is to be fed long term. Dietary therapy should be combined with an increase in physical activity (where possible) and behavioural modifications which aim to produce lifelong habit changes and, therefore, permanent weight loss. A protocol for successful weight reduction in dogs and cats is provided in Table 8.20.

Table 8.20 Dietary management of obesity in dogs and cats

- Counsel the owner on the need to reduce the animal's body weight, stressing the medical implications of obesity.
- Weigh the dog or cat and set a target weight. The planned reduction should represent no more than 15% of the animal's current weight.
- Indicate to the owner how long it is likely to take to reach the target weight safely. The weight loss can usually be achieved in 10–15 weeks in dogs and 16–20 weeks in cats.
- Calculate the amount to feed based on 40–50% (dogs) or 60% (cats) of the maintenance energy requirements at target body weight.
- Stress the concept of feeding the weight reduction diet to the exclusion of all other foods. The discipline and co-operation required of all who come into contact with the animal may be reinforced if they are encouraged to record the total daily food intake on a chart. It may be preferable to confine cats to the home to prevent supplementation from other sources.
- Advise weighing the animal carefully on the same scales at the same time every week or fortnight and encourage the owner to record the weight on the chart supplied. Small and steady weight losses are more evident from the weight chart than from simple observation of the animal.
- Careful monitoring of cats during weight reduction is recommended. Owners should be questioned to check that food intake matches expectations, and clinical examination should be performed at regular intervals. Periodic haematological and blood biochemical evaluation may also be appropriate.
- If satisfactory weight loss is not occurring, then the daily food allowance may be reduced by 10%, whilst keeping a careful watch on the general health of the animal. If such a reduction is necessary, it should be maintained for the rest of the dieting period.
- When a satisfactory weight loss has been achieved, the dog or cat should be changed to a normal high-quality diet. It is important to calculate and regularly reassess the daily amount of food required to maintain the target weight.
- Follow up after 1 and 3 months, and then at six-monthly intervals.
- At all times, give the owner adequate encouragement.

Gastrointestinal disease

Gastrointestinal disorders are common in dogs and cats. In most cases, dietary modification can form an important, sometimes essential, part of managing the condition. Although some acute gastrointestinal disorders can be life-threatening, most cases tend to be self-limiting and respond well to symptomatic treatment. The principle of 'bowel rest' in which food is withheld for 24–72 hours is commonly adopted while fluid and electrolyte status is maintained through the oral or parenteral administration of rehydration fluids. Subsequently, small amounts of a highly digestible, bland diet (such as boiled rice, fish or chicken) may be gradually reintroduced. In contrast, chronic conditions which persist for longer than 3–4 weeks are unlikely to resolve without first identifying a specific cause and implementing the appropriate therapy.

Oesophageal disease

Oesophageal lesions may necessitate feeding via gastrostomy tube to allow the oesophagus to heal, otherwise soft, moist or liquidised foods may be offered. Patients with mega-oesophagus should be fed from an elevated position to allow food to enter the stomach with the help of gravity. Traditionally, slurries have been used but many cases are now thought to cope better when fed a more textured diet.

Gastric dilatation – volvulus

Although cereal-based dry foods have previously been linked this condition in dogs, it is now thought that they may have been falsely incriminated. Gaseous distension of the stomach may result from swallowed air and may be associated with rapid food consumption and excitement or physical activity close to the time of feeding. General dietary recommendations are to feed small frequent meals of a highly digestible, meat-based diet which will encourage gastric emptying and reduce stomach distension. Dogs, particularly those at high risk, should not be fed or allowed to drink large volumes of water within 1 hour of exercise or excitement and should preferably be fed away from other dogs.

Chronic diarrhoea

Diarrhoea may be defined as an increase in frequency, volume or fluidity of faeces, but these characteristics should be considered in the context of the diet being fed. High fibre diets, for example, will lead to a marked increase in faecal volume and frequency of defaecation compared with 'normal' highly digestible foods. Diarrhoea may be classified as 'chronic' if it persists for longer than 3–4 weeks.

Large quantities of water are either consumed or secreted into the gastrointestinal tract every day and in normal circumstances, approximately 95% of this water is reabsorbed from the large intestine. A relatively small decrease in absorption (or increase in secretion) can readily result in increased faecal water content and diarrhoea.

Diarrhoea occurs as the result of one or more mechanisms:

- Interference with the digestion or absorption of nutrients (osmotic diarrhoea). Nutrients retained within the intestinal lumen exert an osmotic effect leading to the retention of water and diarrhoea. Osmotic diarrhoea is most commonly seen with nutritional overload, but it is also associated with any condition in which there is a deficiency of enzymes or enterocytes, including **exocrine pancreatic insufficiency (EPI)**, **small intestinal disease** and **brush border enzyme** (such as lactase) **deficiency**.
- Increased secretion of fluid into the intestine by enterocytes (secretory diarrhoea), which maybe stimulated by bacterial toxins and by the products of bacterial degradation of bile acids and dietary fat.
- Increased intestinal permeability due to mucosal damage, which can result from severe inflammation or conditions (cardiac disease, lymphatic obstruction). If the pore size is large, fluid and plasma proteins escape into the intestinal lumen, creating a protein-losing enteropathy and diarrhoea.
- Altered intestinal motility. Contrary to popular belief, most cases are due to a reduction in segmentation contractions rather than increased peristalsis, resulting in stagnation of intestinal contents, bacterial proliferation and degradation of nutrients. The increased faecal volume stimulates secondary peristaltic contractions which may give the impression of hypermotility.

Small intestinal disease

Diarrhoea of small intestinal origin tends to lead to an increase in faecal volume since this is the main site for digestion and absorption of nutrients and this, in turn, can lead to an increased frequency of defecation. Pale, fatty faeces (steatorrhoea) are seen when there is maldigestion or malabsorption of fat, as in EPI and other small intestinal disorders. Because nutrients are poorly absorbed into the body, weight loss is common, often despite a marked increase in appetite.

Diet plays an important role in the management of many small intestinal diseases, generally in conjunction with appropriate pharmacological therapy. Although no single diet is appropriate for every condition, it is generally accepted that diets for the management of conditions involving the small intestine should be highly digestible since many diseases are likely to interfere with digestive and absorptive function. In most circumstances, therefore, high fibre diets are contraindicated for the management of small intestinal disease.

Restriction of dietary fat is recommended in a range of small intestinal diseases which disturb fat digestion or absorption, including **EPI**, **small intestinal bacterial overgrowth (SIBO)** and **lymphangiectasia**. Pancreatic enzymes are reduced or absent with EPI, whereas SIBO adversely affects bile salts. In addition, bacterial metabolism of undigested fat may promote intestinal secretion and further aggravate the diarrhoea.

In some cases, medium chain triglycerides (MCTs) may form a useful supplemental source of energy, since some MCTs can be absorbed intact from the gastrointestinal tract and can reach the circulation via portal rather than lymphatic channels.

- Restriction of dietary fat is less important in the cat than the dog and some diarrhoeic cats appear to fare better on moderate to high fat diets.
- Moderate to high quantities of good-quality protein are recommended for small intestinal diseases since protein malabsorption or protein-losing enteropathy may be a feature of some cases of chronic small intestinal diarrhoea. Protein deficiency can further compromise a diseased intestinal tract.
- Protein is also important in relation to dietary sensitivity since most 'allergens' are proteins. Gluten, a protein in wheat and other cereals such as barley (not maize), is responsible for a particular enteropathy of Irish setters in which poor weight gain or weight loss is usually accompanied by chronic diarrhoea. Where dietary sensitivity is the cause of diarrhoea, sources of dietary protein should be minimised to one or two ingredients, which are not normally associated with sensitivity reactions.
- Carbohydrate digestion and absorption can be impaired in all conditions that damage the lining of the small intestinal wall. Nevertheless, starch presents a relatively low digestive challenge in comparison with fat and may be used to provide a greater contribution to the energy content of diets which are restricted in fat. Highly digestible sources of carbohydrate, such as rice, are recommended. Simple sugars such as lactose, which is found in milk, should be avoided because the enzymes required for their digestion may be lacking.
- Although dietary fibre is commonly used in the non-specific treatment of acute diarrhoeas, it is generally not

suitable for use in chronic small intestinal diseases. In the short term, fibre may improve faecal consistency, but in chronic cases it may interfere with digestion and absorption, thereby further compromising an impaired gastrointestinal tract. In particular, soluble fibre is contraindicated in EPI since this may interfere with pancreatic enzyme activity.

- Several small intestinal diseases can result in deficiencies of water-soluble B-complex vitamins, especially cobalamin (vitamin B_{12}) and folate.

Large intestinal disease

Animals with large intestinal diarrhoea tend to show very frequent defecation and pass small quantities of faeces on each occasion. This may be associated with urgency, straining or pain on defecation. The presence of fresh blood and copious amounts of mucus are also characteristic of large intestinal problems. Although weight loss is not usually a feature of large intestinal disease, it can occur as a secondary problem if appetite is depressed over a long period of time.

- Dietary fibre may be beneficial in the management of some large intestinal diarrhoeas. Bacterial fermentation of fibres (particularly soluble fibres) within the large intestine yield short chain fatty acids, which are important for maintaining the health of cells of the large intestinal wall and promote acidification of the contents of the colon. Insoluble fibre tends to be non-fermentable and its effects are primarily related to an increase in faecal bulk. This may help to exercise the smooth muscle of the colon and improve contractility and, in addition, may bind faecal water to produce more formed stools.
- Diets containing a mixture of both soluble and insoluble fibres can, therefore, be valuable as non-specific therapy in a number of large intestinal diseases, including certain infections and 'irritable bowel syndrome', which is thought to be associated with stress.
- Since many cases of colitis and inflammatory bowel disease in dogs and cats are thought to be immune-mediated, single protein source 'hypoallergenic diets' may be of benefit in their management, at least in the initial stages of therapy.

Constipation

Constipation may be defined as an inability to pass, or difficulty in passing, faeces. Retained faeces in the rectum and colon become progressively harder as water is reabsorbed and the faecal mass becomes increasingly impacted. High fibre diets are of benefit in the prevention, but not the treatment, of constipation. Insoluble fibre increases faecal bulk which is thought to increase colonic motility by stretching colonic muscles, resulting in more forceful, albeit less frequent, contractions. Soluble fibres may add further to faecal bulk, through their ability to retain water in the intestinal lumen. Fibres combining soluble and insoluble properties may be optimal for the prevention of constipation.

Pancreatic disease

Exocrine pancreatic insufficiency

Exocrine pancreatic secretions (pancreatic juice) are reduced or absent in patients with exocrine pancreatic insufficiency (EPI) resulting in an inability to adequately digest fat and, to a lesser extent, protein and carbohydrate in the diet. Because there is poor digestion and malabsorption of nutrients, especially fat, weight loss is common despite a marked increase in appetite and affected animals produce large volumes of pale, fatty faeces (steatorrhoea).

Although enzyme replacement therapy improves digestibility in patients with EPI, their requirements for energy and nutrients are still higher than in the normal animal. Low fat diets of high digestibility help to reduce the digestive challenge within the gastrointestinal tract and may reduce the daily requirement for enzyme replacer. High fibre (particularly soluble fibre) diets are to be avoided since they interfere with pancreatic enzyme activity, which may be reduced by up to 60%. Requirements for cobalamin (vitamin B_{12}) are often raised with EPI, and those for zinc and copper may also be marginally increased.

Pancreatitis

The initial therapy of acute pancreatitis is aimed at preventing the secretion of proteolytic enzymes from the exocrine pancreas, which promote further tissue damage within the organ. This involves a strict policy of nil by mouth (food and water) for 2–5 days with the parenteral administration of fluid and electrolytes. If vomiting does not occur for 48 hours, oral electrolyte drinks may be given for 1–2 days before the gradual reintroduction of solid food.

High carbohydrate foods (such as rice, pasta or potatoes), which have the least stimulating effect on pancreatic secretions, may be offered initially in several small feeds per day. If this is tolerated, a highly digestible, low fat diet may be offered, in which the protein content is moderately reduced and of high biological value. This type of diet is useful in the recovery period of acute pancreatitis and also to help prevent recurrent bouts of chronic pancreatitis.

Liver disease

Hepatobiliary disease can lead to derangements in both the metabolism and storage of proteins, fats, carbohydrates and certain micronutrients, as well as in the detoxification of potentially hazardous by-products. **Hepatic encephalopathy (HE)** can occur where there is either critical loss of functional hepatic tissue (60–70%) or **portosystemic shunting**. In HE, a number of neurotoxic substances (mainly ammonia) may enter the peripheral and cerebral circulation, giving rise to a complex of neurological signs. These toxins are derived mainly from the alimentary tract, being synthesised by gastrointestinal flora or consumed in the diet, but ammonia is also produced as a by-product of protein catabolism and when amino acids are converted to glucose and energy via gluconeogenesis.

Nevertheless, the liver has a large functional reserve and a phenomenal capacity for regeneration following insult. Nutritional support during the period of hepatocellular repair can help to delay or prevent irreversible progression of the disease. For dogs, this can be achieved by modification of the diet in the following ways:

- Adequate energy provision, using non-protein sources. This limits ammonia production by avoiding the use of amino acids to provide energy and by preventing muscle wastage.
- Moderate restriction of dietary protein to help limit the amount of ammonia generated both in the intestines and from the use of amino acids for gluconeogenesis. However, dietary protein intake must be carefully balanced to meet the individual animal's needs since an inadequate intake will promote the breakdown of structural proteins.
- High-quality proteins are recommended since they tend to be highly digestible and are likely to meet the animal's needs with minimal production of ammonia.
- Careful use of fat as an energy source, which increases the energy density of the diet and improves palatability. Both these effects are beneficial in the management of dogs with liver disease, since inappetence is a common problem. However, moderate fat restriction is indicated in dogs with an impaired ability to digest fat due to a lack of bile.
- Provision of complex carbohydrates, such as starch and fibre, in the diet to improve glucose utilisation by slowing down the delivery of glucose from the gut to the liver.
- Inclusion of dietary fibre, which may assist in the elimination of ammonia and other toxins in the faeces, inhibit ammonia production by bacteria in the colon and prevent constipation, which is also important in the management of HE.
- Supplementation with water-soluble vitamins (B-complex) to compensate for impaired synthesis and increased losses of these nutrients. Supplementation with vitamin E may be beneficial in limiting ongoing liver disease.
- Supplementation with zinc, which is involved in the detoxification of ammonia, can help to improve nervous signs associated with HE. Zinc reduces fibrosis and, by reducing the availability of copper, provides protection against liver injury associated with copper accumulation in the liver. This is particularly beneficial in patients with copper storage liver disease.
- Restriction of dietary copper intake.
- Moderate restriction of sodium intake, especially where liver disease is associated with hypoalbuminaemia or portal hypertension, since an excessive intake can precipitate or exacerbate ascites.

Diets for cats with liver disease must meet the normally high feline requirements for protein and essential amino acids. Protein-restricted diets are not recommended unless the disease is accompanied by HE, although this is rare in cats. The protein content of these diets should be of high biological value and ensure an adequate intake of arginine,

taurine and carnitine. Diets formulated for the management of feline chronic renal failure may be appropriate in this minority of cases.

Most cats with liver disease, particularly those with **hepatic lipidosis**, may have increased protein requirements and the requirements for B-complex vitamins and fat-soluble vitamins K and E may be similarly raised. High fat diets may be detrimental in feline hepatic lipidosis and in cats with other forms of hepatic disease. Highly digestible diets with a relatively high protein content, moderately reduced fat content and enhanced levels of zinc and vitamins B, K and E are likely to be of benefit in most cats with hepatic disease. For cats with hepatic lipidosis, enteral tube feeding will almost certainly be required.

Diabetes mellitus

Animals with **diabetes mellitus** have impaired production or release of insulin which may be combined with a tissue insensitivity to insulin (insulin resistance). See also Chapter 17, p. 457. This results in an imbalance in the metabolism of carbohydrate, fat and protein and is characterised by hyperglycaemia and an inability to regulate blood sugar levels. Successful long-term management of diabetes mellitus involves a combination of appropriate insulin replacement therapy and a suitable dietary regime. The aim is to provide a consistent supply of nutrients to match the activity of exogenous insulin and thereby achieve relatively stable blood glucose levels. Consistency in the feeding regime is essential and involves the standardisation of the quantity of food given, the dietary content (energy density and dietary constituents) and the timing of meals. The exercise routine, which may alter the animal's energy requirements, should also be carefully regulated. A schedule should be established that is compatible with the normal household routine.

Timing of feeding should be arranged such that maximal absorption and metabolism of nutrients coincides with maximal activity of administered insulin and may vary with the type of insulin preparation used. Insulins with an intermediate duration of action (such as lente or isophane preparations in dogs and lente or protamine zinc preparations in cats) are commonly used as single or, where insulin metabolism is faster, as twice daily injections.

Generally, increasing the number of meals daily reduces the degree of post-prandial hyperglycaemia and improves glycaemic control, provided that the meals are fed whilst the injected insulin is still active. In most cases, however, the daily food allowance may be divided into two meals. When insulin is injected once daily, one meal may be fed at the time of injection with the second meal given 6–8 hours later. When insulin is given twice daily, meals should either be given at injection times (2 meals/day) or additionally at times of peak insulin activity (3–4 meals/day).

For **canine** diabetics, modification of the diet can help to improve glycaemic control and may reduce the requirement for replacement insulin therapy:

Simple sugars, such as glucose, sucrose and lactose, are to be avoided (other than in the emergency treatment of hypoglycaemia resulting from insulin overdosage) since they are rapidly absorbed and promote wide fluctuations in blood sugar levels.

- Complex carbohydrates such as starch, however, are digested relatively slowly and result in a more gradual release of glucose into the circulation over a period of hours.
- Dietary fibre further slows down the rate of digestion within the gut lumen and therefore slows the rate of post-prandial nutrient uptake. When combined with the slow digestion of starch, this effect helps to reduce post-prandial glycaemic peaks which facilitates the control of blood glucose levels.
- High fat diets should be avoided since diabetics tend to develop hyperlipidaemia and other lipid-related complications.

The benefits of high fibre, high starch diets have not been demonstrated in diabetic cats, which are poorly adapted to high carbohydrate diets. Current recommendations are to feed diabetic cats a 'normal' feline diet although semi-moist foods, which are high in simple sugars, are contraindicated. As with dogs, meal times and the amount and type of diet must be standardised as far as possible.

If the diabetic animal is also obese, which can exacerbate diabetes, weight reduction measures should be incorporated into the diabetic regimen. Dietary therapy for other co-existing disease, such as chronic renal failure, hepatic disease, congestive heart failure or chronic gastrointestinal disease, may take priority over diets designed for improving glycaemic control, but again, consistency in the feeding regime is the rule.

Chronic renal failure

Chronic renal failure (CRF) is a relatively common syndrome in older dogs and cats and represents the end stage of a number of renal diseases. It is a progressive condition in which existing renal damage is irreversible, but dietary measures can improve the clinical signs of uraemia associated with CRF and may help to slow progression of the condition. Clinical signs of CRF are not apparent until at least 65–75% of renal tissue is destroyed, so unless blood and urine parameters are routinely monitored, early cases often go undetected.

Since many of the clinical signs related to CRF are associated with the accumulation of toxic protein catabolites and failure to excrete phosphorus, the emphasis in dietary therapy is on modification of the phosphorus and protein contents of the diet. However, other dietary components to be considered include calcium, sodium, potassium and water-soluble vitamins, together with the dietary energy content and fat. Maintenance of normal hydration is also important, through the provision of unlimited access to drinking water or via intravenous fluid replacement in cases of persistent vomiting.

- Dietary **phosphorus restriction** is an important part of management of CRF which should be initiated early in the course of the disease. This helps to limit renal mineralisation and secondary hyperparathyroidism, and in dogs has been shown to slow progression of renal damage.
- **Moderate restriction of dietary protein** is of clinical benefit in uraemic patients since this minimises the accumulation of nitrogenous waste associated with protein breakdown; helps to limit the intake of dietary phosphorus; and reduces the protein-related solute load on the failing kidneys, thereby lessening the severity of polydipsia/polyuria. Nevertheless, excessive protein restriction is to be avoided since this can result in protein malnutrition in both dogs and cats. The protein in diets for patients with CRF should be of high biological value.
- For dogs with CRF, a staged approach to management is recommended and early cases may benefit from phosphorus restriction whilst maintaining a protein intake that adequately meets adult maintenance requirements. More advanced cases which are showing clinical signs of uraemia should be fed diets which are restricted in both phosphorus and protein. Where possible, the degree of protein restriction should be individualised according to the dog's clinical and biochemical status.
- The potential risks of dietary protein reduction are greater in the cat than in the dog. It is currently recommended that well-hydrated cats with azotaemia (increased concentrations of urea, creatinine or other non-protein nitrogenous compounds in blood) and hyperphosphataemia should be fed diets which are restricted in phosphorus and moderately restricted in protein.
- Feeding an **energy-dense** diet, in which the energy content is derived from non-protein sources, avoids tissue catabolism and helps to reduce nitrogenous waste production. Appetite is often poor in affected animals, so the energy density of the diet should be high to enable the animal to obtain its nutritional requirements from a relatively small volume of food. Fat is particularly useful in this respect, since it increases energy density and aids **palatability** of the diet. For this reason, canned diets designed to support dogs and cats with CRF tend to be high in fat.
- Many cats with CRF are hypokalaemic and require some degree of dietary **potassium** supplementation. However, some cats (often those most severely affected) are hyperkalaemic so serum potassium levels should be closely monitored in cats with CRF.
- Serum **calcium** levels may be low, normal or high in patients with CRF. Calcium supplementation may be required in hypocalcaemic individuals.
- **Sodium** balance may be disrupted in advanced CRF and systemic hypertension can occur in both dogs and cats. It is currently recommended that dietary sodium levels are either normal or moderately restricted, since excessive sodium restriction may also be detrimental.
- Requirements for **water-soluble (B-complex) vitamins** are increased in dogs and cats with CRF because of reduced intake (inappetence), increased urinary losses in polyuric cases and higher demands during the recuperative processes.

Urolithiasis

Urolithiasis is the disease which results from the formation of calculi (uroliths) within the urinary tract. Urine is normally supersaturated with the mineral components of a variety of uroliths and urolith crystals form when the concentrations of its constituents exceed a critical level. Dietary factors can profoundly influence urolith formation because dietary ingredients and feeding patterns influence the pH, volume and solute concentration of the urine.

Urolithiasis is a common cause of feline lower urinary tract disease (FLUTD), particularly in obstructed cases. Traditionally, struvite urolithiasis has been of greatest importance but although the incidence has declined in recent years, calcium oxalate urolithiasis is now seen with increasing frequency. Uroliths which are commonly found in dogs include struvite, calcium oxalate, cystine and ammonium urate. Mixed calculi may also occur in some cases.

Struvite

Factors which decrease the risk of struvite (magnesium ammonium phosphate) crystal formation in urine include:

- Acidification of the urine (to between pH 6.0 and 6.5 in cats and between pH 5.5 and 6.0 in dogs).
- Increased urine volume to dilute solute concentrations and increase in the frequency of urination.
- Moderate restriction of dietary magnesium and phosphorus.

Diets which achieve these goals may be used to dissolve struvite crystals *in situ* or to prevent recurrence of the condition. Initial relief of obstructed cases may require surgical intervention.

Commercial diets are available which have been designed to achieve urinary undersaturation with struvite although urinary acidifiers may be added to an animal's normal diet to achieve the appropriate effect. Diets of high moisture content and high digestibility are preferred but water may also be added to dry foods if necessary. Moderate supplementation with sodium chloride (salt) may stimulate thirst and promote increased water turnover. Acidified diets are not appropriate for feeding to young animals or to pregnant or lactating females. Furthermore, levels of taurine and potassium should be enhanced when acidified diets are fed to cats.

The main difference between canine and feline struvite urolithiasis is that in dogs, struvite uroliths are usually associated with urinary tract infection whereas most feline struvite uroliths are sterile. Urease-producing bacteria such as staphylococci and *Proteus* spp. create an increasingly alkaline environment and conditions which are ideal for the formation of struvite and, occasionally, other types of urolith. Where infection is present, prolonged antibiotic therapy is essential in addition to dietary and other measures. Dietary protein restriction may also be beneficial in these cases, since this reduces the available substrate in urine for urease-producing bacteria.

Calcium oxalate

It is not possible to dissolve calcium oxalate uroliths *in situ* by dietary or any other means, and surgery is currently the only method of removing them in dogs and cats. Nevertheless, dietary manipulation can help to prevent recurrence of the condition. Achieving a urine which is undersaturated with calcium and oxalate is of major importance, but inhibitors of calcium oxalate crystallisation (such as magnesium and citrate) in urine may also have a significant role.

Diets designed for the management of calcium oxalate urolithiasis should promote increased urine volume, preferably through the addition of water to the food. Although restriction of dietary calcium and oxalate may be beneficial, restriction of only one of these components may increase intestinal absorption of the other. Urine pH may also be important and although calcium oxalate saturation is increased in very acidic urine, studies in cats suggest that saturation is lowest in moderately acidic urine (pH 6.0–6.5). Although increased magnesium intake is sometimes recommended in the prevention of calcium oxalate urolithiasis, care should be taken to ensure that this does not predispose the animal to struvite urolith formation.

Cystine

Cystine urolithiasis occurs in dogs with an inherited defect in cystine metabolism, resulting in impaired reabsorption of the amino acid from the proximal tubule of the kidney and, hence, cystinuria. This leads to cystine urolith formation since cystine is relatively insoluble, particularly in acidic urine. Dissolution and prevention of recurrence of cystine uroliths can be achieved through:

- Increasing water intake to increase urine volume.
- Reduction of dietary protein to reduce cystine production and excretion.
- Restriction of dietary sodium to promote tubular reabsorption of cystine.
- Alkalinisation of urine (with bicarbonate or citrate) to increase cystine solubility.
- Administration of compounds such as D-penicillamine or 2-mercaptopropionylglycine (2-MPG) which convert cystine to a more soluble compound.

Ammonium urate

Urate uroliths occur mostly in Dalmatians and in patients with portosystemic shunts, when hepatic conversion of uric acid (a product of purine metabolism) to allantoin is impaired. Allantoin is highly soluble but urinary increased excretion of uric acid may predispose the dog to urolith formation through the precipitation of ammonium urate crystals.

Surgical relief of obstruction may be required in some cases. In others, dissolution and prevention of recurrence of urate uroliths may be achieved by:

- Restriction of dietary protein to limit purine intake.
- Supplementation with potassium citrate to promote neutral or slightly alkaline urine.

- Increased water intake.
- Administration of allopurinol which inhibits uric acid production.

Idiopathic FLUTD

For a significant proportion of cats with signs of non-obstructive lower urinary tract disease, a specific cause cannot be identified and the condition is classified as 'idiopathic'. Although clinical signs resolve spontaneously within 5–7 days, many cases recur after a variable period. Studies have shown that the rate of recurrence can be reduced by feeding a canned diet formulated for the production of acidic urine, although the equivalent dry formulation had no impact on the natural biological behaviour of the disease.

Skin disease

Deficiencies of essential fatty acids, protein, zinc, vitamins A, E and certain B-complex vitamins may give rise to skin disease which is commonly manifest as seborrhoea. In addition, supplementation with supraphysiological doses of certain nutrients, including vitamins A and E and essential fatty acids, have been used in the treatment of specific skin conditions where no apparent dietary deficiency exists. Essential fatty acids, particularly those of the omega-3 series found in marine fish oils, are currently thought to be of greatest value in the management of pruritic skin diseases associated with hypersensitivity reactions. A third area in which diet is related to skin disease is that of dietary sensitivity which, in dogs and cats, is commonly manifest as a pruritic skin disorder.

Cardiac disease

Congestive heart failure

Congestive heart failure is associated with retention of sodium and water, due to low blood pressure and poor renal perfusion, which results in volume overload and hypertension. Restriction of dietary sodium is a useful dietary strategy which helps to decrease fluid retention and should be implemented early in the course of disease. Renal function is often compromised in cardiac failure and so the transition to a low sodium diet should take place gradually (over at least 5 days) to allow the kidneys to adapt.

Weight loss is common in cardiac patients (**cardiac cachexia**) as a consequence of a number of factors. Patients are often anorectic and malabsorption may occur as a result of reduced intestinal perfusion. Furthermore, energy requirements may be increased which can accelerate the wasting process. It is essential to ensure an adequate energy intake and if voluntary intake is reduced, some form of nutritional support is necessary. Fat may improve palatability and increase the energy density of the diet, but high fat diets may not be appropriate in all cases. Some cardiac patients may be obese and for these, controlled weight reduction can help to improve clinical status.

Some degree of renal and hepatic dysfunction is often associated with congestive heart failure. Diets in which the protein content is moderately restricted and of high biological value should be introduced for these patients, but in other patients with protein energy malnutrition an increase in protein intake may be necessary.

Diuretic agents can have a marked effect on nutritional requirements, particularly for sodium and potassium, and may increase urinary losses of water-soluble vitamins (B-complex). Long-term use of frusemide or thiazide diuretics may cause potassium depletion and may also promote urinary magnesium loss. Conversely, spironolactone tends to conserve potassium but sodium excretion is enhanced and, in this case, low sodium diets should be avoided. Low salt diets should also be used with care when vasodilators such as captopril and enalapril are administered, since these drugs are also associated with sodium loss and potassium retention.

Dilated cardiomyopathy

Low myocardial concentrations of **carnitine** have been associated with **dilated cardiomyopathy** in some dogs, notably Boxers, and dietary supplementation with L-carnitine (not D-carnitine or a mixture of D- and L-carnitine) is recommended as an adjunct to conventional medical therapy. In cats, many cases of dilated cardiomyopathy have been linked to **taurine** deficiency and plasma taurine status should be determined in all cases, prior to supplementation. Where appropriate, the deficient diet should be replaced with a feline diet of adequate taurine content and additional taurine supplementation should be provided as necessary, usually for a period of 12–16 weeks.

Nutrition of small and exotic pets
Small mammals

Basic energy and macronutrient requirements for rabbits and rodents are given in Tables 8.21 and 8.22.

Rabbits

Rabbits are herbivores with a high dietary requirement for fibre. Most domestic rabbits are fed balanced commercial pelleted foods or coarse mixes which may be supplemented with hay (as bedding) and small quantities of a variety of green vegetables, carrots and fresh salad crops. Supervised browsing on grass and other plants may also be encouraged but grass cuttings should not be fed.

Rabbits have an unusual metabolism of calcium which necessitates careful regulation of the dietary calcium content. Excessive dietary calcium can give rise to urolithiasis, whereas dietary deficiency (often exacerbated by a vitamin D deficiency) is a common cause of osteodystrophy with associated skeletal and tooth defects. Problems can arise in some rabbits fed 'rabbit mixes' because rabbits are selective feeders and may reject the pellets and whole grain in the ration. Most vitamin and mineral supplements are

Table 8.21 Basic energy requirements for rabbits and rodents (ME (kcal/day) = 110–440 $W^{0.75}$) (after Tobin, 1996)

	Rabbits	Guinea pigs	Hamsters	Gerbils	Rats and mice
Body weight (W)	0.5–7.0 kg	0.75–1.0 kg	85–140 g	50–60 g	20–800 g
Maintenance	110.00	110.00	110.00	110.00	110.00
Growth	190–210	145.00	145.00	145.00	145.00
Gestation	135–200	145.00	145.00	145.00	145.00
Lactation	300.00	165.00	310.00	440.00	440.00

Table 8.22 Basic macronutrient requirements for rabbits and rodents (after Tobin, 1996)

	Rabbits	Guinea pigs	Hamsters	Gerbils	Rats and mice
ME (kcal/g)	2–2.4	1.7–2.9	2.5–3.9	2.5–3.7	2.2–3
Protein (%)	12–18	18–20	18–22	17–18	13–20
Fat (%)	2–4	2–4	4–5	10–12	1–5
Fibre (%)	10–16	7–11	4–8	4.00	4.00

incorporated in the pelleted portion of the diet and rejection of these can produce a diet which is seriously deficient in calcium, vitamin D and other nutrients. Owners should encourage the rabbit to eat all ingredients in the ration by offering smaller quantities and refilling the pot only when all food has been consumed.

Rabbits tend to adjust their food intake according to their energy requirements and the energy content of the diet, but adults are likely to eat approximately 30–60 g of dry food/ kg BW/day. Free access to clean water in bowls or suspended bottles should be provided and adults may drink 5–10 ml/100 g BW/day.

Guinea pigs

Guinea pigs are herbivorous animals and, like humans and other primates, require a dietary source of vitamin C. A deficiency can result in clinical signs of scurvy within 2 weeks of feeding a deficient diet. The main types of feed are pelleted foods or coarse mixes, but these should be formulated specifically for guinea pigs. Rabbit feeds are unsuitable since they are lower in protein and are not supplemented with vitamin C, and some products contain coccidiostats which can cause liver or kidney damage in guinea pigs. Some pelleted feeds for guinea pigs contain vitamin C at levels which only just meet the minimum requirements and prolonged storage (over 3 months) can deplete vitamin C levels in the food. Supplementary vitamin C may be administered in the drinking water (1 g/litre) or fresh fruit or leafy vegetables, which contain high levels of the vitamin, may be added to the diet. Any dietary changes should take place gradually to avoid gastrointestinal upset.

Relatively high levels of fibre are required and a shortage can cause caecal impaction and fur chewing which may

result in the formation of hairballs. An adequate supply of good-quality hay can usually prevent these conditions. Guinea pigs should be provided with a diet that requires gnawing to promote balanced wear of the teeth. Malocclusion can prevent feeding, drinking and swallowing of saliva (*slobbers*) and can prove fatal within 6 days of signs occurring.

Guinea pigs may eat 5–8 g/100 g BW/day. Food may be provided in open bowls on the cage floor, but may become contaminated with excreta. Average daily water intake is 10 ml/100 g BW but this may increase if no succulent foods are fed and free access to water should be provided. Open water bowls may be contaminated and so inverted water bottles with a small sipper tube are often suspended from the side of the cage slightly above floor level. Fresh water should be provided daily and the water bottle cleaned.

Rats and mice

Rats and mice are omnivorous and will eat almost anything. Their nutritional requirements are well documented and commercial pelleted foods or coarse mixes are widely available. The basic ration may be supplemented with small quantities of a variety of foods including biscuit, apple, tomatoes and chocolate (as a treat) and offering these may encourage handling by the owner. Most rats and mice will adjust their energy intake to match their requirements but overfeeding of highly palatable foods can lead to obesity. As a guide, adult rats require 10–20 g/day of dry food whereas adult mice require 5–10 g/day.

Free access to water should be available from small bowls or suspended water bottles. Adult rats may drink 25–45 ml/day and adult mice may drink 5–7 ml/day.

Hamsters

Hamsters are omnivorous and although specific diets are available, most good-quality rat or mice diets will meet the requirements of the hamster. Commercial pelleted diets or coarse mixes can be supplemented with treat foods such as washed vegetables, seeds, fruits, crackers, and small amounts of cheese or cooked meat. Diets rich in simple sugars (glucose, lactose, sucrose, fructose) are best avoided and hamsters fare better when the carbohydrate source is starch. Malocclusion and overgrowth of teeth can be prevented by providing hard foods that require gnawing, such as dog biscuits or whole cereal seeds, such as maize.

Most adults will eat 5–15 g of pelleted feed and drink 15–20 ml of water/day, although free access to water should be offered. Food and water should be provided in heavy dishes that are not easily overturned or contaminated or, alternatively, hoppers may be used. Stale food should be removed from the cage to prevent hoarding by the hamster.

Gerbils

Gerbils are herbivorous or granivorous and their natural diet is based on grains and seeds which is supplemented with fresh vegetables and roots when these are available. Commercial pelleted foods or seed and grain diets are available for gerbils, although adult gerbils can be fed good-quality rat or mice diets. Some mixes may contain large amounts of sunflower seeds which are very palatable to gerbils but have a high fat and low calcium content. Gerbils may therefore selectively eat sunflower seeds at the expense of other dietary ingredients but an excessive intake can result in obesity and calcium deficiency with associated skeletal problems. The diet should be supplemented with chopped green vegetables, roots and fruit, and if pelleted food is given, an appropriate seed mix should also be provided. Average food consumption in the adult is 10–15 g daily. Like other rodents, gerbils need some hard foods or pieces of wood in their environment to gnaw and so prevent problems with tooth malocclusion.

Gerbils conserve water efficiently through their ability to concentrate their urine. Most of their water requirement is met from succulent foods and from metabolism of the diet. Nevertheless, free access to clean water should always be provided. Food dishes should be ceramic since plastic dishes may be eaten. Water containers with drinking tubes are best placed outside the cage and should be checked regularly to ensure that they are working.

Chinchillas

In the wild, chinchillas eat a wide range of vegetables, but their diet is composed mainly of grasses and seeds. Commercial diets are available but good-quality rabbit or guinea pig diets are also suitable. Good-quality hay should be available *ad libitum* and the diet may be supplemented with small quantities of dried fruit, nuts, carrot, washed green vegetables and fresh grass. However, supplements should be provided in moderation to prevent obesity, bloat,

diarrhoea or other gastrointestinal upsets. Some hard foods or objects should be available to gnaw and prevent teeth malocclusion problems.

Adults may eat approximately 20 g/day. Free access to water should be provided from hanging water bottles, although it may be advisable to offer an additional water dish until the animal is used to drinking from a bottle.

Ferrets

Ferrets are essentially carnivores with high protein and fat requirements. High fibre diets should be avoided. Pelleted diets for ferrets are commercially available, otherwise high quality tinned or dry cat foods may be fed. Dog foods are not appropriate for long-term feeding. Whole carcasses (mice, rabbits, day-old chicks) or chicken heads may occasionally be offered to provide variety or to supplement the diet. Many ferrets will eat other foods, and small quantities of raw carrot or apple, cooked meat, dried fruit and raw liver can be offered.

Food intake in adults may be 20–40 g/day and working ferrets are commonly fed twice daily. Food preferences are established early in life and some individuals may resent dietary change. Water intake is approximately 75–100 ml/day.

Reptiles

Chelonians

Land tortoises are herbivores or omnivores whereas terrapins are mainly carnivores and scavengers. Feeding errors in captive chelonians are a common cause of shell defects and hypovitaminosis A, so vitamin/mineral supplementation is usually required. Newly hatched tortoises start to feed properly once the yolk sac has been absorbed and may be offered a variety of finely chopped fruits, vegetables, cold hard-boiled eggs, sprats, day-old chicks and other sources of animal protein. This should be supplemented with vitamins and minerals and meals should be offered twice daily. Juvenile and adult tortoises may be fed the same range of foods but these do not need to be chopped up and the tortoises can be housed outdoors in summer, with access to grass and other plants. Food intake is reduced or will stop for up to several weeks prior to hibernation, which occurs when ambient temperature and daylight hours begin to decrease. Although most water requirements are met from their food, tortoises should be provided with regular access to water.

Young terrapins feed in water and their diet includes small insects, small crustaceans and amphibian eggs and larvae. Adult terrapins eat amphibians and fish in the wild, so in captivity whole fish or chopped portions of whole fish should be fed to prevent nutritional imbalance. Herring, sprat, whitebait, sardines, minnows, sand eels, tadpoles or froglets, fresh prawns, shrimps and snails are all suitable foods. It is also possible to feed tinned cat or dog foods, hard-boiled eggs, cheese, earthworms or fresh liver or kidney rubbed in a vitamin/mineral supplement occasionally. However, feeding should take place in a separate container from the normal living quarters and the amount of food offered at any one time should not exceed that which can be eaten within 20 minutes.

Snakes

Snakes are carnivorous and in captivity will eat rabbits, rats, mice, gerbils, chicks, earthworms, fish, amphibians, lizards or even other snakes. The whole carcass is fed, to provide a balanced diet. For humane reasons and to prevent injury to the snake, food is generally offered as dead prey, which may be freshly killed or thawed from frozen. Certain types of fish, including whitebait, has high thiaminase activity and prolonged feeding without thiamine supplementation can result in thiamine deficiency. Water requirements of snakes are low but water should always be provided.

The quantity of food and frequency of feeding depends on the bodyweight and surface area of the prey. For example, small garter snakes may require feeding on a daily basis whereas a large python feeding on antelope may only need to feed twice a year. As a guideline, adult snakes should be fed as often as is required to maintain normal bodyweight. Snakes may not eat for long periods of time and although this is normal at certain times of the year or before a slough, this can result in inanition. Regular weighing is advisable and excessive weight loss may indicate that nutritional support is required. Fluids and easily assimilated foods can be administered by stomach tube.

Lizards

The range of lizards kept in captivity are insectivores, carnivores, herbivores, frugivores and omnivores, and consequently eat a wide variety of foods. Some species may change their feeding requirements as they mature. Insectivores (geckos, chameleons, skinks, anoles, lacertids) feed mainly on mealworms, silk moth larvae, crickets, locusts and wingless fruit flies. However, these insects are relatively deficient in calcium and the insects themselves must be fed an appropriate nutritional supplement to ensure an adequate intake of supplement in the lizard. Common iguana are usually fed vegetables, fruit, chicken, pink mice or dog food. Monitors and tegus eat raw eggs, meat, dog food or rodents such as pink mice, mice or rats. Biotin deficiency can occur due to the avidin content of raw eggs. Vitamin and mineral supplementation is usually required in diets for captive lizards. All lizards should have access to fresh water. Some, such as chameleons, will only drink from water droplets on plants and it is important to mist the tank several times a day. Most lizards should be regularly sprayed with water to prevent skin problems associated with low humidity.

Amphibians

Amphibian species include the frogs, toads, salamanders and newts. Most adults are terrestrial but return to the water to breed and the larval stages are aquatic. Adult amphibians are carnivorous and since feeding is initiated by the movement of prey, live prey is usually required. However, some species may adapt to feeding on dead prey, meat, tinned dog food or even commercial pelleted diets. Raw meat must be supplemented with calcium (10 mg/g of meat). Captive amphibians should be fed twice weekly.

Adult frogs and toads feed on insects such as fruit flies, crickets and mealworms and large toads will also eat mice. Aquatic species may eat fish and prepared fish diets. Salamanders eat earthworms, slugs, insects and prepared fish diets. Larval stages are herbivorous and feed on algae initially, or food sprinkled on the water. As they mature, aquatic prey (small crustaceans) and then larger insects or animals are eaten.

Ornamental fish

One of the difficulties in feeding ornamental fish is that, with a few exceptions such as the goldfish, they are rarely kept in a single species environment. Anatomical differences and variations in feeding strategies complicate the formulation of a single diet which will meet all the requirements of a mixed community, which may include representatives of herbivorous, omnivorous and carnivorous fish species. See Table 8.23.

An adequate delivery of nutrients is essential for the optimum health of the fish, but in a closed aquatic environment, overfeeding and poor diet formulation can have a detrimental effect on conditions in the aquarium. Waste, in the form of uneaten food, undigested food and the excreted metabolic breakdown products of protein, will directly pollute the living environment and can pose a serious threat to the health of aquarium fish. To minimise the risk of pollution-induced stress, the diet must be palatable, easily digested, nutritionally balanced and of high biological value. A number of commercial diets are available for ornamental fish. Nutritionally complete diets are marketed as pellets, flakes and granules and other, complementary, foods include certain pond foods and frozen insect larvae, bloodworms and cockles.

Incomplete foods should be fed with care and although they are useful 'treats' for aquarium fish, an excessive intake may result in dietary imbalance. Live aquatic food, such as *Daphnia* or *Tubifex* spp., is sometimes offered but may represent a disease risk and pre-frozen packs are considered safer. Fish kept in an established pond may feed on the pond's natural flora and fauna, so complete diets are seldom required. Species which are kept in relatively bare display ponds, such as koi carp, will require a complete diet.

Of the complete diets available, flake formats offer versatility in that they can be floated on the water for surface feeders or submerged to sink slowly for middle and bottom feeders. Since the flakes are easily broken up into smaller pieces, they provide an excellent single food for a range of species and sizes of fish. Granules offer lower leaching of nutrients because their surface area to volume ratio is larger, and different granule sizes and

Table 8.23 Maintenance feeding requirement of five popular species of ornamental fish (after Pannevis and Earle, 1994)

Fish species	Fish size (g/fish)	Maintenance feeding requirement (% BW food/day)	Maintenance feeding requirement (mg food/(fish.day))
Goldfish	3.60	0.40	14.40
	4.80	0.20	11.50
	8.10	0.30	25.80
	11.70	0.20	18.30
Neon tetras	0.18	1.90	3.80
Leopard danio	0.31	≤2.4	≤7.2
Kribensis	1.10	≤1.0	≤10.2
Moonlight gourami	1.90	≤1.5	≤28.5

densities may be used to target different groups of fish in the aquarium.

As a general guideline, fish kept in a community tank should be fed to satiation 2–3 times per day. This allows close inspection of both the fish and tank on a regular basis. Feeding to satiation involves the continuous addition of small amounts of food to the aquarium until the fish stop feeding eagerly, and normally is achieved in a few minutes or less, depending on the tank size and stocking density.

It should be emphasised that pollution from nitrogenous waste is a considerable threat to the health of fish held in a closed water volume. Correct diet formulation and feeding regimen can improve protein utilisation and help to minimise pollution, but water quality should be maintained through regular water changes or, in the larger aquaria, through the use of filter systems which must be properly maintained.

Cage birds

Passerine bird species, such as the canary and zebra finch, eat a wide variety of insects, fruit and small seeds to obtain a balanced diet in the wild. Captive birds should be fed a mixture of seeds and fruit which mimic the bird's natural feeding ecology. Similarly, **psittacine** birds, such as parrots, budgerigars, cockatoos, cockatiels, macaws and parakeets, seek out a natural diet containing a wide range of insects, fruit and seeds but in captivity they are commonly fed only seed mixes which are composed predominantly of sunflower seeds that are high in fat but low in calcium and vitamin A. This type of diet may predispose the bird to obesity or nutritional disorders and the problem is compounded in some individuals that become addicted to sunflower seeds.

Commercial diets formulated to meet the needs of different types of bird are preferred to home-formulated diets. All-seed diets are unlikely to be nutritionally complete for birds and careful vitamin/mineral supplementation will be required. Although commercial, balanced diets need no supplementation, but supplementary foods such as green vegetables (lettuce, chickweed, parsley, watercress), sprouted seeds, root vegetables, fruit (apples, plums, oranges, grapes, tomatoes) may be offered to provide variety and, in home-prepared diets, nutritional balance. These foods may be mixed with cooked egg, chicken, cheese or milk. Millet sprays are often fed to adult budgerigars, but if soaked in hot water and left for 24 hours, they can also provide a useful toy and food for young budgerigars and canaries.

Small birds have high metabolic rates and energy requirements, so it is important that a continuous supply of food is available. Empty husks should be blown from the top of the food on a frequent basis to avoid mistakes in judging how much the bird has actually eaten. Food may be provided in seed hoppers but young birds may be fed from the floor of the cage until they are familiar with alternative feeding systems. Fresh water or milk and water (for breeding and moulting birds) should be available at all times.

Two types of mineral grit, insoluble and soluble, are frequently offered to companion birds as a dietary supplement. Insoluble grit, such as quartz or other forms of silica, remains in the gizzard where it may assist in the mechanical digestion of food and, thus, improve digestibility of the diet. Soluble grit, such as oyster shell or cuttlefish, is usually completely digested by birds and provides a valuable supplementary source of minerals including calcium and phosphorus. However, oversupplementation with insoluble grit is potentially hazardous and may lead to gizzard impaction and eventual death. Canaries do not appear to need insoluble grit in their diet but a source of soluble grit is essential.

Further reading

Beynon, P. H. and Cooper, J. E. (eds) (1991) *Manual of Exotic Pets*, BSAVA, Cheltenham.

Burger, I. (ed.) (1993) *The Waltham Book of Companion Animal Nutrition*, Pergamon Press, Oxford.

Harper, E. J. and Skinner, N. D. (1998) Clinical nutrition of small psittacines and passerines. *Seminars in Avian and Exotic Pet Medicine*, vol. 7, no. 3, pp. 116–127.

Kelly, N. and Wills, J. (eds) (1996) *Manual of Companion Animal Nutrition and Feeding*, BSAVA, Cheltenham.

Markwell, P. J. (1994) *Applied Clinical Nutrition of the Dog and Cat*, Waltham Centre for Pet Nutrition, Waltham-on-the-Wolds.

Pannevis, M. C. and Earle, K. E. (1994) Maintenance energy requirements of five popular species of ornamental fish. *J. Nutrition*, **124**, S2616–2618.

Tobin, G. (1996) Small pets – Food types, nutrient requirements and nutritional disorders. In Kelly, N. and Wills, J. (eds) *Manual of Companion Animal Nutrition and Feeding*. British Small Animal Veterinary Association, pp. 208–225.

Thorne, C. (ed.) (1992) *The Waltham Book of Dog and Cat Behaviour*, Pergamon Press, Oxford.

Wills, J. and Simpson, K. W. (eds) (1994) *The Waltham Book of Clinical Nutrition of the Dog and Cat*, Pergamon Press, Oxford.

Wills, J. M. (1996) Basic principle of nutrition and feeding. In Kelly, N. and Wills, J. (eds) *Manual of Companion Animal Nutrition and Feeding*. British Small Animal Veterinary Association, pp. 10–21.

9

Genetics and animal breeding

S. E. Long

Genetics is the science of inheritance, i.e. the study of how characteristics are passed on from parents to offspring. These characteristics may be, for example, the colour of the eyes, the length of the fur or the type of enzyme that is produced by a cell. The information for all these factors, and many, many more, is located on special structures in the nucleus. These structures are the *chromosomes*.

Chromosomes

The chromosomes are composed of **chromatin fibres**, which are long molecules of **DNA** and associated protein.

DNA (deoxyribonucleic acid) has a unique structure. It consists of two strands, joined together rather like a ladder. The 'steps' of the ladder are formed by two bases, either adenine (A) and thymine (T) or guanine (G) and cytosine (C). A always links with T and G always links with C. Thus the steps of the ladder are a sequence of **base pairs** and it is this sequence which forms the **genes** (see p. 208). If on one side of the ladder there is a sequence of, for example AGTAACGGC, then on the other side of the ladder the sequence must be TCATTGCCG (Fig. 9.1). The structure of the base pairs is such that they cause the sides of the ladder to twist,

forming a double spiral, or double helix (meaning spiral). The DNA molecule is then very tightly folded and coiled to form the chromatin fibres of the chromosomes.

Each species has a characteristic number of chromosomes. For example, the number of chromosomes in the cell of a cat = 38 (Fig. 9.2), dog = 78, horse = 64. Two of the chromosomes are called the **sex chromosomes** and are designated **X** and **Y**. The female has two X chromosomes (XX) and the male has one of each of the sex chromosomes (XY). The other chromosomes, i.e. those that are not the sex chromosomes, are called the **autosomes**. Chromosomes are usually considered in pairs because one of each pair is inherited from each parent. A chromosome pair is alike, one to another, and therefore said to be **homologous** (meaning 'same'). If you were to weigh all the chromosomes from a cell in each of the different species you would find that the total weight of the genetic material was more or less the same. In other words, they all have roughly the same amount of genetic material, but it is cut into a different number of pieces.

Sex chromosomes and X inactivation

The sex chromosomes are the X and Y chromosomes. The Y chromosome is usually quite small and carries the genes that code for maleness. Very few other genes are carried on the Y chromosome. In contrast, the X chromosome is often one of the largest chromosomes and carries a number of genes that are important in the day-to-day metabolism of the cell. Since females have two X chromosomes (XX), and males have one X chromosome and one Y chromosome (XY), it follows that females must receive twice the number of genes that are carried on the X compared to males. In order to compensate for this, only one X chromosome in each cell of a female is activated and the genes on this chromosome are functional. The other X chromosome becomes highly contracted, and most of the genes are inactivated and non-functional. In some cells this contracted X chromosome is visible in the nucleus as a small dot and is known as the **Barr body** (after the person who first described it) or **sex chromatin**.

Genes

Genes are particular sequences of base pairs along the chain structure of DNA *and it is the genes that code for the characteristic* of the cell and hence the individual. Each gene is located at a particular position on the chromosome which is called the gene locus.

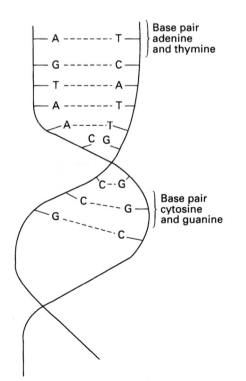

Fig. 9.1 Double helix structure of the DNA molecule.

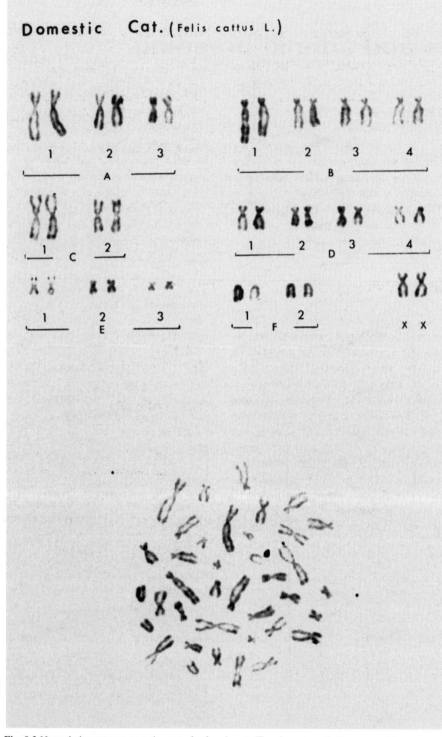

Fig. 9.2 Normal chromosome complement of a female cat. (Top: karyotype; bottom: spread.)

The genes that are located on the sex chromosomes are said to be **sex-linked genes**. There are many more genes on the X chromosome than the Y chromosome, so that sex-linked genes are more likely to be on the X than the Y. The orange coat colour gene in the cat or the gene for haemophilia A in the dog are examples of sex-linked genes on the X chromosomes. Genes that can only be expressed in one sex, such as the genes associated with milk quality, are said to be **sex-limited genes**.

Some genes or gene combinations are not compatible with life and are said to be **lethal factors**. If an individual receives such a gene or genes, that individual dies.

If the chromosome is damaged at the site where the gene is located and there is mis-repair, i.e. the sequence of base pairs is not the same as it was before, then one of two things may happen:

- The sequence is so different that the code no longer exists and so the gene is destroyed.
- The sequence allows coding for the characteristic but in a slightly different way, i.e. there is a **gene mutation**.

Alleles

Two or more genes that occupy the same locus on the chromosome are said to be **alleles**. Alleles arise because of small mutations in genes which make their coded message slightly different from each other. They occupy the same locus because they are just slightly different versions of the same gene. Only one allele can occupy the locus at any one time but, since each animal receives chromosomes from the mother and the father, there will be two loci (one on each homologous chromosome) and thus two alleles in each cell. There can be any number of alleles (in some cases there are literally hundreds) but each cell can only have two because there is only 'space' for two on the chromosomes.

Dominant and recessive genes

If there are two different alleles in a cell, it might be expected that both alleles would be expressed. In fact this does happen in many circumstances and the genes are said to be **co-dominant** (e.g. genes coding for blood groups).

However, some alleles are only expressed if there are two copies of the same allele in the cell. These are said to be recessive genes. Genes that can be expressed when only one copy is present and which can suppress the other allele are said to be **dominant** genes.

The different action of genes are symbolised by a capital letter for a dominant gene and a small letter for a recessive gene. For example, the gene for black coat colour in the Labrador is dominant to the gene that codes for brown. Therefore, the black gene is designated *B* and the brown gene is designated *b*. A black labrador can either have *BB* or *Bb* genes because black is dominant to brown and the *B* gene will suppress the expression of the *b* gene. However, brown Labradors must all be *bb* because brown is recessive and can only be expressed if two copies of the allele are present.

If an animal has two copies of the same allele it is said to be **homozygous** for that allele. If an animal has two different alleles then it is said to be **heterozygous** ('hetero' implies 'different').

Epistasis

Some genes can suppress the expression of other genes that are not their alleles, i.e. they suppress the effect of genes on a different locus (e.g. the albino gene blocks the expression of all the coat-colour genes). These genes are said to show **epistasis**.

Genotype and phenotype

It can be seen, from what has been discussed above, that two animals may look alike but have different genes. What the animal looks like is said to be its **phenotype**, whilst its genetic make-up is said to be its **genotype**.

Cell cycle

When a cell is carrying out its normal functions, it is said to be in interphase. If it wants to replicate itself it has to first synthesise new genetic material and this is called the synthesis (or **S**) stage. This is followed by a resting stage, called **G₂** (G stands for 'gap') and then there is separation of the new genetic material into the two new cells. This is the nuclear division **M** phase. The two new cells can then get on with their jobs so they are again said to be in interphase. There is thus a cell cycle (Fig. 9.3).

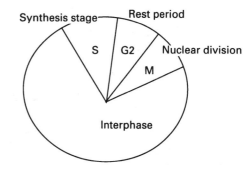

Fig. 9.3 The cell cycle.

Cell replication

Mitosis

When a cell replicates, it is important that the genetic material, i.e. the chromosomes, replicates exactly, otherwise new cells would not be coding for the same characteristics. Many cells are continually replicating (e.g. cells from the lining of the intestine) and it is important that the new cells can carry on the job of the old. The actual separation of the genetic material to the new cells is a dynamic process but for the purposes of description it has been divided into four stages:

(1) Prophase.
(2) Metaphase.
(3) Anaphase.
(4) Telophase.

Prophase (Fig. 9.4). This is the beginning of the division. The nuclear membrane breaks down and the chromatin contracts so that the chromosomes appear as separate

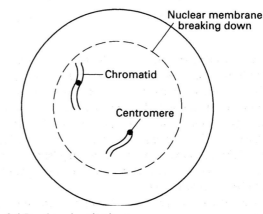

Fig. 9.4 Prophase in mitosis.

objects. Synthesis of the new chromosomes has already taken place (in the S phase of the cell cycle) but they have not separated and appear held together at the centromere. Since they have not separated the two identical chromosomes are called chromatids.

Metaphase (Fig. 9.5). Once contracted down, the chromosomes line up in the middle of the cell and the two chromatids begin to repel each other. This is the stage at which the chromosomes are most easily seen under the light microscope.

Anaphase (Fig. 9.6). The chromosomes become attached to the cell spindle which is a series of fibres. As these fibres contract, the chromatids are pulled apart and the new chromosomes move towards the two poles of the cell.

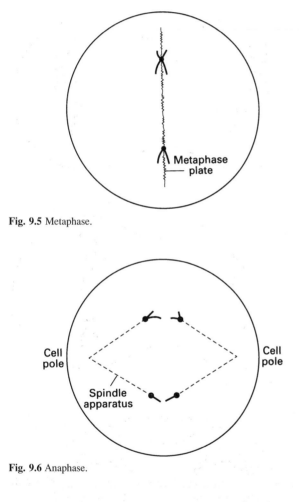

Fig. 9.5 Metaphase.

Fig. 9.6 Anaphase.

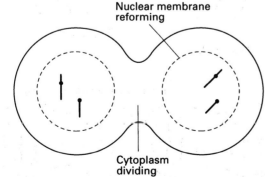

Fig. 9.7 Telophase.

Telophase (Fig. 9.7). Once the chromosomes have reached the poles new nuclear membranes are formed, surrounding each set, and the cytoplasm begins to divide. The resulting two new cells are genetically identical to each other and to the cell from which they originated.

Meiosis

Whereas mitosis is the type of cell division that is undertaken by most cells in the body, a different type of cell division is necessary for those cells (the oogonia and spermatogonia) that are going to develop into gametes (ova and sperm). This is called **meiotic division** and its stages are similar to those of mitotic division. However, it is a longer and more complicated process because the chromosomes have to be separated into different gametes in such a way that the total number is reduced by half and yet there is still one copy of each pair of alleles that was present in the parent cell. In this way, when the two gametes fuse to form a zygote, the new individual has the right number of chromosomes for the species and the right combination of genes in order that each cell can do its job. Thus, each individual receives half its chromosomes (and thus half the genes) from one parent and half from the other.

During the stages of meiotic division, new DNA is synthesised in the S phase of the cell cycle, as with mitosis, and the new chromosomes are held together at the centromeres. However, the prophase in meiosis is much longer than mitosis.

Prophase (Fig. 9.8). The nuclear membrane disappears, the chromosomes contract down and the homologous pairs line up side by side. *(In mitosis, the homologous chromosomes do not lie side by side.)* Effectively, there are four chromosomes lying together (i.e. the homologous pair each comprised of two chromatids held together at the centromere).

The four chromatids become entwined and exchange segments. This is called **crossing over.** The homologous chromosomes then begin to try to pull apart. (Because this is such a long procedure, meiotic prophase is subdivided into five stages: leptotene, zygotene, pachytene, diplotene and diakinesis.)

Metaphase (I) (Fig. 9.9). The homologous pairs of chromosomes line up in the centre of the cell and start to attach to the spindle apparatus.

Anaphase (I) (Fig. 9.10). The spindle fibres contract and the homologous chromosomes are separated and move to the opposite poles of the cell. *(In mitosis, this is the stage where the two chromatids separate.)*

Telophase (I) (Fig. 9.11). The cytoplasm begins to divide but there is no reconstitution of the nuclear membrane. *(In mitosis, the nuclear membrane reforms at this stage.)* In some cells the cytoplasmic division is completed and in others the cell forms a dumb-bell like structure or syncytium.

The cell now immediately goes into a second division which is exactly like a normal mitotic division.

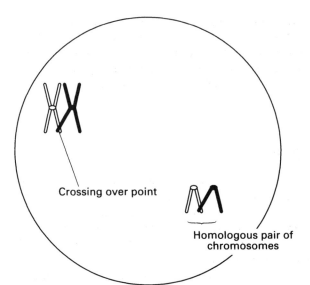

Fig. 9.8 Diplotene of meiotic prophase.

Prophase. This is transitory because the chromosomes are already contracted.

Metaphase (II) (Fig. 9.12). The chromosomes line up in the centre of the cell and attach to the spindle apparatus. The chromatids begin to repel each other.

Anaphase (II) (Fig. 9.13). The spindle fibres contract; the chromatids pull apart at the centromere and move towards opposite poles of the cells.

Telophase (II) (Fig. 9.14). The cytoplasm begins to divide and the nuclear membrane reforms.

Thus from one original cell, four new cells are formed which contain half the original number of chromosomes. The new individual inherits the genetic material from each parent but with some variation because of the crossing over.

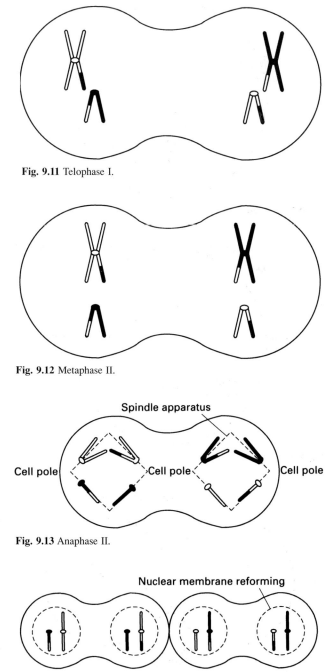

Fig. 9.11 Telophase I.

Fig. 9.12 Metaphase II.

Fig. 9.13 Anaphase II.

Fig. 9.14 Telophase II.

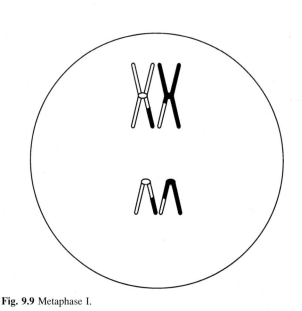

Fig. 9.9 Metaphase I.

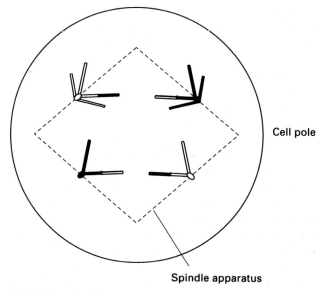

Fig. 9.10 Anaphase I.

Mendel's first law

Mendel's first law describes the outcome of meiosis. Mendel (1822–1884) was an Austrian monk and a biologist. He did not know anything about chromosomes or the mechanism of cell division but he knew that the process was orderly and organised such that one could predict the outcome of different matings.

> ***Mendel's first law states:*** **Alleles separate to different gametes.**

Identification of animals carrying a recessive gene

Animals homozygous for a particular gene will always breed true when bred together but heterozygous animals will sometimes produce offspring which are homozygous for the recessive gene. Usually (but not always), the recessive gene is unwanted so that breeders would like to be able to identify those animals that are heterozygous for a recessive gene and avoid breeding from them. Identification of the recessive carrier can be done by test mating to either a homozygous recessive animal or to a known heterozygous recessive carrier.

Crossing to a homozygous recessive animal

If you have a black Labrador and you want to know whether its genotype is *BB* or *Bb* then you can cross it with a brown (*bb*) or liver pigment Labrador (Fig. 9.15):

- If the black Labrador is *BB* then all the offspring will be black puppies (although with the genotype of *Bb*).
- If the black Labrador is *Bb*, it will still produce black puppies, but it will also produce brown (*bb*) puppies.

Instead of drawing the diagram as in Fig. 9.15, it could be written as a checkerboard (Fig. 9.16).

It can be calculated mathematically that if the black Labrador produces seven black puppies when mated to a brown Labrador then you can be 99% sure that its genotype is *BB*. The more black puppies that are produced the more sure you can be that the genotype is *BB*. Of course, if only

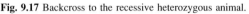

	b	*b*
B	*Bb*	*Bb*
b	*bb*	*bb*

Fig. 9.16 Checkerboard illustrating the genotype of the offspring when heterozygous black (*Bb*) is mated to the homozygous brown (*bb*).

one brown puppy is produced, irrespective of the number of black, then you know the black Labrador must be *Bb*. You do not have to mate your black Labrador to the same brown Labrador to get the offspring, it is the number of offspring that is important.

Crossing to a known heterozygous animal

If there are no homozygous recessive animals available it is possible to carry out the test mating with a known carrier of the recessive gene. For example, if a second black Labrador has previously produced a chocolate puppy, then it must be *Bb*. The first black Labrador (which could be either *BB* or *Bb*) can be mated to the second (*Bb*) black Labrador (Fig. 9.17). The checkerboard for this mating would be as in Fig. 9.18.

This time *16* black puppies would have to be produced before you could be 99% sure that the animal was *BB*. Again, these puppies do not have to be produced from a single mating and the birth of only one chocolate puppy will prove the dog to have been *Bb*.

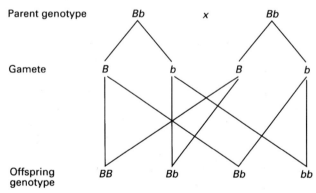

Fig. 9.17 Backcross to the recessive heterozygous animal.

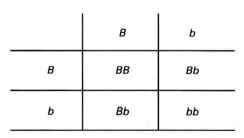

	B	*b*
B	*BB*	*Bb*
b	*Bb*	*bb*

Fig. 9.18 Checkerboard illustrating the genotype of the offspring when a heterozygous black (*Bb*) is mated to a heterozygous black (*Bb*).

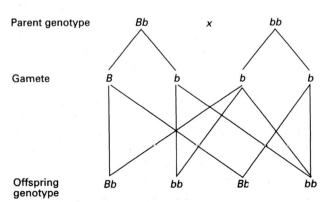

Fig. 9.15 Backcross to the recessive homozygous animal.

Both these matings, i.e. to a homozygous recessive animal or a known heterozygous animal, are called the **backcross to the recessive**. The animals that are mated are the parent generation and the offspring are the filial generation or F_1 generation. If the offspring were to be mated they would produce the F_2 generation and so on.

Inheritance of more than one pair of genes

Animals obviously have a large number of genes but each is inherited without being influenced by the presence of other genes. This is Mendel's second law.

Mendel's second law states: **Each pair of alleles separates independently of every other pair of alleles.**

There are exceptions to this law due to linkage. Genes separate independently because of the processes during meiosis, in particular because of the phenomenon of crossing over. This causes genes on the same chromosome to be separated. However, the closer on the chromosome that two genes lie, the less likely it is that the crossing over will separate them. Therefore, genes lying close to each other on a chromosome are said to be **linked** and if an animal inherits one of the linked genes it is very likely that it will inherit the other gene as well. This is an advantage if both genes are desirable but a big disadvantage if a breeder is trying to retain one gene and eradicate the other.

Multifactorial inheritance and the influence of environment

Some characteristics are governed by single genes but many others are controlled by the combination of a number of genes. Such characteristics are said to be **polygenic** (meaning many genes). Variation in the genes controlling these polygenic traits will cause a variation in the characteristic. Furthermore, the degree to which these genes can be expressed may be influenced by the environment. In other words the final production of a characteristic is **multifactorial** (meaning having many causes). For example, the size of a dog will depend upon its genes but also on the amount of food that is available. There is great scope for variation but such characteristics are difficult to control by selective breeding because of the number of different factors that are involved.

Breeding strategies

When breeders wish to ensure that animals breed true they try to make them homozygous for the genes governing the desirable characteristics. One way of doing this is by **inbreeding**, which is the breeding of two individuals more closely related than the population as a whole.

The reason this is done is because related individuals are more likely to have the same alleles and so more likely to produce offspring which will be homozygous for the genes. The more closely they are related the more likely it is that they will have the same alleles. Therefore, the closer the inbreeding, the more likely is it that the offspring will be homozygous. Inbreeding is a very good way of 'fixing' a characteristic (i.e. creating homozygosity), but *inbreeding will fix the 'bad' alleles as well as the good*. This is why inbreeding is generally regarded as dangerous.

Line breeding is a form of inbreeding. It involves mating within a certain family or line and aims to maintain a relationship with a particular popular ancestor (e.g. show champion). In general, although the animals that are mated are related, they are not so closely related as, for example, father and daughter or brother and sister. They are more likely to be grandparents and grandchildren or cousins. In this way it is hoped that the 'bad' alleles will be different in the two animals to be mated and so not be homozygous in the offspring.

If breeders wish to mask the effects of recessive genes that are considered to be 'bad' then the simplest way is outcrossing or **outbreeding** – the mating of two individuals less closely related than the population as a whole.

The rationale behind this is that such individuals are unlikely to have the same alleles and so the offspring will be heterozygous. Outbreeding masks the effects of recessive genes and results in **hybrid vigour** or **heterosis**. The offspring of an outcross seem to be 'bigger and better' than their parents because they are heterozygous for 'bad' recessive genes which therefore are not expressed. Unfortunately, such individuals will not breed true because they are heterozygous and not homozygous for their alleles.

Parentage analysis

Since an individual inherits its genotype from its parents we can determine whether a putative sire or dam could or could not possibly be the parent by examining each genotype. In the past, this analysis has been carried out by looking at the alleles an individual was carrying, e.g. those governing red cell surface antigens. By looking at a number of different loci, the combination of different alleles creates a unique picture of an individual. This is the basis of **blood typing analysis**. Molecular genetic techniques of parentage analysis now look at the sequence of base pairs in the DNA molecule itself. (This is a little like constructing a bar code in the supermarket!) Patterns of sequences must be found in the DNA of the offspring which could have come from one or other of the parents. However, if enough sequences are examined, no two individuals will have exactly the same patterns and so a **genetic 'fingerprint'** can be made. When a dog breeder requires an analysis to prove the parentage of a puppy this may require several blood samples being submitted to the laboratory, e.g. of the puppy, the two parents and even the grandparents in some situations. Cat parentage can also be determined by similar analysis.

Breed variation

Selection for various different characteristics has resulted in a number of different breeds. This has been more extensive with dogs than with cats. Dogs can be divided into six breed groups recognised by the English Kennel Club:

- Hounds.
- Gundogs.
- Terriers.
- Utility dogs.
- Working dogs.
- Toys.

Cats have not undergone such intensive selection for such a long period of time and are usually just divided simply into long- and short-hair breeds. However, there is considerable variation in the body size, length of head and coat colour. See Chapter 5 (Management of Kennels and Catteries).

Table 9.1 Inherited defects in the dog and cat

Inherited defects in the dog

Hip dysplasia	An abnormality of the hip joint. Multifactorial. Eradication scheme: the BVA/KC hip dysplasia scheme. Minimum age of dog entering scheme is 1 year. Hips are X-rayed by client's own veterinary surgeon and plates are sent to BVA. Panel of scrutineers scores each hip, minimum score 0 to maximum of 53. Mean score for any breed represents overall hip status of that breed. All breeders wishing to control hip dysplasia should breed only from animals with scores well below the breed mean. BVA informs KC of registered dogs with a score of 8 or less, or not more than 6 on one hip.
Elbow dysplasia	A developmental disease affecting large and giant breeds. Lesions include ununited or fragmented coronoid process and osteochondritis dissecans.
Eye defects	Many different defects with different genetic origins. BVA/KC/International Sheepdog Society eye scheme to monitor inherited ocular disease. Conditions considered are: Central progressive retinal atrophy (CPRA) Generalised progressive retinal atrophy (GPRA) Hereditary cataract (HC) Primary lens luxation (PLL) Gonodysgenesis/primary glaucoma Collie eye anomaly (CEA) Retinal dysplasia (RD) Persistent pupillary membrane (PPM) Congenital cataract (CHC) Persistent hyperplastic primary vitreous (PHPV). Different conditions seen in different breeds at different ages. Animals examined by member of eye scheme panel (not by client's own veterinary surgeon) to whom they are referred by client's veterinary surgeon. Recommended that examination be carried out each year. Result is sent to BVA and also (in case of KC registered dogs) to KC and/or ISDS for publication.
Entropion	Inward turning of the eyelid. Polygenic.
Ectropion	Outward turning of the eyelid. Polygenic.
Cryptorchidism	Failure of one testis (unilateral) or both testes (bilateral) to descend into the scrotum. Mode of inheritance unknown but possibly polygenic.
Umbilical hernia	Protrusion of tissue through the umbilical ring. Probably polygenic.
Merle	Incomplete dominant gene. Homozygotes have white coats, blue eyes which are smaller than normal, with a lack of tapetum, and predisposition to glaucoma. Also often deaf. Heterozygotes have white markings on the head and shoulders and dappled coat or normal and dilute markings. Only matings of Merle with normal are to be recommended in order to avoid producing abnormal homozygote.
Scottie cramp	Rigidity of muscles brought on by excitement or strenuous exercise. Autosomal recessive.
Progressive axonopathy	Axon degeneration of motor nerve fibres. Condition confined to Boxers. Due to an autosomal recessive gene.
Haemophilia	Failure in the clotting mechanism of blood. At least nine different types of haemophilia due to different abnormalities of complex cascade of reactions necessary to achieve normal clotting of blood. Haemophilia A (factor VIII deficiency) is most common and is sex-linked.

Some common inherited abnormalities in the cat

Manx	Taillessness. Associated with other abnormalities of conformation of vertebral column. Autosomal dominant. Homozygous is lethal.
Deafness	Due to dominant White gene. Affected cats white with blue eyes.
Polydactyly	Extra toes on feet. Autosomal dominant.
Flat-chested kitten syndrome	Seen in Burmese breed. Affected kittens show breathing difficulties and do poorly. Probably autosomal recessive.
Folded-ears	Incomplete dominant. Heterozygote has folded ears but homozygote also has abnormalities of the epiphyses leading to a thickened tail, swollen feet and disinclination to move.

Deformities and malformations

Any deviation from the normal anatomy is described as a malformation or deformity. These can arise during foetal development or be acquired during life.

Congenital abnormalities

When a malformation is present at birth it is said to be **congenital**. Congenital abnormalities may or may not be genetic in origin. The term simply means that it was present at birth. Sometimes, congenital abnormalities that are not caused by a genetic defect, look exactly like those abnormalities which are inherited. These are said to be **phenocopies** (meaning copies of what the animal looks like). This can make it extremely difficult to determine whether an abnormality is genetic in origin.

Inherited defects

Inherited defects are caused by the genes acquired from the parents. Some common inherited genetic defects are shown in Table 9.1.

Further reading

Nicholas, F. W. (1987) *Veterinary Genetics*, Clarendon, Oxford.
Robinson, R. (1990) *Genetics for Dog Breeders*, 2nd edn, Pergamon, Oxford.
Robinson, R. (1991) *Genetics for Cat Breeders*, 3rd edn, Pergamon, Oxford.

10

Exotic pets and wildlife

J. E. Cooper and C. J. Dutton

'Exotics', sometimes called the 'other' pets, are an important feature of veterinary practice in Britain and many other parts of the world. The definition of 'exotics' is imprecise. Strictly the term means 'foreign, bizarre' but in practice an exotic includes any small pet that is not a dog or a cat as well as wild animals brought in as casualties, and they present an exciting challenge to the veterinary nurse, who is often the first and most immediate point of contact for the client.

Anatomy and physiology

Many exotic pets are **vertebrates** and share various anatomical and physiological similarities. **Invertebrates** such as insects and spiders are substantially different. The main groups of exotic pets and their features are given in Table 10.1.

Mammals and birds are **endothermic**, or 'warm-blooded'. An endothermic animal is able to maintain its own body temperature above that of its surroundings, within certain limits, using internal (physiological) control mechanisms. Thus a rabbit's body temperature is likely to be 39.5°C in both summer and winter.

Reptiles, amphibians and invertebrates are **ectothermic**, or 'cold-blooded'. With very few exceptions they are unable to control their body temperature by intrinsic (internal) means and so it will fluctuate depending upon the ambient temperature. However, an ectothermic animal uses external or behavioural means (e.g. basking, burrowing) to control its body temperature.

Mammals

The mammals that are most commonly kept as pets are set out in Table 10.2. which shows that they fall into three different groups (Orders): the Rodentia, the Lagomorpha and the Carnivora. Most of them can be considered domesticated species and many that have become popular as pets were first used as laboratory animals. Other species are sometimes encountered in veterinary practice, such as the diminutive Roborovski's hamster or the large Shaw's jird, but knowledge of their close relatives means that they can be treated as if they were hamsters or gerbils although they are possibly a little less amenable to handling.

Although small mammals share many anatomical features, there are some differences that are relevant to the biological and veterinary care of these species (Tables 10.3 and 10.4). The veterinary nurse should take every opportunity to become familiar with the normal features, in order to be able to detect ill health or abnormalities more easily.

Having once studied the anatomy and physiology of the dog and cat in detail (see Chapter 11, Anatomy and Physiology), veterinary nurses should be able to note the external features of the herbivorous and omnivorous small mammals (i.e. excluding the carnivorous ferret) where they differ:

- Both the herbivorous and the omnivorous small mammals have chisel-shaped incisors for gnawing; they also have flat tables of cheek teeth for grinding coarse vegetable matter. The rodents have one pair of incisors in both upper and lower jaws. Rabbits have one pair in the lower jaw but two in the upper (one large and a smaller pair directly behind them). All the teeth of rabbits and herbivorous rodents are what is known as **open-rooted**: they grow continually throughout life.
- The joint surfaces of the tempero-mandibular joint are flat compared with those of the dog and cat, allowing both sideways and backwards-and-forwards movement of the lower jaw.
- Lower in the gastrointestinal tract they have a relatively large **caecum**, where bacteria break down the cellulose of plant cell walls to allow the animal to make use of this plant material as food.
- The rabbit and all the small rodents practise **caecotrophy**, which is the eating of faeces. The rabbit passes two different types of faeces: the dry pellets that we consider 'normal', and, at night, **caecal** pellets, which are dark in colour and covered with mucus so that they tend to stick together and emerge in a mass. These caecal pellets are eaten directly from the anus and complete a second passage of the gut so that all possible nutrients are extracted from the food.
- The hamsters have cheek pouches, used for carrying food back to the nest when on extensive foraging expeditions.
- The chinchillas and the small pet rodents tend to hold their food in their front paws while feeding. They are able to do this as they can supinate their front paws – rotating the radius to twist the carpus and manus, as can cats (but not dogs).

There are also certain features to note regarding skin and glands:

- Rabbits have no foot-pads: their feet are covered with hair.
- Female rabbits have a **dewlap** (a large fold of skin under the chin) from which they pluck fur to line the nest.
- Gerbils have a large skin gland on the mid-ventral abdomen, which in old age may become hypertrophied.
- Syrian hamsters have glandular areas on their flanks, where the skin is darkly pigmented. Older hamsters often lose their hair in these areas.

Table 10.1 Main groups of exotic pets and their features

Group	Features	Examples
Vertebrates		
Mammals (Mammalia)	Internal skeleton Endothermic ('warm blooded') Skin bears hairs Lungs Bear live young Feed young on milk Internal fertilisation	Rat (*Rattus norvegicus*) Mouse (*Mus musculus*) Guinea pig (*Cavia porcellus*) Chinchilla (*Chinchilla laniger*) Syrian hamster (*Mesocricetus auratus*) Mongolian gerbil (*Meriones unguiculatus*) Ferret (*Mustela putorius furo*)
Birds (Aves)	Internal skeleton Endothermic Wings Skin bears feathers Scales on legs Lungs Eggs with hard shell Internal fertilisation	Budgerigar (*Melopsittacus undulatus*) African grey parrot (*Psittacus erithacus*) Amazon parrot (*Amazona* spp.) Canary (*Serinus canaria*) Cockatiel (*Nymphicus hollandicus*) Fowl (chicken) (*Gallus domesticus*) Pigeon (*Columba livia*)
Reptiles (Reptilia)	Internal skeleton Ectothermic ('cold-blooded') Dry skin with scales Lungs Oviparous (eggs with hard or soft shells) or ovo-viviparous (live-bearing) Internal fertilisation	Common iguana (*Iguana iguana*) Mediterranean tortoise (*Testudo* spp.) Box tortoise (*Terrapene* spp.) Garter snake (*Thamnophis* spp.) Corn snake (*Elaphe guttata*) Leopard gecko (*Eublepharis macularius*)
Amphibians (Amphibia)	Internal skeleton Ectothermic Moist skin with mucus and sometimes poison glands Oviparous, occasionally ovo-viviparous Lungs in adult, gills in larva (tadpole) Larval form External fertilisation	Common toad (*Bufo bufo*) Marine toad (*Bufo marinus*) European tree frog (*Hyla arborea*) Edible frog (*Rana esculenta*) Great-crested newt (*Triturus cristatus*) European salamander (*Salamandra salamandra*) Axolotl (*Ambystoma mexicanum*)
Fish (Pisces)	Internal skeleton Ectothermic Moist skin with scales Gills Oviparous (eggs without shells) or ovo-viviparous (live-bearing) Sometimes larval form Usually external fertilisation	Goldfish (*Carassius auratus*) Koi carp (*Cyprinius carpio*) Guppy (*Lebistes reticulatus*) Angel fish (*Pterophyllum scalare*) Platies (*Xiphophorus* spp.) Siamese fighting fish (*Betta splendens*) Discus (*Symphysodon discus*) Oscar (*Astronotus ocellatus*) Seahorse (*Hippocampus* spp.)
Invertebrates		
Arthropods (Arthropoda)	External skeleton (cuticle) Paired jointed limbs Segmented Open vascular system Oviparous or viviparous	Indian stick insect (*Carausius morosus*) Red-kneed tarantula (*Euthalus smithii*) Tree bird spiders (*Avicularia* spp.) Tree crabs (*Coenobita* spp.) Emperor scorpion (*Pandinus imperator*)
Molluscs (Mollusca)	Shell but no cuticle Ventral muscular foot Unsegmented Open vascular system Oviparous or viviparous	African land snail (*Achatina* spp.) Garden snail (*Helix aspersa*)

- Guinea pigs have a greasy glandular area just above the tail, which is quite normal and should not be considered pathological.
- Chinchilla fur is very dense. These animals were originally imported to be bred for their pelts (skins). The coat over the body has no guard hairs and there may be up to 70 fine downy hairs per skin follicle. The tail does have a covering of guard hairs and there are fewer downy hairs in this region.

Sexing small mammals

This is more difficult in some species than in others. In all female rodents, the genital and urinary orifices are separate so that there are three orifices (from the most dorsal: anal, genital and urinary); in the male there are only two. However, the genital orifice is not patent much of the time and is often only to be seen as a patch or strip of naked skin. It becomes patent when the animal is in season and prior to

Table 10.2 Small mammal species commonly kept as pets

Order	Sub-order	Family	Species	English name
Rodentia[a]	Myomorpha	Muridae	*Rattus norvegicus* *Mus musculus*	Fancy rat Mouse
		Cricetidae	*Meriones unguiculatus* *Mesocricetus auratus* *Phodopus sungorus* *Cricetulus griseus*	Mongolian gerbil Syrian hamster Russian hamster[b] Chinese hamster[b]
	Hystricomorpha	Caviidae Chinchillidae	*Cavia porcellus* *Chinchilla laniger*	Guinea pig Chinchilla
	Sciuromorpha	Sciuridae	*Tamias sibiricus*	Siberian chipmunk
Lagomorpha		Leporidae	*Oryctolagus cuniculus*	Rabbit
Carnivora		Mustelidae	*Mustela putorius furo*	Ferret

[a] Note the division of the family 'Rodentia', the rodents. The 'mouse-like' rodents are further divided into the rats and mice, and the gerbils and hamsters. All these small rodents are omnivorous. The Sciuromorphs, or squirrel-like rodents, are also omnivores, and the Siberian chipmunk has a lifestyle very like the squirrels of Europe and North America. Hystricomorphs are the third group of rodents; they are herbivores and come from South America.
[b] The Russian and Chinese are the dwarf hamsters. Unlike the Syrian hamster they are social animals, living in family groups in the wild.

Table 10.3 Anatomical differences in small mammals

	Mouse	Rat	Syrian hamster	Gerbil	Guinea pig	Rabbit	Ferret
Teeth	Well developed incisors for gnawing (one upper pair, rodents; two upper pairs – one small, rabbit)						Well-developed canines for tearing
Dental formula	$\dfrac{1003}{1003}$	$\dfrac{1003}{1003}$	$\dfrac{1003}{1003}$	$\dfrac{1003}{1003}$	$\dfrac{1013}{1013}$	$\dfrac{1033}{1023}$	$\dfrac{3131}{3132}$
Ears	Hairless	Hairless	Sparse hair	Hairy	Sparse except tip	Hairy	Hairy
Cheek pouches	Absent	Absent	Present	Absent	Absent	Absent	Absent
Stomach	Simple, two distinct regions	Simple, two distinct regions	Simple, two compartments	Simple, two distinct regions	Simple	Simple	Simple
Intestine	Long	Long	Long	Long	Long	Long	Short
Gall bladder	Present	Absent	Present	Present	Present	Present	Present
Appendix	Small	Small	Small	Small	Large	Very large	No caecum or appendix
Mammary glands	No teats in male	No teats in male	No teats in male	No teats in male	Teats in male	Teats in male	Teats in male
Testes	Retractable	Retractable	Retractable	Retractable	Retractable	Retractable	Not retractable
Scent glands	None	None	On flanks	Ventral midline	Perineal	Perineal	Anal sacs
Tail	No hair, scales	No hair, scales	Hair	Hair	No tail	Hair	Hair

parturition. In any female rodent, the separate orifices make it easy to distinguish whether a discharge or bleeding is urinary or vaginal in origin.

Rabbits, and most rodents, have large, open inguinal rings which allow the testes to be retracted into the abdomen. In all the small pet mammals except the Russian hamster, the descended testes are obvious in the mature male. Otherwise the sexes can be distinguished by the presence of the vaginal membrane in the female and the greater ano-genital distance in the male.

- *Rabbits* are not difficult to sex once the testes have descended, as they lie in scrotal sacs on either side of the penis, which is easily protruded in the adult rabbit, slightly less easily in the young. The vulva of the female is a slit, pointed at the front, whereas the prepuce is more circular.
- *Guinea pigs* are easy to sex from birth: the penis can be protruded with gentle pressure around the relevant orifice or can be felt through the skin.
- *Chinchillas* can be difficult to sex unless one is aware that there is a significant urethral prominence in the female, which may be mistaken for a penis. The ano-genital distance is greater in the male and the female has a vaginal membrane.
- In the *ferret*, the opening of the prepuce is on the belly, near the umbilicus. The testes are only within the scrotum during the breeding season. The penis contains the os penis (a bone) that can be easily palpated.

Table 10.4 General biology of small animals

	Average life expectancy	Maturity	Oestrus	Gestation period	Size of litter	Age at weaning	Adult weight (g)	Temperature (°C)
Rabbit	M 8 years+ F 6 years	3 months+	Induced ovulation Oestrus Jan–Oct/Nov	28–32 days	2–7	6 weeks	varies	38.5
Guinea pig	4–7 years	M 8–10 weeks F 4–5 weeks	15–16 day cycle	60–72 days (average 65)	2–6	3–3.5 weeks	750–1000	38–39
Rat	3 years	6 weeks+	Every 4–5 days	20–22 days	6–12	21 days+	400–800	38
Mouse	1–2.5 years	3–4 weeks	Every 4–5 days	19–21 days	5–1	18 days+	20–40	37.5
Gerbil	1.5–2.5 years	10–12 weeks	Every 4–6 days	24–26 days	3–6	21–28 days	70–130 (M>F)	38
Syrian hamster	1.5–2 years	6–10 weeks	Every 4 days	15–18 days	3–7	21–28 days	85–150	37–38
Russian hamster	1.5–2 years	6–10 weeks	Every 4 days	19–20 days	3–5	21–28 days		
Chinese hamster	1.5–2 years	6–10 weeks	Every 4 days	20–22 days	3–5	21–28 days		
Chinchilla	10 years (up to 15)	8 months	Seasonally polyoestrous Cycle 30–35 days Nov–May	111 days	2 or 3 (1–4)	6–8 weeks	M 400 F 500	38–39
Chipmunk	M 3 years F 5 years	1 year	Seasonally polyoestrous Cycle 14 days Mar–Sep 2 litters/year	28–32 days	2–6	6–7 weeks	80–130	38 (NB: hibernation)
Ferret	5–7 years	6–9 months	Induced ovulation Oestrus Feb/Mar–Sep	42 days	2–6 (up to 10)	8 weeks	500–2000	38.8

Birds

Birds may be kept either as pets (often individually, or in pairs, in cages indoors) or for breeding or exhibition. Larger species and most wild birds are bred in aviaries but the smaller domesticated species, such as budgerigars and canaries, are usually bred in custom-built bird-rooms.

Domesticated species are those that have been bred in captivity for long enough for significant genetic changes to be established – such as the development of different breeds (in domestic fowl and canaries) or different colour mutations (in the budgerigar and the peach-faced lovebird). There are 28 different orders of birds but most of those presented for veterinary attention are likely to fall into one of the following:

- Order Psittaciformes – budgerigar, parrots, etc.
- Order Passeriformes – perching birds, including canary, finches.
- Order Falconiformes – diurnal (not nocturnal) birds of prey such as hawks, falcons.
- Order Strigiformes – owls.
- Order Galliformes – domestic fowl, pheasants, quail.
- Order Anseriformes – ducks, geese and swans.

Table 10.5 describes some of the birds commonly kept in aviculture and also some of the different groups of non-domesticated species. Table 10.6 shows the significance of some of the anatomical features of various species.

Although the anatomy of birds follows the basic verte-brate pattern, it also shows a number of important differences from mammals, including adaptations for flight – especially by keeping weight to a minimum.

Skeleton and muscles

- The bones have thin cortices and some of them (pneumatised) contain an air sac as an extension of the respiratory system.
- Throughout the skeleton the number of joints (Fig. 10.1) is reduced to facilitate flying. The fusion of many of the vertebrae reduces mobility in the trunk region but a long, very flexible neck allows the bird to reach most parts of its body with its beak.
- An enlarged sternum (keel bone) allows the attachment of very bulky flight muscles, which in some species may comprise up to one-quarter of the bodyweight of the bird.

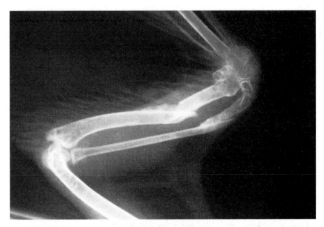

Fig. 10.1 Fractured radius and ulna in a Meller's duck (*Anas melleri*). (Good radiography facilitates diagnosis and treatment of skeletal problems in birds. Note that young growing feathers are visible on this radiograph – their vascular sheath is radiopaque.)

Table 10.5 Bird species commonly kept

Name	Origin	Description
Domestic species		
Budgerigar (*Melopsittacus undulatus*)	Australia	Many colour varieties. 'Show' budgies are much larger than the wild type.
Canary (*Canarius serinus*)	Canary Islands	Many different breeds, some judged on colour, some on colour and 'type' and some on their song.
Cockatiels (*Nymphicus hollandicus*)	Australia	Many colour varieties.
Peach-faced lovebirds	East Africa	In the wild a green bird with a pink/orange face and blue rump. Now in many colour varieties. An aggressive species.
Zebra finches	Australia	A prolific breeder, now in many colour mutations.
Bengali	East Asia	A finch kept in its own right or as a foster parent for species unwilling to care for eggs or young in captivity.

Other species that may now be considered to be domesticated are the Indian Ringneck Parakeet and the Australian Gouldian Finch, both of which are produced in many colour mutations.

Different groups of non-domesticated species commonly kept in aviculture	
Foreign finches	Commonly Australian, African or East Asian species.
Softbills	Such as Pekin robins, mynah birds, various starlings and thrushes.
British birds	It is permitted to keep certain species of British birds in captivity, but they must not be taken from the wild without a licence, and any young that are to be sold or exhibited must have been aviary-bred and close-ringed (ABCR) during the first few days of life.
Grass parakeets	Small Australian parakeets related to the budgerigar. Examples are the Elegant, the Splendid, and Bourke's grass parakeet
Parrots	Many species kept by enthusiasts and others by commercial breeders to supply the demand for English-bred, hand-reared (EBHR) parrots as pets.
Waterfowl and pheasants	Many species are endangered or threatened in the wild and are kept successfully by aviculturists. Birds that are to be kept 'free range' must not be allowed to escape into the wild and so may need to be pinioned or contained in some way.

Table 10.6 Significance of anatomical features in birds

Feature	Significance
Beak – variation in shape and size	Related to feeding habits, e.g. parrots open fruit and nuts, canaries and finches peck at seeds, raptors tear meat. Many psittacine birds also use beak for climbing.
Legs and feet – variation in appearance	Related to habits and habitat, e.g. parrots climb (two toes pointing forwards, two backwards), canaries and finches perch (three toes forwards, one backwards), raptors grasp prey with talons, ducks swim with webbed feet.
Wings – variation in shape and size	Related to flying, e.g. falcons have long pointed wings for hunting prey from a height, hawks have short rounded wings for quick dash through undergrowth. Some birds, e.g. penguin, ostrich, do not fly.
Plumage – variation in colour and structures (e.g. crests)	Related to behaviour, e.g. recognition of own species or a mate, threat or warning to predators. Some species show sexual dimorphism, i.e. plumage differs between male and female.

- The pelvis is modified to allow the passage of a large egg. This is achieved by having an open pubis rather than a symphysis.
- The weight of the skull is reduced by cavities in certain bones, reduction of the maxillary region and there being no teeth.
- In many species the tongue is rigid, containing a lingual bone, whereas in many parrots the tongue is thick, fleshy and very mobile and is used to manipulate food.
- There is a **quadrate bone** lying between the maxilla and each dentary, producing two joints between upper and lower jaw. This allows a variable amount of backwards-and-forwards movement in some species (it is particularly well developed in the parrots). There is also a joint between the upper part of the beak and the rest of the skull – the **cranio-facial hinge** – and again the amount of movement varies from species to species.
- The number of digits in the forelimb (wing) is reduced to two: digit III, and a much reduced digit I which forms the **alula** (bastard wing) that carries a few feathers which are important for control at take-off and landing. In some adult and many embryonic birds there may be a claw on the alula.

Feathers

The plumage, composed of keratin, provides lightweight but strong feathers which help to insulate the bird. The feathers are divided into several groups:

- **Flight feathers** of the wings and tail are long and rigid.
- **Contour feathers** are those that make up the outer layer of feathers over most of the body. They are shorter and more flexible than the flight feathers.

- **Down feathers** and **filoplumes** lie beneath the contour feathers and provide a layer of insulation. (Birds carry very little subcutaneous fat compared with mammals.)

All feathers have the same basic structure. In the majority of birds all the feathers are shed each year during the moulting season, which in most species occurs in late summer, at the end of the breeding season. The developing feather is covered by a keratin sheath; while it is growing, a blood vessel runs up

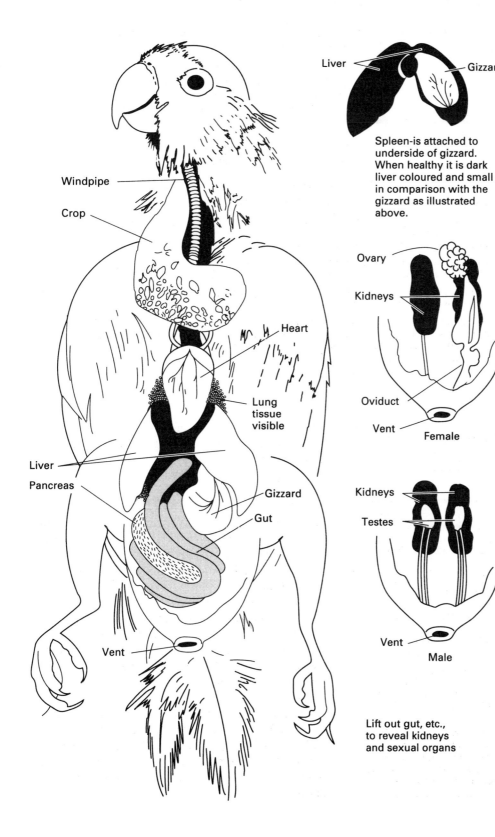

Spleen-is attached to underside of gizzard. When healthy it is dark liver coloured and small in comparison with the gizzard as illustrated above.

Lift out gut, etc., to reveal kidneys and sexual organs

Fig. 10.2 Internal organs of a parrot.

the shaft (the feather is described by aviculturists as being 'in pin', by falconers as 'in the blood'), so that damage to a feather at this stage will result in haemorrhage.

Birds keep their feathers in good order by preening. Most birds use oil from the **preen gland** on the top of the tail to waterproof them although not all birds have a preen gland. Some birds (notably the cockatoos and cockatiel) produce a fine dust from their feathers which helps to keep the plumage in good order. Most birds in the wild bathe regularly and will do so in captivity as well, especially if encouraged.

It is important for all birds, but particularly for falconry birds and racing pigeons, to protect the feathers and to minimise damage to the plumage when a bird is hospitalised.

The gastrointestinal tract

The gastrointestinal tract in birds follows the basic vertebrate pattern of foregut, midgut and hindgut but with certain modifications (Fig. 10.2):

- There are no teeth. Some birds hold food with their feet and tear it with their beaks; others swallow food whole.
- In most species there is a diverticulum of the oesophagus in the ventral neck – the **crop**. This is used as a storage organ. In pigeons and parrots it produces a secretion known as **crop milk** that is used to nourish the young in the nest. There is no crop in the owls or in many diving birds.
- The stomach in most species is divided into a **proventriculus**, which is the glandular stomach, and the **ventriculus** or **gizzard**, which is a thick-walled chamber where food can be ground up and which may contain grit. There is no gizzard in birds that have a predominantly

fluid diet, such as the nectar-eating (nectivorous) sunbirds and hummingbirds.

- The small intestine is short but otherwise unremarkable.
- The large intestine may or may not sport two large **caeca** (sing. caecum) from the junction between large and small intestines. This is the site for bacterial digestion in herbivorous and omnivorous species. Caeca are reduced or absent in carnivorous and nectivorous species.
- The digestive, urinary and genital tracts all open to the outside through one orifice, the **cloaca** or **vent**.

The respiratory system

The respiratory system of the bird is very different from that of the mammal and these differences have implications for anaesthesia in birds.

- The bird has no diaphragm. The main muscles of respiration are abdominal, which should never be restricted during restraint of the animal.
- The lungs are small compared with those of the mammal, and they are non-distensible. They lie close to the dorsal body wall in the cranial part of the body cavity.
- The air is drawn into and expelled from the body by the expansion and contraction of thin-walled air sacs, which are lined with serous membrane and extend throughout the body, even into some of the bones (pneumatisation).
- Air circulates through the lungs continuously, during both inspiration and expiration. This means that changes in depth of anaesthesia are likely to take place much more rapidly in birds than in mammals of comparable size.

Table 10.7 Reptiles and amphibians kept as pets			
	Type	**Species**	
Class Reptilia	Order Chelonia (tortoises and turtles)	*Testudo hermanni*	Hermann's tortoise
		Testudo graeca	Spur-thighed tortoise
		Terrapene spp.	American box tortoise/'turtle'
		Pseudemys scripta elegans	Red-eared terrapin
	Order Squamata (snakes and lizards)	*Natrix natrix*	Grass snake
		Thamnophis spp.	Garter snake
		Elaphe guttata	Corn snake
		Elaphe obsoleta	Black rat snake
		Lampropeltis spp.	King snake
		Python sebae	African rock python
		P. regius	Royal python
		P. molurus	Indian python
		P. reticulatus	Reticulated python
		Lacerta vivipara	Common lizard
		Anguis fragilis	Slow-worm
		Iguana iguana	Common or green iguana
Class Amphibia	Order Anura (frogs and toads)	*Bufo bufo*	Common toad
		Bufo marinus	Marine toad
		Xenopus spp.	Clawed toad
		Rana esculenta	Edible frog
		Rana pipiens	Leopard frog
		Hyla arborea	European tree frog
	Order Urodela (newts and salamanders)	*Triturus cristatus*	Great-crested newt
		Salamandra salamandra	European salamander
		Ambystoma mexicanum	Axolotl

Reptiles and amphibians

Table 10.7 shows some of the species most commonly seen in veterinary practice. Reptiles and amphibians are ectothermic animals: although unable to control body temperature intrinsically, they can do so very effectively by behavioural means. For example, a lizard basks in the sun in order to raise its body temperature but it hides under a log or seeks the shade in order to lower its body temperature.

Ectothermic animals have their own **preferred body temperature** (PBT), which is the temperature range at which they can move about and feed and at which their digestive enzymes, etc. are best able to act. Some species are tolerant of wide ranges of temperature; others come from very stable environments in the wild, where there is very little temperature variation. Examples of PBT for different reptiles are given in Table 10.8.

Some reptiles **hibernate** in cold weather. This is a complex physiological process and should not be confused with torpor induced by a sudden temperature drop. Other species **aestivate**, i.e. they become lethargic and they sleep because the temperature is too high and/or environmental conditions are too dry.

All reptiles have a dry skin, impervious to water and usually covered with scales. All of them shed (slough) their skins as they grow. Some, such as the tortoises, shed it in small parts; others, such as the snakes and some lizards, shed their skins at one time, often in one piece.

Some lizards can shed their tails (**autotomy**) if they are handled incorrectly, e.g. if the tail is grasped. This is a defence mechanism when it occurs in the wild: a predator's attention may be attracted to the discarded tail, allowing the lizard itself to escape unscathed. A new tail will grow but it is a poor cartilaginous replica of the original.

Although the basic anatomy of reptiles is similar to that of other vertebrates, the following special points should be noted:

- **Tortoises** and other chelonians have a modified skeleton: a bony 'box' composed of an upper part (**carapace**) and lower part (**plastron**), fused at the sides. The box consists of a modified vertebral column, ribs and sternum.

- Snakes and certain snake-like lizards have modifications related to their elongated shape: they have no limbs, or only vestigial limbs, and they have elongated lungs (only one functional in snakes), liver and intestine.

Reproduction

Reptiles produce eggs and they are either oviparous or ovo-viviparous:

- **Oviparous** reptiles lay their eggs within a calcareous shell (some are almost as rigid as a bird's egg but others are little more than a parchment-like membrane).
- **Ovo-viviparous** reptiles retain their eggs within the body of the female until the young are fully developed and capable of independent life.

This retention of the egg until hatching is not the same as true **viviparity**, because the developing reptile embryo is nourished only by the yolk of the egg, rather than by the mother via a placenta as is the case with viviparous mammals.

The young reptiles, whether hatched or born, emerge as small replicas of the adult and are immediately capable of feeding themselves.

Amphibians

Amphibians are often grouped and discussed with reptiles but they show many differences. In particular their skin is generally thin, mucous and permeable. Many amphibians can respire through their skin as well as using lungs (adults) or gills (larvae). The larvae metamorphose into adults.

Fish

There are three main groups of fish: the primitive Placoderms, the huge group of Osteichthyes (bony fish) and the Chondrichthyes (cartilaginous fish). Those of most relevance to veterinary practice are the bony fish (e.g. goldfish). Cartilaginous fish, such as sharks, are sometimes kept in captivity.

The type and temperature of water in which fish live are very relevant to their physiology and health, and Table 10.9 gives some examples.

Management and nutrition

Veterinary nurses are often asked for advice on the management of exotic pets, including suitable housing, feeding and general husbandry, and perhaps breeding. They

Table 10.8 Preferred body temperatures of some reptile species (adapted from Cooper and Jackson, 1981)

Species	Activity range (°C)	PBT (°C)
Box turtle (*Terrapene ornata*)	22–35	27
Greek tortoise (*Testudo graeca*)	15–30	24
Green anole (*Anolis carolinensis*)	30–36	34
Green (common) iguana (*Iguana iguana*)	26–42	33
Flap-necked chameleon (*Chamaeleo dilepis*)	21–36	31
Slow-worm (*Anguis fragilis*)	14–29	22
Boa constrictor (*Constrictor constrictor*)	26–37	32
Garter snake (*Thamnophis sirtalis*)	20–35	29

Table 10.9 Water temperatures for fish

Type	Cold (up to 21°C)	Warm (21–29°C)
Freshwater	Goldfish	Guppy
Saltwater	Herring	Seahorse

are also asked which pets might be suitable in various circumstances. It is therefore important to have a good background knowledge on all aspects of pet care, as well as knowing how to handle the animals when they are brought into the practice and how to look after those that become hospitalised.

Choosing a pet

The choice of pet depends upon many factors and Table 10.10 suggests the main questions that should be asked of a potential owner who is considering an exotic as a pet. Clients may want pets for various purposes and these requirements have to be taken into consideration when making a choice. In all cases the animal must be easily handled and managed, relatively robust and unlikely to transmit disease. Examples of specific circumstances are given in Table 10.11.

Mammals

The housing, nutrition, general management and breeding of rodents, rabbits and ferrets are summarised in Table 10.12, and the species are looked at in more detail below. There is also useful information on cages for small mammals in the *How to Choose* ... leaflets produced by the Universities Federation for Animal Welfare (UFAW), copies of which can be given to clients – preferably before they acquire a new pet. Much useful information on the management of small mammals has resulted from their use in laboratories, and contacts with these establishments, especially animal technicians who look after the animals, can prove beneficial.

Rabbits and guinea pigs

The domesticated rabbit is of European origin whereas the guinea pig comes from South America. In addition to being popular pets, both species are used in research and as a source of food – in the case of the guinea pig, primarily in poorer parts of South America and Africa.

Husbandry and housing. Rabbits and guinea pigs are usually kept out-of-doors, although many people now also keep them entirely as indoor pets ('house' rabbits). The standard housing for the rabbit or guinea pig is a hutch, with a covered sleeping area and a wire-fronted 'living' area. Owners should be encouraged to view a grassy outdoor run as essential for these species, or to allow regular 'free-ranging' in the garden.

Rabbits are hardy in the Northern European climate and suffer only if they are unable to keep dry, or from excessively high temperatures. With an underground burrow in the wild, they are always able to escape from the rain and from the heat of the summer sun.

Guinea pigs also dislike very hot weather and may suffer if they cannot stay dry.

Rabbits and guinea pigs may (but by no means must) be taken indoors during the winter, but care should be taken

Table 10.10 Advising on choice of pet: questions to ask

Question	Explanation
Are financial considerations important?	Some species are expensive to keep.
What facilities do you have?	Avoid large pets such as rabbits and parrots if the owner has no garden or lives in a flat.
How much spare time do you have?	Some pets, such as parrots, need considerable attention if they are not to become bored. Others, such as fish and invertebrates, need relatively little attention.
What are your domestic arrangements?	Some pets are unsuitable for young children or elderly persons. Some animals are active at night, others by day.
Are there any significant human health consequences?	People who are sensitive to fur or feathers should be wary of mammals and birds. Immunosuppressed persons should only have contact with pets of known health status.
What other animals do you keep?	Some species may be incompatible or difficult to keep together, e.g. small birds and cats. Commensal bacterial and other organisms of some species may cause clinical disease in others.

Table 10.11 Advising on choice of pet: considerations

Requirement	Considerations
A pet for children	Diurnal.
A pet (companion) for elderly people	Easy to feed. Food readily obtained and affordable. Temperature needs compatible with those of owner(s).
A family pet	No risk to babies. Compatible with family's lifestyle.
For educational studies in the classroom	Weekend and holiday care need consideration. Heating may be switched off. Food supply must be reliable. Continuity in terms of care.
Pets for educational talks and visits	Portability. Resilient to repeated handling. No special legal requirements.

that the winter accommodation is well-ventilated and not overheated, as poor ventilation and overheating may predispose to respiratory disease, particularly in rabbits.

Both species are social, living in colonies in the wild. Rabbits and guinea pigs can be kept together, although in some cases problems are encountered such as rabbits mounting cavies, or the cavies chewing the rabbit's fur. Owners should be encouraged to keep rabbits together, and to keep guinea pigs together, but with certain precautions:

Table 10.12 Small mammal husbandry: a summary

	Rabbits and Guinea pigs	Rats and Mice	Gerbils and Hamsters	Ferrets
Housing	Hutches or floor pens or outside runs	Cages or mouse/rat houses with opportunity to climb	Cages with deep bedding for tunnelling	As rabbit and guinea pig
Bedding	Newspaper plus sawdust or woodchips and hay/straw	Sawdust, shavings, woodchips, well-shredded paper	As rats and mice	As rabbit and guinea pig
	(Avoid synthetic fibres which can wrap around limbs or cause impaction of stomach)			
Diet	Pelleted diets are available for all species but are best supplemented with: vegetables, fruit, seeds			Meat and eggs
	Some rodents will eat and apparently benefit from live invertebrates			
	Rabbits and guinea pigs need hay			
Special care	All species should be kept dry in a draught-free environment. A warm area is needed if rabbits, guinea pigs or ferrets are kept out of doors. Hygiene is important: cages should be cleaned thoroughly at least once a week.			
Vaccines, medicines	Myxomatosis and VHD vaccine may be advisable for rabbits	–	–	Distemper vaccine may be advisable
	Avoid unnecessary use of antimicrobial agents in all species but especially rabbits and rodents			

- Two male rabbits will fight.
- Two female rabbits may live in harmony, or one may start to exert dominance over the other when she comes into season and starts to defend the 'nest burrow' as her own.
- A male and a female rabbit will live together, and either (or preferably both) can be neutered to prevent unwanted offspring. Rabbits in the wild will form pair bonds and so obviously this is the best and most natural arrangement for them in captivity.
- A group of female guinea pigs will live together without fighting.
- Male guinea pigs will live together without fighting if there are no females within sight, sound or smell.

Feeding. As rabbits and guinea pigs are grazing animals, the most important part of their diet is good-quality *roughage* – either hay or grazing. In the absence of sufficient roughage, both species (but particularly the guinea pig) may chew the fur of companions to make up the deficiency.

In the same way that puppies, kittens or breeding or working dogs are fed differently compared with a sedentary pet, so too a young or breeding rabbit or guinea pig requires a different diet from that of a sedentary adult animal. The amount of *protein* in the diet is as important for a young rabbit or guinea pig as it is for a young dog. The pellets used by rabbit breeders usually contain approximately 18% protein; commercial rabbit and guinea pig mixes vary in protein between 12.5% and 16.5%, and the higher level should be regarded as optimum for young and breeding rabbits.

Free access to good-quality grazing can make up a shortfall in the quality of the dry feed. Remember that during the winter the food value and certainly the *vitamin* content in greens that have been standing without growing for months are quite low.

Guinea pigs have a specific requirement for dietary **vitamin C**: animals on free range, especially during the spring, summer and autumn, usually find enough vitamin C in the growing grass but otherwise the diet should be supplemented at a rate of 50 mg per guinea pig per day (more for pregnant and lactating animals). Some guinea pig mixes now contain this vitamin but otherwise it can be given in water, although this poses two possible problems.

- If given in a water bottle, it should be in one with a stainless steel spout, as the soft metal of many drinking bottles will inactivate vitamin C.
- If given in a drinking bowl, vitamin C can be inactivated by organic matter – and guinea pigs are known to deposit their faeces in the bowls.

Some rabbit pellets and mixes contain **coccidiostats** and these should *not* be fed to guinea pigs due to the risks of toxicity. Coccidiosis is not a major problem in guinea pigs (though it can occur) and coccidiostats tend to reduce the efficiency of the gut, and cause poor growth in young animals.

Handling rabbits. Rabbits can be picked up by the scruff and supported under the rump. If they are then tucked under the arm, so that the eyes are covered, they can be carried safely using only one arm and (usually) without any struggling (Fig. 10.3).

(a)

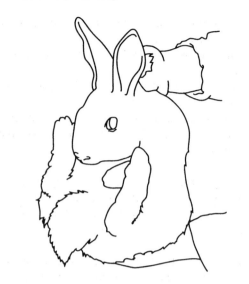

(b)

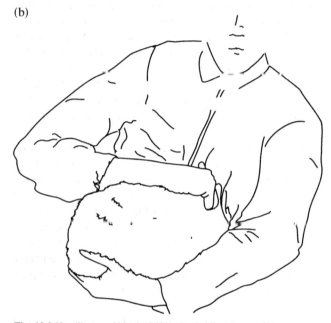

Fig. 10.3 Handling a rabbit. (a) Lifting by holding the scruff in one hand and using the other hand to support the body. (b) Carrying safely under the arm so that the rabbit's head is covered, leaving one hand free to open doors, etc.

Handling guinea pigs. Guinea pigs can be picked up with a hand around the shoulders. They should also be supported under the rump, especially if large or pregnant animals.

Breeding rabbits. Rabbits are seasonally polyoestrous and are induced ovulators. They are mated by taking the female (doe) to the male (buck). She is then removed after mating, which takes place almost immediately. Pregnancy diagnosis by abdominal palpation can be performed at about 14 days. The gestation period is 28–32 days; the larger breeds take longer and have larger litters.

The doe spends very little time with her young, leaving them covered up in the nest and returning only once or twice every 24 hours to feed them. Owners may become anxious at the doe's apparent lack of interest in her litter and have to be reassured that this is normal. In the wild, the young are

in danger every time the doe goes to them, possibly showing predators the way to the nest.

Young rabbits may be weaned from 6 weeks of age, preferably by removing the doe. The litter should then be kept together in familiar surroundings for a further week before they are sold.

Breeding guinea pigs. Guinea pigs have a long gestation period (63 days or more) and give birth to precocious young. Guinea pigs should be bred for the first time before they are a year old, as the large size of the young means that the pubic symphysis must open to allow them to be born. If the sow is too old before her first litter, the symphysis may not open and a caesarean section may be required. The opening of the symphysis, detectable by palpation, indicates that she is likely to give birth within a couple of days.

The age of puberty in the female guinea pig is only 4–5 weeks. The male should be removed in good time so that young females in the litter are not already pregnant by the time they are weaned.

Chinchillas

Husbandry and housing. Chinchillas are native to the Andes mountains but there are very few left in the wild. They were first imported for their skins but are now mainly bred as pets. The wild chinchilla is grey but many other colours have been developed by selective breeding.

Chinchillas are social animals and so are best kept in pairs. Ideally the pairs should be established while the animals are young. Females are more aggressive than males: if adults are to be introduced to one another, they should be kept in adjoining cages for a while and then the female should be introduced into the male's cage.

Although chinchillas can be recommended as pets for older children, they are nocturnal, and are very agile and active after dark. It is better not to house them in bedrooms where people are trying to sleep. They are normally kept indoors and so do not suffer extremes of cold, but with their very dense coats they are susceptible to overheating.

They are usually kept in all-wire cages, which should be as large as possible to allow plenty of exercise, and should include ledges and branches to climb on and chew and a nest-box for sleeping. They are very destructive animals and so all the food and water containers should be of earthenware or metal.

They keep their fur in order by dust-bathing. A shallow, non-chewable pan of commercial 'chinchilla dust/sand' should be put into the cage each day but should not be left there permanently as the animals tend to use it as a litter tray once they have dust-bathed.

Feeding. A commercial chinchilla pellet contains about 18% protein. The animals must also be given good-quality hay; treats such as apple and carrot are acceptable. Too much of any high-fat foods such as peanuts or sunflower seeds may dull the coat and, if given to excess, may lead to fatty changes in the liver.

Handling. Chinchillas should be picked up gently around the shoulders, if necessary using the base of the tail as further support. Breeders who exhibit their animals do not appreciate greasy hands spoiling the fur and a pair of light cotton gloves, a scarf or a towel can be used when handling such animals.

Breeding. The breeding season in Northern Europe is from November to May. The gestation period is 111–114 days and up to three precocious young are born. Owners sometimes ask whether to remove the male or to leave him in with the female and the litter. In most cases the male is very caring and protective but may tread on the young accidentally as he runs around the cage, particularly if no nest-box is provided.

Chipmunks

Husbandry and housing. The Siberian chipmunk has become popular as a pet in recent years. Because the animals can become very stressed in the presence of electrical equipment such as televisions, videos and computers, they should be kept out of doors. They will live outside happily all the year round, as long as they have weatherproof nest-boxes and their enclosure is shaded to protect them from very hot weather. They do not hibernate for long periods but will sleep for short periods during very cold weather, becoming active again on warmer days.

They are usually kept in aviary-like accommodation, built with security in mind and always with a safety door. A weatherproof nest-box stuffed with hay should be provided for each adult, as they prefer not to share sleeping-quarters. They can be kept as a pair or, if the enclosure is large enough, as a group although there may be aggression between males or between females, particularly during the breeding season. They usually have two litters a year, in about April and again in August. The young leave the nest-box at about 6 weeks of age but should be left with the parents for at least another 2 weeks.

Feeding. Chipmunks are omnivorous and should be fed a diet that contains meat protein, fresh fruit and vegetables and a seed-and-nut mix. The animal protein can be provided by a complete cat food; the seed-and-nut mix can be a combination of birdseed with a commercial small rodent mix.

Handling. Unless they have been hand-reared, chipmunks are not easy to restrain and are best captured using a light net or trapped inside a nest-box and moved with the nest-box. If hospitalisation becomes necessary it should be for the minimum time possible; the veterinary surgery is likely to be a very stressful environment for them.

Small mammals (rats, mice, gerbils and hamsters)

The veterinary nurse is sometimes asked for advice about choosing small mammal pets for children and the following facts are worth bearing in mind:

- Hamsters are nocturnal; gerbils are diurnal; rats and mice are active at any time.
- All small mammals need to be handled regularly to keep them tame.
- Gerbils, when alarmed, leap in the air – and out of the owner's hands.
- Hamsters and gerbils are easily injured by falling.
- Rats and mice are climbers; they cling on to clothing, etc., and are less likely to injure themselves if they fall.
- Rats are probably the quickest learning of the small mammal pets. They are more likely to form attachments to their owners. Fancy rats, handled regularly from weaning, are very unlikely to bite.

Husbandry and housing. Syrian hamsters are solitary by nature. Dwarf hamsters will usually live in a pair if put together when young but it is unwise to attempt to introduce two adults to each other. Gerbils are social animals and live in extended family groups – do not attempt to introduce a non-family gerbil to a group, but make up pairs at weaning. Rats and mice are loosely social and very tolerant: two or more female rats or mice will live satisfactorily together; males will tend to fight but sometimes two or more males will live together if there are no females within sight, sound or smell.

Feeding. All these small mammals are omnivores, thriving on a diet containing a proportion of animal-based protein. In the wild, hamsters and gerbils in particular will catch and eat invertebrates, while wild rats and mice will also eat carrion. A comparison of the nutritional content of most commercial 'hamster mixes' with that of a commercial laboratory animal pellet shows how poor the diet is on which these pets live. The diet, and thus their general health, can be improved by giving a daily helping of table scraps plus small pieces of fruit and vegetable.

Handling. Tame hamsters and gerbils can be scooped up into two cupped hands, but be sure to support a gerbil so that it cannot leap away. Gerbils should never be picked up by the tail, as the skin may peel off.

In the case of aggressive small mammals, some authorities recommend scruffing (and this is standard in many laboratories). However, this can be distressing for the watching owner and is not easy to accomplish without being bitten. It may also be injurious for the Syrian hamster, with its protuberant eyes (the problems are similar when handling a Pekingese dog). It is best to pick up potentially aggressive small mammals with the aid of a small net or a towel: they can then be manipulated within the towel to expose the part required for examination or injection. In some cases, light (isoflurane) anaesthesia is helpful.

Mice may be picked up around the shoulders, or by the base of the tail, and then placed on a surface such as a rough towel. Pet fancy rats accustomed to being handled may also be picked up round the shoulders (Fig. 10.4a); a more anxious handler can put the thumb under the animal's lower jaw to hold the mouth gently closed. Awkward animals are best handled using a towel, after initially taking hold of the base of the tail. Rats may be scruffed to restrain them for

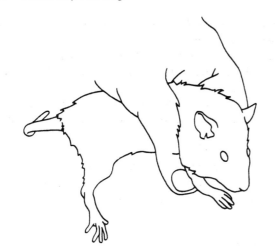

(a)

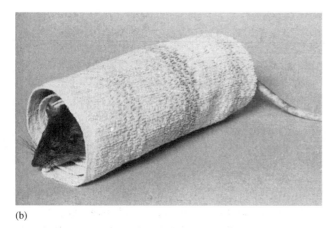

(b)

Fig. 10.4 Handling a pet rat. (a) Holding by grasping the shoulders. (b) Wrapped in a towel while recovering from anaesthesia (in this case, the towel is important in post anaesthetic nursing care as small animals can quickly become hypothermic, but towel-wrapping is also useful as a restraint for an active rat).

injections but being rolled up in a light towel (Fig. 10.4b) is less stressful for an animal that is accustomed to only gentle handling at home.

Breeding. Most small mammals can be induced to breed all the year round but in practice they tend to stop breeding during periods of decreasing day length, from late summer to the turn of the year. They all have a post-partum oestrus, which means that if male and female are kept together or have brief contact after parturition they will probably mate.

The solitary Syrian hamster female will usually be aggressive towards a male except when she is in oestrus, which occurs every 4 days. When ready to mate she exhibits lordosis (ventral curvature of the lower spine), as do most of the small mammals.

The young of most small mammals commonly kept as pets are born naked and blind. Many books, and folklore in general, claim that the young should not be handled for, say, a week after birth because it would induce the mother to eat her young. In practice this depends on such things as the tameness of the mother and her confidence in her usual handler. Many breeders handle young from birth.

Pet owners should be reminded that the mother will require several times as much food as usual while raising a

litter, particularly a large litter. The usual diet can be supplemented with dry complete cat or dog food and baby-weaning foods.

Weaning should not be carried out too early. The young will start to eat solid food some time before they are ready to be weaned. To avoid stress at weaning, the female should be removed and the litter left together in the familiar environment for a few days before being sold or rehoused. In this way they lose their mother, siblings and familiar environment in easy stages rather than all at once.

Ferrets

Housing. For at least 2000 years ferrets have been kept in Europe for hunting. Working ferrets are often kept in hutches or in a 'ferret court' which may be an outdoor enclosure with a shelter, or in an indoor area in a shed or barn where a number of ferrets live together.

Pet ferrets may live indoors (the standard in the US where hunting with ferrets is banned by law) or in a hutch outside. It is important to remember that ferrets are highly active carnivores and supreme escapologists, with an intelligence comparable to that of a cat. All pet ferrets should have regular exercise (mental as well as physical) in a stimulating environment and they have a great capacity for 'play'. Although solitary in the wild, they enjoy company and two or more will usually live together though two males are likely to fight.

Feeding. Working ferrets are often fed on their prey. The ferret's nutritional requirements are similar to those of cats but tinned cat foods tend to produce foul-smelling faeces (complete cat foods make them more acceptable). All ferrets, working or not, enjoy whole carcasses occasionally, such as those that are sold frozen for feeding to snakes and birds of prey. On no account should ferrets be restricted to the traditional diet of bread and milk, but milk alone will often be useful to tempt a sick or anorexic ferret to feed.

Handling. Ferrets can be picked up around the shoulders, with a thumb placed under the lower jaw if there is any suspicion that the animal might attempt to bite (Fig. 10.5). Biting is more often through surprise than aggression, and it

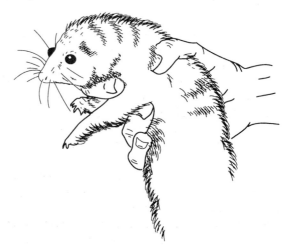

Fig. 10.5 Holding a tame ferret.

should also be remembered that ferrets have very poor eyesight but are highly efficient predators: a tentative finger is assumed to be edible prey. If a ferret does bite, its jaws tend to 'lock' and it can be difficult to remove though there are one or two tricks (including simply letting the animal find its feet if it is dangling in mid-air or immersing the ferret in water).

Breeding. The breeding season for ferrets lasts from spring to autumn in Northern Europe. The testes of the male (hob) are withdrawn into the abdomen during winter and descend into the scrotum at the onset of the breeding season. When the female (jill) comes into season her vulva swells. She is an induced ovulator and is seasonally polyoestrous (like the cat; see Chapter 18); if she is not mated she can remain in season until the autumn, which can be dangerous for her and can produce a potentially fatal anaemia. Unless jills are required for breeding, spaying is recommended. Some ferret keepers who want to postpone breeding in a young jill will 'mate' her with a vasectomised hob to take her out of season and into a pseudopregnancy.

Birds

An understanding of the biology and natural history of birds is important if one is to deal adequately with them in captivity and to provide them with optimum conditions when they are unwell. Some key points for hospitalised birds are as follows.

- *Birds are easily stressed*, especially by close proximity of people, by loud noises and by violent movements:
  - Reduce close contact by keeping birds some distance from people and other animals. An elevated position for the cage is ideal: most birds like to be in a high commanding position with a good view of their environment. Observe the bird from a distance before approaching it.
  - Further reduce the stress of proximity by covering part of the cage or providing vegetation behind which the bird can hide.
  - Reduce light intensity if a bird is frightened but remember that most birds must be able to see in order to feed.
  - Avoid excess noises, including rattling of keys, banging of doors, barking of dogs. Discourage unnecessary visitors.
- *Birds must feed regularly*, especially if they are small species with a high metabolic rate:
  - Encourage feeding by providing the company of other birds or by offering moving or colourful food items such as mealworms, egg or berries (depending upon species).
  - Acceptability may be enhanced if seeds are soaked before being offered, or if novelties are provided, e.g. a teasel head containing seeds.
  - Food and water containers must be the correct shape; for instance, a heron needs a deep water container, not a shallow bowl.
- *Encourage normal behaviour* to promote recovery from illness. For example:
  - Social species will benefit from company.
  - Preening behaviour may be stimulated if the bird's plumage is sprayed.
- *High standards* of hospitalisation facilities promote better care of avian patients. Examples of good features include:
  - Elevated cages.
  - Dimmer switches to alter light intensity.
  - A door that opens inwards (to discourage escapees from coming out) but that also closes naturally.

Choosing birds as pets

A veterinary nurse who is asked to give advice to novice bird-keepers should encourage them in the right direction (for the sake of the birds) with the following suggestions:

- Gain experience by keeping domesticated rather than wild species in the first instance.
- Those who would like a pet parrot but have never kept birds before: start with, perhaps, a pair of hand-reared cockatiels before attempting to keep the larger, non-domesticated species.
- Those who are determined to acquire large parrots as pets: spend a little more and acquire a British-bred, hand-reared parrot rather than an imported, wild-caught bird.
- Bear in mind that each species of large parrot has different inherent characteristics – in exactly the same way that different breeds of dog have different characteristics.
- Consult library books on the subject and talk to experienced bird-keepers before deciding to acquire a bird.
- Remember that a parrot might live for 40 or 50 years, or more.
- The young British-bred parrot that is sold just after weaning is a particularly demanding pet; it requires as much of its owner's time as would a new puppy.
- Most birds, and particularly the parrot species, are social and do much better when they have the company of their own species as well as that of humans. In the absence of contact with their own species, extensive human company is vital.

Cages and aviaries

Accommodation for pet birds can be divided into cages and the larger aviaries. In addition some tame birds may be allowed the freedom of the house, a practice that appeals to many people but the bird may damage furniture or other objects and can expose itself to hazards such as electric wires, ovens, poisonous chemicals and even lead pecked from leaded-light windows or old paint.

Cages. The two main groups of cage are the all-wire type or the box cage (with wire at the front but solid sides, roof and back wall). Their features are described in Table 10.13.

Table 10.13 Cage design: box cages and all-wire cages	
Box	**Wire**
Open on only one side (front).	Open on all sides, unless covered.
Often made of wood, not easily disinfected, subject to chewing.	Easily disinfected, not likely to be chewed.
Bird usually less easily frightened as it feels secure.	Bird easily frightened unless one or more sides are covered.
If illumination poor, inner recesses of cage may be too dark for feeding and other normal behaviour.	Illumination good: facilitates clinical observation and encourages normal behaviour.
Not liable to draughts but ventilation often poor.	Liable to draughts but ventilation good.

All-wire cages are acceptable for tame birds but they should always be placed at the side of the room or in a corner, reasonably high up, to give the bird a sense of security. Box cages are more suitable for wild and more nervous species, which feel less stressed when they cannot be viewed from all sides.

In the UK, any cage used for a captive bird (except poultry) should by law be large enough for the bird to stretch both wings fully in all directions. There is an exemption for birds that are being transported (e.g. to the surgery) or are under treatment by a veterinary surgeon but this does not necessarily apply to any bird in a veterinary practice or under the care of a non-veterinarian.

Cages for pet birds should be as large as possible, allowing room for parrots to climb and for canaries or finches to have a short flight between perches. Most commercial cages are fitted with ridged, plastic perches, which should be replaced by natural perching in several different diameters for the sake of the bird's feet. Fruit trees (unsprayed) and willows are reliable sources of non-poisonous wood but the branches should be scrubbed to remove any wild-bird droppings before they are placed in the cage.

Food and water receptacles should be placed where the bird can reach them easily (bearing in mind whether the bird normally feeds on or off the ground) but cannot defaecate into them. Most parrots, whether large or small, appreciate 'toys' in the form of things to investigate, chew and destroy but there should not be so many toys that there is no room for movement.

Hygiene is most important. Food and water containers should be cleaned daily. Cages should be emptied and thoroughly cleaned at least once a week.

Aviaries. Many people choose to keep birds in aviaries. They may have only one aviary as an ornament in the garden; or they may have a number and be keen aviculturists who try to breed birds in captivity. Most serious aviculturists are well aware of how to build and maintain an aviary but the amateur wishing to have one in the garden may ask for advice at the veterinary practice.

There are two components to an aviary:

● The mesh flight area – open to the air, wind, rain, snow and sun.
● The sheltered area – enclosed (other than an entrance), windproof, warmer, probably with windows to allow some sun to enter.

Each design should suit the intended occupants but the main points to be considered are as follows:

● Is planning permission necessary? In any case, as a courtesy, inform neighbours and do not keep noisy species if the neighbours are close or the garden is small.
● Avoid overhanging trees and strong winds.
● Try to position the aviary away from the road where disturbance and theft may prove a problem. Bird theft is big business. Keep only low-value species or invest in proper security.
● The smallest viable aviary size is about 1.8 m × 0.9 m but at this size it will be very difficult to keep clean.
● All aviaries should be protected against rats and mice by having deep foundations or a solid concrete base and also suitable wire around the room to exclude the rodents (e.g. 1 cm × 1 cm weld mesh).
● A frost-free shelter should be provided for all but the hardiest species. The shelter should have heat and light for any species likely to suffer during the winter without them.
● Roofing over the flight area will reduce the possibility of disease spreading from wild birds.
● Human entrance to the aviary is likely to be through a door. This should always open inwards (to discourage birds from flying out) and it is wise to have a double-door safety porch to minimise escape. At no time should both doors be open simultaneously.
● Seek advice from experienced bird-keepers about stocking densities and compatible species. Usually, only one pair of parrots can be kept in each aviary.
● Large parrot species may require heavy gauge wire to keep them contained (up to 12–14 g).

Disease control can be a problem in aviaries, especially if they cannot be fully cleaned because of the presence of soil, plants, etc. The following routines are important:

● Remove as much faeces, uneaten food, old feathers, soiled leaves and other debris as possible, preferably once a week.
● Ensure that the aviary is well watered and receives ample sunshine.
● At least twice a year turn over or replace soil and have faeces of birds checked for endoparasites.
● Ensure that aviary birds are kept under careful observation and can easily be caught or isolated if they appear to be unwell.

Handling birds

> **All birds, except nocturnal species such as owls, are more easily caught and handled in the dark or in subdued light, which calms them.**

Before removing a bird from a cage, always check that no doors or windows are open and no fans are in operation. Always transport birds in a secure box or basket, even over very short distances.

Small cage birds should be caught within their cage with as little chasing about as possible. Quietly remove toys and perches first.

Large birds, and those inclined to bite, can be caught using a towel or gloves (Fig. 10.6) – a towel is often preferable as it gives better control and does not restrict the handler's fingers once the bird has been caught. The large parrots should be grasped gently at the base of the skull with one hand, the other being used to support body and legs. A bird that clings to the bars of the cage with beak or feet should be detached gently by an assistant, not just pulled away. Pecking can be discouraged by putting an elastic band over the beak (but remember to remove it!) or by covering the bird's head with a light cloth bag.

Whatever the species, the aim when handling a bird should be to restrain its wings so that it can neither fly nor flap. Small birds can be held in one hand, with fingers around the neck, while larger birds are best grasped round the body (Figs 10.7 and 10.8).

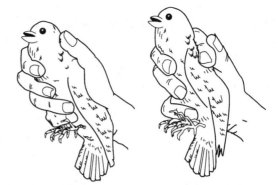

Fig. 10.7 Holding a small bird. Great care must be taken with these delicate animals, and no pressure should be placed on the abdomen.

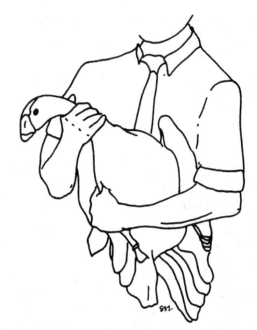

Fig. 10.8 Restraining a large bird: its neck is supported and it is unable to flap its wings.

Most pets are tame. This must be distinguished from **imprinting**, whereby a bird that has been hand-reared becomes imprinted upon humans rather than birds of its own species. Such individuals usually make affectionate and trusting pets but may react adversely to other birds and can develop other behavioural problems.

Feeding

The nutrition of birds is an important subject. Many non-specific diseases are due to or are exacerbated by nutritional deficiencies. Birds may be predominantly vegetarian, predominantly carnivorous or omnivorous (taking a mixture of foods). In practical terms several feeding groups of birds are recognised (Table 10.14).

In the wild, most birds have seasonal changes in their diet. Typical garden 'seed-eaters' often become almost entirely insectivorous during spring and summer and might enjoy a late summer/autumn glut of fruit before the leaner days of winter. Throughout the world, most birds time their breeding season to coincide with peak food availability to rear their young, be it the onset of warmer weather or the rainy season.

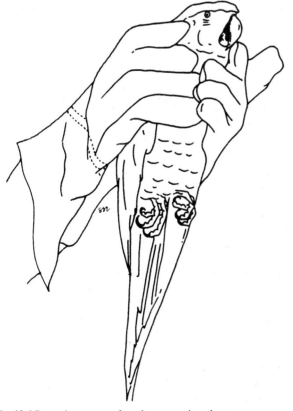

Fig. 10.6 Removing a parrot from its cage, using gloves.

Table 10.14 Features of birds affecting feeding preferences

Group	Predominant food	Characteristic features	Examples
Hardbills	Seed	Strong broad beaks	Finches
Softbills	Fruit and/or insects	Pointed beaks	Thrushes, whydahs
Birds of prey	Dead animals (meat)	Hooked beaks	Falcons, hawks, owls
Nectar-feeding	Nectar, sometimes fruit	Long thin beaks and/or specialised tongues	Sunbirds, hummingbirds, lories, lorikeets

For captive birds, food should be fresh and of good quality and should be replaced regularly. Small birds (e.g. canaries) require ad lib feeding; they may eat 25% or more of their bodyweight per day. Large birds (e.g. owls) may need feeding only once a day and eat only 7–10% of bodyweight.

All captive birds should have a constant supply of clean drinking-water, though some species (e.g. raptors) will only drink infrequently or during certain periods such as egg-laying.

Seed-eaters (hardbills). Dry seeds are a convenient way to supply a very basic diet but there are very few birds that eat only dry seeds in the wild. No bird should be fed on dry seeds alone. However, birds that have been fed on one diet for a long time may be very reluctant to change, so that patience and determination are required to effect this. As with all animals, diet changes should be introduced gradually.

The veterinary nurse should be aware of the different seed mixes that are available for cage birds and should be able to distinguish between mixes for budgerigars, canaries, parakeets and finches, and be able to identify the seeds in them. The different types of seed have different food values, so that birds fed on one mix may be deficient in different nutrients from those fed on another mix.

Basic seed diets for small cage birds may be supplemented with:

- **Soft foods** – egg-based food that can be fed all the year round but particularly during the breeding season or moult or during convalescence.
- **Tonic mixes** – seed mixes giving a greater variety and more fat-rich seeds (useful during the winter when the need is for energy to keep warm, but feeding an excess of fat-rich seeds can lead to problems).
- **Greenstuff** – chemical-free weeds and vegetables from the garden increase the level of fat-soluble vitamins in the diet (always deficient in a seed-only diet).
- **Fruit.**
- **Vitamin/mineral supplements** – if the adequacy of the diet is in doubt.
- **Grit, cuttlefish bone and iodine blocks** – the last of these is essential for budgerigars that are not given iodine-supplemented seed.

Softbills. The softbills are birds that feed naturally on 'soft' foods such as insects and fruit, in contrast to the hardbills that have beaks adapted to feeding on grain, seeds and nuts. Softbills commonly kept as pets include the greater hill mynah and the Pekin robin as well as various indigenous aviary species. They are fed on proprietary softbill foods supplemented with fruit, vegetables, cheese, meat, insects, etc., according to the natural diet of the species in the wild. Those who care for wild bird casualties sometimes breed suitable insects (such as grasshoppers and maggots) to provide a ready supply of fresh food for softbills.

Parrots and parakeets. Different parrot species are adapted to diverse habitats in the wild and so have disparate dietary preferences. None of them eats exclusively dry seeds. Some are nectar feeders (lories and lorikeets) and in captivity they are fed on a variety of commercial and home-made nectar substitutes with the addition of fruit. Most of the large parrots are omnivorous in the wild, eating a mixture of fruit, vegetables and seeds, plus insects and carrion to provide extra protein. A good diet for captive large parrots may include a good-quality parrot mix – but only up to about 20% of the total bulk of the diet. The rest will be made up of fruit, all sorts of vegetables and perhaps meat, dairy produce (yoghurt, fromage frais, cheese), brown bread, etc. Any bird that is not eating a very mixed diet will need a vitamin/mineral supplement.

Some pet parrots are encouraged to consume whatever the rest of the household is eating and, depending on that household's dietary habits, this can result in a well-nourished parrot. Parrots can be resistant to dietary change but are often willing to try foods if they see someone else enjoying them – either another parrot or the owner.

The birds tend to be wasteful feeders, taking one or two bites from a piece of fruit and then discarding the rest. This is sometimes interpreted by the owner as a dislike of a certain food. To minimise waste, it may be best to cut the food into small pieces before offering it.

Raptors

The diurnal (falconiform) birds of prey and owls are often brought into veterinary practices, perhaps as wild casualties or as birds belonging to falconers (kept either for hunting or for breeding). Falconry has become increasingly popular and while many people take a great deal of trouble to gain knowledge before acquiring a bird, others do not. Those who do show an interest should be encouraged by the veterinary nurse to go on a reputable falconry course and to join a falconry association before acquiring their own birds.

Raptors brought into the practice have special requirements that concern legislation as well as general handling and husbandry.

Legal position. In the UK, the Wildlife and Countryside Act 1981 makes it an offence to have in captivity certain falconiform birds of prey unless the bird has been ringed and registered. There is **an exemption for up to 6 weeks** for birds that are under the care of a veterinary surgeon, as long as proper records are kept. The current regulations should be checked with the Department of the Environment, Transport and the Regions (DETR).

Handling raptors. The general rules of handling are as for other birds but owls are usually quieter in bright light rather than darkness. Gloves will protect the handler; alternatively, the bird can be wrapped in a towel. Falconers' birds are often relatively easy to handle, especially if they wear a hood; advantage can also be taken of their jesses and leash, which can be held or pulled tight.

Falconry birds that come to the surgery on the falconer's fist can be restrained for examination by being 'cast' – catching them by both hands around the body from behind, holding the wings against the body. The bird can then be laid on its sternum, preferably on a towel. The bird's head should be covered if it is not already hooded, so that it becomes quieter and more amenable.

Feeding raptors. The majority of birds of prey are wholly carnivorous but the preferred diet depends upon the species. Live food is not needed in captivity and may present legal and ethical problems. Most species will take butcher's meat, dead mice, or dead day-old chicks (hatchery waste) or quail. A regular supply of bone is important as a mineral source, especially for young birds. Feathers, fur and roughage will be regularly regurgitated as a pellet.

Water must be provided but is rarely taken, as the birds obtain moisture from their diet.

Reptiles and amphibians

Housing

Reptiles and amphibians vary greatly in their requirements but the main features of a captive environment are common to all and involve the following considerations:

● Ample *space* for normal behaviour including moving, climbing, swimming as appropriate.
● A *type* of environment matching that of the animal in the wild, e.g. damp areas for toads, pieces of bark (or artificial material) under which lizards can hide. Provision of choices.
● A *temperature gradient* (warmer at one end) so that the animal can select the temperature it favours. The heating element should be attached to a thermostat and monitored with a thermometer (ideally a maximum/minimum thermometer). The vivarium should be maintained at the inhabitant's preferred body temperature.
● Although some snakes can cope with poorer *lighting* conditions, lizards and land Chelonia require good lighting for activity and foraging. Various fluorescent tubes are made specifically for vivaria and will provide a good daylight spectrum, including some ultraviolet light.
● *Humidity* is important. Powerful heaters tend to dry the atmosphere. Regular water-spraying from a plant mister

will maintain a reasonable degree of humidity and this should be done regularly, even for desert species and of course very often for rainforest species.

● *Drinking-water* must be provided, though some species (e.g. chameleons) will drink only drops from moist foliage.
● *Ventilation* is important for maintaining health in the vivarium. If it is poor, it can be improved by introducing an airline powered by a small aquarium pump to encourage the circulation of fresh air, but this should be placed with care so that it does not cause draughts.

Vivaria may be glass aquarium tanks or they may be custom-built, often made from chipboard covered with melamine, the corners sealed with an aquarium sealant. Glass tanks are much harder to maintain at a reasonable temperature and are more difficult to service because the only access is from the top.

The furnishings of a vivarium will vary. Some herpetologists favour a clinically hygienic environment for snakes, with paper on the floor, a hide-box and a climbing branch for arboreal species. Others prefer a more natural design. Common substrates include bark chippings, peat, aquarium gravel and sand; the last of these tends to be used only for desert species of lizard but not for snakes as it can cause scale abrasions. Arboreal species should be given branches for climbing; burrowing species need sufficient depth of substrate for hiding. All species should have hiding areas or hide-boxes.

Hygiene is essential. Faeces should be removed as soon as possible, along with soiled areas of substrate. This is not easy in the 'natural' type of vivarium and tends to be done infrequently. Hypochlorite is a suitable disinfectant for the stripped-down vivarium, which must then be thoroughly rinsed and dried before being refurnished and its inhabitants returned.

Nutrition

Reptiles range from total herbivores (eating only plants) through omnivores (taking a mixture of plants and animals) to total carnivores (eating only animals). Some general guidelines are given in Tables 10.15 and 10.16

Table 10.15 Feeding reptiles

Order

Order Crocodilia	Crocodiles, alligators and caimans: predominantly carnivorous.
Order Chelonia	Land tortoises: predominantly herbivorous but a number of species (e.g. box turtles) take food of animal origin. Freshwater terrapins: predominantly carnivorous. Marine turtles: predominantly carnivorous
Order Squamata	Snakes: predominantly carnivorous. Lizards: predominantly carnivorous but a few species (e.g. iguanas) take food of plant origin.

Table 10.16 Examples of reptile diets	
Species	**Staple diet**
Greek (spur-thighed) tortoise (*Testudo graeca*)	Vegetable material.
Garter snake (*Thamnophis* spp.)	Fish, amphibians, earthworms.

Rodent-eating snakes. These include corn snakes, rat snakes and all the commonly kept pythons and boas. They should be fed on whole dead rodents – it is inadvisable in the UK to feed live vertebrate prey as it may make one liable to be prosecuted under the Protection of Animals Act 1911. As a general rule, feed as much food as the snake will consume and then do not feed again until that meal has been digested and faeces passed. Captive-bred snakes are accustomed to feeding on dead prey; wild-caught snakes are sometimes more difficult to feed.

Fish-eating and invertebrate-eating snakes. These include garter snakes which can be fed on earthworms, small mice and pieces of fish. Frozen fish such as whitebait should be heat-treated in water at 80°C for 10 minutes in order to destroy thiaminase.

Insectivorous lizards. These can be fed on commercially produced insects such as crickets and locusts. It is important to dust the insects with a vitamin/mineral supplement first and to feed the correct size of insect for the animal. Lizards fed an unsupplemented diet tend to develop vitamin A deficiency and osteodystrophy caused by the poor Ca:P ratio in insects. Many insectivorous lizards in the wild also consume pollen, nectar and some fruit. Sweet, fruit substitutes should be offered from time to time.

Large omnivorous lizards. Lizards such as green iguanas are mainly insectivorous when young, becoming omnivorous as they grow. Their diet should contain a good amount of animal protein, as well as a good mixture of fruit and vegetables, and should be supplemented with calcium and vitamin D$_3$.

Basic husbandry

Mediterranean tortoises. Of the two common Mediterranean species, Hermann's tortoise (*Testudo hermanni*) has a horny spur on the end of its tail whereas the spur-thighed or Greek tortoise (*T. graeca*) has a short spur on the caudal aspect of each thigh.

Mediterranean tortoises can spend most of the spring and summer outside, with a shelter to sleep in at night. Indoor heated accommodation should be available for days when it is too cold for the tortoises to be active and feeding out of doors. Some people use greenhouses (heated or unheated) for this purpose.

Tortoises are herbivorous and the best diet for them is what they can find free-ranging over a large garden. If confined to a small pen, more food will have to be provided. Those that are kept over a period on one patch of ground may have high levels of roundworm infestation and need regular worming.

Male Mediterranean tortoises are most persistent in their pursuit of females. Courtship consists of butting the shell of the female and biting at her legs. A great deal of damage can be done to both animals if the female cannot escape from the male. It is best to keep males and females separate except when mating is required.

Mediterranean tortoises hibernate during the winter (and only those clearly unfit to do so should be kept awake). They should not be offered food for 3–4 weeks prior to hibernation, so that the intestines are empty before the animal becomes torpid. It is very difficult to keep a tortoise awake once day length starts to decrease; to keep it awake and feeding it is necessary to maintain artificial heat and also an artificial day length of 12 hours, with 'daylight' quality lighting.

Hibernation should be in a frost-proof and rodent-proof environment with good ventilation. The choice of insulation (e.g. hay, leafmould or shredded paper) does not matter as long as the tortoise is well protected. A healthy tortoise can lose up to 1% of its body weigh per month in hibernation and anxious owners are known to weight their pets regularly throughout the winter to monitor health. A sudden drop in weight indicates that something may be amiss and the tortoise should be awoken.

Young tortoises. Since import controls were applied, the average age of pet tortoises in the UK has been increasing steadily but many people now successfully produce hatchling tortoises. However, these enchanting little animals are very difficult to rear. They should be treated as adults as far as possible, i.e. they should graze outside and have access to sunlight, preferably in a cold-frame without its top to provide a draughtproof grazing area. On cold days they can be kept indoors in a vivarium. They should never be overfed: in the wild they would be active for much of the day in search of food, but in captivity they are inevitably less active and need less food to maintain optimum growth rate. Overfeeding and lack of supplementation of the diet lead to gross shell deformities in young tortoises that have grown much too fast.

Young tortoises would hibernate in the wild and should be allowed to do so in captivity.

Box 'turtles'. In the past the majority of land tortoises kept in the UK and other European countries were of the Mediterranean species. Large numbers were imported, often under unhygienic and inhumane conditions, and the mortality rate was very high.

Tighter controls on the capture and sale of Mediterranean tortoises has led to other species being imported and finding their way into homes and collections. These include the hinge-backed tortoises, *Kinixys* spp., and leopard tortoise (*Geochelone pardalis*) from Africa and the box 'turtles', *Terrapene* spp., from North America. The veterinary nurse should be familiar with the needs of box turtles (or tortoises), of which there are several species and subspecies, some of the latter being difficult to differentiate. It should be noted that their requirements in captivity are very different from those of the Mediterranean tortoises.

There are two main groups of these American tortoises. The Eastern usually has a uniformly dull brown plastron, sometimes smudged with darker brown; the Western has an intricate pattern of dark brown and yellow stripes on the plastron. The Eastern Box comes from the south-eastern states such as Florida and is adapted to a warm climate with a high relative humidity; the Western comes from the more arid states of New Mexico and Arizona and so prefers a drier climate.

In general, box tortoises should be kept all the year round in an indoor vivarium, in a warm environment and moist atmosphere but with good ventilation so that it never becomes stuffy. Species and subspecies vary in their temperature requirements and it is best to provide a temperature gradient of 20–30°C. During the summer, when the temperature is over 21°C, they enjoy being out of doors in a planted enclosure where they have access to water and shade – they do not fare well if left in the full sun.

The box tortoises are more closely related to freshwater terrapins than to true land tortoises. Most of them are omnivores, although youngsters may be largely carnivorous and some subspecies prefer insects. Many captive box tortoises are not given an adequate diet. Only one-third of the diet should consist of plant material, and of that 75% should be vegetable and 25% fruit. The remaining two-thirds of the diet should be of animal material, and examples of good sources of animal protein include crickets, grasshoppers, slugs, caterpillars, mealworms and sardines. Invertebrate food should be dusted with a calcium supplement to minimise the risk of metabolic bone disease. Small amounts of dog or cat food can be given but large quantities may cause nutritional disorders as they are not formulated for these species.

Most (but not all) box tortoises hibernate in the winter, though some can be kept awake in a warm cage with ample lighting. Only healthy box tortoises should be allowed to hibernate. The optimum conditions for hibernation are a temperature of 7–17°C, a draught-free and rodent-proof box and at least 40 cm depth of bedding – dry leaves, good-quality hay or shredded paper.

Health care of box tortoises is important and follows the general guidelines for captive chelonians. However, these animals can prove difficult to examine if they withdraw their head and all four limbs and close the shell.

Terrapins. The terrapin most commonly seen in captivity in the UK is the red-eared terrapin of North America. Hatchlings are sold at 3–5 cm long. The adult male is approximately 17–18 cm long and the female can grow to 28–30 cm.

Young terrapins require a vivarium with heated water and a basking area, with a basking spotlight, to help them dry out and to shed their scutes as they grow. They can be fed on a mixture of trout pellets, complete cat food, meat and fish. The latter should be supplemented with vitamins and minerals before feeding, and frozen fish such as whitebait

should be heat-treated (as described for garter snakes). To minimise fouling of the water, it is best not to feed terrapins in their tank but in a separate container.

Large terrapins do well in an outdoor pond during the summer but it should be enclosed so that they cannot escape.

Mature males can be very aggressive and will attack other males (and sometimes females) if they are kept together in a small tank where the subordinate animal cannot escape.

Snakes. The detailed requirements of snakes in captivity depend on the species. The North American group includes the corn snakes, rat snakes, garter snakes and king snakes.

- Corn snakes and rat snakes are generally easy to maintain in captivity and easy to handle (particularly the corn snake). Captive-bred young of these rodent-eaters are commonly available and there are several colour mutations of the corn snake.
- Garter snakes are relatively small and are good first snakes for well-informed children. In the wild they live in woodland and by watercourses, eating fish and dead invertebrates.
- King snakes are more aggressive and they are reptile-eaters in the wild: they should be kept singly in the vivarium. Captive-bred individuals should have been brought up to eat dead mice but the feeding of wild-caught snakes can be a problem.
- Royal (or ball) pythons are the smallest of the larger snakes commonly available and can be very reluctant to feed in captivity if caught in the wild. Veterinary practices often see long-term anorexics and these require lengthy treatment to rehydrate and then force-feed – some never feed voluntarily in captivity.
- Indian (Burmese) pythons grow up to 4 m or more; they are strong snakes and, though some remain easy to handle, others can be belligerent. Many of them become too much of a handful for their owners, who offer them to zoos that may be already overstocked. Yet they continue to be bred regularly in captivity and hatchlings are commonly available.
- Boa constrictors do not grow as large as Indian pythons: they have a slimmer build but they still tend to grow too large to be accommodated by the average household. They reproduce well in captivity and a snake that has been handled well when young usually remains amenable as it grows.
- Reticulated pythons grow as large and as strong as Indian pythons, and are generally more aggressive.

Small lizards. Most lizards are territorial. There should be only one male of any species in a small vivarium, together with perhaps two or three females. The species generally recommended as a beginner's lizard is the leopard gecko, a nocturnal lizard that has been bred in captivity for many generations and is relatively easy to handle.

Large lizards. The large lizard most commonly kept is the green iguana, often imported as young animals at 30–45 cm long. Many purchasers fail to appreciate that the males can grow up to 150 cm and that the species requires extensive heated accommodation: they are very demanding in time, space and money. In captivity they rarely reach their full potential size and often suffer from fibrous osteodystrophy due to an inadequate or poorly balanced diet.

Handling

Snakes. It is assumed that the snakes brought to a veterinary practice are not venomous. Venomous snakes are kept by some herpetologists, but in the UK many are covered by the strict regulations of the Dangerous Wild Animals Act.

All snakes are susceptible to bruising: they should be handled carefully and never held more tightly than necessary. Those that are normally quiet and easy to handle will become upset in a new and possibly threatening environment or as a result of maltreatment during clinical examination, injection or blood-testing.

Small snakes, unless they threaten and strike at the handler, should be lifted gently by a hand under their broadest part and then supported as they coil around the arm (Fig. 10.9). Aggressive small snakes can be caught with the aid of a towel or gloves and gently restrained behind the head.

To examine the head and mouth, the snake is supported just behind its head and then its mouth opened (if required) by gently inserting a flat instrument in the labial notch at the front of the mouth. Wooden lolly-sticks and pen-tops have been found useful for this task; there are doubtless many other possibilities.

Large snakes should be handled with care and never draped around the neck. Two or three competent people should be present to help with really large snakes. Those known to be aggressive should be sedated before handling.

Lizards. Small lizards should be picked up round the pectoral girdle. Very small and delicate lizards can be trapped against the side of the vivarium with a soft cloth. Never catch a lizard by its tail: the shedding of the tail (autotomy) is a defence mechanism in many species (but not all).

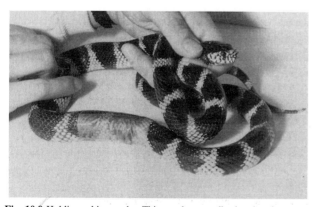

Fig. 10.9 Holding a king snake. This one has an adhesive dressing on a skin lesion, which needs careful nursing to avoid secondary infections.

Iguanas should be handled with care: they can inflict damage with their teeth, their short claws (particularly on the hind limbs) and their long, lashing tails. It is best to use a towel or gloves, unless they can be grasped briskly in two hands with one hand round the shoulders and one holding the thighs along the side of the tail.

Fish

The health and welfare of fish depend very much upon the quality of the water in which they live. Important features of water quality are:

● Temperature (less oxygen is present at higher temperatures).
● pH (6–8 is the usual range for freshwater species).
● Hardness/salinity (hard water is usually preferable).
● Metallic salts in solution.
● Ammonia and nitrate levels (deaths may occur if high – testing kits are available).
● Bacteria levels.
● Some species are very specific in their requirements. Experienced aquarists can advise.

Aquaria

Aquaria are usually made entirely of glass but tanks with frames are still in use. Setting up an aquarium needs planning and patience, and the following points are important:

● Choose a site away from direct sunlight.
● Ensure that the aquarium is properly supported – a tank full of water is heavy. Use pieces of polystyrene under all-glass tanks to minimise uneven pressures.
● Install gravel on floor. It must be several centimetres deep if there is under-gravel filtration.
● Add rocks and ornamental structures as necessary. Clean them first.
● Add plants, ensuring that they come from a reputable dealer. Soak in 2 p.p.m. potassium permanganate for 48 hours before transfer.
● Let the aquarium settle for 2 weeks before stocking with fish. Some people then add 'cheap fish' to test the water before introducing other species.
● Tropical species need heating, either of the tank or of the whole room.

Feeding and maintenance

Proprietary food should be the staple diet, supplemented with live food if necessary, but the latter can introduce disease. Various supplements are available and can be useful. Never overfeed: assess how much is being eaten and give slightly less than this, provided once or twice daily.

Maintenance includes:

● Regular observation of the fish and their environment.
● Weekly cleaning (removal) of gross dirt from the bottom of the aquarium plus 10–15% of the water. Dechlorinate tap water before it is added.

- Installing mechanical, biological or chemical filters for large tanks and the more sensitive species.
- Taking prompt action if fish appear unwell or die or if the water changes in appearance.
- Quarantining all incoming fish for at least 2 weeks.

Invertebrates

Invertebrates are increasingly being kept in captivity (Fig. 10.10). Their management differs according to their species, origin, age and other factors, and some examples are given in Table 10.17.

Wildlife

Space does not permit detailed discussion of the care of wildlife. Nevertheless, some basic information is important. Members of the public have traditionally brought wild mammals and birds that are in need of attention to veterinary practices and in recent years there has been an increased interest in work with such casualties. Wildlife organisations, including bat, badger, fox and hedgehog conservation groups, understandably expect an in-depth knowledge and commitment from practising veterinarians. Specialist rehabilitation centres (some run privately, some by organisations such as the RSPCA) are also well established. An ability to deal with wildlife is, therefore, a useful skill for the veterinary nurse to acquire.

Wild animals are likely to fall into one or more categories:

- Those that have an infectious or parasitic disease (e.g. tuberculosis, tick infestation).
- Those that have an injury (e.g. a broken wing).
- Those that have been poisoned, intentionally or accidentally.
- Those that have been electrocuted or burnt, e.g. on power-lines or following a fire.
- Those that are oiled or have other chemical damage (see Chapter 3, p. 35).
- Those that are, or appear to be, orphaned.
- Those that have been displaced for some reason, e.g. birds that fly off-course on migration.

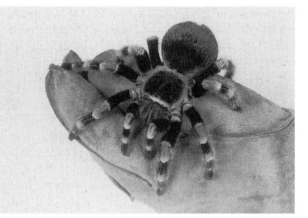

Fig. 10.10 A red-kneed tarantula on the hand. Gloves are not usually necessary but will reduce the risk of irritation from the spider's hairs (setae).

There are several questions that should be asked when dealing with a wildlife casualty:

(1) When and where was it found?
(2) What species is it? Some wild animals, particularly certain birds, are covered by special legislation (birds of prey in particular) and steps may need to be taken to register them or to keep appropriate records.
(3) Does the practice have the necessary facilities and staff to deal with the animal? Some species, such as badgers and herons, require a great deal of personal attention whereas others can be tended with a minimum of specialised accommodation or equipment. If the practice cannot cope, is there a wildlife centre that may be better able to assist?

From the outset it is necessary to ascertain whether it is in the animal's best interests to embark on care and treatment – and this can be a hard decision. Many factors have to be taken into consideration, of which the most important are:

- Is the animal so unwell or badly injured that it is unlikely to survive and is probably in severe pain?
- Even if the animal is likely to survive, will it be possible to return it to the wild when recovered? (With all wildlife casualties this must be the aim and is often a legal requirement.)

Table 10.17 Management and feeding of invertebrates

Species	Management	Main food
Indian stick insect	Well-ventilated containers. Temperate.	Privet leaves.
Giant millipedes	Containers with ample substrate. Tropical	Dead leaves, fruit, vegetables, waste organic material.
Giant snails	As above. Tropical. High humidity.	Fruit, vegetables. Calcium source.
Red-kneed tarantula	Spacious container with some substrate. Tropical. High humidity.	Insects, other invertebrates.

● If it cannot be rehabilitated in the wild, can it properly be retained in captivity? Will it have a reasonable quality of life?

Although the treatment of wildlife is challenging and stimulating, this must not be allowed to obscure the fact that the kindest approach to some casualties is euthanasia. Heroic surgery, expensive drug therapy and dedicated nursing have their place and will yield successful results in a proportion of cases but others, for a variety of reasons, fail to respond and are probably best humanely killed. Euthanasia is an option at each stage, as indicated in Fig. 10.11.

Assuming that the decision is made to attempt to keep the casualty, the following points are important:

● Keep proper records – species, date of arrival, diagnosis, treatment, outcome.
● Carry out all handling, examination and treatment with care – wild animals are easily stressed.
● Remember that nursing plays a very important part in the care of wild animals. Warmth, fluids and feeding, coupled with attention to wounds and discharges, will often go a long way towards keeping the patient alive and facilitating recovery.
● Getting the animal to eat voluntarily can prove difficult and needs a great deal of patience. Force-feeding may be necessary at first.
● Rehabilitation and release can prove time-consuming, difficult and sometimes impossible. Help can be obtained from people who specialise in wildlife care, e.g. those who run the reputable rehabilitation centres.

The British Wildlife Rehabilitation Council publishes a Code of Practice and can give advice.

Pain assessment and welfare considerations

An important part of the veterinary nurse's responsibility is to promote the welfare of the animal and to minimise pain and distress. It is best to assume that all animals are capable of feeling pain (the majority, including invertebrates, are certainly capable of *responding* to it) and to give them the benefit of the nurse's skill in practice.

It is helpful to consider this aspect of welfare under three headings: pain, discomfort and distress.

● **Pain** is a physical phenomenon, with which all humans are familiar. One assumes that exotic (and native wild) species can also experience pain of different degree (mild, moderate, substantial) and of different duration (acute or chronic).
● **Discomfort** is also a physical phenomenon but is milder than pain and may only be an inconvenience or irritation to the animal, e.g. a piece of bandage that has become loose and makes it difficult for the animal to walk or to lie down comfortably.
● **Distress** is a psychological phenomenon and may be associated with pain or discomfort, or can be entirely distinct. It occurs, for example, when a mother is separated from her young, or a social animal is kept alone. These and other 'stressors' can cause 'stress' in the animal. The terminology is important.

There are many ways in which the nurse can contribute to the relief of pain, discomfort and distress in exotic species. For example:

● Ensure that the animal receives the best possible care in terms of good feeding, handling and general management.

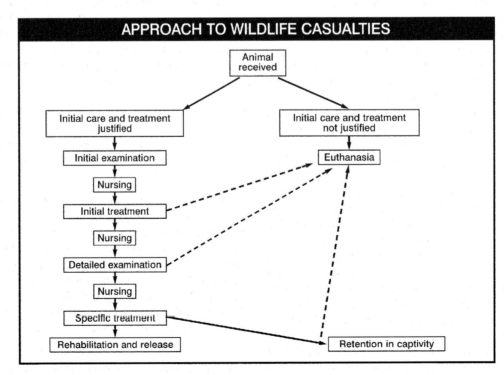

Fig. 10.11 Considerations in dealing with wildlife casualties.

- Provide an environment that is appropriate to both the species and the particular individual.
  - Animals that like to burrow (such as gerbils) or to hide in a damp place (such as toads) should be permitted to do so.
  - Social species should not be kept alone.
  - Species that fight or strongly challenge one another should not be kept together in close confinement.
- Attend promptly to wounds, infections and other problems. Such attention must include supportive care (e.g. cleaning of ocular discharges, and handfeeding) as well as specific therapy.
- Make appropriate changes to management, e.g. use rubber mats to reduce pain and to minimise further damage to a rabbit with 'sore hocks' or a guinea pig with pododermatitis.
- Administer analgesics to prevent or minimise pain. These can include specific agents (e.g. buprenorphine) or general anaesthetics that have an analgesic effect (e.g. nitrous oxide).
- Administer other chemotherapeutic agents that, while not themselves analgesic, reduce the risk of further pain or distress (e.g. tranquillisers to prevent an animal from damaging itself in its cage).
- The question of euthanasia must never be overlooked. As with other species, the exotic or wild animal that is in substantial pain which is likely to persist may need to be killed on humanitarian grounds.

The veterinary nurse is likely to ask: 'But how do I know when an unfamiliar species is in pain?' This is a valid question, to which there are three answers: subjectivity, clinical indications and responses.

- **Subjectivity**. Subjectivity is probably a good guide. If under similar circumstances a human would be in pain, assume that the animal is also. Thus, if *any* species is anorexic and lethargic following surgery, consider postoperative pain as one of the likely causes.
- **Clinical indications**. Certain clinical features are now considered to be indicative of pain in laboratory mammals and it is prudent to apply the same criteria to these same species in veterinary practice. Much has been written about pain assessment in laboratory animals in recent years (see Further Reading) and the veterinary nurse can gain from reading these publications and discussing the matter with experienced animal technicians. A scoring system is often used in laboratory animal work and this can be applicable to small mammals in practice. Clinical features can be common to all species (e.g. anorexia, dehydration, lethargy, weight loss) or may be specific to the type of animal (e.g. failure of rats to groom or a tendency for rabbits to press their heads against the wall of the cage). An observant veterinary nurse will quickly develop the ability to recognise signs that indicate pain, discomfort and distress.
- **Responses**. If in doubt, give the animal appropriate treatment (e.g. an analgesic) and see if there is a response. A ferret, for example, that looks dejected and is reluctant to move or feed following surgery on a broken leg may behave very differently after a subcutaneous injection of buprenorphine or flunixin.

Common problems and diseases

Diseases of exotic species can be infectious or noninfectious. Often there is an overlap and many apparently infectious diseases (e.g. respiratory conditions of rabbits, foot infections of birds) are due to, or precipitated by, poor management or inadequate diet. When taking a history, or discussing a problem with an owner, the veterinary nurse should obtain as much information as possible about the housing, feeding and general management of the patient. Ideally, the client's premises should be visited but in a busy practice this is not always practicable. Owners should therefore be encouraged to produce the animal in its own (uncleaned) cage together with samples of uneaten food. It can prove helpful if they also bring a photograph or drawing of the animal at home, in its own environment.

Common problems and diseases for different groups of exotic pets are summarised in Tables 10.18–10.20. Much useful information on the diseases of small mammals can also be obtained by reference to the literature on laboratory animals (see Further Reading).

Zoonoses

Veterinary nurses should be aware of the potential of some exotic animals to carry and/or transmit zoonoses. See also p. 140 and Chapter 17. A zoonosis can be defined as a disease or infection that can be naturally transmitted from a vertebrate animal to a human. Each part of this definition is important:

- A zoonosis need not cause disease in its host: the organism may be present and transmitted without clinical signs, e.g. a guinea pig can excrete *Salmonella*.
- The disease or infection must be naturally transmitted. Many organisms can be spread experimentally, e.g. by injection, but in that case they are not considered to be zoonoses.
- Only vertebrate animals can be sources of a zoonosis. An organism transmitted from an invertebrate, such as a mosquito or tick, with no involvement of another animal (mammal, bird, reptile, amphibian or fish) is not considered to be zoonotic.

Some zoonotic diseases are common to a wide range of species: bacteria of the genus *Salmonella*, for example, can be acquired from animals ranging from ferrets to frogs. Others are more specific: for example, the virus of lymphocytic choriomeningitis (LCM) is only likely to be contracted from rodents. Animals with zoonotic infections need not show clinical signs of disease, since they may either be incubating the disease or carrying the organisms asymptomatically, and therefore the veterinary nurse's approach to zoonoses must be based upon other factors:

- *Awareness* that such infections exists and that apparently healthy animals may transmit them.

Table 10.18 Some diseases of small mammals

Species	Condition	Clinical signs	Treatment	Comments
All	Skin wounds and abscesses	Skin abrasions and lesions.	Clean with appropriate disinfectant or cleansing agent. Suture where appropriate. Irrigate abscesses.	Wounds may indicate fighting or other management problems. Rabbit abscesses may need to be excised *in toto*.
	Traumatic injuries	Incoordination, collapse, hyperpnoea, etc.	Warmth, fluids orally and/or by injection. Hand-feeding and nursing.	Some species, e.g. hamsters, are prone to fall off surfaces. Damage may also be caused by poor handling (especially by children), cats, etc.
	Fractures	Locomotor disturbances, swelling, pain, etc.	Euthanasia may be necessary. Limb fractures can be fixed (externally or internally) but in small rodents often heal spontaneously. Nursing.	Vertebral injuries are common in rabbits.
	Dental problems	Excessive salivation ('slobbers'), dysphagia.	Clipping of overgrown teeth. Removal of plaque, attention to inflamed gingivae.	Overgrowth of incisors and cheek teeth (malocclusions) is common in rodents and lagomorphs and may be associated with genetic factors, soft food, lack of wear, etc. Dental abscesses and periodontal disease are prevalent in ferrets.
	Ectoparasites (flea, mite, tick or louse infestation)	Vary from inapparent infection to marked pruritus and skin lesions.	Appropriate parasiticidal treatment of skin (and, in case of fleas, environment).	Skin lesions may also be due to environmental factors, nutritional deficiencies, or behavioural traits (barbering).
	Endoparasites (nematode, cestode, trematode, or protozoan infestation)	Vary from inapparent infection to diarrhoea. Rectal prolapse may be indicative of infestation with the pinworm *Syphacia*.	Anthelmintic or antiprotozoal treatment. Various agents can be used orally including mebendazole (10 mg/kg), praziquantel (5–10 mg/kg) and for protozoa, sulphonamides or dimetridazole (1 mg/ml water).	Diagnosis of endoparasites will depend upon careful examination of faeces or (post-mortem) body tissues.
	Respiratory disease	May range from mild respiratory signs, e.g. nasal discharge in rabbits, sneezing in rats, chattering in mice, to dyspnoea. Headtilt, due to labyrinthitis, may be seen.	Antimicrobial agents may be tried. Isolation of affected animals and attention to management (temperature and ventilation) are important.	Difficult, if not impossible, to eliminate from a group or colony of rodents. Many different microorganisms may be involved but the primary pathogen in rodents is usually a virus or *Mycoplasma*. Secondary bacterial infection is common and may respond to chemotherapy.
	Diarrhoea, enteritis (various types)	Loose faeces, fluid loss, electrolyte imbalance, etc.	Specific therapy plus fluids where appropriate.	Many different causes, ranging from changes in diet to bacterial, viral and parasitic infections. Specific therapy will depend on cause, and laboratory investigation of faeces may be necessary. It is wise to check for *Salmonella*.
Mouse, rat, guinea pig and rabbit	Ringworm	Hair loss, occasionally erythema and pruritus.	Oral griseofulvin (25 mg/kg) for 4–5 weeks.	Differential diagnosis in the rabbit includes plucking of hair for nest-building.
Mouse and rat	Mammary tumours	Swollen, usually hard, mammary glands.	Surgical removal.	Often malignant, especially in rats. May be confused with mastitis.

Table 10.18 (Continued)

Species	Condition	Clinical signs	Treatment	Comment
Mouse and rat (continued)	'Ringtail'	Raised corrugated (usually hyperkeratinized) lesions on tail.	Raise relative humidity. Lesions which become infected can be treated topically.	'Ringtail' and certain other non-specific skin lesions are associated with a low relative humidity (<40%).
Mouse, rat, golden hamster, jird and guinea pig (occasionally rabbit)	Tyzzer's disease (*Bacillus piliformis* infection)	Diarrhoea, loss of condition, death.	Rarely successful. Tetracyclines may be tried. Improve management.	Stressors may be responsible for onset of disease.
Golden hamster	Impacted cheek pouch.	Swollen side(s) to face.	Remove impaction manually or by irrigation with saline.	Often caused by artificial foods, e.g. sweets, pellets.
	'Wet tail' (proliferative ileitis)	Diarrhoea and perianal excoriation, especially in newly weaned animals.	Rarely successful. Fluids by mouth or injection. Oral neomycin, kaolin preparations, etc. Nursing.	Cause uncertain, possibly a form of colibacillosis. Often precipitated by stressors, e.g. change of diet or overcrowding. A similar condition may be seen in jirds but is probably not identical.
Jird	'Fits' (epileptiform seizures)	Convulsions, lasting for 10–90 s.	None necessary. Animal should be returned to cage and not disturbed.	Cause and significance are uncertain. Often precipitated by stressors, e.g. handling.
	Sebaceous gland disorders	Swollen gland on ventral surface of abdomen	If inflamed and/or infected use topical antimicrobial agent and/or corticosteroid. If neoplastic – surgical removal.	
Guinea pig	Alopecia	Hair loss, usually without pruritus	Change of environment. Improved diet (including addition of vitamin C and hay).	Cause often uncertain. Common in female animals during pregnancy.
	Scurvy (vitamin C deficiency)	Lethargy, swollen joints, weight loss, death. Often predisposes to infectious or parasitic disease	Vitamin C orally (50–100 mg/day per animal).	May occur even if diet contains vitamin C since deterioration of the latter can be rapid, especially at high temperatures.
	Pregnancy toxaemia	Depression and anorexia during last 1–2 weeks of pregnancy or immediately after parturition.	Corticosteroids by injection. Dextrose by mouth or injection. Avoidance of stress.	Probably associated with heavy and long pregnancy, and obesity. Often only diagnosed post mortem.
Guinea pig and rabbit	Pseudotuberculosis (*Yersinia* infection)	Diarrhoea, weight loss, enlarged mesenteric lymph nodes, death.	Rarely practicable or wise. Culling and disinfection are preferable.	Infection may be introduced by other animals (including wild birds and rodents) or contaminated greenfood.
Rabbit	Ear canker (*Psoroptes cuniculi* infestation)	Inflammation of external ear canal: pruritus and self-inflicted damage.	Soften exudate with liquid paraffin prior to cleaning and application of ear drops, for 5 days.	Regular inspection of rabbit's ears will enable early infestation to be detected. In severe cases light anaesthesia will facilitate cleaning.
	Sore hocks	Hair loss, swelling, ulceration and/or infection of hock(s)	Treat wounds. Provide soft bedding.	Often follows trauma or prolonged periods on hard floor.
	Hairball (gastric)	Anorexia, dehydration, sometimes diarrhoea. Hairball may be palpable.	Liquid paraffin by mouth coupled with manual massage to break up hairball. Surgery may be necessary.	Usually follows self-grooming and this may be due to boredom. Particularly prevalent in long-haired breeds, e.g. Angora.

Table 10.18 (Continued)

Species	Condition	Clinical signs	Treatment	Comment
Rabbit	Hepatic coccidiosis (*Eimeria stiedae* infestation)	Weight loss, anorexia, occasionally diarrhoea. Liver may be enlarged.	Oral sulphonamides (e.g. 0.2% sulphadimidine or 0.3% sulphaquinoxaline) in water for five days.	May be present in subclinical form – oocysts detectable in faeces. In severe clinical cases chronic hepatic damage may persist after treatment.
	Enteritis complex	Depression, diarrhoea, fluid intestinal contents, dehydration, mainly in recently weaned animals (5–10 weeks old).	Food with high fibre content, e.g. hay. Nursing and supportive care. Antimicrobial agents may be helpful.	Cause uncertain – probably multifactorial and associated with bacteria and change of diet. Differential diagnoses include coccidiosis and diarrhoea following a change in diet.
	Myxomatosis	Conjunctivitis, blepharitis, subcutaneous swellings. Anorexia, depression, death.	None specific. Nursing and supportive care, including hand-feeding.	Vaccination can be used prophylactically. Control of the vector – the rabbit flea (*Spilopsyllus cuniculi*) – is also important.
	Viral haemorrhagic disease	Lethargy, anorexia, haemorrhage, sudden death.	None specific. Nursing and supportive care, including hand-feeding.	Vaccination can be used prophylactically. Hygiene and isolation of affected cases.
Ferret	Persistent oestrus	Swollen, sometimes abraded, vulva. May be severe – depression, anorexia, pale mucous membranes, death.	Termination of oestrus by stimulation of vagina, mating (entire or vasectomised male) or hormonal therapy, e.g. proligestone 0.5 ml sc. Ovariohysterectomy and/or blood transfusions in severe cases.	The mild syndrome is common but the more severe condition (oestrus-associated bone marrow depression) has only once been reported in Britain.
	Canine distemper	Respiratory signs, conjunctivitis, diarrhoea, neurological signs, death.	None specific. Nursing and symptomatic treatment.	Vaccination can be used prophylactically.

- *Reducing unnecessary exposure* to animals that may be a source of zoonoses. This may involve not handling an animal unnecessarily; or ensuring that, when it is handled, it is unlikely to bite or scratch or to contaminate wounds.
- *Practising good hygiene* so that infections are less likely to spread. Hand-washing, protective clothing and other standard safeguards are usually adequate.
- *Taking prophylactic action* where this is available. For example, all veterinary nurses should be immunised against tetanus and those who come into contact with zoo animals or captive primates should consider rabies and hepatitis vaccinations.

Common problems in pet mammals

Rabbits

- Overgrown claws.
- Malocclusion of front and cheek teeth – the teeth are not properly worn down, resulting in spikes and grossly overlong teeth that may require clipping or filing.
- External parasites – *Psoroptes cuniculi*, the rabbit ear mite, and *Cheyletiella parasitivorax*, the fur mite.

- Internal parasites – including roundworms (*Passalurus ambiguus*).
- Coccidiosis – most commonly seen in litters reared in unhygienic conditions. Signs are diarrhoea, poor growth, weight loss. Hepatic coccidiosis may be seen in adults.
- Abscesses – usually round the head, sometimes associated with tooth-root infection.
- Gastrointestinal problems – anorexia; diarrhoea; faeces matted around the anus (possibly if rabbit fails to eat its 'night faeces' because it is too obese to reach its anus); furballs; gastric dilatation (an emergency). Rabbits that have been anorexic and had gastrointestinal upset can often be tempted to eat with fresh, coarse greenstuff such as long grass, raspberry or dandelion leaves.
- 'Snuffles' – purulent nasal discharge or pneumonia. Most pet rabbits develop some lung damage during their lives. The incidence of respiratory disease increases in poorly ventilated or too warm an environment.
- Myxomatosis – a viral disease still widespread in the wild population, carried by the rabbit flea, which can reach the pet rabbits via a cat or dog passing through the garden. Vaccination is recommended for all pet rabbits.

Table 10.19 Some diseases seen in birds

Condition	Clinical signs	Diagnosis	Treatment	Comment
Skin wounds	Skin abrasions and lesions, bleeding.	Observation and examination.	Clean with appropriate disinfectant. Control haemorrhage. Suture where appropriate	Wounds may indicate poor cage design, pecking by other birds, or predation (e.g. by cats). *See also* Abscesses.
Traumatic injuries	Incoordination, collapse, hyperpnoea, etc.	Examination.	Warmth. Fluids. Hand-feeding and nursing. Attention to wounds.	As above.
Fractures	Lameness, drooping wing, swelling, pain, etc.	Examination.	External (splints, taping, plaster) or internal (pinning, wiring, plating) fixation. Nursing.	Callus formation is rapid in small birds and fixation may not be necessary after 14–21 days.
Feather conditions (various)	Feather loss or damage. Irregular or abnormal moult.	Observation, examination of feathers.	Depends on cause. If parasites present parasiticidal treatment. If no parasites detected improve diet, change environment, provide company and/or a mate. Some cases are due to hormonal imbalance and may respond to thyroxine or testosterone.	A complex and often frustrating group of diseases.
'Scaly leg' and 'scaly face' (*Cnemidocoptes* infestation)	Raised keratinous lesions on feet and/or cere.	Observation. Examination of crusts for parasites.	Painting with liquid parafin to soften scabs, followed (if necessary) by weekly painting of affected areas with 10% benzyl benzoate or 5% piperonyl butoxide.	Deformity of the beak may be a sequel to 'scaly face'. Ivermectin may be effective against the mites.
'Bumblefoot' (usually *Staphylococcus aureus* infection of foot)	Swollen, painful foot or digit.	Observation. Examination. Aspiraion of pus and bacteriology.	Lancing, removal of pus and irrigation. Dressing of foot. Improved hygiene of perches.	Differential diagnosis can include visceral gout (*see below*) and traumatic injuries.
Articular gout	Swollen, painful joint(s).	Observation. Aspiration of urates.	None, other than removal of urate deposits. Improve renal function by ensuring adequate water intake.	Aetiology uncertain. May be associated with renal damage. Urates are deposited in joints and, in some cases (visceral gout), on the serosae of internal organs.
Skin tumours	External swellings.	Examination. Aspiration for cytology or biopsy for histopathology	Surgical removal.	May be lipomas, fibromas, adenomas, or malignant equivalents. Differential diagnosis includes haematomas, feather cysts (*see below*) and abscesses (*see below*).
Abscesses	External swellings.	Examination. Aspiration for bacteriology and cytology.	Surgical removal or lancing and irrigation.	Pus is usually caseous. Differential diagnosis includes haematomas, neoplasia (*see above*) and feather cysts (*see below*).
'Feather cysts' (*hypopteronosis cystica*)	External swellings, especially on wings.	Incision or excision to demonstrate whorls of keratin.	Surgical removal.	Particularly prevalent in certain strains of canary. May be a genetic predisposition.
Regurgitation	Food is regurgitated. In crop necrosis bird is unwell with fluid around beak and, sometimes, diarrhoea.	Eliminate 'normal' regurgitation (*see Comment*). Swab of crop for bacteriology and mycology (*Candida*).	Nursing. Fluids. Clavulanate-potentiated amoxycillin 12.5 mg/kg orally and/or nystatin orally. Vitamin B supplementation.	Male budgerigars regurgitate food as part of courtship and may do this in captivity, even when kept alone. Crop necrosis is an infectious condition, possibly secondary to a nutritional deficiency or overuse of antibiotics.

Table 10.19 (Continued)

Condition	Clinical signs	Diagnosis	Treatment	Comment
Sinusitis	Swollen periorbital region.	Observation and examination. Swabs for bacteriology.	Parenteral antibiotics. Change of environment. In severe or intractable cases surgical drainage and irrigation of sinuses.	Probably part of an upper respiratory disease syndrome, possibly precipitated or exacerbated by adverse temperature/relative humidity or prolonged exposure to smoke.
Ectoparasites	May be none. Feather loss or damage, pruritus, anaemia	Observation. Examination of birds and cage/aviary for evidence of parasites.	Pyrethrum-based powders or sprays. Dichlorvos strip in birdroom.	In cases of mite infestation treat environment as well as bird. *See also* 'Scaly leg' and 'Scaly face' and Feather conditions.
Endoparasites	May be none. Loss of weight or condition, lethargy, anorexia, diarrhoea.	Examination of bird and laboratory investigation of faeces and/or buccal/crop smears.	Depends on parasite. Nematodes treated with levamisole 10 mg/kg orally or febendazole 100 mg/kg orally. Do not use latter in pigeons.	Some parasites e.g. *Capillaria* may infest upper alimentary tract. High burdens of ascarids can block intestine.
Enteritis	Diarrhoea, loss of weight and condition.	Observation and examination. Investigation of faeces may or may not prove helpful.	Depends upon cause. Change of diet and/or oral antibiotics or sulphonamides (coupled with fluids and nursing) may be beneficial.	'Enteritis' is a general term and probably refers to many conditions. Normal droppings consist of two portions – white urates and brown/black/dark green faeces. Very green faeces are usually indicative of reduced food intake and excess bile production.
Respiratory disease	Noisy, difficult or exaggerated breathing 'Clicking' or other sounds. Nasal or ocular discharge. Swollen sinuses.	Observation and examination. Laboratory investigation.	Depends upon cause. Antibiotics or sulphonamides preferably by injection. Supportive care.	There is a whole range of respiratory diseases. Many are due to or associated with bacteria but fungi and mites may also be involved. Psittacosis (chlamydiosis) must always be considered: laboratory investigations (blood and faeces) will confirm. *See also* Sinusitis.
Poisoning	Usually found dead but may be collapse, diarrhoea, dyspnoea, etc.	Examination of bird and surroundings. Laboratory investigations.	Depends upon cause. Generally similar to treatment in domesticated species. Supportive therapy of prime importance.	Important causes of poisoning in birds include carbon monoxide (car exhaust), polymer fumes (non-stick cooking utensils), pesticides and lead.
Egg binding	Abdominal distension, straining, collapse. Prolapse of oviduct or cloaca may follow.	Observation and examination.	Immediate warmth (30–32°C), calcium borogluconate intramuscularly, manual removal. Surgery. Drainage of egg with syringe.	A relatively common condition. Many cases respond to warmth alone.
Dropsy	Swollen abdomen.	Observation and examination. Radiography, laparoscopy, laboratory examination of fluid aspirate.	Depends on cause. Internal tumours may be operable. Infectious conditions treatable with antimicrobial agents. Ascites can be treated temporarily by paracentesis. Constipation will respond to liquid paraffin.	A variety of causes. Differential diagnosis includes 'egg binding' (*see above*) and obesity.
'Going light'	Chronic loss of weight and condition; sometimes diarrhoea, often fatal.	Examination of bird and aviculturist's records.	Improved nutrition and supportive care may help. Specific therapy where an organism, e.g. a *Toxoplasma*, is implicated.	A term used by aviculturists. The condition is recognised in several species of bird but the aetiologies may differ.

Table 10.20 Some diseases seen in lower vertebrates

Species	Condition	Clinical signs	Treatment	Comment
All (Reptiles, amphibians and fish)	Skin wounds and abscesses	Skin abrasions and lesions.	Clean with suitable disinfectant. Suture where appropriate. Drain abscesses or remove surgically.	Abscesses are best removed *in toto*. Amphibians and many fish can be kept in a 0.6% salt solution to encourage healing.
	Traumatic injuries	Incoordination, collapse. External lesions, haemorrhage.	Optimum temperature. Fluids by sc, iv or ip injection. Hand-feeding and nursing	All lower vertebrates must be handled and transported with care to minimize risk of trauma.
	External parasites	See individual groups.	See individual groups.	See individual groups.
	Hypothermia	Lethargy, anorexia. Colour changes.	Slowly raise temperature to preferred body temperature.	Species vary in requirements – *see text*.
	Bacterial septicaemia	Sudden death. Severe incoordination. Haemorrhage. Ascites. May be associated with skin lesions.	Isolation. Antibiotics. Hygienic precautions to reduce spread.	Gram-negative bacteria usually involved – especially *Aeromonas* spp.
	Obesity	Increase in weight. Sometimes sudden death. Occasionally jaundice.	Reduction of food intake. Increased exercise.	Common in captive animals. Often diagnosed post mortem – fatty change in liver, kidneys, etc.
Reptiles and amphibians	Fractures	Locomotory disturbances, swelling, pain, etc.	External or internal fixation. Dietary changes; some fractures in small species will heal spontaneously.	Keeping an amphibian in shallow water will help to reduce pressure on limbs and facilitate healing. Fractures are often due to a nutritional deficiency (usually calcium).
	Endoparasites	Vary. Often diarrhoea. May be loss of condition and anorexia.	Depends on cause. Anthelmintics. Antiprotozoals. Fluids. Hygiene.	Laboratory examination of faeces necessary for diagnosis. Fresh wet preparations for demonstration of protozoa – e.g. ciliates, entamoebae.
	Inanition	Loss of weight and condition. Anorexia. Exhaustion due to prolonged under nutrition.	Control of parasites. Attention to other diseases. Correction of environment. Tube feeding.	A common problem in captive reptiles and amphibians but not so prevalent in fish (*see* 'Obesity'). Assess condition of Mediterranean tortoises by Jackson ratio.
	Maladaptation syndrome	Loss of weight and condition. Anorexia. Difficulty in sloughing. Skin lesions, etc.	As above. Attention to skin lesions and other secondary signs.	Common in captive animals. Cause often not clear, frequently multifactorial. Some species and some individuals particularly prone to maladaptation – possibly not suited to captivity.
	Dermatitis	Skin lesions. Various: often proliferative in reptiles, ulcerative in amphibians.	Depends on cause. Topical or systemic antibiotics. Antifungal agents. Excision may be advisable.	Biopsies and/or swabs can be helpful in diagnosis. Papillomatous lesions in certain lizards may be viral in aetiology. Lesions in amphibians are often due to fungus.
	Dysecdysis	Difficulty in sloughing or abnormal frequency.	Attention to environment. Soaking of reptiles will facilitate sloughing.	Underlying hormonal disturbances may also be involved.
Amphibians and fish	'Fungus' (*Saprolegnia* infection)	Distinct fungal growth (like cotton wool) on body surface.	Treat underlying factors. Topical therapy with povidone-iodine or malachite green	Usually secondary to other factors – e.g. skin lesions, poor water quality.
	Leech infestation	Leeches visible. Anaemia. Secondary infection.	Sodium chloride baths.	Often introduced with live food or vegetation.

Table 10.20 Continued				

Species	Condition	Clinical signs	Treatment	Comment
Amphibians and fish (continued)	'White spot' (*Ichthyophthirius*) infection	Pinhead-size white foci on skin	Proprietary treatment – usually malachite green.	Parasites can complete lifecycles rapidly in warm water. Often fatal if untreated.
Fish	'Fin rot'	Damaged and necrotic fins and tail.	Depends on cause but attention to water quality essential. Antibiotics. Parasiticides.	Environmental factors often responsible. *Saprolegnia* may supervene (*see* 'Fungus' *above*).
	External parasites: Protozoa, Monogenea, Crustacea	Various. Parasites may be visible on skin or gills. Hyperaemia and/or ulceration may occur.	Depends on cause. Large parasites (e.g. *Argulus*) may be removed manually. Others may require parasiticide baths.	Detection of gill parasites may prove difficult in live fish. Skin parasites can lead to ulceration and bacterial septicaemia (*see earlier*).
	Tuberculosis	Various. Weight loss, skin lesions, ascites.	Best to isolate/cull affected fish but treatment can be attempted. Hygiene.	Common causes are *Mycobacterium marinum* and *M. fortuitum*. Zoonotic. Often only confirmed after death but skin (and other) biopsies may permit ante mortem diagnosis.

- Viral haemorrhagic disease (VHD), first reported in China in 1984, has spread rapidly and reached the UK in 1992. It is highly infectious and can be spread from rabbit to rabbit or mechanically. An inactivated vaccine is available and rabbits should be immunised regularly.
- Traumatic injuries – falls, attacks by dogs/cats. Rabbits have very powerful hindlegs and a sudden leap in fear can result in spinal injury.

Many rabbits bought as pets for young children end up unhandled and largely ignored because of the development of behavioural problems, usually related to the onset of sexual maturity. Males often become aggressive and may bite or urine spray; females will bite and stamp in defence of their 'nest-burrow'. Neutering of both sexes is recommended: it will avoid these problems and will also reduce the incidence of uterine adenocarcinoma, a major cause of death in female rabbits.

Guinea pigs

In the case of any sick guinea pig, ascertain the likely vitamin C status – low dietary levels are likely to hamper recovery from skin and other diseases.

- Malocclusion – occurs but probably less commonly than in rabbits. Salivation may be a sign – commonly called 'slobbers'.
- Skin disease – may be caused by sarcoptic mange mite (*Trixacarus caviae*) and less frequently by ringworm. Lice are also sometimes seen. Poor hutch hygiene may lead to pododermatitis (sore feet). Hair loss may be due to 'barbering' by other guinea pigs.
- Nutritional disease – guinea pigs may 'barber' (chew) each other's hair if there is insufficient roughage in the diet. Vitamin C deficiency shows in young animals as

poor growth, reluctance to move, swollen joints; skin wounds take a long time to heal.
- Diarrhoea – a number of causes.
- Impaction of the anus – quite common, particularly in males. Faeces may be normal or softer than usual and accumulate just inside the anus.
- Cystic and urethral calculi – not uncommon in guinea pigs.
- Respiratory disease – common in guinea pigs.
- Pregnancy toxaemia – quite common in the last 2 weeks of pregnancy; more likely in obese or stressed animals. The disease tends to have a rapid course. Sometimes the animal is found dead by the owner.

Chinchilla

Common problems include malocclusion ('slobbers'), abdominal pain (often gastric dilatation), fur-chewing (where not enough hay is supplied) and, less commonly, ringworm.

Rats, mice, gerbils and hamsters

- Malocclusion may occur in all the small pet mammals.
- Respiratory disease – all are susceptible and they may contract some infections from owners with sore throats and colds.
- Parasitic diseases – including various mange mites (*Demodex* species in hamsters, commonly *Notoedres* in mice and rats).
- Nutritional disease – more likely to be subclinical than an obvious nutrient deficiency, but a great many clinical problems in small mammal pets can be helped by improving the diet. Animals allowed unlimited amounts of sunflower seeds may suffer from osteodystrophy.

- Impacted pouches – all species of hamster may suffer; the pouches may become impacted with either food or unsuitable bedding material (such as cotton wool).
- Traumatic injuries – not uncommon in the small pets (they may be dropped accidentally). The protruding eyes of Syrian hamsters are sometimes damaged and may require enucleation.
- 'Wet tail' disease in hamsters – seen in young, recently weaned animals which develop diarrhoea and quickly become dehydrated; often fatal. If the hamster was recently acquired, owners should not purchase a replacement from the same source.

Many small mammal pets develop behavioural problems, especially as a result of living in an inadequate unstimulating environment – often both too small and inadequately furnished. Gerbils without much to dig in will scrabble obsessively at one corner of the cage. Some will eat too much or drink too much or gnaw at the bars if there is nothing better to chew. Others exhibit stereotypical behaviour, performing a series of actions over and over again. Chipmunks kept in small cages indoors often repeatedly somersault in one corner of the cage.

Ferrets

The most common problems in ferrets are fleas, abscesses (which require veterinary attention) and endoparasites. They can also suffer from distemper (vaccination may be recommended if the disease is locally prevalent) and can catch colds or influenza from humans. Owners might also require advice about oestrous control, spaying, vasectomy and castration. Working ferrets, kept for hunting, tend to be susceptible to different diseases – many of them related to an outdoor life – from those kept as pets. American publications refer only to the latter.

Common problems in birds

Nutrition and environment

General poor health in birds is often associated with suboptimal accommodation and poor nutrition. Only with experience can the distinction be made between a really healthy, fit and active bird with glossy plumage and one that is surviving but in suboptimal health. However, there are certain specific deficiencies:

- Iodine deficiency – common in budgerigars, often presents as respiratory distress caused by pressure of the enlarged thyroid gland on the trachea.
- Vitamin A deficiency – very common in all cage-birds, particularly those that have very little fruit or vegetable in their diet. Clinical signs may be those of mild to moderate upper respiratory disease, with swellings around the eyes, nasal discharge and blocked nostrils. More severe cases have small abscesses on the palate.
- Calcium deficiency – may occur in any species but is a particular problem in African grey parrots. Initially inactivity, drooping wings and general discomfort,

progressing in severe cases to fits. Also seen in birds that have been laying constantly over a period.
- 'Stuck in the moult' – a state of constant moulting. Birds normally moult in response to decreasing day length at one end of the summer but some birds kept indoors moult constantly under the influence of artificial lighting. There may be a nutritional factor as well; increasing the protein content of the diet has helped in some cases.

Infectious and parasitic disease

- Roundworm infestation – common in aviary birds, particularly ground-feeding grass parakeets. Birds should be dewormed twice a year, before the breeding season starts in spring and after the moult in the autumn.
- Trichomoniasis – commonly transmitted to aviary birds (usually budgerigars) via the faeces of wild birds, especially pigeons. It is caused by a protozoan that infects the upper part of the digestive tract, particularly the oesophagus and crop, resulting in inappetence and regurgitation.
- Salmonellosis – not uncommonly diagnosed in birds showing gastrointestinal signs. The serotypes isolated may or may not be those that commonly cause disease in humans. May be spread to aviaries by wild birds.

The two major infectious diseases in birds are psittacosis (chlamydiosis or ornithosis) and PBFD (see below). **Psittacosis** is caused by a *Chlamydia* and may produce either respiratory or gastrointestinal signs. Suspect birds should be isolated. There is a danger to human health: the disease is spread in dry faeces. Nurses caring for such birds should wear gloves and masks, and should dampen the paper at the bottom of the bird's cage before moving it (to minimise the spread of the spores). The disease can be treated but pet birds that are confirmed carriers are sometimes euthanased because of the risk to human health.

Psittacine beak and feather disease (dystrophy) (PBFD), a viral disease affecting the integument, is seen in many different species but most commonly in cockatoos. Birds often present as 'feather pluckers': in severe cases the birds have very few feathers and those that remain are broken and greasy-looking, while the horn of the beak is soft and crumbly. Affected birds eventually die of the effects of secondary bacterial and fungal infection of the damaged skin and feathers. This is a very infectious disease and could pose a serious threat in a breeding colony of rare or valuable parrots. Rapid diagnosis is advisable.

Reproductive disorders

Persistent egg-laying may occur in any species but is particularly common in cockatiels. In the wild, birds continue to lay eggs until they have a full clutch. If an owner removes unfertilised eggs from a captive bird, it will lay more and may suffer severe depletion of stored calcium and protein. If a bird is 'broody' (wishing to lay eggs and then sit on them), it is far better that the owner should give her a nest-tray or box and allow her to sit, not removing the eggs (or putting in dummy eggs) until she has finished with them after a couple of weeks of fruitless incubation.

Egg-binding may occur with a first egg, or after a period of egg-laying. The bird may collapse and become anorexic: it will need supportive therapy as well as specific treatment to remove the egg.

Tumours and 'lumps'

Tumours are common in pet budgerigars. Lipomas occur over the breast in obese pet birds and tumours may also affect internal organs, particularly the gonads. This can result in pressure on the sciatic nerve, causing difficulty in perching. Feather lumps, or feather cysts, are particularly common in canaries. They are caused by deformities of a feather follicle, which eventually forms a large mass.

Behavioural problems

Behavioural problems are common in the larger pet birds. They include:

- Feather plucking.
- Nail chewing.
- Self-mutilation.
- Excessive screaming.

Stress-inducing factors that may contribute to such problems include:

- Poor diet.
- Boredom.
- Lack of companionship (bird or human).
- Lack of privacy.
- Sexual frustration (or wishing to breed).
- Lack of sleep (parrots need 8–10 hours of undisturbed sleep to remain healthy).
- Hot, dry atmosphere (often made worse by cigarette smoke or fumes). Rainforest species in particular prefer a high relative humidity.

Common problems in reptiles and amphibians

Failure to feed (in an otherwise healthy animal) may be because of an inadequate environment (temperature too low, poor lighting) or unsuitable food (a wild-caught snake may not recognise a dead white mouse as food).

Failure to slough (shed the skin) may occur in any reptile but is most important in snakes. When a snake is ready to shed, the skin becomes dull, the eyes appear milky and the animal will not feed. Sometimes the failure to shed is total but more often parts of the shed remain on the snake, including the eyelids or the tip of the tail. It is important that these are removed, and with great care, particularly the 'spectacles' over the eyes. Increasing the humidity or allowing the snake to bathe will often help.

Other problems include:

- Stomatitis ('mouth rot') – infection within the mouth. This is common in snakes and also in debilitated tortoises (particularly after hibernation).
- Necrotic dermatitis ('scale rot') – common in snakes. Predisposing factors may be too low a temperature, or

too moist a vivarium so that the snake cannot dry out after being in water.

- Regurgitation of food – occurs for a number of reasons: the temperature in the vivarium may be too low for digestion; the snake may be suffering from endoparasites or a gastric infection; and some snakes will regurgitate if they are handled too soon after feeding.
- Hypovitaminosis A – not uncommon in lizards and Chelonia. The signs include swelling of the eyes, epiphora and unwillingness to feed. Hypervitaminosis A can also occur, usually as a result of over-supplementation, and causes skin lesions (usually a moist dermatitis).

Land tortoises may develop **post-hibernation anorexia (PHA)**, a blanket term to cover all those that do not start eating within a week or so of emerging from hibernation. They may have stomatitis, liver failure or kidney failure; or they may simply have exhausted their vitamin reserves or be dehydrated. The kidneys barely function during hibernation, so that waste products build up in the circulation and blood tests may reveal a very high blood uric acid. Some tortoises with PHA respond well to basic fluid therapy and vitamin supplementation.

Other land tortoise problems include:

- Roundworms – particularly where a number of tortoises are kept, or where they have been on the same piece of ground for a number of years.
- Infectious rhinitis – a very infectious and debilitating viral disease affecting the spur-thighed tortoise and certain other species; it may take a year or more to clear and carriers may remain.
- Osteodystrophy in young animals fed a diet low in calcium or with a poor calcium/phosphorus ratio.

Nursing and anaesthesia

Animals that are sick and debilitated may need to be hospitalised and nursed within the surgery. Sometimes there is merit in housing the patient in its own cage; at other times special accommodation may need to be constructed. The practice should ensure that it is always prepared for emergencies involving exotic pets by having one or more of each of the following:

- 'Hospital cages' – designed for birds but equally useful for small mammals and sometimes reptiles and amphibians.
- Glass or plastic aquaria – primarily used for fish but easily modified to accommodate other species.
- Other suitable containers, e.g. bird cages (preferably with solid sides), buckets.

Important aspects of nursing exotics include:

- Provision of warmth/maintenance of the patient at its preferred body temperature.
- Maintenance of fluid balance.
- Ensuring adequate nutrient intake.
- Minimising stress.

Table 10.21 Physical methods of restraint

Tools	General	Mammals	Birds	Reptiles
Diminish sense perception	Light if nocturnal. Dark if diurnal. Reduced physical contact. Reduced noise.	Cloth bag over head of (for example) a roe deer.	Hooding a bird of prey/ ostrich.	Lower temperature[a]. Hooding.
Allow safe confinement and examination	Bag. Towel. Net.	Crush cage. Anaesthetic induction chamber.	Guillotine restraint device. Specially designed harnesses, e.g. Velcro swanwrap.	Snake tube. Sandbag.
Lend added strength or extend the arms	Net.	Rope. Snare.		Snake hook or grab[b].
Subdue the animal	Physical restraint (with or without gloves)[c].		Towel wrap.	Lower temperature[a].
Special techniques	Several methods are available[c].	Hypnosis of rabbits.	Tonic immobility (galliforms).	Tonic immobility (dorsal recumbency) in lizards or crocodilians. Vaso-vagal response in lizards[d].

[a] No analgesia.
[b] Care must be taken not to cause injury (do not handle sloughing reptiles).
[c] The greatest protection of all is a detailed knowledge of the biology and behaviour of the species.
[d] Pressure on the eyes causes hypotension and bradycardia – recovery is spontaneous or follows a tactile or sonic stimulus (Malley, 1997).

Anaesthesia of mammals, birds and reptiles

Diagnostic or surgical interventions often require manipulation or restraint. Simple, non-invasive procedures, such as radiography or ultrasonography, may sometimes be possible using physical methods alone, provided humane considerations are met. Examples of such methods are described in Table 10.21 and Fig. 10.12.

More invasive procedures (in terms of duration, levels of pain, etc.) will generally require chemical restraint. Variation in biology, including anatomy, physiology or behaviour, makes anaesthesia of exotic species a particularly interesting and challenging task. Fundamentals, however, remain the same as for domestic species, and it is important to emphasise that the needs and well-being of an animal during the pre- and post-operative periods are an integral part of the anaesthetist's responsibilities. Thought must be given to a

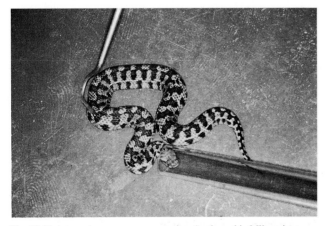

Fig. 10.12 Aggressive or venomous snakes (such as this Milos viper, *Macrovipera schweizeri*) can be safely restrained and examined using a Perspex snake tube.

reduction in pain, distress and mortality rate, as well as to improvements in the speed and quality of recovery.

Pre-operative preparations

Pre-operative assessment is important. The species *must* be identified. It should then be maintained at its PBT. This is particularly vital in reptiles due to their ectothermic nature. The preferred body temperature of an individual reptile can be taken to be its body core temperature (usually measured as the cloacal temperature) at which its heart rate is as close as possible to that calculated by the following allometric formula (Malley, 1997): heart rate (pulse) = 34 (bodyweight $[kg])^{-0.25}$. Temperatures for common species are suggested in a number of texts (e.g. Jackson and Cooper, 1981; McKeown, 1986) and examples are given in Table 10.8. In practice, given a choice, reptiles will select their own preferred body temperature and so it is generally simpler and safer to offer a thermal gradient (Davies, 1981), for example, by use of a heat-lamp or heat-pad at one end of the vivarium.

Patients should be allowed to acclimatise to their environment. During this period, food and water intake, bodyweight, urine and faecal loss, and other biological parameters, can be measured. For the more sensitive patient or where facilities for hospitalisation are inadequate, resulting in increased stress or risk of cross-infection, time away from the normal home environment should be minimised. This biological data may instead be provided by the owner.

Body condition must be assessed. Weight to length ratios (e.g. weight to cube of carapace length in chelonians; weight to ulnar ('carpal') length in birds) are useful indicators, as is the simple evaluation of pectoralis musculature in birds. Blood samples may be taken for routine biochemistry and

Table 10.22 Methods of fluid replacement

Mammals	Birds	Reptiles
Oral administration of proprietary rehydration fluids. Parenteral administration – saline or Hartmann's solution. Given subcutaneously, intraperitoneally, intraosseously or intravenously.	Oral administration of proprietary rehydration fluids. Parenteral administration – saline, dextrose saline, or Hartmann's solution. Given subcutaneously, intramuscularly, intraosseously or intravenously.	Immersion in potable water at preferred body temperature. Oral administration of proprietary rehydration fluids – prepared as for mammals then diluted a further 10% with potable water. Parenteral administration – a mixture of one part each of non-lactated dextrose saline, Ringer's solution, and water for injection. Given epicoelomically, intracoelomically, intraosseously or intravenously.

haematology. It is important to note that reptiles are very susceptible to bacterial infections introduced through the skin and so the site of any injection must first be thoroughly scrubbed with povidone-iodine solution. Hydration status should be assessed and corrected, if necessary (see Chapter 22, Fluid Therapy and Shock). Methods of fluid replacement are described in Table 10.22. All fluids should be given at the preferred body temperature.

Ideally, animals should be free from clinical disease. Subclinical disorders, such as chronic respiratory diseases, are also important because they may cause respiratory depression, leading to anaesthetic complications. Normal liver and kidney function is essential for many anaesthetic agents and should be assessed or such agents avoided.

The duration of pre-anaesthetic fasting (withdrawal of food) depends on the species and is summarised in Table 10.23. Fasting is necessary in some species, e.g. chelonians, to avoid compression of the lungs, and in many other species, particularly some mammals and all snakes, to prevent vomiting (with its associated risks of an aspiration pneumonia). It is also important for some diagnostic procedures. Fasting in small mammals and birds, that have a high metabolic rate, can result in hypoglycaemia and is contraindicated.

Pre-anaesthetic handling and medication

Experienced animal handling is vital. Great care must be taken to minimise stress to the patient at all times,

particularly during anaesthetic induction. Lighting and noise levels should be reduced, mobile phones and pagers switched off. It is often beneficial to minimise physical contact. This may be achieved by use of an anaesthetic induction chamber or by using fast methods of induction. Animals may also be habituated beforehand to the various anaesthetic techniques, e.g. trained to tolerate a facemask.

Pre-anaesthetic medication is often useful. It may allow a reduction in fear or apprehension leading to stress-free induction, a reduction in the dosage of anaesthetic agents, a reduction in salivation or reflex bradycardia, a smoother recovery, and a reduction in pre- and post-operative pain. A variety of agents are used, which include anticholinergics (e.g. atropine and glycopyrronium), phenothiazines, butyrophenones and benzodiazepines.

It is important that all anaesthetic and surgical equipment is prepared and checked prior to the start of any procedure.

General anaesthesia

Methods of induction depend on the species of animal, its size and ability to be physically restrained, its demeanour, for example, whether it is alert and aggressive or sedated and sleepy, the anaesthetic requirements, i.e. whether or not a surgical plane of anaesthesia is required, the presence of any concurrent diseases, the anaesthetic equipment available and the drugs available. Details are given in Table 10.24.

Topical anaesthetic agents (local analgesics) may sometimes be used and can reduce general anaesthetic requirements. Particular care is required in birds, in view of their susceptibility to the toxic effects of these agents.

Once the animal has been anaesthetised, it is important to position it correctly. In general, it is best to avoid dorsal recumbency in birds and reptiles; the weight of viscera on the lungs can reduce the tidal volume and accentuate respiratory embarrassment.

Maintenance of anaesthesia may be achieved by the use of inhalation agents, continuous intravenous infusion or repeated intramuscular injections – the last method being the most variable and unreliable.

Inhalation agents may be administered via a close-fitting facemask, particularly in small mammals and birds.

Table 10.23 Duration of pre-anaesthetic fasting

Species	Time
Mammals (Flecknell, 1997)	Small primates or ferrets – 12–16 hours. Small rodents or rabbits – unnecessary.
Birds (Forbes, In press)	<200 g – rarely required (never more than 3 hours), crop should be empty. Granivorous birds – rarely required. Waterfowl and carnivores – 4–10 hours.
Reptiles (Malley, 1997)	Chelonians or lizards – 18 hours. Snakes – 72–96 hours.

Table 10.24 Common methods and drugs of induction

Species	Oral	Inhalation	Injection Intramuscular	Intravenous
Mammals	Generally unpredictable. Ketamine has been used in primates.	Anaesthetic induction chamber or facemask. Isoflurane (Isoflo; Schering-Plough) or Sevoflurane (Abbott)[a] are agents of choice.	Fentanyl/fluanisone (Hypnorm; Janssen) and midazolam, both given intraperitoneally in small mammals, intramuscularly in large mammals; reversed with butorphanol. Ketamine and medetomidine (Domitor; Pfizer), both given intramuscularly or intravenously; reversed with atipamezole (Antisedan; Pfizer).	
Birds	Rarely used. Tiletamine 5% and zolazepam 5% (Zoletil; Virbac) in birds of prey.	Anaesthetic induction chamber or facemask. Isoflurane (Isoflo; Schering-Plough) or Sevoflurane (Abbott)[a] are agents of choice.	Ketamine and medetomidine (Domitor; Pfizer); reversed with atipamezole (Antisedan; Pfizer). Alphaxalone and alphadolone (Saffan; Schering-Plough). Ketamine with diazepam or xylazine or midazolam. Avoid xylazine in pigeons.	Ketamine and medetomidine (Domitor; Pfizer); reversed with atipamezole (Antisedan; Pfizer). Alphaxalone and alphadolone (Saffan; Schering-Plough). Ketamine with diazepam or xylazine or midazolam.
Reptiles	Not used.	Facemask, isoflurane (Isoflo; Schering-Plough) in lizards only. Tracheal intubation in conscious patient, isoflurane (Isoflo; Schering-Plough) in chelonians, snakes and lizards.	Alphaxalone and alphadolone (Saffan; Schering-Plough). Metomidate in snakes (also intracoelomically). NB: no analgesic properties. Ketamine and medetomidine (Domitor; Pfizer) in Chelonia.	Propofol (Rapinovet; Schering-Plough) commonly used (also intraosseously in Chelonia and saurians). Alphaxalone and alphadolone (Saffan; Schering-Plough).

[a] No product licence in the UK.

High gas flow rates (3–4 times the respiratory minute volume) are usually required. Once asleep, it is preferable to intubate the animal with an endotracheal tube and to use an appropriate anaesthetic circuit. Intubation is particularly important for operations on the head and mouth, or for situations where respiratory monitoring or mechanical ventilation may be required (especially in reptiles). Intubation may be complicated in some species, e.g. it is important not to bypass the lung of small snakes, leading to intubation of the non-absorptive air sac, or not to bypass the carina of chelonians, resulting in insufflation of only one lung. It may also be impossible to intubate very small animals without a significant risk of saliva obstructing the air flow. An Ayre's T-piece is probably the most useful anaesthetic circuit, since most patients will be less than 10 kg in weight. This circuit is best modified with the addition of an open-ended bag to the reservoir tube (Jackson-Rees modified T-piece), thus allowing assisted ventilation. The reservoir volume should be equal to approximately one-third of the animal's tidal volume and the fresh gas flow rate should be about 2–3 times its respiratory minute volume. The use of intermittent positive-pressure ventilation (IPPV) throughout anaesthesia may be necessary in reptiles, especially when premedicants are used. In birds, on occasions where access to the trachea is required, an air sac breathing tube may be inserted through the abdominal wall and used for the maintenance of anaesthesia. In mammals, birds and reptiles, isoflurane (Isoflo; Schering-Plough) or sevoflurane (Abbott) (no product licence) are the inhalation anaesthetic agents of choice.

Total intravenous anaesthesia is possible, e.g. using alphaxalone and alphadolone (Saffan; Schering-Plough) or propofol (Rapinovet; Schering-Plough), but often an additional opioid may be required for its analgesic properties. An infusion pump should be used.

Anaesthetic management

Methods of assessing the depth of anaesthesia are listed in Table 10.25. In addition to the reflexes, it is important to monitor respiration and the cardiovascular system. The depth, rate and pattern of respiration should be recorded. Tools include simple observation of the reservoir bag, use of an oesophageal stethoscope, or use of an electronic apnoea alarm. Cardiovascular parameters, such as the heart rate, rhythm, quality of pulse or tissue perfusion are also important. Tools include observation of a carotid pulse, estimation of the capillary refill time, use of an oesophageal stethoscope, use of an electrocardiogram or use of a Doppler probe to monitor peripheral perfusion. Pulse oximetry is also used to monitor anaesthesia, the lingual clip

Table 10.25 Methods of assessing the depth of anaesthesia

Mammals	Birds	Reptiles (Suborder)
Heart rate	Heart rate	Heart rate
Respiratory rate	Respiratory rate	Respiratory rate
Righting reflex	Pedal reflex	Movement (A)
Response to painful stimuli:	Corneal reflex	Serpentine (slithering) movement (S)
Toe or tail pinch	Cloacal reflex	Muscle relaxation (A)
Ear pinch		Righting reflex (A)
Palpebral reflex (some species)		Tongue withdrawal reflex (S)
Eyeball position		Head-raising reflex (S)
Pupillary dilatation		Response to painful stimuli:
Nystagmus		Skin prick (A)
		Tail pinch (S)
		Pedal (L)
		S-form (strike) posture (S)
		Jaw tone (Ch)
		Bauchstreich reflex (S)
		Laryngeal reflexes in alligators

S = snakes; L = lizards; Ch = chelonians; A = all species.

being applied to the tongue or mucous membranes, or across a toe, footpad or tail, or a small rectal probe being inserted into the rectum, cloaca or oesophagus, as appropriate (Fig. 10.13). Despite such techniques, a good observer (such as a veterinary nurse) is *the* most important form of monitoring.

Body temperature should be monitored, preferably via an oesophageal or rectal electronic thermometer (contra-indicated if using radiosurgery), and kept within the preferred range.

Fluid balance should be maintained. As a routine, fluid should be replaced at a rate of 10–15 ml/kg of bodyweight/hour of general anaesthesia, administered parenterally. Details are given in Table 10.22.

If vomiting or regurgitation occurs, the animal must be placed in a head-down position, and the vomit aspirated from the mouth and the pharynx.

Reversal of anaesthesia

As soon as the procedure is complete, recovery from anaesthesia can begin. In many cases, this simply involves

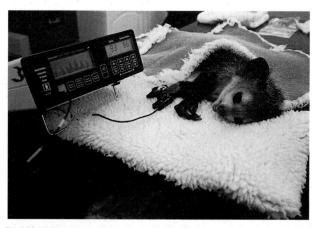

Fig. 10.13 Monitoring anaesthesia is important: use of a pulse oximeter on an anaesthetised patient.

turning off the supply of isoflurane (Isoflo; Schering-Plough), while maintaining oxygen flow. With some of the injectable anaesthetic agents, such as the α_2-agonists (e.g. medetomidine) or the opioids, an antagonist may be used. Rapid recovery is advantageous, especially in patients with high metabolic rates; however, analgesia must be administered where relevant.

Post-operative care

The demarcation between intra- and post-operative care is often not clear, and many of the monitoring procedures and routine therapeutic regimes should be continued until the animal has recovered. In reptiles, this may not be considered to be the case until the righting reflex has fully returned, with normal locomotion.

Warmth and comfort must be provided. The patient should be kept at its preferred body temperature. If possible, an animal incubator should be used. Respiratory depression must be prevented. Cardiorespiratory stimulants, such as doxapram hydrochloride (Dopram-V; Fort Dodge), may be routinely used, particularly in reptiles. Intermittent positive pressure ventilation (with 10% carbon dioxide and 90% oxygen, or with air) can be necessary (and in reptiles, essential) right up until the removal of the endotracheal tube. In mammals, tube removal should occur when the swallowing and cough reflexes return, whereas in reptiles, it may not be appropriate until the animal is fully recovered. Maintained intubation also reduces the risks of an aspiration pneumonia and, in reptiles, where the glottis is normally closed in the relaxed state, intubation can prevent suffocation. Once again, dehydration status should be assessed and corrected, with anticipation of a period of reduced voluntary fluid uptake following anaesthesia. Consideration of analgesia is also important, particularly if agents such as propofol (Rapinovet; Schering-Plough) and isoflurane (Isoflo; Schering-Plough) have been used, with their minimal post-recovery analgesic properties.

The recovery environment is critical. The veterinary nurse must consider potential stressors to the patient and try to eliminate them accordingly. Simple improvements in the surroundings might include: reduced noise and light levels; reduction of draughts; positioning away from busy entrances and passageways; positioning at a suitable height (birds feel more secure in a high position); positioning away from other animals, e.g. barking dogs, birds should not be placed near cats or other predatory birds; provision of a nest box; provision of a suitable substrate; avoidance of unnecessary obstacles and perching before the animal is fully recovered. With careful planning, a number of injuries will undoubtedly be avoided.

Following anaesthesia, food and fluid intake, faecal and urine production, and the animal's demeanour should be monitored. Small patients, with a high metabolic rate, must eat soon after recovery. The total period of starvation should not exceed 3 hours. Low light levels may subdue, but may also prevent feeding. If the patient does not eat voluntarily, gavage feeding should be used. Should *any* problems occur, then assistance from a veterinary surgeon must be quickly sought.

Anaesthesia of amphibians and fish

Common anaesthetic agents of amphibians and fish include dilute solutions of tricaine methane sulphonate (MS222; Sandoz) or benzocaine (Scott, 1991a,b).

For induction, fish are immersed and amphibians submerged up to their nostrils in one of these solutions, preferably within an induction tank (Fig. 10.14). The rate of induction is very variable, and the patient must be carefully monitored. The aim is to reach a stage of minimal activity, essentially sedation, rather than anaesthesia. Once this stage is reached, then the patient is removed from the induction tank and placed on a damp cool towel. Head and tail are covered. Depth of anaesthesia can be varied by syringing either oxygenated water or anaesthetic solution onto the animal and, in particular, its gills, if present. Gills should be

kept wet. For recovery, fish are immersed and amphibians submerged up to their nostrils in clean oxygenated water and, in species with gills, encouraged to move with their mouth open, so that water flows over the gills.

Acknowledgements

The authors would very much like to thank Jackie Belle VN, Paul Flecknell MRCVS, Neil Forbes FRCVS, Dermod Malley MRCVS and Martin Lawton FRCVS for their constructive criticism of, and specialist input into, this chapter.

Further reading

Barnett, J. (1998) Treatment of sick and injured marine mammals. *In Practice*, vol. 20, no. 4, pp. 200–211.

Beynon, P. H., Forbes, N. A. and Harcourt-Brown, N. H. (eds) (1996) *Manual of Raptors, Pigeons and Waterfowl*, BSAVA, Cheltenham.

Beynon, P. H., Forbes, N. A. and Lawton, M. P. C. (eds) (1996) *Manual of Psittacines*, BSAVA, Cheltenham.

Coles, B. H. (1997) *Avian Medicine and Surgery*, 2nd edn, Blackwell, Oxford.

Cooper, J. E. (1986) Animals in schools. *Journal of Small Animal Practice*, vol. 27, pp. 839–850.

Davies, P. M. C. (1981) Anatomy and physiology. In Cooper, J. E. and Jackson, O. F. (eds), *Diseases of the Reptilia*, vol. 1, pp. 9–73, Academic Press, London.

Flecknell, P. A. (1984) The relief of pain in laboratory animals. *Laboratory Animals*, vol. 18, pp. 147–160.

Flecknell, P. A. (1997) *Laboratory Animal Anaesthesia*, 2nd edn. Academic Press, New York.

Flecknell, P. A. (1998) Developments in the veterinary care of rabbits and rodents. *In Practice*, vol. 20, no. 6, pp. 286–295.

Forbes, N. A. (1998) Avian anaesthesia. In *Manual of Anaesthesia*, 4th edn, BSAVA, Cheltenham, in press.

Frye, F. L. (1992) *Captive Invertebrates: A Guide to Their Biology and Husbandry*. Krieger Publishing, Melbourne, FL.

IATA (1993) *IATA Live Animal Regulations*, 20th edn, International Air Transport Association, Montreal, Canada.

Jackson, O. F. and Cooper, J. E. (1981) Nutritional diseases. In Cooper, J. E. and Jackson, O. F. (eds), *Diseases of the Reptilia*, vol. 2, pp. 409–428, Academic Press, London.

Mader, D. R. (ed.) (1996) *Reptile Medicine and Surgery*, W. B. Saunders, Philadelphia.

Malley, D. (1997) Reptile anaesthesia and the practising veterinarian. *In Practice*, vol. 19, no. 7, pp. 351–368.

Mattison, C. (1987) *The Care of Reptiles and Amphibians in Captivity*, 2nd edn, Blandford Press, Poole.

McKay, J. (1989) *The Ferret and Ferreting Handbook*, Rowood Press, Avon.

McKeown, S. (1986) General husbandry and management. In Mader, D. R. (ed.), *Reptile Medicine and Surgery*, pp. 9–19, W. B. Saunders, Philadelphia.

Redig, P. T., Cooper, J. E., Remple, J. D. and Hunter, D. B. (eds) (1993) *Raptor Biomedicine*, University of Minnesota Press, Minneapolis.

Scott, P. W. (1991) Ornamental fish. In Beynon, P. H. and Cooper, J. E. (eds), *Manual of Exotic Pets*, pp. 272–285, BSAVA, Cheltenham.

Williams, D. L. (1991) Amphibians. In Beynon, P. H. and Cooper, J. E. (eds), *Manual of Exotic Pets*, pp. 261–271, BSAVA, Cheltenham.

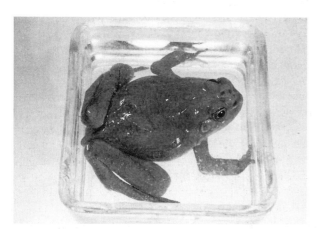

Fig. 10.14 Non-domesticated species may need special equipment or techniques for anaesthesia: this frog is being anaesthetised in water in a glass dish, using a water-soluble agent (benzocaine).

Journals and magazines

Animal Welfare
Aquarist (The)
British Journal of Herpetology
Cage and Aviary Birds
Fur and Feather
Journal of Association of Avian Veterinarians
Racing Pigeon Pictorial
Symposia of the British Wildlife Rehabilitation Council
Tropical Fish Hobbyist

Societies

Bat Conservation Trust
British Chelonia Group
British Falconers' Club
British Herpetological Society

British House Rabbit Association
British Rabbit Council
British Veterinary Zoological Society
British Waterfowl Association
British Wildlife Rehabilitation Council
Commercial Rabbit Association
Federation of British Aquarists' Society
Hawk and Owl Trust (The)
National Cavy Club
National Council for Aviculture
National Fancy Rat Council
National Ferret School (The)
National Hamster Council
National Mouse Club
Royal Pigeon Racing Association
World Pheasant Association

Addresses and details of these can be obtained from the BSAVA *Manual of Exotic Pets* or through the authors.

11

Anatomy and physiology

A. J. Pearson

Introduction

This section is concerned with the anatomy and physiology of the species which most concern the veterinary nurse: the dog and the cat.

Definitions

- **Anatomy** describes the actual structure of the body.
- **Physiology** describes the working of the body.
- **Histology** is the anatomy you can only see down a microscope – the micro-anatomy.
- **Pathology** and **histopathology** describe the diseased states of the body – pathology can be seen with the naked eye, while histopathology (like histology) requires a microscope.

Directions

It is important when describing the structure of a body, be it dog, cat or human, to be able to describe where things lie in relation to one another:

- **Dorsal** and **ventral** mean the sides of the body furthest from and nearer to the ground (in the standing quadruped).
- Within the limbs, the 'top' is still dorsal, but the underneath – the palm of the hand or sole of the foot – are **palmar** (or **volar**) and **plantar**.
- **Cranial** is towards the head end, and **caudal** is towards the tail – except within the head region, where towards the nose is **rostral**.
- Within the limbs, **proximal** is the end of the limb nearer to the body, whereas **distal** is towards the toes – further from the body.
- **Medial** means towards the centre midline of the body, whereas **lateral** means towards the sides.
- **Superficial** and **deep** describe relative distances from the surface of the body.
- **Internal** and **external** refer to relative depths within the organs and body cavities.

It is sometimes necessary to talk about a section through a body and these sections are called **planes**:

- The **median plane** divides the body longitudinally into two equal halves.
- A **sagittal** plane is any plane that lies parallel to the median plane.
- A **dorsal plane** is a horizontal section parallel to the back (or dorsum) of the animal.

- A **transverse plane** or section runs perpendicular to the long axis of the part to be sectioned. For example, a transverse section of the abdomen runs from the vertebral column to the ventral surface of the abdomen, whereas a transverse section of a limb is a horizontal slice across the limb at one level.

The systems of the body

All bodies are made up of a number of systems, each of which has a specific function, e.g.:

- The **respiratory** system takes oxygen into the body and expels waste gases.
- The **digestive** system takes in and processes food and excretes waste.

The systems are divided into three groups: the **structural** systems, the **co-ordinating** systems and the **visceral** systems.

Structural systems

Structural systems make up the basic structure of the body:

- The **skeletal system** consists of the rigid structures that support and protect the soft structures of the body. It is composed mainly of bone and cartilage, plus the tissues that make up the joints.
- The **muscular system** is generally understood to be the skeletal muscle of the body – that which is attached to the skeletal system and under voluntary control. There is muscular tissue elsewhere in the body, e.g. within the visceral systems, but this is not under voluntary control.
- The **integument** is the covering of the body – the skin, hair, claws, etc.
- The **cardiovascular system** carries blood around the body.

Co-ordinating systems

- The **nervous system** carries information to the central nervous system and instructions away from it. Included in this system are the **special senses**.
- The **endocrine system** is also a communication system, carrying the **hormones**, which are chemical messengers, in the blood.

Visceral systems

The visceral systems are all tubular in design and have one or two openings onto the surface of the body.

- The **digestive system** takes in food, digests and absorbs it, and excretes waste.
- The **respiratory system** takes in oxygen and excretes carbon dioxide.
- The **urinary system** removes waste from the body.
- The **reproductive system** enables the organism to replicate itself.

Cells, tissues and systems

Each of the systems of the body is made up of different types of **tissues**, e.g. muscular tissue, nerve tissue, bone. Tissues are made up of three components, which may be present in varying amounts in different tissues.

- The **cells** of the tissue.
- **Intercellular materials** – such as fibres and membranes found between the cells.
- **Fluid** bathing the cells or flowing round them.

The smallest unit of a tissue within the mammalian body is the **cell**. Several different types of tissue may be required to construct an organ such as the kidney, and several organs together make up a **system** within the body, e.g. the urinary system is made up of kidneys, ureters, bladder and urethra.

The structure of the cell

Each cell in the body of a mammal is, in its way, as complex a structure as the whole body. Each cell has the ability to take in nutrients, to expel waste, to grow and to repair itself, to respire and to reproduce. All cells within the mammalian body are specialised to some extent, but they still have all the basic cellular structures and functions (Fig. 11.1).

The cell membrane

The cell membrane surrounds the cell. It is made up of a double layer of **phospholipid**, with **protein** molecules interspersed among them. **Transport** of substances across the cell membrane may be by one of a number of methods:

- Small pores in the membrane allow the passage of very small molecules.
- Some molecules cross the cell membrane by being dissolved in the lipid of the membrane and diffusing through.
- Large molecules depend on what are termed **active transport mechanisms**. Proteins in the cell membrane are able to bind to particular molecules and carry them across the cell membrane. This process requires energy expenditure by the cell, but means that molecules can be moved from an area of low to one of high concentration – which is the opposite of what would occur by simple diffusion. Sodium ions are moved by this method.
- Some substances use **carrier molecules**, but are transported from an area of high concentration outside the cell to a lower concentration inside the cell. Glucose is transported into the cell by this method.

Phagocytosis and pinocytosis

Cells may ingest particles of food or fluid by engulfing them in a vesicle of cell membrane. This process is called **phagocytosis** when applied to solid matter, or **pinocytosis** if fluid is taken into the cell.

The nucleus

The nucleus controls the cell and all its activities. A cell without a nucleus cannot reproduce and will eventually die.

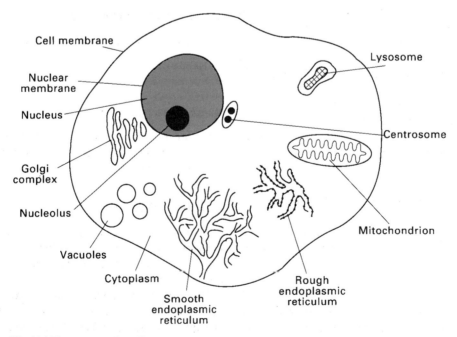

Fig. 11.1 The structure of a cell.

The nucleus of the cell contains its **chromosomes**, which carry the genetic code for the organism and are responsible for coding for the construction of proteins within the cell. The chromosomes are made of **DNA (deoxyribonucleic acid)**. Except when the cell is dividing, the nucleus is amorphous in appearance except for one or more spherical structures called **nucleoli** (singular: nucleolus) which are responsible for the manufacture of **ribosomes**.

Cytoplasm

The cytoplasm is the semi-fluid substance within the cell, which contains protein, salts, glucose and the nucleus and organelles of the cell.

Organelles

Organelles are the various structures visible within the cell, other than the nucleus:

Mitochondria (singular: mitochondrion) consist of an inner and an outer membrane, the inner one of which is folded to increase its surface area. The mitochondria convert energy in food to stored energy within the cell. They do this by using a chemical called **ATP (adenosine triphosphate)** which stores energy in the phosphate group linkage to the rest of the molecule. Energy is released when one phosphate group splits from the rest of the molecule, leaving **ADP (adenosine diphosphate)**. The ADP can then be converted back to ATP and more energy is stored. There may be many mitochondria within a cell.

Lysosomes are membranes within the cytoplasm filled with digestive enzymes. They digest material phagocytosed by the cell, and digest the remains of the cell once it has died. In the case of the phagocytosed matter, the lysosomes are emptied into the **vacuole** containing the engulfed matter.

Endoplasmic reticulum is a network of fine channels running through the cytoplasm. There are two types of endoplasmic reticulum, the rough and the smooth. Rough endoplasmic reticulum has **ribosomes** on it that have been produced in the nucleolus – they give it a rough or knobbly appearance under the microscope. Endoplasmic reticulum and the ribosomes attached to it are responsible for protein synthesis and transport within the cell.

The **Golgi complex** is a series of tubes which store substances such as lysosomal enzymes.

The **centrosome** lies near the nucleus and is made up of two **centrioles** which are important during cell division.

Cell reproduction – mitosis and meiosis

The cells of the body reproduce themselves by a process known as **binary fission** which means that they divide in half. Before this can happen, however, the chromosomes within the nucleus of the cell must replicate themselves, so that there is an identical set of chromosomes for each of the so-called 'daughter cells'. This process of chromosome multiplication and then cell division is called **mitosis** (Fig. 11.2).

Mitosis can be divided into four stages:

- Prophase.
- Metaphase.
- Anaphase.
- Telophase.

What appears to be a resting stage between cell divisions is called **interphase**, during which the chromosomes are duplicated within the nucleus of the cell. By the time the process of mitosis begins, each chromosome consists of two identical **chromatids**, joined together at the **centromere**. The individual chromosomes are not visible in the nucleus during interphase.

During **prophase**, the chromosomes become visible. The long threads of DNA become shorter and fatter, so that they are visible in the nucleus. Also at this stage the centrosome is replicated, and one of the two migrates round to the opposite side of the nucleus.

During **metaphase**, the nuclear membrane breaks down, and all the chromosomes line up along the 'equator' of the cell. The two centrosomes form **nuclear spindle fibres**, consisting of a series of fine tubules that pass from the centrosome on one side of the cell to one of the chromatids of the chromosome.

During **anaphase**, the chromatids separate from one another and move towards the opposite sides of the cell, pulled by the nuclear spindle fibres.

During **telophase**, the cell membrane starts to form a 'waist' and the cell divides into two, leaving one set of identical chromatids on either side of the division. The chromatids then unravel to form a dense nuclear mass and the nuclear membrane reforms, as the cell enters another **interphase**, and replication of chromatids occurs to form complete chromosomes again.

A different type of cell division occurs during the formation of the germ cells – this is called **meiosis** and is dealt with in Chapter 9 on Genetics and animal breeding.

The tissues of the body

There are four types of tissue within the body:

- Muscular.
- Nervous.
- Epithelial.
- Connective.

The structure of muscle and of nervous tissue will be considered under the sections dealing with the muscular and nervous systems.

Epithelial tissue

Epithelial tissue (Fig. 11.3) covers all the surfaces of the body, both inside and out. The skin is epithelial tissue, but so are the linings of all the body cavities and the hollow organs within the body.

The function of epithelial tissue is to protect, but also, depending on its position within the body, to allow absorption across its surface. Where filtration or absorption is required across a layer of epithelium, it has to be as thin

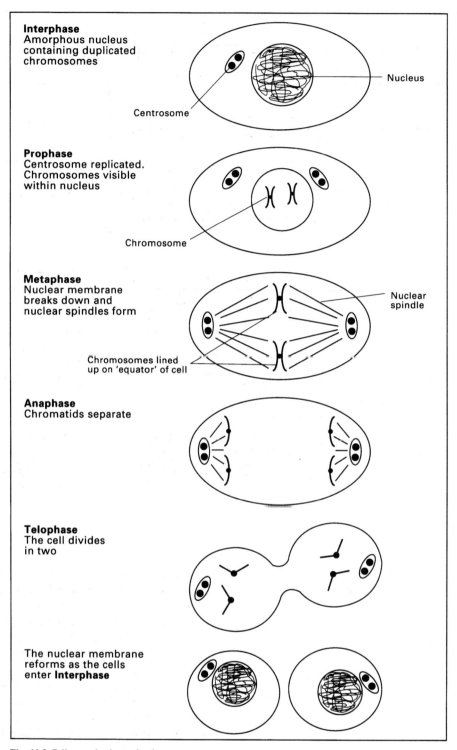

Interphase
Amorphous nucleus containing duplicated chromosomes

Nucleus

Centrosome

Prophase
Centrosome replicated. Chromosomes visible within nucleus

Chromosome

Metaphase
Nuclear membrane breaks down and nuclear spindles form

Nuclear spindle

Chromosomes lined up on 'equator' of cell

Anaphase
Chromatids separate

Telophase
The cell divides in two

The nuclear membrane reforms as the cells enter **Interphase**

Fig. 11.2 Cell reproduction: mitosis.

as possible. **Simple epithelium** is just one cell thick, and the cells may be **squamous** (flattened), **cuboidal** or **columnar** (elongated) in shape. Where a thicker, more protective layer of epithelium is required, there are two or more layers of cells, and the epithelium is known as **stratified** or **compound**.

Mucus and cilia

Many parts of the body are lined with a mucous epithelium or a ciliated mucous epithelium. **Mucus** is a thick proteinaceous fluid secreted by specialised epithelial cells to protect the tissue beneath. (Note: 'mucus' is the noun: 'mucous' is the adjective). **Cilia** are very small hair-like projections on the surface of epithelial cells that move mucus along by constant waves of movement.

Keratinisation

Keratin is a protein that is found in the top layers of a stratified squamous epithelium in positions where a great deal of protection is required, such as the skin. The cells in

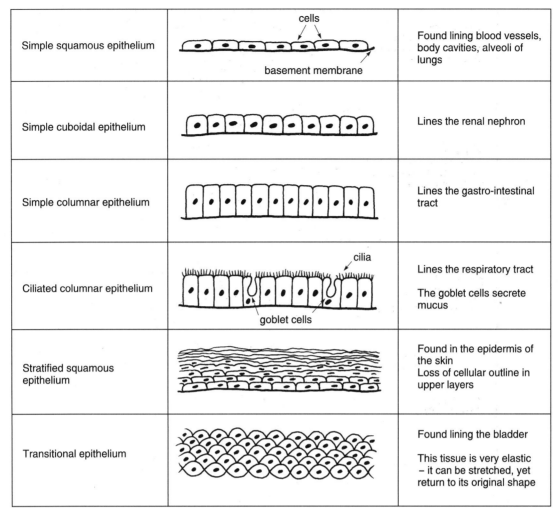

Simple squamous epithelium	cells / basement membrane	Found lining blood vessels, body cavities, alveoli of lungs
Simple cuboidal epithelium		Lines the renal nephron
Simple columnar epithelium		Lines the gastro-intestinal tract
Ciliated columnar epithelium	cilia / goblet cells	Lines the respiratory tract. The goblet cells secrete mucus
Stratified squamous epithelium		Found in the epidermis of the skin. Loss of cellular outline in upper layers
Transitional epithelium		Found lining the bladder. This tissue is very elastic – it can be stretched, yet return to its original shape

Fig. 11.3 Epithelial tissues.

the outer layers of the epithelium dry out and form a tough layer of keratin that protects the underlying tissue from bacterial invasion, drying and physical damage.

Transitional epithelium

Transitional epithelium is a stratified epithelium that is very elastic. It can be stretched to many times its resting size, and then return to its original size. It is found lining the bladder and ureters.

Glands

All the glands in the body are derived from epithelial tissue. Glands may be unicellular or multicellular (Fig. 11.4).

An example of **unicellular glands** is the modified epithelial cells found in the linings of, for example, the digestive tract, secreting mucus to protect the lining of the tract. These very simple glands are called **goblet cells**.

Some **multicellular glands** are quite obviously of epithelial origin, as they lie mainly within the layers of epithelial tissue and have ducts connecting them to the surface of the epithelium, e.g. sebaceous glands in the skin and sweat glands in the paw pads.

Some glands still have ducts connecting them to the epithelial surface, but are found beneath the epithelium, e.g. salivary glands, discharging their secretion into the mouth. Glands with ducts are called **exocrine glands**.

Some glands are not only remote from an epithelial surface, but also no longer have a duct to discharge their secretion. These are called **endocrine glands**. The secretions of **endocrine** glands are called **hormones** and they are carried in the blood to their target organ, which may be in a different part of the body to the gland. Examples of endocrine glands are the thyroid gland and the gonads (testes and ovaries).

Connective tissue

Connective tissue (Fig. 11.5) binds all the other body tissues together. It supports them and acts as a transport system.

Connective tissues often have a lot of intercellular material among the actual cells – this material is called the **ground substance**.

The types of connective tissue are:

- Loose connective tissue.
- Dense connective tissue.
- Bone.

● Cartilage.
● Blood.

Details of the structure of bone will be dealt with in the section on the skeletal system, and that of blood in the section on blood and the circulatory system.

Loose connective tissue

Loose connective tissue is sometimes called **areolar tissue**. It is found between the surrounding organs within the body, and forms the layer between the skin and the tissues beneath.

It consists of a loose network of **collagen fibres** and **elastic fibres** with a few cells such as fibroblasts (which produce the fibrous collagen fibres) and **fat cells**. There are usually blood vessels and nerves within the tissue.

Adipose tissue

Adipose or **fatty tissue** is essentially the same as areolar tissue, but the spaces between the collagen and elastic fibre network are filled up with fat cells. It forms a food reserve and an insulating layer, and in some cases pads of fat support and protect vulnerable organs such as the kidney and the eye.

Dense connective tissue

Dense connective tissue is also known as **fibrous tissue**. It consists of large numbers of collagen fibre bundles with fibroblasts between them. The fibres may be arranged at random, with the fibres all running in different directions, or they may be arranged in parallel, as in tendons or ligaments. This latter arrangement gives the tissue great strength. The

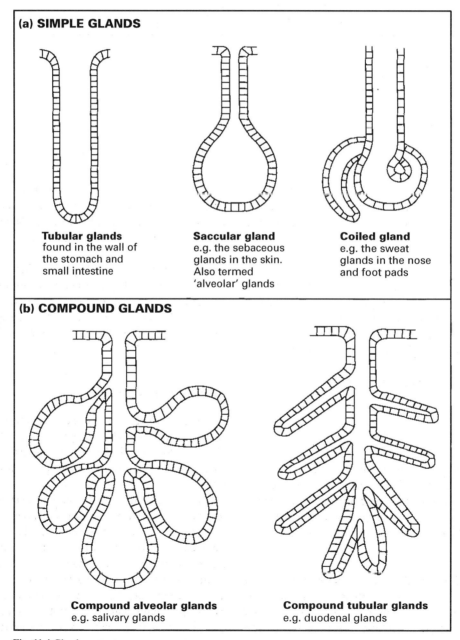

(a) SIMPLE GLANDS

Tubular glands
found in the wall of the stomach and small intestine

Saccular gland
e.g. the sebaceous glands in the skin. Also termed 'alveolar' glands

Coiled gland
e.g. the sweat glands in the nose and foot pads

(b) COMPOUND GLANDS

Compound alveolar glands
e.g. salivary glands

Compound tubular glands
e.g. duodenal glands

Fig. 11.4 Glands.

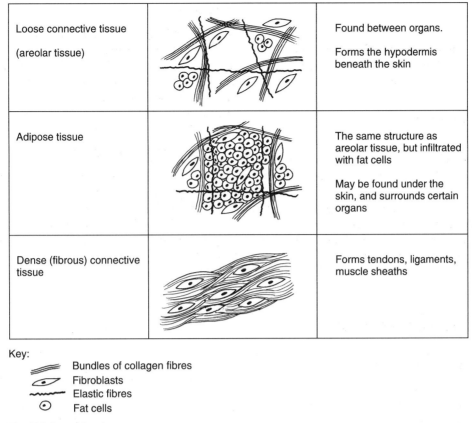

Loose connective tissue (areolar tissue)		Found between organs. Forms the hypodermis beneath the skin
Adipose tissue		The same structure as areolar tissue, but infiltrated with fat cells. May be found under the skin, and surrounds certain organs
Dense (fibrous) connective tissue		Forms tendons, ligaments, muscle sheaths

Key:

- Bundles of collagen fibres
- Fibroblasts
- Elastic fibres
- Fat cells

Fig. 11.5 Connective tissue.

sheaths of **fascia** that support and bind together muscles throughout the body are also made up of dense connective tissue, but this time arranged to form flat sheets of tissue.

Cartilage

Cartilage (Fig. 11.6) is a dense, clear, blue-white substance which is tough and (with the exception of elastic cartilage) quite rigid. It is found principally at joints and between bones. It does not contain blood vessels (unlike bone) but is covered by a membrane called **perichondrium**, from which it derives its blood supply.

There are three different types of cartilage:

- Hyaline cartilage.
- Fibrocartilage.
- Elastic cartilage.

Hyaline cartilage. The cartilage-producing cell is called a **chondrocyte**. Hyaline cartilage consists of chondrocytes lying within a **hyaline matrix**, with a few very fine collagen fibres running through it. It is a very smooth tissue, and forms the rings of the trachea and the articular surfaces of joints.

Fibrocartilage. Fibrocartilage is stronger than hyaline cartilage. It has a similar basic structure, but has more collagen fibres in it, and is therefore stronger. Fibrocartilage surrounds and so deepens the articular sockets of some bones (e.g. the acetabulum of the pelvis and the glenoid

fossa of the scapula). It also forms the intra-articular cartilages (**menisci**) of the stifle, and contributes to the structure of the intervertebral discs of the vertebral column and the cartilaginous parts of the ribs.

Elastic cartilage. Elastic cartilage has a hyaline matrix and chondrocytes, but also numerous elastic fibres within the matrix, which give the tissue its elastic properties. It is found in the pinna of the ear and in the epiglottis of the larynx. It is very flexible and readily springs back into shape when deformed.

The body cavities

There are two main body cavities: the **thorax**, and the **abdomen and pelvis**. (Sometimes the latter cavity is divided into abdominal and pelvic cavities, but this is an unnatural division as there is no physical barrier between them.)

All the body cavities are lined with **serous endothelium**. A serous membrane is a shiny, smooth membrane that produces a watery fluid to act as a lubricant between two surfaces (as opposed to the mucous membrane that produces the thick proteinaceous mucus as a protective layer). Examples of serous membranes are the pleura that lines the thoracic cavity and the peritoneum that lines the abdominal cavity. The fluids within the cavities are called the pleural and peritoneal fluid, respectively. **Endothelium** is simply the term used for an epithelium lining a body cavity.

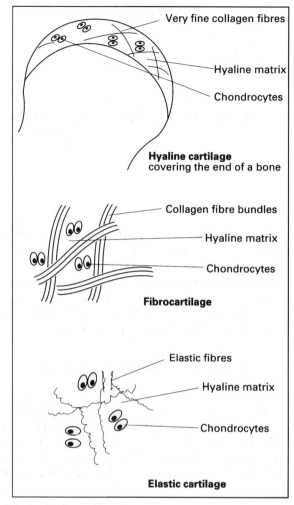

Fig. 11.6 Types of cartilage.

The boundaries of the thoracic cavity are:

● Anteriorly, the thoracic inlet.
● Dorsally, the thoracic vertebrae and hypaxial muscles.
● Ventrally, the sternum.
● Laterally, the ribs and intercostal muscles.
● Posteriorly, the diaphragm.

The boundaries of the abdominal/pelvic cavity are:

● Anteriorly, the diaphragm.
● Dorsally, the sub-lumbar hypaxial muscles.
● Ventrally, the abdominal muscles and the floor of the pelvis.
● Laterally, the abdominal muscles and the lateral walls of the pelvis.
● Posteriorly, the pelvic diaphragm.

The thoracic cavity

The serous lining of the thoracic cavity is called **pleura**. The thoracic cavity is divided into two pleural cavities (Fig. 11.7), between which lies the potential space of the **mediastinum** (a double layer of pleura that separates the two pleural cavities from one another). The lungs lie in out-pouchings of the pleura. The pleural cavities themselves are empty except for a small amount of the lubricating pleural fluid. Different parts of the pleura are given different names

according to their position: so the diaphragmatic pleura covers the diaphragm, the costal pleura covers the ribs, the visceral pleura overlies the lungs themselves and the double layer of pleura that separates the two pleural cavities is called the mediastinal pleura.

The mediastinum varies from species to species in its toughness. In humans, and to a lesser degree in the dog and cat, it is quite strong – it is possible for one lung to collapse yet leave the other functioning efficiently. However in the ruminants, and particularly the horse, the mediastinum is weak and damage to the chest wall may lead to the collapse of both lungs.

The abdominal cavity

The serous membrane lining the abdominal cavity is called the **peritoneum**. All the viscera within the abdominal cavity lie either behind the peritoneum (e.g. the kidney lies against the dorsal body wall in its kidney capsule) or in a fold of mesentery, which is a continuation of the peritoneum. So, although the abdominal cavity is full of viscera, the peritoneal cavity, like the pleural cavity, simply contains a little serous fluid.

The peritoneum that lines the cavity and is attached to the body wall is called **parietal peritoneum**. The layer covering the viscera is called **visceral peritoneum**.

The **pelvic diaphragm** consists of the structures that close the posterior part of the pelvis – mainly the muscles that surround the muscular anal sphincter. The pelvic diaphragm is important as it has to hold its shape against the regular muscular straining involved in defecation. Weakness in this area can lead to 'perineal hernia', with the breakdown of the muscles of the pelvic diaphragm.

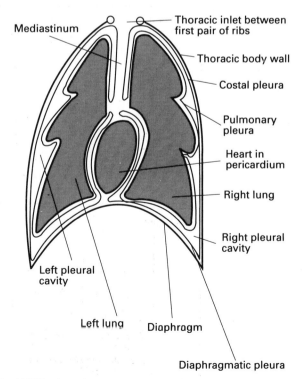

Fig. 11.7 Horoizontal section of thorax, to illustrate pleurae and pleural cavities.

The chemistry of the cell

Although cells may be specialised to perform different tasks, they all share some basic biochemical processes.

Before considering gross anatomical structure, it is useful to consider some of the basic chemical processes within the cell and in the generalised multi-cellular animal. We need to consider respiration, digestion, temperature regulation and water balance at a simple, cellular level, before we can understand how these functions are performed in a complicated mammal.

Inorganic content of the body

The body is made up of organic materials (carbon-based molecules) and inorganic materials.

The **inorganic** content of the body is made up of water, and minerals such as calcium, phosphorus, magnesium, chlorine, iron, copper, manganese and iodine. None of these minerals exists in the body in the form of the pure element (copper in its pure form is a brown metal and chlorine is a gas); they are instead in the form of **ions**.

Ions are positively or negatively charged particles which may be made up of one element, e.g. H^+ the hydrogen ion, or of two or more in combination, e.g. OH^- the hydroxyl ion, or HCO_3^- the bicarbonate ion.

An **electrolyte** is a substance that will split up into ions when it is dissolved in water. Sodium chloride (salt) is an electrolyte; in solution it splits up into Na^+ and Cl^-.

Ions that carry one or more positive charges are called **cations**, ions that carry one or more negative charges are called **anions**.

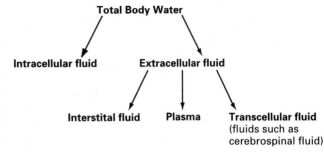

Fig. 11.8 Water in the body.

Water

About 60–70% of the body's weight is water. This is divided between the **intracellular water** and the **extracellular water**.

The extracellular water can be divided into **plasma** (the fluid part of the blood), the **interstitial fluid** that surrounds the cells of the body outside the blood vascular system, and the **cerebrospinal fluid** and **lymph**. See Fig. 11.8.

Diffusion, osmosis and semipermeable membranes

A semipermeable membrane is one that allows the passage through it of small molecules, but not large ones.

Diffusion is the movement of substances from a fluid of high concentration to a fluid of lower concentration, across a semipermeable membrane, in an effort to equalise the two concentrations (Fig. 11.9). Diffusion can only occur if the molecules are small enough to pass through the holes in the semipermeable membrane.

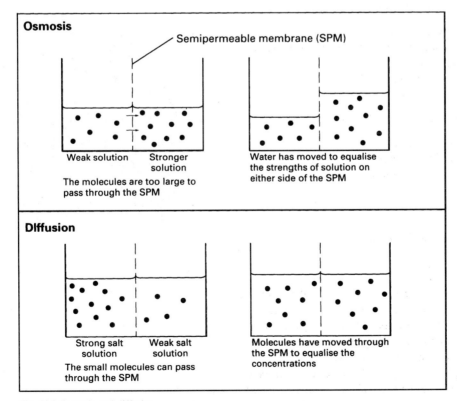

Fig. 11.9 Osmosis and diffusion.

Osmosis is the movement of water through a semi-permeable solution to a stronger (higher concentration) solution.

If the actual molecules in the solution on either side of the membrane are too large to pass through the holes, the water will tend to move instead, in order to equalise the concentration on both sides of the membrane (Fig. 11.9).

Osmotic pressure is the pressure difference that would be required to stem the flow of water across the membrane.

Osmotic pressures within the body are described relative to the osmotic pressure of plasma. A fluid, relative to plasma, is either **isotonic** (the same osmotic pressure), **hypertonic** (a greater osmotic pressure) or **hypotonic** (a lower osmotic pressure).

The osmotic pressure of plasma is maintained largely by the plasma proteins.

Fluid balance. The water in the body is constantly moving. It is taken in through food and drink, and is lost not just through the obvious means, in the urine and faeces, but also through tears, sweat, vaginal secretions and the moisture in expired air. It may also be lost to the body in increased amounts if an animal vomits, has diarrhoea or loses blood after an accident.

It is very important to the body to maintain the correct fluid balance between input and output.

The water content of the body varies with age and obesity – it is slightly higher in young animals (65–70% of bodyweight) and slightly lower in older or obese ones (60–65%).

Typical water losses from the body per 24 hours are:

- 20 ml/kg through respiratory system and sweat.
- 20 ml/kg in urine.
- 10–20 ml/kg as faecal losses.

Thus a healthy animal, eating, drinking and producing urine and faeces, needs between 50 and 60 ml of water/kg bodyweight per day. A vomiting animal, or one with, say, a copious vaginal discharge or diarrhoea, will need much more.

Acidity and alkalinity. It is also important for the body to maintain the correct degree of acidity or alkalinity.

An acid is a substance that liberates hydrogen ions in solution, and an alkali or base is one that accepts hydrogen ions.

For example the following equation:

$$H_2CO_3 \rightleftharpoons H^+ + HCO_3^-.$$

means that carbonic acid (H_2CO_3) in solution gives hydrogen ions and bicarbonate ions. Carbonic acid is an acid because it gives up or produces a hydrogen ion in solution. The bicarbonate is an alkali or base, because, if the chemical reaction is reversed, the bicarbonate will accept the hydrogen ion to form carbonic acid.

The acidity of a solution is measured by its hydrogen ion concentration, on a scale of 1 to 14, and is called the pH value. A neutral pH is 7; acidity increases as the numbers decrease, and alkalinity or basicity increases as the number increases.

Body fluids are at pH 7.35 and it is very important that they are kept stable at this level.

Because the pH scale is logarithmic, an increase or decrease of 1 means a 10-fold increase in acidity or alkalinity.

Other inorganic substances within the body

The most important inorganic substances after water are the minerals **calcium, phosphorus** and **magnesium**. These are stored in the body within the bones and teeth, and give rigidity and strength to these structures. They are also essential for muscle and nerve function, and play a part in blood clotting and in milk production.

It is important not only to have sufficient of these minerals but also, particularly in the case of phosphorus and calcium, to have them in the correct proportions.

Sodium, potassium and **chloride** are important in the regulation of fluid balance between the intracellular and extracellular fluid. Sodium and chloride are found mainly in the extracellular fluid, whereas potassium is mainly found within cells.

Iron and **copper** are found in all tissues but are particularly important in the production of **haemoglobin**, the oxygen-carrying compound within the blood.

Organic compounds within the body

Organic compounds are chemicals built on a carbon base.

Three types of organic compound are important to the body:

- **Amino acids and proteins.**
- **Sugars and carbohydrates.**
- **Fatty acids and lipids.**

These are the main classes of foodstuffs.

Amino acids and proteins

Amino acids are the building blocks of proteins. Two amino acids join together to form a **peptide**; when a larger number join together the new unit is called a **polypeptide**; and when there are several hundred it is called a **protein**. This process of joining together simple units to make complex ones is called **polymerisation**.

Amino acids contain carbon, hydrogen, oxygen and nitrogen, and may also contain sulphur and iodine. There are 20 different amino acids, which are constant throughout nature.

Proteins within the body may be either **structural** (such as collagen and keratin) or **functional** (such as enzymes and hormones).

Dietary proteins must be broken down to amino acids before they can be absorbed by the body.

Sugars and carbohydrates

Sugars are made up of carbon, hydrogen and oxygen. Simple sugars join together in chains to form the **polysaccharides** or **carbohydrates**. Sugars are important as a source of energy for the animal and are stored in the body as **glycogen**, a polysaccharide. Carbohydrates must be broken down to simple sugars before they can be absorbed by the body.

Fatty acids and lipids

Fatty acids are also made up of carbon, hydrogen and oxygen. **Lipids** are important in the formation of cell membranes and steroids, in the insulation of nerves and, in the form of fat, as a food store and insulation against cold. Lipids must be broken down to fatty acids before they can be absorbed by the body.

Enzymes

Enzymes are organic catalysts. A catalyst is a substance that assists or accelerates a chemical reaction without itself taking part in the reaction or being changed by it in any way.

Enzymes are involved in chemical reactions throughout the body – they assist in the breakdown of food in the gut and regulate the chemical reactions going on all the time in every cell.

Chemical reactions within the body

The **Law of Conservation of Energy** states that energy cannot be created or destroyed, but it can be stored as potential energy, or dissipated as heat or electrical energy.

Some chemical reactions need or use up energy, others release it. A chemical reaction requiring energy is called an **anabolic reaction**, whereas one releasing energy is called a **catabolic reaction**.

The body is in a constant state of degradation and repair all the time; throughout the body, there are catabolic and anabolic reactions releasing and using energy. The sum of all this energy use, be it gain or loss, is the **total metabolism** of the body.

The **basal metabolic rate** (BMR) is defined as the rate at which a resting animal produces heat.

All animals require energy. Plants use solar energy and carbon dioxide to produce sugars and carbohydrates. Animals eat plants, or they eat other animals that have eaten plants, and so they in turn have access to the stored solar energy.

The skeletal system

The skeletal system consists of the hard structures that protect and support the soft parts of the body. Usually included in this are the bones, and also the cartilage and the joints that connect the bones and provide for movement between them.

The functions of the skeleton are:

● To support the body.
● To provide leverage for voluntary muscles, and surfaces for their attachment.

● To protect the soft internal organs of the body, especially those inside the chest (the heart and lungs).
● To provide a store of minerals, particularly calcium and phosphorus, for use in the body.

The structure of bone

There are two types of **bone tissue**:

● **Compact bone**.
● **Spongy bone**.

Compact bone (Fig. 11.10) is the hard white substance we think of as bone. It is a complex tissue, in the form of a series of canals running along the length of the bone, surrounded by layers of bone tissue. The canal in the centre of each of these **Haversian systems** carries the blood vessels, nerves and lymphatics that serve the bone.

The bone tissue itself consists of:

● Calcium-containing minerals, chiefly **calcium phosphate**.
● **Collagen** fibres.

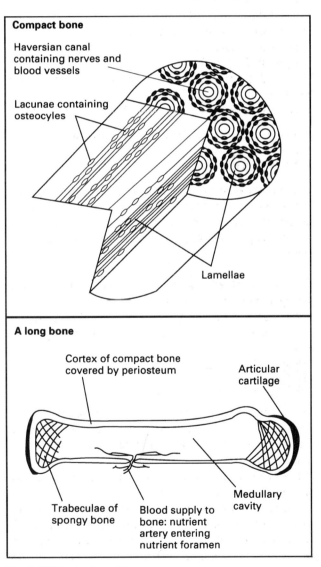

Fig. 11.10 The structure of bone.

- **Mucopolysaccharide polymer**, forming the ground substance.
- **Osteocytes** (bone cells) within **lacunae** or spaces within the bone lamellae.

Compact bone is found in the cortices (the outer layer) of all bones.

In **spongy** or **cancellous bone** the Haversian canal systems are spread widely apart, and the spaces between them are filled with red bone marrow, which is made up of fat and blood cells. This type of bone tissue is found in the ends of long bones, and forms the core in both short and flat bones.

All bones are covered by a tough fibrous membrane called the **periosteum**.

Bones can be classified as one of three types by shape and composition:

- Long bones.
- Flat bones.
- Irregular bones.

Long bones have a shaft and two ends (Fig. 11.10); the proximal end is often called the 'head' of the bone. They have an outer layer of compact bone (a cortex), with spongy bone at the extremities, forming lines of **trabeculae**, which give strength to the bone without adding too much to its weight.

Long bones have a medullary cavity, which is filled with marrow. However, most of the blood cell formation takes place at the ends of the bone, among the spongy bone.

Flat bones consist of two layers of compact bone with a layer of spongy bone between them. Examples of flat bones are those of the vault of the skull, the scapula and the pelvis.

Irregular bones are also made up of two layers of compact bone with spongy bone between them. Examples of irregular bones are those of the vertebral column, and the carpal and tarsal bones. The carpal and tarsal bones are sometimes put in a separate category as 'short' bones.

Sesamoid bones are small bones that develop within a tendon to ease the passage of the tendon over a joint. Examples are the patella, protecting the tendon of the muscle quadriceps femoris as it passes over the stifle, and the proximal and distal sesamoids in the digits.

Development of bone

Bones form by one of two methods:

- Intramembranous ossification.
- Endochondral ossification.

Ossification is the term used for the development of bone.

Membrane bones – those that form by **intramembranous ossification** are formed between two layers of membrane which are the layers of periosteum. An example of membrane bones is the flat bones of the skull.

In the case of **endochondral ossification**, the bone develops from a cartilage model of the bone formed within the embryo (Fig. 11.11).

Centres of ossification appear within the cartilage; there may be as few as two or as many as seven. Centres of ossification start as groups of bone-producing cells called **osteoblasts**, that break down the cartilage and lay down bone instead. The bone tissue gradually extends towards the ends of the bone and a little later from the extremities towards the shaft.

The area of bone development within the shaft of the bone is called the **diaphysis**, and each area that develops towards the ends of the bone is called an **epiphysis**. Between the developing diaphysis and the epiphyses is a strip of cartilage called the **epiphyseal plate** or **growth plate**, which is where the growth continues until the plate is obliterated by bone tissue, at which point the bone no longer increases in length.

The **medullary cavity** of the bone develops by the activity of **osteoclasts**, or bone-destroying cells, which remove bone from the centre of the diaphysis, and the continuing activity of osteoblasts laying down bone on the outside of the shaft as the animal grows.

Bone is a living tissue, and has the potential to remodel and change its shape throughout life. The bone of a young animal is relatively smooth, but that of an old one shows roughened areas where periosteum has been pulled away from bone, and remodelling at the site of damaged tendons, as well as possibly arthritic change.

Joints

Joints are formed wherever two or more bones meet – but not all joints allow movement. Other terms for a joint are an **arthrosis** or an **articulation**.

Joints can be classified in three groups:

- **Synovial joints**.
- **Cartilaginous joints**.
- **Fibrous joints**.

Synovial joints

Synovial joints (Fig. 11.12) occur where the articular or joint surfaces of the bones involved are covered with hyaline cartilage. The whole joint is surrounded by a **joint capsule** consisting of an outer layer, which is the continuation of the periosteum, and an inner layer of **synovial membrane** which lines the joint cavity and secretes **synovial fluid**. This fluid lubricates the joint surfaces and provides nutrients for the articular cartilage; it varies in consistency, being more viscous and plentiful in fit and athletic animals but more sparse and watery in the unathletic.

Synovial joints may have stabilising ligaments associated with them, either on the outside or the inside of the joint capsule. Most commonly the ligamentar support is in the form of 'collateral ligaments' that lie on either side of nearly all hinge joints.

Synovial joints may also have one or more fibro-cartilage **menisci** (singular: meniscus) within them, which increase the range of movement of the joint and reduce wear and tear on the articular surfaces. Examples of joints containing

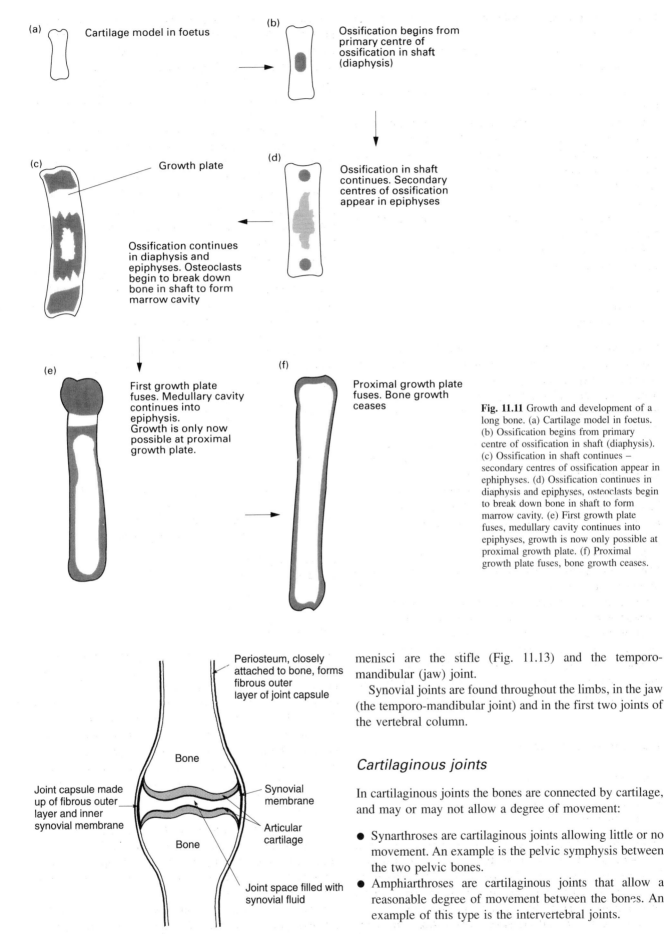

(a) Cartilage model in foetus

(b) Ossification begins from primary centre of ossification in shaft (diaphysis)

(c) Growth plate

(d) Ossification in shaft continues. Secondary centres of ossification appear in epiphyses

Ossification continues in diaphysis and epiphyses. Osteoclasts begin to break down bone in shaft to form marrow cavity

(e) First growth plate fuses. Medullary cavity continues into epiphysis. Growth is only now possible at proximal growth plate.

(f) Proximal growth plate fuses. Bone growth ceases

Fig. 11.11 Growth and development of a long bone. (a) Cartilage model in foetus. (b) Ossification begins from primary centre of ossification in shaft (diaphysis). (c) Ossification in shaft continues – secondary centres of ossification appear in ephiphyses. (d) Ossification continues in diaphysis and epiphyses, osteoclasts begin to break down bone in shaft to form marrow cavity. (e) First growth plate fuses, medullary cavity continues into epiphyses, growth is now only possible at proximal growth plate. (f) Proximal growth plate fuses, bone growth ceases.

Periosteum, closely attached to bone, forms fibrous outer layer of joint capsule

Bone

Joint capsule made up of fibrous outer layer and inner synovial membrane

Synovial membrane

Articular cartilage

Bone

Joint space filled with synovial fluid

Fig. 11.12 A synovial joint. In life, the periosteum, joint capsule and synovial membrane are fused to form one sheet of tissue.

menisci are the stifle (Fig. 11.13) and the temporo-mandibular (jaw) joint.

Synovial joints are found throughout the limbs, in the jaw (the temporo-mandibular joint) and in the first two joints of the vertebral column.

Cartilaginous joints

In cartilaginous joints the bones are connected by cartilage, and may or may not allow a degree of movement:

- Synarthroses are cartilaginous joints allowing little or no movement. An example is the pelvic symphysis between the two pelvic bones.
- Amphiarthroses are cartilaginous joints that allow a reasonable degree of movement between the bones. An example of this type is the intervertebral joints.

The intervertebral disc that separates two adjacent vertebrae consists of two parts: a fibrous outer shell called the annulus

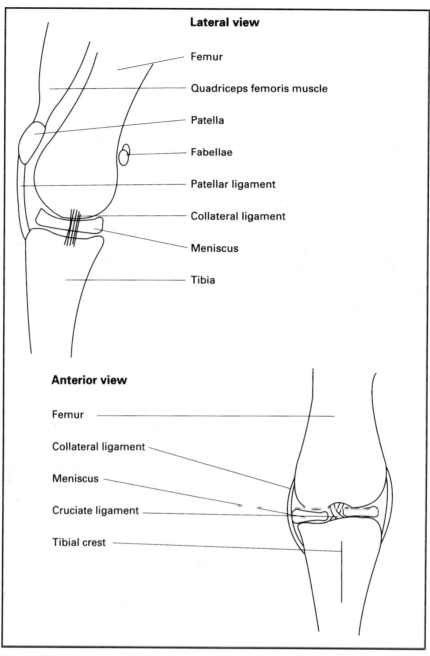

Fig. 11.13 The stifle joint.

fibrosus and a jelly-like inner substance called the nucleus pulposus. These discs form a cushion between the vertebrae that absorbs sudden jarring movements and helps prevent damage to the spinal cord (Fig. 11.14).

Fibrous joints

In fibrous joints the bones are joined together by dense fibrous connective tissue and there is very little or no movement between the bones. An example of fibrous joints is the sutures between the flat bones of the skull.

Both fibrous and cartilaginous joints may eventually become ossified, or may develop pockets of synovial fluid. The latter commonly occurs in the sacro-iliac joint, which tends to relax during parturition.

Movement of joints

The movement of joints can usually be described as being one or more of the following:

- **Flexion** and **extension** – flexion decreases the angle between two bones: extension increases it. Where the movement continues past the straight line, it is called **over-extension**.
- **Abduction** and **adduction** – abduction moves the limb away from the body (as when the male dog lifts his leg): adduction moves it towards or beneath it.
- Inward and outward **rotation** – one end of the bone swivels round in the joint, allowing the other to move in a circle towards or away from the body.
- **Gliding** or **sliding** – when one articular surface slides over the other.

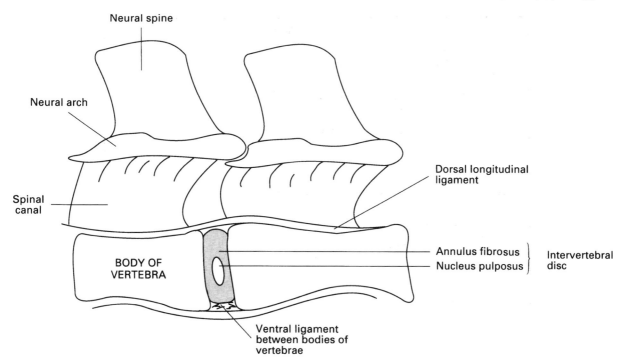

Fig. 11.14 Section through two lumbar vertebrae, showing position of the intervertebral disc.

Anatomists have devised many ways to categorise joints. Here is one relatively simple method:

- **Hinge joints** allow movement in one direction only, e.g. the elbow joint, which flexes and extends again to a (more or less) straight line.
- **Condylar joints** allow flexion, extension to the straight line, then over-extension. An example is the carpal joint.
- **Pivot joints** allow rotation. An example is the radio-humeral joint in the cat.
- **Ball and socket joints** are the most freely moveable of joints. They allow flexion and extension, rotation, and adduction and ɔduction. An example is the hip joint.
- **Plane joints** allow a restricted amount of gliding movement of one bone over another, e.g. the small bones in the carpus and tarsus.

The skeleton

The skeletons of all vertebrate animal – be they mammal, bird, reptile, amphibian or fish – are really very similar. They all have a skull and a vertebral column. They nearly all have four limbs, and each limb has the potential for up to five digits.

They may have different numbers of toes or different numbers of ribs but the basic structure is the same; and the bones have the same names though they may differ in shape from species to species.

The skeleton is divided into three parts:

- **The axial skeleton** – the skull, vertebral column, ribs and sternum.
- **The appendicular skeleton** – the limbs.

- **The splanchnic skeleton** – bony elements that develop in tissue unattached to the rest of the skeleton, e.g. the os penis of the dog and cat.

It is useful when studying the skeleton to have access not only to a skeleton but also to a tolerant live dog, so that each bone can be considered in place, held against the living animal (Fig. 11.15).

The axial skeleton

The bones of the head consist of the skull, the mandible or lower jaw, and the hyoid apparatus.

The skull

Different breeds of dog have very different head shapes, which can generally be placed into one of three categories:

- The long, thin **doliocephalic** head, e.g. the borzoi.
- The short, broad **brachiocephalic** head, e.g. the bulldog.
- The 'normal' **mesocephalic** head.

Although the shapes of the skulls may differ, they all contain the same bones. The skull consists of two parts:

- **The cranium**, which encloses the brain.
- **The maxilla**, which forms the upper jaw and contains the nasal chambers.

The only way to become thoroughly familiar with the skull is to handle one, noting the following points (Figs 11.16 and 11.17):

- At the back and towards the base of the cranium is the **foramen magnum** – the large hole through which the spinal cord enters the cranial cavity.

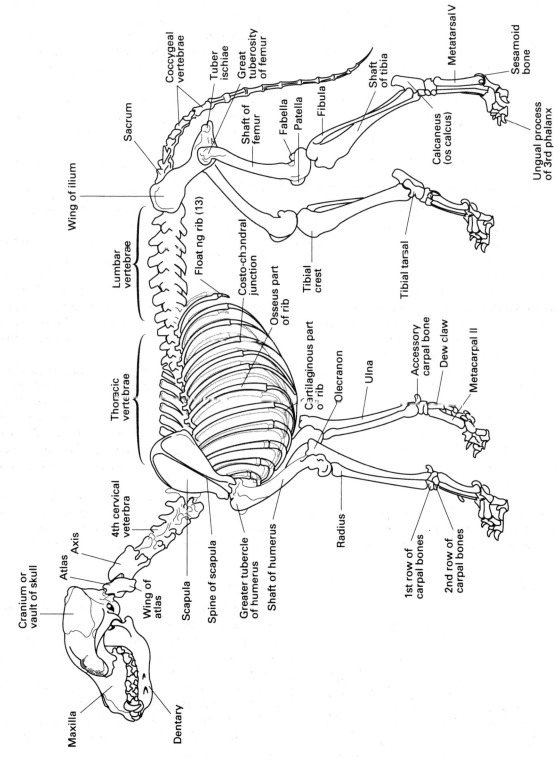

Fig. 11.15 The skeleton of the dog.

Coccygeal vertebrae

Tuber ischiae

Great tuberosity of femur

Metatarsal V

Sacrum

Shaft of femur

Fabella

Patella

Fibula

Shaft of tibia

Sesamoid bone

Calcaneus (os calcus)

Ungual process of 3rd phalanx

Wing of ilium

Floating rib (13)

Costo-chondral junction

Osseus part of rib

Tibial crest

Lumbar vertebrae

Cartilaginous part of rib

Olecranon

Ulna

Accessory carpal bone

Dew claw

Metacarpal II

Tibial tarsal

Thoracic vertebrae

Radius

1st row of carpal bones

2nd row of carpal bones

4th cervical vetebra

Atlas

Axis

Wing of atlas

Scapula

Spine of scapula

Greater tubercle of humerus

Shaft of humerus

Cranium or vault of skull

Maxilla

Dentary

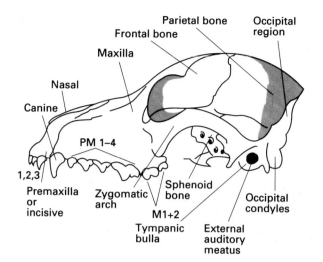

Fig. 11.16 Lateral view of the skull of the dog, showing main bones and permanent dentition.

- At the back of the skull, above the foramen magnum, is a flat area – the **occipital region**. Muscles that support the head on the neck attach here.
- At the base of the skull, on either side of the foramen magnum, are the rounded **occipital condyles**, where the first cervical vertebra articulates with the skull.
- On either side of these are two prominences, the **jugular processes** – again for muscle attachment.
- Just in front of each jugular process is a round protuberance – the **tympanic bulla** – which houses the structures of the middle ear. On the lateral aspect of each tympanic bulla is the **external acoustic meatus** – the opening where the external ear canal attaches to the skull.
- Continuing forward up the ventral midline of the skull, the flat bone enters a canal with walls of bone on either side. This bone forms the roof of the pharynx, and the soft palate is attached between the 'walls' on either side.
- Imagine the soft palate in place, and go up a step on to the **hard palate**, which forms the roof of the mouth. In life, the hard palate is covered with tough, ridged mucous

membrane. It is possible to see on the skull the suture lines between the three bones contributing to the hard palate. These are (from the back) the **palatine**, the **maxilla** and the **premaxilla** (or incisive).

- Now turn the skull on its side, and follow the maxillary bone and the premaxilla on to the side and top of the nasal cavity. One other pair of bones contributes to the maxillary region: the nasals, which run down the top of the nose. Notice that the bones stop well short of where the nose pad (rhinarium) of the dog actually lies. This is because the pad of the nose is supported by cartilage, not bone.
- Two bones make up the vault or top of the cranium. At the front, occupying the 'forehead', is the **frontal bone**, which contains the **frontal sinus**. (A sinus is an air-filled cavity within a bone.) Behind the frontal bones are the **parietal bones**, with the little **interparietal bone** between them.
- Now look at the orbit, which in life contains the eye and eye muscles. See how it is protected on the lateral side by the bony **zygomatic arch**.
- Other bones that lie within the orbit are the little **lacrimal bone**, which carries the lacrimal drainage to the nasal chamber, and the **sphenoid**, a bone near the base of the orbit with many holes, or **foramina**, in it. Foramina are found throughout the skull, particularly on its base. They provide an exit from the cranial cavity for the cranial nerves, and allow blood vessels to enter the cranium to supply the brain.
- The nasal chamber is divided into two longitudinally by a cartilaginous **nasal septum**. In each chamber there are two **nasal turbinates**, which are much-branched, thin, scroll-like bones covered with ciliated mucous epithelium. The dorsal turbinate stops well short of the nostrils, but the ventral turbinate continues forward, forming the **alar fold**, which only terminates just behind the rhinarium (the nose pad).
- On the front of the **mesethmoid bone**, which separates the cranial from the nasal cavities, are some more delicate turbinate bones, the **ethmoturbinates**, which carry smell receptors in their covering mucous membrane.

The mandible

The lower jaw of mammals is made up of two bones, the **dentaries** (Fig. 11.18). They join together at the chin in the **mandibular symphysis**. This is always a point of weakness in the jaw, and a common site for fractures following road traffic accidents, especially in cats.

The lower jaw is divided into two parts, the **horizontal** and the **vertical rami** (singular ramus).

The **coronoid process** provides an area for muscle attachment of the temporal muscle, and the **masseteric fossa** for the masseter muscle.

Teeth

The mammals are unique among the vertebrates in having teeth in different parts of jaw specialised to perform different functions (Figs 11.16 and 11.18). Mammalian teeth

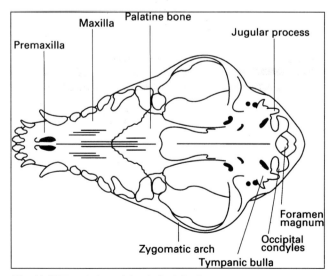

Fig. 11.17 Ventral view of the skull of the dog.

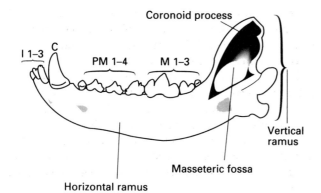

Fig. 11.18 Lateral view of dentary.

can be divided into four groups: **canines (C), incisors (I), premolars (P)** and **molars (M)**. For each species there is a 'dental formula' for the temporary and for the permanent teeth.

The dental formulae for the dog are:

$$\frac{\text{I3 C1 P4 M2}}{\text{I3 C1 P4 M3}} \text{ for the adult and } \frac{3.1.3.0}{3.1.3.0} \text{ for the milk teeth.}$$

There are never any temporary molars.

The dental formulae for the cat are 3/3, 1/1, 3/2, 1/1 for the permanent teeth and 3/3, 1/1, 3/2, 0/0 for the deciduous teeth.

Both of the above are acceptable methods of writing dental formulae. In the example given for the dog, the characters above the line identify the top teeth and those below are the teeth in the lower jaw. For the cat, the formulae have a 'slash' separating top and bottom teeth.

Both pups and kittens lose their deciduous teeth and start to gain their permanent set between (usually) 4 and 5 months old. The process is complete by about 7 months old.

The structure of teeth

- The tooth can be divided into a **crown** and a **root**, the division being at the line of the gum (Fig. 11.19).
- The crown is covered with **enamel**, a very hard, white, calcified substance.
- Beneath the enamel, making up the bulk of root and crown, is **dentine**. Within the dentine is a **pulp cavity** containing the nerves and blood vessels supplying the tooth.
- The root is covered with **cement**, which may overlap with the enamel at the gum margin, and which fixes the tooth firmly in the socket in the bone, via the fibrous **periodontal ligament**.
- The different teeth have different functions.
- The incisors (I) are relatively unimportant in carnivores. They help the canine teeth to hold prey, particularly in the dog.
- The canines (C) are long and sharp, and are the main implement for catching and holding prey.
- The premolars (P) and molars (M) of carnivores are not designed for grinding and crushing (as in the case of

human cheek teeth) but for shearing chunks of meat off bone. Dogs and cats do not chew their food: they swallow pieces, and leave the rest to the digestive juices.

The carnassial tooth

The carnassial tooth is the last premolar in the upper jaw. It is a very large tooth, with three roots, that shears against the first lower molar to form a very efficient scissor-like cutting action.

The hyoid apparatus

The hyoid apparatus is a series of small bones and cartilages that hang down from the tympanic bone of the skull and suspend the larynx below the pharynx. The two arms of the hyoid apparatus move backwards and forwards, allowing the larynx to move back and forth as if on a swing.

The vertebrae

The vertebrae are divided into regions:

- Seven **cervical** vertebrae.
- 13 **thoracic** vertebrae.
- Seven **lumbar** vertebrae.
- Three fused **sacral** vertebrae.
- Up to 20 or more **caudal** or **coccygeal** vertebrae.

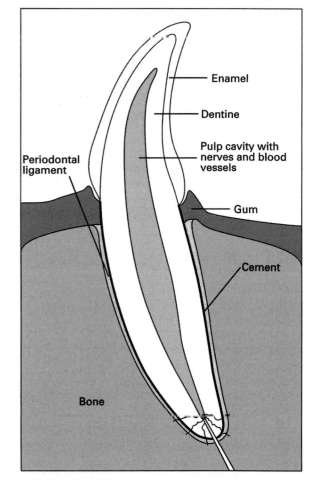

Fig. 11.19 The structure of a tooth.

The vertebrae of each region are distinctive in shape and slightly different in function (Fig. 11.20).

The basic plan of a vertebra is of a **body** or **centrum**, with a **neural arch** above it, topped with a **neural spine**. The spinal cord runs through the neural arch in the **spinal canal**.

There are lateral **transverse processes**. (Where there are ribs, they are called transverse processes, but where there are no ribs they are properly called costo-transverse, to indicate that the rib is incorporated into the process.)

There may also be other processes for muscle attachment.

The cervical vertebrae

The first cervical vertebral is the **atlas**. It has no body, and consists mainly of a canal and a large wing-like pair of transverse processes. In common with all the cervical vertebrae, it has intervertebral foramina running through it, to allow the passage of the vertebral artery to the head. The atlas articulates with the base of the skull.

The second cervical vertebra is the **axis**. It is elongated, has a blade-like neural spine, and a cranially projecting process, the **dens**, attached to its body. The dens (odontoid process) was historically the centrum of the atlas.

Attached to the neural spine of the axis is the **nuchal ligament**, a thick fibrous band that attaches to the neural spine of the first thoracic vertebra, and so helps support the head.

There are synovial joints between the skull, the atlas and the axis, allowing an enormous range of movement. The remaining five cervical vertebrae are similar to each other, with poorly developed spinous processes and fibrous intervertebral joints.

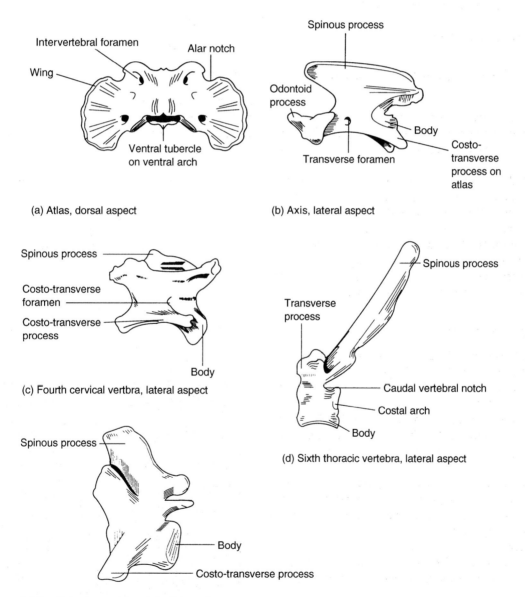

(a) Atlas, dorsal aspect

(b) Axis, lateral aspect

(c) Fourth cervical vertbra, lateral aspect

(d) Sixth thoracic vertebra, lateral aspect

(e) Fourth lumbar vertebra, lateral aspect

Fig. 11.20 Regional differences in vertebral structure. (a) Dorsal view of 1st cervical vertebra (atlas). (b) Lateral view of 2nd cervical vertebra (axis). (c) Lateral view of 4th cervical vertebra. (d) Lateral view of thoracic vertebra. (e) Lateral view of lumbar vertebra.

The thoracic vertebrae

The thoracic vertebrae have short bodies, and tall neural spines that gradually decrease in height throughout the series. They also have articular depressions, or **foveae**, (singular: fovea) on the centra, where they form a synovial joint with the head of the rib, which has a second articulation with the transverse process of the vertebra.

The lumbar vertebrae

The lumbar vertebrae have bulky neural spines and costotransverse processes for the attachment of the powerful lumbar muscles.

The sacral vertebrae

The three sacral vertebrae are fused together to form the sacrum, which forms a support for the pelvis. The joint between the sacrum and pelvis is called the sacro-iliac joint.

The **sacro-tuberous ligament**, which runs from the sacrum to the sciatic tuberosity on the pelvic bone, is a strong band of fibrous tissue that supports much of the musculature of the rump.

The caudal or coccygeal vertebrae

The caudal vertebrae in the dog vary in number from breed to breed, and depending on whether the dog has had its tail docked. They decrease in size as they go down the tail. The first few have a neural arch and costo-transverse processes, but the last few are merely small rods of bone.

The ribs and sternum

The dog and cat both have 13 sets of ribs, which are made partly of bone (the osseous part) and partly of cartilage (the costal cartilage). They have two articulations proximally with the thoracic vertebrae: the **capitulum** articulates with the body of the vertebra, and the **tuberculum** with the transverse process.

The distal ends of the first eight ribs join on to the **sternum**, which is composed of eight **sternebrae**. From the cranial end of the first sternebra projects a bony prominence called the **manubrium**. The last sternebra has a flap of cartilage attached to it called the **xiphisternum**, or **xiphoid cartilage**.

The costal cartilage of ribs 9–12 join on to the cartilage in front of them and form the costal arch. The 13th rib is called the 'floating' rib: it is very short and the end lies free within the muscle of the body wall.

The appendicular skeleton

The forelimb and hindlimb are joined to the body in different ways. The forelimb of the running animal has no pectoral girdle – it is joined to the trunk by muscles. This allows a degree of shock absorption as the limb hits the ground, because the muscular attachment allows the weight of the body to drop between the two forelimbs, instead of

jarring as it would with a rigid bony attachment. The hindlimb, however, has a rigid girdle, because the hindlimb produces the main propulsive force for the body.

It is important to be familiar with the shapes of the bones of the limbs, and to be able to identify them. Most of the long names given to the different features seen on bones are not that complicated once you know the meaning of just a few of the words.

- A tuberosity, a trochanter or a tubercle are all bumps on the bone; they are usually sites for muscle attachment.
- The greater tuberosity is a big bump or protuberance and is usually on the lateral aspect of the bone.
- Most long bones have a head, sometimes a neck, and always a shaft.
- A trochlea is a groove for a pulley (usually a tendon).
- Condyles are rounded articular surfaces. Epicondyles are the bits of the bone lateral to or above the condyles.
- A fossa is a hole or depression in a bone.

The forelimb

The scapula is a flat, roughly triangular bone with an obvious **spine** on the lateral side, that divides the lateral surface into a **supraspinous fossa** and an **infraspinous fossa**. There is a neck, an articular surface called the **glenoid cavity** and an **acromion**, which projects from the distal end of the spine.

The humerus is a classic long bone with a head and a neck, a shaft and greater and lesser tubercles. Proximally it forms the shoulder joint with the scapula, and distally it forms the elbow joint with the radius and ulna.

The clavicle (our 'collar bone') is greatly reduced in the cat and absent in the dog, where it is reduced to a strip of tendon within a muscle. In the cat it is a slim curved bone about 1 cm long embedded in the muscle just anterior to the shoulder, and is easily identified in radiographs of this region.

The radius and ulna lie side by side and are the bones of the forearm.

The ulna has the **olecranon** at its proximal end, and just in front of it the **anconeal process**. It has a deep **articular notch** that holds it close to the humerus.

The radius is a relatively simple rod-like bone that lies on top of the ulna at the elbow joint.

Distally, the ulna lies lateral and the radius medial to the carpus.

The carpus, or wrist, consists of two rows of small bones held together by numerous ligaments. The **accessory carpal bone** projects from the ventral aspect of the carpus, and provides a point for muscle attachment.

The metacarpus of the dog consists of four long metacarpal bones.

There are **five digits** in the forelimb of the dog and cat, the innermost (digit I) being the dew claw, which attaches to the carpus, not to a metacarpal bone.

Each digit (toe) consists of three phalanges (see Fig. 11.27): the proximal (or first) phalanx, middle (or second) and distal (third). The toes are numbered from the medial side in Roman numerals.

The first and second phalanges are relatively simple long bones, but the third phalanx carries the **ungual process** that forms the core of the claw.

Behind the metacarpo-phalangeal joint and the distal inter-phalangeal joint are pairs of small sesamoid bones.

The hindlimb

The pelvis

The two pelvic bones are in fact each formed from three large and one very small bone. The three large bones are the **ilium**, the **ischium** and the **pubis**, and the small bone the **acetabular** bone.

The two pelvic bones are attached to the sacrum, and join each other in the midline at the **pubic symphysis**, so forming the floor of the pelvic cavity.

Lateral to the pubic symphysis on each side is a large hole, the **obturator foramen**, which allows blood vessels and nerves to pass out of the pelvic cavity into the hindlimb.

Parts of the pelvic bone that can be palpated on the live dog include the wing of the ilium and the **ischial tuberosity**, which is the origin of the biceps femoris muscle.

The pelvis articulates with the femur at the **hip joint**, which is a ball-and-socket joint and therefore very mobile – it allows flexion and extension, adduction and abduction and rotation of the femur. The socket for the hip joint is the **acetabulum**. The head of the femur is held in the socket by the **round ligament**, which attaches to the non-articular area in the centre of the acetabulum.

The femur

The femur has a head, a neck, greater and lesser tubercles, a shaft, and lateral and medial condyles. (The hip joint has been discussed above.) **The stifle joint**, at the articulation of femur with tibia and fibula, has been called the most complex joint in the body (Fig. 11.13).

When studying the dry bones, this articulation looks most unstable, but the soft tissues round and in the joint make it very stable, and relatively resistant to injury (considering its position and the stresses put upon it).

The stifle joint is stabilised by four ligaments. The **cruciate ligaments** run across from tibia to femur within the joint, and stop the bones sliding forward and back on one another. The strong **collateral ligaments** on either side of the joint prevent sideways movement.

Two **menisci** cushion the bones, and increase the area for articulation as they move back and forth as the bones move on each other.

Three **sesamoid bones** are also associated with the stifle joint:

- The **patella**, which lies in the tendon of the quadriceps muscle (which inserts on the top of the tibial crest).
- Two **fabellae**, which lie on the caudal aspect of the distal femur, within the origins of the two bellies of gastrocnemius.

The tibia and fibula

The tibia and fibula lie together. The tibia is much the larger bone and has a flat articular surface proximally, for articulation with the femur at the stifle joint. The fibula lies lateral to the tibia throughout its length.

On the front of the tibia is the **tibial crest**, which provides a broad area for muscle attachment.

The tarsus

Like the carpus, the tarsus is made up of a number of small bones closely attached to one another. Two of special significance are the **tibial tarsal** and the **fibular tarsal** bones. These two bones form the articular surface for the tibia and fibula at the hock joint. The fibular tarsal bone, or **calcaneus**, is enlarged to form the point of the hock – the point of attachment for the Achilles tendon.

The metatarsus and digits

The metatarsus and digits of the hindlimb are very similar to those of the forelimb, except that the dew claw is often absent, leaving only digits II to V.

The splanchnic skeleton

The os penis, the bone of the penis, has a groove in it that surrounds the urethra within the penis. In the dog, the groove is on the ventral side of the bone, whereas in the cat (owing to the different position of the penis) the groove is dorsal.

The muscular system

Muscle tissue

There are three types of muscle tissue (Fig. 11.21):

- Skeletal (also called striated or voluntary) muscle.
- Smooth (also called involuntary) muscle.
- Cardiac muscle.

Skeletal muscle is found attached to the bones of the body. It is under the control of the animal and so is also called voluntary muscle.

The cells of striated muscle are called muscle fibres, and they lie parallel to one another in bundles, bound together by connective tissue. Groups of bundles together then make up the whole muscle, which is surrounded by a muscle sheath of fibrous connective tissue.

Smooth muscle is found throughout the body. It is found, for example, in the bowel, in the walls of blood vessels, in the walls of the bladder and uterus and in the respiratory tract. Smooth muscle is not under voluntary or conscious control.

The cells of smooth muscle are spindle-shaped, and have less connective tissue associated with them than does striated muscle.

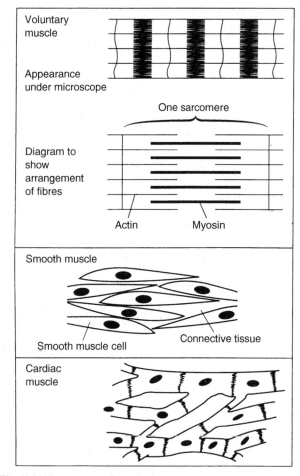

Fig. 11.21 The structure of muscle tissue.

Cardiac muscle, as its name implies, is found only within the heart. The cells are short and cylindrical, and are bound together by connective tissue. The cells are arranged longitudinally, as in voluntary muscle, and contract automatically and rhythmically throughout life – they are not under voluntary control.

Muscle contraction

Muscle contraction occurs as a result of the stimulation of a fibre by a nerve impulse. Muscle fibres are made of thick and thin fibres: the thick fibres are of the protein **myosin**, and the thin ones of **actin**.

In striated muscle the different types of fibres are arranged so that they overlap. Where there are thick myosin fibres, or where the actin and myosin fibres overlap, the tissue looks dark, but where there are just actin fibres, the tissue appears lighter in colour. The alternating light and dark bands give rise to the name striated or striped muscle.

There are numerous attachments between the actin and myosin, and when the muscle contracts the attachments break and reform as the myosin and actin fibrils slide along one another, so shortening the muscle fibre.

All the muscle fibres that are activated by a single nerve fibre are termed a **motor unit**. The size of the motor unit varies throughout the body: a muscle that makes small,

intricate movements will consist of very small motor units, whereas a muscle performing only large movements may have 200 or more fibres innervated by a single nerve fibre.

The control of muscle contraction

The contraction of skeletal muscles is controlled at a number of levels. At the highest level, contraction is stimulated or inhibited via nervous pathways from the brain, down the spinal cord to the muscle groups. Some of these pathways are voluntary, i.e. the animal makes a conscious decision to move a certain muscle group (to scratch an ear, to pick up food in the mouth), but others are involuntary, and are mainly concerned with balance and posture (we stand upright without thinking about it), and with locomotion (once we've initiated a walking movement, we can carry on without thinking about putting one foot in front of the other).

At a lower level, there are receptors in the muscles and tendons that measure the length and tension of a muscle fibre. Through a feedback system, these receptors make small changes in the muscles responsible for maintained posture, and also act to prevent (in most cases) overstretching of muscle fibres.

Muscles are nearly always in a state of slight tension, which is called **muscle tone**:

- **Isometric** contraction increases muscle tone without shortening the muscle.
- **Isotonic** contraction shortens a muscle without changing its tension.

To retain its tone a muscle must be used constantly. Muscles that are not used tend to get weak and lose muscle fibres (**atrophy**), whereas a muscle that is constantly and vigorously exercised will **hypertrophy** (get bigger).

Muscles, tendons, bursae and tendon sheaths

Muscles may be the classic 'muscle shape' or they may be in the form of flat sheets. They may have one origin or starting point and one insertion on bone; or there may be several muscle bellies (the thick, fleshy, central part of the muscle) inserting together at one point, in which case the muscle is said to have two or more heads.

The muscle sheath which surrounds each muscle may be quite delicate, or it may be thick and fibrous. The muscle sheath continues at each end of the muscles into the dense fibrous tissue of the tendons of origin and insertion of the muscle. (To avoid confusion: a ligament runs from bone to bone, whereas a tendon runs from muscle to bone.)

Muscles may have very short tendons, and appear to start or end with the fleshy part of the muscle, or they may have long tendons attaching the belly to the bone. Examples of the latter are the long muscles of the digits of the dog, where the tendon of insertion may be longer than the muscle belly itself.

Where the muscle is in the form of a flat sheet, the tendon is drawn out into a fibrous sheet as well – this is then called an **aponeurosis**.

A **bursa** is a cavity lined with synovial membrane, and filled with synovial fluid, that lies between tendons and bone, or between tendon and tendon, to minimise friction between the structures as they move backwards and forwards. If a bursa wraps itself completely round a tendon, it is called a **synovial sheath**.

'Acquired' bursae may form on, for example, the point of the elbow or hock in large dogs, particularly those that habitually lie on hard surfaces. A bursa forms to protect the bony prominence from the constant friction with the ground.

Skeletal muscle groups

This section deals only briefly with the most important muscle groups in the body. Wherever possible, the text should be related to a skeleton to help understand the muscles' positions, and palpation of the muscles of a good-natured dog will help in appreciating their positions and actions in the live animal.

Intrinsic and extrinsic muscles

Intrinsic muscles lie completely within one region of the body (the head, the trunk or a limb) and alter the position of parts of that region of the body, e.g. they close the eye, bend the spine or curl a toe.

Extrinsic muscles run from one region of the body to another, and alter the position of one region in relation to another, e.g. they turn the head on the neck or pull a limb forward in relation to the trunk.

Muscles of the head

The muscles of the head can be categorised as follows:

- The muscles of facial expression.
- The muscles of mastication.
- The eye muscles.
- Muscles of the tongue, pharynx, larynx and soft palate.
- Extrinsic muscles of the head.

The **muscles of facial expression** are formed from a single sheet of muscle. There are muscles that raise the lips (to snarl), move the ears, move the eyelids and nostrils. All these muscles are innervated by the facial nerve (cranial nerve VII) and damage to this nerve will result in flaccid paralysis of these muscles.

The main **muscles of mastication** are:

- **Digastricus**, the jaw-opening muscle which runs from the mandible to the base of the skull.
- **Temporalis**, one of the jaw closing muscles, which fills the temporal fossa of the skull and inserts on the medial side of the vertical ramus of the mandible.
- **Masseter**, the other jaw-closing muscle, which runs from the zygomatic arch to the lateral side of the vertical ramus of the mandible.
- **Medial and lateral pterygoids**, which produce side-to-side movement of the lower jaw. This is important in the

carnivores for pushing the carnassial teeth against the lower molars so that they can have an effective scissor action. In herbivores these muscles are much larger and produce the grinding action of the molars against one another.

The eye muscles are:

- **Medial, lateral, dorsal and ventral rectus** – allowing dorsal, ventral and lateral movement.
- **Retractor oculi** – enabling the eye to be drawn back into the socket and the third eyelid to move across the eye.
- **Dorsal and ventral oblique** – allowing a small amount of rotatory movement.

Muscles of the tongue may be intrinsic or extrinsic. The intrinsic muscles of the tongue allow it to curl up, flatten out or move from side to side, while the extrinsic muscles draw it forwards or backwards or lift it towards the roof of the mouth.

Muscles of the pharynx, larynx and soft palate allow the movements needed for voice production, respiration and swallowing.

The extrinsic muscles of the head move the head on the neck.

Vertebral column muscles

The vertebral column muscles are divided into:

- **Epaxial muscles** above the vertebral column.
- **Hypaxial muscles** below the vertebral column.

The **epaxial** muscles attach to the pelvis, the sacrum, the vertebrae and the ribs. Some of these muscles are long, running a good proportion of the length of the spine, and some are short, spanning only two or four vertebrae. They support the spine, help to move the spine as the animal runs, support the weight of the head and neck and tail, and allow a certain amount of rotation between the vertebrae.

The **hypaxial** muscles are less bulky than the epaxials – they do not have to support the vertebral column, head and neck. They act to flex the lumbar spine as the animal runs, and to bend the neck downwards.

Muscles of the thorax

The most important muscles of the thorax are the **internal and external intercostals**. These run from rib to rib and are important muscles of respiration.

The diaphragm

The **diaphragm** (Fig. 11.22) separates the thoracic from the abdominal cavity. It is made up as follows:

- A peripheral muscle that occupies the outer part of the diaphragm.
- A central tendon.
- Two muscular crura – the right crus being larger than the left.

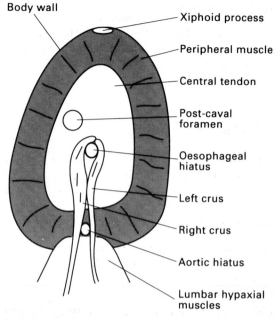

Fig. 11.22 The structure of the diaphragm and the structures that pass through it (viewed as if from the abdomen, with the dog lying on its back).

There are three holes where structures pass through the diaphragm:

- The **post-caval foramen**, carrying the posterior vena cava.
- The **oesophageal hiatus**, carrying the oesophagus and the vagal nerves.
- The **aortic hiatus**, carrying the aorta, the azygos vein and the thoracic duct.

The diaphragm is dome shaped, and bulges forwards into the thoracic region. It is attached dorsally at the level of thoracic vertebrae 9/10, and ventrally to the caudal end of the sternum.

Abdominal muscles

There are four muscles on each side of the body that together make up the abdominal wall:

- **External abdominal oblique.**
- **Internal abdominal oblique.**
- **Transversus abdominis.**
- **Rectus abdominis.**

The main function of the abdominal wall is to enclose and protect the abdominal viscera. The four abdominal muscles are so arranged that all their fibres run in different directions, so giving the abdominal wall great strength.

Each abdominal muscle (except rectus abdominis) ends in a sheet of aponeurosis, and all the sheets join in the ventral midline to form the **linea alba** (white line).

Because of the different origins of the muscles there is a small area in the groin where there is no muscle in the wall, merely a sheet of fascia (part of the aponeurosis of external abdominal oblique). In this area there is a small hole or slit known as the **inguinal ring**, which carries the structures in the spermatic cord to and from the scrotum, and allows blood vessels out of the abdomen to supply the mammary glands and external genitalia. **Hernias** are quite common in this region, as the inguinal ring may enlarge, producing a hole that will let other structures such as bladder and uterus out of the abdomen, to lie subcutaneously in the groin or on the medial aspect of the thigh.

The **rectus abdominis** muscle has its origin on the first rib, and inserts on what is called the pre-pubic tendon on the front of the pubis, next to the pubic symphysis. It supports the abdominal cavity and also helps to flex the lumbar spine.

Muscles of the forelimb

The extrinsic muscles of the forelimb attach the forelimb to the trunk. Among them are:

- **Trapezii** (singular: trapezius) which run from the spine of the scapula to the dorsal midline, and support the limb on the body.
- **Brachiocephalicus**, which runs from the anterior aspect of the humerus to the base of the skull, and either bends the neck or brings forward or protracts the forelimb (depending on the action of other muscles and whether the forelimb is on the ground).
- **Latissimus dorsi**, which runs from the humerus to form a large fan of muscle attached to the dorsal midline – it retracts the forelimb (pulls it backwards).
- **Pectorals**, which run from the humerus round the front of the thorax to the sternum and ribs. The pectorals are adductors: they hold the forelimb in close to the body.

Muscles of the shoulder

- **Supraspinatus** runs from the supraspinous fossa of the scapula to the greater tuberosity of the humerus and extends the shoulder.
- **Infraspinatus** runs from the infraspinous fossa of the scapula to the lesser tuberosity of the humerus and helps support the shoulder joint.

Muscles of the elbow

- **Triceps** is a four-headed muscle that originates from the scapula and humerus, and inserts on the olecranon of the ulna. It extends the elbow joint.
- **Biceps brachii** runs from the bicipital tuberosity of the scapula (also known as the supraglenoid tubercle) and inserts on the ulna. It flexes the elbow.
- **Brachialis** originates just beneath the head of the humerus and inserts with biceps brachii. It too flexes the elbow.

Muscles of the carpus and digits

Although there are many small muscles within the paw, most of the action of flexing and extending the carpus and digits is performed by eight muscles:

- Two carpal flexors.
- Two carpal extensors.

- Two digital flexors.
- Two digital extensors.

To help understand these muscles, look at a forearm (either of a dog or your own) and locate the proximal and distal ends of the radius and ulna. The ulna (starting at the olecranon) starts ventral and ends up lateral, and the radius starts dorsal and ends up medial.

You will notice that there are two masses of muscle – one dorso-lateral, and one ventro-medial.

The dorso-lateral muscle mass consists of the two carpal extensors (originating on the humerus and inserting in the carpal region) and two digital extensors (originating on the humerus and inserting on the third phalanx).

The ventro-medial muscle mass contains the two carpal flexors and two digital flexors. The superficial digital flexor inserts in the second phalanx and the deep digital flexor on the third phalanx.

Muscles of the hindlimb

The very mobile ball-and-socket joint of the hip is moved by a number of relatively short muscles at the top of the leg, among them the **gluteal muscles** that make up the muscle mass of the curve of the rump.

The hamstring group consists of three muscles that lie on the caudal aspect of the thigh, but act together on the hip, stifle and hock joints to extend the whole limb backwards, providing the main propulsive force in the running animal.

The hamstring group consists of:

- **Biceps femoris**, the most lateral of the group.
- **Semitendinosis**.
- **Semimembranosis**, the most medial of the group.

Other important muscles of the upper part of the hindlimb are:

- **Quadriceps femoris**, the bulky muscle that runs down the front of the thigh. It extends the stifle.
- **The adductor group**, on the inside of the thigh, that hold the limb in towards the body. This group is made up of adductor, gracilis and pectineus. They all run from the medial aspect of the femur to the pubis.

The **Achilles tendon** runs down the back of the shank to the point of the hock (the tuber calcis). It includes the tendons of **superficial digital flexor**, which runs over the point of the hock and then on down towards the digits, and also the tendons of **gastrocnemius, biceps femoris** and **semitendinosis**, which all insert on the tuber calcis.

Muscles of the hock

- **Cranial (anterior) tibial** is the main flexor of the hock – it arises from the proximal end of the tibia, on the lateral side of the tibial crest, and inserts on the tarsus.
- **Gastrocnemius** is the main extensor of the hock (along with the hamstrings). It arises from the ventral aspect of the distal part of the femur and inserts on the tuber calcis. It forms the muscular bulge at the top of the calf.

Muscles of the digits

The muscles of the digits of the hindlimb are very similar to those of the digits of the forelimb, except that there are three digital extensors and two digital flexors.

The integument

The integument is the covering of the body. It includes the skin, hair or feathers, and the claws or nails. It blends with the mucous membrane at the various natural openings of the body.

In mammals, the skin has several functions:

- It protects the surface of the body.
- It protects the body against invasion by micro-organisms.
- It plays a part in temperature control.
- It helps prevent excessive water loss (or, in the case of aquatic mammals, water uptake) by the body.
- It manufactures vitamin D.
- The hair and the pigment in the skin protect the body from the harmful effects of ultraviolet radiation.
- It contains pressure, temperature and pain receptors and so can be thought of a sense organ.
- It contains glands (sebaceous and sweat glands) and so has a secretory function.

Epidermis, dermis and hypodermis

There are three distinct layers to the skin:

- The **epidermis**.
- The **dermis**.
- The **hypodermis**.

The epidermis

The epidermis (Fig. 11.23) is the most superficial layer of the skin, and is made of **stratified squamous epithelium**. It consists of four layers, or strata:

- Stratum germinativum.
- Stratum granulosum.
- Stratum lucidum.
- Stratum corneum.

The whole of the epidermis is avascular (i.e. contains no blood vessels at all).

The deepest layer of the epidermis is the basal cell layer, or **stratum basale**, also known as the **stratum germinativum**. In this layer the cells divide rapidly. Between the basal skin cells are the **melanocytes** that give colour to skin. This deep layer of the epidermis rests on the **dermal papillae**, which are deeper and more numerous where the skin is thickest and most liable to trauma (e.g. in the pads).

The next layer of epidermal cells is the **stratum granulosum**, where the cells are starting to flatten and become infiltrated with the protein keratin.

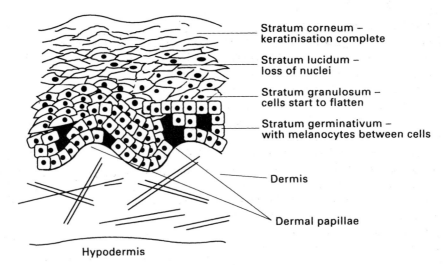

Stratum corneum –
keratinisation complete

Stratum lucidum –
loss of nuclei

Stratum granulosum –
cells start to flatten

Stratum germinativum –
with melanocytes between cells

Dermis

Dermal papillae

Hypodermis

Fig. 11.23 The structure of the epidermis.

Above this is the **stratum lucidum**, where the skin cells start to lose their nuclei. The top layer is the **stratum corneum**, where the process of keratinisation is complete, and the cellular outlines have disappeared.

The dermis

The dermis, deep to the epidermis and firmly attached to it, consists of vascular dense connective tissue. It also contains elastic fibres, nerve fibres and the sensory nerve endings of the skin. It is invaded by hair follicles, sweat glands and sebaceous glands, which grow downwards from the epidermis.

The hypodermis

The hypodermis, beneath the dermis, is not truly part of the skin: it consists of loose connective tissue, often infiltrated by fat.

Hair

Hair is formed from epidermal tissue that firstly extends down into the dermis to form a '**hair cone**' over a piece of dermis called the **dermal** or **hair papilla** (Fig. 11.24). As the hair starts to grow from the hair cone, the epidermal cells around and above it are destroyed, so leaving an open channel or hair follicle for the hair. The hair then grows continuously until it dies and becomes detached from its hair cone. The hair may be shed then, or may stay attached to the skin, supported by hairs around it, until it is combed out.

Associated with each hair follicle is a **sebaceous gland**. This is an alveolar gland that opens off the side of the follicle and secretes sebum. The functions of sebum are:

● To lubricate and waterproof the hairs.
● To produce a smell that is thought to act as a territorial marker (the distinctive smell of a wet dog is due to sebum).
● To produce pheromones, which play a part in attracting the opposite sex.

There are three types of hair:

● Guard hairs.
● Undercoat (wool hairs).
● Vibrissae.

The **guard hairs** are the long hairs of the topcoat and provide the waterproof layer of the coat. Only one guard hair grows from each follicle. Associated with each guard hair is an involuntary **arrector pili** muscle, which raises the hair from its resting position. This happens as a result of exposure to cold or, in the case of the dog, when the hackles are raised. It may also be seen when a cat goes into a threat stance with a 'bottlebrush' tail.

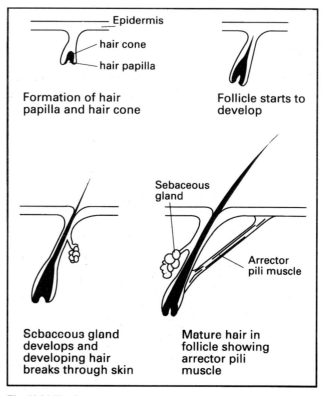

Epidermis

hair cone

hair papilla

Formation of hair
papilla and hair cone

Follicle starts to
develop

Sebaceous
gland

Sebaceous gland
develops and
developing hair
breaks through skin

Arrector
pili muscle

Mature hair in
follicle showing
arrector pili
muscle

Fig. 11.24 The formation of hair.

The **wool hairs**, or undercoat, provide an insulating layer of shorter, softer hairs beneath the topcoat. They trap air between them, and so keep the body warm. Wool hairs make up the main part of the 'puppy' coat, and in the adult there are more of them in the winter than in the summer coat. They grow from small secondary hair follicles that surround the primary follicle. There may be many wool hairs emerging from a single primary follicle with its guard hair.

Density of coat varies over the body and with the individual and breed. Generally, hair is more sparse on the underside of the body, and what there is tends to be mainly guard hairs, with less undercoat than on the top of the body. The scrotum of the dog is often quoted as an area of the body that carries guard hairs and no undercoat.

The **vibrissae**, or **tactile hairs**, are even thicker than guard hairs, and protect beyond the rest of the coat (Fig. 11.25). They grow from specialised follicles that project deep into the hypodermis. At their base they have nerve endings that respond to the movements of the hair. In this way the vibrissae are important sensory organs, particularly in the cat, but also in the dog, and should never be cut without good reason.

Most vibrissae are found round the head – on the upper lip and above the eyes. Dogs also have a substantial tuft on the cheek, and cats have a tuft on the carpus as well.

Moulting

Moulting is the seasonal shedding of hair. Most dogs shed during spring and autumn, although many household pets shed to some extent all the year round. This is due to the effect of household living, with electric lighting upsetting the normal stimuli of seasonal increase or decrease of photoperiod (day length). Cats moult most heavily in the spring, then less heavily throughout summer and autumn.

Pads

The epidermis of the footpads of dogs and cats is very thick and hairless (Fig. 11.26). The dermis is similarly thickened,

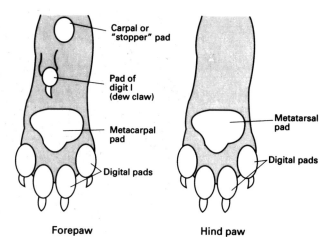

Fig. 11.26 Ventral view of dog's (a) forepaw and (b) hind paw, showing footpads.

is very vascular and contains adipose tissue. This forms a **'digital cushion'** that supports the foot and provides some shock absorption as the feet of the running animal hit the ground.

The **rhinarium** or nosepad is also thick, keratinised and hairless. Like the fingerprints of people, each dog's nose gives a unique print that reflects the pattern of dermal papillae beneath the surface.

Unlike the hairy skin of the dog, the nose and footpads contain sweat glands.

Dogs and cats have on each foot a main pad (or metacarpal/metatarsal pad) and four digital pads. In addition, there is on the forelimb a digital pad on the dew claw (digit I) and a carpal pad covering the accessory carpal bone.

Claws

Claws have different functions in cats and dogs. In cats, the needle-sharp retractable claws are tools for prey capture. In the dog, however, they are used for digging, and give added stability and grip when running down prey – especially if this involves cornering. See Fig. 11.27.

The horny part of a nail is modified epidermis, and grows from a specialised part of the epidermis called the **coronary border** or **coronary band**, which lies underneath a fold of skin, the **claw fold**.

The claw grows in two sheets which form the walls of the claw, and cover the **ungual process** of the third phalanx.

The **sole**, in the groove between the two walls of the claw, is made of softer horn.

The dermis lies between the horn and the third phalanx, and provides the blood and nerve supply to the claw. Trimming of claws should be done with great care so as not to cut into the sensitive dermis.

The claws of the cat are held retracted and are only extended by the action of the digital flexor muscles, which pull the claw forwards against the pull of two little **elastic ligaments** that run from the third to the second phalanx and hold the claws off the ground.

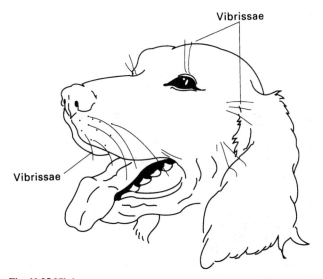

Fig. 11.25 Vibrissae.

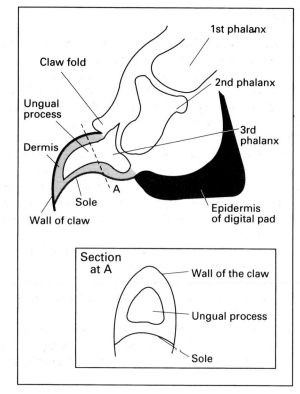

Fig. 11.27 Longitudinal section of dog's toe, showing claw.

The dew claws

The dew claws of dogs and cats are the reduced remnants of digit I, which has become obsolete as the carnivore changed from a plantigrade (walking with 'palm' of hand on ground) to a digitigrade (walking on the toes) posture. Horses, sheep and cattle have taken this reduction in digits to a more extreme state, with, in the case of horses, only one toe remaining.

Dew claws are usually present in the front feet of both dogs and cats, where they are made up of the three phalanges and a claw, as the other digits (but no metacarpal bone). In the rear foot, dew claws are very rare in cats (usually only seen in polydactyl specimens), and variable in dogs – they may have one or two phalanges, and be either firmly or loosely attached to the metatarsus.

Sweat glands

Sweat glands, or sudiferous glands, are epidermal structures but lie deep within the dermis, not alongside the hair follicle. They are coiled glands, and in the dog and cat they are only found on the hairless epidermal areas, i.e. the nose and footpads.

The mammary glands

The mammary glands are modified sweat glands and are dealt with in detail under 'The female reproductive system' (see p. 302).

Specialised sebaceous glands

These epidermal structures include:

- Tail glands.
- Circum-anal glands.
- Glands of the anal sacs.

The **tail glands** are a group of sebaceous glands that lie on the dorsal surface of the tail in the dog. Particularly in middle-aged and elderly dogs, the hair may get very sparse in this area and hypertrophy of the glandular area may occur until the tail looks swollen. The glandular secretion lying on the surface may smell, and cause irritation to the dog.

The **circum-anal glands** are sebaceous glands that form a ring around the anus, where their ducts drain into the ducts of modified sweat glands. It is thought that it is the secretion from these glands that dogs smell when they sniff each other's anal areas.

The **anal sacs** are small sacs with ducts leading to the exterior. They lie beneath the skin on either side and just below the anus. The lining of these sacs contain numerous modified sebaceous glands that produce the foul-smelling anal sac secretion, which in the normal animal is squeezed out a little at a time on to the surface of faeces as the animal defecates, and so acts as a territorial marker.

The respiratory system

Respiration is the gaseous exchange between a living structure (be it plant or animal) and its environment. Respiration may be either external or internal.

External respiration in an animal is the gaseous exchange between the air and the blood. **Internal respiration**, also known as **tissue respiration**, is the gaseous exchange between the blood and the tissues.

The respiratory system transports oxygen-containing air from outside the body into the lungs, where it can be absorbed into the bloodstream.

The composition of inspired air is:

- Nitrogen: 79%.
- Oxygen: 21%.
- Carbon dioxide: 0.04%.
- Water vapour.
- Other gases: traces only.

In expired air the oxygen is down to about 16%, the carbon dioxide has risen to about 4–5% and the water vapour may have increased. The other gases are unchanged.

The respiratory system consists of:

- The nose and nasal chamber.
- The pharynx.
- The larynx.
- The trachea.
- The bronchi.
- The bronchioles.
- The alveolar ducts and alveoli.

The nasal chamber

The nasal chamber extends from the **external nares**, or nostrils, to the **internal nares** where the air enters the pharynx (Fig. 11.28).

The nasal chamber is divided into left and right chambers by a cartilaginous **nasal septum**, and these are partly filled by the dorsal and ventral **naso turbinate** bones, which arise from the dorsolateral wall of the chamber and are covered with ciliated mucous membrane. The function of the nasal turbinates and their coverings is to moisten, warm and filter the air that passes over them, so that it is warm, moist and clean before passing into the lower respiratory tract.

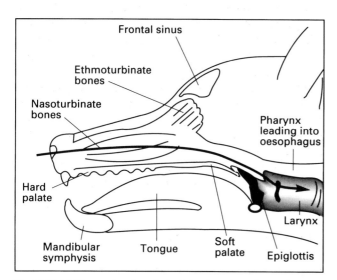

Fig. 11.28 Midline section through dog's head, to show the respiratory passage.

From the nasal chamber the air passes across the pharynx and into the larynx at the top of the trachea. The **pharynx** is the name given to the area at the back of the mouth used by both the respiratory and digestive tracts. The openings into the pharynx are:

- The nasal chamber.
- The mouth.
- The two **Eustachian tubes** from the middle ear.
- The oesophagus.
- The larynx.

Paranasal sinuses

Sinuses are air-filled cavities within a bone, lined with ciliated mucous epithelium and having drainage, usually into the nasal chamber.

The dog has only one true sinus – the **frontal sinus** – within the frontal bone of the skull. The **maxillary sinus** in the dog is not a true sinus, as it is not enclosed within a single bone – it is merely a recess at the caudal end of each nasal chamber, between the maxillary and palatine bones. Other species, particularly the large herbivores (horses and cattle), have many paranasal sinuses that lighten an otherwise very heavy skull.

The larynx

The larynx is a rigid, hollow structure made up of a number of cartilages. It forms the opening to the lower part of the respiratory tract, and is also the 'voice box' for the production of sound. It is attached to the skull by the **hyoid apparatus** (see Fig. 11.39), which allows it to move backwards and forwards between its two arms like the seat of a swing.

The opening at the front of the larynx is called the **glottis**. When the larynx moves forwards (during swallowing) this opening is closed by the elastic cartilage of the **epiglottis**. When the larynx moves backwards to its resting position, the epiglottis falls forward and the glottis is open again.

Within the larynx lie the **vocal cords** or **vocal ligaments**, that are the free borders of two folds of mucous membrane that project from the sides of the larynx. These folds are relaxed or tensed by muscular activity to produce different laryngeal sounds.

In its resting position the tip of the broadly triangular epiglottis lies above the **soft palate**, so that there is a continuous open passage for air from the nasal chambers to the larynx.

The trachea

The trachea is a permanently open tube that runs from the laryngeal cartilages through the thoracic inlet into the thorax, where just above the heart it divides into the right and left bronchi.

It is made up of a series of incomplete rings of hyaline cartilage separated by fibrous connective tissue and smooth muscle fibres, and lined with ciliated mucous epithelium.

The open part of each tracheal ring is on the dorsal aspect and it has been suggested that this enables the oesophagus, lying above it, to expand without hindrance when a large bolus of food passes along it.

The bronchi and bronchioles

The bronchi are similar in structure to the trachea. Each bronchus divides to enter one of the lobes of the lungs, and then the air passages continue to divide throughout the lung substance, getting smaller with each division. In the very small bronchioles the cartilage gets very sparse, and eventually disappears altogether. The structure of air passages formed by this division is called the bronchial tree.

The lungs

The lungs are two large spongy organs that lie in the thorax on either side of the **mediastinum**. Each lung is divided into lobes – the left into three and the right into four lobes (Fig. 11.29). On the right lung these are called:

- The **cranial** (or apical) lobe.
- The **middle** (or cardiac) lobe.

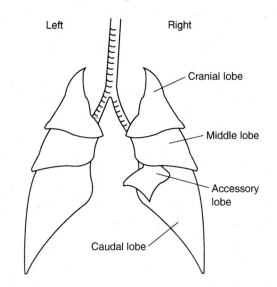

Fig. 11.29 The lobes of the lungs.

- The **caudal** (or diaphragmatic) lobe.
- The **accessory** lobe.

The left lung does not have an accessory lobe.

The terminal air passages

The smallest of the bronchioles are called the **respiratory** or **terminal bronchioles** (Fig. 11.30). They have no cartilage in their walls, and no cilia on their epithelium. Each of them gives rise to two or three **alveolar ducts** and each duct terminates in an **alveolar sac**. Each alveolar sac is divided into **alveoli**, which make up the soft tissue of the lung. The alveoli are where the gaseous exchange takes place, and are very well supplied with blood.

Respiration

The muscles and movements of respiration

The main muscles of inspiration are the diaphragm and the external intercostals. Expiration is mainly passive, caused

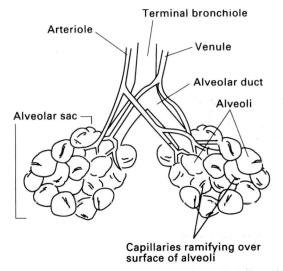

Fig. 11.30 The terminal air passages.

by the relaxation of the muscles of inspiration, but is assisted by the internal intercostals and, in the case of forced expiration, by the abdominal muscles as well.

The lung tissue contains no muscle: it cannot expand on its own. It is, however, very elastic tissue that returns to a collapsed state when there is nothing to expand it forcibly.

The lungs lie within and nearly fill the thoracic cavity. The pleural cavity that lies between them and the body wall contains nothing but a little pleural fluid.

When an animal breathes in, it increases the volume of the thoracic cavity by flattening the diaphragm, increasing the length of the thorax and by swinging the ribs out so as to increase the diameter of the thorax. Because of the vacuum between the lungs and the chest wall, the lungs are forced to expand to fill the enlarged thoracic cavity, and air is drawn into the bronchial tree and so into the lung tissue.

When the animal breathes out, the diaphragm is relaxed (decreasing the length of the chest) and the ribs fall back to their resting position (reducing the diameter of the ribcage). As the lungs collapse to their resting volume, air is expelled from the respiratory tract.

The control of respiration

The **respiratory centres** are in the hindbrain, in the pons and the medulla. One centre is responsible for inspiration (the apneustic centre), one for expiration and one prevents over-inflation of the lungs. **Stretch receptors** in the walls of the bronchioles feed information to these centres on the degree of inflation of the bronchial tree (the **Hering–Breuer reflex**).

The rate of respiration is also controlled by centres in the medulla that monitor the pH of the blood. If respiration is too slow or too shallow, carbon dioxide builds up in the blood and in the form of carbonic acid decreases the pH of the blood. The respiratory pacemaker is then stimulated to increase the rate and depth of respiration to blow off the surplus carbon dioxide and restore the pH of the blood to its correct level.

There are also chemoreceptors in the walls of arteries (the **aortic** and **carotid bodies**) that respond to changing levels of oxygen and carbon dioxide in the blood and influence the medullary respiratory centre accordingly.

Respiratory rate and lung capacity

When animals are at rest and breathing quietly, they are only using a small fraction of their total lung capacity. The **resting respiratory rate** in the dog varies between about 10 and 30 breaths per minute (depending on the size of the dog). In the cat it is between 20 and 30 breaths per minute.

The amount of air breathed in and out during quiet respiration is called the **tidal volume**. If there is a forced intake of breath, the extra air drawn into the lungs in addition to the normal tidal volume is called the **inspiratory reserve volume**. The tidal volume plus the inspiratory reserve volume is called the **inspiratory capacity**.

A forced exhalation after quiet respiration will give the **expiratory reserve volume**, and this plus the normal tidal volume will give the **expiratory capacity**. However, even after the hardest possible expiration, there is still some air left in the lungs – this is the **residual volume**. The **functional residual capacity** is the air left in the lungs after quiet expiration, which allows gaseous diffusion to carry on during expiration.

The **vital capacity** is the total volume of the respiratory tract that can be used during respiration (from the maximum point of the inspiratory reserve volume to the minimum point of the expiratory reserve volume). Vital capacity can be affected by such things as the fullness of the stomach, the presence of an intra-abdominal mass or a gravid uterus and even by the position of the animal (standing or lying). In heart failure, vital capacity may be reduced by the presence of pulmonary oedema, reducing the alveolar volume.

The **total lung capacity** is the total volume of the hollow respiratory tract (if you removed it from the animal and filled it with water, for example).

Dead space is the volume of air drawn in at each respiration that never reaches the alveoli – i.e. it is the volume of the trachea, the bronchi and the bronchioles. During general anaesthesia, dead space is an important consideration, and may be increased (functional dead space as opposed to anatomical dead space) by inappropriate use of anaesthetic apparatus (e.g. using too long an endotracheal tube) to the point where it reduces the ability of the animal to respire effectively.

Blood and the circulatory system

The **blood–vascular** or **circulatory system** is a system of tubes distributed throughout the body to allow the circulation of blood. The **lymphatic system** is closely allied to the blood vascular system and carries lymph, which is essentially excess tissue fluid, from the periphery back to the circulation.

The **heart** is part of the blood vascular system. It is a folded and elaborate piece of muscular tubing that is modified to form a four-chambered pump.

The blood circulation can be divided into **pulmonary** and **systemic** parts. The pulmonary circulation takes deoxygenated blood from the heart through the lungs, where it is oxygenated, and returns it to the heart. The systemic circulation takes oxygenated blood from the heart to the rest of the body, where the oxygen is used by the tissues. It then returns the deoxygenated blood to the heart.

An **artery** is a relatively large vessel carrying blood away from the heart, whether it is in the pulmonary or the systemic circulation (Fig. 11.31). Arteries have relatively thick walls, which contain smooth muscle, and can constrict or dilate to allow a greater or lesser flow of blood to a particular organ.

As the arteries divide they get smaller in diameter. These smaller arteries, called **arterioles**, lie within the organs they are supplying with blood.

Within the tissues themselves the blood vessels become very small and very thin-walled, so as to allow oxygen exchange – these are the **capillaries**. The capillaries form a network (the **capillary bed**) within the tissue.

A **vein** is a relatively large, thin-walled vessel, carrying blood towards the heart. A **venule** is a small vein within an organ, receiving blood from the capillary bed.

As well as being thinner walled than arteries, veins also have valves, which offer no resistance to the flow of blood towards the heart but prevent any back flow. These valves are most numerous in the veins of the limbs, and quite sparse in the veins of the internal organs.

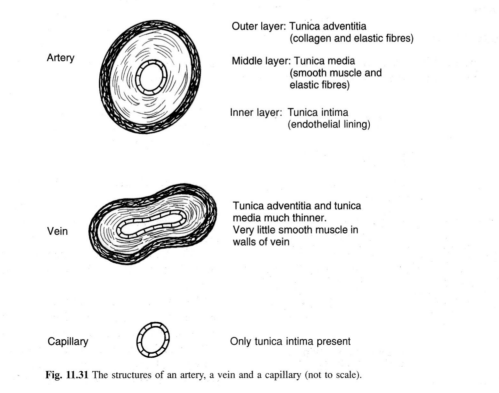

Fig. 11.31 The structures of an artery, a vein and a capillary (not to scale).

Veins and arteries have a similar structure. Both have an outer fibrous coat, a middle layer composed of muscular and elastic fibres, and an inner lining membrane of elastic fibres and flattened epithelial cells.

Although most tissues are supplied by a network of capillaries, there are three organs within the body that have a system of end arteries instead. End arteries are capillaries that branch like the branches and twigs of a tree, getting smaller all the time but never joining up with one another. The organs that have end arteries rather than a capillary bed are the brain, the heart and the kidneys.

The reason for end arteries in these organs is thought to be protection against sudden drops in blood pressure, e.g. after blood loss. All the other organs of the body can survive a period of vasoconstriction and poor blood supply, while the available oxygenated blood is diverted to these three vital organs.

This system does have a disadvantage as well, in that obstruction of a vessel (e.g. with a blood clot) will cause the death of the tissue supplied by that vessel, whereas in a network capillary bed there are many routes for blood to reach each section of tissue.

The functions of blood

The functions of blood are:

- To carry oxygen to and carbon dioxide away from the tissues.
- To carry digested food products to the tissues.
- To supply water to the tissues.
- To carry waste away from the tissues to the kidneys for excretion.
- To help regulate body temperature by distributing heat throughout the body.
- To stop haemorrhage when it occurs, through the blood clotting mechanism.
- To act as a transport system throughout the body for hormones and enzymes.
- To protect the body against infection by the blood-borne cells of the immune system, and by transporting antitoxins and antibodies in the blood.
- To assist in the maintenance of the correct pH of the tissues.

The composition of blood

Blood is a red fluid – it is brighter red in the systemic arteries, where it is rich in oxygen, and darker in the veins after it has given up some of its oxygen to the tissues.

It has a pH of approximately 7.35 and forms about 7% of the total weight of the body. The pH is higher in arterial blood and lower in the relatively deoxygenated venous blood, owing to the amount of carbon dioxide dissolved in it, which increases the acidity.

Blood consists of a fluid part and a solid part. The solids are cells and cellular fragments; the straw-coloured fluid is called plasma.

The composition of plasma

The composition of plasma reflects the different functions of blood:

- **Water**.
- **Mineral salts**. Sodium is the main extracellular cation and chloride the main anion. There are also significant amounts of potassium, calcium, phosphate and carbonate. The mineral salts in plasma act as buffers, maintaining the correct pH of the body fluids.
- **Plasma proteins**. These include albumin, globulin, fibrinogen and prothrombin. They are large molecules that cannot pass out of the circulation to the tissues and so they help to maintain the osmotic pressure of the blood, stopping too much fluid leaking out of the circulation into the tissue spaces. Most of the plasma proteins are produced by the liver, with the exception of the immunoglobulins (part of the immune system) which are produced by plasma cells.
- **Foodstuffs**. The amino acids, fatty acids and glucose that are the end products of food breakdown are carried in the plasma.
- **Gases** in solution. Most of the oxygen for the tissues is carried in the red blood cells as oxyhaemoglobin and only a very little is dissolved in the plasma. However, a significant amount of carbon dioxide is carried in the plasma as bicarbonate.
- **Waste products**. Urea and creatinine are carried to the kidneys for excretion.
- **Hormones** and **enzymes**.
- **Antibodies** and **antitoxins**

Blood cells

Blood cells are divided into three types: two are true cells, the third are cell fragments (Fig. 11.32):

- **Erythrocytes** – red blood cells.
- **Leucocytes** – white blood cells.
- **Thrombocytes** – platelets.

Red blood cells

Red blood cells are very small (diameter 7 micrometres or 0.007 cm) biconcave discs without nuclei. A biconcave disc is like a ring doughnut where the hole has not gone all the way through – a disc with a dent top and bottom. They contain an iron-containing protein called haemoglobin, which is what gives the cells their red colour, and enables them to carry oxygen.

Before birth, red blood cells are produced in the bone marrow, the liver and the spleen, but after birth they are only produced in the bone marrow. They are formed from cells called **erythroblasts**, which have nuclei. These develop into **normoblasts** as they take up haemoglobin and the nucleus shrinks. The nucleus then disappears completely, leaving only a network of fine threads in the cytoplasm. At this stage the cell is called a **reticulocyte**. Finally the network disappears and the mature erythrocyte passes into the bloodstream. It has a lifespan of up to 120 days, after which

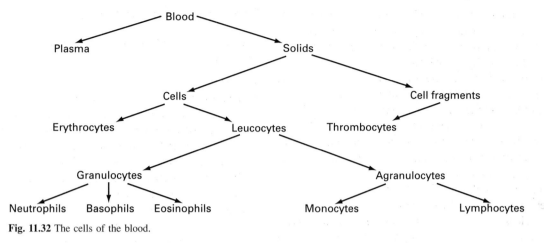

Fig. 11.32 The cells of the blood.

it is broken down in the spleen or lymph nodes. The haemoglobin in spent cells is broken down – the iron is recycled, and waste pigment is converted by the liver into bile pigments. The 'globin' part may be re-used or broken down.

The level of red cell production is regulated by the amount of oxygen reaching the tissues. When there is a low oxygen level the kidney secretes **erythropoietin factor** (or **erythrogenin**), a substance that converts an inactive plasma protein to **erythropoietin**, which stimulates the bone marrow to produce more erythrocytes. In some circumstances, e.g. after anaemia, when there is a significant deficit to be made up – immature reticulocytes will be seen in the blood alongside mature red blood cells.

White blood cells

The white blood cells, or leucocytes, are larger than red blood cells and can be divided into two groups:

- **Granulocytes**, which can be subdivided into:
  - neutrophils
  - basophils
  - eosinophils
- **Agranulocytes**, which can be subdivided into:
  - lymphocytes
  - monocytes

Granulocytes

Granulocytes, also know as **polymorphonuclear leucocytes**, have a granular cytoplasm and a multi-lobed nucleus. They make up about 70% of all the leucocytes in the body and usually spend less than 12 hours in the circulation before migrating into the tissues for 2–3 days before they either die or are lost from the body via an area of infection (e.g. an abscess) or via one of the visceral systems of the body, where they help to guard against infection.

All granulocytes (and monocytes) are produced in the bone marrow from **myeloid tissue**.

The three types of polymorphonuclear leucocytes are classified according to their ability to take up different dyes, which gives them different appearances in the stained blood film:

Neutrophils, which account for over 90% of the granulocytes, take up both acid and alkaline dyes, and the cytoplasm remains clear after staining. They are **phagocytes**, which means that they can move about and ingest small particles such as bacteria and cell debris. Neutrophils increase in number in the presence of bacterial infection, when immature forms, with a banded instead of a segmented nucleus, are seen in the blood. Hence the terms 'bands' and 'segs' in blood counts. An increase in the 'bands' indicates recent bacterial infection.

Basophils absorb alkaline dyes and stain blue. They produce heparin and histamine.

Eosinophils take up acidic dyes and stain red. They increase in number with parasitic infestation.

Agranulocytes

The agranulocytes have clear cytoplasm:

Lymphocytes make up over 80% of the agranulocytes in the body. There are two types of lymphocytes: T lymphocytes and B lymphocytes. They are both produced in the foetus within the lymphoid tissue, but those destined to become T lymphocytes pass to the thymus, and the others to the spleen where they mature into B lymphocytes.

T lymphocytes are long-lived cells, spending between 3 and 7 months circulating between blood and tissues. B lymphocytes are shorter lived, surviving less than a week.

Monocytes are the largest of the leucocytes and are phagocytic. They are produced in the bone marrow from myeloid stem cells, and are in the circulation for up to 12 hours before migrating into the tissues, where they may be active for several months.

Platelets

Platelets (or thrombocytes) are cell fragments that are an essential part of the body's blood-clotting mechanism. They are formed in the bone marrow from cells called **megakaryocytes**.

Blood clotting

When a blood vessel is damaged, a series of reactions take place which result in the vessel being sealed with a 'clot' of blood:

(1) Platelets stick to the damaged walls of the vessel, and broken platelets release an enzyme, **thromboplastin**.
(2) The protein **prothrombin** (normally present in plasma), in the presence of thromboplastin and calcium, is converted to **thrombin**.
(3) Thrombin is an active enzyme, which acts on the plasma protein **fibrinogen** to produce insoluble fibres of **fibrin**.
(4) The fibrin sticks to the platelets to form a firm clot.

After some time, the clot shrinks and serum is released (i.e. serum is plasma minus the clotting factors).

Vitamin K is required for the manufacture of prothrombin and the tendency to bleed is increased if this vitamin is destroyed (as in the case of warfarin poisoning).

The anticoagulant **heparin** is normally present in the blood, and prevents unwanted clots forming in the body.

Blood clotting does not only occur when there is major damage to the body; it deals all the time with minor damage to vessels throughout the body – particularly in areas that are constantly moving or subject to minor trauma, such as the lungs, the lining of the gut and the joints.

The immune system

The **immune system** is the body's mechanism to deal with invasion by foreign matter (most commonly infectious agents such as bacteria or viruses).

The **humoral immune response** relies on the production of antibodies by the **B lymphocytes**. (An antibody is a substance that reacts with a particular foreign body or antigen to render it harmless.) When an antigen enters the body, the particular B lymphocyte that can produce the appropriate antibody multiplies to produce many **plasma cells**, which then produce antibodies against the invader.

The **cellular immune response** relies on the ability of **T lymphocytes** to recognise any cell that does not belong to the body, including cells that have been invaded and altered by viruses. T lymphocytes act within the blood, but also elsewhere in the tissues, such as on mucous surfaces.

The **reticuloendothelial system** is the system of phagocytic cells that move about through the body and consume foreign matter such as bacteria. These cells are given different names when they occur in different parts of the body. In the blood they are the **monocytes**; in connective tissue they are **macrophages** or **histocytes**. They are also found in the lymph nodes, the bone marrow, the spleen and the liver.

The heart

The function of the heart is to pump blood round the body under pressure. It is supplied with blood by the coronary arteries, which are the first two branches of the aorta.

The heart lies within the pericardium, which in turn lies within the mediastinum in the thorax, between the lungs. It is more or less conical in shape. The point, or apex, points downwards, and lies to the left of the thorax, near the sternum, at the level of rib 7. The heart lies at a slight angle, pointing forward.

The **pericardium** consists of a double layer of membrane. The inner layer, a serous membrane closely attached to the heart, is called the **serous pericardium**. The outer layer, a thicker fibrous membrane with serous endothelium on its inner side, is called the **fibrous pericardium**. With this arrangement, the heart lies within a double sac of pericardium with a little serous fluid (pericardial fluid) between the two layers. This fluid acts as a lubricant, allowing the heart to move freely.

When the heart within the thorax is viewed from the side, as in the lateral radiograph, the right side of the heart is more anterior, while the left ventricle is more posterior.

The epithelial inner lining of the heart is the **endocardium** and is continuous with the endothelium of the blood vessels. The muscle of the heart is called the **myocardium**. The outer layer of the heart, the **serous pericardium**, is also known as the **epicardium**.

The heart has right and left sides, and each side is divided into an **atrium**, a thinner walled chamber, and a thicker walled **ventricle** (Fig. 11.33). From shortly after birth there is no connection between the chambers of the left and right sides of the heart.

On each side of the heart, blood enters the atrium, then is forced by the contraction of the wall of that chamber through a valve and into the ventricle, the valve preventing back flow of blood. Contraction of the ventricle then pushes the blood through a second valve and out of the heart into the circulation.

The valves, which consist of fibrous **cusps** or flaps, are as follows:

- The **right atrio-ventricular** or tricuspid valve lies between the right atrium and the right ventricle; it has three cusps.
- The **left atrio-ventricular** or mitral valve lies between the left atrium and left ventricle; it has two cusps.
- The **aortic valve** lies between the left ventricle and the aorta; it has three cusps.
- The **pulmonary valve** lies between the right ventricle and the pulmonary artery; it has three cusps.

The **atrio-ventricular valves** are restricted in their movement by 'guy-ropes' called **chordae tendinae**, which are in turn attached to **papillary muscles**, which extend from the lining of the ventricle.

The conducting mechanism of the heart

Cardiac muscle is able to contract rhythmically without a constant nerve supply (the autonomic nerves to the heart serve only to control heart rate). Co-ordination of the contraction of heart muscle is carried out by a conducting mechanism that involves the following structures:

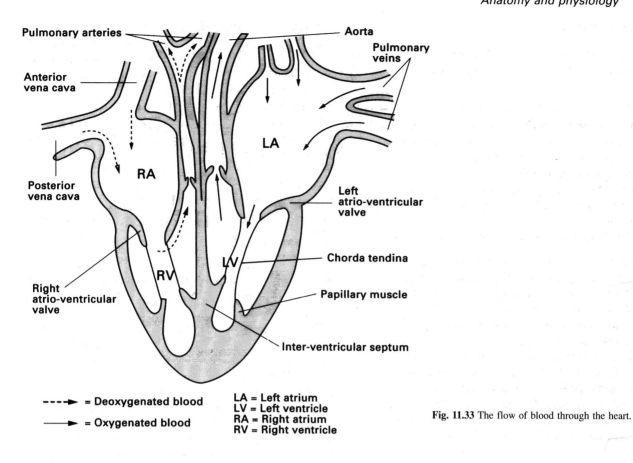

Pulmonary arteries

Aorta

Pulmonary veins

Anterior vena cava

LA

RA

Posterior vena cava

Left atrio-ventricular valve

Chorda tendina

RV

LV

Papillary muscle

Right atrio-ventricular valve

Inter-ventricular septum

- - - ► = Deoxygenated blood

──► = Oxygenated blood

LA = Left atrium
LV = Left ventricle
RA = Right atrium
RV = Right ventricle

Fig. 11.33 The flow of blood through the heart.

- The **sinu-atrial node** (SA node).
- The **atrioventricular node** (AV node).
- The **atrioventricular bundle**, or bundle of His.
- The **fibrous plate**.
- The **Purkinje fibres**.

Before considering the conduction system of the heart (Fig. 11.34), it is important to understand that the exit for blood from the ventricles is at the top of the ventricles, towards the base, not the apex of the heart. The aorta and the pulmonary artery twist round each other as they leave the heart.

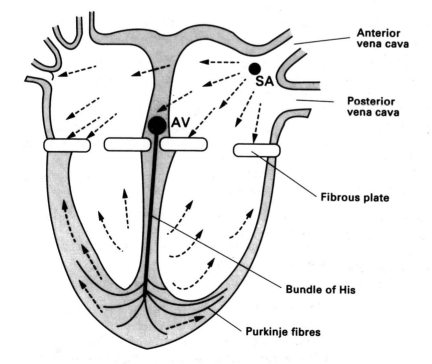

Anterior vena cava

SA

Posterior vena cava

AV

Fibrous plate

Bundle of His

Purkinje fibres

SA = Sinuatrial node
AV = Atrioventricular node
- - - - ► Spread of contraction across the heart

Fig. 11.34 The conduction system of the heart (aorta and pulmonary arteries omitted for the sake of clarity).

The **SA node** is an area of specialised heart muscle situated in the wall of the right atrium, near where the anterior vena cava enters the heart. It is from the SA node that the impulse for a wave of muscle contraction starts and spreads across the atria.

The cardiac muscle of the atria and ventricles is not continuous, but is separated by a fibrous plate, so that the only electrical connection between the atria and ventricles is at the top of the inter-ventricular septum.

The impulse activates the AV node, which lies at the top of the inter-ventricular septum, and passes the impulse down the bundle of His to the apex of the heart, where it spreads out over the ventricles in the network of Purkinje fibres.

In this way the wave of contraction of the ventricles starts at the apex of the heart, and the blood is pushed upwards towards the aortic and pulmonary valves.

The whole cycle of contraction then relaxation of atria then ventricles is called the **cardiac cycle**. Within the cardiac cycle, the period of contraction is called **systole**, and the period of relaxation is termed **diastole**.

The heart sounds

The sound made by a normal heart is usually described as: lup-dup, lub-dup, lub-dup. The first sound is made by the contraction of the ventricles and the closing of the atrio-ventricular valves. The second sound is made by the closing of the pulmonary and aortic valves.

The circulation of the blood

Deoxygenated blood returning from the body to the heart enters the right atrium (Fig. 11.35). It is then pumped through the right ventricle and enters the pulmonary circulation via the pulmonary artery. It then enters the lungs, where it is oxygenated, before returning to the left atrium via the pulmonary vein.

This oxygenated blood is then pumped through the left atrium and ventricle and enters the systemic circulation through the aorta, branches of which supply the trunk, the limbs and the thoracic, abdominal and pelvic viscera. The deoxygenated blood returns to the right atrium via the veins, culminating in the anterior and posterior venae cavae.

The hepatic portal system

The hepatic portal system lies within the systemic circulation.

The function of the hepatic portal system is to enable the products of digestion absorbed by the gut to be transported directly to the liver for storage or use.

The general rule throughout most of the body is that blood passes from the heart through arteries to a capillary bed and then returns to the heart via veins.

In the case of the hepatic portal system, however, the blood passes through two sets of capillaries before returning to the heart:

(1) The blood moves from the heart to the capillaries of the stomach and intestine.
(2) It then moves into the **hepatic portal vein** to the liver, where it enters another capillary bed.
(3) Blood from the liver then drains into the **hepatic vein**, which joins the posterior vena cava.

The arteries

Apart from the pulmonary circulation, the major vessels supplying blood to the body of the animal all arise as branches of the **dorsal aorta**, which runs from above the heart through the thorax and abdomen and into the pelvis (Fig. 11.36).

From the thorax down to the sacrum the aorta gives off pairs of arteries that supply the bones and muscles of the vertebral column and body wall.

After the coronary arteries have been given off the aorta, there are two large branches that come off what is termed the **aortic arch**. The first of these is the **brachiocephalic trunk**, which gives rise to the two **common carotid arteries** that travel up the neck to supply the head with blood. The **brachiocephalic trunk** then becomes the **right subclavian artery**, which continues as the **right axillary**, and then the **right brachial artery** as it supplies the right forelimb with blood. The second large branch off the aorta is the **left subclavian**, which becomes the **left axillary** and then the **left brachial artery** as it supplies the left forelimb.

In the abdomen, several important pairs of arteries are given off the aorta, including the **renal arteries** and the **spermatic or ovarian arteries**. There are also three large unpaired arteries in the abdomen:

- The **coeliac artery** supplies the stomach, the liver and the spleen with oxygenated blood.
- The **cranial mesenteric artery** supplies the small intestine, and anastomoses (joins up with) branches of the third unpaired artery.
- The **caudal mesenteric artery** supplies the large intestine.

In the lower abdomen and pelvis there are aortic branches to supply the hindlimb, in particular the **femoral artery**, and branches to the various pelvic viscera and much of the external genitalia.

The aorta, by now a very slender artery, ends as the **median sacral artery**, running along the ventral aspect of the coccygeal vertebrae.

The pulse in the brachial artery can be felt on the medial aspect of the humerus, distally, just above the elbow. The pulse of the femoral artery can be felt on the medial aspect of the thigh.

The veins

The head is drained by branches of the **jugular veins**, which run down the neck. The forelimbs are drained by a double system: the brachial veins which run with the brachial artery on the medial aspect of the limb; and the **cephalic vein**

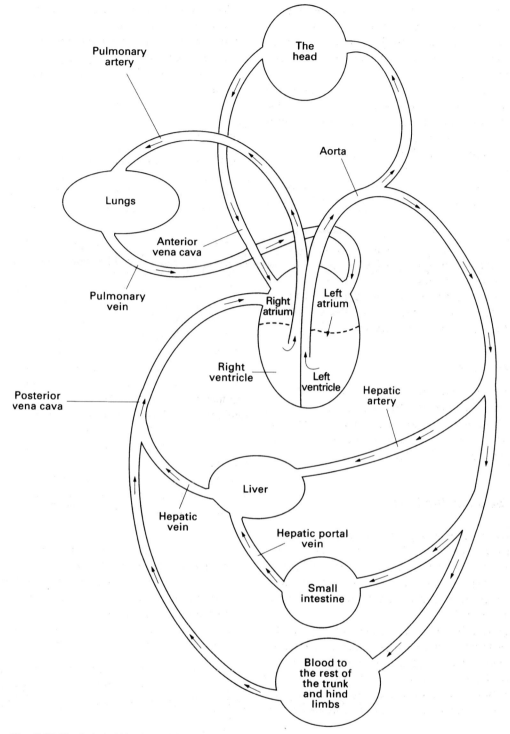

Fig. 11.35 Circulation of blood round the body.

which lies on the anterior aspect of the antebrachium (forearm). All the veins draining the head and forelimbs join the **anterior vena cava**, which in turn empties into the right atrium.

Another vein which may either join the anterior vena cava or empty independently into the right atrium is the **azygos vein**, which runs along the right side of the aorta and collects the venous blood from the intercostal spaces.

The **posterior vena cava** collects all the venous blood from the abdomen, pelvis and hindlimbs, returning it to the right atrium.

The hindlimb, like the forelimb, has a double venous system – the veins that run with the arteries and a more superficial system. The femoral vein runs with the femoral artery, and the saphenous veins lie just beneath the skin.

In the forelimb, the cephalic vein is more superficial than the brachial and therefore more useful for **venepuncture**. One vein in the hindlimb that is occasionally used for venepuncture is the **saphenous**, which crosses the lateral aspect of the limb just above the hock; however, the vein is very mobile under the skin and is therefore rarely a first choice of vein.

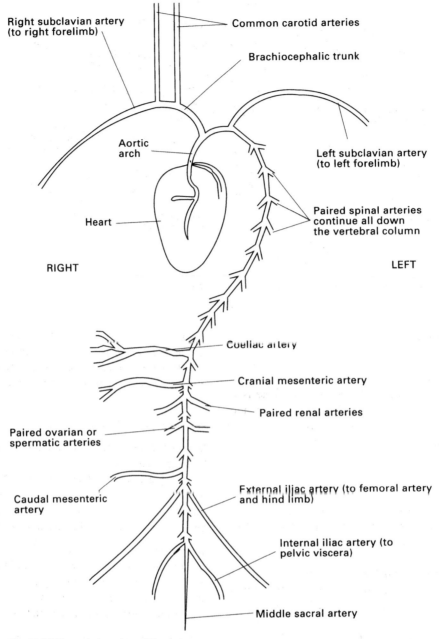

Fig. 11.36 The main branches of the aorta.

The lymphatic system

As the blood passes through the capillary network in the tissues, some fluid leaks out of the vessels into the interstitial spaces between the cells. This is called **tissue fluid**. Some of the fluid is drawn back into the capillaries by osmotic pressure, but much remains in the tissues and must be returned to the circulation by the lymphatic system – a set of fine vessels found almost everywhere throughout the body (Fig. 11.37). The fluid within this system of vessels is called **lymph**.

The functions of the lymphatic system are:

● To return excessive tissue fluid to the circulation.
● To filter bacteria and other foreign substances out of the fluid within the lymph nodes.
● To produce lymphocytes.
● To transport digested food, particularly fat.

The lymphatic system consists of.

● **Lymphatic capillaries**.
● **Lymphatic vessels**.
● **Lymphatic tissues** (the **lymph nodes** and **spleen**).
● **Lymphatic ducts**.

Lymphatic capillaries

The **lymphatic capillaries** are the very fine channels that collect up surplus tissue fluid. They join together to form larger lymphatic vessels. The lymphatic capillaries found within the small intestine, in the intestinal villi, are called **lacteals**; they have a role in collecting fat from the small intestine after a meal, at which time the lymph in all the vessels proximal to the small intestine can appear milky because of the fat droplets within them.

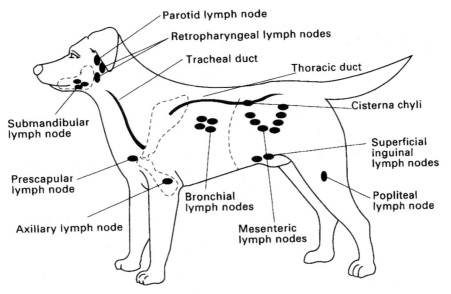

Fig. 11.37 The lymphatic system: major nodes and ducts.

Lymphatic vessels

The **lymphatic vessels** are thin-walled structures rather like veins. However, they are more numerous within tissues than veins, and have valves throughout their length. There is no smooth muscle in their walls: they rely on the movement of their surrounding tissues to 'milk' the lymph along the vessels past the non-return valves.

Lymphatic nodes

As they travel back towards the circulation, lymph vessels pass through one or more **lymph nodes**, which consist of lymphocytes joined together by a network of connective tissue.

They enter the node through **afferent vessels**, which may enter the node from all sides, and leave it through the **efferent vessels**, which are all clustered together at one point.

The functions of the **lymph nodes** are:

- To filter bacteria and other foreign matter from the lymph.
- To manufacture lymphocytes.

Lymph nodes are found mainly at the tops of the limbs, and at what can be called the portals of the body (where the inside meets the outside) in the neck and pharynx, in the mediastinum, on the bronchi, and in the abdomen – particularly within the mesentery of the small intestine.

Some lymph nodes are palpable in the healthy animal, while others are only palpable if they are enlarged as a result of local infection or infiltration by tumour cells.

Lymphatic ducts

After passing through the lymph nodes, the lymphatic vessels enter one of the two large **lymphatic ducts**. The smaller right lymphatic duct drains the right forelimb and the right side of the head and neck. The larger duct drains the whole of the rest of the body; in the abdomen it is called the **cisterna chyli** but once it has crossed the diaphragm it is called the **thoracic duct**. Both lymphatic ducts empty into either the right jugular vein or the anterior vena cava.

Lymphatic tissues

Other structures that contain lymphatic tissue are the tonsils, the spleen and the thymus.

The spleen is made up of lymphatic tissue and lies within the layers of the great omentum, next to the greater curvature of the stomach. It is not essential to life and can be surgically removed. Its functions are:

- The storage of red blood cells.
- The destruction of worn-out red blood cells.
- The production of lymphocytes.
- The removal, by phagocytosis, of bacteria and other foreign matter from the circulation.

The tonsils are masses of lymphoid tissue within the pharynx. They lie within the **tonsillar fossae**, on either side of the pharynx near the root of the tongue, and when enlarged are easily visible when a compliant animal opens its mouth.

The thymus is a lymphoid organ situated in the anterior part of the thoracic cavity. In the first few months of life it is an important site of lymphocyte production, but after this is reduced in size and the lymphoid tissue is replaced by fat.

The digestive system

The digestive system is one of the visceral systems of the body. Its function is to take and break down complex foodstuffs into simple compounds that the body can absorb. The waste is then excreted.

The digestive system starts with the mouth. The teeth, used to prehend (take hold of) food, have been discussed as part of the skeletal system.

The tongue

The **tongue** (see Fig. 11.28) is a muscular organ attached to the base of the pharynx. The functions of the tongue are:

● The manipulation of food.
● Tasting food, by means of the taste buds on its surface.
● Grooming.

In cats, the tongue is covered by many backward-facing papillae, which 'comb' the coat as the animal grooms itself. This also means that the hair which is groomed out by the tongue must be swallowed, as the papillae will not let it be passed forward out of the mouth.

Dogs and cats do not chew their food in the same way that humans do. The food (in the wild, mainly animal prey) is cut up by the shearing action of the carnassial teeth against the lower molars, and is swallowed in lumps.

The paired sublingual veins run along the underside of the tongue, in parallel with the two lingual arteries. The arteries may be used to monitor the pulse during general anaesthesia, and the veins can also be used in an unconscious animal for intravenous injection.

The salivary glands

While it is in the mouth, the food is moistened by saliva from the salivary glands (Fig. 11.38). There are four pairs of salivary glands in both the dog and the cat:

● The **zygomatic**.
● The **sublingual**.
● The **mandibular**.
● The **parotid**.

All the salivary glands have ducts that open into the mouth. The secretion of saliva is stimulated by the sight of food, the smell of food, or even just the anticipation of food (e.g. the sight of an owner wielding a tin opener). The production of saliva is continuous, but may increase or decrease in response to the above stimuli. The salivary glands are innervated by both sympathetic and parasympathetic nerves, which act on the glandular tissue and also on the blood vessels to increase or decrease the flow of blood to the glands.

Saliva has a number of functions:

● It moistens and softens the food, helping to break it up physically, so that the digestive enzymes can then break it up chemically.
● It lubricates the food to ease its passage down the oesophagus.
● It moistens the mouth, helping prevent drying of mucous membranes.
● The smaller salivary glands (zygomatic, sublingual and mandibular) produce mucus to help keep the mouth moist.
● The parotid gland produces a serous fluid which contains the enzyme **ptyalin**, or α-amylase, which starts to digest carbohydrate.

Swallowing

When food is swallowed, the following sequence is performed:

● A bolus (lump) of food is positioned on the tongue and pushed to the back of the mouth.
● The soft palate is raised, blocking off the nasopharynx.
● The hyoid apparatus (Fig. 11.39) moves forward and the epiglottis is pushed backwards to close off the larynx, preventing the entry of food.
● The pharynx is opened.
● The tongue pushes the bolus of food into the top of the pharynx, which closes behind it.
● Waves of muscular contraction (peristalsis) then carry the food from the pharynx to the stomach.

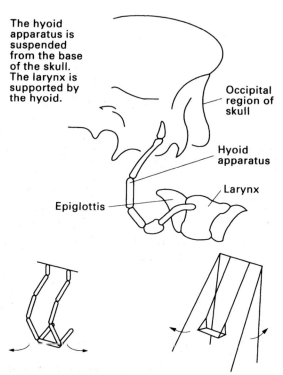

The hyoid apparatus is suspended from the base of the skull. The larynx is supported by the hyoid.

Occipital region of skull

Hyoid apparatus

Larynx

Epiglottis

The movement of the hyoid apparatus – and so of the larynx – is like a swing

Fig. 11.39 The hyoid apparatus.

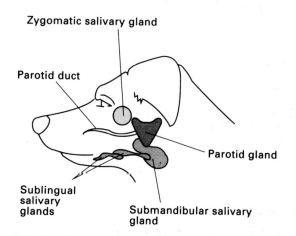

Zygomatic salivary gland

Parotid duct

Parotid gland

Sublingual salivary glands

Submandibular salivary gland

Fig. 11.38 The salivary glands of the dog.

- The soft palate is lowered.
- The hyoid apparatus moves backwards and the epiglottis falls forward, leaving the larynx open again.

The abdominal part of the digestive system

The digestive system within the abdomen can be divided into three parts (Fig. 11.40):

- The **stomach**, where storage and mixing of the food takes place.
- The **small intestine**, the main site of digestion and absorption of nutrients. The small intestine is divided into **duodenum**, **jejunum** and **ileum**.
- The **large intestine**, which is made up of **caecum**, **colon** and **rectum**.

The stomach

The stomach lies on the left side of the abdomen. It is divided into three areas:

- The **cardia**, the area where the oesophagus enters the stomach.
- The **fundus**, or body of the stomach.
- The **pylorus**, where the stomach narrows, and where the food passes into the small intestine.

The stomach is capable of considerable distension. It varies in size a good deal, as the carnivores (particularly the dogs) are able to gorge very large amounts of food at one time. In the wild, the stomach is the storage organ for perhaps several days' supply of food, and the means by which food is carried home to a den full of puppies. This explains the 'bottomless pit' nature of the average dog's appetite. An empty stomach lies tucked up under the ribs, but a fully distended stomach will extend to the ventral body wall and even cause distension of the ribs.

The mucosal lining of the stomach is thrown into longitudinal folds called **rugae,** that flatten when the stomach is filled.

All of the gastrointestinal tract is attached, either firmly or loosely, to the dorsal body wall by a dorsal mesentery. The dorsal mesentery of the stomach is massively expanded to form a double sheet of doubled mesentery which is the great omentum.

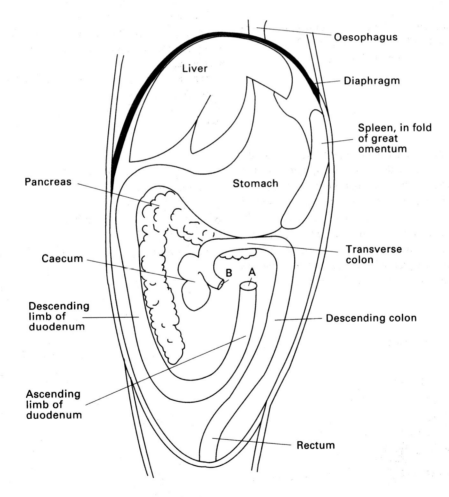

A. Junction of duodenum and jejunum
B. Junction of ileum and ascending colon (ileo-caeco-colic junction)

Fig. 11.40 Position of the gastrointestinal tract within the abdomen. (The view is from the ventral aspect. The jejunum and ileum have been removed.)

The spleen lies within the layers of the **great omentum** which lies over the ventral surface of the small intestine as a covering, and is the first organ to be seen when the abdomen is opened along the mid-ventral line.

Gastric secretions

A number of different secretions are produced by cells in the stomach wall:

- **Mucus** is produced in all parts of the stomach. It protects the lining of the stomach.
- **Hydrochloric acid (HCl)** is produced in the fundus by goblet or parietal cells. A low (acid) pH is required for the enzyme pepsin to act.
- **Pepsinogen** is produced in the fundus and is acted on by the hydrochloric acid to produce pepsin, an active enzyme that breaks down protein.
- **Gastrin** is a hormone produced by what are termed 'G cells' in the fundus. The gastrin is carried in the bloodstream to the goblet cells in the stomach wall, and stimulates the production of hydrochloric acid.
- **Lipase**, an enzyme that breaks down fat, is also produced, but only in small amounts.

The food in the stomach is mixed with the various gastric secretions, then the resulting fluid is passed out of the stomach and into the small intestine. The mixture of food, saliva and gastric secretions that leaves the stomach is called **chyme**.

Vomiting

The entry into the stomach, known as the cardiac sphincter, normally remains closed unless food reaches it from the oesophagus. However, vomiting (the forceful expulsion of gastrointestinal contents through the mouth) does occur as a response to over-distension of the stomach or irritation of the stomach lining (gastritis). The smooth muscle of the stomach wall relaxes, the cardiac sphincter opens and the stomach contents are forced up the oesophagus by the forceful contraction of abdominal muscles.

The small intestine

The small intestine is the site for further digestion and also the main site for absorption of the products of digestion.

The first part of the small intestine is the **duodenum**. It lies on the right side of the abdomen and forms a U-shape. It has three ducts leading into it – two **pancreatic ducts** and a **bile duct**.

The second and third parts of the small intestine – the **jejunum** and **ileum** – are indistinguishable to the naked eye and can be considered together. This is the very long section of the gut that lies loose in the abdominal cavity within the great mesentery.

There are three secretions into the small intestine:

- **Pancreatic juice.**
- **Bile.**
- **Intestinal juice.**

Pancreatic juice

The pancreas is a mixed gland, containing both exocrine and endocrine tissue. It lies between the two arms of the duodenum.

The exocrine secretion of the pancreas is involved in digestion, and enters the duodenum through two pancreatic ducts.

Pancreatic juice contains bicarbonate (HCO_3^-), which is alkaline, and so helps to neutralise the acid within the chyme and produce a suitable pH for the pancreatic enzymes. Pancreatic juice is secreted in response to a variety of stimuli. The hormone cholecystokinin which is secreted by duodenal cells stimulates the pancreas to secrete a wide range of proenzymes and enzymes. The pancreatic enzymes are:

- **Amylase**, which continues the breakdown of carbohydrate started by the salivary amylase.
- **Trypsin**, which acts on proteins and on the products of protein breakdown started by the pepsin in the stomach. It is secreted as **trypsinogen**, which is converted to the active enzyme trypsin by the action of the intestinal hormone **enterokinase**, which is secreted in the intestinal juice.
- **Lipase**, which breaks down fats to fatty acids and glycerol.
- **Peptidases**, which break down polypeptide chains to free amino acids.
- **Nucleotidases**, which break down RNA and DNA.

Bile

Bile enters the duodenum down the bile duct. It is produced in the liver and then stored in the gall bladder, which is attached to the liver, until it is required for digestion. Bile is essential for the breakdown of fats. If too little bile is produced, then there will be fat in the faeces. The two main constituents of bile are:

- **Bile salts**, which act as detergents: they break the surface tension between fats and water so that the fats are broken into small droplets, forming an emulsion. It is easier for the lipase to act on small droplets in an emulsion than on large drops of fat.
- **Bile pigments** are waste produced in the liver from the breakdown of blood pigments. They give the faeces their distinctive colour.

Intestinal juice

Intestinal juice is the third secretion into the small intestine. It is produced by cells in the wall of the **crypts of Lieberkuhn**, which lie between the villi of the small intestine. Like the pancreatic juice, it contains bicarbonate, and also the following enzymes (some of which are also pancreatic):

- **Disaccharidases**, which break down the disaccharides (e.g. maltose, sucrose and lactose) into simple sugars that can be absorbed.
- **Peptidases** to break down peptides into amino acids.
- **Nucleotidase.**
- **Enterokinase.**

Absorption

Absorption of the products of digestion – the amino acids, the fatty acids and the sugars – takes place almost entirely through the villi of the wall of the small intestine. Amino acids and simple sugars are absorbed into the blood capillaries, and are carried in the blood to the liver, via the hepatic portal system. Chyle is the milky fluid taken up by the lacteals from the intestine during digestion.

The fatty acids and glycerol are absorbed into the lacteals (lymph vessels within the villi), where in the form of minute fat droplets they are carried to the cisterna chyli then into the thoracic duct and back into the bloodstream.

The large intestine

The large intestine is composed of the caecum, the colon and the rectum.

The **caecum** is a small blind-ended sac that has no significant function in the carnivores. In herbivores such as the rabbit and guinea pig it is much larger and is a site where bacteria are used to break down coarse vegetable matter so that it can be used by the animal.

The **colon** is attached to the dorsal body wall and has three parts: the ascending, transverse and descending colon.

Water, electrolytes and water-soluble vitamins are absorbed in the large bowel, and the waste products are then passed down towards the **rectum**, where they are held before being excreted.

Defecation

Defecation is a combination of voluntary and involuntary acts. The involuntary movement of the large bowel moving faeces into the rectum produces the wish to defecate. However, the relaxation of the external anal sphincter, which allows faeces to be passed, is a voluntary act.

The liver

Closely associated with the digestive system is the liver, sometimes termed 'the largest gland in the body'. It lies against the diaphragm, in front and to the right of the stomach, and is divided into a number of lobes.

The gall bladder lies centrally on the caudal aspect of the liver, and from it the gall bladder carries bile to the duodenum.

The liver receives blood from two sources: about 20% is normal arterial blood from a branch of the aorta, and the rest comes from the veins carrying venous blood away from the intestine, in the hepatic portal system. This blood, of course, carries many of the products of digestion.

The liver performs many chemical functions for the body:

- **Protein metabolism.** Many of the plasma proteins are synthesised in the liver, as are fibrinogen and other proteins involved in blood clotting.
- **Urea formation.** Ammonia, the toxic waste product of protein breakdown, is converted to the less toxic urea.
- **Carbohydrate metabolism.** Blood sugar levels are kept within narrow limits as surplus is stored in the liver as glycogen, and then released into the circulation as energy is required by the body.
- **Fat metabolism.** Some lipids required by the body are synthesised in the liver, and fatty acids are metabolised to produce energy.
- **Formation of bile.**
- **Detoxification and conjugation of steroid hormones.**
- **Vitamin storage.** The liver is the main store of the fat-soluble vitamins (A, D, E and K). Some of the water-soluble vitamins, particularly B_{12}, are also stored.
- **Production of heat** and regulation of body temperature.
- **Iron storage.**

The urinary system

The urinary system is responsible for removing waste products – including surplus water – from the body (Fig. 11.41). The system consists of:

- The two **kidneys**, which filter the blood.
- The **ureters** that carry the urine from the kidneys.
- The **bladder**, the storage organ.
- The **urethra**.

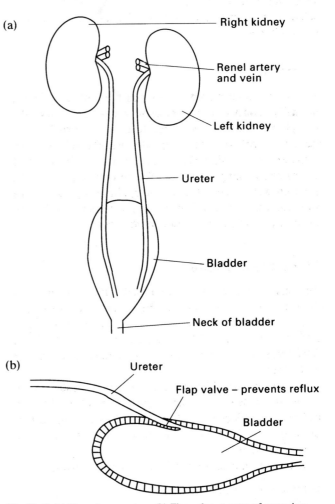

Fig. 11.41 (a) The urinary system. (b) Flap-valve at entry of ureter into bladder – it prevents urine flow back up the ureter.

The kidneys

The two kidneys lie against the dorsal wall of the abdomen, attached to it by a covering or 'capsule' of fibrous tissue. They are, needless to say, kidney shaped (although this is not the case in all species). The right kidney is about half a kidney's length in front of the left.

The indented part of the kidney is called the **hilus**, and is the point at which blood vessels and nerves and also the ureters enter or leave the kidney.

A cross-section of a kidney (Fig. 11.42) shows that the organ can be divided into three main areas: a **cortex**, which is darker in colour; the paler **medulla**; and the hollow collecting area of the **renal pelvis**.

The blood supply to the kidneys comes from the **renal arteries**, which leave the aorta close to the kidneys.

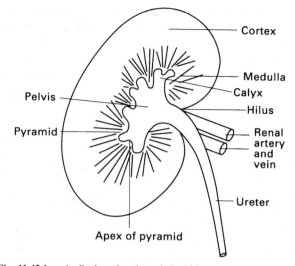

Fig. 11.42 Longitudinal section through the kidney.

The functions of the kidney

- The formation of urine.
- The production of renin.
- The conversion of vitamin D to an active form.
- The production of erythropoietin.
- The maintenance (with other organs) of the correct pH of the body.

The formation of urine involves the excretion of excess and waste materials from the body (including excess water).

The nephron

The **nephron** (Fig. 11.43) is the functional unit of the kidney. There are many thousands of nephrons in kidney tissue and they are the mechanism by which the blood is filtered and urine is produced. The nephron starts in the cortex of the kidney with the cup-shaped **Bowman's capsule**, which contains the **glomerulus**, a knot of capillaries fed by an **afferent arteriole** and drained by an **efferent arteriole**.

As the tubule leaves the capsule, it makes several twists and turns and this part of the nephron is called the **proximal convoluted tubule (PCT)**. The next part forms the long **loop of Henle** that dips down into the medulla then returns to the cortex. There is then another series of convolutions – the **distal convoluted tubule (DCT)** – before the nephron empties into a **collecting duct** that serves a number of nephrons and carries the urine through the medulla to the

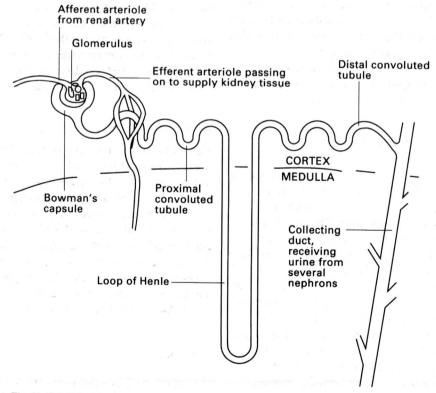

Fig. 11.43 A kidney nephron.

renal pelvis. The collecting ducts all discharge their contents into the renal pelvis at the apex of each pyramid of the medulla.

The indentations of the renal pelvis that lie between the pyramids of the medulla are called **calyces** (singular calyx).

The ureters

The **ureters** (one from each kidney) are thick-walled, narrow tubes that carry urine from the renal pelvis to the **bladder**. They are lined with mucous membrane and have smooth muscle in their walls which undergo peristaltic movements to move the urine on down towards the bladder. The ureters enter the bladder close to its neck, on its dorsal aspect, and there is a simple flap valve that prevents the return of urine up the ureter under the high pressure of a full bladder.

The bladder

The bladder is capable of considerable distension. It is covered with peritoneum, and it has a double layer of smooth muscle fibres in its wall and a lining of **transitional epithelium** which continues into the urethra. The lining of the empty bladder is thrown into folds, which allows for tremendous expansion when it is full.

The area between the ureteral openings and the neck of the bladder is known as the **trigone** of the bladder.

The urethra

In the male, the urethra carries urine from the bladder to outside the body. In the female, it carries the urine from the bladder to the **urethral orifice**, which opens into the genital tract at the junction of vagina and vestibule.

The urethra has two sphincters near to where it leaves the bladder. The **internal sphincter** is involuntary, but the **external sphincter** is under voluntary control.

Renal filtration and absorption

The blood in the glomerulus is under high pressure, and the low pressure in the hollow Bowman's capsule allows some of the constituents of blood to enter the Bowman's capsule. This is known as the **glomerular filtrate**. It can be described as an ultrafiltrate of plasma, as it is very similar to plasma except that the larger protein molecules have remained, with the blood cells, in the circulation.

The difference in pressure between the blood in the glomerulus and the pressure of the fluid in the Bowman's capsule is known as the filtration pressure. Over 100 litres of glomerular filtrate may be produced in a day by a large dog – and as only a fraction of this ends up as urine (1–2 litres), there must be considerable reabsorption down the length of the nephron. Urine volume may be from 0.5% to 15% of the original glomerular filtrate.

Reabsorption and secretion in the renal tubule

Most of the substances in the glomerular filtrate are reabsorbed lower down the nephron either by active transport across the lining membrane or by passive diffusion.

- **Water** is actively absorbed, mainly in the proximal convoluted tubule (PCT) but also in the distal convoluted tubule (DCT).
- **Sodium** is actively absorbed in the PCT, with chloride following by passive diffusion.
- **Glucose** is very efficiently absorbed in the first part of the PCT unless the plasma concentration is very high and exceeds what is called the **renal threshold**, when glucose starts to appear in the urine (e.g. in diabetes mellitus).
- **Amino acids** are reabsorbed completely in the convoluted tubules.
- In the healthy animal, any **protein** that is filtered is reabsorbed in the PCT.
- The waste product **urea** is reabsorbed in the PCT, then re-secreted into the tubule in the loop of Henle.
- **Acids and bases** in the filtrate are selectively absorbed, and **hydrogen ions, bicarbonate** and **ammonia** may be secreted into the tubule to help maintain the correct pH within the body.
- There are some other substances, e.g. **penicillin**, which are also actively secreted into the PCT.

Control of filtration and reabsorption

Water

The reabsorption of water is controlled by **anti-diuretic hormone** (ADH), which is secreted by the posterior pituitary gland. When the body needs to decrease the volume of urine to conserve fluid within the body, ADH acts on the DCT to increase water reabsorption. Conversely, a fall in secreted ADH will decrease water reabsorption in the DCT and allow more urine to enter the collecting ducts.

Sodium

The reabsorption of sodium is controlled by **aldosterone**, which is secreted by the adrenal cortex. When the plasma sodium level falls, the kidney firstly produces the enzyme **renin**, which acts on **angiotensinogen** in the plasma to convert it to **angiotensin I**. The angiotensin I is then converted to **angiotensin II** which stimulates the adrenal cortex to release aldosterone. Aldosterone acts on the DCT to increase reabsorption of sodium and chloride. The angiotensin also increases blood pressure by causing vasoconstriction, and so increases the glomerular filtration rate as the filtration pressure is increased.

Vitamin D

The fat-soluble form of vitamin D is converted to the more active water-soluble form within the kidney.

Erythropoietin

Active **erythropoietin**, the substance that stimulates the production of red blood cells in the bone marrow, is produced from an inactive plasma protein by 'erythropoietin factor', which is produced by the kidney in response to low oxygen levels in the blood.

Urine and micturition (urination)

As the bladder fills with urine, stretch receptors in its wall send messages to the brain giving the animal the wish to pass urine. These stimuli can be suppressed for a certain time, but then when the situation is right or the bladder is very distended, voluntary motor nerves will cause relaxation of the external sphincter and shortening and so dilatation of the urethra, allowing urine to be passed.

A dog passes 20–80 ml urine/kg bodyweight per day, while a cat passes rather less, at 10–15 ml/kg. Analysis of urine is very useful as a diagnostic aid in veterinary medicine, as many disease conditions may be reflected in abnormal urine contents:

* **pH and specific gravity**: The urine of a carnivorous animal when it is fed on a meat-based diet is normally slightly acid, in the range pH 5–7, with a specific gravity of 1.016–1.060 in the dog and 1.020–1.040 in the cat.
* **Protein** should not appear in the urine of a healthy animal, although it may do if there is damage to the urinary tract or increased permeability of the glomerulus. Protein appears in the urine in chronic renal disease and in cystitis.

* **Blood** may appear in urine as a result of physical damage to the urinary tract, or as contaminant from, say, the prostate in the male, or blood-stained discharge from an in-season bitch.
* **Bile** will show up in the urine in certain types of liver disease or blockage of the bile duct.
* **Glucose** in the urine usually reflects an abnormally high plasma glucose, most frequently as a result of diabetes mellitus.
* **Ketones** are produced by the body when fats are being oxidised as an energy source, and may appear in the urine in diabetes mellitus, or when there is insufficient calorie intake.
* **Deposits** in urine may also be useful for diagnostic purposes and may include **cells** from different parts of the urinary tract, **crystals** or larger stones (**calculi**), or **casts** of the inside of renal tubules.

The male reproductive system

The reproductive or genital system of the male is responsible for the production, storage and nourishment of sperm, and for their transport into the genital tract of the female so that the ova of the female may be fertilised (Figs 11.44 and 11.45).

The male reproductive system consists of:

* The testes.
* The epididymides (singular: epididymis).
* The vasa deferentia (singular: vas deferens) or deferent ducts.
* The prostate gland.

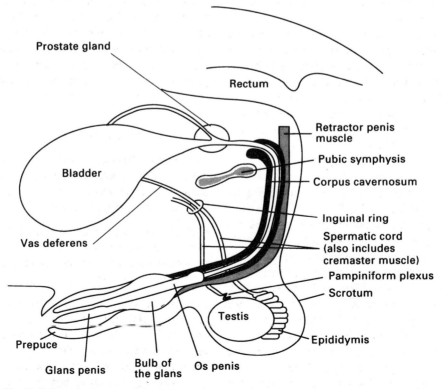

Fig. 11.44 Reproductive tract of the dog.

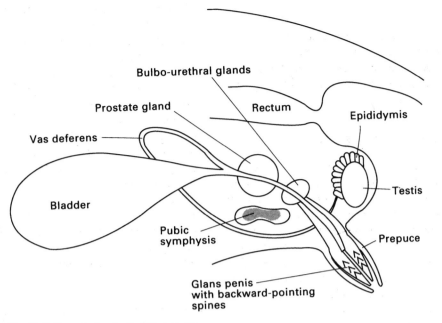

Fig. 11.45 Reproductive tract of the tom cat.

- The urethra.
- The penis.
- The prepuce.

The urethra and penis are common to both the reproductive and urinary tracts, and indeed the systems are often considered together as the urogenital tract.

The testes

The testes of the dog lie in the scrotum, a sac of skin between the hind legs. In the cat the scrotum lies on the perineum, below the anus.

In the foetus, the testes develop from undifferentiated gonads – glands with the potential to be either ovary or testis. These gonads start life in the abdomen, just behind the kidneys. As development proceeds, they move across the abdomen, out through the inguinal ring in the abdominal wall, and so come to lie in the scrotum, surrounded by a double fold of peritoneum – the internal and external tunic of the **tunica vaginalis**. Because the blood supply, nerve supply and ducts that run to and from the testis originate from when the testis was an intra-abdominal organ, they run from the abdomen out through the inguinal ring, taking the same route as the migrating testes.

In some cases the testes do not complete their journey, and may end up either lying just subcutaneously in the inguinal region, or still within the abdomen. A dog with both testes undescended is termed a **cryptorchid** and a dog with only one is termed **monorchid**. In the normal puppy the testes are palpable in the groin by 8–10 weeks of age, though the scrotum may not be fully formed by then, and of course the testes are still small in the prepubertal dog.

The group of blood vessels, nerves and ducts that run from the scrotum through the inguinal ring into the abdomen is called the **spermatic cord**. It also has a thin strip of muscle running with it, called the **cremaster muscle**, which originates from the internal abdominal oblique muscle of the abdominal wall and allows the raising and lowering of the testes within the scrotum, to bring them closer to or further from the body wall.

Surgical removal of the testes is termed castration or neutering. Early castration (before the onset of puberty) can affect the development of the secondary sexual characteristics – the heavier musculature (particularly in the neck) and the development of erectile tissue in the penis in the dog; and the heavier shape and distinctive smell and voice of the tom cat.

The blood supply to the testis is the testicular artery, which originates from the abdominal aorta. As it enters the scrotum and runs alongside the epididymis it becomes massively convoluted, forming the **pampiniform plexus**. The reason for these convolutions is said to be to allow blood to cool and to smooth out the pulsations in the vessel before the blood reaches the gonad.

Structure of the testis

The internal structure of the testis is made up of several hundred convoluted **seminiferous tubules** with supportive connective tissue and cells between them. They are lined with two different types of cell:

- **Spermatogenic** cells, which divide by meiosis to produce spermatozoa.
- **Sertoli cells**, which produce oestrogens and also nutritive fluid for the sperm.

The cells among the supportive connective tissue are called the **interstitial cells**, or the **cells of Leydig**, and they produce the male hormone **testosterone**, which is responsible for spermatogenesis and the development and maintenance of secondary male sexual characteristics.

Testosterone is also responsible for the descent of the testes into the scrotum, and in the young animal it has an inhibitory effect on the hypothalamus in the brain. At puberty, however, it stops being inhibitory, and the hypothalamus stimulates the anterior pituitary gland to produce **interstitial cell stimulating hormone (ICSH)** and **luteinising hormone (LH)**, which stimulate the development of the seminiferous tubules and so sperm production, and also increase testosterone production by the cells of Leydig.

The epididymis

Sperm leave the testis in a series of small ducts, **the vasa efferentia** or **efferent ducts**, which carry them to the **epididymis**, a larger, much coiled duct that lies alongside the testis in the scrotum and is where the sperm are stored.

The vas deferens

The **deferent duct** or **vas deferens** runs within the spermatic cord. It carries the sperm from the epididymis, through the inguinal ring, to the urethra. It empties into the urethra through the prostate gland.

The prostate gland

The prostate gland of the dog lies just below the neck of the bladder. In the cat it lies a little further down the urethra.

The prostate produces a large part of the **seminal fluid** that makes up the volume of ejaculate in the dog. It is a bilobed structure about the size and shape of a peeled walnut, and surrounds the urethra at the level of the pelvic brim. Enlargement of the prostate can cause obstruction to the passage of faeces through the pelvis, or when very large it may move into the abdomen, where it can often be palpated as a mass posterior to the bladder.

The bulbo-urethral glands

The bulbo-urethral glands are found in the cat but not in the dog. They, like the prostate, make a contribution to the seminal fluid. They lie further down the urethra, near to the perineum.

The penis

In the dog, the penis runs from the ischial arch of the pelvis, down the perineum and between the hind legs of the dog. The distal part is contained within the **prepuce**, a sheath or fold of abdominal skin suspended from the midline of the ventral abdominal wall. The prepuce is lined with mucous epithelium. It covers and protects the distal part of the penis, but is pushed back during coitus (mating) to expose the erect glans penis.

The penis itself consists of:

- The urethra.
- The os penis.

- The corpus cavernosum penis.
- The corpus spongiosum penis.
- The retractor penis muscle.

The **corpus cavernosum penis** consists of two **crura** or strips of erectile tissue that originate at the **root of the penis** on the ischial arch of the pelvis and continue down into the body of the penis, although not as far as its tip. The **urethra** runs in a groove between the two crura.

The **corpus spongiosum penis** runs beneath the corpus cavernosum and the urethra, and is expanded proximally into the **bulb of the penis** and at its tip into the **glans penis**, where it completely surrounds the urethra and forms the apex of the organ.

The penis of the cat differs from that of the dog in that it does not lie along the ventral abdomen, but points backwards. It also differs in having a number of backward-facing spines on the glans.

The **os penis** in the dog lies dorsal to the urethra, but in the cat, owing to the different orientation of the penis, it lies ventral to the urethra. In both species the os penis is V-shaped, with the urethra lying along the groove in the bone.

The **retractor penis** muscle originates from the first few coccygeal vertebrae, and its action is to pull the penis back into the prepuce.

The female reproductive system

The female reproductive system (Fig. 11.46) consists of:

- The two ovaries.
- The Fallopian tubes or oviducts.
- The uterus – horns, body and cervix.
- The vagina.
- The vestibule.
- The clitoris.
- The vulva.

The genital system of the female produces eggs, or ova, which are fertilised in the Fallopian tubes, then carried to the uterine horns, where they are implanted. It is here that the foetus grows throughout the gestation period.

The ovaries

The ovaries are situated in the abdomen, behind the kidneys. Each one is attached to the dorsal body wall via the kidney capsule by the ovarian or **suspensory ligament**. The blood supply comes from the ovarian artery, which is a branch of the aorta and is very convoluted as it follows the ovarian ligament to the gonad.

Like all structures within the abdominal cavity, the ovaries lie within a fold of mesentery, in this case called the **mesovarium**, but in this case there is an opening into the fold to allow the ova to escape. This opening is the opening to the **ovarian bursa**.

Within the ovary are many **primary ovarian follicles**, each of which can develop into a ripe ovarian follicle

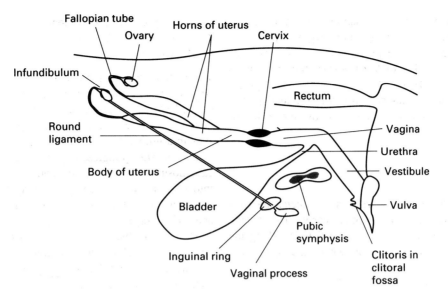

Fig. 11.46 Reproductive tract of the bitch (lateral view).

(Graafian follicle). Some species release just one egg at a time; others, including the dog and cat, release groups of follicles together. Each ripe follicle contains a large amount of fluid, and one ovum.

At ovulation, the follicle ruptures at the surface of the ovary, releasing the ovum, which is taken up by the **fimbria** of the **infundibulum** at the head of the oviduct.

After ovulation there may be some bleeding into the ruptured follicle, but then the cells of the follicular wall proliferate to form a solid corpus luteum.

The oviduct

The oviduct is a narrow, convoluted tube that runs from the horn of the uterus to the trumpet-like infundibulum that encloses the ovary and captures the released ova.

The uterus

In the cat and the dog the uterus consists of two long horns, and then a body leading to a single cervix. It lies within the mesometrium (or broad ligament) of the uterus and is dorsal within the abdomen, except when it is enlarged, when it may hang down under its own weight and lie more ventral within the abdomen.

The wall of the uterus is made up of layers of smooth muscle which together are called the myometrium, and the mucous epithelial lining called the endometrium.

At the base of the body of the uterus is the cervix, a muscular organ that acts as a sphincter to close the uterus except during mating and parturition.

The round ligament runs from the ovary towards and through the inguinal ring, where it terminates in a pad of fat known as the vaginal process. The round ligament is the female homologue of the gubernaculum, which in the male draws the gonad (the testis) through the inguinal ring and into the scrotum. The round ligament lies in a fold of the broad ligament.

The vagina and vestibule

The vagina extends from the cervix to the external urethral orifice, and lies entirely within the pelvis. After the vagina, the genital tract has a sharp bend downwards as the tract passes into the vestibule, which is that part of the tract that is used by both the genital and urinary systems. The muscles in the wall of the vestibule are very strong, and in the bitch they contribute to the 'tie' between bitch and dog during mating.

The vulva and clitoris

The vulval lips form the boundaries of the vertical slit that is the external opening of the female urogenital tract. The clitoris, the erectile tissue that is the female homologue of the penis, lies in the clitoral fossa – a small cavity just inside the base of the vulva. The vulval lips are normally soft, but become enlarged and turgid when a bitch is in season.

Reproductive patterns

Most animal species have particular breeding seasons during the year. The time of the year when an animal chooses to have its young is usually based on there being a plentiful food source at that time. The onset of the breeding season may be triggered by external factors such as increasing or decreasing day length (changes in photoperiod) or the beginning of a wet season, or a rise or fall in temperature.

The domestic dog has two breeding seasons during the year, but these may fall at any time – although more bitches come 'on heat' during the spring and autumn than at other times. The timing of their seasons may be influenced not only by photoperiod but also by other bitches: bitches living in groups all tend to have their 'seasons' at about the same time.

The queen has a breeding season that is dictated by increasing then decreasing day length and runs from early spring (January/February) until autumn (late August or September).

The oestrous cycle

Oestrus is the period during the oestrous cycle when the female is prepared to accept the male, and it varies in length from species to species. Oestrus coincides with the release of ova by the ovary and the female's willingness to mate at this time makes it likely that the ova will be fertilised soon after ovulation.

The general pattern of the oestrous cycle in the mammal is as follows (see Table 11.1):

- **Pro-oestrus** is the period during which the follicles in the ovary enlarge and become mature.
- **Oestrus** is when the follicles rupture and the ova are released.
- **Metoestrus** is the period when the corpus luteum starts to form at the site of the ruptured follicle.
- **Dioestrus** is the time when the corpus luteum is established or, if the ova have been fertilised, a pregnancy may be established.
- **Anoestrus** is a period when there is no ovarian activity.

If there is no pregnancy, then after a time the corpus luteum will degenerate and either there will be a period of anoestrus or the ovary will enter another phase of pro-oestrus as another batch of follicles start to mature. (This subject is covered in detail in Chapter 18, Obstetric and Paediatric Nursing of the Dog and Cat.)

The oestrous cycle in the bitch

The bitch is **monoestrous**: she has only one oestrous cycle in each breeding season. Bitches may come into season for the first time at any time between 6 and 18 months old. Thereafter they usually come into season about every 6 months (although there are plenty of exceptions that have one or three breeding seasons a year.)

Pro-oestrus in the bitch lasts on average about 9 or 10 days. During this time the vulva swells and there is a blood-stained mucous discharge from the vulva. Internally, the ovarian follicles are maturing and the endometrium is thickening and producing the secretion that appears at the vulva. Pro-oestrus is initiated by secretion of **follicle stimulating hormone (FSH)** from the anterior pituitary, which stimulates the development of the mature **Graafian follicle**. **Oestradiol** is secreted from the wall of the developing follicle, and this causes the thickening of the endometrium and the changes in the external genitalia seen at this time.

Oestrus lasts on average 7–10 days, though it may be longer or shorter. During this period the discharge becomes less bloody and the follicles rupture. The follicular fluid contains oestradiol secreted by the cells lining the follicle, and as ovulation occurs there is a sudden surge of oestradiol in the bloodstream that depresses any further production of FSH and stimulates the production of **luteinising hormone (LH)**, which in its turn stimulates the development of the corpus luteum at the site of the ruptured follicle.

The bitch ovulates whether or not she is mated and so is termed a **spontaneous ovulator**.

Corpora lutea form during the period of **metoestrus** whether or not the bitch has been mated, and produce **progesterone**, which maintains the pregnancy if it exists, and may produce the symptoms of **pseudopregnancy** (false pregnancy or pseudocyesis) if the ova have not been fertilised. Some bitches show signs of false pregnancy, such as mammary gland enlargement, milk production, and then nest-making; others show little or no signs.

After the period of **dioestrus**, when the corpora lutea are established and maintaining a pseudopregnancy, or at the end of the true pregnancy, the corpora lutea regress and the bitch goes into **anoestrus** until the next breeding season.

The total length of the 'season' in the bitch is usually quoted as 21 days – but many take much longer than that,

Table 11.1 Summary of the oestrous cycle of the bitch

	Duration	Dominant hormones	Ovarian activity	Other signs
Pro-oestrus	5–11 days	FSH – follicle development. Oestradiol – signs of oestrus.	Maturation of follicles.	Vulva enlarges, blood-stained mucous discharge.
Oestrus	7–10 days	LH – stimulates ovulation, then formation of corpus luteum. Oestradiol surge at ovulation causes dog interest and bitch willingness to be mated.	Rupture of mature Graafian follicles and release of ova. Corpus luteum starts to form on site of ruptured follicle.	Discharge less blood-stained. Bitch will stand to be mated (exhibiting 'lordosis').
Metoestrus	5–15 days	LH – formation of corpus luteum. Progesterone – from forming corpus luteum.	Formation of corpus luteum.	Discharge decreases, dog much less interested, vulva reduced in size.
Dioestrus	6–7 weeks	Progesterone – maintaining pregnancy or producing changes associated with pseudocyesis (false pregnancy).	Mature corpus luteum (or corpora lutea)	Increase in uterine size if pregnant. Whether pregnant or not, mammary development towards end of dioestrus.
Anoestrus	3–5 months	None	None	None

and some will still be willing to stand for a dog on the 21st day or even later.

The oestrous cycle in the queen

The oestrous cycle in the queen is different to that of the bitch: she is **seasonally polyoestrous** and is an **induced ovulator**.

Seasonally polyoestrous means that after one oestrous cycle, instead of going into a period of anoestrus, the cat will return to pro-oestrus and have another oestrous cycle for as long as the breeding season lasts or until she becomes pregnant.

Induced ovulation means that if the queen is not mated, she will not ovulate. Instead, after a period of oestrus, the unruptured follicles will regress, there will be no corpus luteum development, and another batch of follicles will develop between 1 and 3 weeks later.

Young queens become mature between 6 and 12 months of age, and first come into oestrus in the first spring following their maturity.

Pro-oestrus in cats lasts from 1 to 3 days and oestrus up to about 10 days.

Detection of correct time of mating

Many books on dog care suggest that a bitch should be mated on the 11th and 13th day of oestrus. This is a very hit-or-miss method and is only successful in a large number of cases because of the longevity of dog sperm in the reproductive tract of the bitch (up to 7 days).

Other methods that can be used (apart from running the dog with the bitch and letting them decide the best time to have a go. . .) are vaginal cytology and progesterone assay.

Vaginal cytology (smears) can be used to follow the changes in the reproductive tract, but can only detect the time of ovulation by detecting the first day of metoestrus. This means that ovulation has occurred about 6 or 7 days previously – possibly rather late for a successful mating.

Blood tests to detect progesterone are more commonly used, as serum progesterone rises dramatically within a couple of days of the LH surge that initiates ovulation.

Mating

In the bitch, puberty may occur any time between about 6 and 18 months. Small breeds tend to reach puberty earlier than large breeds. The age of puberty in the dog is likewise variable, but most breeders would not use a dog at stud until he was a year old or more and he is sufficiently mature for his quality to be judged.

As a bitch comes into oestrus, she exhibits a number of signs that show her readiness to mate. As part of the pre-mating ritual, the dog will lick round the bitch's vulva and clitoris, and if she is ready to mate the bitch will exhibit '**lordosis**' – arching the back downwards so that the vulva is presented to the dog, while stretching her tail to one side so that it is out of the way. She will also **stand** still to receive the dog's attentions (hence 'standing oestrus'), whereas before she reaches oestrus she will swing round to face him as he attempts to lick her vulva and to mount.

When the bitch is ready she will permit the dog to mount and mate. His erect penis enters her vagina and with a series of thrusting movements he ejaculates. As he ejaculates, the strong vestibular muscles of the bitch tighten behind the erect bulb of the penis, so firmly holding the two animals together in a '**tie**'. After ejaculation the dog will dismount by swinging one hind leg over the bitch's back so they are standing tail-to-tail. They remain in this position for the duration of the tie, which may be anything from a few minutes to more than an hour.

The dog and bitch should not (and indeed cannot) be forced apart during the tie. It is possible to have fertile mating without a tie.

Female cats in oestrus exhibit lordosis by crouching with dipped back and thrusting their perineal area into the air. Stroking down the cat's back at this stage will make the arch even more pronounced and elicit vigorous trampling with the hind feet. They are also very vocal at this time. When cats mate, the procedure is much swifter than in dogs, and as the tom cat withdraws, the backward-pointing barbs on the glans irritate the female to the extent that she will usually turn round and take a swipe at the male.

Pregnancy

Pregnancy in bitches and queens may be diagnosed in a number of ways. Many owners will swear that they know a week or so after mating whether their pet is gravid (pregnant), by a change in attitude and behaviour.

Pregnancy diagnosis by abdominal palpation of the developing embryo can be performed, usually between 21 and 28 days (veterinary surgeons may have different preferred timings).

By 5 weeks there is a degree of abdominal enlargement, and the teats start to enlarge.

When an animal is pregnant for the first time she is said to be primigravid, or to be a primigravida. In later pregnancies she is known as multigravid. An animal that usually has only one offspring at a time is said to be uniparous, but the bitch and queen, with their large litters, are said to be multiparous.

During pregnancy, the position of the uterus within the abdomen changes. As the pups grow, the horns of the uterus increase in length and breadth, and their increased weight causes them to tend to slide down the sides of the abdomen, lateral to the mass of the intestines, until they lie ventrally within the abdomen. The final position will depend on the size of the litter

The mammary glands

Mammary glands (Fig. 11.47) are really modified sweat glands. Bitches usually have five pairs of glands and queens have four pairs, though the number is variable.

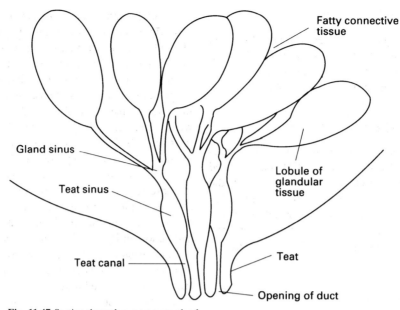

Fig. 11.47 Section through a mammary gland.

Mammary glands develop in the embryo from **mammary ridges** that run from the axilla to the groin. A **teat papilla** develops on the surface of the body, then solid epidermal buds or 'sprouts' grow downwards into the hypodermis and branch. When the branching system has been well established, the epidermal tissue hollows to produce the duct system of the gland. Rudimentary teats are found in the males of most but not all mammal species.

Mammary tissue consists of glandular tissue surrounded by fibrous connective tissue and fat. During pregnancy it becomes active and hypertrophies, and towards the end of the pregnancy it starts to produce mammary secretion. The teats hypertrophy as well, so they stand up proud from the skin by the time the young are born, and are easily found by the pups or kittens.

There are two ways of naming the mammary glands, particularly of bitches, where mastectomy for neoplasia is a common operation. The anatomist's terminology describes two thoracic pairs, two abdominal pairs and one inguinal pair. Some clinicians name them as three thoracic and two either abdominal or inguinal and this terminology relates to the lymphatic drainage of the glands. The front three pairs drain into the axillary lymph node and the posterior two pairs into the superficial inguinal lymph node.

Milk

The first milk produced is the colostrum, which is important in many species as a source of antibodies for the young. In the bitch and queen, antibodies are produced over a period of days, but the bowel ceases to absorb various antibodies at different times. As a general rule, all pups and kittens should have sucked within 8 hours – and preferably 4 hours – of birth. Ideally, the young should find themselves a teat as soon as the mother has finished cleaning them.

Milk contains fats, protein, and carbohydrate as the milk sugar lactose. Solids may make up less than 20% or more than 70% of the content of the milk, depending on species. Milk also contains calcium, phosphate, magnesium, sodium and chloride, vitamins A, E and K, and the B vitamins.

Early embryological development

Fertilisation

The ovum that is released from the ovary is surrounded by a double protective layer (Fig. 11.48). The inner layer, or **zona pellucida**, is glycoprotein; the outer layer, or **corona radiata**, is of small follicular cells.

Fertilisation takes place within the Fallopian tube. The first sperm to burrow through the corona radiata and penetrate the zona pellucida sets up the **fertilisation reaction**, which stops any other sperm entering the ovum. The fertilised ovum is then called a **zygote**.

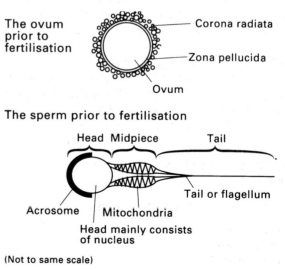

Fig. 11.48 Structure of ovum and sperm.

The zygote

After fertilisation the zygote continues to travel down the Fallopian tube, and as it does so the cells start to divide – first into two, then four, then eight and then irregularly to form a solid ball of cells called a **morula** (see Fig. 11.49).

Formation of germ cell layers

The morula then develops a cavity, with a mass of cells towards one end of the structure. The mass of cells is called the **inner cell mass**, and the cells lining the cavity are the **trophoblast**. The inner cell mass, which at this stage is in the form of a flat plate of cells, will eventually form the embryo.

The next stage is the development of three **germ cell layers** (Fig. 11.49) that will eventually form recognisable parts of the body:

● The **ectoderm**, or outer layer, of the inner cell mass forms the skin and nervous system.
● The **mesoderm**, or middle layer, forms the musculo-skeletal system and other internal organs.
● The **endoderm**, or inner layer, forms the lining of the gastrointestinal tract and other visceral systems.

The **mesoderm** forms as two longitudinal blocks of tissue, beneath which the endodermal cells spread round to line the trophoblast and form the yolk sac (Fig. 11.49). In the mammal there is no yolk within the yolk sac, but in reptiles and birds the yolk sac encloses the yolk of the egg that provides nourishment for the growing embryo.

Mesodermal cells then migrate to lie in two layers – one adjacent to the ectoderm and one to the endoderm – and a cavity starts to develop between them.

The inner cell mass starts to curl round to enclose the mesodermal and endodermal cells that will form its internal organs, leaving the yolk sac and the trophoblast to form **extra-embryonic membranes** – the placenta and the membranes that we see covering the foetus at birth. (In this context 'extra' means 'outside'.)

Implantation

At about this stage the developing embryos reach the uterine horns, where they tend to distribute themselves evenly between the two horns, and then settle against the wall of the uterus to implant.

Implantation takes place in the cat between 11 and 16 days, and in the dog between 14 and 20 days after ovulation. During implantation the zygote invades and partly destroys an area of hypertrophied endometrium so that it can lie within it, well attached to the wall of the uterus.

Formation of the extra-embryonic membranes

The extra-embryonic membranes are:

● The **yolk sac**.
● The **chorion**.
● The **amnion**.
● The **allantois**.

As the early embryo starts to curl up on itself, the top of the yolk sac becomes narrower and narrower as the top part of the endoderm is pinched off to become the primitive gut tube – though at this stage without openings at either end of the body. Then another diverticulum starts to develop from the primitive gut tube, and push its way out beside the yolk sac. This is the **allantois**; it will form the **allantoic sac**, which receives urine from the foetal kidneys via the **urachus**, which is the tube that carries the foetal urine from the bladder of the embryo out of the body.

As the cells of the inner cell mass multiply and then start to curve round underneath themselves, they form the head and trunk of the embryo, and within it the main body cavity, or coelom. In mammals, the coelom is divided into thorax and abdomen by the diaphragm. The diaphragm is formed from contributions of tissue from various structures. These include the caudal part of the mediastinal pleura, the septum transversum (formed during the development of the heart), and folds of tissue that develop from the body wall.

As the embryo continues to develop, the yolk sac contracts and the allantois increases in size and starts to push its way into the mesodermal cavity between the two mesodermal layers.

While the allantois is developing, the trophoblast continues to expand, reaching round the developing embryo so that it forms a double layer of membrane that completely surrounds the embryo. The outer membrane is called the **chorion**, and the inner layer membrane the **amnion** (Fig. 11.49); each consists of two layers – ectoderm and mesoderm.

The allantois continues to expand as foetal urine is produced, and soon the whole cavity between the chorion and amnion is filled with the allantois and its contents. The membrane of the allantois then fuses with that of the chorion above it and the amnion below it and the basic plan of the extra-embryonic membranes is complete. The outer membrane is now called the **chorioallantois** and the inner is simply called the amnion.

The amnion is the inner most membrane enclosing the foetus and is filled with amniotic fluid. The chorioallantois is an extraembryonic structure formed by the union of the chorion and allantois, which forms the placenta. The amnion is recognised as the water bag which ruptures as the foetus moves down the birth canal.

The placenta

The placenta is the thickened area of the extraembryonic membranes by which the mammalian foetus is attached to the endometrium. It is through the placental blood supply that the embryo receives oxygen and foodstuffs, and gets rid of waste products.

The structure and shape of the placenta varies a great deal in the different mammal species. That of the dog and cat is called a **zonary placenta**, as the placental tissue forms a broad belt round the extraembryonic membranes.

In the area of placenta formation the chorioallantois develops folds that form villi, which increase the area of contact with the maternal tissue.

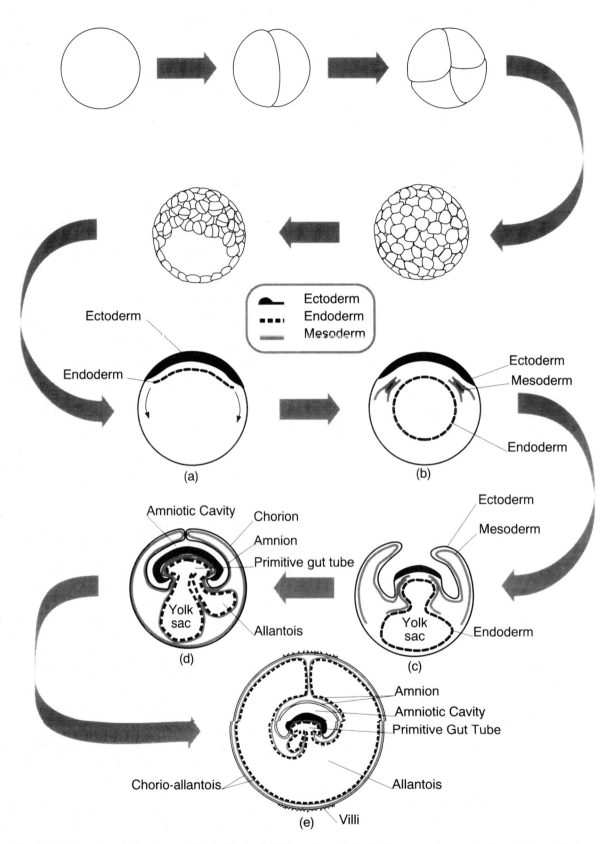

Fig. 11.49 Early embryonic development. The fertilised cell divides to form a ball of cells – a morula; a cavity then develops – this is now a trophoblast (a) A layer of endodermal cells starts to line the trophoblast. (b) The endoderm forms the primitive yolk sac. (c) Blocks of mesoderm start to form as the inner cell mass starts to be pinched off to form the embryo mesoderm. (d) Another diverticulum forms from the primitive gut tube – this is the allantois; the yolk sac starts to regress. (e) Early embryonic development. Developing villi forming a band around the extra-embryonic membranes.

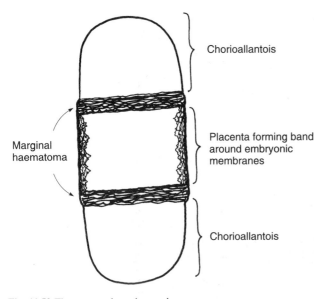

Fig. 11.50 The extra-embryonic membranes.

At the edge of the placenta is the **marginal haematoma**, where there is degeneration of material endothelium, with bleeding into the spaces so formed. Substances secreted by the chorion prevent the clotting of this blood, which is broken down to form (it is thought) a source of iron for the embryo.

It is this marginal haematoma – coloured green in bitches and brown in queens – that gives the colour to the vaginal discharge at parturition.

Later development of the embryo

The following applies to a medium-sized dog. Kittens are slightly in advance of pups at each stage.

- At 3 weeks; the amnion and allantois have formed; the embryo is 5 mm long.
- At 4 weeks; 'limb buds' are visible; the embryo is 20 mm long.
- At 5 weeks; eyelids and pinnae are visible; the embryo is 35 mm long.
- At 6 weeks; digits and external genitalia are well developed; the embryo is 60 mm long.
- At 7 weeks; colour markings and hair are starting to develop; the embryo is 100 mm long.
- At 8 weeks; the embryo is 150 mm long and has hair and pads.
- At 9 weeks (approximately); the pup is born, with eyes and ears closed.

The actual process of birth (**parturition**) is described in Chapter 18 (Obstetric and Paediatric Nursing of the Dog and Cat).

The hormonal control of parturition

Parturition is brought about by a series of changes in hormones within the body.

Pregnancy is maintained by progesterone from the corpus luteum in the ovary, which in turn is maintained by chorionic gonadotrophin, a hormone produced (as its name suggests) from the foetal membranes. Towards the end of pregnancy, when the foetus is ready to be born, the placenta secretes a prostaglandin ($PGF_2\alpha$) which causes regression of the corpus luteum and so initiates the birth process. Other hormones involved in triggering parturition are relaxin which causes softening of the tissues round the birth canal, and oxytocin which causes uterine contraction.

The nervous system

The nervous system is made up of two parts:

- The **central nervous system** consisting of the brain and the spinal cord.
- The **peripheral nervous system** – consisting of all the other motor and sensory nerves throughout the body.

The functions of the nervous system are:

- To receive information about the external environment.
- To receive information about the tissues and organs of the animal's own body.
- To interpret the information received.
- To send impulses throughout the body via the nervous system to stimulate activity of some kind.

Nervous tissue

Nervous tissue is made up of nerve cells (**neurons**) that are able to conduct electrical impulses, and the connective tissue that runs between them (**neuroglia**).

The neuron (Fig. 11.51) consists of:

- A cell body with a nucleus.
- Several short processes called **dendrites**, through which nervous impulses enter the cell.
- A long process, the axon, along which the nerve impulse travels. This may or may not be myelinated (i.e. surrounded by a sheath of a fatty substance called myelin). Nervous impulses travel faster in myelinated than in unmyelinated nerves. The myelin is produced by Schwann cells, which wrap themselves round the axon. Axons vary in length from less than a millimetre to many centimetres.
- The whole axon is surrounded by a sheath of connective tissue, the **neurilemma**.
- There are gaps in the myelin sheath along the axon where the axon is in direct contact with the neurilemma. These points are called the **nodes of Ranvier**. It is thought that at these points the nerve cell can take in oxygen and nutrients from the surrounding tissues.
- At the end of the axon are branching **nerve endings**, which transmit the impulse to the dendrites of the next axon.

Neurons may be unipolar, bipolar or multipolar, depending on the position of the cell body and the number of dendrites. One neuron may have connections with only one nerve cell, or it may exchange information with a number of different nerve cells.

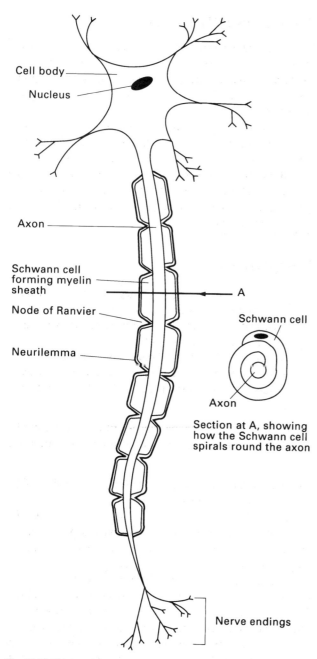

Fig. 11.51 The structure of a neuron.

A nerve is made up of many neurons bound together in a connective tissue sheath.

The nervous impulse

The nervous impulse starts at the dendrites of a nerve cell and is passed down the axon to the nerve endings. From there, it must either pass to another nerve fibre or to a muscle fibre. The junction between two nerve fibres is a **synapse**, and that between a nerve fibre and a muscle fibre is a **neuro-muscular junction**.

The movement of the impulse across the synapse or neuro-muscular junction is not by electrical conduction but by the release of chemical transmitters that diffuse across the gap to stimulate the next nerve or the muscle fibre.

The propagation of the electrical impulse is an 'all or nothing' phenomenon. Either a nerve cell is stimulated or it is not – there is no half-way house of a little bit of stimulation. The varying effects of the nervous system depend on some neurons being inhibitory rather than stimulatory, and also on the number of nerve fibres involved.

The brain

The division of the brain into **forebrain, midbrain** and **hindbrain** is a matter for descriptive convenience, and gives no indication as to the evolutionary age of the different parts of the brain (Fig. 11.52). The divisions are made from observing embryological development, where the brain develops at the anterior end of a hollow tube.

When examining the different parts of the brain, and the brains of lower vertebrates, for clues as to how the brains of the higher mammals developed, the 'oldest' parts of the brain are found to be partly within the forebrain, partly in the midbrain and partly in the hindbrain. For instance, the brains of fish feature very large olfactory lobes (because smell is important under water) and these are part of the forebrain.

Among the higher vertebrates (birds and mammals) other parts of the forebrain become more important – notably the cerebral hemispheres, which are the most obvious and largest part of the brain.

The forebrain includes:

- The **cerebrum**, or **cerebral hemispheres**, which receive and process information from all over the body. The hemispheres are divided by a deep groove, the **longitudinal sulcus**.

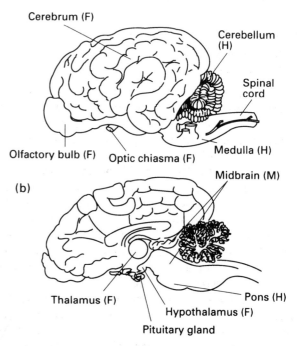

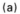

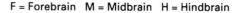

Fig. 11.52 The dog's brain, showing main features and division into forebrain, midbrain and hindbrain. (a) Lateral view. (b) Longitudinal section.

- The **thalamus**, deep within the brain tissue at the base of the cerebral hemispheres; it relays impulses to and from the cerebral cortex.
- The **hypothalamus**, which lies just above the pituitary gland. It has an important role in regulating the autonomic nervous system and the pituitary gland.

The **midbrain** passes on impulses from the hindbrain and the senses of sight and hearing to the forebrain.

The **hindbrain** includes:

- The **pons**.
- The **medulla oblongata**, which contains centres that control the heart and respiration.
- The **cerebellum**, which co-ordinates muscular activity within the body.

The ventricles

The ventricular system of the brain originates from the canal down the middle of the primitive neural tube from which the brain was formed. There are four ventricles, all of which contain cerebrospinal fluid (CSF), and are continuous with the spinal canal down the middle of the spinal cord.

- The **two lateral ventricles** lie within the two cerebral hemispheres.
- The **third ventricle** lies just above the thalamus.
- The **fourth ventricle** lies beneath and in front of the cerebellum.

The meninges

The meninges are the three layers of membrane that cover and protect the brain:

- The **dura mater**.
- The **arachnoid layer**.
- The **pia mater**.

The **dura mater** is the tough, fibrous membrane that lines the cranial cavity in the skull. It is formed from two layers: the outer is continuous with the periosteum, and the inner is mainly in contact with it, though at certain points it folds inwards to make a fold of membrane between different parts of the brain, e.g. the **falx cerebri** between the two cerebral hemispheres and the **tentorium cerebelli** between the cerebrum and cerebellum. The dura extends all the way down the central nervous system to the end of the spinal column. Within the spinal column it is not so closely attached to the surrounding bone, but leaves an **epidural space** that is used as a site for the injection of local anaesthetic in epidural analgesia.

The **arachnoid layer** (so named because it resembles a spider's web) is a delicate membrane that is closely attached to the inner layer of the dura. Beneath the arachnoid layer is the subarachnoid space, which is filled with CSF.

The **pia mater** is a delicate and very vascular membrane that is closely attached to and follows every contour of the brain beneath it.

Cerebrospinal fluid (CSF)

Cerebrospinal fluid fills the ventricles, the spinal canal and the subarachnoid space. It is secreted by structures called **choroid plexuses**, which are found within each ventricle. CSF is a clear liquid, very like plasma but with rather less protein in it.

The function of CSF is to protect the brain against sudden movement and trauma, and to provide a cushion between it and the skull. Samples of CSF for diagnostic purposes can be withdrawn from the **cerebromedullary cistern** (cisterna magna), which lies between the cerebellum and the medulla and, conveniently, can be reached with a needle via the atlanto-occipital space.

The spinal cord

The **spinal cord** (Fig. 11.53) runs from the medulla oblongata to the lumbar region, where it terminates in the **cauda equina** – a group of nerves running together that is supposed to look like a horse's tail.

Throughout its length, the spinal cord gives off pairs of nerves – one pair for each segment, or intervertebral space.

The nerve on each side of the cord is divided into two roots:

- The **dorsal root**, carrying sensory fibres into the cord.
- The **ventral root**, carrying motor fibres away from the cord.

Each dorsal root has a **ganglion**, where the cell bodies of the sensory nerves are found.

The spinal nerves supply the whole of the musculoskeletal system. At the levels of the pectoral and pelvic girdles the spinal nerves are thicker than elsewhere as they have to supply the limbs as well as the trunk.

The spinal nerves are named according to the vertebra in front of where they leave the central nervous system (CNS). The cervical (Ce) region, however, is the exception to this rule, because the first spinal nerve leaves in front of the first cervical vertebra and there are eight cervical nerves (Ce7 in front of the seventh cervical vertebra and Ce8 behind it, then T1 behind the first thoracic vertebra).

The front limb is supplied by nerves from spinal nerves Ce6 to T2, and the hind limb by nerves from spinal nerves L4 to S2 (the fourth lumbar to the second sacral nerve).

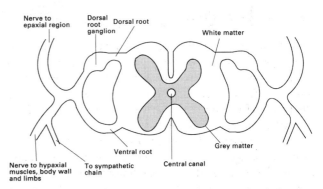

Fig. 11.53 Diagrammatic representation of section through spinal cord.

Motor and sensory; visceral and somatic

Motor nerves are **efferent nerves** – they take impulses away from the CNS to the periphery. Sensory nerves are **afferent nerves** – they carry impulses towards the CNS, taking information to the brain.

There can be a sensory nerve without a motor nerve (nerves from the eye or ear, or the skin) taking information to the brain, but there cannot be a motor nerve without a sensory nerve running with it and carrying information about its effect back to the CNS.

A somatic motor nerve takes instructions to the voluntary muscle of the body, and a somatic sensory nerve reports back on its action.

Visceral motor nerves take instructions to the smooth or cardiac muscle (i.e. the involuntary muscle of the body), and the visceral sensory nerves report back on their action.

Reflex arcs

Reflex arcs are fixed, involuntary responses to certain stimuli. For example, if an animal stands on a sharp thorn the foot is withdrawn suddenly. If a person accidentally touches the hotplate of a cooker, they will withdraw their hand almost before they can register the fact of pain or burning, let alone say 'Ow!'. This is because both of these automatic withdrawals involve spinal reflexes, or local reflex arcs, that involve only the spinal cord and would still work even if the cord were cut through. The 'Ow!' and the consciousness of pain follow after the sensory information has been transmitted to the brain.

The spinal reflex arc works as follows (Fig. 11.54):

(1) The pin-prick pain or heat receptors initiate an impulse in the sensory nerve.
(2) The impulse travels up the nerve and enters the spinal cord through the dorsal root of the nerve.
(3) There is often (but not always) one extra neuron, called an interneuron, between the sensory and the motor neuron.

(4) An impulse is initiated in the motor nerve, which leaves the spinal cord in the ventral root, and instructs the relevant muscles to withdraw the affected paw.
(5) Meanwhile, the information about the assault on the body is carried to the CNS.

Reflexes have been divided into conditional and unconditional reflexes – the first being those that can be 'overcome' by a conscious decision. For example, if we pick up a hot plate, the reflex movement would be withdrawal and the plate would be dropped – but we can over-rule the reflex and make a conscious decision to hold onto the plate till we can put it safely on a table. Unconditional reflexes have been defined as those that cannot be over-ruled. An example is the knee-jerk reflex. In fact, however, even these reflexes can be overcome with practice.

The cranial nerves

The cranial nerves all originate or end within the brain. Some are purely sensory, while others are mixed nerves (motor and sensory). They are numbered in Roman figures I to XII.

A few important facts about the cranial nerves:

Three are purely sensory and supply the special sense organs:

- I   **Olfactory** – the sense of smell.
- II   **Optic** – sight.
- VIII **Vestibulocochlear** (also called auditory) – the senses of hearing and balance.

Three supply motor fibres to the muscles of the eye:

- III   **Oculomotor**.
- IV   **Trochlear**.
- VI   **Abducens**.

Of the other six (all mixed nerves):

- V   **Trigeminal** is sensory to the skin of the face and motor to the jaw muscles.
- VII   **Facial** is motor to the muscles of facial expression.
- IX   **Glossopharyngeal** carries sensory taste fibres from the tongue and carries motor fibres to the pharynx.
- X   **Vagus** carries motor fibres to the larynx, and to the thoracic and abdominal viscera including the whole of the gastrointestinal tract, right down to the descending colon.
- XI   **Accessory** carries motor fibres to the muscles of the neck.
- XII   **Hypoglossal** carries motor fibres to the tongue.

See Table 11.2.

The autonomic nervous system

The **autonomic nervous system** is the name given to the visceral motor system of the body (Fig. 11.55). It supplies motor nerves to all the internal organs of the body and also the blood vessels – all the organs not under voluntary control. The nerve fibres run to smooth and cardiac muscle and also to glands such as the liver and the pancreas.

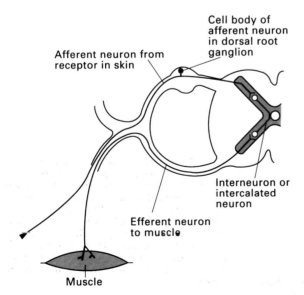

Afferent neuron from receptor in skin

Cell body of afferent neuron in dorsal root ganglion

Interneuron or intercalated neuron

Efferent neuron to muscle

Muscle

Fig. 11.54 The spinal reflex arc.

Table 11.2 The cranial nerves

No.	Name	Sensory or mixed nerve	Function
I	Olfactory	Sensory	Sense of smell
II	Optic	Sensory	Sight
III	Oculomotor	Mixed	Motor to eye muscles
IV	Trochlear	Mixed	Motor to eye muscles
V	Trigeminal	Mixed	Sensory from skin of head; motor to jaw muscles
VI	Abducens	Mixed	Motor to eye muscles
VII	Facial	Mixed	Motor to muscles of facial expression
VIII	Vestibulocochlear	Sensory	Hearing and balance
IX	Glossopharyngeal	Mixed	Sensory from taste buds of tongue; motor to muscles of pharynx
X	Vagus	Mixed	Motor to larynx, and all the viscera of the thorax and abdomen (parasympathetic)
XI	Accessory spinal	Mixed	Motor to some neck muscles
XII	Hypoglossal	Mixed	Motor to tongue muscles

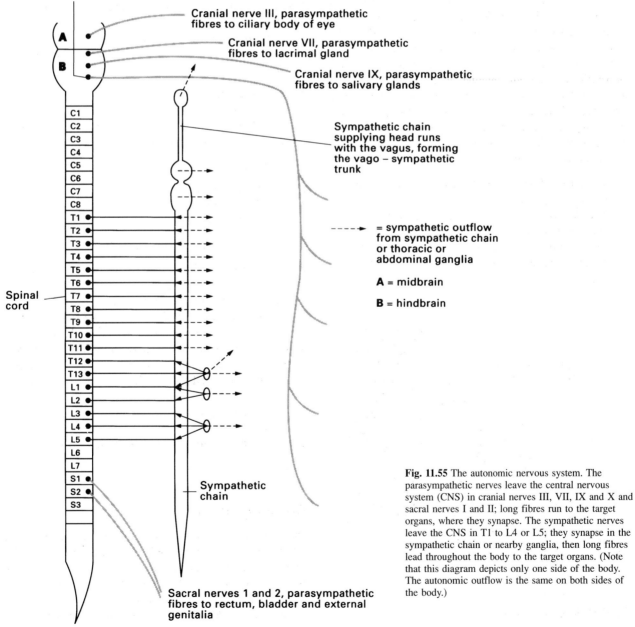

Cranial nerve X, parasympathetic fibres to heart, lungs, bronchi, all abdominal viscera

Cranial nerve III, parasympathetic fibres to ciliary body of eye

Cranial nerve VII, parasympathetic fibres to lacrimal gland

Cranial nerve IX, parasympathetic fibres to salivary glands

Sympathetic chain supplying head runs with the vagus, forming the vago – sympathetic trunk

- - - - ▶ = sympathetic outflow from sympathetic chain or thoracic or abdominal ganglia

A = midbrain

B = hindbrain

Spinal cord

Sympathetic chain

Sacral nerves 1 and 2, parasympathetic fibres to rectum, bladder and external genitalia

Fig. 11.55 The autonomic nervous system. The parasympathetic nerves leave the central nervous system (CNS) in cranial nerves III, VII, IX and X and sacral nerves I and II; long fibres run to the target organs, where they synapse. The sympathetic nerves leave the CNS in T1 to L4 or L5; they synapse in the sympathetic chain or nearby ganglia, then long fibres lead throughout the body to the target organs. (Note that this diagram depicts only one side of the body. The autonomic outflow is the same on both sides of the body.)

Very often the term 'autonomic nervous system' is taken to include the sensory fibres carrying information from these organs to the CNS as well.

The autonomic nervous system can be divided into two parts:

- The **sympathetic nervous system**.
- The **parasympathetic nervous system**.

The two systems tend to have opposite effects, and most organs have both sympathetic and parasympathetic supplies. The control of the organ's function is a balancing act between the two systems.

The sympathetic nervous system quickens the heart and respiration and dilates the bronchi and bronchioles, so increasing the diameter of the airway. It slows the movement of the bowel and stops the secretion of digestive juices. It also dilates the blood vessels in skeletal muscle, so increasing their blood supply, and constricts the vessels supplying the bowel.

The parasympathetic nervous system has the opposite effect – it slows the heart and respiratory rate, and increases the peristaltic movement of the gut and the secretion of digestive juices.

The sympathetic system helps the body respond to stressful situations (the 'fight, flight and frolic' responses) whereas the parasympathetic system dominates when the animal is relaxed and not fearful or anxious.

The sympathetic fibres leave the spinal cord in spinal nerves T1 to L4 or L5. They synapse in the sympathetic chain or in ganglia close to it, then the long post-ganglionic fibres supply the various organs, mainly by taking a route that follows the blood vessels supplying the organs. The sympathetic chain is a nerve trunk that runs along the dorsal body wall and from which the sympathetic nerves arise.

The parasympathetic fibres leave the CNS in the cranial nerves III, VII, IX and X. The first three supply structures within the head, but the vagus supplies all the viscera of the thorax and abdomen. The pelvic viscera are supplied by parasympathetic nerves from S1 and S2. Parasympathetic fibres synapse near their target organ, so have only very short post-ganglionic fibres.

The special senses

The special senses are:

- Smell.
- Sight.
- Hearing and balance.
- Taste.

All these special senses have specialised receptors to receive stimuli from the external environment before they are passed on to the central nervous system.

Smell

The bipolar receptor cells of the olfactory system lie within the mucous epithelium covering the **ethmoturbinate**

bones, at the back of the nasal cavity. From there the fibres pass through the **mesethmoid bone** into the olfactory lobe of the brain in cranial nerve I (**olfactory nerve**).

Sight

The eye, the organ of sight, is situated within the orbit, where it is to some degree protected from injury by the zygomatic arch of the skull. The eyes are also protected by the **eyelids** and the **lacrimal apparatus** (Fig. 11.56).

The eyelids

The eyelids consist of a layer of fibrous tissue (the **tarsal plate**) covered by skin on the outer surface and lined with mucous membrane. At the **medial canthus** (the angle where the upper and lower lids meet) the eyelids are closely attached to the bone, but at the **lateral canthus** they can be moved relatively freely.

Opening on to the edge of the eyelids are the ducts of the **tarsal glands** (or Meibomian glands), which secrete a fatty material that makes up about 10% of the tear film that moistens the eye. Eyelashes, or **cilia**, are thick hairs growing out of the edge of the eyelid that help to protect the eye from dust, etc. The carnivores do not have true eyelashes (although the hairs on the upper eyelids may in some cases give the impression of 'eyelashes' where they are relatively long and overlap the edge of the eyelid) but there may be a few '**ectopic cilia**' growing from the edge of the tarsal plate. Sometimes these 'ingrowing eyelashes' cause irritation to the cornea and have to be removed. Occasionally either eyelid may be curled inwards on to the eye so that the hairs of the skin irritate the cornea (**entropion**); or the lower lid may be too large for the eye and droop, exposing the conjunctiva and making the eye more prone to infection (**ectropion**). Both conditions may have to be corrected surgically.

The **third eyelid** lies below the true eyelids, on the medial side of the eye. It is supported by a piece of cartilage,

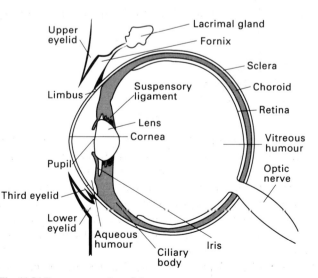

Fig. 11.56 Transverse section of the eye.

but unlike the true eyelids it is covered with mucous membrane on both sides.

The lacrimal apparatus

This consists of the lacrimal glands and the lacrimal ducts.

The main **lacrimal gland** lies between the eyeball and the dorso-lateral wall of the orbit. There is also glandular tissue on the underside of the third eyelid.

Lacrimal fluid is distributed over the surface of the eye by the eyelids, and is then collected by the **lacrimal puncta**, near the medial canthus in the upper and lower lids, where it then drains via the **nasolacrimal duct** into the nasal cavity.

The eye

The globe of the eye itself can be considered as having three layers:

- A fibrous, protective outer layer.
- A middle layer that is vascular and pigmented.
- An inner layer of receptor cells.

The outer layer

The outer layer of the eyeball can be divided into a posterior part, the **sclera**, and an anterior part, the transparent **cornea**. The junction between the sclera and cornea is termed the **limbus**.

The sclera has a white outer surface, which gives the colour of the 'white of the eye'. The conjunctiva is attached to the sclera.

The cornea bulges out slightly from the rest of the globe and allows light to enter the eye. Its shape starts to focus the light onto the retina.

The middle layer

The whole of this vascular, pigmented layer is called the **uvea**, or **uveal tract**. It is made up of the following structures:

- The **choroid**.
- The **tapetum**.
- The **ciliary body**.
- The **suspensory ligament**.
- The **iris**.

The **choroid** is the dark-coloured lining at the back of the eye. The blood vessels supplying all the internal structures of the eye lie within the choroid.

The **tapetum** is the area of light-reflecting cells on the inner surface of the choroid that makes the eyes of dogs and cats shine at night. Its function is thought to be to improve vision when there is very little light, by reflecting light back onto the retina.

The **ciliary body** is the inward projection of the uvea from the lining towards the centre of the eye. It contains smooth muscle, and with the suspensory ligament that supports the lens it changes the shape of and so focuses the lens.

The **iris** contains two layers of muscular tissue. The hole in the centre of the iris is the **pupil**. Opening and closing the iris varies the amount of light that reaches the retina. Dogs have a circular iris, but the pupil of the cat, when fully closed, is a vertical slit.

The inner layer

The inner layer of the eyeball is the retina, which is made up of three layers:

- Closest to the choroid, a layer of **photoreceptor cells** – the rods and cones.
- A middle layer of **bipolar receptor cells**.
- An inner layer of **ganglion cells**, that carry the information into the **optic nerve** (cranial nerve II).

The end of the optic nerve lies within the retina, where it appears as the **optic disc**. It is an area where there are no receptor cells.

The lens and aqueous and vitreous humours

Within the substance of the eye are:

- The **lens**.
- The **aqueous humour**.
- The **vitreous humour**.

The **lens** is held in place by the suspensory ligament, and the muscular ciliary body that it can pull on the lens to change its shape and so the focus of the eye.

The **aqueous** is the watery fluid that fills the space between the lens and the cornea. It provides nourishment for the lens and cornea and helps to maintain the shape of the relatively fragile cornea.

The **vitreous** is a transparent jelly-like substance that fills the space between the lens and the back of the eye.

How the eye works

- Light enters the eye through the cornea, which starts to focus it on to the retina.
- The iris controls the size of the pupil and so the amount of light allowed into the eye.
- The lens, its curvature altered by the ciliary muscle, focuses the light on to the retina.
- The light passes through the retinal layers to the light-receptive cells, where it produces an image upside down.
- Light that missed the rods and cones on the way through the retina is reflected back on to the retinal layers by the tapetum.
- The bipolar receptor cells and ganglion cells then transmit the image through the optic nerve to the brain's optic chiasma, where the two optic nerves join, and some of the fibres cross over from one nerve to the other before continuing on into the midbrain and up to the cerebral cortex.

Hearing and balance

The organ of hearing and balance is, of course, the ear. It can be divided into three parts (Fig. 11.57):

● The external ear.
● The middle ear.
● The inner ear.

The external ear

The external ear is made up of three parts:
● The pinna.
● The vertical canal.
● The horizontal canal.

The **pinna**, or ear flap, varies a great deal in size and shape amongst dogs of different breeds. The 'wild type' of dog ear is upright: it acts to funnel sound towards the ear, and also as a means of expression between dogs (ears up, ears back, ears flat, etc.).

The ear canal extends from the base of the pinna to the tympanic membrane or eardrum.

The shape of both the pinna and the ear canal are maintained by cartilage – a sheet of cartilage in the pinna and a tube surrounding the ear canal.

The ear canal is lined with modified skin, which contains very few hair follicles (except in some hairy-eared breeds

such as miniature and toy poodles), but a large number of modified sebaceous glands (**ceruminous glands**) that secrete wax. There is a bend part way down the ear canal that divides it into vertical and horizontal canals.

The external ear ends at the **external auditory meatus**, where the **tympanic membrane** (ear drum) lies across the entrance to the middle ear.

The middle ear

The middle ear lies within the **tympanic bulla** of the temporal bone. It is an air-filled space, connected to the pharynx by the **auditory (Eustachian) tube**.

A chain of three tiny bones (**ossicles**) lie across the middle ear, and they transmit vibrations from the tympanic membrane to the inner ear. The ossicles are called the **malleus**, the **incus** and the **stapes**.

The malleus is attached to the **tympanic membrane**, and the base of the stapes fills what is called the **oval window**, which leads into the inner ear.

Just below the oval window is the membrane called the **round window**.

The inner ear

The inner ear also lies within the temporal bone, inside a **bony labyrinth** – a cavity within the bone carved out to fit the organs of hearing and balance. Within the bony labyrinth is the **membranous labyrinth**, and between the two is a fluid known as **perilymph**.

Nervous impulses are carried to the brain from the inner ear in the two branches of the eighth cranial nerve – the **vestibulocochlear** or **auditory nerve**.

The membranous labyrinth

The membranous labyrinth contains a fluid called **endolymph**, and consists of:

● The **utricle**.
● The **saccule**.
● The **semicircular canals**.
● The **cochlear duct**.

The **semicircular canals** are three tubes that lie within a cavity of exactly their shape within the bony labyrinth. At their base are two more open cavities, the **utricle** and the **saccule**. The semicircular canals lie in different directions: one is vertical, one is horizontal and the third is transverse.

At the base of each semicircular canal is a bulge – the **ampulla**. With each **ampulla** is a sensory **crista** with hair cells embedded in a jelly-like cupula which swings to and fro as the endolymph moves within the canals, pulling the hair cells whose combined outputs along the **auditory nerve** register turning movements in all spatial planes.

Within the utricle and saccule are two further receptors, the **maculae**, that monitor the position of the head with respect to gravity. Thus the semicircular canals sense the movements of the head, and the maculae sense the position of the head.

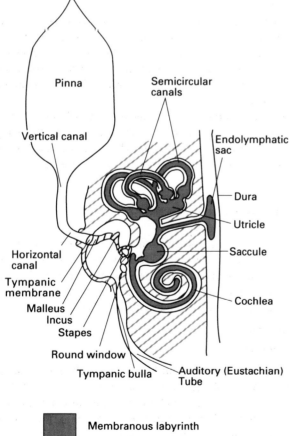

Pinna

Semicircular canals

Vertical canal

Endolymphatic sac

Dura

Utricle

Saccule

Horizontal canal

Tympanic membrane

Malleus

Incus

Stapes

Cochlea

Round window

Tympanic bulla

Auditory (Eustachian) Tube

▓ Membranous labyrinth

▨ Bone

Fig. 11.57 The ear.

The **cochlea** is concerned with hearing. It is in the form of a spiral, like a snail shell, and the internal canal of the spiral is divided into three channels. Within the cochlea is the **spiral organ**, or **organ of Corti**, which contains sensory hairs that react to different frequencies as a sound travels through the endolymph up the spiral of the cochlea.

Taste

Taste buds are found on the tongue and there are also scattered patches of them on the palate, pharynx and epiglottis. Stimuli from the taste buds pass to the brain in cranial nerves VII (facial), IX (glossopharyngeal) and X (vagus).

The endocrine system

The endocrine system is part of the regulatory system of the body. It consists of a number of ductless glands which produce chemical substances (hormones) that are carried round the body in the bloodstream. The target organ for a hormone is often a considerable distance from the gland. See Fig. 11.58.

Not all hormones are produced by the endocrine glands. For example, **secretin** (which stimulates the secretion of pancreatic and intestinal juice) is produced by the wall of the small intestine, in response to the presence of food in the duodenum. **Gastrin** (which stimulates the secretion of hydrochloric acid from the oxyntic cells) is secreted by the stomach wall in response to the stimulus of food entering the stomach. **Chorionic gonadotrophin** is secreted by the ectodermal layer of the chorion during pregnancy and helps maintain the corpus luteum throughout the gestation period.

The thyroid glands

The thyroid glands lie on either side of the midline on the ventral aspect of the first few tracheal rings. Hormones produced by the thyroid glands are:

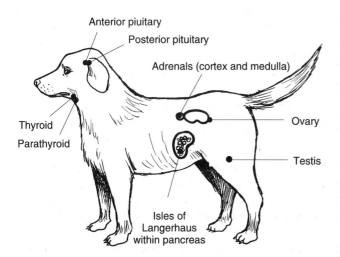

Fig. 11.58 Components of the endocrine system.

- **Thyroxin**.
- **Tri-iodothyronine**.
- **Thyrocalcitonin**.

Thyroxin and **tri-iodothyronine** have a similar effect in the regulation of metabolic rate. Undersecretion of these hormones will produce the condition called **myxoedema**, in which the animal is fat and sluggish, with poor skin and coat, all due to a lowered metabolic rate. Oversecretion causes an increase in metabolic rate, with weight loss, increased heart rate and often overactivity and increased irritability.

Thyrocalcitonin decreases the level of plasma calcium by slowing the resorption of the mineral from bone.

Parathyroid glands

The parathyroid glands lie on either side and very close to the thyroid glands. The hormone produced is **parathormone**, which regulates the metabolism and distribution of calcium in the body. Secretion of the hormone increases as the plasma level of calcium decreases. Parathormone increases the absorption of calcium from the digestive tract and increases the reabsorption of calcium from bone in the kidney.

Hyperparathyroidism may occur in three ways:

- **Neoplasia** of the glands may result in overproduction of parathormone, which may lead to demineralisation of bone.
- **Chronic renal failure** may result in secondary indirect hyperparathyroidism as calcium is lost in the urine and the body tries to compensate by absorbing more from the bone. In this case there is often preferential reabsorption from maxillae and mandibles, producing the condition **rubber jaw**.
- **Secondary nutritional hyperparathyroidism** occurs as a result of a diet so low in calcium that the daily requirement cannot be met. This is most common in young animals fed entirely on butcher's meat.

The pancreas

The pancreas lies in the mesentery of the duodenum. It is a mixed gland: most of its substance is the lobulated exocrine gland that secretes digestive enzymes, but within its substance is the endocrine part of the gland, the **islets of Langerhans**, which secrete two hormones:

- **Insulin**.
- **Glucagon**.

Insulin is secreted by the beta cells, which make up about three-quarters of the cells in the islets. It is secreted in response to a rise in blood glucose (e.g. after a meal) and lowers the blood level by increasing the uptake of glucose into cells, and its storage in the form of glycogen. A shortage of insulin, such as occurs in diabetes mellitus, results in the urinary excretion of glucose and the body using fats and protein for energy.

Glucagon is secreted by the Islets' alpha cells, in response to a fall in blood sugar. It stimulates the conversion of glycogen to glucose, so raising the blood sugar level again.

The ovary

Hormones produced in the ovary are:

- Progesterone.
- Oestradiol.
- Relaxin.

Oestradiol is one of a group of compounds called oestrogens. The function of oestradiol is to prepare the genital tract and external genitalia for coitus and the reception of fertilised eggs. It is produced by the cells of the wall of the developing ovarian follicle, and passes from there into both the bloodstream and the follicular fluid.

Progesterone is essential for the maintenance of pregnancy. It is produced by the corpus luteum that develops in the place of the ruptured follicle after ovulation, and acts on the lining of the uterus and on the mammary tissue.

Relaxin is produced by the corpus luteum in the late stages of pregnancy, and causes relaxation of the sacrotuberous and other ligaments round the birth canal, to ease the passage of the foetus.

The testis

Hormones produced in the testes are:

- **Testosterone**.
- **Oestrogens**.

Testosterone is produced by the **interstitial cells** of the testis (**cells of Leydig**) and is responsible for sperm production, and for the development and maintenance of male secondary sexual characteristics.

Oestrogens are also produced by the testis, from the **Sertoli cells**. Tumours of the Sertoli cells of the testis may result in an increase in oestrogen output, and the feminisation of the dog so that it develops a soft, pendulous prepuce, increased nipple size, and often coat changes resulting in a soft 'puppy' type of coat.

Adrenal glands

The adrenal glands lie close the anterior pole of each kidney. Each has an outer region, the **cortex**, and an inner region, the **medulla**. The cortex and medulla act independently, and can be considered as two different endocrine glands.

Adrenal medulla

The hormones secreted by the adrenal medulla are:

- **Adrenaline (epinephrine)**.
- **Noradrenaline (norepinephrine)**.

They act on the body in a similar way to the sympathetic nervous system, preparing the body to meet emergencies, and are controlled by fibres of the sympathetic nervous system. They increase heart rate and they increase blood glucose level by increasing glycogen breakdown. They also increase the rate and depth of respiration, and dilate the arteries supplying skeletal and voluntary muscle.

Adrenal cortex

The adrenal cortex produces three groups of hormones, each from a different layer of tissue:

(a) **Glucocorticoids**.
  - Cortisol (hydrocortisone).
  - Corticosterone.
(b) **Mineralocorticoids**.
  - Aldosterone.
(c) **Adrenal sex steroids**.

All of these are **steroids** and have a similar structure based on lipid.

The **glucocorticoids**, although present at all times in the bloodstream, are secreted in increased quantities as a response to stress within the body. They increase the blood sugar level by decreasing the use of glucose by cells, stimulating the conversion of amino acids to glucose in the liver (**gluconeogenesis**) and mobilising fatty acids from adipose tissue. In large quantities they depress the inflammatory and so the healing or repair mechanisms of the body.

The **mineralocorticoid aldosterone** regulates the level of electrolytes in the body, particularly sodium and potassium. It stimulates the resorption of sodium in the kidney tubule, and increases the excretion of potassium. The reabsorption of sodium is linked to that of chloride and water.

The **adrenal sex steroids** – male and female sex hormones – are produced in the adrenal cortex. They are not generally considered of great importance, although they may have a significant effect in the spayed or castrated animal.

The pituitary gland

The pituitary gland can be considered as two different glands: the anterior pituitary (or adenohypophysis) and the posterior pituitary (neurohypophysis).

The adenohypophysis

The anterior pituitary produces the following:

- **Thyrotropic, or thyroid stimulating hormone** (TSH).
- **Somatotrophin**, or **growth hormone**.
- **Adrenocorticotropic hormone** (ACTH).
- **Prolactin**.
- **Follicle stimulating hormone** (FSH) a gonadotrophin.
- **Luteinising hormone** (LH) – a gonadotrophin.
- **Interstitial cell stimulating hormone** (ICSH) a gonadotrophin – the male equivalent of LH.

Thyroid stimulating hormone (TSH) regulates the uptake of iodine by the thyroid gland, thyroid hormone manufacture, and the release of the thyroid hormones into the circulation.

Growth hormone, or **somatotrophin**, controls the rate of growth in the young animal. It acts mainly on the bones, controlling the rate of growth of the epiphyses. It is also involved in the production of proteins from amino acids and the regulation of energy use within the body during periods of poor food supply, conserving glucose for use by the nervous system and stimulating the breakdown of fat for use by the rest of the body.

Adrenocorticotropic hormone (ACTH) regulates the secretion of adreno-cortical hormones.

Prolactin stimulates milk production in late pregnancy and lactation.

Follicle stimulating hormone (FSH) stimulates the maturation of ovarian follicles in the ovary.

Interstitial cell stimulating hormone (ICSH) is the male equivalent of FSH and stimulates the production of sperm.

Luteinising hormone (LH) stimulates the development of the corpus luteum in the female after ovulation. In the male it controls the secretion of testosterone.

The neurohypophysis (the posterior pituitary)

The hormones listed as coming from the posterior pituitary are in fact manufactured higher up in the brain by secretory nerve cells, and stored in the posterior pituitary prior to release:

- **Anti-diuretic hormone** (ADH or vasopressin).
- **Oxytocin**.

Anti-diuretic hormone (ADH), also known as vasopressin, increases the absorption of water by the kidney tubules, so reducing the amount of urine excreted and increasing the water retained by the body.

Oxytocin acts during pregnancy and parturition. It causes contraction of the smooth muscle of the uterus and of the ducts in the mammary glands.

Medicines: pharmacology, therapeutics and dispensing

J. Elliott

Pharmacology, the science of drugs, can be divided into two parts. First, it is concerned with the study of the way in which the functions of the living body are affected by drugs (**pharmacodynamics**) and, secondly, with the absorption, metabolism and excretion of drugs by the body (**pharmacokinetics**). Much of our understanding of the pharmacology of drugs is derived from studies in normal healthy animals; the study of **clinical pharmacology** attempts to transpose this information to the diseased clinical patient.

Therapeutics can be defined as the rational and optimal use of drugs in the management of disease states or in the manipulation of physiological functions. In order to use drugs in a 'rational' and 'optimal' way, an understanding of the nature of the disease process and of the pharmacology of the drug to be used is required. Without such an understanding, the clinical use of drugs is 'empirical'.

The subject of **pharmacy** can be defined as the **preparation** of drugs and their formulation into medicines followed by their **dispensing** (giving out) to the owner of a sick animal. Nowadays, most medicines are formulated by the pharmaceutical companies ready for dispensing. In many veterinary practices, medicines are dispensed to owners of sick animals from the practice premises. They can also be dispensed by pharmacists when presented by the owner of the animal with a written instruction (**prescription**) from the veterinary surgeon who is responsible for the care of the animal in question.

Drug classification

Definitions

Drugs are often classified according to:

(a) The way in which they bring about their effect on the body.
(b) Which body system (or infective agent) they affect.

This is the most useful form of classification for the practice pharmacy as, in many instances, it determines what the drugs are used for in clinical cases (i.e. their **major desired effect** on the body). In addition, a knowledge of the mode of action of drugs may enable the prediction of **side effects** (effects which occur in addition to the desired therapeutic effect). However, it is important to recognise that side effects of drugs cannot always be predicted from the way in which they cause their desired effect. When the side effects of a particular drug compromise the health of an animal they are termed **undesirable** or **adverse drug**

reactions. Any suspected adverse drug reactions encountered in veterinary practice should be reported to the Veterinary Medicines Directorate on special reporting forms. Any drug which is administered at dosages above those recommended for therapeutic use (accidentally or deliberately) may cause **toxic effects** in the animal. The **therapeutic index** of a drug is the ratio between the dose which causes toxic effects and the dose required to produce the desired therapeutic effect. The lower this ratio the more dangerous a particular drug may be to use and the smaller the margin of error allowed when determining the dose for a particular animal.

Most drugs produce their desired effects by interacting with a defined target in the body or in the infective organism. This target may be a receptor for a naturally occurring hormone or neurotransmitter, which the drug may **mimic** by stimulating the receptor (receptor agonist) or **block** by occupying the receptor without stimulating it (receptor **antagonist**). Other targets for drugs include enzymes which serve physiological functions in the body or the infective organisms and which may be inhibited by drugs.

The categorisation of drugs set out in the rest of this section is used by both veterinary and medical formularies and would be a logical way of organising a practice pharmacy into groups of drugs. In each case, examples of drugs used in small animal practice are given. The name used is always the **generic** (approved or official) name rather than a **proprietary** (brand or trade) name. Where possible, examples will be given where a product exists which has been approved (**authorised**) for use in small animals.

Drugs used in the treatment of infections caused by micro-organisms

The micro-organisms include bacteria, fungi, viruses and protozoa. Drugs used to treat infections caused by these organisms can be termed **antimicrobial agents**. If the drug is a natural product of another micro-organism (as many are) then it is called an **antibiotic**. These drugs show the property of **selective toxicity**, targeting and damaging processes which are essential to the micro-organism but which do not take place in animal cells.

Antibacterial drugs

These are some of the most commonly used drugs in small animal practice. If they are capable of killing bacteria they are described as **bactericidal**; whereas if they just prevent division of bacteria they are called **bacteriostatic**. An antibacterial drug is described as **narrow spectrum** if it is active against a narrow range of bacteria (usually either Gram-positive or Gram-negative organisms) and **broad spectrum** if it is active against a wide variety of bacteria (or other micro-organisms such as protozoa). Some antibacterial drugs when used in combination produce more than the additive effects of the two drugs when used alone. In these cases, the drugs are said to **potentiate** each other (e.g. *potentiated sulphonamides are a combination of a sulphonamide plus trimethoprim or baquiloprim*). Antibacterial drugs are classified into families of drugs which are chemically related. The family of *penicillins*, for example, have the same mode of action and so are all bactericidal and share common side effects (all can induce allergic reactions in sensitive animals) for the animal being treated. Small changes in structure, however, may change their spectrum of activity. Table 12.1 summarises the main families of antibacterial drugs used in small animal practice, giving examples of each. Selection of appropriate antibacterial drug therapy depends on a number of factors (e.g. the bacterium involved, the site of infection and the immunocompetence of the patient). Good prescribing practice would be to have first-line antibacterial drugs for certain routine uses (e.g. prophylactic use in orthopaedic surgery) and to reserve some drug groups (e.g. the fluoroquinolones) for treatment of difficult life-threatening bacterial infections.

Antifungal drugs

These will kill or stop the growth of fungi (and could be described as **fungicidal** or **fungistatic**). *Griseofulvin* is used to treat dermatophytosis ('ringworm') in the dog and cat and *nystatin* is contained in some topical ear preparations to treat yeast infections.

Antiviral drugs

These are infrequently used in veterinary medicine. *Aciclovir* is used topically in the eye to treat feline herpes virus infection.

Antiprotozoal drugs

These are used to treat infections caused by protozoal organisms such as *Toxoplasma gondii*. Example: *pyrimethamine*.

Drugs used in the treatment of parasitic infections

Endoparasiticides

These are used to treat infections of internal parasites. The majority of such infections in veterinary medicine are caused by helminths (nematodes, cestodes and trematodes) and so

---

Table 12.1 Antibacterial drug families

Family	Example	Spectrum of activity	Bactericidal or bacteriostatic
Penicillins[a]	Benzyl penicillin	Narrow (Gram-positive)	Bactericidal
	Amoxycillin	Broad	Bactericidal
Tetracyclines	Oxytetracycline	Broad	Bacteriostatic
Aminoglycosides	Neomycin	Narrow (Gram-negative)	Bactericidal
Lincosamides	Clindamycin	Narrow (Gram-positives and anaerobes)	Bacteriostatic
Sulphonamides	Sulphadiazine	Broad	Bacteriostatic
Potentiated sulphonamides	Sulphadiazine plus trimethoprim	Broad	Bactericidal
Nitroimidazoles	Metronidazole	Narrow (anaerobes)	Bactericidal
Chloramphenicol	Chloramphenicol	Broad	Bacteriostatic
Fluoroquinolones	Enrofloxacin	Broad	Bactericidal

[a] Penicillins and cephalosporins (e.g. cephalexin) are related chemically and collectively called β-lactams.

Table 12.2 Examples of anthelmintics

Drug	Tape worms			Round worms		
	Echinococcus	Taenia	Dipylidium	Toxocara/ Toxascaris	Hookworms (Uncinaria)	Whip worms (Trichuris)
Fenbendazole	0	2	0	2	2	2
Mebendazole	1	2	0	2	2	2
Nitroscanate	1	2	2	2	2	0
Piperazine	0	0	0	1	1[a]	0
Praziquantel	2	2	2	0	0	0

[a] Effective at 1.5 times the normal dose.
2, excellent activity; 1, very good activity; 0, poor or ineffective.

the drugs are termed **anthelmintics**. The internal parasites of the dog and cat are **nematodes** (round worms) and **cestodes** (tape worms). As with antibacterial drugs, anthelmintics can be broad or narrow spectrum. Table 12.2 gives examples of commonly used drugs and their spectrum of activity.

Ectoparasiticides

Ectoparasiticides are used to treat infestations of fleas, lice, ticks and mites, and are often administered topically in the form of sprays, baths, dusting powders or impregnated collars. The organophosphate compounds (e.g. *dichlorvos*), synthetic pyrethroids (e.g. *permethrin*), *fipronil* and *imidacloprid*, are commonly used in small animal medicine. Other ectoparasitacides are given orally to dogs and cats and rely on the parasites ingesting the drug with a blood meal (e.g. *Lufenuron*). An understanding of the life cycle of the parasite involved is important for the successful treatment of parasitic infestations.

Drugs acting on the gastrointestinal system

These are shown in Table 12.3.

Drugs used in the treatment of disorders of the cardiovascular system

These work primarily on the heart, the blood vessels, the blood coagulation system or the kidney.

Drugs acting on the heart

The heart can be stimulated to beat more strongly by drugs which are called **myocardial stimulants** (or positive inotropes) – examples include *digoxin* and *etamiphylline camsylate*. Other drugs also increase the rate at which the heart beats and may be used in an emergency to treat complete heart block. The **sympathomimetic** *isoprenaline* (mimics the action of the sympathetic nervous system on the heart) is an example of such a drug. When the heart beats very fast with an abnormal rhythm it is said to be *arrhythmic*. Cardiac arrhythmias can be suppressed by **antidysrhythmic drugs** such as *lignocaine* (for ventricular arrhythmias) and *diltiazem* (for atrial arrhythmias). (NB: The preparation of lignocaine used to treat ventricular arrhythmias must not contain adrenaline.)

Drugs acting on the blood vessels

Vasodilators relax the smooth muscle of blood vessels and lower resistance to blood flow, so reducing the work the heart has to do. Some act primarily on arterial smooth muscle (**arterial dilators**; *hydralazine*), some act primarily on venous smooth muscle (**venodilators**; *glyceryl trinitrate*) and others act on both sides of the circulation (**mixed dilators**; *enalapril*). A potential side effect of these drugs is excessive lowering of arterial blood pressure (*hypotension*). Indeed, some are used in man to treat hypertension and are called **antihypertensive** drugs. Recently, hypertension has been recognised as occurring in cats, often secondary to diseases such as chronic renal failure. The vasodilator drug, *amlodipine*, which is a calcium channel blocker with selectivity for vascular smooth muscle, has proved an effective antihypertensive agent in cats.

Drugs acting on the kidney

Diuretics increase the volume of urine produced by an animal and the amount of salt excreted. Many are used in

---

Table 12.3 Drugs acting on the gastrointestinal system

Main drug class	Class	Mode of action	Examples
Antidiarrhoeal agents		*Suppress diarrhoea non-specifically*[a]	
	Adsorbents	Coat the gut wall, adsorb toxins	Charcoal, kaolin, bismuth
	Modulators of intestinal motility	Reduce gastrointestinal motility	Loperamide, diphenoxylate
	Chronic antidiarrhoeals	Anti-inflammatory agents	Sulphasalazine, prednisolone
Anti-emetic drugs		Prevent or suppress vomiting (emesis)	Metoclopramide (vomiting due to gastritis) Acepromazine (motion sickness)
Emetic drugs		Stimulate vomiting	Washing soda (orally) Xylazine (by injection)
Laxatives		*Increase defecation*	
	Lubricant laxatives	Lubricate faecal mass	Liquid paraffin
	Bulk-forming laxatives	Increase volume of faeces	Isphagula husk
	Osmotic laxatives	Hypertonic solutions, poorly absorbed	Phosphate (enemas)
	Stimulant laxatives	Stimulate local reflex gut motility	Danthron
Antacids		Neutralise acid secreted in stomach	Aluminium hydroxide
Ulcer-healing drugs		Inhibit acid secretion in the stomach and allow ulcers to heal	Cimetidine
Pancreatin supplements		Contain protease, lipase and amylase activity to aid digestion in EPI[b]	

[a] Specific treatment relies on identifying the underlying cause. In some cases, for example, antibacterial drugs or anthelmintics may be indicated.
[b] Exocrine pancreatic insufficiency.

the treatment of congestive heart failure because in this condition the kidney tends to retain salt and water which contributes to the problem. The loop diuretics (e.g. *frusemide*) and the thiazide diuretics (e.g. *hydrochlorothiazide*) are most commonly used. Both give rise to excess potassium loss. Use of potassium sparing diuretics (e.g. *spironolactone*) with these drugs will counteract this effect. Angiotensin converting enzyme (ACE) inhibitors, which block the formation of angiotensin II and, thus, the secretion of aldosterone, can be regarded as potassium sparing diuretics, but also have balanced vasodilator activity as mentioned above (e.g. *benazepril and enalapril*).

Drugs acting on the blood clotting system

Anticoagulants prevent blood clotting (*heparin, warfarin*) where as **fibrinolytic agents** break down clots once they have formed (e.g. *streptokinase*). **Haemostatics** arrest haemorrhage and are usually applied topically to local bleeding areas (e.g. *calcium alginate*).

Drugs used in the treatment of disorders of the respiratory system

Inhalation of infective agents or allergens (e.g. pollen) stimulate inflammation and tissue damage leading to reflex stimulation of coughing and bronchoconstriction. The sites at which drugs may counteract some of these disease processes are shown in Fig. 12.1. Examples of the drugs acting at these sites are given in Table 12.4.

Drugs acting on the nervous system

Sedatives

Sedatives produce calmness, drowsiness and indifference of the animal to its surroundings, and are often used as **premedicants** for animals which are to be anaesthetised. Examples include *acepromazine* and *medetomidine*. The action of medetomidine can be reversed by the **sedative antagonist** *atipamezole*. The degree of drowsiness produced depends on the particular agent or agents used, the dose and the route of administration. A mild sedative is sometimes referred to as a **tranquilliser** whereas drugs used to produce deep sedation (*narcosis*) can be called **narcotics**. See also Chapter 23, p. 594.

Opioid analgesics

These relieve pain by acting on opioid receptor sites in the brain and spinal cord. Examples are *morphine* and *buprenorphine*.

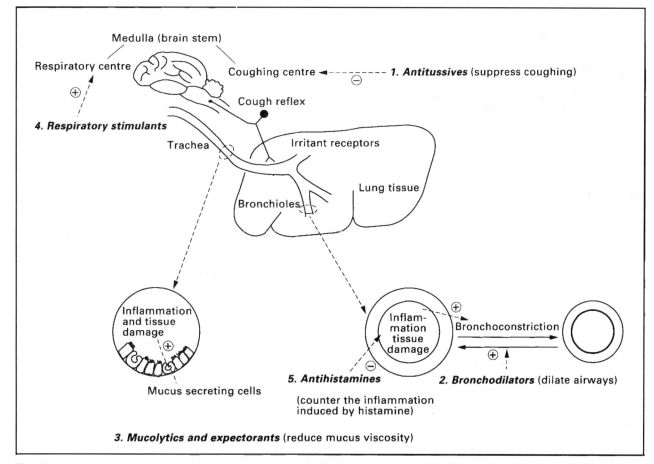

Fig. 12.1 A schematic representation of the respiratory system showing the sites at which drugs act in the treatment of respiratory disorders (⊕ = stimulation, ⊖ = inhibition of the processes indicated). Inhalation of allergens or infective agents initiate inflammation, bronchoconstriction, increased mucus secretion and coughing (via the cough reflex which stimulates the coughing centre in the medulla).

Table 12.4 Drugs used in the treatment of disorders of the respiratory system

Drug class	Example
Antitussive	Butorphanol
Antihistamine	Diphenhydramine
Bronchodilator	Theophylline, terbutaline
Mucolytic/expectorant	Bromhexine/ipecacuanha
Respiratory stimulant	Doxapram

Combinations of sedatives and opioid analgesics can be used to produce deeper and more reliable sedation than sedatives alone. Such combinations are termed **neuroleptanalgesics**, an example being *fentanyl* and *fluansinone*. Sedation can then be reversed using an **opioid antagonist** such as *naloxone*.

General anaesthetics

These produce unconsciousness so that surgical or other procedures can be carried out painlessly. Pre-anaesthetic medication with sedatives and analgesics will allow a reduction in the dose of general anaesthetic required and produce a smoother induction and recovery from anaesthesia. **Injectable general anaesthetics** may be used for induction of anaesthesia (e.g. *thiopentone*) and maintenance of anaesthesia is often achieved by the use of **inhalational** (or **gaseous**) general anaesthetics (e.g. *halothane*).

Antimuscarinic drugs may be given before anaesthesia to counteract the salivation and increased bronchial secretions which, in small dogs and cats, may obstruct the airway. In addition, some surgical procedures may increase vagal nerve stimulation of the heart, reducing heart rate (causing bradycardia). Antimuscarinic drugs will prevent bradycardia. Examples: *atropine*, *hyoscine*.

Muscle relaxants

These prevent the message from the nerve reaching the skeletal muscle and so paralyse the muscle. *Pancuronium* is an example of such a drug which is used with general anaesthesia for intrathoracic surgery. Its effects can be reversed by the **muscle relaxant antagonist** *neostigmine*.

Local anaesthetics

These temporarily prevent conduction of an impulse along a nerve fibre. Tissues are infiltrated with drug around sensory nerve fibres to produce analgesia of an area. Motor nerve fibres can also be affected if the injection is made around them. Vasoconstrictors are often included in such preparations to reduce blood flow to the area and so prevent the local anaesthetic being removed from its local site of action. Example: *lignocaine* with *adrenaline*.

Anti-epileptics

These drugs are used to treat epilepsy, a condition of the central nervous system characterised by the spontaneous occurrence of convulsions or seizures. Examples: *phenobarbitone*, *diazepam*.

Drugs used in the treatment of disorders of the endocrine system

Disorders of the endocrine system result either from lack of production or overproduction of a hormone. Drugs are used either to replace the natural hormone or to prevent overproduction of the hormone in question (Table 12.5). Anterior pituitary hormones (or their analogues) are used in diagnostic tests for endocrine diseases. For example *tetracosactrin* (an adrenocorticotrophin analogue) is used in the

Table 12.5 Drugs used in the treatment of endocrine disorders

Gland	Disease state	Drug class	Example
Adrenal gland	*Deficiency:* Hypoadrenocorticism (Addison's disease)	Adrenal corticosteroids Mineralocorticoids (sodium conserving) Glucocorticoids	Fludrocortisone Prednisolone, dexamethasone
	Excess: Hyperadrenocorticism (Cushing's disease)	Adrenolytic agent Glucocorticoid synthesis inhibitor	Mitotane ketoconazole
Thyroid gland	*Deficiency:* Hypothyroidism	Thyroid hormone replacement	Levothyroxine
	Excess: Hyperthyroidism	Antithyroid agent	Carbimazole
Endocrine pancreas	*Deficiency:* Diabetes mellitus (hyperglycaemia)	Insulin Oral hypoglycaemic agents	Protamine zinc insulin Glipizide
	Excess: Hypoglycaemia (low blood glucose)	Glucose (intravenous) Anti-insulin agents	Dextrose solution Dexamethasone (glucocorticoids)
Posterior pituitary gland	Diabetes insipidus (deficiency of ADH)	Posterior pituitary hormone (ADH analogue)	Desmopressin

Table 12.6 Drugs used in the treatment of reproductive and urinary tracts

	Examples	Uses
Sex hormones – (sex steroids) **Oestrogens**	Diethylstilboestrol, Oestradiol benzoate	Prevent implantation following accidental mating (misalliance). Treat urinary incontinence. Reduce the size of an enlarged prostate gland and anal adenomas.
Progestogens Steroids which mimic the actions of progesterone	Megoestrol acetate, Delmadinone, Proligestone	Postpone or suppress oestrus in the bitch and queen. Management of some behavioural problems (aggression in male dogs).
Androgens Esters or analogues of the male sex hormone, testosterone	Methyltestosterone	Hormonal alopecia in dogs and cats. Deficient libido in males.
Luteolytic agents (prostaglandins) Cause regression of the corpus luteum	Dinoprost	Management of open pyometra in the bitch (unlicensed use). Synchronisation of oestrus in cattle and sheep. Induction of parturition in pigs.
Myometrial stimulants (ecbolics) Stimulate the uterus to contract	Oxytocin (extract of posterior pituitary gland)	Dystocia due to weakness of the uterine muscle (uterine inertia).
Drugs used to treat urinary tract disorders. **Urinary acidifiers** Lower the pH of the urine	Ethylenediamine	Cystitis (aid action of antibacterials and urinary antiseptics). In the management of urolithiasis (struvite calculi).
Urinary alkalinisers Raise the pH of the urine	Sodium bicarbonate	In the management of urate uroliths.
Urinary antiseptics Hydrolyse in acidic urine to release formaldehyde	Hexamine	Prophylaxis and long-term treatment of recurrent urinary tract infection.

ACTH stimulation test which is performed in the diagnosis of both Cushing's disease and Addison's disease.

Steroid hormones share a common chemical structure and are produced by the adrenal cortex (**adrenal corticosteroids**) or by the ovary and testes (**sex steroids** – see below). **Anabolic steroids** are derivatives of the male sex hormone, testosterone, and are used to increase muscle mass and to promote tissue repair in convalescing animals. Example: *nandrolone*.

Drugs acting on the reproductive and urinary tract

Table 12.6 describes sex hormones (sex steroids), luteolytic agents (prostaglandins), myometrial stimulants (ecbolics) and drugs used to treat urinary tract disorders. Drugs used in the management of disorders of urination are presented in Fig. 12.2.

Drugs used to treat malignant disease

Cytotoxic drugs kill actively dividing cells and are used in the **chemotherapy** of some forms of cancer which cannot be removed surgically (e.g. malignant lymphoma). As normal cells in the body are actively dividing, these drugs have a low therapeutic index and need to be used with great care. They are also a hazard to people handling them (as are some other drugs already discussed), a subject which will be dealt with below. Examples: *cyclophosphamide, vincristine*.

Drugs used to treat disorders of the musculoskeletal system and joints

Anti-inflammatory drugs

Anti-inflammatory drugs are considered here although they can be used to reduce or suppress inflammation wherever it occurs in the body. The value of such drugs is to relieve the pain, swelling and fever caused by acute inflammation.

Corticosteroids of the glucocorticoid group will suppress inflammation and, at high doses, can produce **immunosuppression** which is required in the treatment of immune-mediated diseases which sometimes cause polyarthritis in the dog.

Non-steroidal anti-inflammatory drugs (NSAIDs) mostly inhibit the formation of prostaglandins and related compounds, which are important mediators of acute inflammation. These drugs will reduce pain and swelling following surgery or in a number of acquired inflammatory conditions such as osteoarthritis. Examples: *phenylbutazone, flunixin meglumine, carprofen, aspirin*.

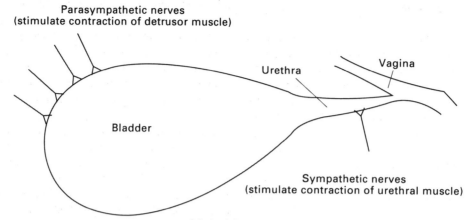

Parasympathetic nerves
(stimulate contraction of detrusor muscle)

Urethra   Vagina

Bladder

Sympathetic nerves
(stimulate contraction of urethral muscle)

Clinical Problems

Clinical problem	Signs	Drug class and action	Example
Atonic bladder	Bladder overfills and may leak (overflow incontinence)	Parasympathomimetic (stimulates detrusor muscle to contract)	Bethanechol
Weak bladder neck (intra-pelvic bladder)	Dribbles urine particularly at rest	Sympathomimetic (increases urethral tone)	Phenylpropanolamine
Urethral spasm	Unable to pass stream of urine	Sympathetic antagonist (lowers urethral tone)	Phenoxybenzamine (α-adrenoceptor antagonist)

Fig. 12.2 The bladder and drugs which affect urination. The process of urination is brought about by parasympathetic stimulation of the detrusor muscle and inhibition of sympathetic tone to the urethral smooth muscle, allowing the bladder to contract and empty through the relaxed urethra. When the bladder fills, the sympathetic nervous system is active, maintaining continence by closing the urethra; the parasympathetic system is inactive, allowing the detrusor muscle to relax and the bladder to fill.

Chondroprotective agents

These prevent further breakdown of cartilage and stimulate the synthesis of new articular cartilage. Example: *pentosan polysulphate sodium.*

Drugs acting on the eye

Antimicrobial and anti-inflammatory agents can be applied topically to the eye in the form of drops or ointments. Local anaesthetics can also be formulated for topical application to the eye. Other drugs with actions on the eye include the following.

Mydriatics and cycloplegics

These dilate the pupil (mydriasis) and reduce spasm in the ciliary muscle. Examples: **antimuscarinic agents**, *atropine*, *homatropine.*

Drugs used in the treatment of glaucoma (raised intra-ocular pressure)

Miotics constrict the pupil and thus open the drainage angle for ocular fluid. Drugs which mimic stimulation of the parasympathetic nerve supply to the eye (**parasympathomimetics**) have this effect. Example: *pilocarpine.*

Carbonic anhydrase inhibitors will reduce the formation of aqueous humour. Examples: *dorzolamide* (given topically), *acetazolamide* (given orally).

Drugs used in keratoconjunctivitis sicca (dry eye)

These replace the tear film, which is deficient in this condition. *Hypromellose* drops are the most commonly used artificial tears. A **mucolytic**, *acetylcysteine*, may be beneficial when the tears are particularly mucoid and viscous. **Parasympathomimetics** (*pilocarpine*) administered by mouth may stimulate lacrimal secretion in some cases.

Drugs acting on the ear

Topical preparations containing antimicrobial, ectoparasiticide and anti-inflammatory agents are all available. **Sebolytics** dissolve wax and cleanse the ear canal. Many different preparations are available using solvents such as *squalene* or *propylene glycol* and incorporating *benzoic acid* and *salicylic acid.*

Drugs acting on the skin

The skin can be treated with drugs given orally or parenterally, which reach the skin via its blood supply, or by topical application of preparations of drugs directly to the affected area. Topical drugs are usually formulated as creams, ointments, lotions, powders, shampoos or sprays. The vehicle or base of these may be selected to suit the type of lesion and location being treated, as described later. The active drugs contained in such preparations may be antibacterials, ectoparasiticides or anti-inflammatory agents. Drugs which have not been mentioned elsewhere which are used for disorders of the skin include the following:

- **Keratolytics** which loosen the horny layer of the epidermis causing it to separate away from the deeper epidermis. Examples: *benzoyl peroxide, salicylic acid.*
- **Astringents** precipitate protein on the surface of the skin to produce a protective coating. Example: *zinc oxide, calamine.*
- **Disinfectants** in the correct concentration can be used topically to cleanse the skin and chemically destroy surface bacteria. Example: *chlorhexidine gluconate.*
- **Essential fatty acids** are given orally to animals and have potential *anti-inflammatory* properties with some evidence of beneficial effects in inflammatory skin conditions. Examples: *gamolenic acid* (GLA), *eicosa-pentanoic acid* (EPA). There are many proprietary preparations available containing these essential fatty acids, some of which also contain vitamins and minerals.

Drugs affecting nutrition and body fluids

Electrolyte and water replacement solutions (crystalloid fluids)

These are used to treat animals suffering from dehydration. **Oral rehydration solutions** consist of mixtures of sodium, potassium, chloride ions and an anion which is metabolised by the liver to form bicarbonate (e.g. citrate). In addition, glucose and amino acids such as glycine are included, not for nutritional purposes, but because they help the transport of sodium and water across the gut wall and into the blood stream. **Parenteral solutions** are used to replace fluid losses in cases where the oral route is unsuitable and a parenteral route (usually intravenous route) is chosen. The composition of the fluid used depends on the type of losses sustained. For example, *replacement* of extracellular fluid volume requires a fluid with plasma concentration of sodium (about 140 mmol/l). When parenteral fluids are given to *maintain* hydration in an animal that is unable to drink, fluids which are much lower in sodium are more appropriate. Isotonicity of such fluids is maintained by the addition of glucose (e.g. 4% glucose and 0.18% sodium chloride). **Concentrated additives** such as potassium chloride, glucose (dextrose monohydrate) and sodium bicarbonate are available for addition to commercially available fluids so that the composition of the fluid can be adjusted to suit the requirements of the animal being treated. Nutrient solutions are available to provide nutrition by the intravenous route (parenteral nutrition). They consist of concentrated solutions of glucose or emulsions of lipid to provide calories and amino acids. They should only be administered through the jugular vein as the risk of phlebitis and infection when given through a small peripheral vein is high.

Hypertonic saline (e.g. 7.0% sodium chloride) is a special type of crystalloid fluid used in the treatment of hypovolaemic and endotoxaemic shock. Small volumes are given for the pharmcological effect this has on cardiac output and arterial blood pressure. Volume replacement with conventional isotonic crystalloid fluids or colloids (see below) should still form part of the treatment of such patients.

Plasma substitutes

Plasma substitutes are large molecular weight **colloids** in solution which are retained in the circulation rather than leaving capillaries and distributing into the whole extra-cellular fluid volume (as is the case with crystalloid fluids). Thus, a smaller volume of such colloid preparations will restore the circulating fluid volume in an animal suffering from haemorrhagic shock when compared with the volume of replacement crystalloid solutions required. Example: *gelatin.*

Vitamins and minerals

These can be used as supplements for sick and debilitated animals, and, as such, would be regarded as medicines. Nutritional deficiencies may occur but are uncommon in the dog and cat nowadays with the use of commercial pet foods. Specific indications for a mineral would be eclampsia in the bitch where *calcium gluconate* would be given intra-venously. *Phytomenadione* (vitamin K_1) is the specific antidote to warfarin poisoning.

Vaccines and immunological preparations

Vaccines are given to animals to stimulate immunity against an infectious disease (e.g. canine distemper). The body responds to antigens in the vaccine and the immunity produced is termed **active immunity**. **Live vaccines** consist of living organisms of a slightly different strain from that which causes the natural disease making them non-pathogenic (no signs of disease result) but still able to stimulate a protective immune response. The organisms in live vaccines multiply inside the host after administration and stimulate a long-lasting immune response. **Inactivated vaccines** contain sufficient antigen to stimulate an immune response and no multiplication of the organism in question is possible following administration of an inactivated vaccine. **Toxoids** (e.g. *Tetanus toxoid*) are forms of inactivated vaccines where toxins produced by organisms have been extracted and heat-treated to render them harmless. Inactivated vaccines usually contain adjuvants such as aluminium hydroxide or mineral oil which help to enhance the immune response to the antigens in the vaccine which is generally not as long lasting as that obtained with live vaccines. An **autogenous vaccine** is prepared from material collected from an individual animal for administration to the same animal.

Immunoglobulins (antibodies, antisera) can be administered to animals to confer **passive immunity**. Example: *tetanus antitoxin*. These consist of serum containing antibodies raised in another animal (usually of the same species). They can have a neutralising effect on the organism or toxin in question and therefore give some immediate protection in the face of infection. Passive immunity only persists for about 3 weeks.

Formulation and administration of drugs

Systemically administered drugs

If a drug cannot be applied locally (topically) to the site at which its action is desired, it must first be administered in such a way that it is **absorbed** into the blood circulation (systemically) from which it **distributes** to the place in the body where it acts. The rate and extent of absorption of the drug from its site of administration will depend upon its route of administration and the physical and chemical form in which it is administered (see below). The body gets rid of (**eliminates**) the drug by converting it into a different chemical compound by a process of metabolism followed by excretion of the drug from the body. The liver is the major organ where drug **metabolism** occurs and excretion of the drug itself or of its metabolites is into the bile or urine. Some volatile agents are excreted from the body via the respiratory tract.

Oral preparations

The oral route is the most convenient route for many drugs used in small animal veterinary practice as owners can dose their own pets at home. There are a number of problems with oral dosing, however, which are listed below:

- The absorption of the drug from the gut into the blood stream is often slower and less complete than when drugs are injected (given by a parenteral route, Fig. 12.3). It may take time for a tablet to dissolve and release its contents: some drugs are absorbed primarily in the small intestine rather than the stomach and so their absorption only occurs once the stomach empties.
- If the animal is vomiting the oral route is not reliable.
- Some drugs are unstable in gastric acid or are destroyed by the enzymes of the gut so the oral route cannot be used (e.g. penicillin G, insulin).
- Some drugs are broken down very rapidly and efficiently in the liver after absorption from the gut and so do not reach the general circulation (e.g. lignocaine, glyceryl trinitrate) or a higher dose is required when the drug is given orally (e.g. propranolol).
- Food in the gastrointestinal tract may affect the absorption of the drug by delaying its entry into the blood

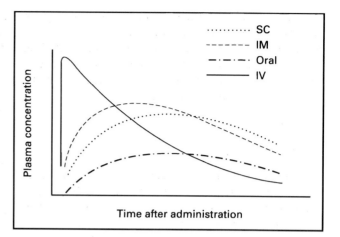

Fig. 12.3 Plasma concentration versus time curve for a 'typical' drug following its administration by: intramuscular injection (IM), intravenous injection (IV), subcutaneous injection (SC) and oral administration.

stream (e.g. digoxin) or reducing the amount of the drug absorbed (e.g. ampicillin). In other cases, fatty food helps the absorption of some drugs across the gut wall (e.g. griseofulvin, mitotane).
- Some drugs are not absorbed when given orally and remain in the gastrointestinal tract. They can be used as a form of local therapy but will not have systemic effects (e.g. neomycin can be used orally to treat enteric infections but not urinary tract infections).

Tablets. Many oral medications are in the form of **tablets** containing the active drug and some inert ingredients (binder and excipients) which bind the compressed mass together. Tablets may be coated for a number of reasons:

- To protect the tablet from the atmosphere, particularly moisture.
- To delay disintegration of the tablet and so protect the active drug from the acidic environment of the stomach or protects the stomach from irritant effects of the drug (e.g. aspirin).
- To hide the bitter taste of the drug and so facilitate dosing (e.g. erythromycin).

Grinding up tablets will destroy the properties which the outer layers of the tablet provide. Before this measure is recommended or undertaken it is important to check with the manufacturer that such action can be taken without altering the properties of the medication. Some tablets are scored to facilitate breaking them in half for dosing.

Capsules. Other oral medications are formulated as **capsules** which contain either powder or granules. The outer case of the capsule is made of hard gelatin and comes in two halves which slot together. The outer case prevents the drug, which may have a bitter taste, contacting the oral mucosa. Some capsule formulations of drugs contain granules of differing sizes and composition which will dissolve at different rates and so provide a sustained release of drug from the gastrointestinal tract (e.g. slow release formulations of *theophylline*). This reduces the frequency of dosing required.

Mixtures. Liquid medication (or **mixtures**) can be given by mouth and may contain the drug completely in solution if it is freely soluble or in suspension if it is insoluble (e.g. *kaolin* in water). Suspensions require thorough mixing before dosing and should always be labelled with the instruction: 'Shake well before use'.

Parenteral preparations

Strictly speaking, a parenteral route of administration means any route other than the oral route. It is generally taken to mean routes by which drugs are injected into the body of an animal. All preparations for parenteral use must, therefore, be sterile and pyrogen free. The most common routes of injection of drugs in small animal practice are:

- Intravenous – directly into venous blood.
- Intramuscular – into muscular tissue, usually of the leg or back.
- Subcutaneous – into the tissue beneath the skin.

Occasionally the intraperitoneal route of injection is used, particularly in small rodents. The peritoneal membrane provides a large surface area for drug absorption.

Intravenous route. The **intravenous route** will provide the fastest distribution of the drug to its site of action that is possible since the drug is placed directly into the blood stream. The peak plasma concentration of the drug achieved is higher than can be achieved by any other route but the drug concentration often decreases rapidly (depending on the rate at which the body metabolises and excretes the drug) as absorption of the drug from the site of administration is instantaneous and does not continue over a period of time as is the case for the oral route and other parenteral routes (Fig. 12.3).

Preparations for intravenous use must be true solutions where the drug to be administered is dissolved in sterile water (aqueous solution) or another type of solvent. It is important to make any intravenous injections slowly as a rapid (bolus) injection can result in a very high concentration of the drug (or solvent) reaching the heart or brain and causing detrimental effects. Suspensions of drugs cannot be administered intravenously as the particles in a suspension may block capillaries in the lungs causing death.

Drugs which may be irritant to the tissues should preferably be administered by the intravenous route as the drug is rapidly removed and diluted in the circulating blood (if the injection is made slowly). If irritant drugs are given (e.g. sodium thiopentone, vincristine) it is important to ensure that the injection is indeed made into the vein. Accidental injection into the tissues around the vein (perivascular injection) may cause severe damage.

Intramuscular route. **Intramuscular injection** of drugs may be more convenient for less co-operative patients and drugs in suspensions can be given by this route. After inserting the needle into a muscle to make the injection, it is important to draw back on the syringe to ensure that the tip of the needle is not in a blood vessel within the muscle.

Intramuscular injections may be painful; the severity of the pain depends on the volume of the injection, the viscosity of the material being injected and the chemical nature of the compound (how irritant it is to the tissue). The drug diffuses from the injection site by dissolving in the tissue fluid surrounding the muscle cells and is then absorbed into the blood capillaries and lymphatics supplying the muscle.

Subcutaneous route. **Subcutaneous injections** can be made into any area of the body where there is loose skin – usually over the neck or back. Formulations of drugs for subcutaneous injection should be approximately of blood pH and body fluid tonicity, and should not be irritant or cause vasoconstriction as this will impede the absorption of the drug into the blood stream. Larger volumes can be administered by the subcutaneous route than by the intramuscular route.

Absorption rates. In general, the rate of absorption of drugs given by the intramuscular route is faster than those given by the subcutaneous route since muscle receives a larger blood supply than subcutaneous tissue (Fig. 12.3). However, the physical and chemical properties of the drug formulation affect the rate of absorption from both of these sites. Formulations of drugs can be produced which contain a combination of different salts of the same drug, one of which is highly soluble (e.g. sodium salt of penicillin G) and so rapidly absorbed from the intramuscular injection site, another which is more slowly absorbed (e.g. procaine salt of penicillin G) and a third which is absorbed very slowly indeed because of its extremely low solubility (e.g. benzathine salt of penicillin G). This principle is used to produce long-acting injections of drugs which are sometimes called *depot preparations*. Insulin is also prepared in different physical forms which give different time to onset of action and duration of effect based on the speed of absorption of insulin from the injection site. Some formulations of insulin (protamine zinc insulin or insulin zinc suspension) may have a duration of action which make them suitable for once daily administration whereas other formulations (Isophane insulin) have a shorter duration of action such that two injections per day may be necessary. *Implants* are an extreme example of a depot preparation where a small disc or cylinder of relatively insoluble drug (often a hormone) is inserted beneath the skin in a sterile manner using a special injection device. The drug can then be released over an extended period of time preventing the need for repeated administration.

Other injection sites. Other sites of injection of drugs include:

- *Intradermal* – into the dermis (allergy testing in dogs).
- *Intra-articular* – into a joint cavity.
- *Intrathecal* – into the cerebrospinal fluid (contrast media for myelography; therapeutic agents are not given by this route in veterinary medicine).
- *Epidural* – into the vertebral canal outside the dura mater (used to produce spinal analgesia when local anaesthetics are injected).

● *Subconjunctival* – under the conjunctival membrane of the eye.

These are all forms of local therapy as the injection site is the site at which the drug is desired to produce its effect.

Other ways of administering drugs to produce systemic effects

Inhalation of drugs into the respiratory tract is a means of supplying drugs to this site of the body and for drugs to be absorbed into the blood stream (e.g. gaseous anaesthetics). Formulation of drugs for inhalation is more difficult for administration to domestic animals than to man, where inhalation is a common way of administering drugs such as bronchodilators. In some university hospitals, drugs in solution can be produced in a very fine mist of liquid droplets which are inhaled by the animal. This process is called *nebulisation* and has obvious safety implications for the operators (see below).

Drugs can be absorbed across other mucous membranes of the body and produce systemic effects. For example, desmopressin is supplied in the form of drops, which in man are instilled into the nose. In the dog, it is more convenient to place these drops into the conjunctival sac. Absorption of the drug from this site into the blood stream occurs and the systemic effects (antidiuretic action) become evident. As this drug is a peptide (small protein), its absorption following oral administration is reduced by enzymic breakdown of the drug within the gastrointestinal tract.

Some drugs are able to penetrate intact skin and so be absorbed from the surface of the skin and have systemic effects. An example used in small animal medicine is the nitrovasodilator, glyceryl trinitrate. This drug cannot be given by the oral route as it is removed so effectively by the liver. The organophosphate insecticide, fenthion, is another example of a drug which, when applied to a discrete area of skin, is absorbed into the blood stream and distributed systemically.

Topically administered drugs

Topical preparations are applied directly to the site at which the drug is required. The most common sites to be treated topically in small animal medicine are the skin, eyes and ears. Enemas could be considered a form of topical therapy where fluids are infused into the rectum to soften the faecal mass. In large animal practice, topical application of drugs are to the mammary gland (*intramammary preparations*), the vagina and uterus (*vaginal suppositories* or *pessaries*). It is important to remember that drugs can be absorbed across mucous membranes and even intact skin – particularly drugs that are lipid soluble (such as corticosteroids) – and so these drugs should not be assumed to be without systemic effects.

Examples of formulations of topical preparations include:

● *Creams* – semi-solid emulsions of oil or fat, and water (which usually contains the drug). They spread easily without friction and penetrate the outer layers of the skin, particularly if the fat used is lanolin. Water-soluble drugs are more active in creams than in ointments.
● *Ointments* – semi-solid greasy, insoluble in water and the drugs are present in a base of wax or fat (usually petroleum jelly). They are non-penetrating and more occlusive than creams and are most suitable for dry chronic lesions.
● *Dusting powders* – finely divided powders for application to the skin containing usually ectoparasiticides or antibacterials.
● *Wettable powders* – applied to the skin as a suspension after mixing with a large quantity of water. The animal is then dried by warmth leaving the powder in the coat (i.e. it is not rinsed off).
● *Lotions* – liquid preparations which consist of solutions of the drugs in water (e.g. calamine lotion).
● *Medicated shampoos* – aqueous solutions or suspensions of drugs which have a detergent base which gives good penetration of the coat. Shampoos are left in contact with the skin for the recommended period of time and then rinsed off thoroughly.
● *Aerosol sprays* – a way of applying liquid solutions or suspensions of drugs in fine droplet form. The liquid is packaged in a metal container under pressure and pressing the nozzle of the container causes the liquid to be expelled.
● *Eye medications* can be in the form of ointments or drops. Ophthalmic ointments tend to be more liquid (than the ointments described above), having a soft paraffin base, and when applied to the surface of the cornea they melt to form a thin film which covers the whole surface of the eye. Eye drops are aqueous solutions of drugs for instillation to the eye. In general, drops tend to be shorter acting than ointments and require more frequent application. Both forms of medication should be sterile and, once opened, should be stored only for the length of time recommended by the manufacturers.

Calculation of drug dosages

The responsibility for ensuring that the correct dosage of drug is administered to an animal under their care lies with the veterinary surgeon in charge of the case. However, veterinary nurses should understand how to calculate dosages of drugs.

Weights, volumes and concentration

The active ingredient in the preparation of a drug is expressed in terms of its weight. The standard units for weight are kilograms (kg), grams (g), milligrams (mg) and micrograms (no abbreviation used). These weights are related as follows:

1 kilogram (kg) = 1000 grams
1 gram (g) = 1000 milligrams
1 milligram (mg) = 1000 micrograms

If the weight relates to a tablet or capsule, then each tablet or capsule contains the stated weight of active drug. When considering liquid formulations of drugs (solutions or suspensions), the weight of active drug is related to a unit of volume of the suspension or solution. Standard units of volume include litres (l) and millilitres (ml) where 1 l = 1000 ml. Some drugs are relatively unstable in solution and so are supplied as a solid in a vial and the solvent (often water for injection) supplied separately. The drug is reconstituted by adding the solvent to the vial. Unless all the drug is used immediately, it is important to write on the vial the concentration of the solution of the drug you have just made (usually in terms of milligrams of drug per millilitre of solution) and the date on which it was reconstituted. The reconstituted drug may be stable if kept in the refrigerator for several days, so it is important to know the concentration of the solution which has been made.

Percentage solutions

Another way of expressing the concentration of a drug in solution is as a percentage of weight (*w*) of the drug per volume of solution (*w/v*). If 1 g of the active drug is dissolved in a total volume of 100 ml this produces a **1% solution**. If this fundamental fact is remembered, percentage solutions can be readily converted into concentrations in terms of milligrams per millilitre, which is usually a more convenient form when it comes to calculating dosages.

Exceptions to standard weights and volumes

Some drugs, such as insulin, oxytocin and heparin, are extracted from animal tissues and are not produced in a completely pure form. The concentration of the drug in the product is determined by is effect in a laboratory test system (bioassay) against an International Standard. In most cases, the concentration of such preparations is given in terms of international units (i.u.) or simply units per standard volume (usually per millilitre). So, for example, all formulations of insulin for human use are produced at a concentration of 100 units/ml. There is now an insulin preparation licensed for veterinary use in this country which contains insulin at a concentration of 40 i.u./ml. Insulin is administered using special syringes which are graduated in units rather than in millilitres. It is important to use a 40 unit syringe for insulin of concentration 40 units/ml and a 100 unit syringe for insulin preparations of 100 units/ml.

Dosages

Drug dosage rates are usually expressed in terms of weight of drug per weight of the animal to be dosed (most often in milligrams of drug per kg bodyweight of the animal). Some drugs (particularly those used for cancer chemotherapy) are dosed on a weight of drug per body surface area (milligram per square metre body surface area). Conversion charts are available which give body surface area from the animal's weight in kilograms. The following worked examples will illustrate some of the principles in calculation of dosages.

EXAMPLE 1

You are asked to dispense enrofloxacin tablets for a dog weighing 20 kg at a dose rate of 2.5 mg/kg twice daily for 7 days. The drug comes in tablet sizes of 15, 50 and 150 mg. Which tablet size would be most appropriate, how many tablets would you dispense and what instructions for dosing would you give to the owner?

Amount of drug required (mg)

= dose (mg/kg) × bodyweight in kg
= 2.5 (mg/kg) × 20 (kg)
= 50 mg

Thus, the most appropriate tablet size to use would be 50 mg and the owners should be instructed to give one tablet twice a day for 7 days. The number of tablets required will be 14 (7 × 2).

EXAMPLE 2

A 6 kg miniature poodle requires digoxin for treatment of congestive heart failure. The dose rate **required** is 0.01 mg/kg each day which should be divided into two equal doses (0.01 mg/kg divided twice daily). The tablet sizes available are 62.5, 125 and 250 micrograms. What tablet size would you use, what would your dosing instructions to the owners be and how many tablets would you dispense for a 30-day course?

Daily dose required (mg)

= dose (mg/kg) × bodyweight in kg
= 0.01 (mg/kg) × 6 (kg) = 0.06 mg

To convert milligrams to micrograms multiply by 1000:

Thus 0.06 mg = 0.06 × 1000 micrograms
= 60 micrograms

This dose should be divided into two equal daily doses, so each dose should contain:

= 60/2 micrograms
= 30 micrograms

Thus, the most appropriate tablet size to use would be the 62.5 microgram tablets, and the owners should be instructed to give half a tablet every 12 hours before food. For a course of 30 days the owners would require 30 tablets.

TIPS

(a) Please note that it is important to be sure of the position of the decimal point in all drug calculations, so always write 0.01 rather than simply .01.

(b) In addition, the dose required in Example 2 is slightly lower than the convenient tablet size. Digoxin is a drug with a low therapeutic index and care should be taken not to overdose an animal. In this case, the inaccuracy was deemed so small as to be of no consequence but judgement should always be made by the veterinary surgeon in charge of the case.

(c) In dosing with digoxin, food can interfere with the rate of absorption of digoxin from the gut, so an instruction to give the medication before meals is important.

(d) In Example 2 the total daily dose rate was given and had to be divided into two equal doses. An alternative way of expressing this would be to say the dose required is 0.005 mg/kg to be given twice daily which was the way the dose rate in Example 1 was expressed.

EXAMPLE 3

For injection, you are given a drug in solution which is 7.5% w/v. The dose required for the dog you are treating is 10 mg/kg and the dog weighs 18 kg. What volume of the drug should be given to this dog by injection?

Concentration of drug in solution
= 7.5 g in 100 ml (7.5% w/v)
= (7.5/100) g in 1 ml
= 0.075 g in 1 ml
= (0.075 × 1000) mg in 1 ml
= 75 mg/ml

Amount of drug required
= dose (mg/kg) × bodyweight in kg
= 10 (mg/kg) × 18 (kg) = 180 mg

Volume of drug required (ml)
= Amount of drug (mg)/concentration (mg/ml)
= 180 (mg)/75 (mg/ml)
= 2.4 ml

TIP

To convert the concentration of a solution expressed in percentages into mg/ml, multiply the percentage figure by 10.

Legal aspects of medicines and prescribing

The legislation which governs the storage, handling, use and supply of medicines in veterinary practice includes:

● The Medicines Act 1968.
● The Medicines (restrictions on the administration of veterinary medicinal products) Regulations 1994.
● The Misuse of Drugs Act 1971.
● The Misuse of Drugs Regulations 1985.
● The Health and Safety at Work Act 1974.
● The Control of Substances Hazardous to Health Regulations 1998.

They have also been considered in Chapters 4 (Occupational hazards) and 7 (The law and ethics of veterinary nursing).

The Medicines Act 1968

The Government ensures the quality, safety and efficacy of medicines for human and animal use by a system of licences approved by the Department of Health and the Ministry of Agriculture, respectively. Before a product can be manufactured, imported and distributed widely, the company or person who devises it has to gain a marketing authorisation by showing that the drug is safe, efficacious (produces the effects which the data sheet claims) and that the manufacturing process ensures a consistent quality of the product. Manufacturers and wholesale dealers of medicinal products require *manufacturer's* and *wholesale dealer's marketing authority*, respectively. As part of the licensing procedure, the company may need to perform a clinical trial of the drug in question and for this purpose they apply for an *animal test certificate*. An exemption to this law is that veterinary surgeons do not require a product licence to prepare a medicinal product themselves (or to request another veterinary surgeon to prepare such a product for them) for a particular animal or herd under their care. The veterinary surgeon is only allowed to stock a very limited supply of a medicine prepared in this way (2.5 kg of solid and 5 l of liquid). It is not permissible for vaccines (other than autogenous vaccines) to be prepared in this way.

Use of unlicensed products in veterinary medicine

The Medicines (restrictions on the administration of veterinary medicinal products) Regulations became law in December 1994. In non-food-producing animals, the regulations state that a product, which has a veterinary marketing authorisation for the species and the condition to be treated, or is authorised for another condition or another veterinary species should, if possible, be chosen before a product which is only authorised for human use. Products authorised only for human use may be used if no veterinary licensed alternative exists. Special products made by the veterinary surgeon or by a pharmacist for the veterinary surgeon, which have no marketing authorisation at all, should be used only if a veterinary or human authorised product does not already exist. These regulations have been produced to protect the consumer of animal products from drug residues. Their application to small animal veterinary practice has been clarified by guidance notes issued by the Veterinary Medicines Directorate (AMELIA 8).

Legal categories of medicines

When granting a marketing authorisation for a drug the licensing body places the medicine into one of three main categories. In order of decreasing strictness of controls over their supply to the public, these are:

- Prescription only medicines (POMs) including Controlled Drugs (CD).
- Pharmacy only medicines (P) including Merchant's List and Saddler's List medicines (PML).
- General sales list medicines (GSL).

More detailed information of these categories and their subdivisions is given in Table 12.7. In summary, the only category of medicine which can be sold direct to the public by a veterinary practice without the owner having consulted with a veterinary surgeon are GSL products. For all other categories of drugs, the animals for which they are intended

should be *under the care of a veterinary surgeon in* the practice and his or her authority should be sought before these drugs can be supplied by a trained veterinary nurse.

Storage of medicines

The manufacturer's recommendations should be carefully followed for each medicine in terms of storage temperature and the sensitivity of the compound to light and humidity. The part of the building in which the medicines are stored should not be accessible to the general public. Well-designed shelves are essential to allow easy access to the drugs required and to reduce the possibility of breakage, spillage or misplacement of stock. There should be a work surface, which should be easy to clean, and adequate refrigeration space.

It is convenient to store the medicines on the shelves in their classification groups. Products in large containers should be stocked near ground level for safety. Effective stock control will save time and money, ensuring that old stock is used before new so that medicines in stock do not exceed their expiry date and that the pharmacy does not run out of a particular medication. In conclusion, a clean and tidy pharmacy makes for efficient and safe dispensing of medications.

Table 12.7 Legal categories of medicines

Legal category	Sub-category	Definition	Examples
Prescription only medicines (POM)	Controlled drugs	A sub-category of POM where the regulations for supply and storage are even more stringent than general POM medicines.	Morphine (S2) Phenobarbitone (S3)
	General POM drugs	Can only be prescribed and dispensed by a veterinary surgeon or dispensed by a pharmacist against a prescription written and signed by a veterinary surgeon.	Many veterinary medicines such as: Antibacterial drugs Vaccines Any drug intended for parenteral administration
Pharmacy only medicines (P)	General P medicines	Any drug in this category may be sold over the counter by a registered pharmacist to the general public. A veterinary surgeon may supply drugs in this category for the treatment of animals under his/her care.	Most P medicines are human products Veterinary examples: Dermisol®
	Pharmacy Merchant's List (PML)	Drugs in this sub-category in addition to the general regulations described for P medicines may also be sold by agricultural merchants registered with the Royal Pharmaceutical Society to persons whose business involves animals (e.g. farmers).	Large animal anthelmintics Ectoparasiticides
	Saddler's List (PML)	Saddlers who are registered with the Royal Pharmaceutical Society may sell certain anthelmintics to horse owners.	Anthelmintics for horses
General sales list (GSL)	–	Medicinal products where the hazard to health or the need to take special precautions is sufficiently small that they can be sold without a prescription by pet shops or merchants who are not subject to special regulation. A number of veterinary products are GSL only when produced for external use or, when formulated for oral administration, a maximum strength which may be sold is stipulated.	Piperazine citrate Permethrin flea spray Pipronyl butoxide

---

Table 12.8 Recommended containers for different medicines

Container	Medicine
Coloured flute bottles	Medicines for external application. Examples: shampoos, soaps, lotions. Enemas and eye and ear medications should be similarly dispensed if not already packaged in a suitable plastic container.
Plain glass bottles	Oral liquid medicines.
Wide-mouthed jars	Creams, dusting powders, granules.
Paper board cartons/ wallets	Sachets, manufacturer's strip or blister-packed medicines.
Airtight glass, plastic or metal containers (preferably childproof)[a]	All solid oral medicines (tablets and capsules).

[a] Discretion can be exercised with childproof containers. Some aged and infirm clients may request plain screw-top containers.

Table 12.9 Example of label, including information required by law and additional desirable details

Essential

Owner's name, pet identification and address

Date

For Animal Treatment Only
For Mrs Jones' cat 'Boris'
85 Sister's Avenue,
Battersea, London SW11 3SN
18/9/99

Optional

Quantity and strength of drug

21 × 50 mg Ampicillin tablets

Instructions for dosing

One tablet to be given three times daily before food

Essential

Name and address of veterinary surgeon

Keep all medicines out of reach of children
P.J. Barber MRCVS
Veterinary Surgeon
12 St John's Hill, London SW18 1JL

Dispensing and labelling of medicines

The containers listed in Table 12.8 are recommended by the Council of the Royal Pharmaceutical Society for the dispensing of medicines from bulk packs. Note that paper envelopes and plastic bags are unacceptable forms of container.

The Medicines Act and the Medicine Labelling Regulations state the legal requirements for labelling of dispensed medicines. These regulations apply whether the medicines are dispensed in the manufacturer's original container or dispensed from bulk into smaller packages. Labels should be legible and indelible (written in biro or felt pen not washable ink or pencil). Printed labels can be generated by computers used in modern practices. The specimen label shown in Table 12.9 indicates essential information which has to be provided by law and also optional (but desirable) information.

If the medication is for external use the words 'For external use only' should appear on the label. In addition, any safety precautions the owners should take when handling the drug should be added. When the drug is to be used in food-producing animals, the label must also include the withdrawal period (the time between the last dose of the drug and the use of meat, milk or eggs from the animal for human consumption).

The Misuse of Drugs Act 1971 and The Misuse of Drugs Regulations 1985

This legislation controls the production, supply, possession, storage and dispensing of drugs where the potential exists for abuse by humans. These are the controlled drugs (CD), a special category of POM products, and there are five schedules:

- Schedule 1 (S1) – addictive drugs such as *cannabis* and hallucinogens *mescaline* and *LSD*.

- Schedule 2 (S2) – the opiate analgesics *morphine*, *etorphine*, *fentanyl* and *pethidine* plus *cocaine* and *amphetamine*.
- Schedule 3 (S3) – the barbiturates *pentobarbitone* and *phenobarbitone* plus the opiate analgesics, *buprenorphine* and *pentazocine*.
- Schedule 4 (S4) – benzodiazepines such as *diazepam* and *chlordiazepoxide*.
- Schedule 5 (S5) – certain preparations of cocaine, codeine and morphine that contain less than a specified amount of the drug. (Examples: *codeine cough linctus, kaolin and morphine antidiarrhoeal suspension*.)

A veterinary surgeon does not have any general authority to possess or supply drugs from Schedule 1. Some of the other controlled drugs are subject to more stringent regulations than general POM medications, as detailed below:

Purchase. Purchase of S2 and S3 drugs requires a written requisition to a wholesaler, manufacturer or pharmacist which include the veterinary surgeon's signature, their name and address and profession, the purpose for which the drug is required and the total quantity of the drug required. If a messenger is sent to collect the drug, written authority has to be given by the veterinary surgeon for the messenger to receive the drug on their behalf.

Storage. S2 drugs and buprenorphine (from S3) must be kept in a locked cupboard which is attached to a wall. The veterinary surgeon is responsible for the key to such a cupboard which should only be opened with his or her authority.

Records. A bound register of all transactions involving S2 drugs must be kept. Details of incomings (purchases) of S2 drugs and their outgoings (drugs given to animals on the practice premises or dispensed to an owner to give to their

Table 12.10 Example of prescription form for a controlled drug

Mr J. Fishwick, MA, Vet MB MRCVS
50 High Street, Comberton, Cambridge CB4 1RL
Tel: 01223 849623

25th September 1999
Mr J. R. Fox's dog "Smarty"
23 The Green,
Barton, Cambridge.

Rx
Tablets Pethidine 50 mg
Send 10 (ten)

Label: Give half a tablet twice a day for 5 days

For Animal Treatment Only

This animal is under my care

No repeats

---

animal) should be recorded in separate parts of the register, with a section for each individual drug in both parts of the register (i.e. the records for pethidine should be separated from those for morphine). Such registers for controlled drugs are available commercially. In addition, any S2 drug which is no longer required by the veterinary practice can only be disposed of in the presence of a Home Office Inspector. A record has to be made in the register which the Inspector is required to sign.

Special prescription requirements for controlled drugs. These apply to those drugs in S2 and S3. An example of a prescription is shown in Table 12.10. The format is the same for any drug which the veterinary surgeon would like a pharmacist to dispense to one of his/her clients. In the case of S2 and S3 drugs, the name and address of the client, the date and the quantity (in numbers and words) and strength of the preparation should be written in the veterinary surgeon's own handwriting.

The Health and Safety at Work Act 1974 and The Control of Substances Hazardous to Health (COSHH) Regulations 1998

When common sense is used and a few general ground rules followed, the medicines used in most veterinary practices present a relatively small hazard to the health of employees. All data sheets of licensed medicines will discuss any hazards the medicine might pose to the operator (the person dispensing and administering the drug). The practice you work for should also have produced a COSHH Assessment for the substances (including drugs) which you come into contact with during the working day (see Chapter 4, Occupational Hazards). It is important that these documents are read and the safety measures followed to contain any risk to the absolute minimum.

Drugs can get into the body by accident and have systemic effects in the operator in a number of ways.

Absorption across the skin

This can occur with certain drugs such as prostaglandins (luteolytic agents), insecticides, nitrovasodilators and compounds containing the solvent DMSO (dimethyl sulphoxide) which aids penetration of substances which are dissolved in it across the skin. When handling such substances or when handling any substances when you have cuts or abrasions on your hands, gloves should be worn to prevent absorption across the skin. As a general principle, hands should be washed after handling any veterinary medicine and splashes or spills of medicines should be washed from the skin immediately.

Absorption across mucous membranes

The membranes of the eye (conjunctiva), nose and oral cavities are sites where drugs may reach if aerosols from liquid formulations or dust from powders containing the drug are formed. An aerosol is formed by very fine droplets of liquid which can be accidentally sprayed into the eyes or mouth. They are formed most often when reconstituting (dissolving) drugs for injection in the diluent supplied and when expelling air bubbles from a syringe. Care should be taken not to pressurise the contents of vials when reconstituting drugs. In addition, if the needle cover is kept on the needle when expelling air bubbles from the syringe, potentially dangerous aerosols will be avoided. Cytotoxic drugs should only be reconstituted by trained personnel and this should be carried out in designated areas. Should accidental contamination of the eyes, nose or mouth occur, washing or flushing with copious amounts of water should be the initial first aid measure and further medical help should be sought depending on the drug involved.

Accidental ingestion of drugs

This can occur through aerosols or dust, as described above, or through eating contaminated food. Food and drink must not be consumed or stored in areas where drugs are being handled, including areas where topical sprays (e.g. flea sprays) are applied to animals. Smoking should also be prohibited from these areas.

Inhalation

Inhalation of volatile substances such as gaseous anaesthetics (e.g. halothane), dust from powders and droplets from aerosols may cause irritation of the respiratory tract or the drugs can be absorbed and cause systemic effects. Hazards from inhalational anaesthetics can be minimised by the use of an adequate scavenging circuit attached to the anaesthetic circuit and by providing good ventilation of the operating room. Dust masks and eye protection should be worn when dispensing powders from bulk packs where a large amount of dust is inevitable, and insecticidal sprays should only be used in well-ventilated areas.

Accidental injection

This is the final way in which drugs may get into the body. This risk may be minimised by keeping all needles covered until the injection is made and disposing of the used needle in a safe way immediately after use. The quantity of drug which enters the body following penetration of the skin with a needle is very small. Oil-based vaccines can, however, produce very severe reactions. Some drugs, such as etorphine, are extremely toxic to man such that even these minute quantities are hazardous.

Hazardous drugs used in veterinary practice

The groups of drugs mentioned below carry special risks and so are worthy of note. It is important to realise that whilst some drugs may produce acute effects on the operator which are obvious shortly after exposure, other drugs can have cumulative effects, when exposure to small quantities occurs over a long period of time, which can be just as detrimental. For this reason it is good practice to keep your exposure to all drugs you handle to an absolute minimum by following the ground rules mentioned above.

- **Etorphine** – highly toxic following accidental injection or exposure of skin or mucous membranes to the drug.
- **Halothane** – repeated inhalation may damage the liver and has been incriminated in increasing the risk of miscarriages.
- **Cytotoxic drugs** – many are mutagenic (damage genetic material), carcinogenic (cause cancer) and teratogenic (damage the unborn foetus).
- **Prostaglandins** – may cause asthma attacks, have serious effects on the cardiovascular system and cause uterine contractions. Should not be handled by asthmatics or women of child-bearing age. The British Veterinary Association has drawn up a code of practice for using prostaglandins in cattle and pigs.
- **Antimicrobial agents**
  - *Griseofulvin*, the antifungal drug is teratogenic and should not be handled by women of child-bearing age. Protective clothing, impervious gloves and a dust mask should be worn when handling the powdered form and adding this to feed.
  - *Penicillins and cephalosporins* may cause hypersensitivity on exposure in operators who are allergic to

these drugs. The reaction can range from mild skin rash to swelling of the eyes, lips and face with difficulty breathing, symptoms which would require immediate medical attention. You should not handle drugs in these two families if you have a history of allergy to them.
  - *Chloramphenicol* can cause a fatal aplastic anaemia in man, a reaction which is not related to the dose received and occurs in a very small number of people exposed to the drug when prescribed for them by doctors. Nevertheless, it is wise to avoid unnecessary exposure to this drug by taking the precautions mentioned above, including avoiding direct contact of the drug with the skin.

It can be seen from the above discussion that hazards are greatest from drugs which are formulated in a liquid or powder form where aerosols, accidental injection or dust can lead to significant exposure of the operator. Many capsules and tablets can be safely handled with minimal or no contact with the drug, provided they are not broken or ground up to release the contents in a powdered form. For all tablets it is good practice to wear gloves when handling them (e.g. cyclophosphamide, mitotane and griseofulvin). The use of a triangular metal or plastic tablet counter facilitates the counting of tablets and reduces any contact between the operator and the tablets to a minimum.

Further reading

AMELIA 8 (1995) *The Medicines (restrictions on the administration of veterinary medicinal products) Regulations 1994. Guidance to the Veterinary Profession*, The Veterinary Medicine's Directorate.

Animal Medicines: A Users Guide (1995) Published by the National Office of Animal Health (ISBN 09526638 2 1).

Bishop, Y. (ed.) (1998) *The Veterinary Formulary*, 4th edn, The Pharmaceutical Press, London.

Brander, G. C., Pugh, D. M., Bywater, R. J. and Jenkins, W. L. (1991) *Veterinary Applied Pharmacology and Therapeutics*, 5th edn, Baillière Tindall, London.

BVA Code of Practice for sale or supply of animal medicines by veterinary surgeons (1990) *Veterinary Record*, vol. 127, pp. 236–240.

Wilkins, S. (1991) Hazards of handling veterinary medicines: Part 1. *Veterinary Nursing Journal*, vol. 6, pp. 15–17.

Wilkins, S. (1991) Hazards of handling veterinary medicines: Part 2. *Veterinary Nursing Journal*, vol. 6, pp. 53–55.

13

Clinical pathology and laboratory diagnostic aids

P. A. Bloxham

Introduction

Veterinary nurses are now able to provide the practice with the technical skill and ability to operate a small in-house laboratory. They need to understand the equipment currently available and know how to use it to produce good-quality, reliable results. They must perform basic diagnostic tests safely. The RCVS's Guide to Professional Conduct, relating to Practice Standards, advised that the practice must:

> Either provide laboratory facilities; or have access to one or more other laboratories which are adequately equipped to perform routine clinical pathology rapidly and accurately.

If the practice provides laboratory facilities it must ensure that:

- Laboratory procedures are performed in a room or a designated area used specifically for that purpose.
- Laboratory procedures are undertaken only by designated persons or persons under their supervision.
- Persons designated to undertake laboratory procedures are adequately trained for the tasks performed by them.
- Local rules are drawn up to cover cleanliness, tidiness, disinfection, first aid boxes, outbreaks of fire, the safe handling of equipment and clothing, the dispatch of specimens by post, the disposal of laboratory waste, and that the rules are displayed on a notice board in the laboratory.

This chapter is divided into two parts. The first section ('running a small animal practice laboratory') considers the management of a practice laboratory and the understanding, use and maintenance of its equipment. The second section ('diagnostic tests') explains how to collect and examine specimens, or how to prepare them for submission to a pathology laboratory for professional examination.

Running a small animal practice laboratory

Laboratory apparatus

Cleaning and disposal

Chemically clean glassware is essential and although more glass is being replaced by disposable plastic it is important to know how to clean and dry glassware. The use of commercial laboratory detergents is advisable and instructions should be followed carefully.

As a matter of routine, put all reusable glassware into disinfectant containers as soon as it has been used.

The cleaning procedure is as follows:

- Soak any dirty glassware in suitable disinfectants.
- Using disposable gloves, remove any surface material with the aid of test-tube brushes or other soft bristle brushes so as not to scratch the glass.
- Transfer to fresh solution of detergent and leave to soak, or use ultrasonic bath.
- Once the glassware is physically clean, rinse it thoroughly in distilled/deionised water, with two or three changes of fresh water, to ensure complete removal of any residue detergents.
- Allow to drain.
- Then dry in a drying oven or in air, ensuring that the atmosphere is free from dust and chemicals.

CHECKLIST

- Soak in detergent.
- Soak in disinfectant.
- Rinse 2–3 times in distilled/deionised water.
- Drain and dry.

It should be routine practice to clean all equipment and work-surfaces daily following use. Equipment should be wiped down with suitable disposable cloths impregnated with disinfectant. Any tubes, curettes and pipes should be flushed through with disinfectant solutions. Some manufacturers recommend and supply special cleaning and flushing solutions for their machines and they should be used as appropriate.

Put disposable 'sharps' into sharps bins and all other disposable waste into yellow bin bags as soon as they have been used. They should then be disposed of as clinical waste.

Pipettes

Graduated pipettes have a series of lines or marks engraved on the side to indicate the volume of their contents. A 10 ml pipette of this type is graduated in 1 ml divisions; each 1 ml is subdivided into 10 0.1 ml units. The meniscus of the fluid in the pipette should be at the level of the line required.

One-mark volumetric pipettes have only a single mark on them, indicating the level for a specific volume.

Both of these pipettes are usually filled by attaching a rubber tube and applying gentle suction. Care is needed not to suck up the fluid beyond the mark. Cotton plugs may be inserted into the top of the pipettes to restrict fluid into the tube. For safety reasons, it is preferable not to 'mouth-pipette' but to use a large-volume, flexible rubber bulb to create the suction.

Micro-pipettes come in various styles, with single or adjustable volumes and disposable pipette tips. For some (particularly the very small volume types), positive displacement is achieved using a probe which comes into contact with the fluid; other micro-pipettes operate on the principle of air displacement. The disposable tips are usually colour coded for the various volumes. Accurate and reproducible pipetting requires care and practice. Tips should be discarded into sharps bins and most pipettes have an ejection system so that the tips do not need to be handled.

Automatic pipettes are becoming more common and two basic types are in use:

● **Single-shot reservoir** – dial the volume required and fill the reservoir; an electronic button then dispenses the required volume, one shot at a time.
● **Multi-head pipettes** – often used for ELISA (enzyme-linked immunosorbent assay) plate work and normally have eight tips so that eight wells can be filled at the same time (electronically) with the same amount of fluid from a single reservoir.

Pasteur pipettes were originally made from soda glass tubes pulled to a fine point over a Bunsen flame. They have a rubber bulb on the other end. The technique is to press the bulb and then immerse the tip in a liquid; as the bulb is released, fluid passes up the capillary section of the pipette into the lumen of the tube. The fluid in the tube can then be released into a separate container by squeezing the bulb again. This system was commonly used for the removal or separation of serum or plasma from a blood sample. Currently most Pasteur pipettes are of moulded flexible plastic with integral bulbs.

Bottles

Chemicals and reagents are often supplied in plastic containers or in glass bottles. The original amber glass Winchester, a tall bottle, has been replaced by a more dumpy, wider based bottle with a lower centre of gravity, which is less likely to be knocked over. Many acids are supplied in this type of bottle and should be kept in a metal safety cupboard with lockable doors and at floor level. Never put concentrated acid bottles on high shelves.

Common reagent bottles for use in the laboratory have either a screw top or a glass stopper and are made from clear glass, clear or opaque plastic, or amber glass. If making up reagents it is important to label the bottles clearly (using a waterproof marker) showing details of contents and date made, together with any storage details. Any hazardous substances should be clearly identified with the correct symbols and stored in accordance with the Control of Substances Hazardous to Health (COSHH) regulations. Various adjustable volume dispenser systems are available to aid in the transfer of fluid from the bottles.

Smaller reagent bottles with integral pipettes in the lid are used for dispensing reagents and stains. Some dropping bottles have grooved glass stoppers so that drops can be dispensed. Many modern versions of the dropping bottle are of polythene, with an elongated, tapering nozzle that may be cut at the tip to allow a single drop at a time or, if cut lower down at a wider diameter, to dispense a stream.

Universal bottles are small, wide-mouthed, screw-top plastic or glass 30 ml bottles, often used for urine or faeces samples. They are usually supplied as sterile containers.

Microscopes

A good compound microscope (Fig. 13.1) is an essential piece of equipment for every veterinary practice. It is advisable to use a **binocular microscope** with an integral light source (usually a 6 volt halogen filament bulb) in the **base** or **foot**. A **transformer** controlled by a **rheostat** modifies the intensity of the light source. The light passes through a **lens** and **field diaphragm** to a **mirror** that directs the light up from the foot to the **sub-stage condenser**. The condenser consists of two lenses that focus the light source on the object being viewed: the condenser is moved up or down by turning the **condenser knob.** Before the light reaches the condenser it passes through the **iris diaphragm**, which is a lever-controlled aperture that modifies the amount of light passing through the condenser. Below the iris there are often glass filters, e.g. a blue daylight filter to

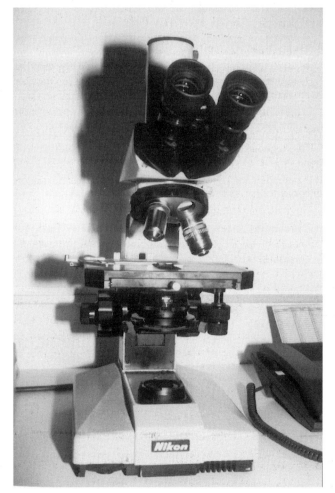

Fig. 13.1 The compound microscope.

reduce the amount of red or yellow components of the light spectrum.

Above the sub-stage condenser is the **stage**, which holds the slide being examined. It is mounted on a mechanical assembly referred to as the **mechanical stage**. This enables the slide holder to be moved left or right, up or down.

> **TIP**
>
> When viewed through a compound microscope an object appears to be upside down and reversed. Movement of the mechanical stage is also reversed, so that as the stage is moved to the left the image moves to the right.

Each **axis** (there are two of them) has a **vernier scale** on it so that the position of any particular item on the object slide may be recorded. Tradition demands that the position is recorded in the same way as grid references on a map.

Above the stage is the **nose piece**, with a **rotating turret** holding normally three or four **objective lenses**, each with a different magnification. The most common objective lenses are: $\times 4$ (scanning), $\times 10$ (low power), $\times 40$ (high dry) and $\times 100$ (oil immersion). The stage is racked up and down by means of an outer **coarse focus** and an inner **fine focus** knob on the **limb** of the microscope.

As light passes through the selected objective lens it travels up the **optical tube** mounted in the **body** of the microscope to a series of **prisms** in the **binocular head (body)** which deflect the light path through the **ocular lenses** mounted in the **eye-pieces**. The eye-pieces may be adjusted to the inter-pupillary distance of the person using the microscope and one of the ocular tubes in the eye-pieces is adjustable to correct for individual differences between the two eyes. The **inclined binocular head** may increase the actual magnification $\times 1.5$ and the factor is engraved on the head. The lenses in the eye-pieces are usually low powered with a magnification of $\times 4$ or $\times 6$, while $\times 8$ is the maximum for practical use.

Some binocular microscopes have interchangeable bodies so that a monocular photographic tube can be attached. Others have a permanent photographic tube as well as the binocular head. Specially designed teaching heads have two binocular sets.

The purpose of a microscope is to magnify and the size of the object can be measured if a measuring scale is put into one of the eye-pieces. The amount of magnification is calculated by the magnification of the eye-piece $\times$ magnification of the binocular head $\times$ the objective magnification.

Care, cleaning and maintenance of microscopes. The microscope is a precision instrument.

- It should be located in a convenient position and not moved unnecessarily.
- If it does have to be moved it should be carried in both hands, one under the base or foot and the other holding the limb.

- Do not place it near centrifuges or other sources of vibration, and keep it away from sinks and direct sunlight.
- Keep it covered when not in use.
- To maximise the life of the bulb, turn the rheostat down before switching it off or if the light is left on for any period when not in use.
- Keep extra light bulbs in stock but do not handle the actual bulb when replacing it.
- Only lens paper should be used to clean the lenses and eye-pieces. It is designed for the job and will not scratch the lenses.
- Remove oil from the oil immersion objective after use and ensure that solvents do not remain in contact with the objective as they may loosen the cement holding the lens in place.
- When finished with the microscope, turn off the light (after turning down the rheostat), then lower the stage and turn the lowest power objective into position. Clean the oil immersion lens and cover the microscope.
- If dirt appears in the field of study it is likely to be on the eye-piece. Rotate it: if the dirt also rotates, clean the eye-piece with a lens paper.

Using the microscope

(1) Check that the lowest objective is in position and that all lenses and eye-pieces are clean.
(2) Check that the rheostat is down low.
(3) Place the slide or counting number chamber firmly into the mechanical stage and centralise below the object lens.
(4) Switch on and then turn up the rheostat to increase the brightness.
(5) Adjust the distance between the two eye-pieces so that each field appears identical and that both fields are viewed as one.
(6) Using the coarse and fine focus knobs, bring the object into clear view.
(7) Adjust the position of the condenser and diaphragms for optimal illumination.
(8) Using the mechanical stage travelling knobs, examine the field on the slide under low power.
(9) If a specific area under view requires higher magnification, rotate the objective nose turret until the $\times 40$ high dry objective lens clicks into place and then adjust the fine focus to obtain a clear image. The diaphragm and condenser may require readjustment as more light may be needed at the higher magnification.

To view under oil immersion:

(1) First view the field under low power.
(2) Then place a drop of immersion oil on the field and rotate the oil immersion objective into position.
(3) If the field does not come into view, stop looking down the eye-pieces and look directly at the position of the oil immersion lens in relation to the surface of the slide and the oil. The lens of the objective should be in the oil but not touching the slide.

(4) Slowly adjust the position with the fine focus knob so that the slide is moved away from the lens but the lens remains in the oil. Careful focusing while returning to view the object via the eye-pieces should bring the field into view.

(5) Adjust the iris diaphragm and condenser to ensure adequate illumination.

Never allow the high dry or other non-oil immersion lenses to come into contact with the oil. When finished with the oil immersion viewing, lower the stage, rotate the lenses so that the lowest power is in position, turn the light down and then off, clean the oil immersion lens and remove the slide from the stage.

Colorimeter

Colorimetry is the measurement of light **absorbed** or **transmitted** by a substance. A colorimeter is the apparatus or analyser which measures the light absorbed (inverse colorimetry) or transmitted (direct colorimetry) by a solution at a wavelength. The selection of a wavelength in a colorimeter is achieved by use of filters; however, most modern analysers are in fact spectrophotometers, which use prisms or monochromatic gratings to separate the light path into a single wavelength. This is then passed through the solution (normally held in a cuvette) and the emergent light is then detected and converted into electrical energy and displayed by means of an analogue meter or, more commonly, by means of digital read-out.

Colorimeters and spectrophotometers are 'wet' chemistry systems that require the use of various liquid reagents which are commercially available in kit form. Detailed methodology for use of the kit in conjunction with a particular analyser is provided by the manufacturer or supplier. The analysers normally found in a veterinary practice are of the manual or semi-automated type allowing one test to be performed on one sample at a time. The systems used in commercial laboratories are larger automated ones allowing a variable number of tests to be performed on batches of samples.

More recently, 'dry' chemistry systems have become available for practice use. With these a sample is put on to a prepared slide or reagent strip and the analyser determines the **reflective light** (usually as the reaction occurs) and displays the results. Whichever system is used, it is important to follow the manufacturer's operating rules fully and to ensure that the machine is kept clean and is serviced regularly.

Temperature control. Enzymes are totally dependent on temperature. In the veterinary world, the recommended temperature for performing determination of enzyme activity is 30°C; however, almost all laboratories have moved to the temperature of 37°C, as most chemical reagent systems are optimised at this temperature. It is essential that the temperature is controlled. Machines should not be placed in positions with direct exposure to sunlight and the ambient operating temperature must be maintained constantly.

Quality control. Storage of kits, reagents and samples must be carefully monitored and regular use of internal quality control samples and external quality assessment samples is essential if the practice is to comply with the RCVS ATAC (approved training and assessment centre) standards. Operators should be adequately trained by the supplier and if necessary receive further professional training in order to become and remain competent.

Centrifuges

These machines spin at speed to produce a high gravitational force referred to as the **relative centrifugal force (RCF)**, which is measured in g **forces**. Acceleration due to **gravity** (g) is 981 cm/second/second. The objectives are:

- To separate the cells from fluid.
- To partition different density (size and mass) of material.
- To concentrate the material.

The deposit is termed the **sediment**; the fluid is the **supernatant**.

Standard centrifuges are of two types according to the style of **rotor head**: a **swing-out** and an **angle-head**.

A swing-out head consists of a rotor with specimen buckets suspended vertically from the arms of the rotor. As the rotor turns, the buckets swing out into a horizontal position. When the rotor slows down and stops, they fall back into a vertical position. The swing-out head generates air friction and it heats up at speed, which may be a problem and restricts the speed at which the centrifuge may be operated. The swinging is likely to remix the samples slightly at the end of centrifugation.

An angle-head rotor has a series of holes drilled around the rotor at a fixed angle (normally 52° from the perpendicular). Samples are placed in these holes. The angled head can be operated at higher speeds without heat build-up but the deposit is laid down at the fixed angle of the head and may be disturbed as the tubes are removed and stood upright in test tube racks.

The inner bowl of the centrifuge is a very solid piece of metal designed as a guard to retain the rotor buckets and samples should they become detached, or should metal fatigue lead to fracture of the rotor. It is good laboratory practice to wipe out, clean and disinfect the entire bowl as a matter of routine.

Modern centrifuges have a number of inbuilt safety devices, including an integral lid-lock that prevents opening of the centrifuge while the rotor is still spinning; nor can the rotor begin to operate until the lid is securely closed. A safety plate is present on many machines either as a separate screw-on lid behind the main lid or as an integral part of the main lid; like the guard bowl, it prevents penetration from inside in case of accidents.

Samples, usually in glass or plastic tubes, are put into buckets or carrier tubes which have rubber cushions at the bottom to prevent the bases of the sample tubes from damage or breakage. For safety, the buckets should be able to be removed for washing (and if necessary autoclaving) in case of breakage or spillage. To prevent aerosol dissemination, especially from potentially pathogenic samples, always use bucket guards or lids (these are autoclavable). It is important to ensure that buckets are balanced and so tubes of equal volume and weight should be placed opposite each other. Water-filled tubes may be used to balance the buckets if necessary.

Most centrifuges now have variable speed control and a gauge to show the speed, a timer to dial up the required period of centrifugation and a brake to slow down the rotor once the timer switches off. To increase the gravitational force, the rotor's turning speed is controlled and so is the duration. If the radius of the centrifuge from the centre of the shaft to the tip of the bucket is R (cm) and the number of revolutions of the rotor per minute (r.p.m.) is N, then relative centrifugal force (RCF) in g forces is calculated using the following equation:

$$\text{RCF (in } g) = 1.118 \times 10^{-5} \times R \times N^2$$

Routine cleaning, lubrication and general service maintenance are essential for reliable and safe operation and the manufacturer's instructions should be followed. The motor is powered by electricity and it is important that the wiring (including the plug and correct fuse) is checked regularly under the Health and Safety rules for the inspection of electrical apparatus. The motor's brushes should be replaced when they wear down. It is advisable to keep a log of the usage of the centrifuge and to relate this to regular servicing by the manufacturer, in the same way that vehicles are serviced on the basis of mileage.

Microhaematocrit. A microhaematocrit is a special type of centrifuge (Fig. 13.2) for separating whole blood in capillary tubes to enable assessment of **packed cell volume (PCV)**. It has a special type of rotor consisting of an almost flat, horizontal surface with slots for capillary tubes. There is a rubber cushion on the outside of the lip of the rotor. A safety plate is screwed down on top of the rotor to hold the tubes in place and then the lid is closed to operate. Sometimes capillary tubes do not seal properly and sometimes there may be breakages, so that the rubber cushion is likely to be covered with blood and may be damaged by fragments of capillary glass. It should be wiped clean after use and the rubber replaced regularly. The entire head, rubber cushion and the safety plate should be disinfected as a matter of routine.

Incubator

Electric incubators are used to culture bacteria. These enclosed units of various sizes have removable shelves and impervious smooth surfaces of metal or plastic. They are well insulated with a gasket sealed door so that the air inside is maintained at a set temperature (37°C is the optimal temperature for almost all pathogenic bacteria). It is important to check the wiring and thermostat and to maintain a daily record of the temperature to ensure that the operation is as desired. Because potentially dangerous bacteria may be grown, it is essential to have a set procedure for cleaning and disinfecting or perhaps fumigating the incubator.

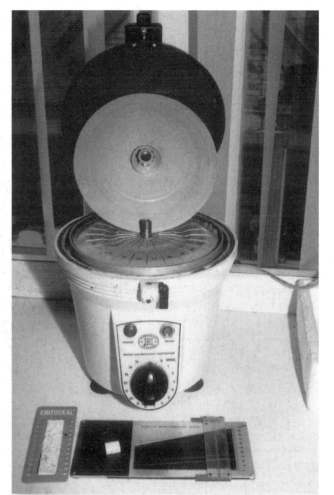

Fig. 13.2 Microhaematocrit centrifuge.

Safety in the laboratory

The laboratory is a dangerous place.

- It should be accessible only to authorised people.
- Smoking, eating or drinking must never be allowed in the laboratory.
- Protective laboratory coats should be donned on entry and removed on departure from the laboratory area.
- Disposable gloves should be worn.
- Surfaces should be kept clean and tidy.
- Books and papers should be kept away from the working bench area and should be kept separate from any samples or reagents being handled.

Training and complete understanding of the Health and Safety at Work Act 1974 as it relates to laboratories is essential, as is knowledge of the Control of Substances Hazardous to Health (COSHH) regulations (discussed in Chapters 4 and 7). Health and safety training courses are available and every person should have attended such courses and also be familiar with simple first aid procedures. See Chapter 4, p. 101.

If glass is broken or liquid spilled, it is essential to know how to protect everybody from risk. Take appropriate action and record what happened. If in doubt, report to a senior person and follow instructions.

ACCIDENT BOOK

The minimum information to be recorded in relation to accidents at work, in order to satisfy the regulations in the Management of Health and Safety at Work Regulation 1992 cover emergencies and Reporting of Injuries, Diseases and Dangerous Occurrences Regulations 1995 (RIDDOR).

(1) Give full name, home address and occupation of the person who had the accident.
(2) The person filling in the book must sign and date it. If they did not have the accident then they must also give their name, home address and occupation.
(3) Record time and date of accident and where it happened.
(4) State how the accident happened. Give the cause if you can. If any personal injury, state what it is.
(5) If the accident is reportable under RIDDOR then employer must initial and report.
(6) Accident books must be retained for 3 years after the date of the last entry.

IN CASE OF ACCIDENTS

- If something is splashed in the eye, wash it out immediately with a deionised water eye-bath (which should be readily to hand).
- Acid or alkaline spillage must be correctly neutralised.
- Any infectious agents must be killed by means of bacterial or viricidal disinfectants.
- All accidents should be reported to a responsible person and entered into an accident book in a standard format such as that shown in the previous box.

Disposal of clinical waste

Because it is possible that significant pathogens may be isolated in the practice laboratory, attention to Health and Safety codes is important at all times when working with bacterial samples in particular. Attention to the control and disposal of clinical waste is very important and current legislation places the responsibility for it on the person who generates the waste. See also pp. 100 and 128.

- Glassware should be soaked in suitable disinfectants and detergents to kill micro-organisms.
- Disposable plastic items should be put into discard bins or sharps bins, as appropriate.
- Culture plates should be placed into autoclave bags and sterilised in an autoclave before being put into yellow clinical waste bags for incineration.

- Samples should also be autoclaved where possible before being placed in the yellow clinical waste bags.

It is the responsibility of the staff in a practice laboratory to ensure that the material is made as safe as possible and that the yellow bags are collected regularly and transported by licensed clinical waste carriers to approved incineration facilities and disposed of correctly under the legislation. Record-keeping and adherence to the regulations are important.

One final aspect of laboratory practice is to ensure at all times that the staff:

- Keep the laboratory neat and tidy.
- Follow the local Health and Safety rules.
- Dispose correctly of clinical waste (used reagents and equipment).
- Clean up and disinfect working surfaces.
- Act immediately to control spillage.
- Record any accident.
- Ensure adequate training.
- If in doubt – ask.

These aspects are very important. Quality results depend on good working practices; safety and care in the laboratory also depend on adherence to standard operating procedures.

Diagnostic tests

Collection of specimens

Quality laboratory results start with the collection of quality samples (remember the old adage: rubbish in means rubbish out). It is essential to collect the correct sample and that it should be in a suitable condition.

Blood

To collect blood by means of venipuncture, using a needle and syringe, first ensure that the animal is safely and securely restrained (see Chapter 1). Next, select a suitable vein. In the dog this is likely to be the cephalic vein in the foreleg; in the cat the jugular may be more suitable. Part the hair (or clip the site) and clean and swab with a topical alcohol wipe.

For the **cephalic**, raise the vein with the left hand under the leg and the thumb on top, or apply a quick-release tourniquet, and approach the vein from the side, using a 1 inch 22 gauge needle. Penetrate into the lumen and up the inside of the vein. Slowly pull back on the syringe and let the blood flow into it. It is important not to apply too much pressure and to ensure that the needle remains in the lumen of the vein. For most practical purposes a 10 ml syringe is preferred but a 5 ml syringe may be used if the correct volume anticoagulant tubes are available.

When sufficient blood has been collected release the pressure on the vein and remove the needle from it. Place a swab of cotton wool on the venipuncture site and apply direct light pressure. Tape the swab in place to stem any bleeding.

Collection from the **jugular** is best achieved with the cat on its side or back and the head extended. The vein is raised by pressure below the point of venipuncture and the pressure should be removed before removing the needle from the vein.

Vacutainer systems. A 'vacutainer' is an evacuated tube (i.e. with a vacuum) as part of a complete system incorporating a double-ended needle screwed into a holder. The small vacutainers have a 3 ml volume but only a 2 ml draw, in order to minimise the amount of pressure put on the red cells. It is important to collect blood with the complete vacutainer system.

If the sample is collected with syringe and needle, remove the needle before slowly allowing the blood to be discharged gently from the syringe into the sample tube. If this happens to be a vacutainer, remove its bung. Do not inject blood from a syringe into a vacutainer.

It is also possible to insert a needle into the vein and collect the blood directly into a container drop by drop. In this case the animal should ideally be standing and the collection tube is held beneath the shank of the needle.

Type and condition of blood. When blood clots and clot retraction takes place, the fluid is referred to as **serum**. **Plasma** is that fluid separated from non-clotted blood. To prevent clotting **anticoagulants** are used, the most common being heparin, ethylene diamine tetra-acetic acid (**EDTA**), oxalate fluoride and sodium citrate.

If the red cells become broken or lysed they release their contents into serum or plasma. This is referred to as **haemolysis**. If serum or plasma is reddish in colour after separation, then haemolysis has occurred. This might result from:

- Excess pressure when pulling back the syringe plunger.
- Too vigorous mixing of samples.
- Osmotic pressure because the skin or the needle/syringe has water on or in it.
- The use of too fine a needle, damaging red cells.
- Leaving the plasma unseparated in transit.

Lipaemia is the presence of lipids/fats in the blood. This is often a physiological condition which occurs after feeding (especially ingestion of fatty foods) and so it is advisable to sample fasted animals, not ones just fed. Lipaemia may also be a pathological condition associated with metabolic conditions.

Icteric samples are those with significant amounts of bilirubin in the blood. The level of 'normal range' bilirubin varies between species: equine serum, for example, will always appear more icteric than feline because of the much higher level of bilirubin in the horse due to the lack of gall bladder.

Chromatins are colour agents and they may interfere with colorimetric or spectrometric biochemical determinations by influencing the colour of serum and plasma. They include the carotene intake in the diet: the serum and plasma colour of grazing animals ingesting high carotene levels, such as dairy cattle, is more yellow than in other species.

Coagulants and colour codes. Table 13.1 shows the colour codes used in vacutainers and the appropriate anticoagulants for specific tests. The general principle is that **EDTA** whole blood is used for haematology. **Oxalates** are usually used as either sodium, potassium, ammonium or lithium salts, but currently the only useful routine salt is the potassium oxalate salt with sodium fluoride (**OXF**) which is used for glucose determination. **Heparin whole blood** is used for lead determination, while **sodium citrate** is used for clotting times and special coagulation studies. **Clotted blood with serum taken off** is used for most routine biochemistry or serology but **heparin plasma** may be used in many (but not all) cases, as an alternative to serum.

Storage of serum and plasma. If serum or plasma is to be stored rather than immediately tested or posted to a laboratory, label the sample clearly with indelible marker and then store at –20°C in a suitable deep-freeze. Do not keep at room temperature for any length of time, but samples can often be retained in a reasonably stable state for a few hours at +4°C in a refrigerator.

Serum and plasma should never be exposed to extremes of heat. If frozen, samples that have been thawed should not be frozen again: they should only be frozen and thawed once.

Urine

Collection of urine should be a routine procedure, as the simple examination of urine is a practical and valuable diagnostic tool. Use a sterile universal container to collect voided urine or urine that is expressed by means of gentle

Table 13.1 Vacutainer colour codes, their anticoagulants and applications

Colour	Anticoagulant	Type of sample	Application
Red	None	Clotted blood/serum	Biochemistry, Serology
Green or yellow/green	Heparin	Whole blood	Biochemistry, Lead, GSHPx and Transketolase
		Plasma	Biochemistry
Lavender	EDTA	Whole blood	Haematology
Grey	Oxalate fluoride	Whole blood	Glucose
Light blue	Sodium citrate	Whole blood/plasma	Coagulation tests
Dark blue	None	Clotted blood/serum	Trace elements

COLLECTION OF SERUM

(1) Using the vacutainer system, select the red-topped tube to collect blood which, because no anticoagulant is added, will clot.

(2) Leave these tubes upright (out of the sun) and undisturbed until clotting and clot retraction occur.

(3) Centrifuge the sample at 2500 r.p.m. for 5 minutes in a swing-head centrifuge.

(4) When this has switched off, carefully remove the tube without shaking and place upright in a test-tube rack.

(5) Take Pasteur pipette (see p. 338), squeeze its bulb and insert the fine tip into the serum near but above the surface of the clot. Do not touch the clot with the tip.

(6) Gently release the pressure on the bulb and suck up the serum into the Pasteur pipette.

(7) Transfer the serum into a suitable plastic or glass tube by gently applying pressure on the bulb again.

(8) Immediately label this tube (or do so in advance).

(9) If the serum is to be sent away, the type of tube or container for the sample must be suitable for postage and have a secure top to prevent leakage, as well as being clearly labelled with the owner's name, the animal's name or identification and the date and time of collection.

COLLECTION OF HEPARIN PLASMA

(1) Take a blood sample into a heparin vacutainer and gently roll and invert the sample to ensure adequate mixing. The benefit of vacutainer systems is that better mixing is easily achieved.

(2) Centrifuge the heparin sample as soon as possible after collection.

(3) The supernatant is plasma and may then be removed with a Pasteur pipette (as for serum) but do not insert the fine tip of the pipette so far down.

(4) Be careful to avoid disturbing the sedimented red and white blood cells as the pressure is carefully reduced by releasing the bulb.

(5) On withdrawing the pipette, ensure that fluid is not dispensed back into the tube.

(6) It is always better to transfer a little plasma and then go back for more, rather than trying to collect all at once and sucking up some red cells at the same time.

Table 13.2 Urine preservatives and their applications

Hydrochloric acid	Biochemical analysis of urea, ammonia, calcium, total nitrogens and uric acid (mix well before testing, as deposits form).
Acetic acid	For ascorbic acid determination.
Boric acid	Similar to HCl.
Chloroform	Cannot use for glucose, is a COSHH risk.
Toluene	Is a COSHH risk.
Formalin	As above but not glucose.
Sodium bicarbonate	For porphyrins.
Refrigeration	The most satisfactory method.

All urine preservatives are used to prevent bacterial action or chemical decomposition, or to stabilise constituents.

pressure on the bladder. It is important to allow the initial urine to pass out (and with it any surface/skin bacteria) before collecting a reasonably sterile **mid-stream** sample. Mid-stream sampling is also more representative of the urine in the bladder, rather than the first few drops which may contain mucoid material from other parts of the urinogenital tract.

Animals may be put into special 'metabolic' cages in order to collect all urine voided over a 24-hour period but these are not usually found in general practice.

Collection of a sterile sample by means of a **urethral catheter** (see Chapter 16) may require sedation of the animal. A suitable sterile catheter should be selected. It is passed up the urethra slowly and gently into the bladder and urine is collected aseptically as it flows out of the catheter into a sterile universal container.

Table 13.2 lists the preservatives used in urine and details the reasons for using them. However, in a practice laboratory it is better to test a urine sample immediately rather than use any preservative. Urine should not be stored frozen but kept at refrigerator temperature, unless some specific analytic requirement calls for freezing.

Spun-down (centrifuged) sediment should be examined as soon as possible, but formalin may be used to preserve the material.

Faeces

Use a wide-mouthed universal container or faeces pot, which must be sterile, and bear the following points in mind:

- It is preferable to collect fresh faeces per rectum with a gloved finger or hand rather than use a stale defecated sample picked up from the ground or litter tray.
- Ensure that the animal is securely restrained so that it is unable to bite, scratch or wriggle while the procedure is carried out.
- It is best to collect urine before collecting faeces, as collection per rectum may cause voiding of urine.
- Long fingernails may damage the mucosa.
- Do not use force to collect faeces from the rectum.

- It is important that the area around the anus is cleaned and lubricated to prevent skin flora being introduced into the faeces sample, and to prevent damage to the anal/rectal mucosa.
- The faeces should fill the pot, to prevent too much air getting into the sample (which may kill off any anaerobic bacteria or lead to desiccation of the faeces and any parasites present).

Faeces should be kept at room temperature for only a short period before being examined, and should be kept out of sunlight. If examination of the faeces has to be delayed for a few hours, take a transport swab of the sample for bacteriology and place the labelled pot, with its lid screwed on securely, in the refrigerator. Do not freeze it. Be aware that stored faeces may ferment in the pots: lids may blow off if not secured.

To summarise:

- Collect fresh rectal samples.
- Fill sterile screw-top universal containers.
- Examine immediately.

Skin

Collection of **plucked hairs** for examination for ringworm infection should be made at the active edge of the lesions. Pluck individual hairs, including the root.

A **tape technique** may be used to examine an area of skin for surface mites:

(1) Take a section of clear adhesive tape.
(2) With the sticky face down, press the tape against the hair and skin.
(3) Pull off and repeat over the area to be investigated.
(4) Place the tape on to a microscope slide for examination.

To obtain samples of **coat brushing** for mite examination, use a toothbrush or similar bristle brush (this method is unlikely to identify ringworm, which affects the root shaft):

(1) Work a small area at a time in the one direction, brushing the coat.
(2) Tap the brush into a Petri dish or on to a glass slide.
(3) Use forceps or tweezers to pick out the hairs.
(4) Do not put hair samples into plastic bags, as static electricity builds up and the samples are then very difficult to handle and examine.

For **skin scrapes**, use a scalpel blade to remove the surface layer of skin. It is important to go sufficiently deep to achieve **petechial** blood oozing (pinpoint clusters of surface capillary bleeding) (see Chapter 15).

(1) Place a drop of paraffin oil on the clipped skin area to be examined.
(2) Gently squeeze the skin into a fold to bring any bacteria or parasites nearer to the surface.
(3) Scrape with the scalpel blade.
(4) Carefully scrape the scalpel on to a microscope slide for examination.

If the sample is to be submitted to a laboratory, put a clear warning that a scalpel blade is included (especially if it is unprotected).

To prevent desiccation, if a sample is to be looked at later:

(1) Place some filter or blotting paper in the lid of a Petri dish and wet it with sterile water.
(2) Place two stick applicators or matchsticks on top.
(3) Suspend the slide on the sticks.
(4) Put the base on as a lid, seal with tape and label the dish.
(5) Place in a cool, dark place.

Some refrigerators may be suitable for storage but be warned that some of them extract moisture as they cool and therefore the period of storage should not be too long (as the seal on the dish is not totally airtight).

For longer storage, use airtight jars with a moist bed – but all must be prepared aseptically. For material under a cover slip on a slide, the area may be protected from desiccation by sealing the edges with nail varnish or epoxy resin.

Pustules may be sampled with a sterile needle on a small 1 or 2 ml syringe:

(1) Suck the contents of the pustule into the needle.
(2) Express on to a glass slide.
(3) Make either a **squash preparation** (by placing a second slide on top at right angles to the first and squashing) or a **smear** (by use of a spreader).
(4) Samples may then be examined fresh under low power or stained and examined under high power.

Cerebrospinal fluid (CSF)

The examination of CSF may be very useful in diagnosing some neurological conditions. The animal must be anaesthetised before the fluid is collected. The area of the spine that is tapped is normally either the atlanto-occipital or the lumbosacral space.

- Prepare the selected area by shaving and full sterile/aseptic precautions, as for any surgical procedure.
- Insert a suitable spinal tap needle into the subarachnoid space of the spinal column, taking care not to advance the needle too far (which could damage the spinal cord).
- Normally the animal is placed in lateral recumbency and the fluid is collected into an EDTA tube for cytology, by means of free flow.
- Do not aspirate the fluid.
- It is possible to collect a second, plain tube sample (with no anticoagulant added) for biochemical tests after the sample has been centrifuged to spin down any cellular material.

Synovial fluid

Synovial fluid is collected by means of **arthrocentesis** from the joint in order to investigate a particular joint problem such as arthritis or in some cases of shifting lameness. Collection may be made on an unanaesthetised animal or following anaesthesia, depending on the animal and the joint. Arthrocentesis is made aseptically with a syringe and needle after the site has been prepared as for any surgical procedure.

Thoracic fluid

The pleural cavity contains only enough fluid for adequate lubrication of the intrathoracic organs and the cavity lining. The main reason for collection and examination of thoracic fluid (by means of **thoracocentesis**) is to find the cause of an increase in fluid volume. Collection is performed aseptically into EDTA tubes and plain tubes.

Abdominal fluid

The amount of peritoneal fluid in the abdominal cavity is only sufficient to provide lubrication of the abdominal organs and peritoneum. Any increase in volume may be investigated by means of **abdominocentesis**. Aseptic collection is usually performed via the most dependent part of the ventral midline in the standing animal following normal skin surgical preparation. Some of the fluid sample is transferred into EDTA for cytology while the rest should be transferred into plain tubes or sterile containers for biochemistry and perhaps bacteriology.

Tissue samples, tumours and abdominal organ biopsy

Biopsy techniques relate to the sampling of a section of tissue, tumour or organ for cytological or histopathological examination.

> ### FORMALIN
>
> Formalin is a strong antiseptic and disinfectant that has the ability to preserve tissue samples by '**fixing**' or hardening them. It is commercially prepared from a pungent gas, formaldehyde, as a solution of 40% strength in water, i.e. a **40% formaldehyde solution**. Formalin is a hazardous substance (it gives off a gas that irritates eyes and nose) and it is important that local COSHH and Health and Safety rules are understood and adhered to.
>
> Containers or pots for formalin-fixed tissues should be wide-mouthed and screw-topped: the fixing process hardens the tissue, so that its removal from a narrow-mouthed container becomes awkward or impossible.

For routine cases, tissues for histopathology are fixed in **10% formal saline**, which is made by diluting formalin in a buffered saline solution so that it contains 10% formalin (Table 13.3). This buffered solution is preferred but it is possible to use normal saline (sodium chloride in sterile

Table 13.3 Buffered 10% formal saline: to make 1 litre	
Formalin (40% formaldehyde solution)	100 ml
$NaH_2PO_4.2H_2O$	4.5 g
Na_2HPO_4	6.5 g
Distilled water	900 ml

distilled water), though the specimen is likely to be affected by cellular and histochemical changes because, with the lack of a buffer, there is no control of pH.

Fresh tissues need to be transferred immediately into the fixative, as the process of **necrosis** (cell death and lysis) can occur very rapidly. The container should be of an adequate size to allow a minimum of 10 parts fluid to one part tissue, by volume, which will ensure sufficient formalin penetration into the tissue for rapid fixation.

When submitting tissue to a laboratory, ensure that the container is labelled and securely sealed, and that there is an indication of the original location of the tissue.

Toxicology specimens

- All specimens should be collected free from any extraneous contamination. They should not be washed.
- Each sample must be collected and submitted in separate leak-proof, airtight, sterile and chemically clean plastic or glass containers.
- Each container must be labelled with the owner's name, animal identification, type of sample, date of collection and the name and address of the practice.
- All samples must then be placed together in one large container.
- Unless tissues are to be examined histologically, samples are best collected fresh and then frozen. They should then be dispatched to the toxicology laboratory on ice. Consult the laboratory prior to packing and submitting as they may have special requirements in certain cases.
- In cases of poisoning, it is essential that accurate records are kept at all stages, as evidence may be needed for possible litigation.

Submission of pathological samples to laboratories

In order to maximise the potential for diagnostic information, the intention is that material should arrive at the laboratory in a condition as similar as possible to that when it was actually collected. Correct preservation, properly completed paperwork, clear labelling and good packaging are all essential.

Preservation for transit

Tissue, once it has been removed from an animal, immediately starts to die. Cell membranes break down, leading to destruction or lysis of cells, and this process of

autolysis is hastened by increased temperatures and humidity. 'Fixing' and freezing are methods of preventing or reducing autolysis. Tissues for standard histological examination should *not* be frozen.

Haemolysis is a form of cell degeneration in blood cells. Red blood cells are likely to be damaged if exposed to heat, cold or violent shaking. If possible, separate serum from the clot by centrifugation before dispatch. Whole-blood samples should be gently but adequately mixed with the correct amount of anticoagulant to avoid clotting (which would make them unsuitable for examination). Pack whole-blood samples and serum in a way that minimises temperature variation and physical damage in transit.

Labelling and paperwork

If samples are being sent away, the name of the veterinary surgeon and the practice's name and address should be recorded. All request forms should also contain:

- Name of owner.
- Name of animal (or some reference number relating to that animal).
- Animal's species, breed, age, sex, and whether intact or neutered.
- Date of sampling and time of collection.
- List of samples collected, including type of anticoagulants used (if applicable).
- Clinical history, including any specific presenting signs and any current treatment.
- Details of site or sites (if swabs, skin scrapings or biopsy material are submitted) with a schematic diagram to show the position.
- Indication of tests or examinations required.

Submit the completed forms in plastic envelopes to protect them from possible contamination. Each sample relating to the case should be individually and clearly labelled with the name of the owner and the animal, and should be in agreement with details on the submission form.

Packaging

Most commercial laboratories supply special postal packs for submitted samples. All samples must be packed in compliance with postal regulations (Table 13.4).

Always assume that if something can be broken in transit, it will be. Packing should be such that:

- Sample material is not damaged.
- Containers do not break or leak.
- Samples do not contaminate each other or the accompanying paperwork, or anybody who handles the package in transit or on receipt.

Containers should be secure, leakproof and protected from breaking but not so bound up in cling-film, cotton wool, bubblepack and sticky tape that the laboratory staff are unable to open them on receipt.

Transport swabs should be used with the correct media in them to prevent desiccation of microbial material. Fixed tissue should be in secure formal saline containers.

Table 13.4 Postal regulations and packaging requirements for pathological specimens

Packaging requirements for pathological samples (from January 1999):

Any diagnostic specimen sent through the Royal Mail has to be packaged in containers conforming to United Nations Regulation 602. The main points concerning the packaging are as follows.

(1) Water-tight primary container(s) such as a glass tube. This has to be surrounded by sufficient absorbent material and placed inside a secondary container. The secondary container and absorbent material must be capable of containing all the contents of the primary container(s).
(2) An itemized list of contents, and details of the sender, must be attached to the secondary container.
(3) The secondary container must be placed inside a UN approved outer container – usually cardboard. This must be labelled with an appropriate hazard designation.
(4) The packaging has to meet UN requirements with regard to pressure and impact. Because of this it is likely to be more expensive than current packaging used to send diagnostic material through the post.

In addition, the following postal regulations should be adhered to:

(1) Use First Class or Datapost. DO NOT USE PARCEL POST.
(2) Label the outside with the words:
PATHOLOGICAL SPECIMEN – FRAGILE. WITH CARE.
As well as the laboratory address it must show the name, address and telephone number of the sender who will be contacted in case of leakage or damage.
(3) Every specimen must be in a primary container which is securely sealed. Maximum of 50 ml volume unless Post Office approved multi-specimen packs.
(4) Primary container must be wrapped in sufficient absorbent material to absorb all of the sample if leakage or breakage occurs.
(5) The container and absorbent material must be sealed in a leak-proof plastic bag.
(6) The plastic bag must then be placed in one of the following:
(a) Plastic clip-down container.
(b) Cylindrical lightweight metal container.
(c) Strong cardboard box with full depth lid.
(d) Two-piece polystyrene box with special grooved join.
(7) It is recommended that this complete package is placed in a padded (Jiffy) bag.
(8) Other packaging systems must be Post Office approved.

Haematology

Blood smears

Clean, washed, oil-free glass microscope slides are required for the preparation of blood smears (Fig. 13.3). The most useful slides have a frosted area at one end on which sample identification can be recorded.

(1) Place a drop (10 microlitres) of well-mixed EDTA whole blood at one end.
(2) Place a spreader slide just in front of the drop of blood and angle the slide at about 25–30° with the surface of the first slide.
(3) Draw the spreader slide back into the drop of blood, causing the blood to run along the interface between the two slides.
(4) Push the spreader slide steadily with an even, rapid motion towards the far end of the other slide. This will

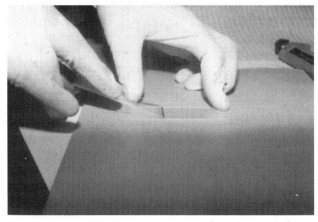

Fig. 13.3 Making a blood smear.

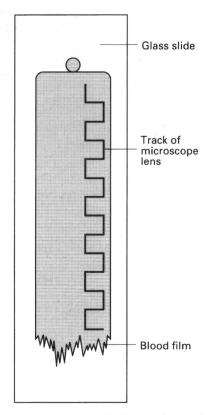

Fig. 13.4 The battlement technique for differential blood films.

draw the blood along behind the spreader slide and make a thin, even blood film.

(5) Allow to air dry.

(6) Clean the edge of the spreader slide.

(7) Once the film is air-dried, it may be stained using Romanowsky stains (various alkaline methylene blue stains combined with eosin) such as Wright's, a modified Wright's/Giemsa or Leishman's stains. Table 13.5 shows the staining protocol.

Examination of blood films

The blood film is used to perform a **differential white blood cell count (WBC Diff.)**. The aim of this important procedure is to estimate the relevant proportions (as percentages) of the different types of white cells in a sample.

(1) The film should be scanned under low power to note the quality of the film and stain and the cell numbers.

(2) Then scan the far end of the film for platelet clumps and large abnormal cells.

Table 13.5 Giemsa staining protocol for differential blood films

Solution 1:	Methyl alcohol, absolute (Analar)
Solution 2:	Giemsa stain consisting of:
	Azure 11-eosin 3 g
	Azure 11 0.8 g
	Glycerol 200 ml
	Solution 1 300 ml
Solution 3:	Buffer solution (pH 7.0) consisting of:
	Disodium hydrogen orthophosphate 9.47 g
	Potassium dihydrogen orthophosphate 9.08 g
	Distilled water 1 l
Protocol	(1) Air-dried films fixed in solution 2 for 3 minutes
	(2) Dilute one volume of solution 2 with nine volumes of solution 3. Flood slide and stain for 15 minutes.
	(3) Wash and differentiate with solution 3, until cells are identifiable microscopically.
	(4) Drain and air dry.

---

(3) Finally, under low power, select an area of the film at least one-third from the end of the film at the side edge which is to be examined under high power oil immersion for cell counting.

(4) Swing out the low power objective, place a drop of oil on the area and then swing in the oil immersion lens; focus and count using the battlement technique.

Battlement technique. Rather than count each cell of each type (though the greater the number counted, the greater the accuracy), technicians often use the battlement technique (Fig. 13.4) to cover a reasonable area of the sample and to counteract distribution bias.

(1) Move two fields along the edge of the field, two fields up, two fields along and two fields down.

(2) Continue the sequence until 100 cells have been counted.

(3) Record the numbers of each type of cell.

(4) Express these as percentages of the total WBC count or in absolute numbers.

The total WBC count is determined by means of an automated haematology analyser or a microscopic counting chamber. Many manual types of commercial differential counters are available to keep tally of the differential cells and there are also several electronic systems. Table 13.6 shows the normal reference haematology data for a number of species.

Poor-quality films – either too thick (so that it is impossible to identify the cells due to poor separation) or too thin (so that insufficient cells are found) or of uneven

Table 13.6 Haematology reference ranges for domesticated animals

Parameter	Units	Canine	Feline	Equine	Thoroughbred	Bovine	Ovine
RBCs	$\times 10^{12}/l$	5.0–8.5	5.5–10.0	5.5–9.5	7.0–13	4.5–9.0	5.0–10.0
Haemoglobin	g%(100 ml)	12–18	9.0–17	8.0–14	10–18	9.5–14.5	8.0–14
PCV	%(1/1)	37–57	27–50	24–44	32–55	30–40	22–38
MCV	fl	60–77	40–55	39–52	37–50	40–60	23–48
MCH	pg	19–23	13–17	15.2–18.6	13.3–18	14.4–18.6	9–13
MCHC	g%(100 ml)	31–34	31–34	30–35	31–38	26–34	29–35
WBCs	$\times 10^9/l$	6–15	4–15	6–12	7–14	3.5–10	4–10
Lymphocytes	$\times 10^9/l$	1–4.8	1.5–6.5	1–6	1.7–9.8	1–4.6	2.6–7.2
	%	12–30	25–33	15–50	25–70	40–60	65–72
Mature	$\times 10^9/l$	3.6–10.5	2.5–12.5	2.1–9	2.1–9.1	0.7–4.9	0.7–3.2
Neutrophils	%	60–70	45–75	35–75	30–65	21–49	18–32
Band	$\times 10^9/l$	0–0.3	0–0.45	0–0.24	0–0.28	0–0.2	0–0.1
Neutrophils	%	0–2	0–3	0–2	0–2	0–2	0–1
Eosinophils	$\times 10^9/l$	0.1–1.5	0.1–1.8	0.1–1.4	0–1.5	0–1.6	0–1.0
	%	2–10	4–12	2–12	1–11	0–16	0–10
Monocytes	$\times 10^9/l$	0.18–1.5	0–0.6	0.12–1.2	0–1	0–1	0–1
	%	3–10	0–4	2–10	0.5–7.0	2–10	0–10
Basophils	$\times 10^9/l$	0	0	0–0.3	0–0.4	0	0–0.2
	%	rare	rare	0–3	0–3	rare	0–2
Platelets	$\times 10^9/l$	200–500	200–600	90–500	100–300	200–300	200–700

Source: Bloxham Laboratories Ltd, Teignmouth, Devon.

thickness due to poor spreading technique – need to be remade. The stains should be filtered, as often debris and deposits prevent adequate staining and cellular differentiation. Production of good-quality smears requires practice. Uniform staining may best be achieved by use of autostaining machines.

When examining the WBCs seen in a blood film, it is important to remember that red cells are also present and that they too should be looked at and commented upon. Figure 13.5 shows the various aspects of red cell development and morphology.

Red cells: morphology and terminology

- **Erythrocytes** (red blood cells, RBCs) are non-nucleated biconcave discs that are pale greenish-yellow when unstained. They take up eosin when stained by Romanowsky stains, and become pinkish.
- **Proerythroblasts** are the first stem cells of **erythropoiesis** or red cell production. They have a large nucleus with nucleoli and a rim of blue stained cytoplasm. Haemoglobin synthesis commences on cell division within the cytoplasm and the cells become smaller. These are referred to as **nucleated RBCs (NRBCs)**. NRBC cytoplasm changes from purple to greyish pink as

the cells get smaller through stages of cell division (**normoblasts**). When the cell is completely haemoglobinised, the small dense nucleus is extruded leaving a greyish-blue or polychromatic cell with a reticular structure which stains blue with supravital stains such as brilliant cresyl blue or new methylene blue. These cells have no nucleus and are referred to as **reticulocytes**. Within normally 12 days in the peripheral blood stream, these lose their polychromasia and are adult red cells.

- **Crenation** is a term applied to cells showing irregular margins and prickly points due to shrinkage. It is usually found in association with too slow air-drying of blood films.
- **Howell–Jolly bodies** are basophilic nuclear remnants seen as the NRBCs change to young erythrocytes. They are found in response to anaemia and splenic disorders or after splenectomy.
- **Target cells** are RBCs with a central rounded area of haemoglobin surrounded by a clear zone, with a dense ring of haemoglobin around the perimeter of the cell due to increased membranes or decreased volume. They are often found in non-regenerative anaemia.
- **Rouleaux** is a type of red cell arrangement used to describe grouping of RBCs in stacks. This is common in

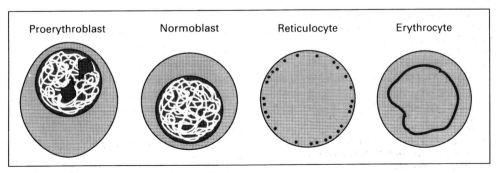

Fig. 13.5 Erythrocyte development and morphology.

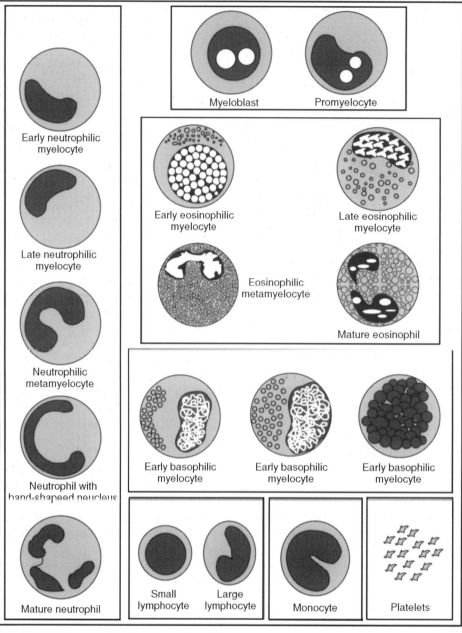

Fig. 13.6 White blood cell development and morphology.

healthy horses but is otherwise associated with increased fibrinogen or globulin concentration in the blood.

● **Supravital stains** are used to detect inclusions and other cellular material such as blood parasites including *Haemobartonella* spp. and *Babesia* spp.

White blood cells (leucocytes). WBCs are nucleated cells consisting of various types (Fig. 13.6) which may be classified into three morphological forms: **polymorpho-nuclear (PMNL) granulocytes**, **lymphocytes** and **monocytes**.

PMNL granulocytes have a single nucleus consisting of a number of lobes. They have granular cytoplasm and can be differentiated by the staining reaction of these granules into neutrophils, eosinophils and basophils.

The nucleus of a **neutrophil** will stain purple-violet. The immature or juvenile cell is shaped first like a kidney-bean

and then like a horseshoe, at which stage it is often termed a **metamyelocyte**. As the cell matures it forms lobes, the number of which increases with increasing maturity. The cytoplasm stains a light pink; the granules are violet.

Neutrophilia is an increase in neutrophils and is found in infectious inflammatory conditions and under 'stress' or conditions induced by steroids.

Eosinophils are similar to neutrophils but they do not usually become as multilobular and their cytoplasmic granules will stain orange-red. In each species of animal, the shape and colour of stained eosinic granules are slightly different: some are small and oval, others are larger (such as in the horse), while cats tend to have large rod-shaped granules.

Eosinophilia is an increase in the number of these cells and is often found in association with allergy and parasit-ism. **Eosinopenia** is a lack of these cells and is often found in the dog in association with steroid usage and Cushing's disease (hyperadrenocorticism).

Basophils are often slightly smaller than neutrophils (8–10 micrometres in diameter). The nucleus is usually shaped like a kidney-bean and the cytoplasm contains a mass of large granules that stain deep purple and may obscure the nucleus. They contain histamine and heparin, which are released at the site of inflammation. They are rarely found in normal films for most animal species but may be present in conditions of chronic tissue damage and myeloid leukaemias.

Lymphocytes are of two types. The nucleus of the smaller (7–10 micrometres in diameter) is round and will stain deep purple; it occupies most of the cell so that the cytoplasm, which stains a pale blue, is seen only as a rim around the nucleus, often only to one side. This is the most common form. The nucleus of the larger type (12–20 micrometres in diameter) stains slightly lighter and has more light blue cytoplasm, which may contain a few reddish granules.

Lymphocytes play an important protective role and are associated with the production of antibodies and recognition of 'foreign' substances such as bacteria and viruses, or the body itself in autoimmune conditions. **Lymphocytosis** is found in some viral conditions and leukaemias. **Lymphopenia** is a decrease in lymphocyte cells that is found in some viral conditions, after steroid use and in some chemotherapy patients. It is important to note that many lymphomas and other neoplastic conditions do not produce a lymphocytosis and may in fact show up as a lymphopenia.

Monocytes are large cells (16–20 micrometres in diameter) and they contain many pink granules. They are involved in the repair of damage to blood vessels: they adhere to the damage and to each other to plug the 'leak' and are then involved in the clotting process (coagulation) to produce fibrin.

Thrombocytopenia, a reduction in the number of platelets, may result in internal or external haemorrhage, while an increase (**thrombocytosis**) may follow haemorrhage or surgery.

Packed cell volume (PCV). The PCV, also referred to as the **haematocrit**, is that percentage of whole blood composed of red blood cells. For whole blood collected in EDTA vacutainers:

(1) Mix adequately by hand or on a roller mixer.
(2) Fill a plain capillary microhaematocrit tube to about three-quarters full by capillary action.
(3) With a finger on the top, seal or plug the bottom end with a clay or plastic material.
(4) Place in a microhaematocrit centrifuge with the plugged end facing out and resting on the rubber rim cushion. Give 5 minutes' centrifugation. (Fresh blood samples, collected directly from the patient by means of a lancet-type puncture or from a drop of blood at the time of venipuncture, contain no anticoagulant and it is necessary to use a **heparinised microhaematocrit capillary tube**. These tubes are internally coated with heparin: as

the blood flows up the tube, the anticoagulant mixes with the blood to prevent clotting.)
(5) After centrifugation, place the tubes in a **haematocrit reader**. This has a linear scale: the bottom of the tube contents is at zero and the top of the plasma meniscus is at 100. From the scale, read off the level of the top of the RBCs (the **red supernatant layer**). This percentage is the **PCV**.
(6) A white-to-grey layer sitting on top of the red cells and below the plasma is referred to as the **buffy coat** and consists of white blood cells and platelets.
(7) The clear-to-yellow layer at the top is the **plasma**.

Normal PCV ranges for various species are shown in Table 13.6. A decrease in PCV is often found in anaemia, haemorrhage, etc., while increases may be found in cases of dehydration.

Total red and white cell counts. Manual or machine total cell counts are an essential part of the haematological examination. Manual cell counting is still required for avian and reptile bloods because their nucleated red cells are not differentiated readily by automated machine counting systems. The procedure for performing manual cell counts involves diluting the blood and counting in a special microscopic chamber, using specific chemical diluents to lyse red cells in order to count the white cells. Refer to standard haematological texts for details of these procedures.

Haemoglobin and calculated RBC parameters. Haemoglobin estimation is a routine part of any haematology examination, generally by colorimetric or spectrophotometric chemical reactions and calculated either manually or by an automated haematology analyser. Calculated values include mean corpuscular volume (MCV), mean corpuscular haemoglobin (MCH) and mean corpuscular haemoglobin concentration (MCHC).

Biochemistry

This section covers the main biochemical tests involved commonly in practice laboratory investigations using simple wet or dry chemistry systems.

Urea and BUN

Urea is a nitrogenous waste product that is formed in the liver from two molecules of ammonia as the end product of amino acid utilisation. It is then transported in the plasma fraction of the blood to the kidneys, where it is excreted in the urine.

The term **blood urea nitrogen (BUN)** expresses the amount of nitrogen atoms in the blood incorporated to urea. Laboratory analysis and measurement of the concentration of BUN and of urea have been used in the evaluation of renal function but are not the same. There is a difference of 2.144 times in magnitude between the weight (in mg/100ml plasma or serum) of urea and that of BUN.

In the international system (SI) of units, these substances are expressed in terms of **molecular** or **molar**

Table 13.7 Biochemical reference ranges for domesticated animals

Parameter	Units	Canine	Feline	Equine	Thoroughbred	Bovine	Ovine
Albumin	g/l	25–37	21–39	23–38	21–34	27–37	24–32
T. Protein	g/l	54–77	54–78	57–84	43–67	70–88	65–78
T. Globulin	g/l	23–52	15–57	16–50	22–50	32–56	27–50
Urea	mmol/l	1.7–7.4	6–10	2.5–8.3	2.8–6.1	2–6.6	3–8
Creatinine	µmol/l	0–106	80–180	60–147	106–168	44–165	44–150
T. Bilirubin	µmol/l	<16	<10	10–40	10–40	<9	<8
Glucose	mmol/l	2–2.5	4.3–6.6	2.8–5.5	3.4–5.9	2–3	2–3
Cholesterol	mmol/l	3.8–7	1.9–3.9	2.3–3.6	2.3–3.6	1–3	1–2.6
ALT	U/l@30°C	<25	<20	<25	<25	<40	<50
SAP	U/l@30°C	<80	<60	40–120	40–160	<80	<40
γGT	U/l@30°C	<20	<20	<25	<40	<15	<20
CK	U/l@30°C	<100	<80	<150	<150	<50	<50
AST	U/l@30°C	<25	<35	<130	<212	<100	<50

Source: Bloxham Laboratories Ltd, Teignmouth, Devon.

concentration, a **mole** (mol) being the unit of amount of the substance. The multiplication factors to convert the old units, expressed in mg/100 ml, to the SI units of millimoles per litre (mmol/l) are 0.17 for urea and 0.36 for BUN.

Increased urea may be associated with several conditions:

- High levels of urea in serum or plasma are usually assumed to be due to renal failure but there are other considerations.
- Chronic heart failure combined with poor renal perfusion will reduce the amount of urea taken to the kidney in the circulation and hence lead to an increase of the amount in the blood. Obviously if severe renal hypoxia occurs due to the poor circulation, renal failure will ensue and urea levels will rise even more.
- High-protein diets may increase the level of urea.
- Low carbohydrate diets may lead to breakdown of body proteins or catabolism and then increase in urea.
- Dehydration may cause an apparent increase in urea.
- Urethral obstruction and ruptured bladder both may lead to increased urea concentrations.
- Other systemic and metabolic conditions may also increase urea.

Table 13.7 shows the normal reference values for urea and a number of other biochemical parameters.

Table 13.8 Conditions associated with increased and decreased blood glucose

Increased glucose	Decreased glucose
Post-feeding sample	Hepatic disorders
Increased glucocorticoids (stress, Cushing's)	Insulin treatment or Insulinoma
Administration of corticosteroids	Starvation/malabsorption
	Hypothyroid/hypoadrenal
Diabetes mellitus	Severe renal glucosuria
Pancreatitis	Idiopathic in some toy breeds
Glucose treatment	Artifact in old sample
Use of morphine	

Blood glucose

Most laboratories continue to refer to 'blood glucose' but the correct term now is 'plasma glucose'. Modern glucose methods are performed on plasma, whereas in the past whole-blood samples were used. As the level of glucose in RBCs is low, blood glucose values quoted in older texts may be lower than those found by current methods.

The level of glucose in the blood is an indication of carbohydrate metabolism and a measure of the pancreatic endocrine function, as it is controlled by insulin and glucagon:

- **Insulin** increases the cellular utilisation of glucose from blood.
- **Glucagon** production causes an increased production and release of glucose from tissue in the blood.

Table 13.8 shows some of the conditions that cause increase or decrease in plasma glucose.

In the practice, it is possible to determine glucose by means of reagent strips or dip-stick methods. Newer reagent strips use whole blood: glucose levels can then be reliably measured by means of a small reflectance meter or by comparing the colour change on the pad with reference colours that indicate the relevant concentration. A number of systems are available and the manufacturer's methodology supplied with the system should be followed.

When sending a sample (plasma) to the laboratory by post, the standard anticoagulant to use for glucose is oxalate fluoride (OXF).

Other biochemical estimations

Determination of total serum protein, albumin, globulin, creatinine, cholesterol, bilirubin and various enzymes assists in the diagnosis of several common conditions (Table 13.9). Various 'dry' or 'wet' chemistry systems are available and a refractometer might be used to determine total serum protein as well as urine specific gravity.

In determining enzymes, controlled temperature conditions are important: in animal biochemistry a temperature of 30°C is recommended. However, it should be noted that some laboratories and some texts quote enzyme activity at

Table 13.9 Conditions associated with increased and decreased blood biochemistry values

Parameter	Increased values	Decreased values
T. Protein	Dehydration, lactation, infection and neoplasm	Liver disease, renal disease, malabsorption, immunodeficiency
Cholesterol	Hypothyroidism, Cushing's, post-feeding, diabetes mellitus, pancreatitis, nephrotic syndrome	Liver disease, lipoprotein deficiency
Bilirubin	Intra- and extra-hepatic icterus, pre-hepatic icterus or haemolysis	Of no diagnostic significance
ALT	Hepatic anoxia, metabolic disorders, hepatoxins, hepatitis	Of no diagnostic significance
SAP	Liver and bile duct damage, bone growth in young, steroids (in dogs)	EDTA sample, haemolysis / No diagnostic significance
GT	Cholestasis and cirrhosis	No diagnostic significance
CK	Myositosis, muscular trauma, myopathy, haemolysis, myocardial infarct	No diagnostic significance
AST	Myopathies, hepatic damage and haemolysis	No diagnostic significance

Table 13.10 Identification of ectoparasites*

		Eggs	Nymphs	Larvae
Lice	Dorsoventrally flattened, wingless / Sucking lice — Biting lice / Grey to red — Yellower / No eyes / Membranous abdomen with hair on segments / Pincer claws — Clasping or running legs / Elongated head — Rounded head / Piercing mouthparts — Mandibular mouthparts	(Nits): Oval white, plug/operculum at one end	Similar to adults but smaller and no reproductive organs	
Fleas	Small wingless (4–5 mm long) / Laterally compressed body / Large hindlegs / Adults have piercing/sucking mouthparts	(Cat flea): Oval, white, glistening, 0.5 mm long		White to brown (creamy yellow on hatching); small, maggot-like; very active, light-shy; 2–5 mm long; sparse hairs. Pupae: very sticky.
Flies (Diptera)	Large adults with wings	Small (1 mm long), elongated, creamy white.		House fly maggots can grow up to 12 mm long in less than 1 week.
Mites	Almost circular body / Four pair short legs, perhaps with suckers (only front two pairs project beyond body) / Adult female 400–600 × 300–400 µm / *Cheyletiella* larger, less rounded; legs longer; horn-like hooks either side of head	Oval	Four pairs of legs	Three pairs of legs; 'orange-tawny'

*See Chapter 15, p. 377.

either 25 or 37°C. In the last few years most laboratories have now moved to the use of 37°C, as the commercial reagents have become optimised for this temperature.

Examination of the skin

Examination of samples for external parasites such as insects (fleas and lice) and arachnids (ticks and mites) depends on collection of suitable samples by means of skin scraping, pustular collection, ear wax collection or hair brushing. The samples are mounted on slides and examined under the microscope.

As the insect may be present in the sample in the form of eggs, larvae, nymphs or adults, or only its faeces may be detected, it is important to understand the parasite's life cycle and to recognise the various stages of development. These are described in Chapter **15**. Table **13.10** gives some of the features to look for in identifying evidence of lice, fleas, Dipteran maggots and mites.

Ringworm

Ultraviolet light from a Wood's lamp may be used to examine hair samples from animals possibly infected by dermatophyte fungi such as *Microsporum* spp. (see Chapter

15). Affected material may fluoresce a bright yellow-green. However, only about 60% of cases of *M. canis* show this fluorescence and its lack does not rule out ringworm infection. It should be noted that non-specific bluish-white fluorescence is not due to ringworm but is commonly found due to scales of flaky skin, mud, dirt, nail surfaces and any petroleum-based materials, including many detergents and paraffin oil.

> ### WARNING
>
> Ultraviolet light is potentially dangerous and can damage the conjunctiva of the eye. Long exposure burns the skin, rather like sunburn (which of course is due to UV rays). Both the operator and the animal must be protected by careful use of the Wood's lamp.

Microscopic examination should be made of any specific fluorescing hairs by plucking them out. If none are seen:

(1) Take hairs plucked from the edge of the lesion, together with a skin scraping, and place on a microscope slide with a few drops of 10% potassium hydroxide (KOH). Place a cover slip over.
(2) Heat the slide over a Bunsen flame, for a few seconds only, to assist in clearing the hairs so that details of the hair shaft may be seen with the microscope under high dry.

In cases of ringworm, the fungal spores or arthrospores will appear as small, spherical, refractile bodies occurring in chains or as a complete sheath around the hair shaft and totally invading the keratinous epithelium. **Hyphae** may be seen as filaments infecting the hair from which the arthrospores are produced. A 20% KOH digest may be used but this is often too strong and damages the hairs too much.

The standard medium for ringworm culture is Sabouraud's dextrose agar, which is incubated at 25°C for up to 2 weeks. Plucked hairs or skin scrapings are pushed into shallow cuts made in the agar. Dermatophyte identification is based on colony morphology and pigmentation together with microscopic examination of the macroconidia or macroaleuriospores (Table 13.11).

There is also a modified commercial Sabouraud's agar with added pH indicator (phenol red): the pathogenic fungi usually grow faster than saprophytes and they produce alkaline metabolites, so that the indicator in the agar turns from yellow to red. Cultures should be examined at 7, 10 and 14 days if an indicator is used.

Faecal examination

The first stage of any faecal examination is to note:

- Consistency (hard, soft, fluid).
- Colour (yellow; brown; green; red, due to blood; or black, due to digested blood).
- Whether fatty or mucoid.
- Presence of any specific obvious material such as worms (round or tape), bones, hair, fur or some other foreign bodies.

Following this macroscopic examination, a direct smear of the faeces may be made for microscopic examination. This enables a rapid assessment of any parasitic burden by looking for worm eggs and protozoan oocytes (Fig. 13.7) and also an initial examination of partially digested or undigested material in the faeces. For **direct wet preparation:**

(1) Place a drop of saline on to a microscope slide.
(2) Add an equal amount of faeces.
(3) To assist in contrast, add stains such as Lugol's iodine (which stains starch granules blue-black) or new methylene blue (which will show up undigested meat fibres).
(4) Mix thoroughly, make a thin smear and place a cover slip on top.
(5) Use low power to examine the field for the presence of worm eggs.
(6) Use medium power to look for protozoa.

Alternatively, instead of putting on a cover slip, allow the slide to dry; then flame-fix and stain for more detailed high-power or perhaps oil immersion examination.

Faecal flotation

Faecal flotation is based on differences in specific gravity. Water has a specific gravity of 1.000; parasitic eggs are heavier at 1.100–1.200; and many solutions of salts or sugar

Table 13.11 Morphological identification of dermatophytes

Dermatophyte	Colony identification	Microscopic identification
Microsporum canis	Flat, white and silky centre. Bright yellow edge. Reverse of culture yellow	Eight to fifteen celled macroconidia or macroaleurospores, knobby end. Thick walled.
Microsporum gypseum	Flat powdery irregular fringe. Brown colour with reverse yellow/brown.	Symmetrical thin-walled three to eight cell macroconidia. Pointed ends. Boat-shaped.
Trichophyton mentagrophytes	Flat, granular, tan coloured or heaped white colony. Reverse yellow-red/brown.	Cigar-shaped two to six celled. Heaped colonies may have no macroconidia.
Trichophyton verrucosum	Small velvet white.	Macroconidia seldom seen.

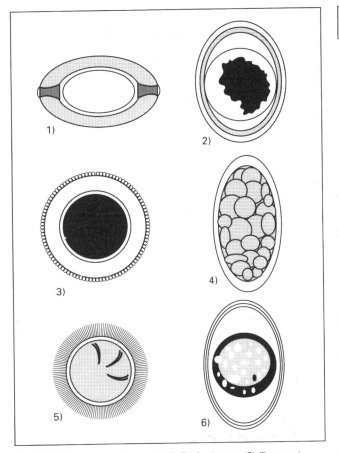

Fig. 13.7 Worm eggs and oocysts: (1) *Trichuris* spp., (2) *Toxascaris* spp., (3) *Toxocara* spp., (4) *Uncinaria* spp., (5) *Taenia* spp. and (6) *Isospora* spp.

Table 13.12 Modified McMaster's protocol

(1) Weigh 3 g faeces. Put into 120 ml wide-mouthed glass-stoppered bottle with glass beads. Add 42 ml tap water and shake well.
(2) Pour faeces suspension through wire mesh screen, collecting filtrate in clean bowl.
(3) Mix and transfer to 10 ml centrifuge tube. Fill to within 10 mm of top.
(4) Centrifuge for 2 minutes at 1000 r.p.m. (800 g).
(5) Discard supernatant and emulsify packed sediment.
(6) Fill to within 10 mm of top with saturated NaCl.
(7) Invert tube several times until even suspension.
(8) Fill both McMaster counting chambers.
(9) Count oocysts and worm eggs under 10× objective and 10× eye piece.
(10) Count/gram of faeces = total number from both chambers ×50.

Faecal sedimentation

Faecal sedimentation concentrates eggs by centrifugation in water but microscopic detection is difficult because of the presence of faecal debris.

(1) Mix about 2 g of faeces with tap water and then strain.
(2) Half-fill a centrifuge tube with the strained fluid.
(3) Spin for about 5 minutes at 1500 r.p.m.
(4) Pour off the supernatant.
(5) With a Pasteur pipette, transfer some of the sediment on to a microscope slide and put on a cover slip.
(6) Lugol's iodine may be mixed with the sediment prior to examination under low power.

McMaster technique

The standard quantitative technique used to determine the number of eggs per gram of faeces is the McMaster technique, which requires a special counting chamber. Table 13.12 describes one of several modified methods based on this technique (see Chapter 15, for various parasite ova found in dog and cat faeces).

Occult blood

Occult ('hidden') blood is evidence of insidious chronic bleeding from ulcers, neoplastic lesions or parasitism in the digestive tract. Dramatic bleeding is usually obvious: faeces are either black (melaena), containing partially digested blood, or they show frank blood (haematochezia). Confirmation of the presence of occult blood requires biochemical detection. The reagents orthotoluidine or benzidine react with haemoglobin peroxidase in faeces with occult blood to yield a colour change which is detected visually. However, both reagents are so sensitive that they will react with any dietary haemoglobin or myoglobin; hence the animal must be placed on a totally meat-free diet for 3 days before its faeces are collected for occult blood testing. Commercial test kits are available.

Other procedures that may also be carried out as part of a faecal examination include:

---

have a higher specific gravity of 1.200–1.250. Faeces placed in such solutions will partition: heavy debris will sink but the lighter eggs will rise to the surface. The most common solutions used for this procedure are sugar solution, zinc sulphate, saturated sodium chloride or sodium nitrate.

The standard flotation method is as follows:

(1) Mix faeces and the solution to break them up.
(2) Push the mixture through a fine sieve or muslin cloth or gauze.
(3) Transfer to a test tube so that the solution fills the tube completely, forming a meniscus at the top.
(4) Place a cover slip on and leave to stand upright, undisturbed for 10–20 minutes.
(5) Carefully lift the cover slip off vertically and place it on to a microscope slide, ensuring that the fluid is trapped between the slide and the coverslip.
(6) Examine the slide under a low-power microscope objective.

Centrifugal flotation is normally performed rather than standard flotation. The tubes are spun at low speed (1000–1500 r.p.m.) in a centrifuge for 3–5 minutes, then the top fluid meniscus is removed and examined.

Commercial kits are based on the standard flotation technique but they consist of a plastic vial containing a filter, so that the sample does not need to be filtered or sieved in advance.

- Faecal trypsin (protease) tests to determine presence or absence of pancreatic trypsin faecal activity.
- Special stains such as Sudan IV to detect undigested fats.

Urine examination

Gross examination should start with the amount produced. The normal dog will produce 25–60 ml/kg bodyweight while a cat normally voids 10–20 ml/kg bodyweight every 24 hours. **Polyuria** is production of excess urine; **oliguria** is a reduction in the amount voided. Other factors to be checked include colour, turbidity, odour and specific gravity.

Colour

The colour of urine is normally yellow. The intensity of the colour may give some indication as to the specific gravity or concentration of the urine: the darker it is, the more concentrated.

- If the urine is browny-yellow and on shaking a slight greenish foam appears on the surface, then bile pigments are likely to be present.
- Red or red-brown coloration is likely to indicate the presence of red blood cells, haemoglobin or myoglobin.
- Drugs may alter the colour of the urine and so will some foods, such as beetroot.

Turbidity

Normal urine should be clear. If it is cloudy or turbid, sediment is likely to be present and this should be harvested by centrifugation for microscopic examination.

Red and white blood cells, crystals, epithelial cells, casts, bacteria, yeasts and fungi may cause increased turbidity of urine and can be identified microscopically.

Odours

Ammonia is produced in stale urine, due to bacterial activity, and an odour is given off.

- This same odour in freshly voided urine may be due to urease-producing bacteria involved in cystitis.
- Male cats tend to produce a strong odour – the males of many species similarly produce strong urine odours to mark their territory.
- The typical sweet acetone smell of peardrops is found in urine from ketotic animals.

Specific gravity

Specific gravity is the density or weight of a known volume of a fluid compared with an equal amount of distilled water. Water has a specific gravity of 1.000.

Refractometer. The specific gravity of urine may be determined by using a refractometer to assess the fluid's refractive index: the higher the concentration, the higher the refractive index. Density is also influenced by temperature and the determination should be made at a constant temperature, or the refractometer should be corrected to compensate for the operating temperature.

Only a few drops of urine are required for determination using a refractometer. They are placed on the glass of the chamber and the lid is closed. The refractometer is held up to the light and the specific gravity is read from the scale. If the reading goes off the top end of the scale, the urine is very concentrated: dilute it with an equal volume of distilled water and measure again. In this case multiply the actual scale reading after the decimal point by 2 to give the correct final specific gravity of the urine.

Hydrometer. Specific gravity may also be determined by means of a hydrometer, which floats in water. The bottom of the meniscus reads zero on the scale of the stalk. The urine volume required may be 10–15 ml and the accuracy is not as good as that of the refractometer. Temperature is much more critical using a hydrometer.

Factors affecting specific gravity. Dehydration increases the specific gravity of urine, as does fluid loss. Other causes of increase include reduced water intake, acute renal failure and shock.

Excess water intake (**polydipsia**), diabetes insipidus, pyometra and some liver and chronic renal conditions exhibit reduced urine specific gravity.

Chemical determination

Reagent urine dip-stick methods have been developed and are commercially available, but they are not reliable for specific gravity measurement of animal urine. They may have limited value for human use but the variations in pH and other chemical constituents in all types of dog and cat urine produce inconsistencies that make dip-sticks unacceptable for reliable determination.

Commercial reagents strips are plastic strips mounted with a variable number of test reagent pads. For example, a 10-determination urine stick can be used for determination of pH, specific gravity, blood, protein, glucose, bilirubin, ketone (acetoacetic acid), urobilinogen, nitrate and leucocytes. These sticks are best used on fresh urine and should never be used on preserved samples. Stale samples are likely to have bacteria growth from the environment or skin or faecal contamination which may affect glucose pH and blood determination. The older the sample, the more the ketones, bilirubin or urobilinogen present will decrease in the urine. Some strip systems enable a reflectometer

Table 13.13 Reference ranges for urine pH and specific gravity

Species	pH	Specific gravity
Canine	5.2–6.8	1.018–1.045
Feline	6–7	1.020–1.040
Equine	7–8.5	1.020–1.050
Bovine	7–8.5	1.005–1.040
Ovine	7–8.5	1.020–1.040

determination of the end result rather than relying on visual determination.

Table 13.13 gives reference values for pH and specific gravity in the urine of domestic animals.

Determination of pH. The pH of a solution is the expression of its hydrogen ion concentration. A pH above 7.0 is alkaline, while below 7.0 is acidic. Stored samples tend to become more acid as CO_2 is lost to the air and false results may occur if the samples are not kept cool and covered.

● Urine pH is affected by diet: vegetarian diets produce more alkaline urine, while carnivorous animals have acid urines.
● Acidic urines (decrease in pH) may be due to pyrexia (fever), starvation, acidosis, high protein diets, muscle catabolism or some drugs.
● Alkaline urines (increase in pH) may be due to high vegetational content of the diet, urinary retention, urinary tract infections, alkalosis or certain drugs.

The pH may be determined simply by means of pH papers or with multi-reagent dip-sticks/strips. It is important to realise that the colour of urine may itself colour the detection strip and cause an artifact in the visual determination. Electrode pH meters are available as small stick-type instruments with digital readout: they are inexpensive and should be considered as a more reliable method.

Blood in urine Blood in urine is detected by means of a similar principle to the detection of occult blood in faeces. Red blood cells, haemoglobin and myoglobin cause oxidation of the reagents, turning them from yellow-orange to green and then to dark blue as the amount of haemoglobin or myoglobin increases. Spots of green are likely to indicate whole RBCs, while solid colour suggests the presence of haemolysed blood. Ascorbic acid may inhibit the detection, giving false negatives, and high specific gravity and high protein levels in the urine may reduce the reactivity. Oxidising agents such as hypochlorites and bacterially produced peroxidases may give false positives. Myoglobin from muscle breakdown will also yield a positive reaction. Any positives found on dip-sticks should be examined microscopically to confirm the presence of blood.

Haematuria is the presence of whole blood in the urine. The presence of lysed blood is referred to as **haemoglobinuria**; and **myoglobinuria** indicates the presence of myoglobin in the urine.

● The most common causes of haematuria are cystitis and associated infection or inflammation of the urinary tract, urolithiasis, acute nephritis, thrombocytopenia and various coagulopathies which cause bleeding.
● Haemoglobinuria is associated with haemolysis of blood in the blood stream or haemoglobinaemia. Conditions such as autoimmune haemolytic anaemia (AIHA), systemic lupus erythematosus (SLE), *Leptospira haemorrhagica* infection, babesiosis and poisoning should be considered as causes.
● Myoglobinuria occurs due to muscle breakdown in cases such as azoturia (rhabdomyolysis) in horses.

● If no haemoglobinaemia is detected in blood but the urine is red-brown and the dip-stick indicates the presence of blood in the urine, then it is more likely to indicate myoglobinuria than haemoglobinuria. Haemoglobin precipitates in ammonium sulphate while myoglobin does not and so confirmatory testing is possible.

Protein in the urine. Protein in the urine is normally present in only very small amounts but collection methods associated with free collection or expressing of the bladder are likely to contain more due to production of secretions from the urinogenital tract. The main cause of increased proteins, however, is associated with decreased reabsorption of proteins by the tubules and leakage from the glomerular part of the kidney. The dip-stick protein reagent primarily detects albumin, not total proteins, and is less sensitive to globulins, mucoproteins and monoclonal proteins. Alkaline urines, and those contaminated with some antiseptic or detergents, may show up as false positive for protein.

True **proteinuria** is found in acute and chronic nephritis, congestive heart failure, other causes of renal damage or nephrosis, cystitis, urethral inflammation, vaginitis and other conditions of the genital tract and traumatic catheterisation. Following parturition or during oestrus the level of protein may rise and be detected but normally any protein detected by the dip-stick is suggestive of **urogenital damage**.

Glucose in the urine Glucose in the urine is referred to a **glucosuria** and the amount present depends on the amount in the blood and the ability of renal filtration and reabsorption. The so-called **renal threshold** is the blood level of glucose above which the normal kidney cannot filter or reabsorb (see Chapter 17).

● Strip-test reagents use a double enzyme reaction system to detect glucose and the test is very specific.
● Tablet reagent systems use a copper reduction method, which is less specific and detects any sugars.

The normal minimum detection level is around 5.0 mmol/l. Ascorbic acid may give false negative results and the presence of ketonuria may reduce the detectable level of glucose in such urine. Stale or bacterially contaminated urine may also have false negative glucose due to the presence of glucose-using organisms.

Glucosuria may occur in diabetes mellitus and occasionally in cases of adrenal hyperplasia (Cushing's disease), hyperthyroidism, chronic liver damage, stress, general anaesthesia and in a specific renal condition in which the tubules are unable to resorb glucose.

Ketones in the urine (ketonuria). Ketones are detected by means of dip-stick or reagent tablets, but these primarily detect one ketone body – that of acetoacetic acid – and are less sensitive to acetone, while they do not detect beta-hydroxybutyric acid (BHB).

Ketonuria may indicate liver damage, diabetes mellitus or ruminant ketosis.

Bile pigments. **Bilirubinuria** is the presence of bile pigments (urobilinogen and conjugated bilirubin) in the urine. It is found in a number of conditions including obstruction of bile flow into the intestine, bowel changes, cholangitis, bile duct obstruction, liver damage due to release of conjugated bilirubin from hepatocytes and in cases of haemolytic anaemia. Bilirubin may be detected by the multi-strip dip-stick but this is not as sensitive as reagent tablets which incorporate a diazo reagent:

(1) Urine is placed on a supplied pad.
(2) A tablet is placed on the pad.
(3) Two drops of water are placed on top of the tablet so that they run down on to the pad.
(4) If the area of the mat around the tablet turns blue, bilirubin is present in the urine.

Urobilinogen is an intestinal bacterial breakdown product of bilirubin. Some of it is absorbed from the intestine into the blood stream and then small amounts are excreted from the kidney into the urine. It is therefore normal to find some urobilinogen in the urine (urobilinogenuria) and a lack of it may indicate bile duct obstruction. However, oxidation occurs rapidly and the oxidised form is not detected. It is essential to test fresh samples of urine. Increased amounts occur in haemolysis and some cases of hepatocyte damage.

Microscopic examination of urine

Normal urine does not contain much sediment, but a few epithelium cells, some mucus and blood cells may be found. Bacteria may be present due to contamination at the time of collection or during subsequent storage. Reagent sticks provide some information but examination of spun-down sediment in urine is potentially a very useful diagnostic aid.

(1) Place 5 ml of fresh mixed urine into a conical centrifuge tube and spin at 1500 r.p.m. (around 100 *g*) for 5 minutes.
(2) Pour off the supernatant, leaving the sediment with a little urine in the bottom of the tube.
(3) Flick the base of the tube to re-suspend the sediment and withdraw some by Pasteur pipette.
(4) Make an unstained wet preparation by placing a drop on a slide and placing a cover slip on top.
(5) Examine by microscope with the condenser down and the iris diaphragm partially closed so that only a little light passes through.

It is possible to add a stain such as 0.5% new methylene blue to aid examination prior to putting on the cover slip. If high-power oil immersion examination is required, make a smear similar to a blood film; air-dry and then stain by Gram stain for bacterial examination, or by Giemsa or modified Wright's stain for cellular study.

Commercial urine microscopic analysis chambers similar to McMaster worm-egg slides and manual blood cell counting chambers are available and these may be used instead of the standard microscope slide and cover slip method.

- **Pyuria** is the presence of large numbers of WBCs (usually neutrophils) in urine and suggests inflammation in the urinogenital tract.
- **Haematuria** is the presence of large numbers of RBCs in urine and indicates bleeding into the urinogenital tract. In concentrated urine the cells shrivel up and are crenated. In dilute urine they swell and lyse, leading to haemoglobinuria – the empty cells are referred to as ghosts and must be distinguished from yeasts, fat globules or crystals.
- **Epithelial cells** are flat, irregular squamous cells with a small nucleus. They are shed from the surface of the urethra, vagina or vulva in naturally voided urine.
- **Transitional cells** are rounder and smaller; they come from further up the tract and in voided urine they indicate cystitis or pyelonephritis. Catheterised samples are likely to have higher numbers than voided urine.
- **Tubular epithelial cells** are the same size as WBCs and are easily confused with them. They tend to be round with a large nucleus and their presence is suggestive of tubular damage.
- **Casts** are formed in the tubules and consist of precipitated proteins due to the acidic condition of the lower (distal) collecting tubules of the kidney. They are defined into various types depending on the other material incorporated with the protein. They dissolve in alkaline urine and should be looked for in fresh urine. High speed centrifugation may break them up and so it is important to prepare the sediment carefully.
- **Hyaline casts** are clear, cylindrical, colourless and refractile and they rapidly dissolve in alkaline urine. An increased number is found with mild tubular inflammation, pyrexia and poor circulation.
- **Cellular casts** may contain RBCs, WBCs, epithelial cell, or a mixture of cell types.
- **Granular casts** are hyaline casts with granules in them. These granules are remnants of epithelial cells and WBCs. They are associated with significant inflammatory change.
- **Waxy casts** are more opaque than hyaline casts and usually wider with square rather than round ends. They are often found in more chronic degenerative renal tubular changes.
- **Mucus threads** are thinner, without definite walls, and are usually twisted strands or ribbons. They are not casts and are normal products of the lower urinogenital tract.
- **Spermatozoa** may be found in entire male urine and are of no diagnostic significance.
- **Bacteria, fungi** and **yeasts** may be found as contaminants of urine but their presence is only likely to be significant if accompanied by large numbers of leucocytes and if the sample was collected aseptically by catheterisation or mid-stream void and examined fresh. Yeasts in particular are likely to be urine contaminants from the external genitalia.

Crystals

Crystals in urine may be associated with clinical conditions such as cystitis, urolithiasis and haematuria, but may also be found in apparently normal animals.

Alkaline urines tend to contain phosphates and calcium carbonates, which dissolve in acid urine. Acid urine may

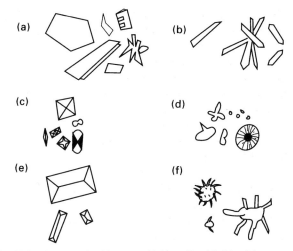

Fig. 13.8 Urine crystals: (a) urates, (b) hippuric acid, (c) calcium oxalate, (d) calcium carbonate, (e) struvite and (f) ammonium urate.

contain urates, oxalates, cystine, leucine and tyrosine crystals.

Crystals are more likely to be found if freshly collected urine is allowed to stand and cool. Figure 13.8 shows the typical morphological pattern of some common crystals seen microscopically in urines.

Uroliths are calculi composed of crystals in the urine and they may cause blockage or damage to the urinary tract. The condition is referred to as **urolithiasis** and chemical analysis of the 'stones' may be performed to identify the materials involved and to assist in the treatment and control of them.

Bacteriological examination

Bacteria may be examined by means of microscopic study using stains. They may be grown on culture media plates (usually a mixture of nutrients and blood in agar): their colony growth may assist in identification and their particular fermentation ability may be used alone or in conjunction with serological tests to confirm their identity.

Sampling

The first stage in any bacterial examination is to obtain suitable samples. Swabs from open wounds, pus or orifices such as the buccal cavity, vagina and ears may be obtained using commercial sterile cotton-tipped swabs.

● If these are to be posted to a laboratory, it is essential that they are placed into **transport media**. Most commercial laboratories supply the transport media and swabs for postal submission.
● For use in the practice, dry swabs may be perfectly acceptable, especially in the preparation of smears.

The collection of body fluids has been described earlier in this chapter. **Vesicles** and **abscesses** are best sampled by means of a needle and syringe. Sampling of **post-mortem organs** is best achieved by heat-searing the surface with a spatula that has been flamed over a Bunsen and placed on the surface to sterilise it. The surface is then cut with a sterile scalpel and a swab of the cut internal surface is taken.

In all cases, it is important to ensure aseptic collection of microbiological samples.

Smears

The making of bacterial smears requires only a thin application of material on to a slide.

For **direct smears from swabs**, lightly roll the end on to the middle of a clean microscope slide.

For **fluid samples**, a drop of the fluid is transferred aseptically with a Pasteur pipette or by means of a flamed and cooled bacterial wire loop.

Colonies from agar plates may be picked off individually by a wire loop and mixed with a drop of sterile saline on the slide.

It is also possible to smear directly from tissue or pus.

Heat-fixing. When the sample has air-dried, the smear is passed through a Bunsen flame 2–3 times with the sample side up. This achieves heat-fixing and prevents the sample from being washed off, provided that the smear is not too thick. It kills the bacteria but preserves the cell morphology. It is important not to overheat: the back of the slide should feel warm but should not burn the back of the hand. When the slide has cooled it is ready for staining.

Staining

Methylene blue. Methylene blue is a simple stain which will show up the presence and morphology of bacteria. A specific aged and oxidised version referred to as polychromatic methylene blue is used for staining anthrax bacilli in blood smears and for demonstrating McFadyean's reaction. Freshly made or **new methylene blue** should never be used when polychromatic methylene blue is required.

Gram stain. The Gram stain is the standard staining method that basically separates bacteria into two types: Gram-positive and Gram-negative organisms, based on the structure of the cell wall. This stain consists of a primary stain of crystal violet which is treated with a mordant iodine (1.0 g iodine crystals, 2.0 g potassium iodide and 200 ml of distilled water). The next stage is to decolorise with alcohol and then counterstain with carbol fuchsin.

● **Gram-positive** bacteria resist decolorisation and remain blue-violet in colour.
● **Gram-negative** bacteria are decolorised; they take up the counterstain and become red in colour.

A procedure for performing a Gram stain is illustrated in Table 13.14.

Lugol's iodine. Lugol's iodine is more concentrated than Gram's iodine: the same amount of stain is combined with only 100 ml of distilled water. Lugol's is used rather than Gram's for a darker colour, giving less chance of excessive decolorisation.

Table 13.14 Gram-stain protocol

Solution 1:	Oxalate crystal-violet solution (containing 2% crystal-violet, 20% ethyl alcohol and 0.8% ammonium oxalate).
Solution 2:	Stabilised Lugol–PVP complex (containing 1.3% iodine, 2% potassium iodide and 10% PVP).
Solution 3:	Decolorise (containing 50% alcohol (95%) and 50% acetone).
Solution 4:	Safranin solution (containing 0.25% safranin and 10% alcohol (95%)).
Protocol	(1) Cover smear with solution 1 for 1 minute. (2) Rinse in tap water. (3) Cover smear with solution 2 for 1 minute. (4) Rinse in tap water. (5) Decolorise with solution 3. (6) Rinse in tap water. (7) Cover smear with solution 4 for 1 minute. (8) Rinse in tap water. (9) Dry. (10) Examine microscopically under oil immersion lens.

Ziehl-Neelsen stain. This is another commonly used stain, which detects acid-fast bacteria such as **mycobacteria** (tuberculosis and Johne's disease). They are stained with carbol fuchsin and heated; they are then resistant to decolorisation with acid alcohol and so retain the red colour when counterstained with methylene blue.

Shape

The other aspect of microscopic examination of bacteria is to define their shape. Round bacteria are **cocci**; they may be single or in pairs (**diplococci**), clusters or bunches (such as staphylococci) or chains (streptococci). Rod-shaped bacteria are termed **bacilli**; some are rods with enlarged round ends (**coccobacilli**) and others may be spiral in shape. Bacteria that have variable shapes are referred to as **pleomorphic**.

Culture media

Culture media for routine bacteriology are available from various commercial suppliers, as either prepoured plates, dry powder or dehydrated media. Some of the most commonly used media – blood agar, MacConkey's, selenite broth and Sabouraud's agar – are described in Chapter 14 (Elementary microbiology and immunology) along with simple (basal) and enriched media, and biochemical media.

After a bacterium has been cultivated and identified as a potential pathogen involved in a disease process, antimicrobial treatment of the animal is ideally based upon *in vitro* sensitivity of the bacterium, so that the most relevant antimicrobial agents can be selected. A specific medium is preferred for performing sensitivity testing and is usually an agar-based medium such as Mueller–Hinton or Sentest agar.

(1) The specific bacterium is plated out to cover the agar.
(2) Antimicrobial discs containing various antimicrobial agents are placed on the surface of the agar. The discs may be placed individually by means of sterile tweezers or loaded into commercial cartridge disc dispensers that can dispense up to eight different antimicrobial discs at a time on to the inoculated plate.
(3) Following incubation, zones of inhibition around some discs indicate that the antimicrobial substance has prevented the growth of the bacterium and the isolate is therefore sensitive to that drug.
(4) If the bacteria grow to the edge of the disc, they are resistant to the particular agent on that disc.

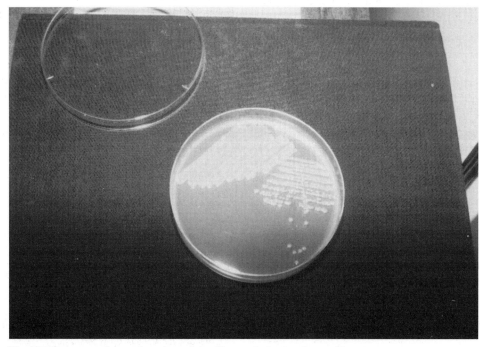

Fig. 13.9 Plating out of a sample: culture plate with growth showing the streaking pattern.

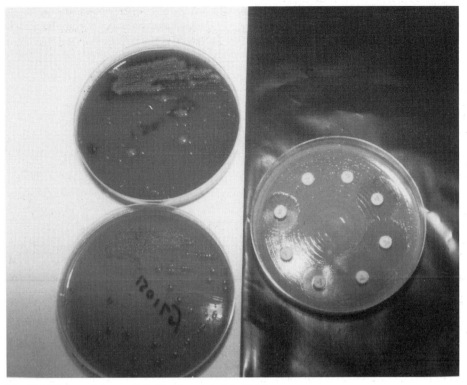

Fig. 13.10 Culture plate growth (left) and sentest plate (right).

Inoculation of agar plates. Whatever the origin of the sample, once it has been aseptically collected and put on to a point of the agar near the edge of the dish it must then be spread on the plate and diluted so that individual colonies are produced. The most common procedure is the **streaking method** (Fig. 13.9):

(1) Take a platinum bacterial loop; flame it until it is red-hot and then allow it to cool. Touch it on to the agar to ensure that it has cooled.
(2) From the point of application of the sample on the plate, streak in a zigzag over one-third of the plate.
(3) Remove the loop and flame it again, using a hooded Bunsen to prevent dissemination of bacteria.
(4) Cool, and then place the loop on agar.
(5) Streak through the previous pattern and over a different third of the plate.
(6) Flame again, and repeat the process a third time, commencing the streak from the previous zigzag.
(7) The loop should then be flamed and put away. Place the Petri dish lid on top of the inoculated agar dish.

Incubation of cultures. Culture plates should be placed upside down in an incubator to prevent moisture accumulating on the bacteria and agar surface. Most common pathogenic bacteria can be grown aerobically at 37°C. The incubator temperature must be constant and the correct temperature must be maintained at all times.

Following incubation (usually for 18–24 hours) the growing bacteria should be seen as separate colonies at the end of the streak (Fig. 13.10). Any growth that is not associated with the streak lines is likely to be due to contamination of the media, either when being poured or

while inoculation was taking place. There may be many airborne yeasts and fungi in the environment and these can become contaminants of the culture plates if sufficient care is not taken.

Identification of bacterial growth on blood agar starts with recording the colony characteristics, such as:

● Any zone of haemolysis in the blood agar around the colony (haemolytic or non-haemolytic).
● The size of the colony – pinpoint, medium, large – and the measurement in millimetres (mm).
● The colour of the colony (grey, cream, yellow, white, etc.).
● If opaque, translucent or transparent.
● The shape and consistency (either irregular or circular, raised, flat, convex, mucoid, flaky, sticky, hard and crusty).
● The odour (sweet, musty, pungent, etc.).

The important subject of disposal of clinical waste, including culture plates, is discussed earlier (p. 342).

Further reading

Baker, F. J. and Silverton, R. E. (1998) *Introduction to Medical Laboratory Technology*, 7th edn, Butterworth-Heinemann, Oxford.

Cowell, R. L. and Tyler, R. D. (1989) *Diagnostic Cytology of the Dog and Cat*, American Veterinary Publications, Santa Barbara.

Doxey, D. L. and Nathan, M. B. F. (1989) *Manual of Laboratory Techniques*, BSAVA Publications.

Hawkey, C. M. and Dennett, T. B. (1989) *A Colour Atlas of Comparative Veterinary Haematology*, Wolfe Medical Publications, London.

Jain, N. C. (1993) *Essentials of Veterinary Hematology*, Lea & Febiger, Philadelphia.

Kaneko, J. J. (1989) *Clinical Biochemistry of Domesticated Animals*, 4th edn, Academic Press, London

Pratt, P. W. (1992) *Laboratory Procedures for Veterinary Technicians*, 2nd edn, American Veterinary Publications, Santa Barbara.

Soulsby, E. J. L. (1982) *Helminths, Arthropods and Protozoa of Domesticated Animals*, 7th edn, Baillière Tindall, London.

Willard, M. D., Tvedten, H. and Turnwald, G. H. (1989) *Small Animal Clinical Diagnosis by Laboratory Methods*, W. B. Saunders, Philadelphia.

14

Elementary microbiology and immunology

M. Fisher and H. Moreton

Disease-causing organisms

The group of living things known as micro-organisms or **microbes** includes the bacteria, viruses, fungi, algae and protozoa. Micro-organisms are generally thought of as those organisms which are too small to be seen clearly with the naked eye. Microbiology is the study of these microscopic organisms, deriving its name from the Greek words: *mikros* (small), *bios* (life) and *logos* (science). Most micro-organisms are **unicellular** (i.e. they consist of only one cell which carries out all the functions necessary for life (but a few, e.g. some fungi, are **multicellular**). Viruses differ from other micro-organisms in that they have no cellular structure. Micro-organisms vary in size from the relatively large Protozoa to viruses that can only be seen with an electron microscope (Fig. 14.1).

The most common concept that people have of micro-organisms is their disease-causing ability; those that cause disease are called **pathogens**. With few exceptions, pathogens are parasites, living on or in the host and interfering in some way with the host's metabolism, to cause clinical signs of disease. The parasite may feed on the host's tissues or body fluids or it may use the host's own food supply.

- **Health** – a state of physical and psychological well-being and productivity.
- **Disease** – an abnormality of structure or function that impairs performance and has a recognisable syndrome of clinical signs.

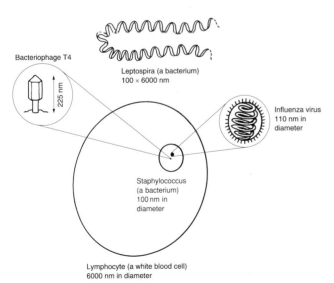

Fig. 14.1 Relative sizes of various micro-organisms, plus a white blood cell for comparison.

Parasites can be divided into three main categories: pathogenic, commensal and mutualistic.

Pathogens harm the host, causing disease, but parasitism is not always harmful. In fact, the more successful parasites cause little or no damage to the host because if they are to survive then the host must survive too. Micro-organisms which lead a parasitic existence but neither harm nor benefit the host are called **commensals**. The surfaces of animal skin, gut and respiratory tracts carry large numbers of commensals which are harmless as long as they are confined to these places. The host's normal defence mechanisms keep these commensals in check. Many commensals are, however, potential or opportunistic pathogens and will cause disease if the natural body defence mechanisms are breached or weakened. For example, the bacterium *Escherichia coli* is normally a harmless resident of the gut but will cause infection in a wound or in the urinary tract. Even within a species of bacterium some strains may be much more pathogenic and/or virulent than others, as the recent food poisoning outbreaks involving *Escherichia coli* 0157 have illustrated.

Some parasitic associations are of actual benefit to both the host and the parasite. These are called **mutualistic** relationships. For example, ruminants such as cattle are unable to digest cellulose but their rumen contains micro-organisms which can break down cellulose into simple substances which the animal can then absorb. In return, the micro-organisms gain a warm environment with plenty of food. The term **symbiosis**, meaning 'living together', is sometimes used to describe any close, permanent association between different organisms, both beneficial and harmful. Therefore, commensalism, mutualism and parasitism are all examples of symbiotic relationships. The macro-organisms affecting cats and dogs that are commonly referred to as parasites are covered in Chapter 15.

When a micro-organism invades a host and starts to multiply, it establishes an infection. If the host is susceptible to the infection then disease results.

In order to cause infectious disease, a pathogen must:

- Gain entry into the host.
- Establish itself and multiply in the host tissue.
- Overcome the normal host body defences for a time.
- Damage the host in some way.

Some micro-organisms cause disease by secreting or releasing poisonous substances called **toxins** which disrupt specific physiological processes in the host. Others invade tissue cells and damage or destroy them. Viruses, for example, cause cell damage because they interfere with the normal cell metabolism and many leave the host cell by rupture of the cell membrane. Once they have entered the tissues of the host, some micro-organisms are localised and remain at the site of entry. For example, *Staphylococcus intermedius*, which causes skin disease, generally attacks in this way. Others spread through the body (systemic spread), usually via the lymphatic system and blood circulation.

Many produce toxic enzymes to assist in the process of invasion and tissue destruction. For example, the enzyme hyaluronidase helps the pathogen to penetrate the tissues of the host by breaking down the 'tissue cement' which holds the cells together. Another enzyme, lecithinase, lyses or disintegrates tissue cells, especially red blood cells. Once they have invaded the host, some micro-organisms can grow and multiply in any tissues of the body but many are more selective and localise in a particular tissue or organ. If these more demanding organisms do not reach the particular cells in which they can live, they will not produce disease. Viruses in particular often have an affinity for a specific tissue or organ. In some diseases symptoms occur because of an over-reaction of the host's own defence mechanisms. This can lead to cell damage or an allergic reaction.

- **Bacteraemia** is used to describe the presence of bacteria in the blood.
- **Viraemia** denotes the presence of viruses in the blood.
- **Toxaemia** indicates the presence of toxins in the bloodstream.
- **Septicaemia** is used when bacteria are actively multiplying in the blood.
- **Pyaemia** describes the presence of pus in the blood.

Parasites vary greatly in their ability to cause disease, or their pathogenicity. Some will almost always cause serious disease while others are less pathogenic and cause milder illnesses. Whether disease develops or not depends on various factors such as the ability of the host to resist infection and the virulence of the pathogen, i.e. the degree of pathogenicity.

Virulence is determined by factors such as:

- The ability of the parasite to invade particular cells and tissues and cause damage (its **invasiveness**).
- Its ability to secrete toxins which disrupt physiological processes in the body (its **toxigenicity**).

Toxins

Toxins are poisonous substances that have a damaging effect on the cells of the host. The effects of the toxin are not only felt in the affected cells and tissues but elsewhere in the body as the toxin is transported through the tissues.

Two types of toxin are recognised:

- **Exotoxins** which are manufactured by living micro-organisms and released into the surrounding medium.
- **Endotoxins** which are part of the micro-organism and only liberated when it dies.

Exotoxins

Exotoxins are proteins produced mainly by Gram-positive bacteria during their metabolism. They are released into the surrounding environment as they are produced. This can be into the circulatory system and tissues of the host or, as in food poisoning, into food that is then ingested. Microbial toxins include many of the most potent poisons known to man and may prove lethal even in small quantities.

EFFECTS OF TOXINS

The effects of toxins are usually very specific. For example, when spores of the anaerobic tetanus bacilli, *Clostridium tetani*, get into a wound which provides favourable conditions, they may germinate and grow in the tissues. The bacteria do not spread through the tissues but secrete an exotoxin which travels along peripheral nerves to the central nervous system where it interferes with the regulation of neurotransmitters that control the relaxation of muscle. This leads to uncontrollable muscle spasms and paralysis. Tetanus toxin is called a neurotoxin because of its activity in the nervous system. Unlike tetanus, which is caused by exotoxins produced while the organism is growing within the host, botulism, caused by the saprophytic bacteria, *Clostridium botulinum*, is the result of ingestion of food containing the toxins. In botulism, the exotoxin affects the nervous system leading to paralysis; it too is therefore a neurotoxin. Other exotoxins formed outside the body include those produced by the bacteria which cause staphylococcal food poisoning, *Staphylococcus aureus*. This is an enterotoxin because it functions in the gastrointestinal tract causing vomiting and diarrhoea.

The body responds to the presence of exotoxins by producing antibodies called antitoxins that neutralise the toxins, rendering them harmless. Exotoxins, as they are proteins, are destroyed by heat and some chemicals. Chemicals such as formaldehyde are used to treat toxins so that they lose their toxicity but not their ability to elicit an immune response. These treated toxins are called toxoids and if injected into the body will stimulate the production of antitoxins. For example, tetanus toxoid is used to provide immunity to tetanus.

Endotoxins

Endotoxins are part of the cell wall of certain Gram-negative bacteria and are released only when the cells die and disintegrate. Compared with exotoxins, they are less toxic, cannot be used to form toxoids and are able to withstand heat. Blood-borne endotoxins are responsible for a range of non-specific reactions in the body such as fever.

They also make the walls of blood capillaries more permeable, causing blood to leak into the intercellular spaces, sometimes resulting in a serious drop in blood pressure, a condition commonly called endotoxic shock. They are also responsible for the change in capillary blood flow in equine hooves that leads to laminitis.

Aflatoxin

Toxins are not made exclusively by bacteria. The saprophytic fungus, *Aspergillus flavus*, produces a toxin called aflatoxin. The fungus grows in warm, humid conditions and contaminates a variety of agricultural products such as peanuts, cereals, rice and beans. Aflatoxin has been implicated in the deaths of many farm animals that have been fed on mouldy hay, corn or on peanut meal.

Bacteria

Size and shape

Bacteria (singular: bacterium) are single-celled organisms and most range in size from 0.5 μm (micrometre or micron; 1000th of a millimetre; 10^{-6} m) to 5 μm in length, though there are some exceptions. Three basic shapes are generally recognised, and these are sometimes used as a means of classification and naming of bacteria (Fig. 14.2):

- Cylindrical or rod-shaped cells called **bacilli** (singular: bacillus). Some bacilli are curved and these are known as **vibrios**.
- Spherical cells called **cocci** (singular: coccus). Some cocci exist singly while others remain together in pairs after cell division and are called **diplococci**. Those that remain attached to form chains are called **streptococci** and if they divide randomly and form irregular grape-like clusters they are called **staphylococci**.
- Spiral or helical cells called spirilla (singular: spirillum) if they have a rigid cell wall or spirochaetes if the cell wall is flexible.

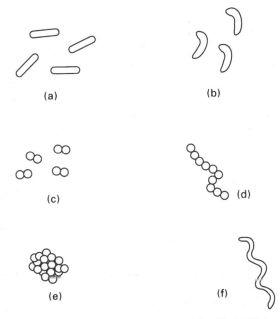

Fig. 14.2 Classification of bacteria by shape. (a) Bacilli. (b) Vibrios (curved bacilli). (c) Diplococci. (d) Streptococci. (e) Staphylococci. (f) Spirochaete.

Structure

As already mentioned, the morphology of bacteria can affect their physiology and pathogenicity. Figure 14.3 shows the structure of a generalised bacterial cell; Table 14.1 gives a summary of bacterial cell structures. Some of the structures are common to all cells; others are only present in certain species or under certain environmental conditions. Table 14.2 shows the shapes of some bacteria that cause disease in dogs.

Cell wall

Most bacteria have a cell wall; this is a rigid structure made mainly of a substance called peptidoglycan (sometimes called murein). It maintains cell shape and prevents the cell from bursting. Cell walls vary in thickness and in composition and it is these differences which help to explain the different response to Gram's stain.

NAMING BACTERIA

All bacteria, in common with plants and animals, are named according to the binomial system; the first word, the generic name, starts with a capital letter and indicates the genus to which they belong, such as *Escherichia*, followed by a species name, that is specific, such as *coli*. Thus *Escherichia coli* is one of the species of the genus *Escherichia*, *Homo sapiens* (modern man/woman) is one of the species of the genus *Homo*. The generic name is frequently shortened, e.g. *(Escherichia) E. coli* and *(Staphylococcus) Staph. aureus.*

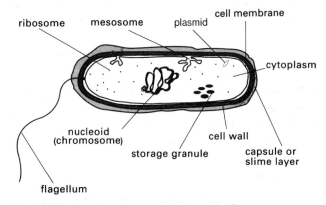

Fig. 14.3 Cross-section of a generalised bacterial cell.

Table 14.1 Summary of bacterial cell structures

Structure	Functions
Cell wall	Maintains shape of cell Protects cell from bursting and from damage
Capsule/slime layer	Protects cell from environmental hazards Aids adherence to surfaces Aids in prevention of phagocytosis Contributes to virulence of some pathogens May act as food reserve
Cell membrane	Controls passage of substances into and out of cell Site of enzyme activity
Cytoplasm	Site of synthesis processes
Chromosome	Carries hereditary information of the cell
Flagella	Movement
Pili and fimbriae	Attachment to surfaces Involved in transfer of genetic material

The cell wall is chemically unlike any structure found in animal cells and is therefore the target for some antibacterials that can attack and destroy bacteria without harming the host. For example, the antibiotic penicillin prevents the synthesis of the cell wall especially in Gram-positive bacteria. During growth of the bacterial cell a deformed cell wall allows the cell to take up water, swell and burst.

Capsules and slime layers

Some bacteria secrete a gelatinous capsule outside the cell wall. These capsules can vary considerably in thickness. Other species produce a more fluid secretion called a slime layer which adheres less firmly to the cell. Capsules and slime layers can serve a number of functions. They act as a barrier between the bacterium and its environment, protecting the cell from hazards such as drying out and chemicals. The presence of a capsule may protect pathogenic bacteria from being engulfed by the host's phagocytic white blood cells because the phagocyte is prevented from forming close enough contact with the bacterium to engulf it. The chances of infection are therefore increased. Capsules assist the adherence of bacteria to surfaces and may also serve as a food reserve.

Cell membrane (plasma membrane)

This lies just inside the cell wall. It is selectively permeable and controls the passage of substances into and out of the cell. In many bacteria, folds of the cell membrane called mesosomes project into the cytoplasm. This folding gives the membrane a larger surface area which is important since mesosomes are thought to be the site of cell respiration. Mesosomes may also be involved in cell division by serving as the site of attachment for the bacterial chromosome.

Cytoplasm

Inside the cell membrane is the cytoplasm, a thick fluid containing dissolved substances such as nutrients, waste products, and enzymes. Within the cytoplasm are numerous small rounded bodies called ribosomes which contain ribonucleic acid (RNA) and are the site of protein synthesis. It also contains various inclusion granules, some of which function as food reserves.

Bacterial chromosome

Suspended within the cytoplasm is the genetic material of the bacterium. A bacterial cell, unlike the cells of other organisms, lacks a distinct membrane-bound nucleus. Instead, the nuclear material or nucleoid consists of a single chromosome. The chromosome is a circular, extensively folded molecule of deoxyribonucleic acid (DNA) and contains the hereditary information of the cell.

Plasmids

Many bacteria also contain one or more plasmids. A plasmid is a small, 'extra' piece of DNA which can replicate independently from the chromosome. The importance of plasmids will be discussed later.

Flagella, pili and fimbriae

Some bacteria also possess various appendages which are found outside the cell wall. Many species of bacteria move by means of one or more thread-like structures called flagella (singular: flagellum). Flagella are long, hollow tubes of a contractile protein which extend from the plasma membrane and through the cell wall. They function by rotating in a corkscrew fashion, moving the bacterium through liquid. Flagella can propel bacteria through liquid

Table 14.2 Bacterial diseases of dogs

Name of bacteria	Disease caused	Gram stain	Shape	Aerobic?
Salmonella spp.	Diarrhoea, etc.	−ve	Rod/bacillus	Yes
Campylobacter spp.	Diarrhoea, etc.	−ve	Curved rods	Yes (but prefer less oxygen than in air)
Bordetella bronchiseptica	Kennel cough	−ve	Short rods/bacilli	Yes
Leptospira spp.	Leptospirosis	−ve	Helically coiled (spirochaete)	Yes
Staphylococcus spp.	Pyoderma	+ve	Cocci	Yes
Clostridium tetani	Tetanus	+ve	Long rods (bacilli)	No

sometimes as fast as 100 μm per second or about 3000 body lengths per minute.

Many bacteria, particularly those that are Gram-negative, have numerous straight hair-like appendages called **pili** (singular pilus) or fimbriae (singular fimbria) which have nothing to do with movement. Different types of pili have different functions. Some play an important part in enabling bacteria to stick to host cells. For example, in infection, pili help pathogenic bacteria to attach to the cells lining the respiratory, intestinal or urinary tracts, thus preventing them from being washed away by body fluids. Other pili, sometimes called sex pili, are involved in the transfer of genetic material from one bacterial cell to another during bacterial conjugation. Some microbiologists now use the term fimbriae to refer to the appendages involved in attachment and restrict the term pili to those involved in the transfer of DNA during conjugation.

Endospores

Some species of bacteria produce dormant forms called **endospores** (or simply spores), that can survive unfavourable conditions. They are formed when the vegetative (growing) cells are deprived of some factor, e.g. when the supply of nutrients is inadequate. It is important to note that endospore formation (or sporulation) is not a method of reproduction; one vegetative cell produces a single spore which, after germination, is again just one vegetative cell. Spore formation is most common in the genera *Bacillus* and *Clostridium*. These genera contain the causative agents of tetanus, anthrax and botulism. These diseases are zoonoses, commonly affecting domestic and farm animals. Species susceptibility to each varies, e.g. dogs do not generally suffer from tetanus, whilst horses are very susceptible and require routine vaccination, as do humans.

Many endospore-forming bacteria are inhabitants of the soil but spores can exist almost everywhere, including in dust. They are extremely resistant structures that can remain viable for many years. They can survive extremes of heat, pH, desiccation, ultraviolet radiation and exposure to toxic chemicals such as some disinfectants. The reason why endospores are so resistant is not completely understood but heat resistance is thought to be due to the fact that a dehydration process occurs during spore formation which expels most of the water from the spore. The spore develops within the bacterial cell and under the microscope appears as a bright, round or oval structure.

The fact that they are so hard to destroy is the principal reason for the various sterilisation procedures which are carried out in veterinary practice. Common techniques employed to kill spores include **autoclaving**: moist heat 121°C under pressure 6.9 kPa for more than 15 minutes; **Tyndallisation**: repeated steaming; **dry heat**: 160°C for at least 2 hours.

Conditions necessary for bacterial growth

Bacteria can grow and reproduce only when environmental conditions are suitable. The essential requirements for growth include:

- A supply of suitable nutrients.
- The correct temperature. The temperature at which a species of bacteria grows most rapidly is the optimum growth temperature. Most mammalian pathogens grow best at normal body temperature.
- The correct pH. The majority of mammalian pathogens grow best at pH 7–7.4.
- Water.
- The correct gaseous environment. Many species of bacteria can grow only when oxygen is present. Bacteria which must have oxygen for growth are called strict or obligate aerobes. Some, the **obligate anaerobes**, can only grow in the absence of oxygen, while others, the **facultative anaerobes** grow aerobically when oxygen is present but can also function in the absence of oxygen. A few species, the **microaerophiles**, grow best when the concentration of oxygen is lower than in atmospheric air.

Reproduction of bacteria

If their environment is suitable, bacteria can grow and reproduce rapidly. The sequence of events in which a cell grows and divides into two is called **the cell cycle** and the time interval between successive divisions is called **the generation time**. In some bacteria the generation time is very short; for others it is quite long. e.g. under optimum conditions the generation time of *E. coli* is 20 minutes, whereas for the tuberculosis bacterium, *Mycobacterium tuberculosis*, it is approximately 18 hours.

Bacteria reproduce asexually by simply dividing into two identical daughter cells, a process called **binary fission**. Prior to cell division, the cell grows; once it has reached a certain size, the circular chromosome or nucleoid replicates to form two identical chromosomes. As the parent cell enlarges, the chromosomes are separated and the cell membrane grows inwards at the centre of the cell. At the same time, new cell wall material grows inwards to form the septum and this divides the cell into two daughter cells (Fig. 14.4). These may separate completely, but in some species e.g. streptococci and staphylococci, they remain attached to form the characteristic chains or clusters. Replication of pathogenic bacteria usually takes place outside the host's cells unlike in viruses where reproduction is intracellular.

Conjugation

The process of conjugation involves the passage of DNA from one bacterial cell, the donor, to another, the recipient, while the two cells are in physical contact. The cells are pulled together by an appendage called the sex pilus which is formed by the donor cell. Once contact has been made, the pilus retracts so that the surfaces of the donor and recipient are very close to each other. The cell membranes fuse forming a channel between the two cells and DNA then passes from the donor to the recipient (Fig. 14.5).

Frequently, a plasmid is transferred from the donor to the recipient but sometimes part of the donor cell chromosome, or even the whole chromosome, is transferred. Conjugation is important because the recipient acquires new character-

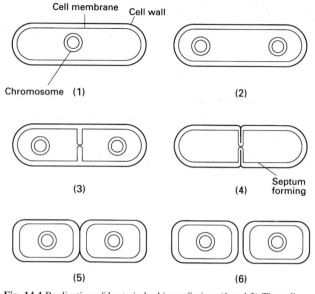

Fig. 14.4 Replication of bacteria by binary fission. (1 and 2) The cell grows and the chromosome replicates to form two identical chromosomes. (3) As the cell enlarges, the chromosomes are separated and the cell membrane grows inwards at the centre of the cell. (4) At the same time, new cell wall material grows inwards to form the septum. (5 and 6) The cell divides into two daughter cells.

istics. For example, one plasmid, the R plasmid, carries genes for resistance to antibiotics.

Conjugation is rare among Gram-positive bacteria but common among those that are Gram-negative. It is sometimes regarded as a primitive type of sexual reproduction but this is misleading because unlike sexual reproduction in other organisms, it does not involve the fusion of two gametes to form a single cell.

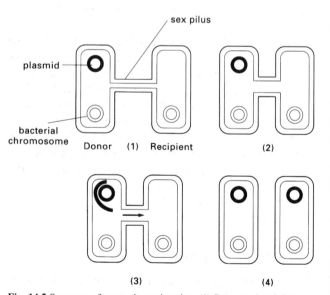

Fig. 14.5 Sequence of events in conjugation. (1) Donor and recipient cells are pulled together by the sex pilus, which is formed by the donor cell. (2) The pilus retracts, bringing the two cells very close to each other, and the cell membranes fuse to form a channel between the two cells. (3) The plasmid replicates and one strand passes through the channel to the recipient. (4) The two cells separate. The recipient becomes a donor because it now has the plasmid.

Staining of bacteria

The identification of bacteria can be helped by their division into groups on the basis of their reaction to certain stains. There are two basic types of microbial staining procedures: simple and differential.

Simple stains such as methylene blue merely colour the cell and can be used to obtain a quick, general picture of the size and shape of the bacteria.

Differential stains involve more than one dye solution and are used to show differences between bacterial cells or their internal structures. One of the most widely used differential stains is the **Gram's stain** developed by Christian Gram in 1884. Gram's method of staining enables bacteria to be divided into two groups:

- Gram-positive which stain purple;
- Gram-negative which stain red.

Bacterial cultivation in the laboratory

The cultivation of bacteria in the laboratory requires an appropriate nutrient material or culture medium. This term is used to describe any solid or liquid on or within which bacteria can be grown. A culture medium must contain a balanced mixture of the essential growth requirements, namely carbon, nitrogen and water. Culture media can also be used as a method of bacterial identification as many bacteria need specific individual requirements for optimal growth. Table 14.3 summarises the uses of common media, and their role in diagnosis is described in Chapter 13 (Clinical pathology and laboratory diagnostic aids).

Media are of two basic types:

- Liquid media or **broths** in which all the required nutrients are included in a fluid.
- Solid media which consist of a nutrient solution hardened to a jelly-like consistency by the addition of a substance called agar (this is used as bacteria cannot utilise it as a food source), a substance which is derived from seaweed.

Solid media are usually used in flat dishes with lids called Petri dishes; a Petri dish containing the solid medium is called a plate. Solid media have the advantage that differences in size, shape and colour of bacterial colonies (i.e. a visible growth of bacteria) can be used for identification and individual colonies can be separated.

Types of media

Simple media (basal media). As the name suggests, this media provides the basic growth requirements for bacteria. Examples of simple media include, **nutrient broth, nutrient agar** and **peptone water**.

Enriched media. Some more fastidious bacteria will not grow in simple media but will do so if it is supplemented with substances such as serum, blood or egg. For example, **blood agar**, produced by adding 5–10% blood to the nutrient medium, supports the growth of most mammalian

Table 14.3 Summary of the uses of common bacterial media

Medium		Use
Plates	Nutrient agar	Growth of nutritionally undemanding species, e.g. *E. coli*
	Blood agar	Enriched medium to support the growth of most pathogens and to detect haemolysis
	Chocolate agar	Enriched medium which is more suitable for certain pathogens, e.g. *Neisseria* species
	Deoxycholate-citrate agar	Selective medium for growing *Salmonella*
	MacConkey's agar	Selective and differential medium used to distinguish those enteric species which ferment lactose (e.g. *E. coli*) from enteric species which do not (e.g. most strains of *Salmonella*)
	Sabouraud's agar	Selective medium for growing fungi
Broths	Nutrient broth	Standard broth for growth of bacteria in fluid
	MacConkey's broth	Selective medium used to isolate enteric from non-enteric bacteria
	Selenite broth	Enrichment medium for growing *Salmonella*

pathogens and is also used to distinguish certain haemolytic bacteria. **Chocolate agar** is made by heating blood agar to 80°C until it becomes chocolate brown in colour. This ruptures the red blood cells, releasing the haemoglobin, therefore making the blood more nutritious.

Selective media. Selective media are designed to inhibit the growth of certain bacteria while not affecting the growth of others. An example is **MacConkey's broth**, which contains bile salts that inhibit non-enteric bacteria but do not affect the growth of enteric species. It is therefore used to isolate enteric from non-enteric bacteria when both are present in a sample. Deoxycholate-citrate agar (**DCA**), another selective medium, inhibits the growth of many non-enteric bacteria but most strains of *Salmonella* will form colonies on it.

Differential media. A differential medium is used to distinguish between different species of bacteria on the same agar plate. **MacConkey's agar** is a typical example of a differential medium. It contains a pH indicator (neutral red) as well as the carbohydrate, lactose. Any lactose-fermenting bacteria such as *E. coli* (a normal inhabitant of the gut) produce acidic products which affect the pH indicator and form red colonies. On the other hand, many enteric bacteria, such as most strains of *Salmonella*, do not ferment lactose and these give rise to colourless colonies.

MacConkey's agar also contains bile salts which inhibit the growth of non-enteric bacteria. It is therefore selective as well as differential.

Enrichment media. An enrichment medium (not to be confused with the enriched media discussed previously), is used when a required species of bacteria is only present in very small numbers in a mixed sample. It favours the growth of the wanted species, allowing it to become dominant. Unlike a selective medium, no inhibitory agent is used to prevent the growth of the unwanted species. For example, selenite broth is an enrichment medium which enhances the growth of *Salmonella* organisms.

Biochemical media. These are used to distinguish between different species of bacteria, by detecting differences in their biochemical reactions with the media. For example, in some genera the different species can be distinguished from each other by the types of sugar which they can ferment. To determine which sugars a particular organism can utilise they are grown in a series of media, usually peptone water or nutrient broth, each containing a different sugar and a pH indicator. If a particular sugar is fermented by the bacteria, acid will be produced and this is detected by the indicator.

For example, bacteria which produce the enzyme **urease** can be detected by growing them on solid media containing urea and a pH indicator. Urease-producing bacteria hydrolyse urea to carbon dioxide and ammonia. The ammonia raises the pH and causes the indicator to turn red.

Transport media. The taking of samples from diseased animals is frequently used to aid diagnosis in veterinary practice. If a micro-organism is suspected of causing an abscess, for example, a sterile swab will be used to collect a sample of the suspected pathogen for laboratory analysis. As many pathogens do not survive long outside their host, a suitable environment must be provided until laboratory culture can be initiated. Transport media are used for the transport or temporary storage of samples such as swabs. Their function is not to support growth, but to ensure the survival of any organisms present until the material can be examined.

Respiratory requirements

The different respiratory requirements of bacteria can be used to help identify bacterial pathogens, as can their detailed biochemical pathways used to provide energy. A lot of bacteria will grow in the amount of oxygen in the air, so may be cultured in an incubator; others will not grow in oxygen (anaerobes). Petri dishes containing appropriate culture media can be placed in an **anaerobic jar** to minimise atmospheric oxygen and encourage the growth of anaerobes. Respiratory mechanisms of any particular bacteria can be identified in a similar way to that mentioned for sugar fermentation, by testing for the presence of **enzymes** involved in oxidative processes, such as the enzymes **catalase** and **cytochrome oxidase**.

The smaller organisms

Infections can be caused by a number of organisms that are a little or a lot smaller than most bacteria. In order of decreasing size these are:

- Rickettsias, mycoplasmas and chlamydias.
- Viruses.
- Prions.

The first three organisms, rickettsias, mycoplasmas and chlamydias, are classified as bacteria and will be considered here. The following sections will examine viruses and prions, and the diseases that they cause.

Both rickettsia and chlamydia possess a cell wall like other Gram-negative bacteria but both of these organisms need to live inside other cells, that is they are obligate intracellular organisms. These bacteria are responsible for a number of diseases in animals including:

- Chlamydia: Various strains of *Chlamydia psittaci*: the cause of psittacosis in psittacene birds (parrots, parakeets) and mammals. Psittacosis is a zoonotic infection which humans can acquire by inhaling chlamydia in the airborne dust or cage contents of infected birds. Feline pneumonitis is caused by *Chlamydia psittaci* and the organism may be the cause of conjunctivitis in the cat. They are transmitted by inhalation of infectious dust and droplets and by ingestion. There is also evidence to suggest that vector-borne infection may occur.
- Rickettsias: They are transmitted by vectors such as the tick, louse, flea and mite from an infected individual. For example *Haemobartonella felis*: infectious feline anaemia.

Generally, the identification of rickettsia and chlamydia is more difficult and thus more specialised than that of most bacteria. Diagnosis of infection may be based on demonstration of the organisms themselves or on the demonstration of increased titres in paired serum samples (see later section on Immunity). The rickettsiae are smaller than most bacteria and are barely visible under the ordinary light microscope. They can only be cultivated in tissue culture or in the yolk sac of embryonated eggs. Typically, they are rod shaped, about 0.8–2.0 μm long.

Mycoplasma are tiny bacteria-like organisms but unlike other bacteria do not possess a cell wall. They include:

- *Mycoplasma felis* – a cause of chronic conjunctivitis in cats.
- *Mycoplasma cynos* – a component of **kennel cough syndrome** in dogs.

Mycoplasma will grow on agar based media but, as they are so fragile, isolation and identification are specialised skills.

More information about the diseases caused by these small bacteria may be found in Chapter 17.

Viruses

Structure and naming

Viruses are extremely small and are sometimes not classified as living organisms as they are incapable of reproduction without a host cell. A virus particle or virion is little more than a package containing instructions for the re-creation of further virus particles. Each virus particle is composed of two parts:

- **Nucleic acid**: RNA or DNA (never both) forming a central core.
- **A protein coat**: the capsid (Fig. 14.6).

Together, these two parts form the nucleocapsid. For some viruses, this is all that an individual virus particle will consist of. Various shapes of virus nucleocapsid have been identified:

- Helical (Fig. 14.7a and b).
- Icosahedral (Fig. 14.7c and d).
- Complex (poxvirus)
- Composite – some bacteriophages (Fig. 14.1)

Some viruses have an additional envelope around the outside, often formed of the host cell membrane (Fig. 14.6c). Each of the helical or icosahedral shapes of the nucleocapsid could be enveloped or non-enveloped (Fig. 14.7), giving four possible basic shapes for viruses. In fact, there are no animal viruses (only plant viruses) that are helical and non-enveloped, so cat or dog viruses can be grouped by and large into the other three types. Viruses have

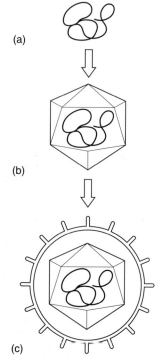

Fig. 14.6 General virus components: (a) central core of nucleic acid; (b) capsid surrounding the nucleic acid to form the nucleocapsid with isosahedral symmetry; (c) in addition, some viruses possess an outer envelope.

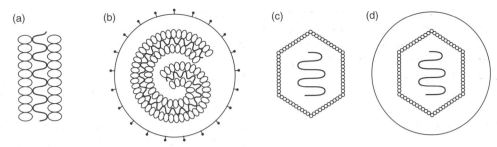

Fig. 14.7 Four types of viral structure: (a) helical naked; (b) helical enveloped; (c) icosahedral naked; (d) icosahedral and enveloped.

been classified together on the basis of structural similarities so, for example, the group of viruses causing true 'flu are the influenza viruses (unlike equine and human 'flu, the disease that we call cat 'flu is caused by two viruses, neither of which is influenza virus), and horse 'flu is caused by equine influenza virus.

Viral replication

A virus is only able to attach to cells that carry a compatible receptor. So, for example, influenza viruses can only attach to ciliated epithelial cells in the respiratory tract. This specificity of viruses for specific tissues is known as tissue trophism. Viruses normally have only one or two host species that they are able to infect. So, parvovirus in dogs does not infect cats and measles virus will only infect humans and apes. Once attached, virus particles are taken into the host cell [Fig. 14.8(2)] by fusing the virus envelope with the host cell membrane or, in the case of non-enveloped viruses, by causing the host cell to engulf the virus particle into the cell. Once inside the cell, the virus is able to switch the cell's normal metabolism to obey the instructions of the virus. The virus may cause this to happen immediately, so the cell begins to produce the constituents of new virus particles within hours of infection [Fig. 14.8(4)]. Alternatively, as in the case of AIDs, the virus may join with the host cell's own nucleic acid for an extended period before making any changes to cell metabolism (more details of retrovirus replication may be found in Chapter 17). New virus particles are then assembled and released from the cell [Fig. 14.8(6)]. Depending on the virus, this may leave the host cell intact or may cause its rupture and destruction.

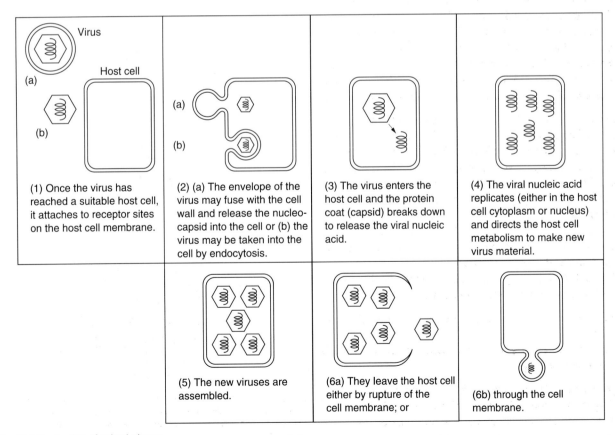

Fig. 14.8 Replication of animal viruses.

Transmission

Viruses are transmitted from host to host either directly (e.g. by a cat licking feline calicivirus in nasal secretions off the face of another cat) or indirectly (e.g. a dog licks the floor of a kennel that had been occupied by a dog with parvovirus infection and that had not been adequately cleaned). Different viruses have adapted their means of transmission according to their structure (which affects their ability to survive in the environment) and their location in the host. So, for example, a respiratory tract virus is often transmitted by sneezing virus particles from one host into the air breathed in by another host. This is ideal for influenza virus as these enveloped viruses are not very robust so do not survive for extended periods in the environment. An ability to survive in the environment for longer periods is beneficial for canine parvovirus. The virus must be licked up and ingested by another dog for infection of the gastrointestinal tract to occur.

Think about the viral diseases that you know that infect dogs, cats and other species, and work out how they are likely to be transmitted. Transmission of disease is discussed in more detail in Chapter 17.

Incubation

Once a host animal has been infected with a small number of virus particles, there is a time lag before the symptoms that are associated with the infection are seen; this is the incubation period. During this time, the virus reaches the cells that it can invade and initially infects a small number of cells in order to increase the number of virus particles. Symptoms are seen once large numbers of virus particles infect a large number of cells.

Viral diseases

The infections in dogs and cats that are caused by viruses are shown in Tables 14.4 and 14.5. More details of each of the diseases caused may be found in Chapter 17.

Diagnosis of viral infections

Viral infections may be diagnosed on the basis of their symptoms and the animal's history. Often, however, there are several infections that may cause similar symptoms and it may be important to be able to confirm the particular virus present. This may be carried out in a number of ways, e.g.

- Virus particles are too small to be seen with the light microscope but they may be seen with an electron microscope
- Large numbers of virus particles may clump together in cells; the clump may then be seen with the light microscope. Large groups of rabies virus are seen in cells of animals infected with rabies; these are known as Negri bodies. An animal can only be examined for these and a number of other virus-related changes at post mortem.
- Serology may be carried out to detect virus antigen or the antibody produced by the host in response to infection.

Treatment of viral infection

Virus infections are generally difficult to treat, as once the virus has infected the animal, it is difficult to kill the virus particles without harming the animal. Treatment of animal

---

Table 14.4 Some viral diseases of dogs

Name of virus	Disease caused	Nucleic acid type	Shape of nucleocapsid	Enveloped
Parvovirus	Parvovirus	DNA	Icosahedral	No
Canine adenovirus 1 (CAV-1)	Infectious canine hepatitis	DNA	Icosahedral	No
Canine adenovirus 2 (CAV-2)	Infectious canine tracheo-bronchitis	DNA	Icosahedral	No
Canine distemper virus	Distemper	RNA	Helical	Yes
Canine parainfluenza virus	Part of kennel cough syndrome	RNA	Helical	Yes
Rabies virus	Rabies	RNA	Helical	Yes

Table 14.5 Some viral diseases of cats

Name of virus	Disease caused	Nucleic acid type	Shape of nucleocapsid	Enveloped
Feline parvovirus (panleucopenia)	Feline infectious enteritis	DNA	Icosahedral	No
Feline herpesvirus	Feline rhinotracheitis ⎫ cat 'flu	DNA	Icosahedral	Yes
Feline calicivirus	⎭	RNA	Icosahedral	No
Feline coronavirus	Feline infectious peritonitis (FIP)	RNA	Helical	Yes
Feline leukaemia virus	Retrovirus causing feline leukaemia	RNA	Icosahedral	Yes
Feline immunodeficiency virus	Retrovirus	RNA	Icosahedral	Yes
Rabies virus	Rabies	RNA	Helical	Yes

virus infections normally involves supportive nursing, for example:

- Fluids to prevent dehydration in the case of canine parvovirus infection.
- Tempting foods for cats with cat 'flu.
- Antibacterials to limit secondary infection.

There are now a few specialised treatments for a few viral infections in humans, such as AIDs, the shingles form of chickenpox and herpes simplex (the cause of cold sores).

Prevention of viral infection

As virus infections are difficult to treat once the animal is infected, control has been aimed at preventing infection, particularly of severe virus infections. This can be done at a number of levels:

- A country can have a border policy to prevent entry of diseases that are not present in a country, e.g. countries seek to prevent entry of rabies by quarantine or vaccine policies.
- Catteries may be designed so that airborne viruses are not readily transmitted from cat to cat.
- Suitable disinfectants can be used to kill viruses that may be present in animal cages in between occupants.
- Individual animals may be protected by vaccination, e.g. **canine distemper** and **parvovirus, feline leukaemia**, etc. More details about vaccination may be found in Tables 17.3 and 17.5 and in the section on Immunity.

Table 14.6 shows the major similarities and differences between the different types of micro-organisms.

Prions

These are very small protein infectious particles that cause infections within the central nervous system that lead, eventually, to the death of the affected animal. The incubation period is usually long – taking from 2 months to 20 years before signs of disease become apparent. Until relatively few years ago, the study of prion diseases was extremely specialised work carried out by a few people. Animal research had investigated scrapie, a prion infection of sheep that has been recorded in Europe for the last 200 years. Interest and research in prion infections increased greatly following the outbreak of BSE (bovine spongiform encephalopathy), which was first identified in the UK in 1985. It is feared that BSE may be transmissible to humans as a result of eating infected beef. Around twenty cases of a similar disease in cats (FSE, feline spongiform encephalopathy) have been recorded in the UK since 1990. Affected cats exhibit incoordination. It is thought that FSE may be derived from scrapie. A lot of research effort is aimed at being able to confirm disease in the live animal. At present, diagnosis is based on the appearance of brain tissue at post mortem examination.

Immunity

With all the potential for injury and infections to cause disease in animals, it may seem amazing that animals have survived until now. The fact that they have is an indication of the effectiveness of their defences against the things in their environments that may be injurious. Innate (natural) defences include:

Table 14.6 Major similarities and differences between different types of micro-organism

Characteristic	Bacteria	Viruses	Fungi	Protozoa	Algae
Size	0.5–5 μm	20–300 nm	3.8 μm (yeasts)	10–200 μm	0.5–20 μm
Cell arrangement	Unicellular	Non-cellular	Unicellular or multicellular	Unicellular	Unicellular or multicellular
Cell wall	Present; mainly peptidoglycan	Absent	Present; mainly chitin	Absent	Present; mainly cellulose
Nucleus	No true membrane-bound nucleus	Absent	Membrane-bound nucleus	Membrane-bound nucleus	Membrane-bound nucleus
Nuclei acids	DNA and RNA	DNA or RNA	DNA and RNA	DNA and RNA	DNA and RNA
Reproduction	Asexual by binary	Replicate only within another living cell	Asexual and sexual by spores, budding in yeast	Asexual and sexual	Asexual and sexual
Nutrition	Mainly heterotrophic – can be saprophytic or parasitic; A few are autotrophic	Obligate parasites	Heterotrophic – can be saprophytic or parasitic	Heterotrophic – can be saprophytic or parasitic	Autotrophic
Motility	Some are motile	Non-motile	Non-motile except for certain spore forms	Motile	Some are motile
Toxin production	Some form toxins	None	Some form toxins	Some form toxins	Some form toxins

- Barriers such as skin, hair, tears, saliva.
- Lysozyme in saliva and tears kills Gram-positive bacteria.
- Phagocytic cells that are specialised at identifying and removing foreign material, e.g. neutrophils and macrophages.

All of these defence mechanisms are designed to protect the animal from foreign or 'non-self' invasion. Throughout early gestation, the foetus learns to recognise what constitutes itself so that later in life it can identify foreign material, in order to eliminate it. The most specific mechanisms that each animal has are termed **acquired immunity**. Acquired immunity, as its name suggests, is not present at birth but is acquired through life. The process begins with the presentation of foreign material or antigen to lymphocytes in lymph nodes. Some lymphocytes will recognise the material and will respond in a number of ways. B lymphocytes react by producing specific antibodies that bind tightly to antigens in the foreign material (Fig. 14.9c). Once covered with antibody, the rest of the immune system can readily remove the foreign material (Fig. 14.9e).

ANTIGEN

An antigen is a foreign material that the immune system can recognise. Not everything that is foreign to the animal will be recognised as foreign, e.g. a metal implant such as a pin or plate will be accepted.

The process of recognition and antibody production is a process that goes on continuously, so that an animal acquires, through exposure to infections, a repertoire of antibodies to protect it from the range of infections in its environment – this is termed **natural immunity**. The process takes a little time to become fully effective against any particular infection. During this time lag, some very pathogenic (an organism that is capable of causing severe disease) organisms may have already caused irreversible damage to the animal (e.g. rabbit myxomatosis or distemper in a dog) or even caused its death (e.g. parvovirus infection in a puppy). There are several ways in which the animal may be assisted to acquire an immune response to infection:

- The animal's mother can pass antibodies to its offspring. This protects the very young animal during the period immediately after birth and prevents it from succumbing to infection. In most domesticated mammals these antibodies are passed in the first milk or colostrum and there is a limited period after birth when the newborn animal's intestine allows the antibodies to pass into the bloodstream. In humans, the structure of the placenta allows transfer of antibodies to occur before birth, thus colostrum is not so important for human babies. This type of transfer of immunity is known as **passive**

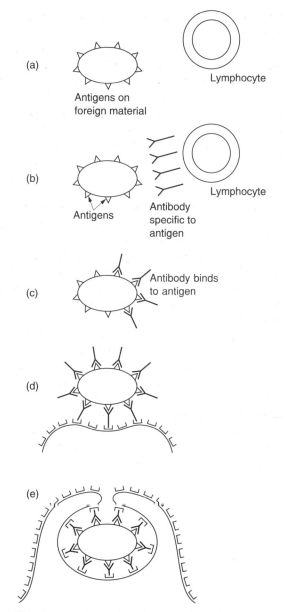

Fig. 14.9 Antibody production following recognition of antigen by B lymphocyte. (b) The lymphocyte produces specific antigen. (c) Antibody binds to antigen. (d) Antibody facilitates adherence to phagocytic cell. (e) Foreign material engulfed by phagocytic cell.

immunisation as the recipient is not producing its own antibodies. In order to maximise the antibody levels in maternally derived immunity, the dam can be vaccinated just before pregnancy or perhaps even during pregnancy, depending on the recommendations of an individual vaccine.

- Another type of passive immunisation is carried out to protect an animal temporarily from an infection or toxin. Here, **antisera** or **antitoxins** to the specific infection or toxin are administered. The antibodies within the preparation bind to the infectious agent or toxin in the animal and stop its damaging effects. Examples of the use of antitoxins include administration of tetanus antitoxin to a horse that is suspected of having tetanus or to a horse that is not protected from tetanus and that had been cut. Antiserum may be administered to a dog that has been bitten by an adder to prevent the venom exerting its adverse effects on the dog.

- **Active immunisation** is carried out more commonly. Here, the animal is presented with a specific antigen in a safe form – this may be in the form of a killed virus, a modified or attenuated virus or bacteria, heat treated toxin (toxoid), just the part of a virus that is recognised by the immune system without the pathogenic part or a bacterial strain that is without virulence. The antigen (or vaccine) is administered when the animal is healthy so that its lymphocytes can respond to the antigen by producing antibody. Importantly, in addition to producing antibody, some **memory lymphocytes** are stored so that the next time the animal meets the same antigen it can respond rapidly and effectively.

- A vaccination schedule for a young pup or kitten usually starts when the pup or kitten is about 8–10 weeks of age. Before this the presence of colostrally derived immunity may prevent the animal from producing its own antibodies.

- A vaccination schedule often consists of two initial priming doses (in pups and kittens spaced 2–3 weeks apart, and in horses 4–6 weeks apart), then regular boosters to keep reminding the memory cells of the antigen. Some antigens, thus vaccines, are very effective at producing a long-term memory (such as distemper vaccine or tetanus); the memory of others fades more quickly (particularly influenza vaccine in horses) so may need boosting more frequently.

- Because vaccines may contain viruses or bacteria and because it is imperative that the animal is presented with undamaged antigen, it is important that vaccines are stored as directed on the data sheet and that they are not used past their expiry date. It is also important that they are administered as directed and not mixed with unrelated products, e.g. other vaccines or antibacterials, as these may adversely affect the integrity of the vaccine.

- Vaccination **certificates** are used to demonstrate that an animal has received appropriate vaccine. It may be used locally to demonstrate that a pet is vaccinated before entry into kennels or may be used to verify that an animal has been appropriately protected prior to export.

Diagnostic use of antibodies

Antibody–antigen binding is recognised to be highly specific; it has therefore been utilised in a number of diagnostic tests, to detect, for example:

- The presence or absence of an antibody.
- The level of an antibody.
- The presence of an antigen (Fig. 14.10).

Pregnancy diagnosis kits commonly utilise this technology as well.

In veterinary practice, enzyme-linked immunosordent assay ELISAs are used to assess the success of transfer of passive immunity in neonates such as calves or foals. Test kits may also be purchased for diagnosis of feline leukaemia.

Epidemiology

Epidemiology is the study of the occurrence and distribution of a disease. It can be used, for example, to identify the cause or the source of an infection, to monitor the number of cases of disease and to monitor the effectiveness of a control policy. All of these applications have been used throughout the BSE epidemic.

Terms that are used in epidemiology include:

- **Endemic** – a disease is present at a normal level in a country or area, e.g. myxomatosis is endemic in wild rabbits in the UK, as is cat 'flu in the cat population.
- **Epidemic** – a pronounced increase in the level of infection. Recent examples of epidemics include parvovirus infection in dogs after its first appearance, BSE in the UK and AIDs infection of humans world-wide.
- **Epizootic** – more specifically, an animal disease 'epidemic'.

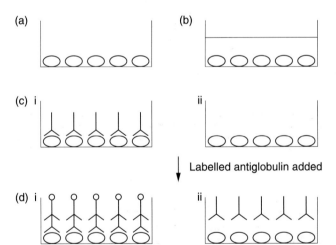

Fig. 14.10 Diagrammatic representation of ELISA. (a) Antigen in base of well; (b) test serum added; (c) (i) test serum contains specific antibody which binds to antigen, (ii) does not contain antibody therefore no binding; (d) labelled antiglobulin added, (i) binds to antibody and produces colour change, (ii) no binding thus no colour change.

15

Elementary mycology and parasitology

M. Fisher

Fungi

There are many different fungi – as one can see by looking at a mouldy slice of bread. Only a few specific fungi, however, are able to infect animals. Fungi can be divided into unicellular yeasts and multicellular moulds, and the fungal pathogens seen in small animal veterinary practice include both categories:

● Moulds (Fig. 15.1a): the 'ringworm' dermatophytes ('skineaters').
● Yeasts (Fig. 15.1b): *Candida albicans*, the 'thrush' yeast, is often present in the intestinal tract of animals without causing disease but it can become pathogenic in certain circumstances.

Fungi grow aerobically and gain their energy from the organic substances on which they grow.

Dermatophytes

Fungal infections of **keratin** (the horny tissue that forms nail, hair and skin) can affect cats, dogs, rabbits and guinea pigs. The condition broadly known as **ringworm** is caused by dermatophytes, such as the species *Trichophyton mentagrophytes* (dog, cat, rabbit and guinea pig) and *Microsporum canis* (dog and cat), amongst others.

In its most obvious form, ringworm appears as circular areas of hair loss with active fungal infection around the edge of the lesion. The lesions may be small and discrete or large and coalescing, with an irregular outline. Some infections are not very inflamed and cause little irritation, whilst others may cause severe inflammation. A more marked reaction is common in dogs.

Transmission may be directly from affected animal to animal, or to humans (many dermatophytes are zoonotic). Long-haired cats, in particular, may appear normal but may

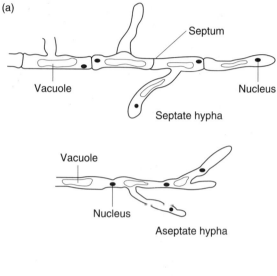

(a)

Septum

Vacuole

Nucleus

Septate hypha

Vacuole

Nucleus

Aseptate hypha

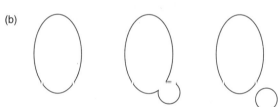

(b)

Fig. 15.1 Different forms of fungi; (a) moulds; (b) yeast, e.g. *Candida albicans*, showing budding.

be carriers of infection. There may also be indirect transmission via bedding, cages, etc. Ringworm spores can remain viable in the environment for prolonged periods. See Chapter 13, p. 354.

Diagnosis

● Place hair pluck or skin scrape on a slide and stain with lactophenol cotton blue or Quink. Affected material, including hair shafts, will stain blue (Fig. 15.2).
● Use a Wood's lamp in a darkened room. Once the lamp has warmed up sufficiently, it produces ultraviolet light and some 60% of *Microsporum canis* isolates will usually fluoresce and appear apple-green in colour. (Other things, e.g. surface scale, may fluoresce but it will not be apple-green.)
● Culture a sample of the suspect hair and/or scale on specialist medium, e.g. Sabouraud's or dermatophyte test medium (DTM). The latter contains a colour indicator that turns from yellow to red in the presence of dermatophytes. The culture should be incubated at room temperature and any dermatophytes should grow within 2 weeks.

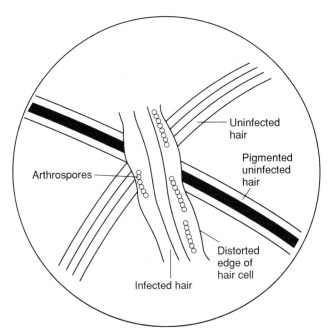

Fig. 15.2 Fungus-infected hair.

Treatment

Topical

- Fungicidal wash such as enilconazole.
- Paint the affected area with povidone-iodine.
- Chlorhexidine shampoo.

Topical treatment is usually repeated after an interval to effect a full cure. It may be possible to treat the area of a discrete lesion only or it may be necessary to wash the whole animal. In severe or non-responsive cases, e.g. some long-haired cats, it will be necessary to clip the entire animal to facilitate treatment.

Systemic. Griseofulvin is administered in tablet form and has to be given for a prolonged period as the levels build up gradually in the skin. Care, including the wearing of gloves, should be taken when handling griseofulvin as it is **teratogenic** (i.e. it can cause malformation of a foetus).

Candida albicans

Candida infections are usually opportunistic, that is they take advantage of a young, debilitated or immunocompromised animal and cause infection. Infection may be seen after prolonged antibacterial treatment. The infection is known as 'thrush' and commonly is seen on mucous membranes, e.g. in the mouths of puppies or kittens.

Identification is by means of the appearance of a white growth on the affected area. Infection of the mouth in a puppy or kitten may be associated with unwillingness to suck and therefore a whimpering animal.

Very rarely they may infect the skin, though *Candida* is not usually included in the dermatophytes.

Malassezia pachydermatitis is a yeast that may be found on normal skin. In some situations it may cause dermatitis.

Table 15.1 Diagnosis and control of insect ectoparasites (See Table 17.32 p. 464)

	Diagnosis	Control
Lice	Demonstration of the eggs attached to hairs. Visualisation of the adult louse. The adult lice may be seen with the naked eye on close examination of an animal's haircoat or may be seen in a skin scrape/brush.	Thorough cleaning. Topical surface treatment with an insecticidal wash or spray.
Fleas	Demonstration of an adult flea or their faeces in the coat of a dog or cat by combing the coat thoroughly, preferably with a very fine toothcomb (ideally a human louse comb). The animal may be brushed over a sheet of damp white paper. Flea faeces will be seen on the paper as small black dots. Since they contain a large amount of undigested blood, a ring of red is seen around the black spot when moistened. There is also a skin test for allergy to fleas.	Control of the environment stages: – Hoovering, particularly around where the pet sleeps. – Applying an environmental insecticide and/or an insect growth regulator such as methoprene to kill the immature stages. Chitin synthesis inhibitor (lufeneron) given orally to the dog or by injection to the cat. It prevents egg hatching and/or larval development. Control of adult fleas on the animal: – Thorough grooming, e.g. using a human louse comb. – Applying an insecticide in the form of, for example, a spray, impregnated collar, powder, shampoo or spot-on. There is also an insecticide that comes in tablet form. The active ingredient in insecticides is often an organophosphate, a carbamate, a synthetic pyrethroid, a phenylpyrazole (Fipronil) or a chloronicotinyl nitroguanidine (imidacloprid).
Dipteran fly larvae	An affected animal will often stop eating and appear restless and later depressed. The animal should be thoroughly examined to find the larvae and thus diagnose the problem.	In order to treat the infestation, the first step is to remove the larvae: – wash the affected area with a mild antiseptic solution, ensuring that the larvae are removed in the process; – lightly towel-dry the area. Apply antiseptic ointment. Any underlying problem (e.g. diarrhoea) that may have predisposed the animal to becoming 'fly blown' should be investigated and treated.

Ectoparasites

Except for certain important fungi mentioned previously, most ectoparasites belong to the animal kingdom and have a hard outer shell or exoskeleton. They include:

- **Insects**, where the adult has three pairs of legs and the body is divided into head, thorax and abdomen (e.g. lice, fleas).
- **Arachnids**, where the adult has four pairs of legs and the body is divided into two parts only: cephalothorax and abdomen (e.g. mites, ticks).

Usually it is the adult stage, often together with the immature stages, that is parasitic. There are two cases where it is only an immature form that is parasitic: the first is a mite, *Trombicula autumnalis,* and the other is the larvae of the blowfly. See Chapter 17, p. 463.

Insects

The diagnosis and control of insect ectoparasites are given in Table 15.1.

Lice

Infection with lice is also known as pediculosis. Lice are subdivided into biting and sucking lice (Figs 15.3 and 15.4), reflecting their manner of feeding.

Infection is transmitted by close contact as the louse spends its entire life cycle on the host. Alternatively infection may be transferred by eggs collected onto grooming equipment. However, lice are highly **host specific** and will not survive if transferred to another host. (Other parasites, such as the cat flea, are more ubiquitous and will be found on a number of different hosts.)

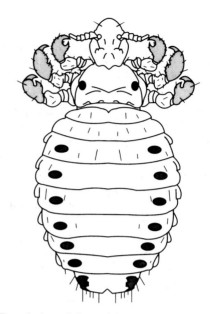

Fig. 15.4 Dorsal view of the sucking louse (approximately 2 mm long). *Linognathus setosus* is the sucking louse of the dog.

Cats, dogs, rabbits, rodents and birds may be affected with lice. Often young or debilitated animals are the worst affected. Large numbers of lice cause intense irritation and concomitant self-inflicted injury. In addition, the sucking lice may cause anaemia if they are present in large enough numbers.

Life cycle

Adult female lice lay their eggs individually and cement them to hairs. The eggs ('nits') are just visible to the naked eye (Fig. 15.5). When these hatch, immature lice that are identical to the adult emerge and, after several moults, become adults. The whole life cycle takes about 2–3 weeks.

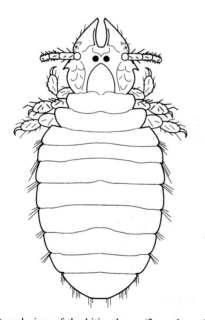

Fig. 15.3 Dorsal view of the biting louse (2 mm long, light to dark brown in colour). If viewed from the side, the louse would appear dorsoventrally flattened. This is the cat louse, *Felicola subrostratus.* The species of biting louse found in dogs is *Trichodectes canis.*

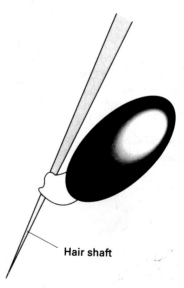

Fig. 15.5 Louse egg ('nit') attached with 'cement' to the shaft of hair.

Fleas

Adult fleas bite the host in order to take a blood meal. The area that has been bitten shows an inflammatory reaction and causes some irritation. A heavy flea infestation may cause anaemia.

Some animals become sensitised to **allergens** (particles that an individual may become sensitised to on repeat exposure) in the flea saliva and develop severe lesions after just a few bites. This is known as **miliary dermatitis** in the cat and **flea allergic dermatitis** in the dog.

The species of flea may be identified by the appearance of the head (Fig. 15.6). Most fleas on cats and dogs are the 'cat flea' *Ctenocephalides felis felis* (often abbreviated to *C. felis*) but dogs in a dog-only situation (e.g. greyhound kennels) may be infected with the dog flea *Ctenocephalides canis*. Infrequently other fleas, e.g. hedgehog fleas, are found on cats or dogs.

Birds have their own species of flea, the immature stages of which live in the nest.

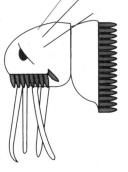

Fig. 15.6 Lateral view of the head of a cat flea, showing combs whose absence or presence and appearance are used in species identification.

Life cycle of the cat flea

The life cycle of the cat flea is shown in Fig. 15.7. The adult is laterally compressed, which allows the flea to move readily between the host's hairs. The female flea mates on the host and then lays eggs. These are smooth and fall off into the environment, particularly around where the animal usually lies. After 2–14 days these hatch out into larvae that look like small maggots. These feed on skin debris, the faeces of adult fleas and other organic matter in the environment. After about a week, each matured larva spins a cocoon and pupates. The outside of the cocoon is sticky and so bits of debris from the environment stick to it. After a further 10 days (though this can be considerably longer in cold or dry conditions) the adult flea is fully developed inside the pupa. Before it emerges, it waits for signs of a host being available, e.g. pressure. (This is one explanation for the stories that occur of occupants going into an empty house and being bitten by fleas within hours). Once emerged from the pupal case the flea will locate a host and jump onto it.

Dipteran flies

Myiasis is defined as parasitism by larvae of the dipteran flies (green-, blue- and black-bottles).

The life cycle is shown in Fig. 15.8. The flies lay their eggs on a suitable site, which might be, though is not necessarily, on an animal, e.g. in the fleece of a sheep or around the anus of a rabbit. Flies are particularly attracted to a smelly animal, such as those that are soiled with diarrhoea, etc.

The larvae (maggots) hatch after as little as 12 hours and begin to traumatise the skin surface and feed off the

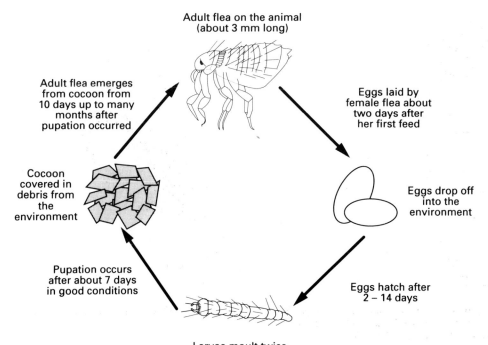

Fig. 15.7 Life cycle of the cat flea.

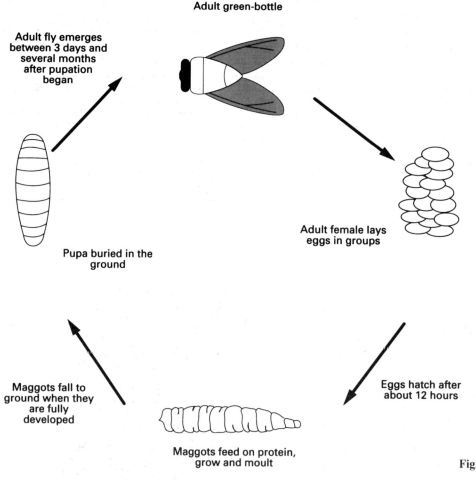

Adult green-bottle

Adult fly emerges between 3 days and several months after pupation began

Adult female lays eggs in groups

Pupa buried in the ground

Maggots fall to ground when they are fully developed

Eggs hatch after about 12 hours

Maggots feed on protein, grow and moult

Fig. 15.8 Life cycle of the blow fly.

damaged tissue. After several moults the larvae drop to the ground. Here they may overwinter as larvae before pupating or they may pupate immediately. Eventually the adult fly emerges from the pupal case.

Arachnids

The arachnids that are of veterinary importance are the ticks and the mites. The immature larvae that emerge from the eggs appear like a smaller version of the adult, except that they have only three pairs of legs, whereas the nymph and adult stages each have four pairs of legs.

Mites

The mites are all **permanent ectoparasites** (they spend their entire life cycle on the host), except for *Trombicula autumnalis,* where only the larva is sometimes parasitic. Mites may be subdivided into the burrowing and the surface mites. Both types of mite cause dermatitis, which may or may not be itchy, depending on the type of mite present. Diagnosis is usually by inspection of coat brushings or skin scrapes; specific guidance on diagnosis and treatment of each mite is given in Table 15.2, see also Table 17.32.

Burrowing mites

Burrowing mites live in small tunnels within the surface layers of the skin. They lay their eggs within small nests within these tunnels. There are three genera of burrowing mites typically seen in domestic pets:

- *Sarcoptes scabiei* var. *canis.*
- *Notoedres* sp.
- *Cnemidocoptes* spp.

Sarcoptes scabiei var. *canis.* This mite affects dogs and, very rarely, cats. (*Sarcoptes* species may also cause mange in rodents.) Often the tips of the ears and then the face are the first areas affected but large areas of the body may be infected in severe cases. Affected areas become hairless, thickened and inflamed. This is partly due to the effect of the mites themselves and partly due to the trauma that the animal causes by rubbing and scratching the affected area – the condition is very itchy. *Sarcoptes* infection in dogs will infect humans but normally the lesions are small and self-limiting. A separate type of *Sarcoptes* is responsible for causing scabies in humans, and another species may cause mange in rodents. See Fig. 15.9.

Notoedres. This, the burrowing mite of the cat (Fig. 15.10), is seen very rarely but it causes similar signs to

Table 15.2 Diagnosis and treatment of mites

Diagnosis	Presence of mite in:	Treatment
Sarcoptes scabiei	Skin scrapes	Mite infections may be treated with a suitable acaricide. Where no licensed product is available, treat with e.g. Fipronil, selenium sulphide or an organophosphate preparation. Where no prolonged activity, repeat treatments after 10–14 days to ensure all immature stages killed. Also treat the environment in *Cheyletiella* infection.
Notoedres	Skin scrapes	
Cnemidocoptes	Skin scrapes	
Demodex	Skin scrapes	
Cheyletiella	Coat brushings (adult mite and/or eggs)	
Otodectes cynotis	Ear wax	Clean the ear canal; instil ointment containing suitable acaricide, often in combination with antibiotic. Also treat in-contact animals to clear reservoir of infection.

SKIN SCRAPES

● Collection: hold a scalpel blade at right angles to the skin surface and draw it repeatedly across a part of the edge of the affected area until the scraped area bleeds slightly. Debris will be collected in front of the scalpel blade: transfer it into a container such as a pill pot. Also place the scalpel blade in the container.

● Preparation: place the material gathered into the container, along with any debris attached to the blade, into a drop of liquid paraffin or 10% potassium hydroxide (KOH) on a microscope slide. Liquid paraffin helps to separate debris from parasites and the parasites may move in the liquid, thus aiding their detection. KOH helps to break down the skin and hair, thus allowing parasites to be spotted more readily. The KOH also helps to 'clear' the parasite to make its features more readily identifiable. The preparation may be heated to speed up the process. A coverslip is then placed over the preparation. Use either KOH or liquid paraffin – not both together!

● Examination: the preparation is initially scanned under the low power (×4) objective to look for evidence of large parasites. It is then examined under the ×10 objective to search for smaller parasites such as *Demodex*.

Surface brushings are most readily examined in a Petri dish under a low power dissecting microscope. A portion of the sample may also be prepared and examined as detailed above for skin scrapes.

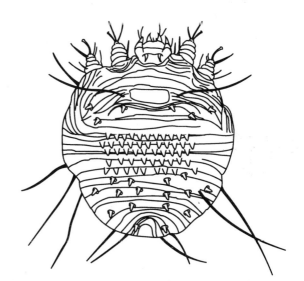

Fig. 15.9 Dorsal view of an adult *Sarcoptes* mite (0.4 mm long). Note the short, stubby legs that barely project beyond the body, spines and pegs, terminal anus, and pedicles at end of legs with suckers on ends.

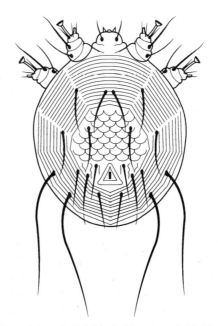

Fig. 15.10 Dorsal view of adult female *Notoedres* mite (0.36 mm long) showing concentric circles on body; dorsal anus.

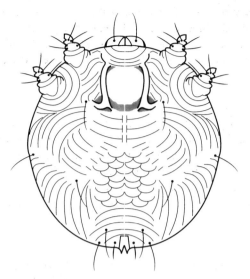

Fig. 15.11 Dorsal view of a *Cnemidocoptes* mite (0.2 mm long)

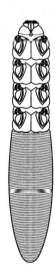

Fig. 15.12 Ventral view of *Demodex* mite showing cigar-shaped body (0.2 mm long).

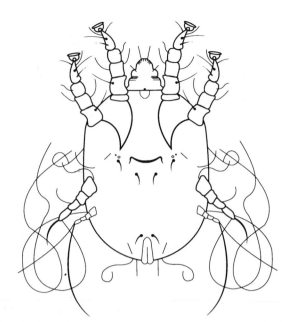

Fig. 15.13 Dorsal view of *Otodectes* mite (0.4 mm long). Note the longer legs protruding from the body and unjointed pedicles with suckers on the ends.

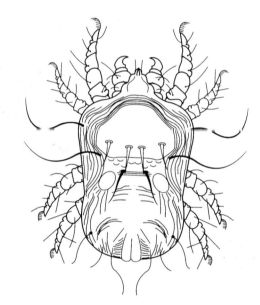

Fig. 15.14 Dorsal view of *Cheyletiella* mite (0.4 mm). Note the 'comb' on the end of each leg and the large palps on either side of the head, each with a large claw.

Sarcoptes in the dog. *Notoedres* species infection also occurs in rats.

Cnemidocoptes **spp.** These mites (Fig. 15.11) are the cause of 'scaly leg' and 'scaly face' in birds, particularly budgerigars.

Demodex. This small, cigar-shaped mite (see Fig. 15.12) may be found in normal hair follicles without necessarily causing any problem. In some individuals, particularly young dogs belonging to short-haired breeds, the number of *Demodex* increases dramatically and causes a dermatitis that is characteristically an area of non-itchy alopecia. Often the area around the eyes is first affected. It can be trickier to find than the other burrowing mites as it is smaller and dwells deep within the hair follicle.

Demodex may also cause mange in hamsters and gerbils. The burrowing mite found in the guinea pig is *Trixacarus caviae*.

Surface mites

Otodectes cynotis. These are the small ear mites in dogs and cats. They live within the ear canal, often stimulating a dark brown waxy discharge. Mites may be seen on the surface as small white moving dots. Secondary bacterial infection may result in a pus-like discharge.

Many cats are infected, often without showing clinical signs. Some cats and most dogs show clinical signs of head shaking and ear rubbing when infection is present. This may result in trauma to the ears and haematoma formation in the ear flap.

Ear canker in rabbits is caused by *Psoroptes cuniculi*.

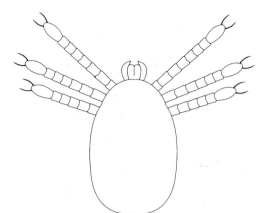

Fig. 15.15 *Trombicula autumnalis* (Harvest mite) larva (1 mm long, orange-brown in colour). Note that there are only three pairs of legs.

Cheyletiella. Animals affected with this fur mite are often said to be affected with 'walking dandruff' since infection often leads to the production of excess scale and since the mites are just visible with the naked eye (they are almost 0.5 mm long). Infection does not usually cause any marked loss of hair. Often the mites will move onto humans handling the animals and, though they will not survive for long periods, they will often bite. Small raised red spots appear in the affected areas of the human body. See Fig. 15.14.

Trombicula autumnalis. This mite (also known as *Neotrombicula autumnalis*) normally becomes a problem in late summer and autumn, particularly in chalky areas of southern England. The larval mites (Fig. 15.15) attach themselves to the legs of passing animals, including dogs or cats, and feed, causing intense irritation to the host.

Dermanyssus. This is the 'red mite' that sucks blood of chickens and occasionally other animals. All stages live off the host, e.g. in the eaves of poultry houses. The mites visit chickens to feed, particularly at night. Infection causes irritation and debility, with anaemia in heavy infections. Control is by cleaning the hen-house and treatment with an acaricide.

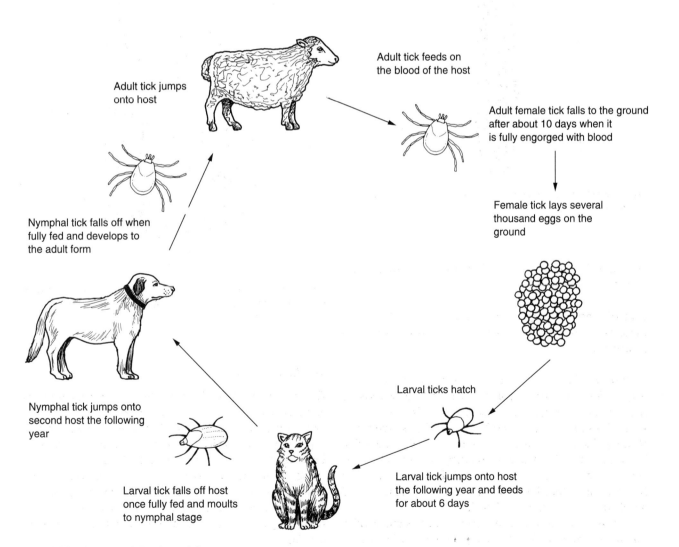

Adult tick feeds on the blood of the host

Adult tick jumps onto host

Adult female tick falls to the ground after about 10 days when it is fully engorged with blood

Nymphal tick falls off when fully fed and develops to the adult form

Female tick lays several thousand eggs on the ground

Larval ticks hatch

Nymphal tick jumps onto second host the following year

Larval tick falls off host once fully fed and moults to nymphal stage

Larval tick jumps onto host the following year and feeds for about 6 days

Fig. 15.16 Life cycle of the sheep tick.

Ticks

Ticks on livestock are important in many parts of the world as carriers or vectors of disease. (A **vector** is a carrier of disease where no development of the disease occurs in the carrier – it simply transfers the infection from one host to the next.) A heavy tick burden may cause anaemia. In small animal practice it is more usual to encounter just one or two ticks on a cat or dog, with an owner who is concerned about how to get rid of them.

Several species of ticks may affect dogs in the UK and one of these *(Ixodes canisuga)* is host specific to the dog. However, by far the most common ticks seen on small animals are the sheep tick *(Ixodes ricinus)* and the hedgehog tick *(Ixodes hexagonus)*. These ticks are remarkably cosmopolitan and will attach to many different hosts. Initially all that is visible is a small greyish swelling, firmly attached to the animal. Inspection reveals pairs of legs close to the attachment with the host; the mouth parts are buried into the animal's flesh. Once the tick has fed fully it will drop off its host. The life cycle of the sheep tick is shown in Fig. 15.16. It should be noted that some other ticks, such as the dog tick, remain on the host from larva to adult and only drop off once they are fully fed adults.

Diagnosis is based on finding the ticks. The identification of the species of tick is a specialised skill.

Individual ticks may be removed by dabbing a cotton wool bud that has been treated with an acaricide (substance that is toxic to ticks). Once dead they can be gently removed. A number of tick removal devices are also available.

> **WARNING**
>
> Never try to pull off a live tick unless using an effective 'tick remover', as its mouthparts may be left embedded in the animal and may become a focus for infection.

Endoparasites

Endoparasites may be further subdivided into helminths and protozoa. The **helminths** are the worms and are further subdivided into three types: the **flukes** (which are found in the livers of sheep and cattle but do not normally affect dogs or cats in the UK), the tapeworms or **cestodes**, and the round worms or **nematodes**. The **protozoal parasites** are small unicellular organisms. Table 15.3 lists the species in each category seen in small animal veterinary practice.

Helminths

Cestodes (tapeworms)

A cestode is tape-like and has no alimentary tract. It is composed of three parts: the head or scolex, an area behind this where segments or proglottids form and finally the maturing segments (Fig. 15.17).

Table 15.3 Species of endoparasite

Helminths		
Flukes		
Cestodes	*Echinococcus granulosus*	Dogs
(tapeworms)	*Dipylidium caninum*	Dogs/cats
	Taenia spp.	Cats/dogs
Nematodes		
(roundworms)		
Ascarids	*Toxocara canis*	Dogs
	Toxascaris leonina	Cats/dogs
	Toxocara cati	Cats
Hookworms	*Uncinaria stenocephala*	Dogs
	Ancylostoma caninum	Dogs
Whipworm	*Trichuris vulpis*	Dogs
Heart worm	*Dirofilaria immitis* (not UK)	Dogs
Capillaria	*C. plica*	Dogs
	C. hepatica	
Lungworms	*Aelurostrongylus abstrusus*	Cats
	Angiostrongylus vasorum	Dogs
	Oslerus osleri	Dogs
Protozoa		
Coccidia	*Eimeria intestinalis*	Rabbits
	E. flavescens	Rabbits
	E. stiedae	Rabbits
Isospora		Dog/cats
Cryptosporidium		Dog/cats
parvum		
Sarcocystis spp.		Dog/cats
Toxoplasma		Cats
gondii		
Neospora caninum		Dogs
Hammondia		Cats
Giardia		Dogs

> **TAPEWORM DEFINITIONS**
>
> Adult tapeworm
>
> - **Scolex**: head of a tapeworm – used for attachment to the host's intestine using suckers and the rostellum (where present) for attachment.
> - **Strobila**: the chain of individual segments.
> - **Rostellum**: the anterior part of the scolex, present in most tapeworms. It is a protrusible cone and is armed with hooks in some species.
> - **Proglottid**: name for each individual segment that makes up the strobila.
>
> Immature tapeworms (**metacestodes**)
>
> - **Cysticercus**: fluid-filled cyst containing a single invaginated scolex attached to the cyst wall.
> - **Cysticercoid**: single evaginated scolex (this is the form found in invertebrate intermediate hosts).
> - **Hydatid cyst**: large cyst containing many scolices, some loose in the fluid inside and some contained within 'brood capsules'.
> - **Coenurus**: a cyst with many invaginated scolices attached to the cyst wall.

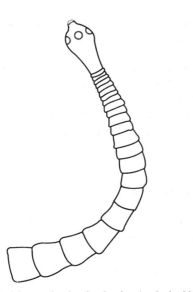

Fig. 15.17 Typical adult cestode, showing head or 'scolex' with ring of hooks on the rostellum and suckers for attachment to the wall of the intestine. Behind this is the neck, where new segments are formed. Further back is the strobila, consisting of maturing segments and, at the posterior end, the gravid segments full of fertilised eggs. These individually drop off the end of the worm and are passed in the faeces.

Each tapeworm has an immature stage that develops in a separate or intermediate host; the exact structure varies according to the species of tapeworm.

The tapeworms in cats and dogs are *Echinococcus granulosus* (dogs), *Dipylidium caninum* (dogs and cats) and the *Taenia* species (one species in cats and several species in dogs). Their presence is not normally any problem to the final host, though the sight of tapeworm segments is repugnant to owners. There is more often a problem with infection of the intermediate host, either because the presence of the tapeworm cysts cause disease or because affected meat is condemned as unfit for human consumption.

Dipylidium caninum. This is probably the most common tapeworm of cats and dogs in the UK. The intermediate host is the flea, and the biting louse in the case of the dog. It is normally diagnosed by the presence of motile segments (shaped like rice grains) around the anus or in the faeces of a cat or dog. See Fig. 15.18.

Control depends on treating the existing infection then eliminating any flea or louse problem to break the transmission cycle.

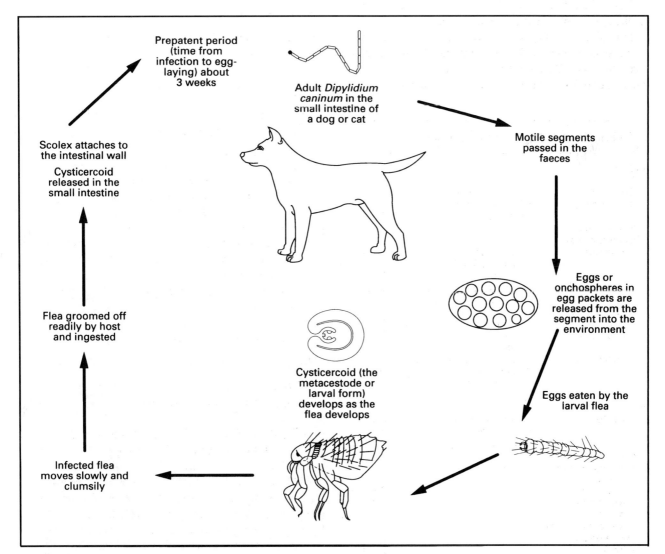

Fig. 15.18 Life cycle of *Dipylidium caninum.*

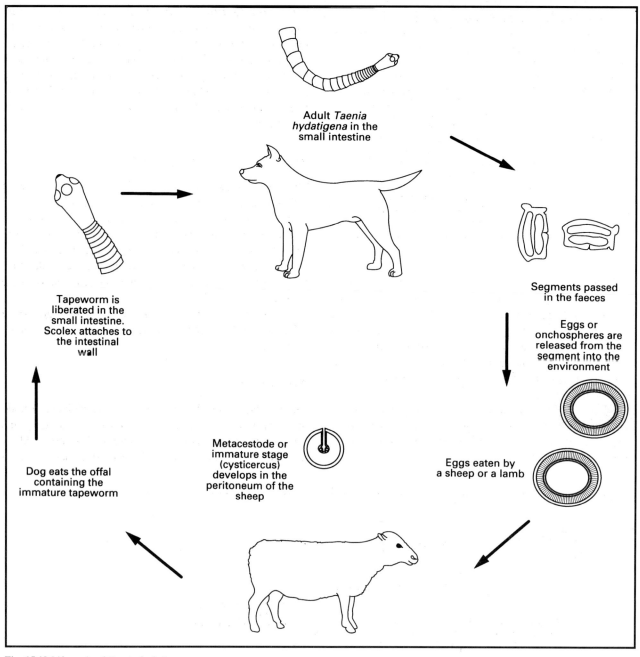

Fig. 15.19 Life cycle of *Taenia hydatigena*.

Taenia spp. Dogs and cats are affected with the taeniae tapeworms when they eat raw meat, either in the form of uncooked meat or offal or through catching and eating prey containing the intermediate stages. The life cycle of *Taenia hydatigena* is shown in Fig. 15.19, and the names of the specific tapeworms with their final and intermediate hosts are shown in Table 15.4.

Diagnosis is based on seeing segments passed by the animal. More rarely eggs, liberated from the segments, are seen during microscopic examination of a faecal sample. These are smaller than *Toxocara* eggs (see Fig. 15.23). Taenia eggs measure about 40 µm in diameter.

Control is based on treating the current infection then preventing the animal having access to uncooked meat – which is something that is easy to do where the animal is fed by the owner but more difficult if the infection is derived from wild prey.

Echinococcus granulosus granulosus. This organism has a dog-to-sheep life cycle (Fig. 15.20). It is an important zoonosis that occurs in the UK but is fortunately fairly rare – it is most common in rural areas, such as parts of Wales, where dogs have the opportunity to feed on sheep carcasses on the hills.

The adult parasite is very small, only about 6 mm long, and several thousand may be present in the intestine of a single dog. Dogs in affected areas should be regularly treated with an effective anthelmintic and denied access to sheep carcasses.

Table 15.4 Hosts of *Taenia* tapeworms		
Name of *Taenia* species	Final host	Intermediate host
T. taeniaeformis	Cat	Rat or mouse (*Cysticercus fasciolaris* in the liver)
T. serialis	Dog	Rabbit (*Coenurus serialis* in connective tissue)
T. pisiformis	Dog	Rabbit (*Cysticercus pisiformis* in the peritoneum)
T. ovis	Dog	Sheep (*Cysticercus ovis* in muscle)
T. hydatigena	Dog	Sheep/cattle/pig (*Cysticercus tenuicollis* in the peritonium)
T. multiceps	Dog	Sheep/cattle (*Coenurus cerebralis* in the central nervous system)

It a human ingests a proglottid or individual eggs, then a hydatid cyst may develop in the liver or lungs in the same way as it will develop in the sheep. This forms a space-occupying lesion that may grow to some considerable size. Treatment of affected people is based on anthelmintic treatment followed by draining the cyst then surgically removing the wall of the cyst. This is quite a hazardous procedure for the patient.

Echinococcus granulosus equinus is a separate tapeworm that has a dog-to-horse life cycle. It occurs particularly where hounds are fed on horse offal. It is not believed to pose a zoonotic risk.

Cestode infections in other animals. Birds and other animals such as rabbits, mice, rats and hamsters may all be infected with adult tapeworms specific to the host species. In most cases infection has no effect on the host. Occasionally a heavy tapeworm burden in hamsters may be associated with weight loss and perhaps intestinal blockage. In each case the intermediate host is an invertebrate such as a beetle or mite.

Treatment of cestode infections

The adult tapeworm can be killed with a number of anthelmintics; these may be products that only have activity against tapeworms, in which case they are known as cestocides. Alternatively the preparation may have activity against other helminths, particularly nematodes, as well as tapeworms; these are known as broad-spectrum anthelmintics. The active ingredients that have cestocidal activity are shown in Table 15.5.

It is much more difficult to kill the immature tapeworm infections in the intermediate hosts and this is not usually carried out.

Nematodes

Nematodes are round worms with a proper digestive tract. Most have a direct life cycle, though some (e.g. the lungworms) have a slug or snail intermediate host. Others may be carried by a **paratenic host** (one that acts as a

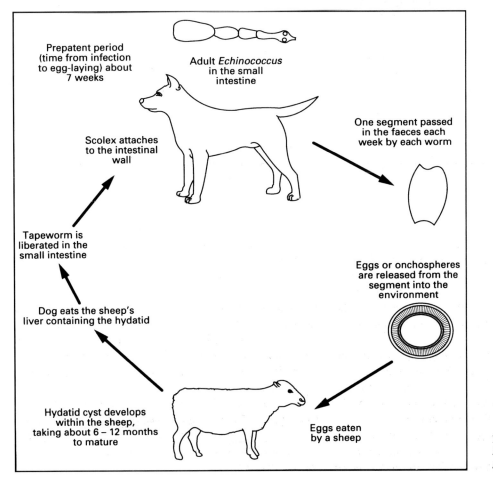

Fig. 15.20 Life cycle of *Echinococcus granulosus granulosus*.

Table 15.5 Anthelmintics

Name of active ingredient	Trade name	Animal	Activity
Dichlorophen	Numerous	Dog, cat	C
Praziquantel	Droncit	Dog, cat	C
Fenbendazole	Panacur	Dog, cat	NC
Mebendazole	Telmin	Dog	NC
Nitroscanate	Lopatol	Dog	NC
Piperazine	Numerous	Dog, cat	N
Pyrantel	Strongid	Dog	N
Pyrantel/praziquantel/ febantel	Drontal plus	Dog	NC
Pyrantel/praziquantel	Drontal cat	Cat	NC

N, nematodes; C, cestodes. This indicates that those preparations have activity against some, though not necessarily all, nematodes or cestodes. The reader is directed to the NOAH Compendium for further details on individual products.

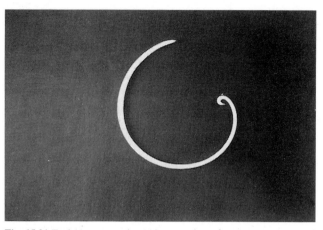

Fig. 15.21 Typical appearance of adult ascarid (approximately 6 cm long).

carrier only – no development of the parasite occurs in this host).

Major groups of nematodes

Important nematode groups seen in small animal veterinary practice include:

- Ascarids (especially *Toxocara canis*, *Toxascaris leonina* and *Toxocara cati* in dogs and cats). Large, fleshy worms (Fig. 15.21), most numerous and frequent in young animals. Ascarids occur commonly in other animals including reptiles (e.g. tortoises) and birds (especially parakeets); in each case the ascarid species is host specific. Heavy burdens may be associated with poor growth or intestinal impactions.
- Hookworms (*Uncinaria stenocephala* and *Ancylostoma caninum*).
- Whipworm (*Trichuris vulpis*).
- Heart worm (*Dirofilaria immitis*) (not in UK).

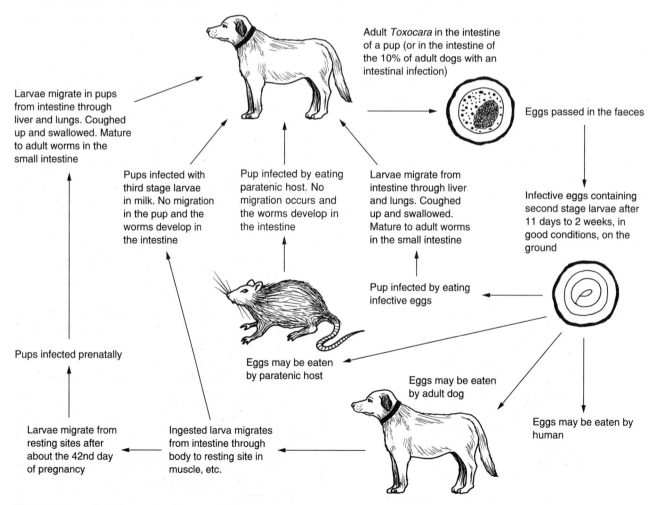

Larvae migrate in pups from intestine through liver and lungs. Coughed up and swallowed. Mature to adult worms in the small intestine

Adult *Toxocara* in the intestine of a pup (or in the intestine of the 10% of adult dogs with an intestinal infection)

Eggs passed in the faeces

Pups infected with third stage larvae in milk. No migration in the pup and the worms develop in the intestine

Pup infected by eating paratenic host. No migration occurs and the worms develop in the intestine

Larvae migrate from intestine through liver and lungs. Coughed up and swallowed. Mature to adult worms in the small intestine

Infective eggs containing second stage larvae after 11 days to 2 weeks, in good conditions, on the ground

Pup infected by eating infective eggs

Pups infected prenatally

Eggs may be eaten by paratenic host

Eggs may be eaten by adult dog

Eggs may be eaten by human

Larvae migrate from resting sites after about the 42nd day of pregnancy

Ingested larva migrates from intestine through body to resting site in muscle, etc.

Fig. 15.22 Life cycle of *Toxocara canis*.

- Bladder and liver worms (*Capillaric* spp.)
- Lungworms (*Aelurostrongylus abstrusus*, *Angiostrongylus vasorum* and *Oslerus osleri* – formerly known as *Filaroides osleri*).

Toxocara canis. This is a very important worm since it is a zoonosis and can also cause disease in young pups. Its life cycle is shown in Fig. 15.22.

Pups are first infected before birth by **larvae** that pass from the bitch's muscles to her uterus after about the 42nd day of pregnancy. These larvae migrate through the liver and lungs of the young pups and are then coughed up and swallowed. They remain in the small intestine where they develop to **adult worms** by the time that the pups are 3 weeks of age. The pups can also receive further infection from infective eggs in the environment and by infective larvae that pass in the mother's milk. Usually the majority of the infection will have occurred across the placenta. Pups that have a heavy *Toxocara* burden will typically be stunted with distended bellies; they may vomit and/or have diarrhoea, and severe infections may lead to a total blockage of the intestine.

The pups begin to expel their *Toxocara* infection spontaneously from about seven weeks of age. Most have expelled all of their adult worms by 6–7 months of age. Further larvae that are ingested pass from the intestine to muscle where they enter a resting state.

Adult worms pass large numbers of **eggs** (as many as several thousand eggs per gram of faeces in a 3-week-old pup). Each egg is surrounded by a thick wall (Fig. 15.23) which is very resistant to either physical or chemical damage. The eggs are not immediately infective but require time for a larva to develop inside. In ideal conditions this will take about 14 days, but may take much longer in low temperatures. Since the larva remains in the shell until eaten by an animal, the eggs may remain infective in the environment for at least 2 years.

Larvae that are accidentally eaten by **other animals** (including humans) migrate from the intestine and enter a resting state in other tissues. If a **human** ingests a large number of infective eggs and these all migrate together through the body, a condition known as 'visceral larval migrans' may develop, associated with signs of damage to the organs through which the larvae are migrating. If only a few larvae are ingested, they will usually migrate through the human body without any signs of illness, except in the rare case where they come to rest in the eye, when blindness may result. Infection is usually seen in children, as they are the most likely to have unhygienic habits. If the animal that ingests the eggs happens to be a *bitch*, the larvae remain in this resting state until she becomes pregnant; some of the larvae will migrate to infect her pups; and others will remain to infect her subsequent litters.

To perpetuate their life cycle, dormant larvae in the tissues of birds or animals other than dogs depend upon their temporary host being eaten by a dog.

In about 10% of **adult dogs**, for one reason or another, adult worms will develop in the small intestine and have a patent infection in the small intestine. Lactating bitches are particularly likely to have a patent infection, probably due to the change in their hormonal status. This infection may come from a number of sources including young worms that are passed by the pups and that the bitch ingests as she cleans up around the nest. Usually the bitch expels her remaining infection shortly after the pups are weaned.

CONTROL OF *Toxocara canis*

This is based on:

- Control of infection in the dog to prevent disease in pups and eggs put into the environment.
- Prevention of infection in children.

Prenatal infection in the pups may be controlled by treating the bitch, prior to whelping, with a product that will kill the migrating larvae, e.g. fenbendazole from the 42nd day of pregnancy to 2 days post-whelping.

Alternatively the pups may be treated at regular intervals with a suitable anthelmintic, starting from 2 weeks of age; the bitch should be treated at the same time.

Reducing the number of eggs in the environment is very difficult once the eggs are present. Scorching with a flame thrower has been found to be the most effective method, but education of the dog-owning public is the best way to reduce egg output in the future.

The most important methods of preventing children from becoming infected are to ensure that:

- Dogs defecate in specified areas in parks.
- Children wash their hands before eating.
- Children are discouraged from handling young pups unless the animals have been thoroughly wormed.
- Use 'pooper scoopers'.

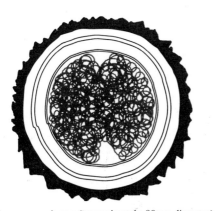

Fig. 15.23 *Toxocara canis* egg (approximately 80 μm diameter). Note the rough outer wall.

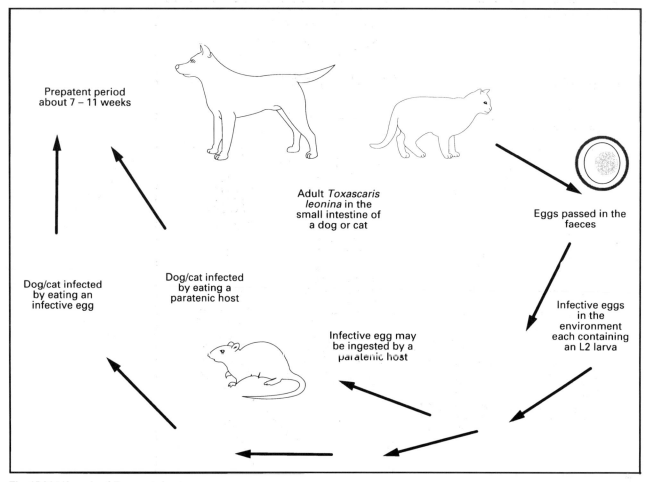

Prepatent period
about 7 – 11 weeks

Adult *Toxascaris
leonina* in the
small intestine of
a dog or cat

Eggs passed in the
faeces

Dog/cat infected
by eating an
infective egg

Dog/cat infected
by eating a
paratenic host

Infective eggs
in the
environment
each containing
an L2 larva

Infective egg may
be ingested by a
paratenic host

Fig. 15.24 Life cycle of *Toxascaris leonina*.

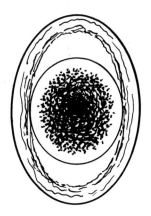

Fig. 15.25 *Toxascaris leonina* egg (approximately 85 μm long). Note the smooth outer wall. Contents are paler than those of *Toxocara* species.

Toxascaris leonina. This ascarid will infect both cats and dogs. Its life cycle is shown in Fig. 15.24. It has not been implicated as a zoonosis.

There is no prenatal infection; therefore infection is usually first seen in adolescent animals. The worm is not usually associated with clinical signs, since large burdens are reasonably well tolerated.

The egg (Fig. 15.25) can be distinguished by the smooth outer wall to the shell.

Toxocara cati. This organism is responsible for ascarid infection in cats, particularly kittens. It is transmitted to kittens by their mothers' milk; infection also occurs through infective eggs in the environment and through ingestion of paratenic hosts (Fig. 15.26). A heavy infection may cause stunting of kittens and a pot-bellied appearance.

The adult worm can be distinguished by the appearance of the alae or 'wings' either side of the head end (Fig. 15.27). The egg is grossly indistinguishable from that of *T. canis.*

Control is by regular treatment of kittens from 2–3 weeks of age until they are several months of age.

Hookworms. Hookworms are short, stout worms (Fig. 15.28) with hooked heads. *Uncinaria stenocephala* and *Ancylostoma caninum* occur in the small intestine of the dog. *U. stenocephala* is the more common of the two in the UK and is known as the northern hookworm; it is particularly seen in greyhounds or hunt kennels.

The two species may be distinguished by the appearance of the head: *A. caninum* has large teeth (Fig. 15.29), while *U. stenocephala* has plates in the mouth cavity. The life cycle is shown in Fig. 15.30.

The worms attach to the intestinal mucosa by their mouthparts. They use their teeth to damage the surface and

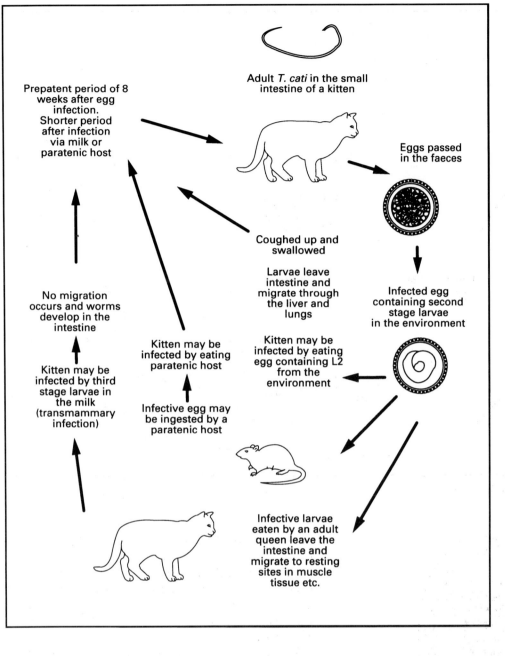

Prepatent period of 8 weeks after egg infection. Shorter period after infection via milk or paratenic host

Adult *T. cati* in the small intestine of a kitten

Eggs passed in the faeces

No migration occurs and worms develop in the intestine

Coughed up and swallowed

Larvae leave intestine and migrate through the liver and lungs

Infected egg containing second stage larvae in the environment

Kitten may be infected by third stage larvae in the milk (transmammary infection)

Kitten may be infected by eating paratenic host

Kitten may be infected by eating egg containing L2 from the environment

Infective egg may be ingested by a paratenic host

Infective larvae eaten by an adult queen leave the intestine and migrate to resting sites in muscle tissue etc.

Fig. 15.26 Life cycle of *Toxocara cati*.

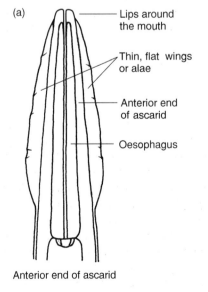

(a)

Lips around the mouth

Thin, flat wings or alae

Anterior end of ascarid

Oesophagus

Anterior end of ascarid

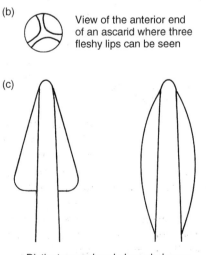

(b) View of the anterior end of an ascarid where three fleshy lips can be seen

(c)

Distinct arrow head shaped alae on the left of *Toxocara cati* compared with more tapered alae of *Toxascaris leonina* on the right

Fig. 15.27 Anterior end and alae of adult ascarid.

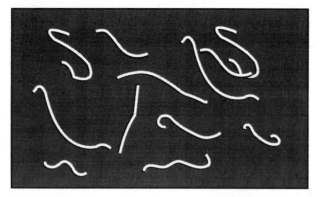

Fig. 15.28 Adult hookworms (*Uncinaria stenocephala*, approximately 1 cm long).

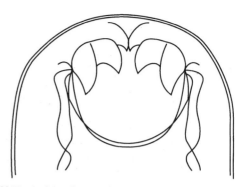

Fig. 15.29 Head of *Ancylostoma braziliense*, showing two pairs of teeth at the entrance to the buccal capsule. *Uncinaria stenocephala* has a similar sized buccal capsule but with cutting plates instead of teeth. *A. caninum* has three pairs of teeth.

then eat the damaged tissue. A heavy *Uncinaria* spp. burden may cause a dog to be thin and *Ancylostoma* spp. may cause anaemia. Eggs (Fig. 15.31) produced by the adult female worms are passed in the faeces.

The infective larvae of both worms may penetrate the skin. *Uncinaria* spp. larvae simply cause a dermatitis as the larvae are incapable of travelling further, whereas *Ancylostoma* spp. larvae may travel to the intestine and develop to adults. Bitches may infect their pups with *Ancylostoma* spp. larvae via their milk.

Whipworm. *Trichuris vulpis*, the whipworm of the dog, has a whiplike appearance (Fig. 15.32). The worms burrow into the mucosa of the large intestine, leaving the thicker caudal end in the intestinal lumen. A low burden is well tolerated but a heavy infection may be associated with a bloody, mucus-filled diarrhoea.

The eggs in which the larvae develop are characteristic (Fig. 15.33) and are covered in a thick shell which makes them resistant to damage in the environment. Eggs containing infective larvae may survive for several years in the

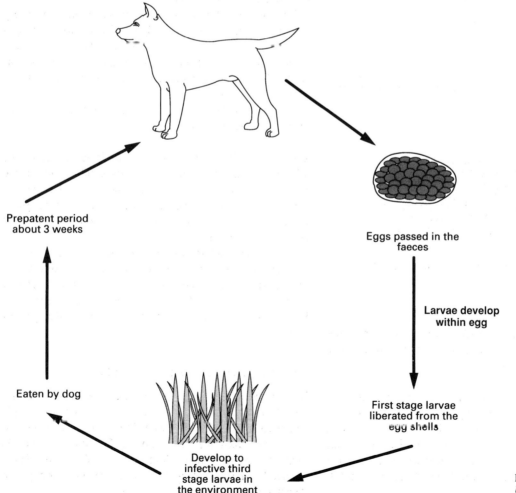

Prepatent period
about 3 weeks

Eaten by dog

Develop to
infective third
stage larvae in
the environment

Eggs passed in the
faeces

Larvae develop
within egg

First stage larvae
liberated from the
egg shells

Fig. 15.30 Life cycle of
Uncinaria stenocephala.

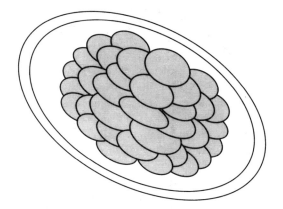

Fig. 15.31 Hookworm egg (approximately 70 μm long).

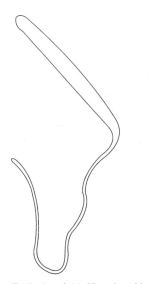

Fig. 15.32 Whipworm (*Trichuris vulpis*). Note the wide posterior end and the narrow anterior end normally buried in the mucosa of the large intestine (1–3 cm).

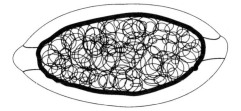

Fig. 15.33 *Trichuris* egg (approximately 70 μm long). Note plugs at both ends.

ground. *T. vulpis* therefore tends to cause problems when dogs have access to permanent grass runs but clinical signs are rarely seen in the UK.

The heart worm. *Dirofilaria immitis* does not occur in the UK but may be seen in dogs that are imported from warmer countries. The adult worms live in the heart and the immature larvae are known as microfilariae. These are dispersed in the host's blood and transmission occurs when a mosquito transfers the microfilariae from one host to another.

Bladder and liver worms (Capillaria spp.). Adult worms of *Capillaria plica* live in the bladder and so the eggs are passed in the urine of affected dogs. The eggs appear very like *Trichuris* eggs, but are smaller with less distinct plugs. Infection is rarely seen in the UK.

Capillaria hepatica is a parasite of rats, particularly wild rats. The adult worm lives in the liver of the host, where it lays its eggs. These are only released when the rat dies or is eaten by another animal. Cats, dogs and man may be infected, but this occurs very rarely.

Other *Capillaria* species specific to birds may cause diarrhoea in pigeons.

Lungworms. Aelurostrongylus abstrusus (cat lungworm). Cats become infected by eating a slug or snail containing the infective larvae. The adult worm lives within the lung tissue of the cat. Infection with many worms may cause coughing, but a few worms often go unnoticed.

Adult females produce larvae (rather than eggs) that are coughed up and swallowed. Diagnosis is confirmed by finding larvae in the faeces using the Baermann technique.

Angiostrongylus vasorum. Infection is acquired when a dog eats a snail containing the infective larvae. Transmission of this infection in England was confined to Cornwall and South Wales, but it is now being seen in southern England as well.

The slender adult worms live in the pulmonary artery of the dog and may cause signs of coughing and dyspnoea. The adult females produce eggs that travel to the alveoli, hatch and then penetrate through the alveolar walls. The larvae are then coughed up, swallowed and passed in the faeces.

Faeces may be examined for presence of the larvae using the Baermann technique.

Oslerus osleri (formerly Filaroides osleri). The adult worms live in small nodules at the bifurcation of the trachea (in dogs, particularly greyhounds). The nodules can be seen on endoscopy and they may cause coughing in some dogs but others tolerate their presence without showing symptoms.

The adult female worms produce larvae that are coughed up and swallowed. The life cycle is direct (i.e. the parasite passes directly from one host to the next without having to infect an alternative or intermediate host) and the bitch may infect her pups as she grooms them.

Diagnosis of nematode infections

It is important that faecal samples are fresh and are quickly picked up from the ground, otherwise the sample can become contaminated with free-living nematodes and their eggs from the environment. The main diagnostic methods are modified McMaster techniques to detect nematode eggs in faeces and the Baermann technique to detect larvae.

Treatment of nematode infections

Treatment of nematode infections is carried out in three main situations:

- Regular treatment to remove any infections that may have accumulated since the animal was last wormed. A broad-spectrum anthelmintic with additional cestocidal activity is often used. Adult dogs and cats will usually be treated at 3–6-month intervals.
- Control of *Toxocara* infections in puppies and kittens. Since these infections occur in the vast majority of litters it is normal to treat all puppies and kittens regularly.
- Treatment of an animal where the presence of an nematode infection has been diagnosed as the cause of a clinical problem. Here the product with the best activity against that infection will usually be chosen.

Protozoal parasites

Major protozoal parasites

Coccidia. Coccidia may cause marked diarrhoea in young animals, particularly lambs, birds and rabbits.

Rabbits may be infected with three *Eimeria* spp., all of which have the typical coccidian life cycle (Fig. 15.34).

- *Eimeria intestinalis* and *E. flavescens* infect the caecum, causing diarrhoea and emaciation.
- *E. stiedae* infects the bile ducts in the liver causing wasting, diarrhoea and excess urine production.

Diagnosis is based on finding oocysts present in the faeces (Fig. 15.35). Small rod-like organisms may be found in the faeces of sick rabbits; these are not coccidia and are not believed to be significant.

Treatment may be given in the rabbits' drinking water, for example using a sulphonamide. Control is based on making sure that the rabbits have clean bedding and that droppings and/or diarrhoea are not allowed to build up in the feeding area.

Isospora. This protozoan is also known as *Levineia*. Two species infect cats and another two infect dogs.

The animals are infected when they ingest either sporulated oocysts (oocysts are not sporulated until a few days after they were passed in the faeces) or infected intermediate hosts. Reproduction occurs in the cells lining the small intestine.

Infection usually associated with few clinical signs – but there may be transient diarrhoea. May cause severe diarrhoea in puppies and kittens.

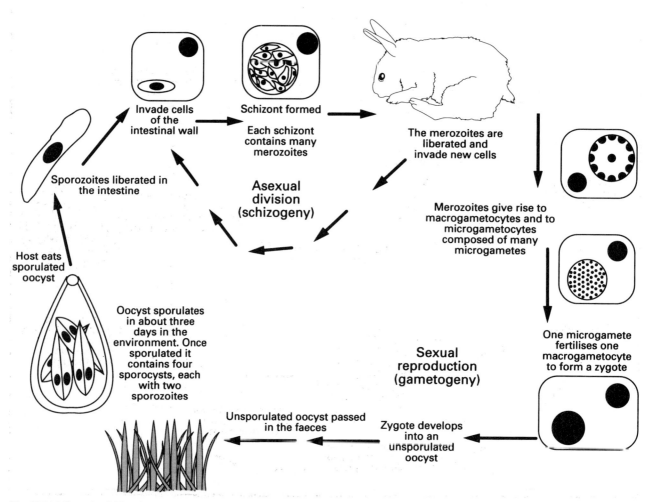

Fig. 15.34 Life cycle of *Eimeria* spp.

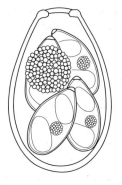

Fig. 15.35 Oocyst of *Eimeria* spp.

Cryptosporidium parvum. This is a small protozoan that parasitises epithelial cells in the small intestine. Both asexual and sexual reproduction occurs in the intestine and small oocysts, the result of sexual reproduction, are passed in the faeces. Infection occurs by ingesting sporulated oocysts; this has been associated with diarrhoea in young puppies and kittens and the young of other domestic animals. Humans may be infected, usually only causing a transient diarrhoea, though severe diarrhoea may be associated with infection in immunocompromised individuals.

Diagnosis is based on finding the oocysts (4.5–5 μm diameter) in the faeces. Identification may be assisted by staining with Ziehl–Neelsen, as the oocysts are acid fast, or by immunofluorescence techniques. There is currently no treatment for the infection.

Sarcocystis. This organism has a more complex life cycle than the coccidia and therefore is classified separately.

The intermediate hosts are ruminants, pigs or horses. Large unsightly cysts are formed in muscle, so infected meat is condemned. The final host for each species is the dog or the cat and the species name reflects the two hosts in the cycle: in *Sarcocystis ovicanis*, for example, sheep are intermediate hosts and dogs are final hosts.

Reproduction occurs in the small intestine without clinical signs. The oocysts, measuring approximately 10 × 15 μm, are already sporulated when passed.

Toxoplasma gondii. The final host for *T. gondii* is the cat (Fig. 15.36). Sexual reproduction occurs in the epithelial cells of the small intestine. Oocysts are produced that are passed in the faeces. The cat usually shows no sign of infection and normally, after excreting oocysts for about 10 days, becomes immune and stops production.

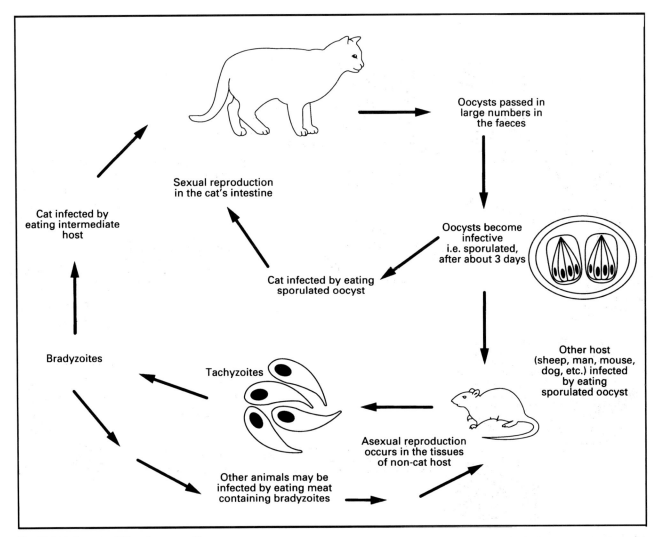

Fig. 15.36 Life cycle of *Toxoplasma gondii*.

Asexual reproduction occurs in the extra-intestinal (outside the intestine) tissue of almost any animal. Following ingestion of oocysts or asexual stages the sporozoites leave the intestine and travel to tissue, particularly muscle or brain. Here they divide to form **tachyzoites**. Once an immune response is started by the host these undergo slower division; they are then known as **bradyzoites**. These remain in the tissue in the hope that they will one day be eaten by a cat.

These cysts in tissue are minute and cause little problem except in certain circumstances:

- A ewe is infected for the first time during pregnancy. Some cysts may occur in the placenta and may cause abortion.
- A woman is infected for the first time during pregnancy, e.g. by eating meat containing bradyzoites or accidentally swallowing sporulated oocysts. Infection of the foetus may result and, depending on the stage of pregnancy, this may result in abortion, severe abnormalities or no clinical signs at all. Fortunately, infections during human pregnancy are not common. Further information and information leaflets can be obtained from the Toxoplasmosis Trust.
- Infection in humans may be associated with malaise and 'flu-like symptoms that vary in severity from individual to individual.
- Cysts in immunosuppressed individuals may once again begin to undergo rapid division and cause severe tissue lesions.

In order to try and prevent these infections occurring:

- Farmers are advised to prevent cats, particularly young cats, from getting into food stores intended for sheep. There is now a vaccine against *Toxoplasma* for sheep.
- Pregnant women are advised to take precautionary measures. For example, they should not clean out cat litter trays, they should wear gloves when gardening and they should ensure that all meat is thoroughly cooked before eating it.

There is no effective treatment to prevent oocyst shedding in the cat. Children that have been infected prenatally are treated with antibacterials to prevent any long-term effects.

It is now recognised that there is a separate parasite, *Neospora caninum*, that may cause incoordination in young dogs and abortion in cattle. In the past, infection was

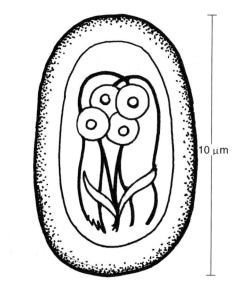

Fig. 15.37 Cyst of *Giardia* spp.

normally ascribed to *Toxoplasma gondii*. It is believed that the dog may be the final host for this parasite.

Hammondia. This is another protozoan parasite where the cat is the final host. Infection is not normally associated with clinical signs. Sexual reproduction occurs in the intestine of the cat and oocysts are produced that appear similar to those of *Toxoplasma*. The intermediate hosts for *Hammondia* are rodents, so the presence of these oocysts does not provide a human health risk.

Giardia spp. This flagellate protozoan may parasitise the small intestine of man and domestic animals. It is still unknown how important *Giardia* infection in pet animals is as a source of human infection, but it may cause death in cage birds such as cockatiels and budgerigars.

Infection may be asymptomatic or may be associated with transient or chronic diarrhoea. Diagnosis is based on demonstration of the cysts (Fig. 15.37), which are small (approximately 10 μm) and may be passed intermittently in the faeces. Even when a sample is positive, cysts may be present in low numbers, so a sensitive detection technique is used, such as centrifugal flotation using saturated zinc sulphate solution. The cysts can then be stained with Lugol's iodine to increase visibility. It is suggested that collecting samples for 3 days and pooling the sample may help overcome the intermittent excretion.

16

General nursing

S.Chandler

Artificial feeding

The importance of maintaining nutrition during recovery of patients from surgery or disease cannot be overemphasised, though in the past it has been sorely neglected. Convalescent periods can be radically reduced when adequate nutrition is provided. As relatively cheap feeding tubes are now readily available, tube feeding should be used more frequently when natural nutrition is impossible or contraindicated. It is important that the veterinary nurse be familiar with their management.

Artificial feeding (which is sometimes referred to as forced feeding) should only be instigated when all attempts to induce the animal to eat voluntarily have failed.

Anorexic patients may be tempted to eat by:

● Warming the food.
● Hand-feeding.
● Offering highly odorous foods.
● Offering favourite food (liaise with owners).
● Smearing food on their lips.
● Liquidising food.

Reasons for forced feeding are:

● Failure to entice voluntary eating.
● Physical inability (e.g. fractured jaw).
● Following injury or surgery to oral cavity, or where feeding is contraindicated (e.g. oesophageal trauma).

Methods of artificial feeding

Methods include:

● Placing food on back of tongue and encouraging the animal to swallow (Fig. 16.1), as in per os administration of medicines.
● Syringe feeding of liquid food.
● Tube feeding.

WARNING

Aspiration pneumonia is a real risk with syringe feeding. Ensure that the patient's head is in a natural position – *not* raised – and that the animal swallows between the administration of each bolus. Give 0.5–5 ml at a time, depending on the size of the patient.

Tube feeding

● Pharyngostomy tube (Fig. 16.2).
● Naso-oesophageal tube.
● Naso-gastric tube.
● Gastrostomy tube, surgically placed in the stomach (Fig. 16.3).
● Enterostomy tube (either duodenostomy or jejunostomy tube).

See also Chapter 8, p. 192.

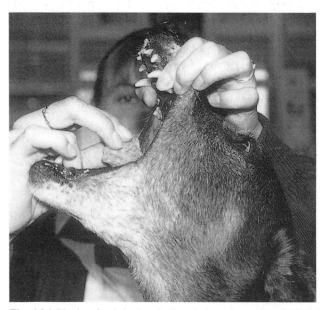

Fig. 16.1 Placing food, by hand, directly into the oral cavity may encourage animals to begin eating after a period of illness or major surgery.

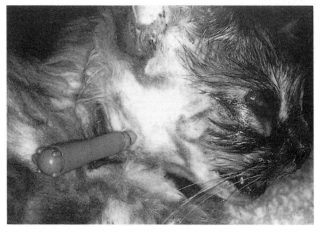

Fig. 16.2 A pharyngostomy tube (placed under general anaesthesia) in a cat with a fractured jaw.

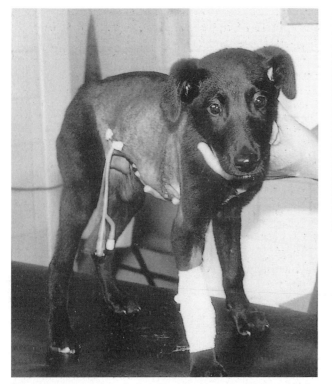

Fig. 16.3 A gastrostomy tube in a 12-week-old puppy after removal of an oesophageal foreign body. Partial thickness oesophageal damage necessitated tube placement. Tube feeding (including all water requirements) were maintained for 5 days. Antibiotics were also given by this route.

METHOD OF FEEDING USING A PHARYNGOSTOMY TUBE

(1) Restrain the patient.
(2) Remove the bung and flush the tube with 2–10 ml of water to ensure patency.
(3) Administer liquid diet. Initially, in the cat, 5–10 ml per feed. This may be increased up to 30 ml after the first 24 hours.
(4) Flush with a further 5–10 ml of water to clean the tube of food and ensure blockage does not occur before next feed.
(5) Replace bung, clean skin and re-bandage.

This procedure should be repeated at regular intervals. It is bad practice to administer the patient's total food requirement at one time since in many cases this would induce vomiting. Always ensure food is at least at room temperature, since cold food can also induce vomiting. Avoid this by feeding warm food little and often.

Diets should be balanced so that they supply the correct amount of all nutrients (including water) and meet the patient's calorific requirement (see later).

For all tube feeding, it is very important to keep the tube free from blockage. In practice the complete milks cause the

Management of these tubes is basically the same. All are indwelling and, with the exception of the naso-oesophageal and naso-gastric tubes, all are placed surgically under general anaesthesia.

Stomach tubing is not recommended for artificial feeding due to its repetitive nature and the stress caused to the patient.

Management of a pharyngostomy tube

This is a soft rubber or plastic tube. The tip of the tube usually lies in the caudal oesophagus, passing through the pharynx, and exits just caudal to the angle of the jaw. The tube is stitched in place and is bunged when not in use. It is bandaged to the patient's neck to prevent both patient interference and contamination of the tube.

Pharyngostomy tubes are most commonly used for cats with fractured jaws. If the injury is at, or caudal to, the pharynx, there is no indication for the use of a pharyngostomy tube. One of the other tubes would be more appropriate.

Equipment

● Use only liquid food (Table 16.1 and Fig. 16.4).
● Generally an adapter is required to attach the syringe to the tube, e.g. a spigot or a nozzled syringe.
● Water for flushing the tube (either sterile or, in some cases, tap water).

Table 16.1 Foods suitable for tube feeding

Food	Manufacturer
Concentrated liquidised tinned food	Various: Hills p/d Waltham concentration diet Iams/Eukanuba nutritional recovery diet
Semi-solid foods (need liquidising)	Hills a/d

Liquid complete foods:
  Reanimyl
  Concentrated Milk
  Fortal
	
	Virbac
	Waltham
	Arnolds

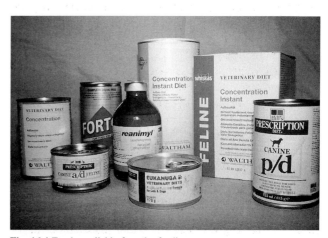

Fig. 16.4 Foods available for tube feeding.

fewest problems, having the added advantage of less preparation time, less mess and higher digestibility.

Some veterinary establishments recommend carbonated drinks to flush tubes, the 'bubbles' helping to loosen any solid food particles that collect on the inside of the feeding tube. This method should be used cautiously as large amounts of fizzy fluid can make patients feel unwell and possibly induce vomiting.

All liquidised foods should be the consistency of whole-fat milk to ensure easy passage down the tubes. Most tinned foods require a large amount of water added to them.

All the diets in Table 16.1 are concentrated and easily digested. This is important because normal dog and cat food when liquidised becomes bulk limiting, i.e. the amount of fluid food that needs to be fed to reach the patient's daily kilocalorie (kcal) requirement is enormous and cannot physically be administered over a 24-hour period without the risk of vomiting.

Calculation of kilocalorie requirements

This should be carried out for all tube-fed patients. The basic energy requirement (BER) is measured in metabolisable kcal/day (see Chapter 8, Nutrition) and calculations depend on the patient's bodyweight (in kg):

- Patients over 5 kg: BER = 30 × bodyweight + 70.
- Patients under 5 kg: BER = 60 × bodyweight.

Taking disease factors into the calculation:

- BER × disease factor = kcal requirement.

The factors are:

- Cage rest: 1.2.
- Surgery/trauma: 1.3.
- Multiple surgery: 1.5.
- Sepsis/cancer: 1.7.
- Burns: 2.0.

Geriatric nursing

Geriatric nursing involves nursing the ageing animal in both health and disease. Geriatric patients must be treated with extra care, for whatever reason they are admitted. They are less able to adapt to change and recover from medical or surgical interference more slowly (for each 5 years of a pet's age, allow 24 hours longer to recover).

The key to nursing the geriatric patient is good information (history, drugs), the provision of security (own blanket, etc.), comfort (soft bedding), the correct type of food and an adequate source of water.

The changes of old age can be physical or mental (Table 16.2). Many of the mental alterations are related to physical change, e.g. disorientation is made worse when the patient is blind or deaf. Ageing changes and the accumulation of any injuries the patient may have sustained result in a loss of functional reserve, i.e. organs of the body become less capable of dealing with extra demands placed on them for repair of tissue, assimilation of substances, etc.

Table 16.2 Physical and mental changes in geriatric animals

Physical	Mental
Greying of muzzle, etc.	Lowered response to stimuli
Thickening of the skin	Less adaptable
Coarse coat	Fussy about food
Loss of musculature	More likely to develop food
Loss of stamina and strength	preferences
Weakening of bone	Lower sensitivity to pain
Lowered tolerance to change	(questionable)
Loss of sight	Less interested in activity
Loss of hearing	Less obedient
Poor tolerance to lack of fluid intake	Disorientation
Impaired temperature regulation	
Arthritis and joint stiffness	
Higher susceptibility to infection	

Disease

Changes due to disease must be carefully distinguished from those of old age, although disease can become more obvious or affect a patient more rapidly when they become old. Very few sick, elderly patients suffer from a single disease. Many conditions are subtle and multiple. Commonly found disorders of geriatric animals include:

- Cancer.
- Chronic renal disease.
- Cardiac disease (cardiomyopathy).
- Osteoarthritis (degenerative joint disease – DJD).
- Cataracts.
- Dental disease.
- Constipation.
- Incontinence.

Incontinence is not always truly incontinence but rather where patients lose bladder muscle/sphincter tone. These patients cannot be left alone for long periods without the opportunity to urinate. They urinate in the house or while asleep and may appear incontinent to their owners.

Nursing considerations

Ensure that the patient's history is known. This includes any current treatment, the preferred food and conditions they suffer from. Remember that they may be suffering from diseases other than those for which they have been admitted. Specific conditions are dealt with in Chapter 17 (Medical Disorders and their Nursing). The following points are general guidelines.

Drugs

All patients should be weighed but it is particularly important to weigh the geriatric patient so that accurate drug dose calculations can be made. Drug dosage is the veterinary surgeon's responsibility but anaesthetic drugs may well be prepared by nursing staff and accurate calculations are essential. Young patients may have the capacity to survive mild anaesthetic overdosage; **geriatrics do not**.

Feeding

Geriatric patients generally need fewer calories but simply feeding them less can result in a lowered intake of protein, vitamins and minerals.

In the absence of any disease that requires dietary management, it is best to feed a highly digestible, well-balanced proprietary food. There are many available and some companies produce diets specifically formulated for the older dog. Cats tend to stay more active for longer and special diets are less available. To avoid digestive upsets, any changes in diet should be introduced gradually. Lack of interest in food is rarely due to true anorexia in the hospitalised geriatric patient. It is more likely that the patient finds the amount offered too great, has dental disease resulting in pain or has difficulty in standing when eating. All can be simply resolved. Split total intake into two or three small meals, check teeth and assist food intake by hand-feeding or supporting the patient.

Obesity

This is common in the geriatric patient and its treatment is usually a case of client education. Stress to the owners that excess weight is potentially *dangerous* to their pet because extra strain is placed on the heart, kidneys, liver and musculoskeletal system in obese patients. Try to persuade owners that their pet would be happier and healthier if it lost weight. Give them target weights to aim for but be careful to check all diets with a veterinary surgeon to ensure that increased exercise (if possible) and diet changes are not contraindicated.

Water

> **WARNING**
>
> *Do not restrict water intake in the geriatric patient unless they are vomiting.* This is particularly important in relation to the withdrawal of fluids prior to surgery.

No patient should be deprived of water for more than an hour before induction of anaesthesia. Water does *not* need to be withdrawn the night before; this can be extremely dangerous. Younger patients will tolerate the insult but geriatric patients can be pushed over the fine dividing line of renal compromise and may well suffer irreparable damage to renal function that will only be noticeable weeks later.

If vomiting is present, ensure that intravenous fluids are administered.

Exercise

Little and often is recommended. Elderly dogs enjoy 'pottering'. Even hospitalised dogs should be given time to wander, maybe in an outside run. Frequent walks will help to exercise stiff joints and ensure plenty of opportunities to urinate (which might save time on cleaning out kennels).

Take special care if the patient is blind or deaf.

Defecation and urination

Check frequency of defecation. Constipation is more common in the elderly dog and cat.

Observe urination to ensure adequate production of urine, with normal colour and passage (i.e. no straining). Report any difficulty in urination and defecation to a veterinary surgeon as well as any concern about urine production in relation to water intake (e.g. lots being drunk with little urine excreted).

Bedding and kennelling

Blankets and soft bedding should be provided, along with foam mattresses for those with osteoarthritis. Keep geriatrics out of draughts and if possible somewhere not too noisy.

Geriatrics may become cold easily, especially their extremities. If in doubt, check their rectal temperature.

Grooming

Groom elderly patients regularly, as they are less likely to keep themselves clean. It helps to give a feeling of well-being and provides an opportunity to check the coat, skin and to clean discharges from eyes and nose. The human contact is also beneficial.

If the patient has lost its sight or hearing, move slowly and talk reassuringly at all times. This will help to prevent the bite of surprise that elderly dogs so often attempt when suddenly touched or frightened.

Vaccination

Geriatric animals are less responsive to vaccination – they probably have sufficient acquired immunity. However, annual boosters are still advisable.

Convalescence

This will take more time and effort than in younger patients. Have patience and allow a longer period for convalescence.

Maintenance of normal body temperature is especially important pre-, intra- and post-operatively. Thermoregulation in geriatrics is often compromised.

If patients are discharged before they have fully recovered, inform the owners that it will take some time for a pet to complete its recovery. Adequate water intake is very important; ensure that patients can reach water bowls and add water to food if necessary. Exercise should be gentle. Physiotherapy, especially massage, may be used to improve circulation to the extremities.

Care of the vomiting patient

Vomiting (**emesis**) is the forcible ejection of contents of the *stomach* through the mouth. It should not be confused with regurgitation, which is the return of undigested food from the *oesophagus* (see Chapter 17, p. 440 Medical disorders and their nursing).

Nursing of the vomiting patient can be very straightforward (e.g. in the case of scavenging) or much more complex (e.g. as a result of metabolic imbalances). Some of the common causes of vomiting are shown in Table 16.3.

Mechanical and functional disorders

Patients suffering from mechanical or functional disorders are usually admitted for surgical correction of the condition. Dietary management is usually simple.

Foreign bodies

Food is generally withheld until surgery has been carried out. If water induces vomiting, it too should be withheld but replaced by intravenous fluids. Most vomiting patients have some degree of dehydration and in these cases an intravenous drip is set up to provide fluid.

The reintroduction of food and water after surgery will vary in each individual case but the following are basic guidelines.

In some cases nothing will be allowed by mouth for 24–48 hours. Intravenous fluid therapy must be continued to supply calculated daily requirements. Feeding during this time should not be neglected and hopefully some form of enteral feeding will be available, e.g. gastrostomy tube (Fig. 16.3), naso-oesophageal tube or jejunostomy tube (surgically placed into the small intestine).

Tube feeding allows the surgical site a chance to heal whilst still providing a route for nutrition, which is essential to rapid recovery.

If fluids by mouth are allowed, initially offer small amounts frequently (50–100 ml every hour). If these are not vomited, then the amounts can be increased slowly over the next 8 hours. Intravenous fluids may be continued during this time as total fluid requirements will not be achieved initially.

Reintroduction of feed begins once fluids are retained, usually over 24–72 hours. Food offered will vary: usually it will be a bland diet of liquidised or semi-moist chunks of food, offered little and often. Bland foods include chicken, fish or a commercially prepared diet.

Similar protocol is used in the management of pyloric stenosis. In this case food will initially be very well liquidised.

Megaoesophagus

Patients with megaoesophagus regurgitate rather than vomit. Food becomes lodged in the oesophagus cranial to a stricture or narrowing, so that only a limited amount of food reaches the stomach.

Dietary management (even after surgery, if performed) will involve liquidised/semi-solid food fed from a height (Fig. 16.5). Feeding from a height helps to prevent

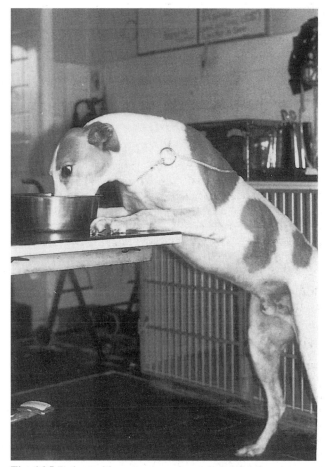

Fig. 16.5 Patient with a megaoesophagus being fed from table-height to aid passage of food to the stomach.

Table 16.3 Causes of vomiting

Mechanical/functional disorders	Metabolic disorders	Miscellaneous
Pyloric stenosis	Kidney disease (nephritis)	Motion sickness
Pyloric stricture	Liver disease	Scavenging
Gastric foreign bodies	Metabolic alkalosis	Pain
Other gastrointestinal	Electrolyte imbalances,	Drug reactions
foreign bodies	e.g. hyponatraemia, hypokalaemia	Neurological disorders
Intussusception	Diabetes mellitus	Food allergies
	Toxaemia	Distasteful smells
	Poisoning	

Table 16.4. Recognition of dehydration*		
Grade	**Percent dehydration**	**Clinical signs**
Slight	<5%	Not detectable
Mild	5–6%	Slight decrease in skin turgor
Mild	6–8%	Delay in skin fold return Slight increase in capillary refill time (CRT) Dry mucous membranes Sunken eyes
Moderate	10–12%	Tenting of the skin Sunken eyes Increased CRT Tachycardia Cold extremities Early signs of shock
Severe	12–15%	Clinical signs of shock, i.e. tachycardia, weak pulse, pale mucous membranes and cold extremities. These may lead to coma and death.

*See also p. 572.

regurgitation and the possible development of aspiration pneumonia – gravity helps the passage of food to the stomach. Passage of food can also be aided after feeding by gentle coupage whilst the patient is in an upright position (see p. 407).

Metabolic disorders

Patients that vomit due to metabolic disorders are generally more challenging to the nurse. If vomiting has been prolonged, they will be dehydrated and require fluid therapy in combination with other treatment. The percentage of dehydration can be estimated clinically (Table 16.4).

It is pleasant for the patient to have moist cotton wool wiped around the mucous membranes of the mouth, especially if water has been withdrawn. This not only freshens the mouth but also removes excess saliva.

If water is not vomited, oral electrolyte fluids may be useful (Chapter 22 gives more details about fluid therapy).

Anti-emetic drugs, such as metaclopramide, are frequently prescribed. They must be administered by intravenous administration as per os is usually contraindicated in these patients. For continuous effect, the veterinary surgeon may request drugs to be placed in the drip fluid.

When vomiting ceases, water and then food can be reintroduced.

Reintroduction of food

The following is a general plan for the reintroduction of food to a patient that has been vomiting. It assumes that water does not cause vomiting. *If at any stage vomiting reoccurs, return to the previous day's protocol.*

Day 1
Offer small amounts of bland food 3–4 times daily. Total amount offered should equal one-quarter to one-half of normal daily requirement.

Day 2
Offer small amounts of bland food frequently, to total one-half to three-quarters of daily requirement.

Days 3–6
As for days 1 and 2 but total amount offered should be equal to normal requirement.

Days 7–14
Reintroduce normal diet by mixing increasing amounts with the bland diet.

Patients that have had a single acute vomiting episode due to scavenging will need to be starved for 24–48 hours before the reintroduction of food. In these cases the above regime can be followed and can be given as advice to owners over the telephone. For any other reason it is only a guideline. Specific types of food may be required, or longer periods of starvation may be necessary. A veterinary surgeon will give instructions on the course to be followed.

General points to remember

- Nausea is unpleasant. It can be identified in dogs and cats by:
  Restlessness.
  Salivation.
  Repeated swallowing.
  Retching.
  Bring these signs to the attention of the veterinary surgeon.
- Clean away any excess vomitus and clean the mouth. If not contraindicated, offer small amounts of cool, fresh water (10–15 ml) to allow rinsing of the mouth.
- Handle gently. Lift only if absolutely necessary, ensuring that no pressure is placed on the patient's abdomen.
- Hand-feeding and encouragement may be required during the recovery period.
- If syringe feeding of fluids is instituted at any time, remember the potential for the development of aspiration pneumonia. It is surprisingly easy to cause pneumonia, especially in smaller dogs and cats.
- When patients are discharged, give the owners **written** instructions regarding the type of food, the amounts to be offered, its consistency and the method of feeding.

The soiled patient

Many hospitalised patients become soiled at some time during their stay. It is the nurse's responsibility to ensure that all soiling is cleaned efficiently, effectively and quickly.

Regular walking of in-patients may seem time consuming but it may conserve time spent in cleaning kennels and soiled patients. Cats must be supplied with litter trays; check with owners regarding types of litter used, as some cats are fussy.

Animals may become soiled by:

- Urine.
- Faeces.
- Blood.
- Vomit.
- Food.
- Other body fluids.

Reasons for soiling include:

- Confinement to a small area.
- Disturbed routine.
- Medical or surgical condition.
- Untrained puppies.
- Recumbency.

Action when soiling occurs

(1) Clean as quickly as possible.
(2) Choose shampoos carefully. Take into consideration patient's coat length, reason for hospitalisation and area to be cleaned or bathed. Chlorhexidine gluconate or povidone-iodine are preferable if the patient has any surgical or open wounds. Dry dog shampoos are available, but they are inadequate if soiling has occurred.
(3) Once the area has been cleaned, dry it thoroughly. Most patients will tolerate a hair dryer after a towel rub down. All knots in the coat should be removed since they may harbour faeces. Conditioners will make the process much less tiresome for nursing staff and the patient, especially in long-haired breeds.
(4) Whilst grooming, check for any area of soreness, especially if the patient is recumbent. If necessary, clip hair away from these areas.
(5) It is best to clip heavily contaminated areas, especially if further contamination is expected (e.g. under drainage tubes). Ensure that client permission has been given. White petroleum jelly can be applied around these areas after clipping, preventing soreness and to make cleaning easier.
(6) Cats generally keep themselves very clean. If bathing is necessary, use mild shampoos and avoid products based on coal tar (phenol is poisonous to cats – see Chapter 3 dealing with poisons). Regular grooming of hospitalised long-haired cats is essential.
(7) Cats with oral lesions or fractured jaws are unable to clean themselves and regular cleaning of the lips, chin and paws will be required.

Enemata

An enema is a liquid substance placed into the rectum and colon of a patient. The enema is not intended to flush colonic contents but to distend the rectum and distal colon gently, initiating normal expulsive reflexes.

Reasons for performing an enema

Emptying the rectum

- To relieve constipation or impaction.
- As preparation for radiographic studies. The colon and rectum overlie abdominal structures and will obscure them if they are not emptied.
- As part of a radiographic contrast study.
- To enable the administration of drugs.

As a diagnostic aid

Barium sulphate enemata can be given to outline the rectal and colonic walls. Remember that the patient needs to evacuate the barium after radiography – a quick retreat to the outside is strongly advised!

Administering drugs

The colon has a large capacity for absorption. For this reason it is a good route for the administration of soluble drugs. Although, it is rarely used in veterinary medicine due to lack of patient co-operation.

Solutions used for enema administration

The choice of solution depends on the purpose of the enema.

Water

Warm tap water is the preferred solution. It is cheap, readily available, non-toxic and non-irritant. In addition, any cleaning of the perianal area is reasonably straightforward.

Liquid paraffin

This is readily available and quite cheap. Cleaning the patient after the enema can be difficult since liquid paraffin is oil-based and not water-soluble. The patient needs to be bathed with shampoo to remove this substance.

Mineral oil

This suffers the same disadvantages as liquid paraffin and is more expensive. However, oil-based substances are an advantage when treating a constipated patient. The oil helps to soften and lubricate the faecal masses and allows easier evacuation of the bowel.

Saline (phosphate enema)

This is usually available as manufactured sachets with phosphate included. They promote defecation by being osmotically active, promoting water retention in the colon. These enemata should be used with care in small (below 15 kg) and young patients because their excessive use can result in unwanted absorption of certain ions resulting in system toxicity.

Ready-to-use mini enemata

A proprietary brand of miniature enema is introduced into the rectum by an attached nozzle. It is extremely useful in cats, the procedure being no more stressful than using a rectal thermometer.

Miscellaneous substances

- Glycerine and water.
- Olive oil and water.
- Obstetrical lubricant.

These variations are all more expensive and have no advantages over solutions already mentioned.

Equipment

The basic equipment is shown in Fig. 16.6. It includes enema solution, gloves, lubricant (e.g. K-Y jelly) and any of the following: can and tubing, Higginson syringe, prepared barium bag, syringe and catheter.

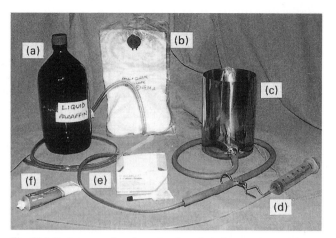

Fig. 16.6 Basic range of equipment and products for carrying out an enema. (a) Liquid paraffin. (b) Prepared barium. (c) Can and tubing. (d) Syringe and catheter. (e) Microlax. (f) Lubricating jelly.

ADMINISTRATION OF AN ENEMA

Table 16.5 gives guidance of the volumes of solution. The method for dogs, which requires two people, is as follows.

(1) Prepare all equipment
(2) The assistant restrains the patient in a suitable area, preferably outside where cleaning will be easier.
(3) Lubricate the end of the tube or nozzle.
(4) Elevate the patient's tail and place the tube into the anus. Twist gently until access to the rectum is achieved (this is easy in the dog but occasionally more difficult in the cat).
(5) Advance the tube into the rectum.
(6) Stand to the side of the patient and allow fluid to run into the rectum by gravity.
(7) Allow the patient free exercise to evacuate bowels.

Table 16.5 Enema solutions and volumes

Solution	Volume used (ml/kg)	Frequency
Water	5–10	Every 20–30 minutes if necessary
Liquid paraffin	2–3	Every 1–2 hours
Saline solution	1–2	Do not repeat for 12 hours
Barium sulphate	5–10	Not necessary

The recumbent patient

An animal that is lying down and unable to rise is described as recumbent. A large number of conditions might result in recumbency, the more common being:

- Fractures (e.g. pelvis, limbs).
- Spinal trauma (e.g. disc protrusion).
- Electrolyte imbalances, head injuries, shock.
- Weakness due to medical disease (e.g. Cushing's syndrome, cardiac disease).
- Neurological disease (e.g. coma).

Kennelling

Bedding

Bed the patient on thick, waterproof (PVC-covered) foam mattresses, with 'Vetbed' or similar on the top. If these are unavailable use thick layers of newspaper with blankets on top. Beanbags, although very comfortable, become soiled very easily and are difficult to clean; they are normally impractical in the hospital situation.

Size

Previously active animals attempt to drag themselves around (especially fracture and spinal cases in which pain has been relieved). The kennel should be large enough for such a patient to lie in lateral recumbency comfortably, but not so big that it has room to cause damage to itself.

Position

Most recumbent patients benefit from being nursed in a kennel sited in an area of activity. This stimulates them and relieves boredom since nursing staff inevitably talk to them more frequently. Ensure kennels are not in direct sunlight, since these patients may be unable to move to a shady area.

Food and water

Ensure that both food and water are within easy reach. Patients who are recumbent due to a medical condition may well be depressed and hand-feeding may be necessary.

Patients who fail to drink sufficiently can have water added to their food or be encouraged to drink by syringing water into the side of their mouths.

Most recumbent patients require a concentrated, highly digestible diet to meet the extra nutritional needs of stress due to kennelling or continuing tissue repair. Highly digestible diets have the added advantage of producing less faecal material. The energy requirement supplied by carbohydrates is generally lower during recumbency and the amount of carbohydrates offered may need reducing. Note, however, that ill animals may have an *increased* nutrient requirement, since these are necessary for tissue repair.

If the recumbent patient fails to eat, seek advice from the owner regarding preferences and favourite foods.

Obesity may be an existing problem or weight may be gained during the period of recumbency due to less energy being used. It may be necessary to introduce reducing diets, but only in consultation with the veterinary surgeon.

Urination and defecation

If possible, recumbent patients should be taken outside. The change of environment and fresh air are beneficial to their mental attitude. In addition, natural urination and defecation are always preferable to catheterisation and enemata. Help patients to stand since many are unwilling to urinate lying down. Towel support is useful (Fig. 16.7); even tetra/quadraplegics can be managed in this way, using crossed towels to support the chest. When an animal is supported, apply gentle pressure to the bladder to encourage urination (Fig. 16.8).

Indwelling catheters can be used. They are beneficial in keeping the patient dry by preventing soiling from urine overflow 24 hours a day.

In bitches, Foley catheters with a bag attached have the added advantage of enabling urine output to be measured.

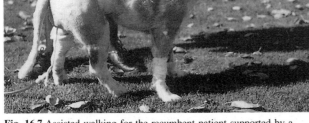

Fig. 16.7 Assisted walking for the recumbent patient supported by a towel. This method can be adapted using crossed towels over the chest when tetraplegia is present.

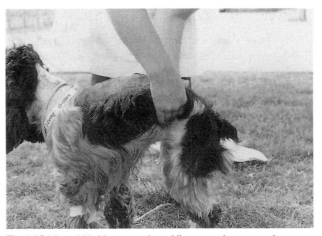

Fig. 16.8 Manual bladder expression whilst supporting a recumbent patient

In dogs, plastic dog catheters can be sutured to the prepuce or catheterisation can be carried out 2–3 times daily. There are also Foley catheters made from silicone that can be passed up the male urethra and remain in the bladder in exactly the same manner as the latex Foley (see p. 414) The silicone is so smooth that the catheter advances up the curved male urethra without the aid of a stylet, although wire guide stylets are available and may make the procedure even easier.

Cats' bladders can generally be manually expressed although catheterisation may also be performed.

Ensure a record of defecation is kept. It is easy for 3–5 days of non-production to go unnoticed. If the patient becomes constipated, a laxative may be required.

Any diarrhoea in the recumbent patient increases the risk of sores, infection in any wounds, fly-strike in the summer and discomfort to the patient. Inform the veterinary surgeon. Clip excess hair in the perianal/anal area.

Decubitus ulcers and urine scalding

Prevention

It is better to prevent both decubitus ulcers (bed sores, Fig. 16.9) and urine scalding, rather than treat them after they have occurred.

- The use of soft bedding with absorbable blankets (e.g. 'Vetbed'), together with regular turning of the patient (every 4 hours), will help to lessen the occurrence of sores.
- Bony prominences are most likely to suffer (e.g. elbows and ischial wings). These areas can be padded with foam rings from the top of tablet pots (Fig. 16.10) or the patient can be encouraged to lie laterally for *short* periods (a balance between lateral and sternal recumbency needs to be found – see Hypostatic pneumonia, below).
- Massage is beneficial and can be performed while the patient is recumbent.
- Slings to raise patients for longer periods are used in the US and at larger veterinary establishments in the UK (Fig. 16.11).

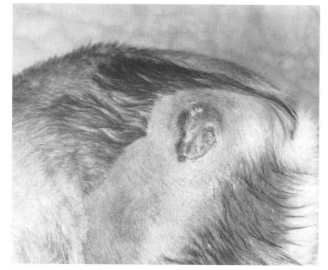

Fig. 16.9 Decubitus ulcer on the skin overlying the ilium.

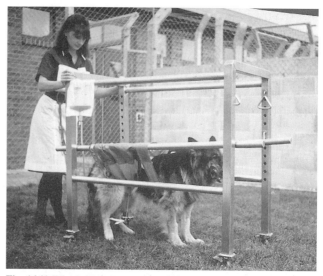

Fig. 16.11 Wheeled 'total support' walking frame systems assist mobility of heavier patients and enable effective physical therapy with the patient in a normal walking position. (The urinary catheter in this figure has been clamped during motion to prevent back-flow of urine whilst the collection bag is suspended above the bladder!).

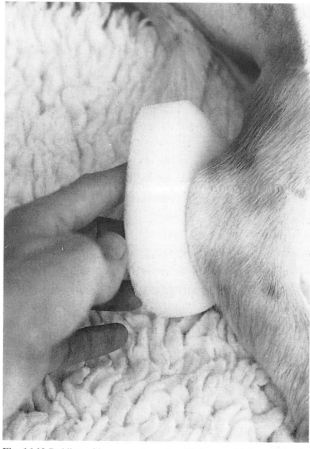

Fig. 16.10 Padding of bony prominences with foam can help to prevent occurrence of decubitus ulcers.

- Catheterisation (indwelling or repeated) enables bladder drainage without soiling. Otherwise assisted walking is essential to provide opportunities for urination.
- Waterbeds may be useful but are rarely used in the UK.

Action

Any patients which are dirtied by urine should be checked for the presence of urine scalds. They begin as innocent-looking red patches and, if treated at this stage, are very easily managed. There is no excuse for them getting worse if nursing care is adequate.

Urine scalding is relieved by:

- Regular washing with a mild antiseptic shampoo (e.g. dilute chlorhexidine gluconate or povidone-iodine). Both must be rinsed off thoroughly.
- Catheterisation.
- Clipping of hair and the application of soothing healing or barrier creams.

Decubitus ulcers are far more serious and can be extremely difficult to resolve.

Treatment:

(1) Clip the area around the sore.
(2) Clean with a mild antiseptic solution (e.g. dilute povidone-iodine or chlorhexidine gluconate).
(3) Dry thoroughly.
(4) Apply an appropriate cream.
(5) If it is summer, and the position of the ulcer allows, cover with a dressing to prevent fly strike and contamination.
(6) Consider using a full-length Robert Jones bandage.

WARNING

Hardening of areas prone to decubitus ulcers with spirit is *not* recommended.

Hypostatic pneumonia

Hypostatic pneumonia is caused by the pooling of blood and a consequent decrease in viability of the dependent lung. It is more likely to occur in an old, sick and debilitated animal that has been in lateral recumbency for a long period. Turning the patient at least every 4 hours – 24 hours a day – is essential nursing. Encourage sternal recumbency by using sandbags, water/sand-filled containers or X-ray cradles and remember to support the head.

Regular **coupage** (the external slapping of the thorax with cupped hands) 4–5 times daily for 5 minutes will improve thoracic circulation; by promoting coughing it also aids removal of secretions that build up in the bronchial tree. *Check with a veterinary surgeon before using coupage* to ensure that there are no contraindications such as fractured ribs.

WARNING

It is important to realise that serious secondary chest infections may result if hypostatic pneumonia is allowed to develop. This alone can cause *death*.

If hypostatic pneumonia with a secondary infection is present, continue all the above guidelines for prevention. In addition, treatment (e.g. antibiotics) will probably be prescribed.

Signs of hypostatic pneumonia are:

● Fast/frequent shallow breathing.
● Increased respiratory effort.
● Moist noises when breathing, possibly even gurgling.
● Depressed attitude.

If you suspect hypostatic pneumonia inform a veterinary surgeon immediately. Auscultation of the lung fields and radiography may be required to confirm the diagnosis.

Passive physiotherapy

Physiotherapy helps to maintain and improve peripheral circulation. It is of benefit to all recumbent patients, even if only for the extra human contact and attention.

Massage

This is particularly useful for the limbs. Massage from the toes towards the body to encourage venous return to the heart.

Supported exercise

Towel-walking is the most common (and cheapest) method. Make sure that adequate staff are available, as both the patient and the staff member can be injured if the patient is heavy.

Hydrotherapy

Swimming is very useful physiotherapy for dogs (cats generally do not appreciate it!). Small dogs can be swum in large sinks and baths in the hospital; larger patients need pools. Swimming enables patients to move their limbs freely without weight-bearing forces.

Check the temperature of the water before immersing the patient. *Constant* support and observation are essential to prevent panic and possible drowning.

Passive joint movement

Manually moving joints within their normal range helps to prevent stiffness and improves circulation.

Coupage

As previously described.

Body temperature

Recumbent patients expend very little energy; therefore heat production is lower than normal. Body temperature will frequently fall to a subnormal level. Blankets to cover the patient may be sufficient. Other heating methods include:

● Veterinary duvet-type covers with reflective filling.
● Veterinary instant heat pads, which should be wrapped initially: when activated, they heat to 52°C.
● Hot water-bottles, which should be wrapped to prevent burning of the patient.
● Heated waterbeds – use only if the patient is very debilitated and will not bite or scratch. They are expensive pieces of equipment.
● Bubble packaging – cheap and effective.
● Silver foil is good for extremities. Remove if patients become active, especially young ones (it is 'edible').
● Infrared lamps.
● Incubators (see p. 11).

WARNING

Electrically heated beds are *not* recommended unless the patient is under *constant supervision*. Some varieties have been implicated in causing serious burns when patients were placed directly on top of them. A blanket should always be between the heated pad and the patient.

Home nursing

Recumbent patients are generally managed in a hospital environment. Some will inevitably be recumbent for a longer period and may be nursed at home. Most owners are quite capable of learning how to nurse their own pet but remember that tasks which come automatically to a nurse need to be pointed out to an owner. It is helpful to write clear instructions to which owners can refer once they are home. Reassure owners that they can phone at any time if they are worried. Arrange weekly checks at the surgery to check for signs of decubitus ulcers, urine scalding or hypostatic pneumonia.

Comatosed patient

In this context, 'comatosed' is interpreted as a long-term coma rather than simple recovery from anaesthesia. This may occur in conditions such as tetanus, neurological disease or after major convulsions. In reality these patients are rarely nursed in general practice – they really need an intensive care unit and a large number of personnel.

The nursing of a comatosed patient is essentially similar to that for a recumbent one and all the nursing points made for the care of the recumbent patient can be implemented for the comatosed patient – with the exception of eating, drinking and exercise. In addition, the following points should be considered when nursing the comatosed patient:

- Keep a patent airway – pull the tongue forward and consider endotracheal intubation.
- Clean any secretions from the oral cavity – use a sucker or swabs or lower the head to encourage drainage by gravity.
- Monitor at 15-minute intervals:
  - temperature, pulse and respiratory rate and rhythm; mucous membrane colour;
  - capillary refill time;
  - urine output;
  - drip rates;
  - drug administration.

Constant 24-hour observation is essential for the comatosed patient.

Urinary catheterisation

A catheter is a tubular, usually flexible instrument passed through body channels for the withdrawal of fluids from (or the introduction of fluids into) a body cavity.

Reasons for urinary catheterisation

To obtain a (sterile) urine sample when:

- A patient will not micturate when required (this may be because the patient is only at the surgery for short periods, e.g. at consultation, or timed urine samples are required, e.g. water deprivation test).
- Obtaining a midstream urine sample (MUS) is impossible because the amount produced during exercise is little (e.g. the male dog that squirts 2 ml at every tree).
- A culture and sensitivity examination is requested (it is essential that urine is collected in a sterile manner for this examination: MUS samples become contaminated at the prepuce and vulva and provide meaningless results).

To empty the urinary bladder:

- Before abdominal, vaginal and urethral surgery.
- Before a pneumocystogram.
- When there is a partial obstruction or inability to urinate but a catheter can be passed into the bladder (e.g. due to prostatic enlargement).

To introduce contrast agents for radiographic procedures.

To maintain constant, controlled bladder drainage (indwelling catheters):

- In the recumbent or incontinent patient to prevent soiling.
- After bladder surgery, to avoid over-distension of the bladder, thereby reducing tension on the suture line and helping to provide optimum healing conditions for the operative site.

In **hydropropulsion** (the use of water pressure to dislodge particles causing an obstruction: a urinary catheter is placed caudal to the particle and water pressure is used to dislodge the calculi from the urethra back into the bladder). Hydropropulsion can be used to relieve a partial blockage in an emergency situation. It is nearly always followed by surgery (e.g. cystotomy or urethrostomy).

To maintain a patent urethra:

- In male cats suffering from feline lower urinary tract disease (FLUTD) – (a catheter may be placed to maintain bladder drainage whilst treatment or diet is initiated; catheter placement also allows flushing of the bladder with solutions which may dissolve struvite crystals, e.g. Walpole's solution, although this is an older technique which is now rarely used).
- Where dysuria or anuria is present but surgery is delayed due to the patient being in a poor condition for surgery (e.g. raised blood urea levels, electrolyte imbalance, etc.).

To monitor urine output:

- Where a patient with renal compromise is on large volumes of intravenous fluids.
- If the patient is in intensive care.
- After renal surgery to ensure adequate production of urine.

N.B. Minimum urine output = 1–2 ml/kg bodyweight/ hour.

- Introduction of drugs.

Complications associated with catheterisation

Complications which might arise include infective cystitis, reactive cystitis, urethral damage, failure to catheterise the urethra, resistance by the patient, blockage of indwelling catheters or removal of indwelling catheters by the patient. Reasons for these complications are described below, and Table 16.6 outlines methods of preventing them and the action to be taken should they arise.

Infection

Urinary tract infection (UTI) can easily be caused by catheterisation if bacteria present in the urethra are pushed into the bladder by the catheter. In most circumstances the bacteria are rapidly eliminated and cause no further concern. The risk of infection is increased when:

- The bladder is traumatised.
- A preputial or vaginal discharge is present.

Table 16.6 Complications associated with catheterisation

	Prevention	Action
Infection	Use only new or re-sterilised catheters. Plastic catheters should only be re-sterilised once. Use sterile gloves to handle catheters or employ the 'no touch' technique described for dog catheterisation. Use sterile lubricants. Clean penis or vulva thoroughly before catheterisation; clip surrounding hair if necessary. Catheterisation should be carried out in a clean environment, not in the patient's kennel. Ensure that systemic antibiotics are prescribed by the veterinary surgeon. A single (long-acting) dose may be sufficient after just one catheterisation of a healthy patient. Patients with indwelling catheters should receive systemic antibiotics whilst catheterised and continue the course for 5–10 days after removal.	If infection becomes evident, treatment will consist of systemic antibiotics and, in some cases, soluble antibiotics flushed directly into the bladder.
Cystitis after catheterisation	Gentle introduction of the catheter – no force should be necessary. Use of lubricants is beneficial – they help to limit the epithelial damage to the urethral mucosa, thereby reducing inflammation. Trauma is less likely if an experienced person catheterises debilitated patients.	With indwelling catheters there is inevitably some degree of cystitis after removal of the catheter. If it is significant: * Encourage the patient to increase its fluid intake, either as water or by adding water to the food. * Walk the patient frequently to allow urination; observe colour and amount of urine passed.
Urethral damage	*Never* use force. Use adequate lubrication. If an obstruction or difficulty occurs, stop and inform a senior member of staff.	If trauma caused by catheterisation is suspected, a veterinary surgeon will have to decide what further action is to be taken. Minor trauma will be treated with a course of antibiotics.
Failure to catheterise the urethra in the bitch	The only prevention is to gain experience in bitch catheterisation, which can only be achieved with practice. The easiest way for the student nurse to appreciate the position of the urethral orifice is the use of a lighted speculum to provide viewed introduction of the catheter.	If catheterisation of the cervix does occur, remove the catheter and begin again with a new one.
Patient resistance		Sedate or, in extreme cases, anaesthetise the patient.
Blockage of indwelling catheters	General hygiene and cleaning. Encourage increased water intake (this helps to maintain a continuous flow of urine through the catheter). If bags are attached, check regularly to ensure that urine is able to drain freely.	Flush with sterile saline or water.

- Indwelling catheters are used.
- The patient is immunosuppressed, i.e. its immune system is compromised in some way and the body's natural defences are not operating correctly.

WARNING

Any urinary tract infection is potentially serious. Prevention is better than cure!

Cystitis after catheterisation

This is associated with indwelling catheters. It is rarely seen otherwise, unless repeated catheterisation has been carried out.

Urethral damage

This is most likely to occur in the male dog, due to the ischial curve of the urethra – some epithelial damage is inevitable as the catheter is passed around the curve. (This is why a small amount of blood may be present in the tip of the catheter on removal from the urethra.)

Failure to catheterise the urethra

Failure to catheterise the urethra may occur in the bitch if the urethral orifice is passed and the catheter cannot be advanced because it meets the cervix. Catheterisation of the cervix is a rare occurrence and is easily identified:

- By viewing the urethral orifice with a lighted speculum.
- Because no urine flows through the catheter – but note that catheters can be placed correctly and still not produce urine, due to either an empty bladder or an obstruction to urine flow (e.g. excessive lubricant blocking the drainage holes).

Patient resistance

This is common in bitches, queens and tom-cats. Sedation or general anaesthesia may be required.

Blockage of indwelling catheters

Urine will cease to flow from the catheter. Flushing of catheters at regular intervals (2–3 times per day) is advisable.

Removal of indwelling catheters by patients

Adequate suturing (tom-cat, dog) and the application of Elizabethan collars should prevent catheter removal by the patient.

Types of urinary catheter

All catheters (Table 16.7) manufactured for the veterinary market, with the exception of the metal bitch catheter, are supplied individually, double wrapped, with an inner nylon and outer paper or plastic sleeve. The catheters are ready for use, having been sterilised by either ethylene oxide gas or gamma radiation.

Urinary catheters are designed for *single use only*. The cleaning and re-use of these catheters is not recommended, though single re-use might be acceptable if thorough cleaning and proper sterilisation techniques are employed.

Re-sterilisation often costs *more* in respect of nursing time (cleaning and packing) and money (cost of packaging, running an autoclave or an ethylene oxide system acceptable to the COSHH regulations) than it would to use a *new* catheter.

Dog catheters

Plastic dog catheters. These have a rounded tip behind which are two oval drainage holes (one at each side) (Fig. 16.12a). They are designed for single use in the male dog and can be used as indwelling catheters.

Choose the largest gauge appropriate for patient size. If too small a catheter is used, the tip of the catheter has a tendency to 'catch' in the urethral epithelium and bend. This may cause significant urethral trauma.

The only exception is where the urethra is narrowed due to a partial obstruction such as enlarged prostate, or a stricture. In these cases, there is no option other than to use a catheter that would otherwise be too small for the patient.

A second disadvantage of using small catheters in large patients is that the patient is stimulated to urinate when the catheter is introduced into the urethra, and urine will flow around the catheter as well as down the lumen.

In recent years, dog catheters have been used to catheterise bitches. They have no curved tip but are much firmer, providing more control for insertion into the urethral orifice, particularly when digital catheterisation is used. This extra rigidity far outweighs the advantage of the Tieman's catheter curved tip.

Table 16.7 Types of urinary catheter

Type	Species	Sex	Material	Indwelling	Sizes (FG)	Length (cm)	Luer fitting
Dog catheter	Dog	Male (or female)	Flexible grade of nylon (polyamide)	No but can be adapted to be indwelling	6–10	50–60	Yes
Silicon Foley	Dog	Male (or female)	Flexible medical grade silicon	Yes	5–10	30 and 55	No
Tieman's	Dog	Female	PVC (polyvinyl chloride)	No	8–12	43	Yes
Foley	Dog	Female	Teflon-coated latex	Yes	8–16	30–40	No
Cat catheter	Cat	Male and female	Flexible grade of nylon	No	3 and 4	30.5	Yes
Jackson cat catheter	Cat	Male and female	Flexible grade of nylon	Yes	3 and 4	11	Yes
Silicon cat catheter	Cat	Male	Medical grade silicon	Yes	3.5	12	Yes
Slippery Sam catheter	Cat	Male	PTFE (teflon)	Yes	3–3.5	14 and 11	Yes
Metal	Dog	Female	Plated brass	No	Various	20–25	No

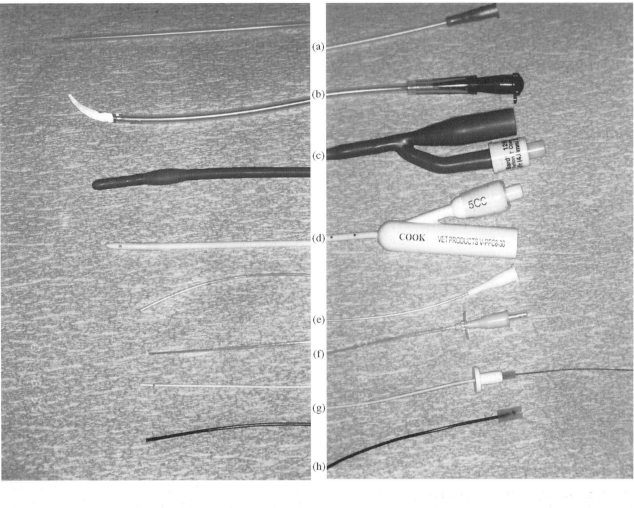

(a)
(b)
(c)
(d)
(e)
(f)
(g)
(h)

(i)

Fig. 16.12 Types of catheter: (a) dog; (b) Tieman's; (c) latex Foley; (d) silicon Foley; (e) cat; (f) Jackson cat; (g) silicon cat; (h) teflon cat; (i) metal bitch catheter.

Foley silcone catheter. In design these catheters (Fig. 16.12d) are exactly the same as a standard latex bitch Foley. For dogs a longer length is obviously selected. The catheter is very flexible but despite this will advance up the curved male urethra into the bladder where the retaining balloon can be inflated, thus creating an indwelling male dog catheter. Wire guide stylets are available to assist in catheter introduction if required. Silicone catheters have the added advantage of being autoclavable and therefore can be re-used (this may make their relatively high cost more acceptable). It is the microscopic 'smoothness' of the medical grade silicone that enables these catheters to be passed up the male urethra. Silicone is inert and causes no mucosal irritation.

All lubricants are compatible with these catheters.

Bitch catheters

Tieman's catheter. Designed for catheterisation of the human male, these catheters (Fig. 16.12b) became popular for use in the bitch due to their curved tip. The moulded tip was found to be advantageous when placing it into the urethral orifice. However, the rest of the catheter is so soft and flexible that the amount of control over the tip is negligible. This makes placing the catheter into the urethral orifice a very difficult task. The excessive length of the catheter is a further disadvantage.

Foley indwelling bitch catheter. Foley catheters (Fig. 16.12c) incorporate an inflatable balloon behind the drainage holes at the tip of the catheter.

The balloon is inflated after placement of the catheter into the bladder, making it an indwelling catheter.

Foley catheters are produced for the human market, but suitable sizes are available for use in most bitches except very tiny puppies. They cannot be used in cats or the male dog (unless in conjunction with a urethrostomy). The balloon is inflated (usually with sterile water or saline) via a channel built into the wall of the catheter which ends in a side arm and a one-way valve. The catheter is removed by deflating the balloon through the same side arm.

These catheters *must not be re-used*: the balloon is weakened after use and cannot be relied upon to function correctly if re-used.

Foley catheters are very flexible – this provides maximum patient comfort but causes a problem when introducing them. Placement is achieved by the use of a rigid metal stylet or probe laid beside the catheter with the point secured in one of the drainage holes at the catheter's tip. The stylet is removed once the balloon is inflated.

WARNING

The stylet *is not* placed up the middle of the Foley catheter (Fig. 16.13).

Latex Foley catheters must not be lubricated with petroleum-based ointments or lubricants, which will damage the latex rubber so that the balloon may burst on inflation.

The absence of a Leur mount in this catheter may cause problems for continuous collection of urine but urine collection bags with appropriate connectors are available from medical suppliers. If these bags cannot be supplied, the catheter must have an adapter placed so that drip bags can be used for urine collection (Fig. 16.14a). Unless 3-litre drip bags are employed, frequent emptying will be required in most dogs. It would be unwise to leave a large dog with only a litre collection bag attached overnight.

An alternative is to bung the catheter and drain the bladder at regular intervals with a spigot (Fig. 16.14b). This method may be acceptable for a recumbent patient but not, for example, after bladder surgery.

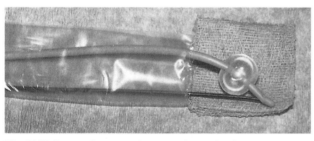

Fig. 16.13 Correct placement of the stylet in the tip of the Foley catheter. The balloon is inflating correctly and therefore the catheter is ready for use.

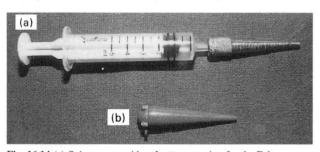

Fig. 16.14 (a) Spigot: to provide a Leur connection for the Foley catheter to enable empty drip-bag attachment (to collect urine) or to allow bladder drainage with a syringe. (b) Bung: to prevent continuous drainage and therefore soiling of the patient, when a urine collection bag is not in use.

Silicone indwelling Foley. These can be used in the bitch (at shorter lengths) as for the male (Fig 16.12d). They still require a stylet for correct placement in the bitch. Their use in bitches is still low due to their cost, the existing latex Foley being adequate in nearly all cases. The silicone Foley is inert, causing little mucosal irritation and may be preferable for use in patients with wounds near to the urethral opening.

Metal. Metal catheters (Fig. 16.12i) are rather outdated and are rarely used in modern veterinary establishments. Their rigid construction may result in considerable trauma unless the operator is very experienced. Even then some urethral damage is inevitable. The use of metal catheters is not recommended.

Cat catheters

Conventional. These straight catheters (Fig. 16.12e), with a Leur connection are compatible with all lubricants and are for single use. They are basically a small version of the dog catheter.

Jackson. Jackson catheters (Fig. 16.12f) were designed primarily for use in male cats suffering from feline lower urinary tract disease. They can be used in any male or female cat.

A fine metal stylet, lying in the lumen of the catheter, gives extra rigidity and provides better control for insertion into the urinary bladder. It also helps to displace any loose obstruction (e.g. protein plugs or struvite crystals in the urethra). A normal catheter would be too flexible to achieve this. The stylet is removed once the catheter is in place.

The Jackson is much shorter than the other cat catheters. This is to enable the entire length of the catheter to be placed in the patient, thereby allowing the flange to be sutured to the prepuce. The circular plastic flange is present just behind the Leur fitting of the catheter. In this way the catheter becomes indwelling.

Silicone tom-cat catheters. A silicone catheter with distal side holes (Fig 16.12g), very similar in design to a standard Jackson cat catheter. A wire guide is supplied to assist introduction. The proximal fitting enables syringe attachment, and suture holes in the baseplate allow suturing to the prepuce.

Teflon tom-cat catheters. In appearance is very similar to the conventional cat catheter (Fig 16.12h). The highly lubricous catheter shaft material ensures ease of catheter placement. The material is also inert and causes no mucosal irritation. Suture holes in the silicone hub allows securing of the catheter to the prepuce. It is therefore an excellent choice for a blocked cat that requires a longer-term indwelling catheter. These catheters are designed for single use only.

All lubricants are compatible. Re-use is not recommended.

Equipment

Specula

A speculum is an instrument which assists cavities to be viewed. Specula assist catheterisation of bitches by holding back the vaginal tissue and allowing good visualisation of the urethral orifice. This is of great aid to the student nurse: digital catheterisation can be difficult without a visual knowledge of the urethral position.

It is preferable for all specula to be sterile and it is often cheaper in the long run to invest in a metal speculum that can be autoclaved, rather than using the home-made variety that needs gas sterilisation. If no specula are available, bitch catheterisation is still possible digitally.

There are several varieties of speculum, most of which are not specifically designed for catheterisation.

Nasal speculum. There are many slight variations, the adult size being the most appropriate. All have two flat blades which separate when the handles are closed together (Fig. 16.15a). Some have a retaining device; others have to be held open. A light source may be attached to one of the blades to illuminate the vagina. If this is not available, a pen torch held by an assistant is an effective alternative.

Rectal speculum. This is used rarely, mainly due to expense. Rectal specula (Fig. 16.15b) are conical in shape and, once in place, a section of the conical arm slides out to allow viewing of the urethral orifice. The main problem is to align the removable section with the urethral orifice – easy in theory, but difficult in practice.

Auroscope. This is a normal auriscope handle and light but the attachment used has a section removed from its wall (Fig. 16.15c).

Home-made speculum. Monojet syringe packing cases are ideal rigid plastic specula and they are cheap. Simply remove one section of the cover, file the edges and use an external light source (Fig. 16.15d).

Batteries and transformers

Ensure that these are electrically tested and working correctly. Spare batteries should always be in stock. Transformers are usually away from the vulva and do not require sterilisation.

Speculum bulbs

These are best stored separately as they break easily. They cannot be sterilised in the autoclave and therefore need gas or, more realistically, chemical sterilisation.

Stylets

Stylets can be made or bought. Ensure that they are long enough for easy use – they need to be at least the length of the longest Foley catheter stocked (approximately 40 cm). Stylets can be packed and autoclaved or chemically sterilised.

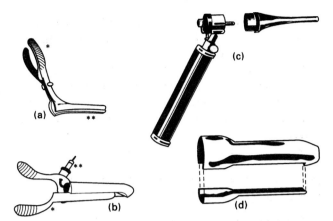

Fig. 16.15 (a) Nasal speculum, suitable for use as a bitch vaginal speculum. Pressing together the handles* causes the blades** to move apart and open the vestibule. (b) Rectal speculum, suitable for use as a bitch speculum. The lower sliding panel* is removed after insertion into the vestibule to expose the urethral opening. The lighting attachment**, which is connected to a battery, provides a self-contained light source. (c) Catheterisation speculum for attachment to an auroscope resembles an ear speculum except that a segment of its wall is absent. (d) A speculum made from the container of a Monojet disposable syringe by cutting away a segment of the plastic.

Urine collection bags

Manufactured varieties come prepacked and sterile; they are designed for single use.

Previously used drip bags can be used with a giving set attached. Ensure that the end of the giving set is thoroughly cleaned and chemically sterilised before being attached to the urinary catheter. Attach a needle to the end of the giving set during storage to keep it clean from dust and dirt.

Bungs and spigots

Plastic bungs come prepacked but are rarely sterile. They are best sterilised chemically. Metal spigots can be autoclaved or placed in chemical sterilising solution until needed.

Three-way taps

These are invaluable when draining bladders via a catheter. They avoid mess by controlling urine flow whilst syringes are emptied.

Catheter storage and checking

Catheters should be stored in a dry environment and laid flat without any pressure on top of them. Unless a suitably long drawer is available, urinary catheters are best left in their boxes and removed only when required.

All catheters have a shelf-life, after which sterility is no longer guaranteed by the manufacturer. Make regular checks, especially if the practice's use of catheters is infrequent. If catheters are re-sterilised, it is advisable to re-

Table 16.8 Methods for urinary catheterisation

	Equipment	Method
Dog catheterisation	Catheter Lubricant Swabs for cleaning Syringe to assist urine drainage Three-way tap (if required) Sample pot Gloves Urine bag or a bung Kidney dish *If the catheter is to be made indwelling:* Suture material Zinc oxide tape	1. Wash hands and put on gloves. 2. Clean prepuce. 3. Extrude penis; if not experienced, get an assistant to do this two-handed (Fig. 16.17). 4. Clean prepuce. 5. Remove catheter from the outer wrapping and cut a feeding sleeve from the inner sterile packaging (Fig. 16.18). This allows easy feeding of the catheter from the packaging into the urethra using a no touch technique. 6. Lubricate the catheter and insert the tip into the urethra (Fig. 16.17). 7. Advance the catheter up the urethra. Resistance may be met at the os penis, where there is a slight narrowing of the urethra, at the ischial arch and area of the prostate gland if enlarged. Steady but gentle pressure should overcome this resistance. If the catheter cannot be passed, re-evaluate catheter size. 8. Proceed according to reason for catheterisation (e.g. drain bladder, collect sample, hydropropulsion). To provide an indwelling dog catheter (Fig. 16.19): 1. Place zinc tape around catheter near to prepuce. 2. Stitch to prepuce; or 3. Stick to prepuce. Neither of these options is ideal because dog catheters are not designed to be indwelling.

Bitch catheterisation
Method 1:
Urethra viewed in dorsal
  recumbency
	Speculum (with or without
	  light source)
	Alternative light source if
	  required
	Catheter
	Lubricant
	Swabs for cleaning
	Gloves
	
	*If a Foley catheter is being
	placed:*
	Stylet
	Sterile water/saline to
	  inflate cuff
	Urine bag
	Syringe
		1. Wash hands and put on gloves.
		2. Ensure the bitch is in a straight dorsal recumbent position with the hindlimbs flexed and drawn forward (Fig. 16.16). The tail needs to be under control too.
		3. Clean vulva.
		4. Remove catheter from outer wrapping and expose tip only from inner sleeve.
		5. If a Foley catheter is being used, insert the stylet.
		6. Place speculum blades between the vulval lips as caudally as possible to avoid the clitoral fossa (Fig. 16.20).
		7. Insert *vertically* into the vestibule and turn handles cranially (Fig. 16.20).
		8. Open the blades of the speculum. The urethral opening will be visible on the cranial side of the vertically oriented vestibule, approximately half way between the vulva and cervix (Fig. 16.21).
		9. Insert the tip of the catheter into the urethral orifice (Fig. 16.21). **Draw the hindlimbs backwards.** This straightens the urethra, making it easier to push the catheter into the bladder.
		10. Proceed depending on reason for catheterisation. If a Foley catheter is being used, inflate balloon, withdraw stylet, attach bag and place Elizabethan collar (Fig. 16.22).

Bitch catheterisation Method 2: Urethra viewed standing	As in Method 1 Generally only one assistant is required	1. Wash hands and put on gloves. 2. Ensure tail is well restrained. 3. Clean vulva. 4. Place speculum between vulval lips and advance at a slight angle towards the spine, then horizontally (Fig. 16.23). 5. Open blades and identify urethral orifice. This will be on the ventral floor of the vestibule. 6. Insert catheter at a slightly ventral angle so as to follow the direction of the urethra into the bladder. 7. Proceed as for Method 1.

use them as quickly as possible – prolonged storage can result in further degradation.

Check that:

- There are no splits, tears, holes, etc., in the packing.
- No kinks are visible.
- The balloon inflates before placement of a Foley catheter.
- The stylet moves freely in the lumen before using a Jackson cat catheter.

Cleaning and sterilisation of catheters

Practice policy regarding re-use of catheters is rarely the nurse's decision; however, the process of cleaning and sterilisation is time-consuming and is *not* recommended for urinary catheters.

Cleaning

(1) Flush, with force, copious amounts of cold water through the catheter immediately after use. This is

Table 16.8 (Continued)

	Equipment	Method
Bitch catheterisation Method 3: Digital	Sterile gloves Catheter Lubricant Swabs for cleaning Collection pots *If a Foley is being placed,* additional equipment is as in Method 1	1. Restrain in preferred position, lateral or standing (standing is generally easiest). 2. Scrub hands and put on sterile gloves in an aseptic manner. 3. Ask an assistant to clean the vulva (gloved member having sterile hands). 4. Assistant removes outer wrapping from catheter and the inner package is removed by the scrubbed member. 5. Holding the sterile part of the packaging, place stylet if necessary. 6. Lubricate first finger of *non-writing* hand. 7. Place finger into vestibule and feel along ventral surface for a raised pimple (Fig. 16.24). 8. Place finger just cranial to this raised area, which is the urethral orifice (Fig. 16.24). 9. Raising hand and finger dorsally, digitally guide catheter, tipped slightly ventrally (as in Method 2) into the urethral orifice. The catheter will run past the fingertip if the orifice is missed. 10. Proceed as for Method 1.
Tom-cat catheterisation	As for dog catheterisation	1. Wash hands and put on gloves. 2. Restrain patient and have control of the tail. 3. Prepare feeding sleeve as for the dog catheter and lubricate tip. 4. With one hand extrude penis by applying gentle pressure each side of the prepuce with two fingers (Fig. 16.25). 5. Introduce catheter into the urethra. 6. Collect sample or drain bladder. 7. If a Jackson catheter is being placed for continuous drainage, stitch flange to prepuce.
Queen catheterisation This is rarely carried out but is quite straightforward if required (e.g. for contrast studies)	As for dog catheterisation	1. Restrain patient. 2. Wash hands and put on gloves. 3. Remove outer wrapping and cut a feeding sleeve. 4. Lubricate tip of catheter. 5. The catheter is placed between the vulval lips and 'blindly' introduced into the urethra. Angle the catheter ventrally, placing gentle pressure until the catheter slips into the urethra. 6. The catheter is not designed to be indwelling.

usually done with a syringe. Cold water prevents coagulation of any protein that may be present.

(2) Remove any blockage with a wire stylet and repeat step (1).

(3) Wash the exterior and interior of the catheter with a mild detergent. Rinse thoroughly, as in (1).

(4) Check catheter for kinks, holes, etc. If any damage is found the catheter *must* be discarded.

(5) Dry in a warm, dust-free atmosphere.

Sterilisation

Pack appropriately (autoclave bags or ethylene oxide). Autoclaving is the best method for nylon catheters. The COSHH Regulations have made the use of ethylene oxide in most practices difficult and expensive. There are no short cuts and therefore it is unlikely that any but the largest of veterinary establishments will continue to sterilise equipment by this method on their own premises.

WARNING

Boiling is not acceptable – it is *not* a method of sterilisation.

Methods for urinary catheterisation

Actual procedures for urinary catheterisation of dogs, bitches (three methods), tom-cats and queens are set out in Table 16.8. Several general points apply to all methods.

Physical restraint

Most patients will allow urinary catheterisation under gentle physical restraint without resistance. If necessary, use a muzzle on a dog. Ensure that the patient is at a comfortable working height.

- Dogs and cats can be restrained in a standing position or in lateral recumbency.
- Bitches can be restrained in dorsal recumbency (Fig. 16.16).

Chemical restraint

Sedation

- Dog: rarely required unless the patient is aggressive or very nervous.
- Bitch: most bitches will accept catheterisation more readily if lightly sedated, especially if dorsal recumbency

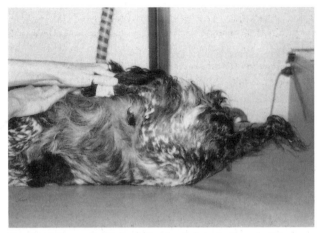

Fig. 16.16 Correct hindlimb position for the introduction of a Foley catheter with the patient in dorsal recumbency.

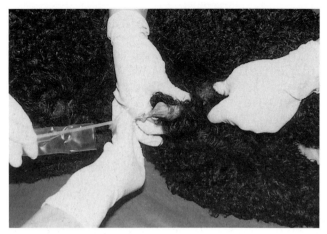

Fig. 16.17 Two-handed method for penis extrusion for introduction of a catheter into the urethra.

is chosen. Standing catheterisation is best done without sedation, otherwise the patient tends to keep sitting down – which can be tiring for the assistant.

- Cat: catheterisation of the cat is generally less stressful for all concerned if the cat is sedated.

General anaesthesia (GA). This is rarely indicated or necessary unless the patient has sustained other trauma which makes catheterisation under sedation humanely unacceptable (e.g. fractured pelvis, vaginal mass). It is sensible to catheterise during general anaesthesia if this is required for other treatment (e.g. catheterise a paraplegic patient whilst under GA for a myelogram).

Equipment preparation

Prepare all equipment *before* restraining the patient. Patient co-operation will be greater if prolonged restraint is avoided.

Lubricants

There is some debate over the necessity for the use of lubricants. Urinary catheterisation can be done without but lubricants aid passage of the catheter and help to avoid abrasive trauma.

- Check contents of lubricants before using them with Foley catheters; most are water-based and are compatible with commonly used catheters.
- Make sure that lubricants are sterile. Xylocaine gel (Astra) and K-Y jelly (Johnson and Johnson) are ideal choices. Xylocaine gel has the added advantage of desensitising the urethra, penis or vestibule.

Cleaning

- Clean the area with an antiseptic solution to remove any discharges and surface dirt.
- Clip around the area if necessary, especially in long-haired breeds. (Remember to check that permission for this has been obtained from the owner.)

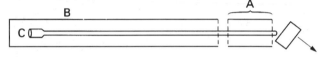

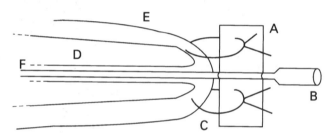

Fig. 16.18 Creating a feeding sleeve for easy introduction of urinary catheters. A: feeding sleeve; B: outer packaging; C: catheter.

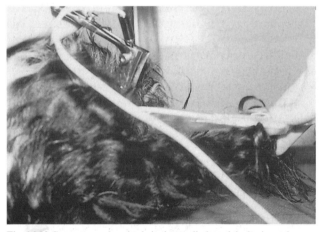

Fig. 16.19 Suturing of catheter to prepuce, to create an indwelling male urinary catheter. A: zinc tape butterfly; B: Leur tip catheter; C: suture; D: penis; E: prepuce; F: catheter in urethra.

Fig. 16.20 Correct speculum angle in the vestibule and the horizontal position of the Foley catheter as it is advanced into the bladder.

Gloves

The use of gloves is recommended for health and safety. In general, multiple packs of non-sterile gloves are adequate because the catheter will be fed from its package using a 'no

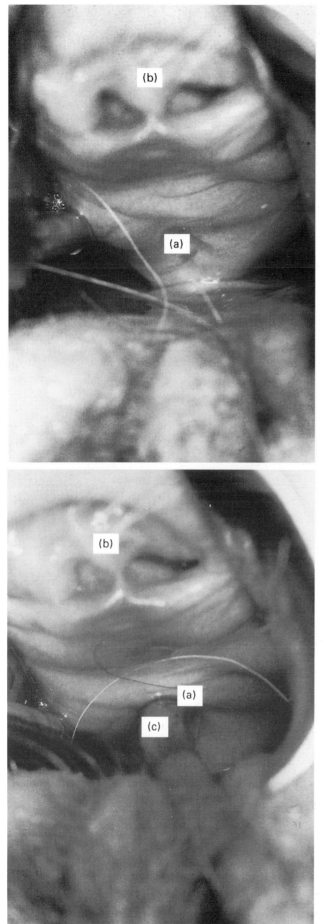

Fig. 16.21 Close-up view of the position of (a) the urethral orifice, (b) clitoral fossa and (c) catheter in position.

touch' technique. Gloves are therefore used to prevent contamination of staff with urine, rather than protection of the patient from infection.

Sterile gloves will be required when digital catheterisation is performed, as the catheter tip is inevitably touched by the finger.

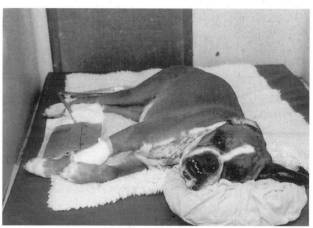

Fig. 16.22 Recumbent patient with Foley catheter in place and urine collection bag attached. (This patient was unable to raise her head; therefore no Elizabethan collar was necessary.)

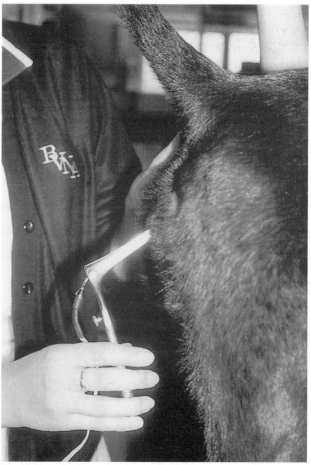

Fig. 16.23 Angle of speculum for introduction between lips of vulva in standing bitch. The speculum handle is then raised to insert the blades fully into the vestibule, avoiding painful interference with the clitoral fossa.

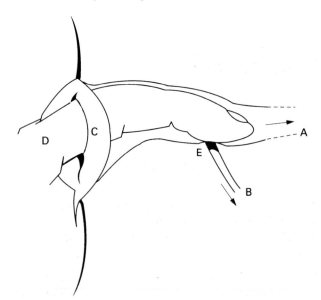

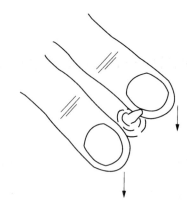

Fig. 16.25 Extrusion of tom-cat penis.

Fig. 16.24 Digital catheterisation: A: to cervix; B: to bladder; C: vulva; D: finger; E: raised area (urethral orifice).

Length of catheter

Measure a dog or cat catheter against the patient before unpacking the catheter. This measurement gives a rough estimate of the length of catheter to insert into the patient.

Stop inserting once urine flows. Over-insertion can result in the catheter bending and re-entering the urethra or, even worse, knotting in the bladder and requiring surgical removal.

Other methods of emptying the urinary bladder

Natural micturition

This is non-invasive and usually easy to achieve by nurse or owner. In most circumstances it is the preferred method for emptying the bladder but there are several disadvantages:

- The sample is always contaminated and therefore useless for culture and sensitivity evaluation.
- If the patient is unable to urinate normally, another method has to be employed.
- Patients often refuse to produce urine when convenient and required.

If not required for culture, then collection of samples from the environment may be acceptable in some cases, e.g. urine can be retrieved from litter trays that have been left empty.

Manual expression of the bladder

In cats this is probably the most common method. Dogs, especially recumbent ones, can also be encouraged to urinate in this way.

As long as the bladder is of a reasonable size, this task becomes easier with practice. Pressure should be applied steadily and slowly – do not use sudden pressure as this may cause trauma to the bladder. Generally very little pressure will initiate a free flow of urine. Excessive pressure should never be required.

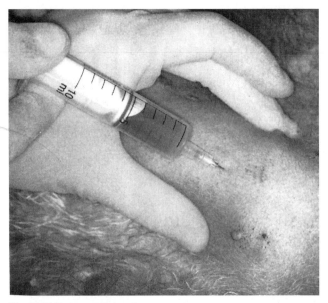

Fig. 16.26 Cystocentesis in a dog.

Cystocentesis

This should only be carried out when the bladder is of a palpable size (Fig. 16.26). The method is as follows:

(1) The patient is restrained in a position between lateral and dorsal recumbency.
(2) Clip an area about 5 × 5 cm on the midline caudal abdomen.
(3) Prepare the skin aseptically, and manually immobilise the bladder, through the abdomen wall.
(4) Using a syringe (5–20 ml) with a needle attached (23 gauge × 1 inch), insert through the abdominal wall and into the bladder.
(5) Remove urine.
(6) Apply gentle pressure at the injection site as the needle is quickly removed. The use of larger gauge needles is to be discouraged because it increases the possibility of urine leakage from the bladder after needle removal.

This technique is fairly straightforward and generally without complications, as long as an aseptic technique is used. It may be the only method available for urine drainage in an obstructive emergency. The procedure must only be carried out by a veterinary surgeon.

17

Medical disorders and their nursing

J. Simpson

Prevention and the spread of infection

The purpose of this section is to explain how infectious diseases are transmitted from one animal to another. There are basically three steps in the process:

- How the infection may leave the infected animal.
- How the infection may pass from one animal to another.
- How the infection can enter the new host.

The actual mode of transmission varies with each disease as does the speed at which the whole process occurs and examples will be used to illustrate the different stages of transmission. Before discussing the transmission of disease, it will be necessary to define some terms commonly used when discussing infectious diseases.

With an understanding of how infectious diseases are transmitted from one animal to another, it is possible to discuss ways in which we can control the spread of disease, often termed **preventive medicine.** In modern medicine the aim is to try and prevent animals becoming ill in the first place, rather than trying to treat life-threatening conditions. For dogs and cats, prevention involves:

- Vaccination programmes.
- High levels of hygiene.
- Use of isolation/quarantine facilities.
- Improving environmental conditions for dogs and cats.

Infectious and contagious disease

An **infectious** disease is one which is caused by micro-organisms, which can successfully invade, establish and grow within the host's tissues. The commonest infectious agents encountered in small animal practice are:

- Bacteria: *Salmonella* spp., *Campylobacter* spp.
- Viruses: Canine parvovirus, cat 'flu (FHV/FCV).
- Fungi: *Aspergillus* spp.
- Protozoa: *Giardia lamblia, Toxoplasma gondii.*

A **non-infectious** disease is one which does not involve micro-organisms, e.g. diabetes mellitus, renal failure or warfarin poisoning.

A **contagious** disease is a disease which is capable of being transmitted by direct or indirect contact from one animal to another. In this category are all the infectious diseases listed above, together with internal and external parasitism.

For a contagious disease to spread by **direct contact** it is necessary for the affected animal to come into physical contact with another susceptible animal. This might be achieved by:

- Animals being housed together in the same kennel.
- Sexual contact during mating.
- Licking or grooming behaviour between animals.
- Biting.

Disease spread by **indirect contact** infers that the affected animal and susceptible animal do not come into direct physical contact (Fig. 17.1). In this context 'indirect' refers to the affected animal **contaminating** the environment in some manner, usually by body secretions such as faeces, urine, saliva or other discharges. A contaminated environment might include, for example, bedding, feed bowls, public parks or consulting-room floors.

The contaminating micro-organism must remain viable away from the host until another susceptible animal contacts the contaminated material. The length of time micro-organisms may remain viable off the host varies considerably.

Some of these micro-organisms can live on **inanimate** objects (such as bedding or feed bowls), in which case the contaminated objects are termed **fomites** (singular: fomes). Other micro-organisms are carried by **animate** agents referred to as **vectors**.

Fomites

Examples of the indirect spread of disease by fomites include parvovirus and ringworm. The organisms that cause these diseases are capable of living on inanimate

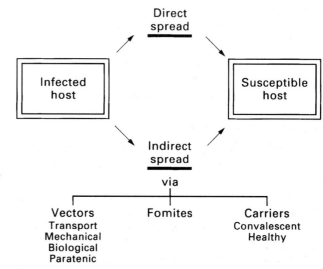

Fig. 17.1 The spread of infection.

objects for long periods, ready to infect any susceptible host that happens to come into contact with the contamination. The vomitus or diarrhoea from a dog with parvovirus can contaminate a public park in this way; the virus is resistant and remains viable off the host for long periods, providing plenty of opportunity for a suitably susceptible dog to become infected.

Ringworm (a fungal infection of dogs and cats) may be spread by direct contact, or by indirect contact following contamination of the animal's environment; again, the fungus can live on inanimate objects for long periods.

Vectors

Another indirect method of spreading disease involves **vectors**, which are animate carriers of disease and include insects (flies), ticks or mites. There are various types of vectors:

- Biological vectors or intermediate hosts.
- Non-biological or mechanical vectors, subdivided into: transport hosts and paratenic hosts.

Biological vectors act as intermediate hosts in the life cycle of micro-organisms or parasites. Good examples are the fleas, rabbits and sheep that act as intermediate hosts in the life cycle of tapeworms. The biological vector or intermediate host varies with each tapeworm in the dogs and cats but some of the organism's development must occur within the intermediate host, which is then ingested by the definitive host – in these cases the dog or cat.

Mechanical vectors transmit disease without playing any role as an intermediate host. They simply transfer infection from the affected animal to the susceptible animal.

Transport hosts pass on infection to a susceptible host at any time. The transport host is unaffected by the infectious agent and acts only to maintain the viability of the micro-organism and to then pass it on directly to another animal. Examples might include the flea carrying feline panleucopenia virus or *Haemobartonella felis*. In each case the infection is passed on when the flea bites a susceptible animal.

Paratenic hosts must be eaten by the host in order to pass on infection because the organism lives within the tissues. There is no development of the micro-organism or parasite in the paratenic host; it simply remains in the tissues until consumed. An example of this might be *Toxoplasma gondii*: to become infected, a cat must eat uncooked meat (e.g. from hunting mice).

Routes of transmission

In considering how an infection can be passed from one animal to another, there are three factors to bear in mind:

- The routes by which organisms may leave the animal.
- The routes of transmission from one animal to another.
- The routes of entry into a new host.

Routes by which organisms leave the animal

The commonest routes by which micro-organisms may leave an animal are via natural body secretions:

- Oral, nasal and ocular discharges.
- In urine.
- In faeces.
- In vomitus.
- In blood.
- Via the skin.
- In milk.
- Venereal contact, semen and parturition.
- From dead animals.

Oral, nasal and ocular discharges. An increase in secretion from the nose and eye, together with a change in its character, may result from infections such as cat 'flu, canine distemper and kennel cough. These secretions are rich in micro-organisms which are released into the environment in the form of an aerosol when the infected animal coughs or sneezes.

In rabies and FIV infection the saliva of infected animals contains large amounts of virus. Aerosols play no major role in the transmission of disease but if these animals bite a susceptible animal the disease will be inoculated into the new host.

In urine. In some infections the kidney is specifically targeted by the micro-organism and consequently the urine may contain large numbers of the micro-organisms concerned. *Leptospira canicola* and infectious canine hepatitis virus are examples of diseases which behave in this way where infection is disseminated via the urine.

In vomit and in faeces. The gastrointestinal tract may be targeted by micro-organisms. This invasion results in dysfunction of the gastrointestinal tract, usually manifest as vomiting and diarrhoea. Both these secretions are heavily laden with micro-organisms which can result in significant contamination of the environment. Examples of this method of spreading disease include canine and feline parvovirus infection.

In blood. Vectors are important in this method of spreading disease. A flea feeds off a cat infected with *Haemobartonella felis*; and in so doing picks up the micro-organism and carries it without becoming infected. When the flea moves to a new host it feeds again and passes on the infection.

Via the skin. This is principally associated with the spread of external parasites including ringworm, lice, fleas and mites. Direct contact is required in order to transmit lice as they cannot live off the host, while fleas and mites are not host specific and may live off the host for some time. Fomites may also be important in the dissemination of parasitism, particularly where ringworm and fleas are concerned as they can live off the host on inanimate objects (e.g. grooming equipment).

In milk. The milk produced by the lactating bitch or queen is an excellent media by which to spread disease from one generation to the next. Feline leukaemia virus and *Toxocara* larvae may be spread by this method.

Venereal, semen, parturition. Disease may be spread during mating or via the foetal fluid and placenta at parturition. *Brucella abortus* is an example of a disease which may be spread in this manner.

From dead animals. All dead animals, unless cremated, decompose and may become a source of infection to others. In particular, animals which die of anthrax (a notifiable disease) may seriously contaminate the environment unless the carcass is carefully disposed of. Dead sheep must not be allowed to lie around in fields as they can be a source of tapeworms. Dogs which eat contaminated sheep may acquire *Echinococcus granulosus*.

Routes of transmission from one animal to another

These routes include:

- Direct contact.
- Indirect contact.
- Aerosol transmission.
- Contamination of food and water.
- Carriers.

Direct contact. Direct spread requires physical contact between the infected and the susceptible animal where body secretions or ectoparasites may be passed directly from one animal to another.

Indirect contact. Diseases which are spread from one animal to another via fomites (e.g. bedding, feed bowls and kennel runs) or by vectors (e.g. fleas, mice or sheep).

Wherever environmental contamination occurs this may allow transfer of infection from one animal to another. Hookworms may contaminate kennel runs and other dogs may receive infection when using the same run. The soil is also a source of infection: *Clostridium tetani* spores can cause tetanus in dogs and *Toxocara canis* eggs remain viable in soil for a considerable time.

Aerosols. Aerosols are particularly important in the transmission of respiratory disease. When the infected animal coughs and/or sneezes this creates an aerosol which carries large numbers of water droplets loaded with micro-organisms into the atmosphere. Other susceptible animals within the same air space inhale this aerosol and may become infected.

Contamination of food and water. Ingestion of contaminated food or water is an important method of spreading disease. In addition to the well-recognised organisms associated with **food poisoning** such as *Salmonella* and *Campylobacter*, other micro-organisms may also be spread in this way. Urine contamination of food or water

is an important method of spreading Leptospirosis. Cats may become infected with *Toxoplasma gondii* by eating uncooked meat or catching infected mice. Sewage contamination of water supplies may also be a source of infection.

Carriers. Occasionally an animal may come into contact with a micro-organism; it may harbour the disease without showing clinical signs. These animals are called **carriers** and may excrete the micro-organism without showing any clinical signs or evidence of ill health (Fig. 17.1). There are two types of carrier: the convalescent and the healthy.

The **convalescent carrier** is an animal which has recovered from the clinical disease. These animals may shed large numbers of micro-organisms into the environment for variable periods of time after recovery. There are many good examples of this situation including cat 'flu (FHV and FCV infection), canine infectious hepatitis and leptospirosis.

A **healthy carrier** is an animal which has been exposed to an infectious disease but has never shown clinical signs of that disease, yet carries the micro-organism and sheds it into the environment. These animals are usually immune to the infection and tolerate the presence of micro-organisms without showing signs of ill health. Examples of this type of carrier include *Campylobacter* infection and *Haemobartonella felis*.

Both types of carrier may harbour the micro-organism without shedding it into the environment (**closed carriers**) or may continuously shed micro-organisms into the environment (**open carriers**).

Routes of entry into a new host

These routes include:

- Ingestion.
- Inhalation.
- Through the skin.
- Via mucous membranes.
- Congenital route.

Ingestion. Ingestion is one of the most common routes by which infections may establish. Whether clinical disease occurs will depend on the dose of infective agent ingested and the susceptibility of the host. Examples of ways in which micro-organisms may be ingested include:

- Food.
- Water.
- Eating faeces of other animals (coprophagia).
- Consuming vectors following grooming – fleas.
- Direct licking and grooming of other animals.
- Fomites – including feed bowls, bedding, chewing sticks or playing with balls.
- Ingestion of other body secretions.

Inhalation. This involves the inhalation of aerosols containing large numbers of water droplets loaded with micro-organisms. In some cases dust or other debris rather than water droplets may be inhaled. Animals housed within the same air space are at risk from both types of medium. The risk is further increased if there is a large number of animals within a small air space or there is an inadequate air turnover. In such cases the infective load or amount of aerosol present is very high and this increases the chance of disease spreading.

Through the skin. Both primary skin disease and systemic diseases can enter through the skin. The likelihood of disease successfully establishing depends on the type of infection and the physical condition of the skin itself. There are several means of establishing infection by this route:

- Penetration of intact skin by hookworm larvae or sarcoptic mites. (Mercury absorption by this route, which acts systemically, is not an infection but is considered in Chapter 3 under Poisoning.)
- Where the skin is physically damaged and the barrier to infection is destroyed, e.g. if the animal cuts its foot, undergoes surgery, receives burns or traumatises itself, then secondary bacterial infection can establish. This may remain localised or become systemic.
- Inoculation following the use of dirty hypodermic needles, insect bites (fleas), bite wounds (rabies) or scratching. In these cases the skin is healthy but the physical barrier is breached and infection establishes itself.
- Transference from one host to another by direct or indirect contact. Lice, mites and fleas may be transferred in this manner.

Via mucous membranes. The importance of the mucous membrane of the digestive and respiratory systems as routes of entry to the body has been discussed. There are other mucous membranes which may also act as points of entry for infection:

- The conjunctiva – *Chlamydia psittaci* infection.
- The vaginal mucous membrane – bacterial and fungal infections.
- The prepuce/penis – balanitis and venereal diseases.

Congenital route. During pregnancy micro-organisms can pass from the bitch or queen to the foetus via the placenta. This is a very important method of transmission which is often termed **vertical transmission** of disease. Examples include:

- *Toxocara canis.*
- Feline leukaemia virus infection.
- Feline panleucopenia virus causing cerebellar hypoplasia in kittens.
- *Toxoplasma gondii* infection.

In some of these cases the foetus will survive although clinically infected but in others transplacental transmission of disease results in stillbirth, abortion or resorption of the foetus.

Modes of transmission of the major organisms

Viruses

In most cases viruses accumulate in large numbers in the secretions produced by the infected animal. In particular saliva, nasal and ocular discharges, faeces and urine. Aerosols created from respiratory secretions are an effective method of spreading respiratory disease. Urine and faeces often contaminate the environment and may induce disease following ingestion. Saliva plays a special role in the transmission of rabies where biting inoculates the virus into a new host.

Bacteria

Although bacteria can cause primary infections, they are often associated with secondary infection following initial invasion of the tissues by viruses. For example, cat 'flu is primarily caused by a viral infection but secondary bacterial infection is common.

Some bacteria are called **commensals**. These bacteria can live in harmony with the host without causing disease but under the right conditions they have the potential to become pathogenic. A good example is some of the *Pasteurella* spp.: these are often 'normally' present in the oral cavity of cats but cat bites will inoculate the bacterium into the skin, often resulting in cellulitis. *Pasteurella* spp. can also act as a secondary invader in feline respiratory infections.

Other bacteria are **obligate pathogens** – these always cause ill health. *Clostridium tetani* is a good example as it is never present in animals without causing tetanus.

Ectoparasites

This group includes mites, fleas and lice which are found in or on the skin. They are readily spread by direct and indirect contact between animals. Some ectoparasites (i.e. ticks) must live off the host for a period of time to complete their life cycle before finding another suitable host. Some ectoparasites of dogs and cats are not host specific, e.g. fleas and sarcoptic mange mites.

Endoparasites

This category includes tapeworms, round worms, lung worms and coccidial parasites. The majority of endoparasites enter the new host by ingestion. Hookworms are an exception as they can penetrate intact skin and migrate to the tissues. Some ectoparasites, especially tapeworms, require an intermediate host to complete their life cycle.

Incubation of disease

The **incubation period** is the interval of time between the animal coming into contact with a micro-organism and the development of clinical signs of disease. The actual time span varies with each disease and is normally given as a range of days rather than an exact number, because the

Table 17.1 Average incubation periods for infectious diseases of the dog and cat

Dogs	Incubation period	Cats	Incubation period
Canine distemper	7–21 days	Feline enteritis	4–5 days
ICH	5–9 days	Cat 'flu	2–10 days
Leptospirosis	5–7 days	FIP	Months
		Chlamydia psittaci	4–10 days
Kennel cough	5–7 days	FeLV	Months/years
Parvovirus	3–5 days	FIV	Months/years

speed at which infection establishes depends on several factors:

- The dose of micro-organisms.
- The immune status of the animal.
- The general health of the animal.
- The age of the animal.
- The route of entry.

The incubation periods of the common infectious diseases of dogs and cats is shown in Table 17.1.

In the majority of cases an infectious agent will initially invade the mucous membrane of the respiratory and digestive tracts. The mucus and cilia of the respiratory tract and the mechanical movement and secretions of the digestive tract will prevent the micro-organisms from becoming established, unless the animal is susceptible and the dose of micro-organisms is great.

Initially the micro-organism will invade the cells of the mucous membrane and possibly the local drainage lymph nodes. It then replicates in these tissues. If the host fails to mount an adequate immune response, the infectious agents will leave the initial site of invasion and spread to other target tissues.

The presence of virus particles in the circulation is called **viraemia**. This is the usual way by which viruses spread to specific target organs that include the intestine, bone marrow and lymphoid tissue, which are all associated with rapidly dividing cells. When these target tissues have been invaded, clinical signs associated with dysfunction of the affected system are observed (Table 17.2).

Methods of disease control

With a sound knowledge of how disease is transmitted, it is possible to devise methods to reduce the risk of disease spread. These include:

- Avoiding direct contact between animals (isolation or quarantine).
- Maintaining very high levels of hygiene, preventing formation of fomites and infestation with insect vectors.
- Reducing the number of animals kept within the same air space or improving the efficiency of air movement.
- Providing early and effective treatment of infected animals.
- Routine vaccination, ectoparasite and endoparasite control.
- Maintaining strict import controls to avoid entry of disease into the UK.

Client education

Client education is the key to achieving these goals. The veterinary surgeon and veterinary nurse are ideally qualified to provide this information and so help prevent rather than treat disease. In modern veterinary practice there are many examples of how preventive medicine is being employed to good effect. The veterinary nurse plays a vital role in this process in helping to educate clients by:

- Running obesity clinics.
- Sending out vaccination reminders.
- Providing dietary advice.
- Advising on worming policy.
- Providing general advice and redirection to the veterinary surgeon.

Table 17.2 The body systems most frequently targeted by viral infections and the clinical signs exhibited following infection

Digestive tract	Vomiting
	Diarrhoea
	Dehydration
	Weight loss
	Abdominal pain
Respiratory tract	Coughing
	Sneezing
	Ocular and nasal discharge
	Tachypnoea
	Dyspnoea
	Exercise intolerance
Bone marrow	Immunosuppression
	Anaemia
	Thrombocytopenia – bleeding tendency

Isolation and quarantine facilities

When dogs or cats are brought together in a confined space the risk of introduction of infection then rapid spread is greatly increased. For this reason animals should be kept physically separate and a close watch kept for early signs of disease. Any animal that shows signs of ill health should be moved to an isolation unit immediately.

Isolation is the physical separation of animals so that direct and indirect contact become very difficult. Healthy dogs and cats that are hospitalised or kennelled should be kept in separate cages so that direct contact is impossible. This will help prevent the spread of some infectious diseases. The facilities should not only ensure physical separation but also ensure that as few animals as possible share the same air space. Where large numbers of dogs or cats have to share the same air space, air turnover should be adequate to ensure the removal of infective aerosols. Several important management points are relevant:

- All new arrivals to a breeding unit should be adequately vaccinated before entry.
- They should then be isolated for at least 21–28 days to ensure they are not incubating disease which could be introduced to the entire group.
- The isolation unit should always have its own equipment so that cross-contamination cannot occur with the main group.
- Special precautions should also be taken by staff servicing the isolation unit with regard to protective clothing and personal hygiene.

Quarantine is a term which is usually reserved for compulsory education. At present all dogs and cats must undergo 6 months' quarantine to prevent rabies from entering the country. In these premises, animals must not come into contact with other quarantined animals nor with any animal outside the quarantine station. The subject of quarantine and kennel management is covered in greater details in Chapter 5.

Hygiene

Avoiding primary contact between animals, maintaining small groups to reduce aerosol spread and keeping infected animals in isolation units are all important factors in preventive medicine, but these barriers will be of little value unless very strict levels of hygiene are practised. The isolation of an infected animal is ineffective if those who care for it do not wash themselves after handling the animal, or if equipment used in the isolation unit is not kept separate to ensure that fomites do not spread infection back to the main group of animals.

In any hospital or kennelling facility where any animal might be incubating disease, the risk of transmission will be reduced if the level of contamination is kept as low as possible by practising the following good hygiene routines:

- All equipment should be thoroughly washed and disinfected as a matter of daily routine.
- All surfaces should be regularly cleaned and disinfected, including work tops, kennel runs, sleeping areas and food preparation areas.
- Do not rely on disinfectants to kill infective agents. If the environment is physically dirty then disinfectants are

often unable to destroy pathogenic micro-organisms. It is therefore essential to *wash* the premises thoroughly with hot water and soap on a regular basis. This will remove the dirt and many of the micro-organism at the same time. Those that remain can be destroyed by disinfection.

- All bedding should be either disposable or made of materials that can be thoroughly washed.
- Personal hygiene should be of a high standard and suitable protective clothing should be worn.
- Always prepare food at a different location to the area handling waste. All foods used should ideally be commercially produced and home-made diets should be kept to a minimum. Do not use uncooked or raw foods; if home-made diets are used ensure they are thoroughly cooked first. No food for human consumption should be prepared or stored in the same areas as for animals.
- Keep all vermin under control. They can act as carriers of infection, especially mice and rats. Insect vectors may also spread disease by transferring infection from waste material to food preparation areas.

Treatment

The veterinary nurse should be vigilant and constantly observing animals for early signs of ill health. The illness may initially present as very subtle changes such as partial anorexia, polydipsia, depression, occasional sneezing or coughing. More obvious signs may then follow such as vomiting, diarrhoea, dehydration or collapse. Keep careful records so that early signs may be noted and acted on before the disease seriously affects the animal or spreads to others.

Quickly remove and isolate any suspect animal. Thoroughly wash and disinfect the kennel including feed bowls, disposing of all bedding material.

A veterinary surgeon should then examine, diagnose and treat the affected animal. The diagnosis should predict whether the disease is likely to spread. It may then be possible to improve the protection of other animals in the group by vaccination or prophylactic treatment.

Prevention and vaccination

Disease prevention is far more effective than having to treat affected animals. All animals, especially those entering a hospital or kennelling facility, should have up-to-date vaccinations against the common infectious diseases. In addition they should have been recently wormed and treated for ectoparasites. The risk of disease can be greatly reduced by maintaining the animals free from infectious disease and parasites.

Zoonoses

A **zoonosis** is a disease which can be transferred from animals to humans, for whom diseases such as leptospirosis and rabies can have fatal consequences. Many other canine and feline diseases and disease-causing organisms may also infect humans, including:

- Salmonellosis
- Leptospirosis.
- Toxoplasmosis.
- *Toxocara canis.*
- Echinococcus granulosus.
- Ringworm.
- Fleas.
- Sarcoptic mange.
- *Chlamydia psittaci.*
- Rabies.

Those working in veterinary practice have a much greater risk of contracting a zoonotic disease than a member of the general public. For this reason nurses and veterinary surgeons in particular should try to minimise the risk of personal infection by taking the following precautions on behalf of themselves and others:

- Always wash hands thoroughly after handling animals with *any* disease. It might turn out to be zoonotic even if it appears unlikely at first.
- Do not allow animals to lick human faces or mouths. This is especially important when children are playing with animals.
- Never let animals eat or drink off utensils used for serving food to humans.
- Wash all dishes and prepare all food for animals in a separate area from those intended for human use.
- Those who are pregnant must take special care if handling animals.
- Keep gardens and kennel runs clear of faeces and prevent animals from contaminating children's sandpits with faeces.
- Ensure the very young and very old are not exposed to animals with possible zoonotic infections.
- Wear protective clothing at all times. Upgrade the amount of such clothing depending on the degree of risk anticipated.
- Seek medical advice quickly if you think you have been exposed to a zoonotic disease.

Canine infectious diseases

Five important canine diseases are considered in this section:

- Distemper.
- Infectious canine hepatitis.
- Canine contagious respiratory disease.
- Canine leptospirosis.
- Canine parvovirus.

The clinical signs, diagnosis and control for each disease are given in Table 17.3.

Distemper

Canine distemper is a common infectious disease of the dog and other species, including fox, badger, mink and ferret. It has a high morbidity rate and a variable mortality rate depending on the body systems affected and how quickly therapy is provided. Distemper is most frequently observed in dogs between 3 and 9 months of age following the fall in maternal immunity where acquired immunity has not been established. However, distemper can occur in susceptible dogs of any age.

Most outbreaks of disease occur in cities, housing estates, rescue centres and where dogs are kept in high density populations. The severity of clinical signs depends on:

- The degree of maternal antibody protection present in puppies.
- The nutritional status of the dog.
- Concurrent infections including parasitism.
- Level of viral challenge.

Both acute and sub-acute forms of distemper are recognised with clinical signs of inflammation of the respiratory and gastrointestinal tracts. Dogs may develop nervous signs following recovery from the acute disease; and in a small number of cases, only nervous signs are observed. Distemper virus may also be responsible for the many cases of **old dog encephalitis (ODE)** observed in middle to old-aged dogs.

Aetiology and pathogenesis

Canine distemper virus (CDV) is caused by a morbillivirus which is related to measles and rinderpest. The virus is labile off the host and is very susceptible to ultraviolet light, desiccation, heating and disinfection.

Virus is shed in the urine, vomitus, saliva, nasal and ocular discharge and faeces of infected dogs. Inhalation is thought to be the most important route of entry following either direct dog-to-dog contact or droplet/aerosol spread between dogs in close contact. Ingestion is not thought to be of significance in transmitting the disease because gastric acid and bile salts effectively destroy the virus. Carriers of infection rarely occur but virus may be retained in the central nervous system for long periods.

Distemper virus has an affinity for macrophages and lymphocytes and this is where initial viral replication occurs following exposure to infection. Only after replication in these cells will the virus target epithelial cells of the gastrointestinal and/or respiratory tracts. Whether epithelial cell invasion occurs depends on the immune response of the dog. A good immune response will prevent epithelial invasion while a poor response will allow the virus to invade these cells.

Sites of initial replication include the lymph nodes of the respiratory tract, after which infected macrophages and lymphocytes enter the circulation via lymphatic vessels and invade other lymphoid tissue and the bone marrow. Virus may be found within the central nervous tissues within 10 days of exposure to infection and may remain there for long

Table 17.3 Canine infectious diseases: clinical signs, diagnosis and control

	Clinical signs	Diagnosis	Control
Distemper	Incubation period – 7–21 days (a) *Mild* or *sub-acute*: rarely diagnosed, may present simply as transient period of depression, anorexia and mild pyrexia (<40°C). Recovery rapid; secondary bacterial infection rare. Some cases remain subclinical and unreported by owner. (b) *Acute*: typical clinical signs associated with CDV infection. Within 7 days of exposure, dog becomes depressed, anorexic and pyrexic (<40°C) due to viraemia. Within 48 hours temperature may have returned to normal but in susceptible dogs rises again ('diphasic temperature rise' – Fig. 17.2) due to epithelial invasion, immunosuppression and secondary bacterial infection. Clinical signs include some or all of: ● Persistent depression, anorexia, pyrexia. ● Tonsillitis, pharyngitis with a dry cough. ● Conjunctivitis, rhinitis initially associated with serous discharge changing to mucopurulent discharge (secondary bacterial infection). ● Exudative pneumonia associated with *Bordetella bronchiseptica* with tachypnoea and dyspnoea. ● Vomiting, diarrhoea, dehydration, loss of body condition. ● Hyperkeratosis of nose and foot pads (hard pad – foot pads painful, thickened with irregular fissures and eventually exfoliate). ● Mortality can be high but many dogs survive if treatment is provided quickly. ● If acute disease developed at less than six months old, may show changes to subsequent permanent dentition: damage to enamel and exposure of dentine (particularly canine teeth) – 'distemper rings'. (c) *Nervous disease*: approximately 50% with acute disease subsequently develop nervous signs, type and severity of which vary individually (Table 17.4). Nervous signs occasionally observed without any previous acute disease. In all cases onset of nervous signs leads to grave prognosis but in some, signs are not detected until years after acute infection, when ODE develops in old age due to latent CDV infection in nervous tissue.	History and clinical signs confirmed by: ● Presence of eosinophilic inclusion bodies in epithelial cells. ● Rising antibody titre of at least 4-fold. ● Immunofluorescence for virus in lymphoid tissue. ● Detection of antibody in CSF. ● Post-mortem changes.	Vaccination using modified live vaccine – allows virus to multiply in lymphoid tissues and stimulate good immune response. Measles vaccine also available to provide unweaned puppies with passive immunity without interference with maternal immunity. Puppies safely vaccinated from 9 weeks of age, primary vaccination programme complete by 12 weeks. Boosted annually.

ICH	Incubation period – 5–9 days
	(a) *Sudden death*, more common in neonatal puppies – most die without showing any clinical signs, other very short period of anorexia, depression, pyrexia (>40°C), collapse and shock before death. Occasionally haemorrhagic diarrhoea, abdominal pain and crying prior to death.
	(b) *Acute* ICH is most common form – sudden onset of depression, anorexia, pyrexia (>40°C) and shock. Pallor of the mucous membranes followed by jaundice as disease progresses. Tonsilitis, generalised lymphadenopathy, abdominal pain, haemorrhagic diarrhoea and hepatomegaly are common. Most dogs reluctant to move and may appear tucked up and occasionally assume praying position due to abdominal pain and crying prior to death
	(c) *Sub-acute* form – signs may include depression, anorexia, mild pyrexia; occasionally transient corneal oedema.
	(d) *Complications* – blue eye;
	  – interstitial and glomerular nephritis;
	  – nervous signs.
		History and clinical signs together with laboratory analysis:
		● Haematology – leucopenia.
		● Biochemistry – elevated SALT, bilirubin and blood urea.
		● Urine analysis – proteinuria.
		● Rising antibody titre.
		● Intranuclear inclusion bodies found within hepatocytes.
		● Virus isolation from tissues such as liver and kidney.
		● Post-mortem findings.
			Maintain high levels of vaccinal protection.
			Most vaccines now use live CAV-2 virus rather than CAV-1 to avoid risk of blue eye.
			Primary vaccination can start at 6–9 weeks of age in combination with distemper vaccination; programme can be completed by 12 weeks.
			Boosted annually

Table 17.3 (Continued)

	Clinical signs	Diagnosis	Control
CCRD	*Incubation period* 5–7 days following inhalation of micro-organisms. Hallmark is dry non-productive cough; coughing often induced by excitement, change of environmental temperature or exercise; paroxysms of coughing frequent, may induce retching and occasionally vomiting. Owners often believe 'something stuck in dog's throat'. Initially serous nasal discharge but may become mucopurulent if significant secondary bacterial infection establishes. Dogs usually remain bright and retain appetite. Lower respiratory disease (bronchopneumonia) rare. Recovery usually uneventful, within 14 days, but a few may be refractory to treatment and infection may persist for months.	History of recent kennelling and clinical signs. Diagnostic tests rarely carried out as patients respond well to symptomatic therapy. Collect pharyngeal swabs for culture or serology to confirm diagnosis.	Vaccines available against *Bordetella bronchiseptica*, CAV and CPIV. Vaccination against CPIV using primary course of two injections given 2 weeks apart; a boost annually. Ideally vaccinate 10–14 days prior to kennelling. Live vaccine against *B. bronchiseptica* also available, administered intranasally, gives high level of immunity within 5 days, maintained for up to 6 months. Booster vaccinations every 6 months.

Canine leptospirosis	As the clinical signs observed in leptospirosis vary it may not be possible to differentiate between the sero-types on clinical signs. However in general the clinical picture with each sero-type may be described as follows:
	● *L. icterohaemorrhagiae*
	Peracute: sudden death in young puppies without any previous signs of ill-health.
	Acute: sudden onset of pyrexia, anorexia, marked depression and jaundice, followed by vomiting, polydipsia, haemorrhagic diarrhoea and petechial haemorrhages on mucous membranes. More generalised bleeding including epistaxis in individual cases. Dehydration, shock and collapse follow rapidly, and can result in death within a few hours even if treatment provided early.
	● *L. canicola*
	Acute: sudden onset of pyrexia, depression and polydipsia, followed by vomiting, oligiuria, dehydration together with swelling and pain involving kidneys. Rapidly become azotaemic, develop halitosis and eventually oral ulceration. In a few cases hepatic involvement results in jaundice.
	Sub-acute: Vague illness associated with anorexia, lethargy and pyrexia lasting only a few days; rarely diagnosed.
		Suspected from history and clinical signs and confirmed by:
		● Serology to detect a rising antibody virus.
		● Urine or blood culture.
		● Clinical chemistry
		  – elevated blood urea and creatinine.
		  – hyperphosphataemia.
		  – elevated SALT, bile acids, bilirubin.
		● Urine analysis
		  – proteinuria, haematuria, granular casts.
		● Leucocytosis.
		● Post-mortem changes.
			Good vaccines available containing killed sero-types of *L. canicola* and *L. icterohaemorrhagiae*.
			Primary course of two injections given 2–3 weeks apart, can be completed by 12 weeks of age.
			Annual boosters essential as immunity is short-lived.

Canine parvovirus	Depend on age of dog, and body system targeted by virus. Sudden deaths or puppies showing signs of heart failure. ● *Myocarditis* – now rarely seen due to presence of adequate levels of maternal antibody. Sudden deaths or puppies showing signs of heart failure. ● *Gastroenteritis* – depression, anorexia and persistent vomiting; initially vomitus contains food but eventually only bile-stained or bloody fluid. Within 24 hours a profuse liquid diarrhoea, red/brown in colour, foul-smelling; marked dehydration, shock and subnormal temperature. If left untreated, death occurs within short period.	Most are severely immunosuppressed with total white blood cell counts less than 1.0×10^9/l. Highly susceptible to secondary bacterial infections involving any body system. CPV antigen capture CITE assay. Histopathology of affected tissue.	Vaccination: live vaccine in some cases given to puppies at high risk of infection as early as 6 weeks of age, repeated at 12 weeks, followed by annual booster. Booster at 16–20 weeks less essential as vaccines improve.

periods. The virus now invades epithelial cells resulting in typical clinical signs and in particular the virus targets the following tissues:

● Respiratory system, conjunctiva.
● Gastrointestinal system.
● Nose and pads of the feet.
● Nervous system.

Some degree of **immunosuppression** is associated with distemper and this assists in the establishment of secondary bacterial infection. In particular *Streptococci* spp., *Staphylococci* spp., *Mycoplasma* spp. *and Bordetella* spp. are most often involved and result in a significant increase in the severity of clinical signs. Concurrent infection with infectious canine hepatitis, Leptospirosis, parvovirus or Toxoplasmosis may also occur.

Treatment

There is no specific therapy for CDV infection so treatment remains symptomatic:

- Broad-spectrum antibiotics – secondary bacterial infections.
- Intravenous fluid therapy – water and electrolyte losses.
- Anti-emetics and anti-diarrhoeal drugs.
- Anti-convulsants – for nervous signs.
- Hyperimmune serum is of little value in clinical cases.

Nursing care

- Disinfect the consulting room and associated areas to which the patient had contact.
- Change protective clothing and thoroughly wash hands after handling clinical cases.
- Isolate infective patients from other dogs to prevent the spread of infection, especially with regard to public places.
- Advise owners on the nursing care required by the patient:
    (1) Keep patient in a warm but well ventilated room with washable impervious floors.
    (2) Keep the nose and eyes free of caked discharge.
    (3) Remove vomitus/diarrhoea and clean the patient.
    (4) Administer therapy prescribed by veterinary surgeon.
- Advise regarding the examination and vaccination of all in contact dogs.
- Make future appointments to allow the veterinary surgeon to monitor progress, taking into account the need to ensure minimal contact with other clients during consulting hours.

Infectious canine hepatitis (ICH)

Infectious canine hepatitis, once known as Rubarth's disease, is a virus disease of dogs and foxes which targets three types of tissues:

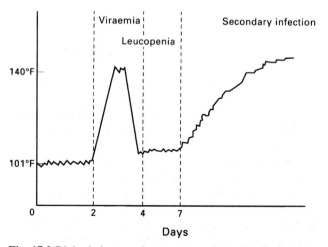

Fig. 17.2 Diphasic increase in temperature in canine distemper.

Table 17.4 Possible nervous signs which may occur in dogs with canine distemper virus infection	
Cranial nerve defects	Poor light reflex. Blindness.
Cerebral	Ataxia. Circling. Pacing. Seizures.
Cerebellar	Ataxia. Dysmetria. Hypermetria. Head tilt. Nystagmus.
Spinal	Weakness. Paresis or occasionally paralysis of hindlimbs. Faecal and/or urinary incontinence. Chorea or twitching associated with any group of muscles, often those of the limbs or flanks.

- The liver.
- The lymphoid tissue.
- Vascular endothelium.

Complications associated with ICH infection include:

- Nephritis.
- Corneal oedema or 'blue eye'.

Mortality can be high, especially in unweaned puppies where ICH often presents as sudden death. However, the severity of clinical signs declines with the age of the dog infected and sudden deaths are rare in dogs over 2 years of age.

Aetiology and pathogenesis

There are two adenoviruses which cause disease in the dog:

- Adenovirus 1 or (CAV-1) – which is associated with ICH.
- Adenovirus 2 or (CAV-2) – which is associated with contagious respiratory disease and possibly enteritis in dogs.

Adenoviruses are more resistant than CDV and can survive off the host for up to 10 days. This means that dogs may become infected from a contaminated environment as well as direct dog-to-dog contact. In spite of this increased resistance the virus is readily destroyed by heat, desiccation and disinfection.

Virus is excreted in the saliva, faeces and urine of infected dogs. Dogs which have recovered from infection may continue to excrete virus for up to 6 months in their urine (convalescent carriers). Transmission of infection requires either direct dog-to-dog contact or contact with infected material. Ingestion is the main method of entry for CAV-1 infection, while aerosol spread is more important in

CAV-2 infection (see section on canine contagious respiratory disease, below).

Following ingestion the virus replicates in local lymph nodes and possibly intestinal Peyer's patches and mesenteric lymph nodes. A viraemia follows within 5–9 days associated with infected lymphocytes. If the animal fails to mount an immune response, the virus targets the bone marrow, liver, other lymphoid tissue and vascular endothelium resulting in typical clinical signs.

When the dog mounts an immune response to acute infection, antigen–antibody complexes form in the circulation and may be deposited in the renal glomeruli leading to glomerular nephritis. At the same time virus invasion of the renal tubular cells occurs leading to an interstitial nephritis in about 70% of cases.

Following recovery, about 20% of dogs develop unilateral or bilateral corneal oedema or 'blue eye'. This represents a local immune reaction associated with interaction between the virus and corneal endothelium leading to leakage of fluid into the aqueous humour. The corneal changes are transient in the majority of cases but occasionally corneal changes become permanent leading to visual impairment.

Although some degree of immunosuppression does occur it is unlikely to result in significant secondary bacterial infection.

Treatment

There is no specific therapy for ICH and clinical cases are treated symptomatically:

- Intravenous fluid therapy.
- Where bleeding has been severe whole blood transfusions can be of great value.
- Antibiotics.
- B-vitamin therapy.

Nursing care

- Check vaccinal status of in-contact dogs.
- Disinfect infected premises.
- Advise owners of the importance of vaccination.
- Assist in therapy devised by the clinician.

Canine contagious respiratory disease (CCRD)

Aetiology and pathogenesis

CCRD, tracheobronchitis or '**kennel cough**' is a highly infectious disease of dogs which is particularly prevalent where large numbers of dogs are kept within the same air space – such as in kennels, breeding establishments and rescue centres.

The canine upper respiratory tract normally harbours many micro-organisms including: *Streptococcus* spp., *Staphylococcus* spp., *Klebsiella* spp., *Pasteurella* spp., *Pseudomonas* spp. and *Bordetella bronchiseptica*. Of these only *Bordetella bronchiseptica* is now considered to act as a primary pathogen, together with some viruses including:

- CAV-1 (canine adenovirus 1).
- CAV-2 (canine adenovirus 2).
- CPIV (canine parainfluenza virus).
- CHV (canine herpes virus).
- Reovirus.

Both CAV-1 and CAV-2 can be associated with respiratory disease. However, CAV-1 induces systemic disease while CAV-2 only results in respiratory disease.

CHV and Reovirus may cause a mild respiratory infection in adult dogs and much less important in the aetiology of the kennel cough than CPIV and CAV-1 and CAV-2.

CPIV acts in a similar manner to CAV-2 and can induce marked respiratory disease. It is very likely to be implicated in the aetiology of kennel cough but it is likely to act together with other agents such as *Bordetella bronchiseptica* in order to induce disease.

Infection follows either direct dog-to-dog contact or aerosol transmission of micro-organisms, especially where dogs are housed within the same air space. It is now clear that kennel cough is not normally caused by one micro-organism but probably by both viral and bacterial agents acting together on the respiratory epithelium. Following inhalation the micro-organisms rapidly colonize the respiratory epithelium leading to an acute inflammatory reaction within 4 days of transmission. The severity of the resultant tracheobronchitis depends on which micro-organisms are involved in the process, the most severe being associated with CPIV and *B. bronchiseptica* (Table 17.3).

Treatment

Symptomatic treatment is usually provided and helps to reduce the duration of clinical signs:

- Use of antibiotics in order to reduce the risk of secondary bacterial infection.
- Anti-tussants such as codeine and butorphanol.

Nursing care

- Advise owners regarding the need to vaccinate in-contact animals.
- Prevent spread of infection, warning owners of the highly infectious nature of the disease.
- Ensure hospitalised cases are kept in isolation, especially with regard to sharing the same air space as other patients.
- Clean and disinfect consulting rooms and other areas where the dog has been hospitalised.
- Ensure the treatment prescribed by the clinician is carried out.
- Advise owners regarding the factors (sudden changes in air temperature, excitement, exercise) that induce coughing so that they may be avoided.

Canine leptospirosis

Aetiology and pathogenesis

Leptospira is a Gram-negative bacteria recognised throughout the world as an important zoonotic organism. Although there are many sero-types, only two are of significance in the dog:

- *Leptospira canicola,* associated with acute interstitial nephritis.
- *Leptospira icterohaemorrhagiae,* associated with inflammation of the liver, vascular damage and haemorrhage. This form of Leptospirosis in man is known as Weil's disease or 'the yellows' (because it causes jaundice).

The clear-cut distinction between the two forms of leptospirosis indicated above does not exist in reality as both sero-types can cause hepatic disease and nephritis.

Infected dogs continue to shed leptospiral organisms in their urine for long periods following recovery. Although the acid pH of urine tends to destroy the organisms, urine contamination of water often results in their survival for long periods of time. Leptospiral organisms are readily destroyed by desiccation, disinfection and ultraviolet light.

Urine from infected dogs is the main source of infection. Rats may also play an important role in the transmission of disease as they may harbour the organism and excrete it in their urine. Routes by which leptospira may infect dogs include:

- Penetrating intact skin.
- Through cuts and abrasions in the skin.
- Transplacental and venereal transmission.
- Through intact mucous membranes of gastrointestinal or respiratory tracts.

Entry via one of the routes described above is followed by a leptospiraemia which persists for about 7 days. At this time the organism invades its target organ (Table 17.3):

- *L. canicola* invades the proximal tubules of the kidney causing tubular cell death and local inflammatory cellular infiltration. This causes marked swelling of the kidneys.
- *L. icterohaemorrhagiae* invades the liver resulting in hepatocellular destruction and perivascular haemorrhage. The vascular damage usually involves the lungs and gastrointestinal tract. Occasionally this sero-type may target the renal tubules in a similar manner to *L. canicola.*

Treatment

Intravenous fluid therapy is essential in both forms of leptospirosis, although dogs with *L. icterohaemorrhagiae* will benefit from whole-blood transfusions. Antibiotics (especially penicillin, streptomycin and tetracyclines) form an essential part of therapy.

Nursing care

> **WARNING**
>
> Remember that this disease is transmissible to man. It is therefore extremely important to take great care in handling dogs with leptospirosis. Disinfection of all contaminated areas is essential. *Always* wear gloves and other suitable protective clothing when handling the patient or body fluids.

- Examine and vaccinate all in-contact dogs.
- Help in the provision of therapy as directed by the veterinary surgeon.
- Inform the owner that the dog has a zoonotic disease and will require careful handling. This is especially true where there are children in the household. Owners should be advised to seek medical advise.
- Advise owners regarding disinfection of kennels and home, and the need to control rats, if present on the premises.
- Liaise with veterinary surgeon regarding re-visits out of normal consulting hours to avoid contact with other dogs.

Canine parvovirus

Canine parvovirus infection (CPV) is a relatively new disease first recognised in 1978 which is thought to have resulted from a mutation of the feline parvovirus associated with feline panleucopenia. It causes two distinct disease syndromes in dogs:

- Acute myocarditis, which occurs in puppies.
- Acute gastroenteritis, which occurs in weaned puppies and adult dogs.

Aetiology and pathogenesis

There are two canine parvoviruses. CPV 1 which has been known for many years and is associated with mild diarrhoea. CPV 2 is antigenically distinct and was not previously recognised before 1978. In 1981 a second mutation is thought to have occurred making the virus even more host specific for dogs.

The virus is highly resistant to destruction compared with the other canine viruses discussed so far. It can remain viable off the host for up to one year, facilitating spread of infection by indirect contact. This virus resists many of the established disinfectants such as phenols and quaternary ammonium compounds but is destroyed by hypochlorite and formalin. Following the recognition of canine parvovirus in 1978 a new series of disinfectants were especially designed to destroy parvoviruses.

Large numbers of virus particles are shed in the faeces of infected dogs and constitute the main source of infection for other dogs. Transmission of disease may occur either by direct or indirect contact between a susceptible dog and an infected dog or faecal contamination.

Following ingestion, the virus replicates in the local lymph nodes and induces a viraemia within 3–5 days following infection. The virus targets rapidly dividing cells in which to replicate, in particular those in the intestine, lymphoid tissue, myocardium and bone marrow. The tissue targeted and subsequent clinical signs depend on the age of the dog.

Prenatal and neonatal puppies have rapidly dividing myocardial cells and infection at this time results in myocarditis. This myocardial development ceases after 7 weeks of age and so the virus invades the rapidly dividing cells of the intestine. Lymphoid tissue and the bone marrow are also targeted in both neonates and adult dogs, resulting in severe immunosuppression.

In 1978 the entire canine population was susceptible to CPV 2 infection. Therefore both myocardial disease and gastroenteritis were commonly observed. However, breeding bitches have now acquired good levels of immunity to CPV 2 and this has been passed onto their puppies, and resulted in a marked reduction in the incidence of myocarditis. It is now more common to observe gastroenteritis in weaned puppies following the loss of maternal antibody protection or in adults which have not been adequately vaccinated (Table 17.3).

Following ingestion the virus replicates in local lymph nodes and induces a viraemia within 3–5 days following infection. The virus targets specific tissues including the myocardium, intestine, lymphoid tissue and bone marrow, depending on the age of the dog.

Treatment

Treatment for myocardial CPV is rarely successful and carries a very guarded prognosis. Where cases do show clinical signs, symptomatic therapy should be provided including: cage rest, diuretics and nutritional support.

Treatment for enteric CPV requires intensive intravenous fluid therapy. Where the dog is severely shocked, whole blood or plasma expanders should be considered. Antiemetics such as metaclopramide will reduce fluid and electrolyte loss and the weakening effects of persistent vomiting. Once vomition ceases, careful introduction of oral fluids may be attempted and if this is tolerated small amounts of low-fat veterinary diets may be provided. Return to normal diet slowly as these dogs have varying degrees of malabsorption.

Nursing care

- As the virus is resistant and survives off the host thorough cleaning of contaminated areas must be carried out using a modern parvocidal disinfectant (see Chapter 5).
- Isolate all clinical cases and ensure strict hygiene to prevent spread of infection to other hospitalized cases. Protective clothing should be used when handling dogs and individual food and water bowls should be used. Careful disposal of infected material is also required.

- Advise the owner regarding the effects of the virus on the dog including the need for a good vaccination programme, especially for any in-contact dogs. The need for careful dietary management through the convalescent period because of the degree of intestinal damage and malabsorption present.

Feline infectious diseases

The following feline infectious diseases are considered in this section:

- Feline panleucopenia.
- Feline upper respiratory disease.
- Feline pneumonitis.
- Feline infectious anaemia.
- Feline infectious peritonitis.
- Feline leukaemia virus.
- Feline immunodeficiency virus.

Clinical signs, diagnosis and control are outlined in Table 17.5.

Feline panleucopenia

This highly contagious disease of the cat family is variously known as feline infectious enteritis, feline distemper, feline parvovirus, as well as feline panleucopenia. Although a disease of young kittens, cats of all ages may be infected. The disease has high mortality and morbidity, especially in kittens.

Aetiology and pathogenesis

Feline panleucopenia is caused by a parvovirus similar to canine parvovirus. The virus can survive for many months off the host and is resistant to heating, phenols, acids and alkalis. Modern parvocidal disinfectants are effective in destroying the virus.

Large amounts of virus are shed in the saliva, vomitus, faeces and urine of infected cats and excretion may persist for months following recovery. Transmission is thought to occur by ingestion following direct or indirect contact and may also be spread by fleas. The highest incidence of disease occurs where susceptible cats are intensively housed such as in rescue centres, breeding establishments and boarding catteries.

A viraemia occurs after ingestion of the virus and replication in local lymph nodes. The virus then targets the rapidly dividing cells of the small intestine, lymphoid tissue and the bone marrow. Following invasion of these tissues the cat shows signs of severe gastroenteritis, and immunosuppression. Unlike canine parvovirus infection, there are *no* cardiac signs with feline panleucopenia.

As the virus can cross the placenta, infection during pregnancy results in viral damage to the cerebellum of the growing foetus, leading to cerebellar hypoplasia. As the cerebellum is still developing at birth, infection up to 2 weeks post-partum can also cause cerebellar hypoplasia.

Table 17.5 Feline infectious diseases: clinical signs, diagnosis and control

	Clinical signs	Diagnosis	Control
Feline panleuco-penia	Four clinical syndromes associated with feline panleucopenia (a) *Peracute* – sudden death in young kittens without any obvious signs of ill-health. Owners may suspect kitten has been 'poisoned' because of speed of death. (b) *Acute* more common – sudden onset of marked depression and anorexia, quickly followed by persistent vomiting of food and subsequently bile-stained fluid. Cats often assume pathetic 'hunched up' appearance with nose resting on floor. Often cry in pain when handled or picked up and abdomen may feel distended. No diarrhoea initially but often appears after 2–3 days of clinical disease – often liquid, yellow–brown and may contain blood. (c) *Sub-acute* usually many of clinical signs observed in acute but less severe. (d) Cerebellar hypoplasia – kittens show dysmetria and hypermetria, muscle tremors, weakness and ataxia.	History of poor vaccinal status, together with typical clinical signs. Definitive diagnosis from: ● Routine haematology revealing marked leucopenia. ● Detection of virus in the diarrhoea. ● CITE test.	Killed and modified live vaccines available. Initial course with injection as early as 9 weeks and a second at 12 weeks of age, then boosted annually. Maintain high levels of hygiene in catteries and isolate all new arrivals.
FURD	Incubation period 2–10 days. Generally acute disease observed but severity varies considerably between individuals. Clinical disease appears more severe in very young or old and in purebred cats, especially Siamese. Paroxysmal sneezing and conjunctivitis with serous ocular and nasal discharge are first clinical signs, followed by anorexia, depression and pyrexia, then signs of nasal and ocular ulceration, hypersalivation, loss of voice and coughing. Secondary bacterial infection results in viscous mucopurulent ocular and nasal discharge – often causes eyelids to stick together (risk of keratitis and corneal ulceration); nasal passage become blocked, loss of olfaction makes it necessary to breathe through mouth. Anorexia and salivation may be due to pyrexia, oral ulceration, loss of olfaction. Clinical signs normally resolve within 7–21 days depending on the breed, age and degree of secondary infection.	From typical clinical picture; can be confirmed by virus isolation from oropharyngeal swabs.	Many cats which recover become carriers and excrete both FCV and FHV-1. FHV-1 is not a resistant virus but FCV remains viable off the host and therefore essential to reduce the level of environmental contamination: ● Good hygiene. ● Isolation of sick cats and new arrivals. ● Keeping the number of cats sharing same air space as low as possible. ● Ensure at least 20 air changes/hour in catteries. ● Ensure cats unable to come into direct contact. ● Establish good vaccination policy: injectable and intranasal vaccines available; modified live vaccine can be used intranasally to provide good local immunity with rapid onset of action (protection usually achieved within 5 days). Occasionally mild signs of upper respiratory disease following this form of vaccination. Dead vaccine useful for pregnant queens. Initial vaccination 2 injections at 9–12 weeks of age, must be boosted annually.
Feline pneumonitis	Initially serous ocular discharge with some degree of blepharospasm, hyperaemia and chemosis, progressing to nasal discharge and sneezing, mucupurulent discharge. Cats initially pyrexic but generally remain bright and continue eating. Improvement expected within 2–3 weeks but persistent infections last many months. May be concurrent FCV and FHV-1 infection.	Confirmation by conjunctival swabs for culture and blood samples detect rising titre.	*Chlamydia psittaci* very difficult to eliminate if endemic with cattery. If not endemic, all new arrivals should be isolated and carefully observed for evidence of infection. If they have no serological titre to *Chlamydia psittaci* it is unlikely they have been exposed to infection. Modified live vaccine available for all cats except pregnant queens. Initial course can start at 9 weeks of age. Two injections 3–4 weeks apart; boost anually.

Table 17.5 (Continued)

	Clinical signs	Diagnosis	Control
Feline infectious anaemia	Sudden onset of weakness, lethargy and anorexia. Often pyrexic, marked pallor of mucous membranes; associated tachycardia, tachypnoea and splenomegaly.	Routine haematology reveals high reticuloctye count indicating regenerative anaemia. Definitive diagnosis from examination of Giemsa-stained blood smears to showing the parasites attached to the red blood cells, but several blood smears may have to be examined before the parasite is detected, due to fluctuating parasitaemia.	Flea control. Use of tetracyclines.
FIP	Early signs vague, including pyrexia, anorexia, weight loss, diarrhoea. Failure to grow is common in kittens. Possible chronic unresponsive diarrhoea with prolapse of third eyelid. Progresses to more specific signs of two clinical forms within few weeks or may take months: (a)*Effusive FIP* (Some 60% of all cases – much shorter duration of ill health): fluid accumulates in the abdomen (and in 25% of cases within the thorax as well); pericardial effusion not uncommon. (b)*Non-effusive FIP* No effusions; granulomatous lesions on any abdominal organs, particularly spleen, liver and kidneys; organs often become swollen, palpable; eventually organ failure. In about 50%, only central nervous signs: generalised and progressive neurological defects including ataxia, paresis, paralysis, disorientation and convulsions. Eye lesions associated with retinitis and uveitis; may be unilateral or bilateral.	Difficult interpretation of serology. Biopsy collection and histopathological examination of granulomatous lesions is only method currently definitive. Other non-specific findings include: ● Examination of ascitic or thoracic fluid – yellow, viscous, sterile and may clot on standing. Protein content usually high (> 35 g/l). ● Anaemia. ● Hyperglobulinaemia. ● Jaundice. ● Lymphopenia. ● Concurrent FeLV and/or FIV infection.	Vaccines available in USA, none at present in the UK.
Feline leukaemia virus	May remain asymptomatic for years. When clinical signs occur, may be associated with either neoplastic disease (20% of cases), or non-neoplastic diseases associated with immunosuppression (80% of cases). Clinical picture with FeLV-related disease varies but may include any of conditions shown in Table 17.6.	Suspected from the history and clinical picture; confirmation by examination of serum, and/or white blood cells or bone marrow cells for viral protein. Infected cells produce protein P27, released in large amounts along with new virus particles. ELISA test detects this protein antigen and provides very reliable method of confirming FeLV infection. False positive and negative results rare as long as test procedure carried out carefully. Virus isolated from plasma.	*Multi-cat households*: testing all cats and isolate those which are positive. Repeated at 3-month intervals, removing any new positive cases, until all cats remain negative on at least two separate occasions. Colony can then be considered FeLV negative; isolate all new arrivals and carefully screen for infection. *Single-cat households*: confining cats to reduce the risk of infection. Cell culture and genetically engineered vaccines are now available in UK. Initial course two vaccinations 2–3 weeks apart; annual boosting. Ideally test cats for FeLV before vaccination, no beneficial effect on cats already infected.

Table 17.5 (Continued)

	Clinical signs	Diagnosis	Control
Feline immuno-deficiency virus	Transient pyrexia and generalised lymphadenopathy after exposure to virus, followed by asymptomatic phase which may last for years before clinically detectable immunodeficiency syndrome develops. Many different clinical conditions associated with immunosuppression and secondary bacterial infections, varying individually. Lethargy, weight loss and anorexia always present; clinical signs associated with either respiratory or digestive tract. Most common forms include: ● Chronic rhinitis. ● Lymphadenopathy. ● Chronic diarrhoea. ● Chronic gingivitis. ● Chronic skin disease. ● Uveitis. ● Neurological disease (behaviour changes, convulsions). ● Neoplasia, especially lymphoid tumours. Most of these associated with secondary opportunist organisms which establish because of FIV-induced immunosuppression. History of chronic or recurring infections which respond poorly to treatment, in a lethargic thin cat, strongly suggestive of FIV infection.	Detection of antibodies to viral protein: commercial ELISA test (CITE and SNAP) kits available and generally very reliable. Immunofluorescence Western blot test is more reliable. Viral isolation from lymphocytes confirms infection.	No vaccines available in UK; prevention involves avoiding situations where cats are likely to become infected: ● Keep indoors or limit outdoor exposure. ● Castrate males to prevent aggression and fighting. ● Control free roaming.

Treatment

There is no specific therapy available so treatment remains supportive:

● Intravenous fluid therapy to reverse dehydration and the electrolyte losses.
● Broad-spectrum antibiotics to protect from secondary bacterial infection due to the immunosuppression.

Once vomition ceases, oral fluid may be provided and assuming no relapse occurs a slow return to normal oral fluid and food intake may be made but *care* is required in the speed at which this occurs and the type of food offered. Most cats have severe small intestinal damage (and therefore some degree of malabsorption) and it is therefore essential to provide highly digestible low-fat diets to prevent chronic diarrhoea and weight loss.

Nursing care

● Ensure that treatment prescribed by the veterinary surgeon is carried out.
● Provide a comfortable environment for clinical cases.
● Careful disposal of clinical waste.
● Discuss with the owner the need to have all in-contact cats examined and vaccinated.
● Ensure strict hygiene when handling infected cats.

Feline upper respiratory disease (FURD)

FURD, or cat 'flu, is a highly contagious disease of the cat which is the traditional scourge of catteries, where a sneezing cat can herald the beginning of a major outbreak of cat 'flu. The morbidity rate is high but the mortality rate is generally low.

Aetiology and pathogenesis

Cat 'flu is caused by two viruses:

● Feline calici virus (FCV), a fragile RNA virus that is easily destroyed once it is off the host.
● Feline herpes virus 1 (FNV-1), a more resistant DNA virus that can survive for up to 8 days off the host; it has also been known by the descriptive name of feline viral rhinotracheitis (FVR) virus.

Reovirus has also been suggested in the primary disease although its role is considered minor compared to FCV and FHV-1. In addition to primary viral infection, secondary bacterial infection can play an important role in the severity of clinical signs and speed of recovery (Table 17.5).

Transmission of infection is associated with inhalation of virus aerosols created by sneezing cats. Chronic carriers of both FHV and FCV may be an important source of infection. However, each of the viruses behave differently in this situation. FHV-1 can remain latent with intermittent shedding of virus associated with stress, steroid administration or concurrent infection, while FCV carriers excrete virus continuously. Detecting carrier cats can be difficult especially with regard to FHV-1. The only effective method of detecting these cats is repeated oropharyngeal swabbing. Ideally this should be carried out once shedding starts as cats often exhibit mild upper respiratory tract signs at these times.

Following inhalation the viruses replicate in local lymph nodes before invasion of the epithelial cells of the respiratory tract and conjunctiva. FCV has a greater tendency than FHV-1 to cause ulceration of mucous membranes which may permit secondary bacterial infection to establish. The complications which may follow infection include:

- Prolonged recovery.
- Keratitis and corneal ulceration.
- Lower respiratory disease – bronchopneumonia.
- Chronic rhinitis – 'snufflers' (chronic FHV-1).
- Latent carrier of FHV-1.
- Persistant excretors of FCV.

Treatment

Treatment of cat 'flu is mainly supportive and includes:

- Correction of dehydration and maintenance of hydration using intravenous fluid therapy.
- Use of broad-spectrum antibiotics to control secondary bacterial infection.
- Enteral nutrition.
- Good nursing care.

Nursing care

Nursing care is especially important in cat 'flu as most cats are unable to smell their food and find eating painful because of oral ulceration: so they stop eating and drinking leading to dehydration and weight loss.

- Ensure that fluid therapy maintains adequate hydration.
- Bathe the eyes and nose of discharge; to aid breathing, improve olfaction and prevent corneal damage.
- Use inhalants prior to feeding.
- Encourage eating by offering highly aromatic, warmed foods.
- Maintain high levels of hygiene to prevent spread of disease.
- Discuss vaccination programmes with the client.
- Advise on examination and vaccination of in-contact cats.

Feline pneumonitis

Feline pneumonitis is caused by *Chlamydia psittaci* and is one of the commonest causes of conjunctivitis in cats. The infection is recognised throughout the world and accounts for over 30% of conjunctivitis in the UK. Kittens appear to be the most severely infected.

The organism targets the conjunctiva of cats but may also be an cause of infertility. Abortions have been recorded and although the organism has been isolated from the reproductive tract, no cases of infertility have been proved.

Pathogenesis

The actual method of transmission is not known but direct contact between cats, especially any ocular or nasal discharge, appears to be important. It also seems likely that long-term carriers may exist without evidence of clinical disease and may act as a source of infection. The organism may also be harboured in the gastrointestinal and genital tract. The incubation period lasts between 4 and 10 days (Table 17.5).

Treatment and nursing care

The most effective treatment for *Chlamydia psittaci* infection is local (topical) and systemic use of tetracyclines. Doxycycline is the drug of choice and all cats within the household should be treated at the same time. Treatment should be maintained for 2 weeks after clinical signs have ceased.

Feline infectious anaemia

Aetiology and pathogenesis

Haemobartonellosis or feline infectious anaemia (FIA) is associated with the rickettsial parasite *Haemobartonella felis* and is an extracellular parasite of red blood cells. FIA can occur in all age groups but appears more common in male cats. Infection may be transmitted by:

- Cat bites.
- Flea infestations.
- Vertical transmission *in utero*.
- Via the queen's milk.

It is thought that many cats may be exposed to the parasite without showing signs of clinical disease. Some of these cats may become carriers and only develop clinical disease if stressed, immunosuppressed or suffering concurrent disease. In particular, there is an association between FIA and FeLV/FIV infection.

Following infection, cycles of parasitaemia develop and are associated with profound anaemia which can occasionally be fatal (Table 17.5). The parasitaemia may be recurrent interspersed with periods of complete remission; in spite of these remissions cats may remain chronically infected. This may be due to a complex relationship between the parasite and the cat's immune system.

Treatment

Assuming there is no evidence of concurrent FeLV or FIV infection, tetracyclines are the drugs of choice in the treatment of *Haemobartonella felis*. The use of prednisolone is now thought to be of value, due to the immune-mediated nature of the disease. Cats with severe anaemia may require a blood transfusion. Where the cat has a flea infestation, this should also be treated.

Nursing care

- Assist in the administration of treatment directed by the veterinary surgeon.
- Discuss with the owner the need to examine other cats within the household, including treatment for fleas.

- Careful observation and monitoring of hospitalised cats, with particular reference to their cardiac and respiratory function.
- Reduce stress and providing a good environment for recovery.
- Ensure the cat maintains adequate fluid and nutritional intake.

Feline infectious peritonitis (FIP)

This disease was first recognised in the early 1960s and now has a world-wide distribution in both domestic and wild cats. The incidence of infection is low (1–5%) and prognosis is very poor. FIP is more common in multi-cat households and among pedigree cats, especially the Burmese (20% of cases). There is no sex predisposition and although clinical cases can occur in any age group those less than 2 years of age are most often affected.

Aetiology and pathogenesis

FIP is caused by a coronavirus similar to the enteric coronavirus (FECV) commonly encountered in cats. Recent research suggests that FIP may arise from a mutation of FECV. The virus is labile and readily destroyed by modern disinfectants.

Direct contact between susceptible and infected cats does not seem to be important even though virus is shed in urine and faeces (this only occurs for a short period of time). However, carriers may be important in the epidemiology of disease and may carry the virus for years. This may have significance with regard to the queen passing on infection to her kittens.

The mode of transmission is not understood and the incubation period appears to be extremely variable. Entry is thought to occur via the oronasal mucosa. When cats are exposed to coronavirus some 90% develop transient gastro-intestinal disease and in about 10% of cats viral replication then develops in macrophages. Infected macrophages reach the general circulation and then target vascular beds such as the peritoneum, pleura, eye, meninges or kidneys.

A cell mediated immune response appears to be important in determining the outcome to viral challenge. If a good cell mediated immune response occurs, the cat eliminates the virus (90%) but a poor response leads to FIP infection.

Antibodies to coronavirus may result in formation of perivascular antigen/antibody complexes, which cause vasculitis, leading to fluid leakage from peritoneal or pleural blood vessels.

Two forms of FIP occur:

- A wet or effusive form which is thought to be associated with a very poor immune response.
- A dry form which may occur following a partial immune response.

Treatment and nursing care

The prognosis remains very guarded and there is no specific treatment for FIP. Concurrent FeLV or FIV results in a further deterioration in the prognosis.

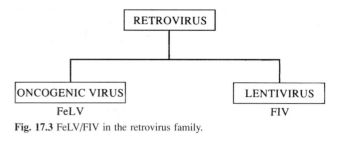

Fig. 17.3 FeLV/FIV in the retrovirus family.

Symptomatic therapy using antibiotics and corticosteroids may result in temporary remission.

Feline leukaemia virus (FeLV)

Aetiology and pathogenesis

FeLV is a species-specific retrovirus (Fig. 17.3) of world-wide distribution affecting both domestic and wild members of the cat family. It has also been suggested that two out of every three cats have been exposed to infection sometime during their life and it is estimated that 18% of sick cats and 10% of healthy cats are FeLV positive. In multi-cat households up to 30% of cats may be FeLV positive.

Susceptibility to infection appears to depend on the age of the cat. Kittens infected *in utero* will become persistently viraemic and die. Exposure at less than 8 weeks old gives a 70–80% chance of becoming permanently viraemic whilst adults have only a 10% chance of becoming persistently viraemic.

Infection can be transmitted vertically from the queen to her kittens either *in utero* or via the milk. Horizontal transmission can also occur following direct contact between cats. The virus is present in saliva, mucus, urine, faeces and milk. Saliva contains high levels of virus, so cat bites may be an important method of transmitting infection.

Table 17.6 Some of the clinical conditions which may be associated with feline leukaemia virus infection	

Neoplastic disease	Lymphosarcoma
	    Multicentric.
	    Thymic.
	    Alimentary.

Non-neoplastic disease	Myeloproliferative disease.
	Non-regenerative anaemia.
	Immunosuppression
	    FIP.
	    FIV?
	    Cat 'flu.
	    Feline enteritis.
	    Toxoplasmosis.
	    Oral infections.
	Immune diseases
	    Glomerular nephritis.
	    Polyarthritis.
	    Polyneuritis.
	Reproductive
	    Stillbirths.
	    Foetal resorption.
	    Abortion.

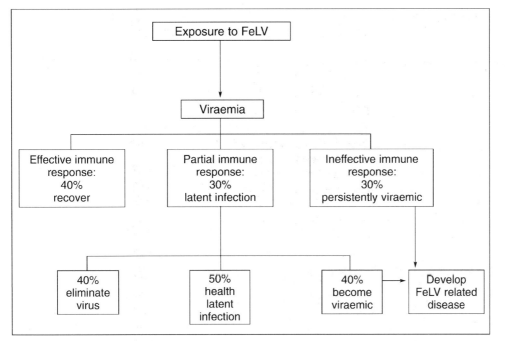

Fig. 17.4 FeLV flow chart.

Following oral infection the virus replicates in the local lymph nodes. A viraemia results and disseminates the virus to distant lymphoid tissue. A second viraemic phase leads to dissemination of virus to the bone marrow and other tissues.

Several outcomes are now possible depending on the cats immune response to the virus (Fig. 17.4; see also Table 17.6). Some 40% will eliminate the virus completely and recover. In the 30% where the immune response is poor, the virus is likely to invade the following tissues:

- The bone marrow – leading to anaemia, leukaemia, immunosuppression.
- The crypts of Lieberkühns of the intestine – enteritis.
- Salivary, lacrymal and pancreatic glands – excretion of virus.
- Urogenital system – abortions, stillbirths, infertility.
- Remain viraemic.

Occasionally FeLV may invade host cells and remains dormant (30%) – this is termed **latent infection**. Over a number of months or years this latent infection may be slowly eliminated. However, in a small number of cases viral replication may be switched on again. This may occur during:

- Periods of stress.
- Concurrent infection.
- Use of corticosteroid therapy.

Treatment and nursing care

There is no specific therapy for FeLV infection. Symptomatic therapy is aimed at reducing the effects of secondary bacterial infection, however, the prognosis remains very guarded.

Feline immunodeficiency virus (FIV)

Aetiology and pathogenesis

FIV is an RNA retrovirus which was first recognised in 1986 in the USA. However, stored blood samples have revealed that it was present in blood samples taken as early as 1968. The infection is now known to have a world-wide distribution and affects both domestic and wild cats. Originally FIV was known as feline T lymphotrophic lentivirus (FTLV) but this name is no longer used.

Infection is rare in cats less than 1 year old but increases with age to a peak at around 8 years old. The disease is 30 times more common in outdoor cats and 3 times more common in males than females. This is probably because cat bites are thought to be the main mode of transmission: saliva contains significant amounts of virus and transmission is by biting. Simple direct contact between cats appears to be unlikely to cause infection but sexual transmission may be important. As the virus is labile, environmental contamination and therefore spread by indirect contact seems highly unlikely.

Recent work suggests that 13% of sick cats are positive for FIV while only 4% of healthy cats are FIV positive. The highest incidence appears to occur in Northern Ireland, Scotland, the south and south-east of England.

It appears that FIV infection cannot be eliminated by a normal immune response. Within 2 weeks of being bitten the infected cat will show evidence of antibody production and virus may be detected in circulating lymphocytes. After a further 4 weeks the cat may develop pyrexia and generalised lymphadenopathy which can last for many weeks (Table 17.5)

Many cats appear to 'recover' and remain asymptomatic for years before a clinically detectable immunodeficiency syndrome develops.

Treatment and nursing care

There is no treatment for FIV at present although symptomatic treatment can be offered. This treatment consists of antibiotics for secondary bacterial infection. However, the prognosis must remain very guarded.

Rabies

Rabies is a disease of the nervous system. It is recognised worldwide, although countries such as Norway, Sweden, Portugal, Japan, Eire and Iceland have managed to remain free of infection. The main risk to the UK lies in importation of dogs from Asia, Latin America and Africa. Foxes appear to be an important reservoir host in Europe, while the skunk, racoon and bat are important in the USA.

Rabies is a very important disease because of some unique characteristics of the virus:

● The virus has the ability to infect many different species.
● It is a zoonosis.
● The effects on the CNS often result in aggression so animals bite each other and increase the chance of spreading the disease.
● Once clinically manifest, the disease is fatal.

Rabies can spread within either the wildlife, domestic dog or cat populations. **Sylvatic rabies** is the term used to describe spread of infection in wildlife while **urban rabies** describes the spread of infection in domestic dogs or cats. Domestic cats are more resistant to rabies than are dogs.

Aetiology and pathogenesis

Rabies is caused by a rhabdovirus which has an affinity for cells of the nervous system. The virus is present in the saliva of infected animals and is readily transmitted by biting. Usually rabid dogs or cats will be showing clinical signs when they have bitten someone but the saliva may contain virus for up to 14 days before clinical signs develop. So being bitten by an apparently normal dog or cat in an endemic area should be viewed with suspicion.

The virus cannot penetrate intact skin but it can cross the oral or nasal mucous membrane. Therefore infection following ingestion and inhalation (via aerosol) is possible although a very large dose of virus is required. The virus is very labile and survives poorly off the host.

The incubation period can vary from 2 weeks to 4 months, with a mean incubation period of 3 weeks. The speed at which clinical signs develop depends on:

● The site of infection (virus reaches the CNS more rapidly if bite is to the head or neck).
● The severity of the bite.
● The dose of virus.

Once a dog or cat is bitten the virus remains at the site of inoculation during the incubation period. Viral replication takes place in the muscle tissue and eventually virus penetrates the neuromuscular tissue and so gains entry into the nervous system.

Infection now rapidly spreads to the central nervous system by axonal flow along nerve fibres. No lymphatic or blood-borne dissemination of infection occurs. Once in the CNS the virus replicates within the neurons and infection then spreads centrifugally to the peripheral nervous system. Eventually peripheral nervous tissue and the organs they supply will become infected. This is how the salivary glands become infected and contain large amounts of virus.

Normally there is inadequate virus production in the muscle tissue to provoke an immune response and subsequently antibody production. However, if the patient is vaccinated, an immune response will be produced and protection given *before* the virus enters the nervous system. Once in the nervous system antibody is unable to provide protection.

> The virus is *only* vulnerable while in the muscle tissue and *before* it enters the nervous system. Therefore speed is essential.

Clinical signs

There are two recognised forms of clinical rabies:

● Furious rabies.
● Dumb rabies.

Initial clinical signs include pyrexia and a change in temperament. Dogs may become more placid and seek affection or they may hide away in corners or under beds. The site of infection may become intensely pruritic. As virus may be present in saliva before these signs develop, it is very important to isolate dogs which have been bitten and observe them for these changes in temperament.

In **furious rabies** the animal will now become progressively hyperexcitable. These episodes may last only a short period of time or may last many hours. During the episodes they may become aggressive, snap and bite at even imaginary objects, they may develop a depraved appetite and chew and eat anything. If they are free to do so, dogs will walk or run many miles before trying to return home. In between these periods the dog or cat may be friendly, placid and calm.

As the disease progresses signs of paresis of the legs and tail occurs. There may be difficulty in swallowing and asymmetry and distortion of the face. In dogs and cats there is *no* evidence of hydrophobia that is a feature of human rabies. Eventually they will die during a violent seizure.

Dumb rabies is much more common with little or no evidence of the signs described above. In dumb rabies there is a progressive paralysis involving the limbs and distortion of the face with drooping of the jaw, eyelids, squinting of the eyes, drooling of saliva and difficulty in swallowing. Great care should be exercised when examining such dogs which may initially appear to have some oral or pharyngeal foreign body. If the examiner has any cuts or abrasions, particularly on the hands, this will allow easy access by the virus. In dumb rabies the animal will eventually become comatose and die.

Although these descriptions indicate there are two clear-cut forms of rabies, it is important to emphasise that such clear-cut divisions do not always occur in reality. Cases may occur with features of both forms of the disease. In all cases death occurs usually within 7 days following the onset of clinical signs.

Where rabies is suspected the dog should not be killed but kept in isolation and prevented from escaping or injuring someone. The Ministry of Agriculture Fisheries and Food (MAFF) should be contacted immediately. If the dog cannot be caught safely other appropriate action will be decided and in such circumstances great care is required to ensure the brain is not damaged.

Diagnosis

Once the dog has died or been destroyed the head is removed by a MAFF veterinary officer and transported to a Ministry laboratory. The diagnosis of rabies is achieved by examining the brain for Negri bodies which represent accumulations of virus protein in the neurons. A fluorescent antibody test is also available which can detect disease in neurons at a much earlier stage. Virus isolation can also be carried out by inoculating mice with brain suspension.

Treatment

Although there are reports of dogs and cats recovering from rabies, such situations are very rare. Generally there is no treatment for rabies and because of the serious risk of human infection, all dogs and cats should be destroyed if rabies is suspected.

Control

Control is achieved by vaccination. Inactivated and live vaccines are available but in the UK only the former is used. There are reports of live rabies vaccination causing disease in cats which have concurrent FeLV or FIV infection (due to immunosuppression). Initial vaccination involves a single injection. Puppies of 3–4 months of age can be vaccinated and boosted regularly.

Foxes are the most important reservoir host in Europe. In order to control the spread of rabies in Europe, oral vaccines have been produced which allow foxes to be vaccinated by using baits. This form of vaccination appears to have been effective in controlling the spread of rabies.

Safe human inactivated vaccines are also available for persons considered to be at risk of infection. Personnel should receive an initial vaccination course followed by regular booster vaccination to maintain protection. See Chapter 5, p. 140.

Diseases of the alimentary tract

Changes in eating behaviour are common reasons for owners to seek veterinary advice. These changes may include an increase or decrease in appetite, a depraved appetite or inability to eat. This subject is covered in greater detail in Chapter 8 (Nutrition).

DEFINITIONS

- **Dysphagia** is the physical inability to eat food, usually as a consequence of mechanical or neurological disorders. The animal is often hungry but is simply unable to eat or swallow food. Dysphagias are usually classified into problems with the oral cavity, pharynx or oesophagus. Owners often refer to this as **inappetence**.
- **Anorexia** is the loss of the desire to eat, while retaining the physical ability to do so. This is also sometimes described as inappetence by the owner. Cases are associated with systemic diseases and nausea.
- **Polyphagia** is an increased appetite beyond the amount the animal would normally consume. In some cases animals not only consume all their food but may steal food or become scavengers. Disorders such as exocrine pancreatitis insufficiency, Cushing's disease and diabetes mellitus may exhibit polyphagia.
- **Pica** describes a depraved appetite. Examples include animals eating their own faeces (**coprophagia**), eating soil or licking concrete. This often distresses owners, who may be reluctant to discuss the problem. The behaviour is often associated with some form of nutritional deficiency.

Anorexia

There are specific instances where anorexic animals should not be fed (such as acute pancreatitis) but most animals should be encouraged to eat, although the final decision rests with the veterinary surgeon. Prolonged anorexia will result in the utilisation of body fat and protein stores for energy. This will lead not only to a loss of adipose tissue and lean body mass but also:

- Poor immune response to infection.
- Poor wound healing.
- Slower recovery.
- Increased metabolic load on the kidneys and liver.

Treating the underlying cause of the anorexia will have the greatest impact on appetite but owners should also be encouraged to improve the nutritional intake of their pet by using a highly palatable and digestible diet. This can be achieved by:

- Warming the food.
- Using strong-smelling foods.

- Providing a moist food rather than a dry food.
- Using high-fat diets.
- Liquidising the food.
- Hand-feeding while talking to the animal.
- Offering several types of fresh food to determine preference.

Where these methods fail, the veterinary surgeon may use drugs to stimulate the appetite or insert a feeding tube into the alimentary tract and initiate further feeding.

Conditions of the oesophagus and stomach

Although owners may present their pets with a history of 'vomiting', sometimes this does not truly reflect what the animal is actually doing. Careful collection of the history may reveal the animal is actually regurgitating its food rather than vomiting. Such a differentiation can provide important information regarding the location of the problem.

Regurgitation is a passive process in which food and fluid are passed back up the oesophagus and out through the mouth. It is always associated with undigested foods or liquids and often occurs shortly after feeding. No abdominal contractions are involved in this process.

Regurgitation may be associated with oesophageal disease (Table 17.7) such as **megaoesophagus**. In this condition there is a failure of peristaltic contractions to move a food bolus from the pharynx to the stomach. The food remains in the oesophagus, which rapidly becomes a large flaccid sac. Eventually the volume of food and fluid in the oesophagus stimulates regurgitation through the mouth.

Vomiting is an active process involving cessation of breathing, closure of the epiglottis, fixation of the diaphragm and contraction of the abdominal muscles. This squeezes the stomach and ejects food along the oesophagus and out of the mouth. Frequent retching precedes actual vomition. The vomitus may contain food, bile-stained fluid, water, blood or intestinal contents. Vomiting may be the result of primary gastric disease or may be secondary to a systemic disease (Table 17.7).

Persistent regurgitation or vomiting can lead to serious complications:

- Loss of water and electrolytes – dehydration.
- Inhalation of food – aspirational pneumonia.

Persistent vomiting leads to excess loss of water and electrolytes. As the animal cannot drink to replace this loss, it becomes **dehydrated**. The degree of dehydration can be determined in the laboratory by measuring the packed cell volume (PCV) and total plasma protein levels. Clinically, the degree of dehydration can be detected by testing skin elasticity:

- 5%: slight loss of skin elasticity.
- 10%: skin inelastic, stays 'tented' for a few seconds and slowly returns to normal. Oral mucous membrane dry; eyes lacklustre.
- +12%: skin stays tented permanently. Eyes become sunken; oral mucous membrane very dry; animal collapses.

Aspiration pneumonia occurs when some food is inhaled during regurgitation or vomiting. As food is not sterile, this can result in a serious infection of the lungs. It is common in animals with persistent regurgitation and can occasionally be fatal.

Treatment

The treatment prescribed for the vomiting patient depends on the underlying cause. In general, vomiting will cease once the underlying cause has been identified and treated. Symptomatic therapy for primary gastric disease includes:

- Complete dietary rest.
- Promotion of fluids by intravenous route. Avoid oral fluids while still vomiting.
- Treat the underlying cause.
- If required, feed intravenously.
- Anti-emetics may be of value in specific cases.
- Antacids (cimetidine) to prevent gastric acid production.
- Surgery (foreign bodies, neoplasia).
- Protectants such as bismuth preparations.

Table 17.7 Some of the conditions which may be associated with regurgitation or vomiting in dogs and cats

Regurgitation	Vomiting	
	Primary disease	Secondary vomiting
Oesophageal FB	Acute gastritis	Azotaemia (renal disease)
Megaoesophagus	Chronic gastritis	Pyometra
Vascular ring	Gastric ulceration	Drug toxicity (morphine, digoxin)
Oesophageal stricture	Gastric neoplasia	Motion sickness
Reflux oesophagitis	Gastric foreign body	Colitis
		Pancreatitis
		Hepatitis

Primary vomiting is associated with gastric disease; in secondary vomiting there is no gastric pathology.

Table 17.8 Some of the causes of enteritis or diarrhoea in the dog and cat (in some cases diarrhoea is secondary to disease of other organs)

Life-threatening	Acute	Chronic	Secondary
HGE	Dietary	Malabsorption	Addison's disease
Parvovirus	Worms	Neoplasia (lymphoma)	Liver disease
Distemper	Colitis	Colitis	Pancreatic disease
Salmonellosis	Giardiasis	Dietary hypersensitivity	Kidney disease

Conditions of the small intestine

Diarrhoea may be defined as the passage of unformed faeces of increased bulk or fluid content. Diarrhoea may be life-threatening, acute, secondary to systemic disease or chronic (Table 17.8). When diarrhoea is associated with intestinal disease, the character of the diarrhoea can often indicate whether it originates from the small or large intestine (Table 17.9).

Blood is occasionally observed in the faeces. When this is due to large intestinal disease it is usually fresh blood that is passed. **Melaena** describes the passage of changed blood in the faeces, which may be black or tarry-looking. This blood has usually originated from the stomach or small intestine.

In **life-threatening diarrhoea** the animal is usually systemically ill and will exhibit clinical signs which include persistent vomiting, marked dehydration, anorexia, abdominal pain and the passage of faeces which may contain blood. Any animal exhibiting these signs should be examined as soon as possible. Aggressive therapy is required if the animal is to be saved. Intensive intravenous fluid therapy together with antibiotics and nil by mouth may be followed by the use of oral and anti-diarrhoeal drugs once vomition ceases. Oral fluids followed by a low-fat veterinary diet and a slow return to normal feeding can be permitted as long as the diarrhoea does not recur.

Chronic diarrhoea may be associated with maldigestion or malabsorption of nutrients:

● **Maldigestion** is usually associated with failure of the exocrine pancreas to produce adequate levels of digestive enzymes.
● **Malabsorption** is associated with damage to the small intestinal villi, preventing adequate absorption of nutrients.

Table 17.9 Some clinical features which may permit differentiation between diarrhoea originating from the small or large intestine

Clinical sign	Small intestine	Large intestine
Faecal volume	increased	normal/reduced
Faecal frequency	increased	increased
Faecal fat	present	absent
Tenesmus	absent	may be present
Blood	black/tarry	fresh
Mucus	absent	present
Weight loss	present	absent

In either case the clinical signs are very similar, so that the conditions cannot be differentiated on clinical signs alone. They include:

● Chronic diarrhoea, often containing undigested/absorbed food.
● Marked weight loss.
● Polyphagia.

Animals with malabsorption require a single protein veterinary diet fed at least twice daily. Anti-inflammatory drugs and occasionally antibiotics may be required. In the case of exocrine pancreatic insufficiency a low-fat veterinary diet should be fed, supplemented with proprietary enzyme replacer.

Colitis is another common cause of chronic diarrhoea, especially in dogs. Weight loss is not a feature of colitis but tenesmus, urgency and the passing of faeces containing blood and/or mucus are common. Treatment involves the use of a non-steroidal anti-inflammatory drug and dietary correction. Both high-fibre diets and hypoallergenic diets have been recommended in the treatment of colitis.

Nursing care in vomiting and diarrhoea

● If an infective disease is suspected, provide isolation facilities and maintain high levels of hygiene to prevent the spread of infection.
● Ensure that the prescribed treatment is carried out.
● Monitor and maintain intravenous fluid therapy.
● Ensure that the patient is not allowed to lie in its vomit or diarrhoea and that any such clinical waste is disposed of properly.
● Record all incidents of vomiting or diarrhoea on a kennel sheet.
● Ensure that the animal receives nil by mouth initially.
● Be responsible for the careful introduction of oral intake once this has been approved by the veterinary surgeon.
● Advise owners regarding the animal's progress and treatment.
● Report any deterioration to the veterinary surgeon.

Foreign body obstruction

Foreign bodies are relatively common in the dog and cat, although the type of foreign body and location vary according to the species involved. They may be found in the oral cavity, pharynx, oesophagus, stomach and small intestine. The large intestine is the least likely site for such

Table 17.10 Foreign bodies obstructing the alimentary tract

	Clinical signs	Treatment
Oral foreign bodies	Sudden onset of excess salivation. Pawing the mouth. Champing the jaw. Possibly bleeding from the mouth.	Remove with care under sedation or general anaesthetic.
Pharyngeal foreign bodies	Sudden onset of choking, retching, gagging. Pawing at mouth. Salivation. Possible difficulty in breathing.	Must be removed under general anaesthetic but great care needed to ensure that a patent airway is maintained at all times.
Oesophageal foreign bodies	Regurgitation of food associated with recent feeding. Possible aspiration pneumonia.	Remove by mouth under general anaesthetic using fibre-optic endoscope or rigid endoscope. Gently pushing foreign body into stomach, or by thoracotomy.
Gastric foreign bodies	May remain asymptomatic if pylorus not obstructed. Persistent vomiting where the pylorus is involved. Occasionally clinical signs will present intermittently when foreign body moves in and out of pylorus.	Remove by fibre-optic endoscopy or gastrotomy.
Small intestinal foreign bodies	Persistent vomiting if duodenal. Dehydration and electrolyte loss. Abdominal pain.	Remove by enterotomy.
Rectal foreign bodies	Pain on defecation. Tenesmus. Blood may be present in the faeces.	Remove foreign body by endoscopy from rectum after sedation or general anaesthesia.

obstructions although rectal foreign bodies involving bone fragments do occur.

Examples of possible foreign bodies in cats include:

- Fish bones stuck at tooth/gum margins or the oral cavity.
- String looped round the tongue and passing down the oesophagus.
- Needles and fish hooks in the pharynx, oesophagus or stomach.
- Chicken bones lodged in the oesophagus.
- Fur balls in the stomach.
- Needles lodged in the stomach with string attached and trailing along the intestine, creating the classical linear foreign body.

Examples of possible foreign bodies in dogs include:

- Stick wedged across the hard palate.
- Balls, bone or hard food lodged in the pharynx.
- Chop bones, potatoes, chicken bones lodged in the oesophagus.
- Balls, bones and almost anything within the stomach.
- Stones, plastic and balls in the intestine.
- Bone fragment lodged in the rectum.

The clinical signs (Table 17.10) depend on the site and degree of the obstruction. Complete obstructions will lead to the most severe signs; partial obstruction may be better tolerated. The diagnosis is based on a thorough examination of the patient and radiographic examination. Treatment depends on the type and location of the foreign body (Table 17.10).

Constipation

Constipation is associated with impaction of the colon and rectum with faecal material. Many animals with constipation will strain in an attempt to pass faeces and this is often referred to as **tenesmus**. The causes of constipation and tenesmus are similar (Table 17.11).

Treatment for constipation depends on the underlying cause. Many cases require surgical correction, including castration for prostatic hyperplasia, rectal strictures, perineal hernias or rectal neoplasia. In cases of simple impaction, the animal may be sedated or given a general anaesthetic so that the colon can be emptied manually.

Table 17.11 Some specific causes of constipation and tenesmus, with conditions that may cause both to occur at the same time(*)

Causes of constipation	Feeding bones* Perineal hernia* Inability to posture Fractured pelvis* Prostatic disease* Rectal neoplasia* Rectal foreign body* Rectal stricture Fur/hair balls Neurological disease Megacolon Anal sac disease
Causes of tenesmus	Inflammation of the rectum Colitis Whipworm infection

It is important to ensure that further access to agents causing impaction is prevented, i.e. the feeding of bones should be discontinued. Prevention of impaction can also be achieved by providing bulking agents or softening agents in the diet, including methlylcellulose, psyllum and dietary fibre.

THE FEEDING OF BONES

Veterinary nurses are quite often asked for advice about giving bones to pets. Although some dogs (and cats) tolerate eating bones, others do have problems. Chicken and chop bones have sharp edges which can tear the alimentary tissue or cause obstruction. Marrow bones can be beneficial but the consumption of too much bone can lead to an accumulation in the large intestine and constipation. Marrow bones may also irritate the large intestine, leading to tenesmus and haemorrhagic diarrhoea.

Administration of enemata

An **enema** is a liquid preparation which is passed into the rectum and colon and is most commonly used for the purpose of treating constipation. Details of administration are given in Chapter 16 (General Nursing).

Conditions of the liver

Hepatitis may be defined as inflammation of the liver. It is usually associated with micro-organisms such as adenovirus or leptospiral infection but may also follow toxic damage to the liver (e.g. copper acccumulation, anticonvulsant drugs, pesticide ingestion, etc.)

Jaundice and **icterus** are terms used to describe elevated levels of bilirubin in the circulation, which leads to a yellow discoloration of the mucous membranes and skin. There are three possible causes of jaundice:

- Pre-hepatic – following excessive breakdown of red blood cells.
- Hepatic – primary liver disease leading to stasis of bile flow.
- Post-hepatic – associated with obstruction of the bile duct.

Cirrhosis of the liver develops when healing occurs by fibrous tissue formation rather than by production of new liver cells. The result is a loss of functional liver, interference with bile flow (causing jaundice) and portal hypertension, leading to ascites. The liver is reduced in size and ultimately there is liver failure.

Ascites refers to a fluid accumulation within the abdominal cavity. Several different types of fluid may accumulate, including blood, transudates, exudates, urine and gut contents. It is usual to determine the type of fluid present by inserting a sterile needle attached to a syringe through the abdominal wall and withdrawing some of the fluid for analysis. This procedure is called **paracentesis**.

Signs of liver disease

The liver has a massive functional reserve and considerable powers of regeneration, even following major damage. Over 70% of the liver must be lost before signs of liver failure develop.

Many of the clinical signs associated with liver disease are non-specific – vomiting, diarrhoea, anterior abdominal pain, weight loss – but more specific signs may include jaundice, ascites and pale faeces.

The final diagnosis of liver disease relies heavily on blood biochemistry, radiographs, ultrasound and ultimately biopsy of the liver.

Diseases of the pancreas

The pancreas is composed of exocrine and endocrine tissues. Diseases of the endocrine pancreas will be considered later in this chapter. Diseases of the exocrine pancreas include: pancreatitis, exocrine pancreatic insufficiency and neoplasia.

Signs of acute pancreatitis

The exocrine pancreas produces and stores large amounts of digestive enzymes. They are normally stored in an inactive form within small granules called zymogens, so that they cannot become active in the gland and digest the pancreatic tissue. Occasionally the protective mechanisms fail and pancreatic enzymes become activated within the gland, leading to the condition called acute pancreatitis.

The clinical signs associated with acute pancreatitis include:

- Persistent vomiting.
- Anterior abdominal pain.
- Dehydration and shock.
- Anorexia.
- Occasionally diarrhoea.
- Varying degrees of ascites and peritonitis.

A diagnosis of acute pancreatitis is usually made by detecting the following changes:

- Localised peritonitis in the anterior abdomen, often revealed by abdominal radiographs.
- Serum amylase and lipase levels are usually elevated, although in some cases only one of these enzymes may be increased in value at any given stage of the condition.
- A leucocytosis, often revealed by routine haematology.
- Raised trypsin-like immunoreactivity test (**TLI test**).

Treatment of pancreatis includes:

- Nil by mouth for 3–5 days.
- Intravenous fluid therapy using Hartmann's solution.

- Antibiotics.
- Analgesics.
- Initiation of low-fat veterinary diet with replacement enzymes.
- Restore bodyweight to normal.
- Maintain long term on low-fat diets.

Signs of exocrine pancreatic insufficiency (EPI)

EPI is associated with congenital atrophy of the exocrine tissue of the pancreas in dogs and is thought to be hereditary in some breeds. In older dogs and cats, EPI is thought to follow severe pancreatitis where there is an inflammatory destruction of exocrine tissues. In either case the result is a significant loss of exocrine tissue which in turn means a lack of digestive enzyme leading to maldigestion. The animal exhibits signs of polyphagia, chronic diarrhoea and marked weight loss. EPI is diagnosed by the laboratory measurement of the TLI in serum. Treatment requires the animal to receive a low-fat veterinary prescription diet together with replacement digestive enzymes supplied as powder or granules for incorporation in the food.

Diseases of the respiratory tract

Nasal discharge

Rhinitis is inflammation of the nasal mucous membrane. **Sinusitis** is inflammation of the sinuses, in particular the maxillary and frontal sinuses of the skull.

Nasal discharge is a common manifestation of rhinitis and sinusitis. It is often described as being **serous**, **mucoid** or **mucopurulent** in character. Occasionally the discharge involves the passage of blood and this is referred to as **epistaxis**:

- Serous nasal discharges are a feature of early infections involving viruses. Secondary bacterial infection is a common complication, when the discharge frequently becomes mucopurulent.
- Fungal infection (particularly *Aspergillus* spp.) usually starts as a mucoid discharge which rapidly becomes mucopurulent due to secondary bacterial infection and haemorrhagic due to ulceration of the mucosa.
- Epistaxis may be associated with trauma, neoplasia, clotting disorders or ulceration of the mucosa following infection.

Nasal discharges are usually **bilateral** when associated with viral and bacterial infection but may be **unilateral** when associated with fungal infection, neoplasia and trauma. Occasionally discharges are initially unilateral but become bilateral with the passage of time.

Inflammation

Inflammation of other parts of the respiratory tract is described according to the region involved:

- **Tonsillitis**: inflammation of the local lymphoid tissue at the entrance to the pharynx.
- **Pharyngitis**: inflammation of the pharynx.
- **Laryngitis**: inflammation of the larynx.
- **Tracheitis**: inflammation of the trachea.
- **Bronchitis**: inflammation of the bronchi.
- **Pneumonia**: by strict definition, inflammation of the lungs, but often used to describe invasion of the lung by micro-organisms.
- **Pleurisy**: inflammation of the pleural lining between the lungs and the thoracic wall; may be 'dry' or 'wet' according to the absence or presence of effusions.

Coughing

Coughing is a classical clinical sign associated with inflammation of the respiratory tract. Conditions which may be associated with coughing include:

- Cardiac failure.
- Neoplasia.
- Foreign bodies.
- Tonsillitis.
- Tracheal collapse.
- Pulmonary oedema.
- Pulmonary haemorrhage.
- Lungworm infection.
- Infections leading to pharyngitis, bronchitis, tracheitis, pneumonia.

Treatment of the coughing patient relies on determining and treating the underlying cause. The types of treatment which may be employed depend on the diagnosis but include:

- Anthelmintics for lungworm.
- Antibiotics for primary and secondary bacterial infections.
- Bronchodilators.
- Anti-tussants to suppress the cough.
- Corticosteroids to reduce inflammation.
- Environmental adjustments such as even air temperature, reduction of exercise, avoidance of airborne irritants.

Respiration

Various terms are used to describe the character and rate of breathing:

- **Dyspnoea**: laboured, or difficulty in, breathing.
- **Tachypnoea**: an increased rate of breathing.
- **Apnoea**: cessation of breathing, usually due to depression of the respiratory centre.
- **Orthopnoea**: breathing through an open mouth (the animal assumes sternal recumbency with the neck extended and elbows abducted).

Acute respiratory failure

Acute respiratory failure represents a true emergency requiring urgent medical treatment. It implies that the lungs are no longer able to oxygenate the blood or allow exchange

Table 17.12 Some causes of acute respiratory failure	
Trauma	Ruptured diaphragm. Pneumothorax. Haemothorax.
Airway obstruction	Foreign body, Pulmonary oedema, Laryngeal paralysis.
Pulmonary embolism	
Neoplasia	Primary or secondary metastasis.
Overdose of anaesthetics	Depressing the respiratory centre.
Pneumonia	Viral or bacterial.
Pleural effusions	Hydrothorax.
Paralysis of respiratory muscles	Tetanus. Botulism
Laryngeal paralysis	
Poisoning	Paraquat.
Pressure on diaphragm	Gastric torsion.

Table 17.13 Action in case of respiratory failure	
Establish and maintain a patent airway	Suction to remove mucus or other secretions. If required, intubate patient. Carry out a tracheotomy.
Provide oxygen via	Endotracheal tube. Nasal tube. Face mask. Oxygen cage.
Drug therapy	Diuretics to correct pulmonary oedema. Bronchodilators to improve ventilation. Respiratory centre stimulants if depressed. Cardiac drugs in heart failure.
Thoracocentesis	To relieve hydrothorax or pneumothorax.

of carbon dioxide in order to sustain life. There are many causes of acute respiratory failure, including those shown in Table 17.12.

Clinical signs associated with respiratory failure vary according to the specific condition involved but may include:

- Cyanosis.
- Tachypnoea, dyspnoea, orthopnoea.
- Tachycardia, weak pulse.
- Assuming a 'dog sitting' position with abducted elbows.
- Eventual collapse and unconsciousness.

Rapid and effective treatment (Table 17.13) is essential if the patient's respiratory function is to be improved and in some cases to save life.

Nursing role

- Ensure that therapy is carried out.
- Monitor patient's vital signs.
- Keep careful records of patient's condition.
- Advise owner regarding patient's condition.

Pneumothorax and hydrothorax

Pneumothorax describes the accumulation of air within the pleural cavity. In **open pneumothorax** air moves freely in and out of the pleural cavity through an opening in the thoracic wall. A **closed pneumothorax** occurs when there is physical damage to the lung leading to the escape of air into the pleural spaces as the animal breathes. In this case the air cannot escape from the pleural cavity during respiration (tension pneumothorax) and accumulates, causing increased breathing difficulties and eventual lung collapse.

Hydrothorax is the accumulation of fluid within the pleural cavity. The various types of fluid which may so accumulate are indicated by specific names:

- **Haemothorax**: accumulation of the whole blood in the thorax, usually associated with trauma, bleeding disorders or neoplastic states.
- **Chylothorax**: accumulation of lymphatic fluid or chyle in the thorax, resulting from rupture of the thoracic duct.
- **Pyothorax**: accumulation of purulent material in the thorax, associated with bacterial infection.
- **Exudates** may also be associated with pleurisy rather than pyothorax, depending on the type of organism involved.
- **Transudates** are serum-like fluids often associated with congestive heart failure or hypoproteinaemia.

The clinical signs associated with pneumothorax and hydrothorax, which depend on the amount of air or fluid

Table 17.14 Pneumothorax and hydrothorax

Clinical signs (varying degrees)	Diagnosis	Treatment
Dyspnoea and tachypnoea Hypoxia and cyanosis Tachycardia and weak pulse Orthopnoea Sucking sounds on inspiration Collapse and unconsciousness Pallor of the mucous membranes	Careful examination of thoracic wall for injuries. Percussion of chest. Radiographs. Thoracocentesis.	Provision of therapy as for acute respiratory failure. Closure of any thoracic injury. Aspiration of fluid and/or gas from pleural space. Monitoring of vital signs. Keep owners informed of current situation. Surgical correction of any lesions. Provide oxygen therapy.

Table 17.15 Fluid samples collected by thoracocentesis classified by certain parameters to aid in diagnosis

Parameter	True transudate	Modified transudate	Exudate	Chyle
SG	≤1.015	≤1.015	>1.015	<1.015
Colour	clear/pink	pink	red	milky
Protein	<30 g/l	30 g/l	>30 g/l	<30 g/l
Bacteria	–	–	yes	–
Clotting	–	–	may clot	–
Cells	–	some	many	some

accumulating in the pleural cavity, are shown in Table 17.14 along with diagnosis and treatment.

Thoracocentesis involves placing a thoracic drain into the chest or using a needle and syringe on a three-way tap to aspirate the pleural space. This procedure yields valuable diagnostic information regarding the type of fluid accumulation (Table 17.15). It also assists in relieving the clinical signs by removing the air or fluid which is interfering with breathing.

Diseases of the circulatory system

Congenital heart disease

Although not common causes of heart disease, specific inherited or congenital cardiac conditions that are most likely to be encountered include:

- Patent ductus arteriosus.
- Pulmonary stenosis.
- Aortic stenosis.
- Ventricular septal defects.
- Mitral and tricuspid dysplasia.
- Tetralogy of Fallot.
- Persistent right aortic arch.

Patent ductus arteriosus

In this condition the fetal blood vessel that connects the aorta with the pulmonary artery fails to close after the animal is born. Normally all that remains is a ligament called the ligamentum arteriosus. Where the vessel remains open, blood shunts from the aorta to the pulmonary artery. Whether the animal exhibits clinical signs depends on the degree of blood shunting from the left to the right side of the heart. Some puppies die suddenly after birth; others show signs of heart failure at some time between birth and adulthood. Clinical signs include weakness, exercise intolerance, coughing and dyspnoea because of left heart failure, and cyanosis only if there is a right–left shunting of blood. On auscultation a classical machinery or continuous murmur is heard throughout systole and diastole.

Pulmonary stenosis

Blood leaves the right side of the heart via the pulmonary artery and its semi-lunar valve. Narrowing or stenosis of

this valve leads to high pressure in the right heart and thickening or hypertrophy of the right ventricle wall. Lung perfusion may be adequate but the right ventricle has to work much harder than normal in order for this to be maintained. Where this compensatory mechanism fails, right-sided congestive heart failure develops.

Aortic stenosis

Blood leaves the left side of the heart via the aorta for the general circulation. Narrowing at the aortic valve causes high pressure in the left ventricle and poor cardiac output. Rarely this may lead to left-sided congestive heart failure. More commonly there will be episodes of fainting (syncope) on exercise and occasionally animals may die suddenly without developing signs of cardiac failure.

Ventricular septal defects

This describes an interventricular defect between the left and right ventricles. The size of the hole varies and will determine the degree of heart dysfunction that may occur. Generally blood shunts from left to right, leading to mixing of venous and arterial blood in the right ventricle. Congestive heart failure is again a likely outcome.

Mitral and tricuspid dysplasia

This is a relatively common cause of heart disease in young dogs and especially in the retriever. Deformity and incompetence of these valves leads to regurgitation of blood and a systolic murmur. The result of these changes is a progressive development of cardiac failure.

Tetralogy of Fallot

In this condition several heart defects are present at the same time. Usually there is a combination of pulmonary stenosis, interventricular septal defect, dextraposed aorta and thickening or hypertrophy of the right ventricular wall due to outflow resistance. The clinical signs depend on the severity of the lesions but are likely to include cyanosis, weight loss, exercise intolerance, harsh systolic murmur and heart failure.

Persistent right aortic arch

Occasionally, during the development of the major blood vessels supplying the heart, the right aortic arch persists instead of the left aortic arch. This leads to the ligamentum arteriosus lying across the dorsal part of the oesophagus while the remainder of the vascular ring around the oesophagus is formed by the pulmonary vein lying to the left, the aorta to the right and the heart base ventrally (Fig. 17.5). The stricture thus formed interferes with swallowing and food becomes trapped in front of the vascular ring. This leads to the development of megaoesophagus and regurgitation of food. Aspiration pneumonia is a likely complication.

Acquired heart disease

Acquired heart diseases include:

- Pericarditis: inflammation of the serous membrane covering the heart.
- Cardiomyopathy: disease of the cardiac muscle.
- Myocarditis: inflammation of the heart muscle, usually associated with infection (e.g. parvovirus); now very rare.
- Endocarditis: inflammation of the inner lining of the heart, particularly the heart valves.
- Endocardiosis: progressive nodular thickening of the heart valves.

Pericarditis

Pericarditis is usually accompanied by pericardial effusion, which may result from tumours such as haemangiosarcomas but many are described as idiopathic in origin. The effusion itself is often serosanguinous in nature. The clinical signs exhibited depend on the amount of effusion, which compresses the heart and impedes its function. The heart sounds are muffled on auscultation and some degree of right-sided congestive heart failure develops in the majority of cases.

Myocardial disease

Cardiomyopathy may be primary, or secondary to some systemic disorder. The cause of primary cardiomyopathy is rarely determined but secondary cardiomyopathy can be associated with malnutrition (taurine deficiency in cats), hyperthyroidism, hypertension and viral infections.

The two forms of cardiomyopathy are:

- **Dilated** (more common in dogs), in which the heart muscle becomes thinned, with a loss of contractibility.
- **Hypertrophic** (more common in cats), in which the heart muscle becomes excessively thickened, reducing the size of the ventricular lumen and so reducing cardiac output.

Clinical signs are those of congestive heart failure.

Endocarditis

This condition is associated with bacterial infection which has spread to the heart valves from some other septic focus. Septic emboli dislodge from the damaged valves and migrate to other sites, including the myocardium, resulting in myocarditis. Clinical signs exhibited by animals with endocarditis include pyrexia, heart murmur, coughing, dyspnoea and signs associated with the original septic focus. These animals are systemically unwell and may show other signs, such as lameness.

Endocardiosis

There is often confusion between endocarditis and endocardiosis. In the latter condition, the progressive nodular thickening of the heart valves in due course renders them physically unable to function correctly and they leak severely when they should be closed. Congestive heart

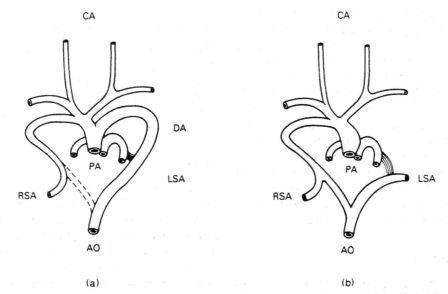

(a)   (b)

Fig. 17.5 (a) Normal aortic position and (b) persistent right arch. (Reproduced with permission of Blackwell Scientific Publications.)

failure often follows. It appears to be more common in males, especially in middle to old age, and there may be a genetic predisposition in Cavalier King Charles spaniels, poodles, Pekingese and schnauzers. Clinical signs are those of congestive heart failure.

NORMAL HEART RATES

Many factors may influence the heart rate in normal dogs and cats, including the breed, age, fitness and general health, as well as excitement, stress of being examined and environmental conditions. The following figures are a guide to the range of normal heart rates for adult dogs and cats:

- Dogs: 60–180 beats/minute.
- Cats: 110–180 beats/minute.

Bradycardia, a very slow heart rate (usually less than 60 beats/minute) may be associated with conditions such as Addison's disease and excessive vagal tone.

Tachycardia, an excessively rapid heart rate, is a frequent finding in congestive heart failure, feline hyperthyroidism and some forms of adrenal tumour.

Cardiac output failure

This occurs as a consequence of:

- Some congenital defects.
- Myocardial disease.
- Electrical disturbance (**arrhythmia**) including: ventricular fibrillation, heart block and excessive vagal tone.

See Chapter 3, p. 86

Table 17.16 Treatment of cardiac output failure and cardiac arrest

(1) Establish and maintain patent airway;
  – insert endotracheal tube.
  OR – Carry out tracheotomy.
  OR – Owners should stretch out head/neck, and pull the tongue forward and remove any obvious obstructions (warn them of being bitten).

(2) Initiate ventilation at 12 ventilations/minute.
  – Use oxygen with carbon dioxide – stimulates breathing.
  OR – Blow down the ET tube.

(3) Cardiac massage at 60 compressions/minute.
  – Apply pressure from lateral sides of the thorax, against table or floor.

(4) Administration of drugs by veterinary surgeon.
  – Adrenaline directly into heart.
  – Possibly calcium salts intravenously.

(5) Defibrillation to restart heart.

(6) Fluid therapy using lactated Ringer's or saline and bicarbonate.

Cardiac arrest, which is rare in dogs and cats, is associated with severe arrhythmias that develop when there is severe myocardial disease, excessive sympathetic stimulation or toxaemic state. Hypoxia is the most common cause and may be associated with anaesthetics or airway obstruction.

Clinical signs of cardiac failure are usually of sudden onset and occur when the animal is excited or exercising. It is unusual to have had warning signs prior to the acute episode. The animal is likely to collapse into unconsciousness, often described as **fainting** or **syncope**. This is often flaccid (unlike a fit) and is due to cerebral anoxia associated with reduced cardiac output. Animals usually recover spontaneously from these episodes and return to normal very rapidly after the event, with no lethargy or drowsiness. The clinical signs associated with cardiac arrest include lack of detectable pulse, collapse and either pallor or cyanosis of mucous membranes.

Treatment of cardiac output failure and cardiac arrest is described in Table 17.16.

Nursing care

In cardiac output failure, the nurse may have a vital role to play if the veterinary surgeon is unavailable when a case is presented. The nurse can:

- Ensure that a patent airway is established.
- Administer oxygen therapy as required.
- Carry out cardiac massage to save life.
- Call for veterinary assistance.

Congestive heart failure (CHF)

When the heart fails to function efficiently, it will compensate by changing its rate and possibly strength of contraction. If the condition progresses, clinical signs will be observed eventually and the animal will be said to have **decompensated** by developing congestive heart failure. Failure in compensation leads to pooling of blood (**congestion**) in the vascular beds. The clinical signs depend on whether the animal has left- or right-sided heart failure:

- Right-sided heart failure: poor venous return to the heart; congestion of the liver, spleen, and other viscera; ascites is likely.
- Left-sided heart failure: poor venous return from the lungs; pulmonary congestion and oedema; tachypnoea and coughing.

The reduced cardiac output also leads to reduced blood flow to the kidneys. They respond by producing **renin**, which in turn activates **angiotensin**, which stimulates **aldosterone** release from the adrenal glands. Aldosterone retains water and salt, causing further venous congestion by overloading the circulation.

Congestive heart failure may occur following cardiomyopathy, valvular stenosis, valvular incompetence, pulmonary or aortic stenosis or cardiac arrhythmias.

The clinical signs observed in CHF include:

- Tachycardia.
- Weak pulse.
- Pallor of mucous membrane.
- Cyanosis if pulmonary oedema develops.
- Coughing.
- Tachypnoea.
- Ascites.
- Hepatomegaly.
- Exercise intolerance and general lethargy and weakness.
- Weight loss.

Nursing care

- Provide a quiet, stress-free environment for the patient.
- Ensure that the patient receives cage rest only.
- Restrict exercise as appropriate.
- Carry out treatments prescribed by the veterinary surgeon:
  - diuretics for pulmonary congestion/oedema;
  - glycosides for improving heart-muscle function;
  - bronchodilators to improve breathing;
  - vasodilators to reduce preload and afterload;
  - potassium supplements following use of diuretics.
- Ensure that the animal receives an appropriate veterinary diet, low in salt and containing a high biological value protein.

Diagnosis of heart disease

The four main aids in the diagnosis of heart disease are auscultation (listening), radiography, electrocardiogram (ECG) and echocardiogram.

Auscultation

By carefully listening to the heart with a stethoscope, the veterinary surgeon will detect heart murmurs due to valvular defects, persistent ductus arteriosus or ventricular septal defects. The heart rate may be counted and compared with the pulse rate. Any abnormal rhythms may also be detected.

Radiography

This is a valuable method of assessing the shape and size of the heart. In CHF the heart is often enlarged and this may be indicated by elevation of the trachea, and by the heart occupying more than 3.5 rib spaces. Radiographs are also useful for detecting pulmonary oedema and pericardial effusions (which cause the heart to appear globular). Ascites and hepatomegaly may also be confirmed by abdominal radiographs.

Electrocardiogram (ECG)

The ECG records the electrical activity of the heart and is therefore only useful where an arrhythmia is suspected.

Where CHF is due to electrical disturbance such as tachy or brady arrhythmias the ECG will record the type of disturbance and allow a diagnosis to be made. It also allows an accurate assessment of the heart rate to be calculated.

Care and use of the ECG

- Before using the ECG, ensure that it contains adequate recording paper.
- Check the setting, including the speed chart (which should be 2.5 cm/second but may be increased to 5 cm/second). Centre the pen(s) on the chart paper.
- Record a 1 mV trace on the recording paper, for calculation of ECG voltages following recording.
- Initially select leads 1, 2 and 3, followed by AVR, AVL and AVF.
- Apply electrode gel to the skin and then clips to hold the recording leads. The clips should be attached just below the elbow and above the hocks. The clips should hang directly downwards to stop excessive movement during recording.
- Lead positions:
  - Red – right foreleg.
  - Yellow – left foreleg.
  - Green – left hindleg.
  - Black – right hindleg.
- Carry out the ECG recording in a quiet, stress-free room to avoid the animal moving about or shaking, as this would affect the quality of the trace produced.
- Do not sedate the animal, as this might affect the ECG trace.
- Once the recording has been completed, the leads and clips should be thoroughly cleaned and the gel should be removed from the animal.
- Always label the ECG recording with the owner's name, the case number, the breed, age and sex of the animal, together with the date.

Echocardiogram

The echocardiogram allows the activity of the heart muscle or myocardium to be assessed, which is useful in cardiomyopathy. It will detect pericardial effusions and enlargement of the heart. The function of the heart valves may also be visualised using ultrasound.

Care and use of ultrasound equipment (see also Chapter 21, p. 563.)

- Sedatives or general anaesthetics should not be used when examining cardiac patients. However, such restraint may be useful where ultrasound is used for collecting biopsy samples. (Ultrasound is now used to guide needle biopsy of organs such as the liver and kidney. This helps to prevent damage to any vital tissue and ensures that abnormal tissue is collected.)
- Shave the coat next to the area to be examined so that the probe can make good contact with the skin.
- Apply ultrasound gel to the probe and carry out the procedure.

- Always clean the gel off the patient and the probe following the examination.
- Apart from care of the probe, there is little other routine attention needed in the care of this equipment.

Anaemia

Anaemia may be defined as a decrease in the numbers of red blood cells (RBCs) below the reference range for the species concerned. Anaemia is *not* a diagnosis but a clinical sign indicating a reduction in the RBCs and the oxygen-carrying capacity of the blood. It is traditional to classify anaemia into the categories shown in Table 17.17, which also describes clinical signs (usually sudden in onset) associated with anaemia and the basis of diagnosis and therapy. Long-term symptomatic therapy is rarely satisfactory; a definitive diagnosis is required so that specific therapy can be provided – usually specific drug therapy together with measures to alleviate the symptoms.

In general, **regenerative** anaemias are associated with haemolytic episodes or blood loss; **non-regenerative** anaemias are associated with bone marrow hypoplasia, chronic inflammatory disease, drug interactions or renal disease.

Table 17.17. Anaemia

Categories	Clinical signs	Diagnosis (based on establishing category of anaemia)	Treatments (used singly or in combination)
Haemorrhagic: (i) Acute blood loss: – RTA trauma to major vessels. – Rupture of an internal organ; spleen, liver and kidney. – Clotting disorders; warfarin poisoning, haemophilia. – Neoplasia, haemangiosarcoma. – Haemorrhagic gastroenteritis. (ii) Chronic blood loss: – Haematuria – Gastrointestinal bleeding; ulceration, hookworms. – Ectoparasites, lice. Haemolytic: – Immune mediated haemolytic anaemia. – Pyruvate kinase deficiency. – Haemobartonella infection – Drugs; sulphonamides, anti-convulsants. Non-regenerative: – Bone marrow hypoplasia; FeLV, FIV, toxaemias, drugs such as chloramphenicol, oestrogens. – Nutritional; iron deficiency – Renal disease – erythropoietin deficiency. – Leukaemia, lymphosarcoma, myeloma. – Poisoning – lead.	Pallor of the mucous membranes. Jaundice. Haemorrhage either: – External, oral, nasal, body surface. – Internal, into the thorax or abdomen. Lymph nodes, liver or splenic enlargement. Weakness, collapse, exercise intolerance. Tachycardia and tachypnoea.	History for knowledge of trauma, access to lead, use of drugs known to cause anaemia, detection of bleeding. Physical examination to establish evidence of haemorrhage. Routine haematology to determine number of RBCs, PCV and haemoglobin levels together with white blood cell count and platelet count. Reticulocyte count to determine if anaemia is regenerative. Coombs' test to confirm immune-mediated anaemia. Bone marrow biopsy when anaemia is non-regenerative.	Whole blood transfusions to provide immediate help in restoring oxygen-carrying capacity. Ideal donors have blood groups A1 and A2 (nearly 60% of dogs). Up to 40% are ideal recipients. Single blood transfusions likely to be successful without cross-matching the blood but follow-up transfusions may be dangerous. Plasma expanders very useful where whole blood not available. They expand circulation but do not restore oxygen-carrying capacity; useful where blood transfusion unavailable and there has been major haemorrhage. Surgical correction of haemorrhage following intravenous fluid therapy to stabilise patient. Splenectomy in immune-mediated disease. Vitamin K$_1$ for warfarin poisoning. Prednisolone therapy for immune-mediated anaemia. Erythropoietin for anaemia induced by renal disease. Stop administration of drugs known to cause anaemia. Dietary supplementation to aid red cell production – haemotinics which include high-protein diet, iron and B vitamins. Cage rest and stress-free environment. Anabolic steroids may help in non-regenerative anaemia especially associated with chronic renal disease.

Diseases of the urinary system

Renal diseases

DEFINITIONS

- **Nephritis.** A general term used to describe inflammation of the kidney. It does not indicate whether the parenchyma, interstitial tissue or vascular tissue is involved. Nor does it indicate whether the inflammation is acute, chronic or progressive.
- **Glomerulonephritis.** An inflammation associated with the capillary bed within the glomeruli with some degree of secondary tubular and/or interstitial inflammation.
- **Pyelonephritis.** An inflammation directly associated with bacterial infection of the kidney, especially the renal pelvis. It is uncommon in dogs and cats, but when present is often associated with inflammatory cells and healing by fibrosis.
- **Polyuria.** The formation and excretion of increased amounts of urine. Usually associated with a compensatory increase in drinking (**polydipsia**).
- **Oliguria.** A decreased production of urine below the values expected for the species of animal concerned.
- **Anuria.** Cessation of urine production which is most often associated with obstruction of the urinary tract or in acute renal failure.
- **Dysuria.** Difficulty in passing urine or pain on urination.

- **Haematuria.** Passage of red blood cells in urine. Usually indicating bleeding into the urinary tract without specifying the location of the bleeding.
- **Isosthenuria.** When the kidney cannot form urine with a higher or lower specific gravity than that of a protein-free plasma. The urine will remain at 1.010 irrespective of fluid intake.
- **Azotaemia.** An increase in the waste nitrogen level in the circulation, usually measured as blood urea (BU) and creatinine. Elevations in values occur when more than 75% of the nephrons are damaged. The actual values do *not* correlate with the degree of kidney damage.

Acute renal failure

Acute renal failure is a condition which results in complete or almost complete cessation of renal function. The clinical signs, which occur suddenly and dramatically and vary depending on the underlying cause, are given in Table 17.18, which also classifies the causes of acute renal failure into groups and describes diagnosis and treatment. The latter requires a major commitment by the veterinary surgeon and nurse in order to save life.

There are generally three phases. Initially an oliguria phase occurs and occasionally anuria. This leads to retention of water, the development of acidosis and retention of potassium (**hyperkalaemia**). These changes occur because more than 75% of the nephrons are not functioning and can be fatal.

Table 17.18 Acute renal failure

Classifications	Clinical signs	Diagnosis	Treatment

Acute interstitial nephritis:
  Leptospira canicola
  infection.
Acute tubular necrosis,
Nephrotoxins:
– mercury poisoning.
– ethylene glycol poison.
– gentamicin.
– sulphonamides.
– phenylbutazone.
Ischaemic:
– (results whenever renal
  perfusion is reduced)
– prolonged anaesthetics.
– acute haemorrhage.
– congestive heart failure.
– Addison's disease.
– dehydration and shock.
	Lethargy.
	Anorexia.
	Vomiting and diarrhoea.
	Dehydration.
	Halitosis.
	Oral ulceration.
	Enlarged or swollen kidneys,
	  which are usually painful.
	Oliguria or anuria.
		History of access to poisons,
		  drugs or failure to
		  vaccinate against
		  Leptospirosis.
		Clinical signs.
		Serum biochemistry (usually
		  reveals elevation in BU,
		  creatinine, phosphorus,
		  and potassium in the
		  presence of isosthenuria).
			Monitor and record vital
			  signs regularly.
			Monitor urine production.
			Initiate intravenous fluid
			  therapy but watch for signs
			  of overhydration.
			Treat any identifiable
			  underlying cause.
			Antibiotics for leptospirosis.
			Stimulate kidneys to produce
			  urine once animal is
			  adequately hydrated by
			  veterinary surgeon using
			  frusemide or mannitol
			  solution (**osmotic diuresis**).
			Provision of comfortable
			  stress-free accommodation.
			Provision of veterinary diet
			  low in protein (14–16%
			  DM) and in phosphorus.
			  Protein must be of high
			  biological value.
			Peritoneal dialysis.

Assuming that the animal receives prompt therapy, the oliguria phase is followed by a polyuric phase during which renal function has not been restored but fluid retention declines, together with a loss of sodium, which can lead to dehydration.

The final phase may be described as recovery when there is a gradual restoration of renal function. This may take several weeks and does not always result in the total restoration of normal renal function.

PERITONEAL DIALYSIS

Where osmotic diuresis fails to stimulate the kidneys to produce urine, peritoneal dialysis can be used to filter waste products from the blood and so reduce azotaemia. The procedure should be carried out under strict aseptic technique as there is a real risk of inducing peritonitis and shock.

The technique involves infusion of a sterile fluid into the abdomen, which will permit nitrogenous waste to leave the rich vascular bed of the peritoneum and enter the fluid. After a specified time the fluid is withdrawn (usually less than was infused) along with the nitrogenous waste, so improving the animal's condition. This may be repeated until the BU and creatinine levels fall.

Equipment required for peritoneal dialysis includes:

- Small surgical pack with drapes.
- Local anaesthetic.
- Peritoneal catheter and giving set.
- Special dialysis fluid which *must* be warmed to body temperature.

The procedure is as follows:

- The hair is clipped from the ventral abdomen.
- The site is then surgically prepared.
- Local anaesthetic infiltrated into the mid line behind the umbilicus.
- The site is draped and a small incision made through the skin.
- The catheter is then inserted with the aid of a trocar into the abdomen.
- Once in place the giving set with dialysing fluid prepared to body temperature is introduced.
- The fluid is removed under gravity after 30 minutes. Occasionally this may prove difficult and the animal may have to be moved around to permit the fluid to flow.
- The procedure should be repeated as required to lower the blood urea level.

Chronic renal failure

Chronic renal failure may be described as a condition where there is a progressive loss of functional tissue over an undefined period. It is characterised by a slow insidious onset of clinical signs. Occasionally the owner may suggest there was a sudden onset, in which case the animal has probably had subclinical disease for some time, with the sudden development of clinical signs when the number of damaged tubules is in excess of 75%.

The numerous causes of chronic renal failure are given in Table 17.19 which also describes the clinical signs – these vary according to the underlying cause and many are non-specific, while others are more suggestive of renal failure. The diagnosis may be suspected from clinical signs, history and may be confirmed from blood tests and urine analysis (Table 17.19). Techniques for urine analysis are given in detail in Chapter 13 (Diagnostic Aids).

Wherever possible, the underlying cause of chronic renal failure should be determined and specifically treated. In the majority of cases this is not possible and treatment remains symptomatic. *Renal failure only occurs when more than 75% of nephrons are damaged.* Restoration of these nephrons is not possible and so recovery depends on the remaining healthy nephrons' ability to increase their workload. When this occurs, the animal is said to have **compensated** with restoration of renal function. If the condition progresses, eventually the animal will **decompensate** or develop renal failure again. Ultimately the kidneys will have so few healthy nephrons left that compensation cannot occur and the animal will have to be euthanased.

Symptomatic treatment which may help the kidneys to compensate is given in Table 17.19.

Nephrotic syndrome

Nephrotic syndrome may be considered as an end-stage disease and is often associated with progression of glomerulonephritis. It is characterised by a severe proteinuria which leads to hypoalbuminaemia and subcutaneous oedema and ascites. The latter are due to retention of fluid which, because of the low plasma albumin, leaves the circulation for the tissue spaces. When this occurs, circulating volume falls which stimulates aldosterone release and further water and salt retention.

Clinical signs, diagnosis and treatment are described in Table 17.20. Treatment is aimed at trying to reduce the loss of protein in the urine by means of drugs and dietary management. Progress is assessed by monitoring the levels of BU, creatinine, serum proteins, sodium and potassium.

Cystitis

Cystitis may be defined as inflammation of the urinary bladder, usually associated with a bacterial infection. It is common in dogs and cats and particularly in bitches (due to the shorter urethra). Underlying causes, clinical signs (varying with the cause), diagnosis and treatment are shown in Table 17.21.

Table 17.19 Chronic renal failure

Causes	Clinical signs	Diagnosis	Treatment
Nephrotoxins. Ischaemia. Pyelonephritis. Congenital and hereditary disease. Idiopathic. Dietary? SLE (systemic lupus erythematosus). Glomerulonephritis.	Anorexia. Weight loss. Lethargy. Anaemia (non-regenerative). Vomiting Halitosis. Oral ulceration and occasionally necrosis of the tip of the tongue. Polydipsia and polyuria.	Blood urea (BU), serum creatinine and phosphorus all elevated to some degree. Calcium : phosphorus ratio often changes from 1.5:1 to 1.4. Urine analysis may reveal proteinuria, granular casts, low specific gravity and sometimes haematuria.	Anti-emetics such as metoclopramide. Intravenous fluid therapy to correct dehydration and electrolyte loss. Antibiotics for primary or secondary infection. B-vitamin therapy to compensate for loss in polyuria. Dietary management – by providing veterinary diet low in protein and phosphorus may be possible to halt the progression of renal failure (protein offered must be of high biological value to allow its efficient use in repair). See Chapter 8, p. 199. Anabolic steroids and erythropoietin may help stimulate the bone marrow and correct anaemia.

Table 17.20 Nephrotic syndrome

Clinical signs	Diagnosis	Treatment
Lethargy, marked weight loss, ascites, subcutaneous oedema of limbs and ventral abdomen and prepuce, polydipsia and polyuria.	Detection of a severe proteinuria on urine analysis and hypoalbuminaemia. High protein: creatinine ratio (>5.0). Elevated blood urea and creatinine.	Dietary management involves feeding veterinary diet with very high biological value protein in reduced amounts, and low in salt and phosphorus. Aim to give as much high quality protein as possible to restore the albumin levels, without causing elevation in BU levels. Plasma expanders have been used to help correct oedema but difficult to achieve when protein loss from kidneys is so great. Anabolic steroids and corticosteroids to correct protein loss and reduce glomerular inflammation. Diuretics occasionally needed to reduce oedema if this interferes with other organ function.

Table 17.21 Cystitis

Underlying causes	Clinical signs	Diagnosis	Treatment
Trauma Calculi Diabetes mellitus Cushing's disease Obstruction Neoplasia Bacterial infection	Increased frequency of urination. Urinary tenesmus (straining and difficulty in urination, often accompanied by pain on urination). 'Wetting' in the house. Apparent incontinence. Haematuria.	By urine analysis – urine collection under strict aseptic technique so that sample can be submitted for culture and sensitivity testing. Collection by either cystocentesis or catheterisation. Bacteria most often associated with cystitis include *E. coli*, *Pseudomonas* spp., *Proteus* spp. and *Klebsiella* spp.	Selection of antibiotic from the sensitivity testing. Where this is not available sulphonamides, trimethoprim, cephalosporins and synthetic penicillins are excreted in urine and may prove useful. Additional symptomatic therapy: ● Increase water intake and thus urine production. ● Acidify urine. ● Prevention of urine scalding by application of barrier creams. ● Frequent walks to encourage urination.

Incontinence

Incontinence is the inability to control the passage of urine. Animals which are incontinent may pass urine whilst walking around or whilst resting. They are particularly likely to develop **urine scalding** (inflammation of the skin of the perineum or around the prepuce). Nursing care should include:

- Use of barrier creams to prevent urine scalding.
- Use of incontinence pads on bedding to reduce soiling.
- Frequent opportunities to attempt normal urination.
- If catheterisation is routinely required, great care must be taken to avoid introduction of infection (cystitis). For this reason an indwelling catheter may be useful.

Calculi

The most common types of urinary tract calculi are shown in Table 17.22. Common sites for obstruction of the urinary tract by calculi include:

- The renal pelvis.
- Ureters.
- Urethra (ischial arch or at the os penis).

Feline lower urinary tract disease (FLUTD)

This disease was previously known as feline urolithiasis syndrome (FUS). It may be caused by the formation of **uroliths** within the urinary tract, though the aetiology of urolith formation is determined in fewer than 50% of cases. Urethral plugs (22%) and uroliths (21%) account for many cases but urinary tract infection only accounts for 1–2%. Uroliths develop in the presence of adequate magnesium and phosphates. Many cases therefore remain idiopathic.

The clinical signs of FLUTD are given in Table 17.23, which also describes treatment. Many cases are presented as medical emergencies, with total obstruction to urine passage, and it is essential to establish normal urine excretion in the first instance.

Diseases of the nervous system

Fits

Several terms are used to describe the fitting animal. **Convulsions** are violent or uncoordinated contractions of the muscles due to abnormal cerebral stimulation. The muscle activity is described as **clonic** when the contractions are interspersed with periods of relaxation or **tonic** when the muscle contraction is sustained without periods of relaxation.

Epilepsy is a central nervous disorder in which an irritable focus within the brain causes disorganised electrical activity which results in convulsions. **Status epilepticus** occurs when the convulsions are continuous or where one fit follows directly upon another.

There are many causes of fits. Those described as primary are directly associated with disorders of the brain. Secondary disorders include conditions of other body organs which influence the brain in some way. Some of the most likely causes of fits include:

- Viral or bacterial infections.
- Intracranial trauma.

Table 17.22 The types of urinary tract calculi are shown together with the likely urinary pH and degree of radiodensity observed in each case

Type of calculi	Likely urinary pH	Radiodensity	Species
Struvite	Alkaline	Radiodense	Dogs/cats
Oxalates	Acid/alkaline	Radiodense variable	Dogs/cats
Urates	Acid/alkaline	Radiolucent	Dogs
Cystine	Acid	Radiolucent	Dogs

Table 17.23 Feline lower urinary tract disease (FLUTD)

Clinical signs	Immediate treatment (emergency cases)	Long-term control
Cystitis Urethritis Urethral obstruction Urinary tenesmus Anuria Haematuria Enlargement of the abdomen Azotaemia with total obstruction	Cystocentesis to relieve urinary bladder tension. Catheterisation of urethra with Jackson cat catheter. Leave catheter indwelling until other therapy has been established. Antibiotic therapy if infection is suspected.	Urinary acidification using DL-methionine or ammonium chloride (both drugs can be toxic and must be used with care by veterinary surgeon). Dietary management – provide a diet with low magnesium and low phosphate to reduce mineral availability, high sodium to increase urinary production and thirst, and a urinary acidifier to change pH to <6.5.

- Brain tumours.
- Hydrocephalus.
- Cerebral anoxia.
- Idiopathic epilepsy.
- Portosystemic shunts.
- Hypocalcaemia.
- Hypoglycaemia.
- Chronic liver disease.
- Hypokalaemia.
- Poisons (cyanide, metaldehyde, lead).
- Renal disease.

Phases

The clinical signs exhibited by animals having a fit are divided into three phases:

- An initial phase before the fit actually occurs: pre-ictal phase.
- The actual fit: ictal phase.
- The behaviour immediately after the fit: post-ictal phase.

In the **pre-ictal phase**, animals may be asleep or resting just prior to a fit and may wake suddenly and appear restless or anxious, or seek attention.

In the **ictal phase (collapse)**, the animal collapses onto its side, champing its jaws, salivating, vocalising, urinating and defecating. The eyes usually remain open and staring. In addition the limbs often start to 'paddle' or may exhibit tonic or clonic contractions. The animal is unaware of its environment and is unable to prevent injury to itself during the fit.

In the **post-ictal phase** immediately after the fit, the animal may appear dazed, exhausted and anxious again before returning to normal over a variable period.

Anticonvulsants

Long-term therapy for fits depends on finding and correcting the underlying cause. For example, there is little point in providing anticonvulsive therapy for a patient with renal disease when control of renal function will prevent the fits from continuing.

If the fit is due to idiopathic epilepsy, anticonvulsive drugs can be of considerable value. The majority of these drugs are available in tablet form and are therefore of little use during a fit. In these circumstances intravenous anticonvulsants are required. Ideally diazepam should be given by the veterinary surgeon directly into a vein with the assistance of the nurse. Rectal diazepam is an alternative route. If this drug is unavailable, pertobarbitone sodium may be used instead. Both these drugs will normally control the fit and calm the animal.

Long-term therapy requires the use of oral anticonvulsants such as primidone phenobarbitone. Anticonvulsants are generally not provided if fits occur less frequently than every 3–6 months. This is because the interval between fits is so long that more problems exist from daily drug administration than from the fits. The dose required by any individual is variable and trial doses must

---

IMMEDIATE ACTION AND ADVICE

If an owner telephones the practice for help whilst their pet is 'fitting', it is important for the nurse to be able to offer the following sound advice:

- The owner will be distressed. The nurse must take control and remain calm, giving positive advice.
- The owner should *not* touch the animal but should:
  - move items away from the animal to prevent injury.
  - clear the room of people.
  - reduce the noise and draw the curtains to provide a quiet environment.
  - stay with the animal until the fit is over and then offer comfort and reassurance.
- The owner should never:
  - try to move or handle the animal, as there is considerable risk of personal injury.
  - attempt to drive to the surgery with a fitting animal in the car, as there is a serious risk of causing an accident.
- When the animal has recovered, it should be brought to the surgery for examination by the veterinary surgeon.
- If the animal has status epilepticus, the veterinary surgeon and nurse may have to attend the owner's home to provide treatment.

The same routine should be used if a patient starts fitting in the surgery, until a veterinary surgeon can be called to administer intravenous anticonvulsant therapy.

---

be used in order to find the level of drug which just prevents fits from occurring. This approach will prevent unnecessary overdosing and allow early detection of progression as the threshold for fits tends to increase with time.

Although anticonvulsants are safe and may be used over a long period, they can have an initial sedative effect and a long-term effect on the liver. In addition owners must be particularly careful about keeping these powerful drugs away from children, as improper use can have fatal consequences.

Owners should be asked to watch for signs of the fits recurring which might change in character following drug therapy and include:

- Sudden episodes of seeking affection, restlessness or anxiety.
- Short-duration fits which may only be manifest as muscle tremors ('petit mal' fits).
- Sudden recurrence of typical fits, indicating loss of control.

Loss of consciousness

Syncope, or fainting, is a transient loss of consciousness due to generalised cerebral ischaemia, secondary to a major reduction in cerebral perfusion.

Unconsciousness may be defined as a state of insensibility or a loss of awareness. Animals are usually unresponsive to external stimulation during these episodes.

The clinical signs associated with unconsciousness must *not* be confused with convulsions. With unconsciousness there is *no* clonic or tonic muscle contractions. The animal usually collapses and lies still without signs of abnormal motor activity.

Additional clinical signs, which depend on the underlying cause of unconsciousness, are shown in Table 17.24 along with the most common causes.

When confronted with an unconscious patient, take the following action:

- Try to obtain help from a veterinary surgeon as quickly as possible.
- Monitor vital signs.
- Ensure that the animal has a patent airway:
  - Remove harness or collar and extend the head and neck.
  - Clear any obstructions observed in upper airway.
  - If the obstruction cannot be removed, carry out emergency tracheostomy.
- Supply oxygen once airway is patent. This may be carried out by face mask, endotracheal tube or oxygen cage.
- Artificial respiration should be provided if the animal fails to breathe for itself. Inflate lungs 12 times per minute, either via an anaesthetic machine or by decompression of the chest.
- If the heart has stopped, apply cardiac massage at 60 lateral compressions of the lower third of the thorax per minute.

Chapter 3 (First Aid) gives more detail of these procedures.

Paresis or paralysis

Injury to the spinal cord or brain may result in limb weakness (**paresis**) or inability to move (**paralysis**). **Paraplegia** usually describes paralysis of the hindlimbs. **Tetraplegia** (or quadriplegia) describes paralysis of all four limbs. Paralysis that involves a forelimb and a hindlimb on the same side is called **hemiplegia**.

Clinical signs such as these occur most commonly following trauma to the brain or spinal cord. In the latter case this is most often because of an intravertebral disc protrusion. The problem can be recognised by observing:

- The animal's inability to walk, support its weight or move its limbs.
- A loss of sensation in the affected limb(s).
- In tetraplegia or paraplegia, there may also be a loss of control over urination and defecation. In other cases there may be retention of urine or faeces.

Neurological tests, carried out by the veterinary surgeon to gauge the extent of nerve damage and also to act as a baseline from which to monitor progress, might include those shown in Table 17.25.

Emergency transport

If owners telephone for emergency help regarding an animal with a possible spinal injury, they should be warned not to lift the animal directly into a vehicle but to slide it gently onto a board or similar structure to keep its spine straight and prevent further injury (see Chapter 3, First Aid). Then the animal can be loaded into the vehicle on the board and brought to the surgery for examination.

Nursing care of a paraplegic patient

- Help the veterinary surgeon to carry out a baseline neurological examination, repeated at regular intervals to monitor progress.

Table 17.24 Unconsciousness

Common causes
  Cerebral anoxia.
  Trauma to the brain.
  Circulatory collapse – heart disease.
  Hypoglycaemia.
  Hypokalaemia.
  Barbiturate poisoning.
  Heat stroke.
  Airway obstruction.
  Hypocalcaemia.
  Narcolepsy.

Additional clinical signs
  Association with exercise.
  Very sudden onset with no pre- or post-ictal phases (as
    occurs with fits).
  Flaccid, no muscle activity.
  Unaware of surroundings.
  Cyanosis of mucous membranes possible.
  Stridor – increased inspiratory noise, with airway
    obstruction.
  Spontaneous, rapid and complete recovery.

Table 17.25 Neurological tests in cases of paresis or paralysis

Withdrawal reflex	Lay animal on its side and prick foot with needle. Limb should be withdrawn immediately and animal consciously aware of your action.
Anal reflex	Gently insert thermometer into rectum. Normal animals will respond with pronounced contraction of anal sphincter.
Tail sensation	Prick the skin of tail and observe for signs of recognition.
Patellar reflex	Hold the hindlimb partially extended with animal lying on its side. Tap patellar ligament with patellar hammer. Limb should extend and return to normal position.
Panniculus reflex	Sensory reception along flanks manifests as twitch of skin to pin prick.

- Regularly monitor the temperature, pulse and respiratory rates. These animals are prone to secondary infections.
- Place the animal in a comfortable, clean and dry cage.
- Keep the spine straight and prevent unnecessary movement.
- Assist in the provision of any specific treatment required (usually surgical intervention).
- Ensure that the animal receives adequate nutrition.
- Assist in the passage of urine and faeces, manually if required or by assisting the animal to posture by supporting with a blanket under its abdomen. It may be necessary to catheterise the patient regularly to prevent urine retention, infections and development of an atonic bladder.
- If the animal is incontinent, steps must be taken to prevent urine scalding by applying barrier creams and regularly changing the bedding. Incontinence pads are useful in this situation.
- Turn the animal regularly to prevent development of pressure sores or hypostatic congestion. Ideally place patient in sternal recumbency.
- Physiotherapy of limbs may be beneficial in some cases.

Muscle disorders

Muscle conditions observed in dogs and cats include:

- **Myositis** – inflammation of muscle tissue.
- **Polymyositis** – a diffuse inflammatory disorder of skeletal muscle often associated with autoimmune diseases. Results in weakness, lameness and pain on movement and palpation.
- **Metabolic myopathy** – muscular disorders associated with such conditions as Cushing's disease, hypothyroidism, glucocorticoid use, hypokalaemia, leading to weakness and muscular atrophy.
- **Muscular dystrophy** – a rare condition that may be inherited and is characterised by progressive degeneration of skeletal muscles in dogs. Clinical signs include weakness, dysphagia and muscle atrophy.

Electromyography (EMG) may be used to identify disease of muscle fibres, neuromuscular junctions, spinal nerves and peripheral nerves:

- Normal muscle is electrically silent. Normally the introduction of a needle into muscle tissue evokes electrical activity which stops when the needle stops moving.
- Where there is damage to a peripheral nerve supply to a muscle, the electrical activity on introducing the needle is prolonged.
- Similar changes occur in primary muscular disease such as myositis.

Diseases of the endocrine system

Diabetes mellitus (DM)

Diabetes mellitus is a condition most commonly seen in middle-aged entire bitches, especially of the terrier breeds. Animals with diabetes mellitus have problems with carbohydrate metabolism. The blood sugar level increases (**hyperglycaemia**) because the cells are unable to take up **glucose** from the circulation due to a deficiency in **insulin** (Table 17.26). When hyperglycaemia reaches the renal threshold, glucose appears in the urine.

The most common cause of DM is degeneration of the beta cells of the endocrine pancreas, leading to insulin deficiency. There are other causes:

- DM often occurs shortly after the bitch has been in season. This is due to the effect of **progesterone**, which stimulates growth hormone which is diabetogenic and causes insulin resistance and hyperglycaemia.
- In **Cushing's disease**, cortisol also causes hyperglycaemia and signs of DM.
- **Obesity** causes insulin resistance and may lead to DM.
- The use of **progestagens** to control oestrus may act in a similar way to natural progesterone and induce DM. This is especially important in cats.
- Excess **glucagon** activity which is also produced by the pancreas to antagonise insulin.

Table 17.26 Common disorders of the endocrine glands

Condition	Gland	Hormone deficiency
Diabetes mellitus	Pancreas	Insulin-deficiency
Diabetes insipidus	Pituitary Kidney	ADH deficiency Fail to respond to ADH
Cushing's disease	Pituitary Adrenal tumour	Excess ACTH → cortisol Excess cortisol
Addison's disease	Adrenal	Deficiency of aldosterone Cortisol deficiency?
Hyperthyroidism	Thyroid	Excess thyroxine
Hypothyroidism	Thyroid	Deficiency of thyroxine
Hyperparathyroidism	Parathyroid	Excess parathormone

● Administration of **glucocorticoids** causes hyperglycaemia, which can be confused with DM although the blood sugar level is usually lower than the renal threshold.

The clinical signs exhibited by animals with diabetes mellitus depend on the duration of the condition. Initially animals will be presented with polydipsia, polyuria and polyphagia but remain bright and active. The clinical signs change as the condition advances, with the development of anorexia, vomiting, diarrhoea, dehydration, weakness and lethargy. These symptoms develop because the animal needs an energy source but cannot utilise glucose. Therefore it starts to break down protein and fat as alternative energy sources. This results in a metabolic acidosis and a toxic build-up of ketones, called **ketoacidosis**.

The initial treatment of diabetes mellitus depends on the clinical signs exhibited. Therapy can be divided into:

● Emergency treatment for ketoacidosis.
● Standard treatment for diabetes mellitus.

Emergency treatment of ketoacidosis

These animals require urgent treatment with intravenous fluids (see Chapter 22), initially using Hartmann's solution to correct the metabolic acidosis and 0.9% saline for maintenance. In addition they should receive a short-acting soluble insulin administered intravenously to provide good control. The veterinary surgeon will be responsible for this therapy, which must be given with care to avoid the development of hypoglycaemia. Once the clinical signs of ketoacidosis improve and the animal starts eating, the standard therapy for diabetes mellitus can be instigated.

Standard treatment for diabetes mellitus

This requires the establishment of a strict daily routine:

● Collection of a urine sample first thing each morning and measurement of the glucose level.
● A *strict* dietary regime. Feed a high-fibre veterinary diet in exact amounts and at the same time each day.
● Subcutaneous injections of insulin each day.
● Female diabetics should be spayed before their next oestrus, to prevent instability of their condition.

Urine samples. The daily routine should start with collection of a free-flow urine sample each morning using a clean container (free from any chemical contamination). The glucose level is measured with ketodiastix, which also have a strip to measure ketones. Once the animal is stabilised, owners should be advised to observe the ketone strip: it will not change colour unless the animal has become unstable. If this occurs, owners should seek veterinary assistance immediately.

Calculation of insulin dose. The amount of insulin should be calculated from the level of glucose in the urine each day. The calculations are based on an initial dose of 0.5 IU/kg of body weight.

● Glucose >1%: give previous day's dose plus 2 IU.
● Glucose 0%: give previous day's dose less 2 IU.

● Glucose 0.1% (one-tenth per cent): give previous day's dose.

Injection of insulin. Before injection, the animal should be fed one-quarter of its daily ration. *Only if this is consumed should the animal be injected with insulin.*

● Insulin is supplied in bottles containing 100 IU/ml as a suspension. (Some veterinary insulins contain 40 IU/ml.)
● The insulin must be kept at +4°C and gently mixed but not shaken before use.
● Insulin syringes for human use are graduated in 50 divisions from 0 to 1.0 ml, so that each division is equivalent to 2 IU of insulin.
● The correct dose of insulin is injected under the skin anywhere along the animal's back. A new site is selected each day to reduce localised pain.

Diet

The remaining three-quarters of the daily ration should be given 8 hours after the insulin injection, so that the timing of the meal coincides with the peak effect of the insulin on the blood sugar level.

Diabetics should receive a high-fibre diet for the following reasons:

● Many animals with diabetes mellitus are obese and need to lose weight. The diet assists in a weight-control programme.
● High-fibre diets slow the rate of gastric emptying, reduce the speed of glucose absorption from the small intestine and prolong the time during which glucose is absorbed. This reduces the surges in blood glucose which can follow a meal and therefore assists insulin in controlling blood glucose levels and tissue uptake of glucose.
● It is very important that the diet is not changed from day to day and that no additional food is offered. Either situation may result in instability.

See Chapter 8, p. 198.

Hypoglycaemia

The most likely complication associated with the standard routine for diabetes is the occurrence of hypoglycaemia. This may be as a result of:

● Injecting too much insulin.
● Injecting the right amount of insulin but the animal fails to eat (this is why it is important to feed the animal before giving the insulin).
● The peak effect of insulin occurs before the animal receives the main part of the daily ration.

The most likely time for hypoglycaemia to occur is when the peak insulin effect is expected, some 8 hours after feeding. Owners should be advised to watch for the signs of hypoglycaemia – including muscle tremors, anxiety, weakness, ataxia, collapse and coma.

Therapy for hypoglycaemia depends on whether the animal is still conscious:

- If the animal is conscious, it should immediately be given sugar, chocolate, honey or similar food to counteract the low blood sugar level.
- If the animal is unconscious, the owner should take it to a veterinary surgeon urgently for an intravenous infusion of glucose.

Over-exertion of an animal with diabetes mellitus may lead to hypoglycaemic crisis and instability. The animal should be permitted to enjoy a moderate amount of exercise but this should be regular and of the same type and duration each day.

Diabetes insipidus (DI)

Diabetes insipidus occurs when there is failure in the production of antidiuretic hormone (ADH) from the pituitary gland or failure of the kidneys to respond to ADH – hence the terms **central diabetes insipidus** and **nephrogenic diabetes insipidus**, which describe the location of the problem.

Normally ADH is produced by the pituitary gland in order to concentrate the urine when the body needs to conserve water. If the animal conserves excessive amounts of water, ADH production falls and a more dilute urine is produced. In this way, water balance within the body can be controlled.

WATER DEPRIVATION TEST

This must always be carried out by a veterinary surgeon and with *great care*. Animals with suspect DI will be deprived of water and can become seriously dehydrated. Constant monitoring is required and the test *must* be stopped if the animal becomes distressed. The procedure is as follows:

- Ensure that the animal is well hydrated and has a normal blood urea level.
- Empty the animal's bladder of urine and measure its specific gravity.
- Weigh the animal and calculate 5% of its body weight.
- Place the animal in a kennel without food or water.
- Every 60 minutes: empty the bladder, measure the specific gravity of the urine and weigh the animal again. Repeat until 5% of the body weight has been lost.
- After 5% of the body weight is lost, the normal animal will have concentrated its urine to > 1.020. Animals with DI will continue to produce dilute urine (<1.007).
- Once the test is completed the animal should be allowed free access to water.

The clinical signs associated with diabetes insipidus are marked polydipsia and polyuria. They occur often because the animal can no longer conserve water due to a defect in the ADH system. Consequently the animal produces very dilute urine all the time, and requires a compensatory increase in water intake to correct the loss. The amounts of water ingested can be dramatic: for example, a dachshund may drink up to 7 litres of water a day.

Urine analysis in animals with DI will be negative except for a very low specific gravity (in the order of 1.000 to 1.007). Repeated measurements of urine specific gravity will confirm that the animal is unable to concentrate its urine. The diagnosis is based on confirming that the animal is unable to concentrate its urine, by carrying out a water deprivation test.

Treatment of diabetes insipidus depends on which form is present:

- In central DI, the administration of ADH by nasal drops will result in a restoration of normal water balance.
- In nephrogenic DI, there is adequate ADH but the kidneys will not respond to the hormone and so replacement hormone therapy will not work. Paradoxically, thiazide diuretics may reduce urine output by 50% in some cases. However, the prognosis for this form remains guarded.

Cushing's disease

Cushing's disease, or **hyperadrenocorticalism**, is associated with the production of excessive levels of cortisol from the adrenal glands. This may occur because there is:

- A tumour of the adrenal gland, with excess production of cortisol.
- A pituitary tumour, resulting in too much ACTH, which stimulates the adrenal glands to produce excess cortisol (this form of Cushings disease is more common).

Clinical signs and treatment are given in Table 17.27. The diagnosis is based on hormone tests such as the ACTH test and the dexamethasone screening and suppression tests, which determine whether Cushing's disease is present and, if so, in which form so that the appropriate treatment can be given.

Hypothyroidism and hyperthyroidism

Over 80% of naturally occurring cases of **hypothyroidism** are associated with autoimmune disease or atrophy of the thyroid glands. Hypothyroidism is the most common cause of endocrine disorder of dogs (usually 6–10 years of age, either sex) but is rare in cats.

Hyperthyroidism, on the other hand, is extremely rare in dogs but is now quite commonly diagnosed in cats (usually over 6 years of age, either sex). Benign thyroid tumours account for over 95% of clinical cases and lead to excess thyroid hormone production.

Thyroid hormone is important for the function of many body organs and deficiencies or excesses result in numerous possible clinical signs, as set out in Table 17.28, which also describes diagnosis and treatment of both diseases.

Table 17.27 Cushing's disease

Clinical signs
  Polyphagia
  Polydipsia and polyuria.
  Pot-bellied because of enlarged liver, loss of abdominal
    muscle tone and fat deposition in abdomen.
  Bilateral alopecia of flanks.
  Change in coat colour in some cases.
  Muscle wasting and weakness in some cases.
  Calcium deposit in the skin (*calcinosis cutis*).

Treatment	
Adrenal tumour	Usually only one adrenal gland involved, which should be removed surgically; other gland will slowly start to function again in most cases.
Pituitary form	Oral mitotane given daily to suppress adrenal function – must be given with food for adequate absorption, and gloves must be worn when handling tablets. Animal must also be carefully monitored to determine when adequate amount of drug has been given: measuring water intake and use ACTH test. Drug therapy to reduce water intake to 50 ml/kg/day; when target is reached, once-weekly mitotane therapy to maintain control.

Skeletal system

Calcium, phosphorus and vitamin D

The majority of calcium and phosphorus in the body is found in the bones and teeth (>90%). Apart from their importance in forming the skeleton, calcium and phosphorus have other important functions:

- Calcium: blood clotting; nerve and muscle function.
- Phosphorus: involvement in enzyme systems throughout the body.

Although there are individual dietary requirements for calcium and phosphorus, the relationship between the two minerals is also very important – as explained in Chapter 8.

Vitamin D is synthesized in the skin by action of ultraviolet light. There may also be a dietary requirement which is to some extent dependent on the dietary content of Ca:P. Following formation in the skin, vitamin D is modified by the liver and kidney to produce the physiologically active form which plays an important part in calcium:phosphorus metabolism by:

- Increasing the absorption of both calcium and phosphorus from the intestine.
- Decreasing excretion of calcium and phosphorus from the kidney.
- Increasing mineralisation of bone or bone resorption.

Hyperparathyroidism

An imbalance in the Ca:P ratio will result in the stimulation of the parathyroid glands and a marked increase in circulating parathormone (which is secreted by the parathyroid and controls the metabolism of calcium and phosphorus). This response may be induced secondary to nutritional deficiency or renal disease.

Secondary nutritional hyperparathyroidism is also known as **juvenile or nutritional osteodystrophy**. A dietary deficiency in calcium or an excess in phosphorus, most commonly associated with feeding all-meat diets, results in hyperphosphataemia and hypocalcaemia and leads to hyperparathyroidism. A similar response may occur when other unbalanced diets are fed or following inappropriate use of dietary supplements. The animal responds by increasing renal excretion of phosphorus and retaining

Table 17.28 Hypothyroidism and hyperthyroidism			

	Clinical signs	Diagnosis	Treatment
Hypothyroidism	Cool feel to the skin. Poor appetite in spite of increasing weight gain.Lethargy and increased sleeping time. Muscle weakness. Loss of temporal muscle mass. 'Tragic' facial expression. Bilateral alopecia especially of the flanks of hindlimbs.	Suggested by low thyroxine (T4) levels and confirmed by carrying out a **TSH test**. TSH normally stimulates thyroid gland to produce more thyroid hormone. This fails to occur in hypothyroidism, with little or no increase in T4 levels after administration of TSH.	Hormone replacement therapy: ideally thyroxine (T4), rather than T3, given daily and treatment continued for minimum of 12 weeks before assessing effectiveness. Response in most cases good but treatment required for life. Thyroid extract may also be used but varies from batch to batch and so tends to give poor results.
Hyperthyroidism	Restlessness, overactivity, aggressive behaviour. Polyphagia. Tachycardia. Weight loss. Diarrhoea. Poor coat and skin condition. Palpable mass in neck (goitre).	Measure basal T3 or T4 levels (elevated). Unilateral or bilateral disease assessed by scanning thyroids after giving technetium-99M intravenously. Over-active glands take up radioactive isotope, which can be photographed with gamma camera.	Surgical removal of over-active thyroid glands gives best results. Radiotherapy using iodine-131 destroys thyroid tissue. Long-term drug management using carbimazole (CBZ) tends to result in problems with maintaining control long term.

calcium, together with resorption of calcium from the bones.

Secondary renal hyperparathyroidism is also known as **renal osteodystrophy, rubber jaw** and **renal rickets**. Animals in renal failure retain phosphorus, which accumulates in the circulation resulting in a change in the Ca:P ratio from 1.5:1 to values as high as 1:4, effectively causing hypocalcaemia. This stimulates the parathyroid glands to produce parathormone. In addition the renal disease may result in failure to activate vitamin D, which in turn compromises Ca:P metabolism. Parathormone attempts to correct the imbalance by improving absorption from the intestine and liberating calcium from the bones. Although all bones are affected, demineralisation most severely affects the mandible and maxilla.

Clinical signs associated with hyperparathyroidism (which depends on whether nutritional or renal hyperparathyroidism is present and on the age of the animal) are given in Table 17.29.

Hypervitaminosis A

This condition is clinically more important in cats than dogs and is associated with feeding diets rich in vitamin A. This may result from feeding cats a diet rich in liver. Excessive quantities of vitamin A are absorbed and accumulate until toxic changes are observed.

Vitamin A is required for normal endochondrial ossification but excessive amounts provoke periosteal new bone formation. Changes associated with vitamin A toxicity are characterized by the development of multiple exostoses, especially involving the cervical and thoracic vertebrae and the forelimbs in young growing animals. They are particularly common around articular surfaces, leading to ankylosis at the attachments of ligaments and tendons.

Typical clinical signs (Table 17.29) are observed in adult cats after ingesting vitamin A rich foods for several months.

Chronic pulmonary osteoarthropathy

Chronic pulmonary osteoarthropathy is also known as hypertropic pulmonary osteoarthropathy or **Marie's disease**. In this condition limb swelling due to periosteal new bone formation along the distal bones of the forelimbs occurs secondary to a mass within the thorax and more rarely the abdomen (especially bladder tumours). The reason for the association between a space-occupying lesion in the thorax and bone changes in the limbs is not fully understood. There is no joint involvement and it is rare to observe bony changes in the hindlimbs. Clinical signs are given in Table 17.29.

Metaphyseal osteopathy

This is also known as **Möller–Barlow's disease, juvenile scurvy** and hypertrophic osteodystrophy. In all cases clinical signs are associated with the metaphysis of long

Table 17.29 Skeletal diseases: clinical signs	
(1) Hyperpara-thyroidism	(a) *Nutritional forms* most common in growing puppies fed diets with incorrect balance of calcium and phosphorus: usually depressed, lame and exhibit pain on moving. Incomplete and compression fractures lead to additional clinical signs.
	(b) *Chronic renal failure*: tend to be middle-aged or older. In addition to signs associated with renal failure, may develop rubber jaw due to demineralisation of mandible, which becomes pliable. Teeth may become loose and in some cases fall out; spontaneous fractures due to osteoporosis (demineralisation).
(2) Hypervitamin-osis A	Signs include, lethargy, poor coat condition (due to inability to groom), reluctance to move, lameness and pain on moving especially neck and head.
(3) Chronic pulmonary osteo-arthropathy	Classically bilateral, painful soft tissue swelling occurs in the distal forelimbs leading to varying degrees of lameness. These clinical signs may occur BEFORE those associated with changes in the thorax.
(4) Metaphyseal osteopathy	Mild to severe lameness together with limb pain, in some cases leading to collapse and inability to walk. Joints of distal fore- and hindlimbs usually involved: painful, hot and swollen. Puppies usually depressed, anorexic and often pyrexic (106°F). Clinical signs may wax and wane, with periods of complete remission. Risk of limb deformity requiring surgical correction. Clinical signs often disappear as dog matures but many are euthanased due to the severity of the condition.
(5) Rickets	Obvious enlargement of growth plates, bowing of the limbs and enlargement of the costochondral junctions ('rickety rosary'), often lead to varying degrees of lameness, fractures, lordosis and loss of teeth.

bones in rapidly growing dogs of large breeds. Although the true cause is not known, vitamin C deficiency, overnutrition and excessive dietary supplementation have been implicated. In particular there appears to be an association between high levels of dietary protein, energy, calcium and vitamin D and metaphyseal osteopathy. Great care is needed in feeding puppies and it is undesirable to feed for maximum rate of growth in large breeds of dog.

A necrotic band of tissue develops adjacent to the growth plate followed by the deposition of a band of osseous material in the soft tissue along the metaphysis. There is periosteal new bone formation and infiltration with many inflammatory cells. Eventually the necrotic tissue is replaced by healthy bone.

Clinical signs, which are most frequently observed in rapidly growing puppies between 3 and 7 months of age, are described in Table 17.29.

Osteochondrosis

This general term is used to describe disturbances in endochondrial ossification. It is sometimes further defined as degeneration of bone and cartilage but this is misleading as only cartilage is primarily involved. Various conditions are considered to be manifestations of osteochondrosis, including osteochondritis dissecans involving the shoulder joint, medial humeral condyle, lateral femoral condyle, cervical intravertebral joints and un-united anconeal process.

Normal epiphyseal growth takes place by proliferation of chondrocytes near the surface of the joint. This is followed in time by degeneration and calcification of the chondrocytes, a condition called **endochondrial ossification**. In osteochondrosis this differentiation of chondrocytes is disturbed and the cartilage becomes thicker than normal. At points of high pressure in the joint, poor vascularisation occurs and the basal layer of the thickened cartilage becomes necrotic. This leads to cracks and fissures in the cartilage. Once these fissures reach the surface of the joint, **osteochondritis dissecans** is said to be present. This is confirmed by joint pain due to a marked inflammatory reaction. A flap of cartilage often forms or breaks off, forming a 'joint mouse' which floats around in the joint space.

Rapid growth appears to be very important in the aetiology of osteochondrosis – hence the increased number of cases seen in males. Overnutrition and dietary supplementation leading to imbalances in calcium, phosphorus and vitamin D have also been implicated. Genetic predisposition may also be important.

Rickets

This term usually describes the disease in young animals – in adult animals the term **osteomalacia** is used. In this condition, mineralisation of newly formed osteoid tissue (and of cartilage matrix in young animals) does not occur around the growth plate.

The cause of these changes remains controversial. Some studies suggest that there is a deficiency in dietary vitamin D while others suggest that there may be deficiencies in dietary calcium and phosphorus. In any case it appears that the relationship between calcium, phosphorus and vitamin D is upset.

Osteomyelitis

This condition may be defined as an inflammatory condition of bone which involves both the cortex and the medulla. Osteomyelitis can be classified as follows:

- Infectious: bacterial infection (Staphylococci, Streptococci, *Escherichia coli, Pseudomonas* spp., *Proteus* spp.) and fungal infections (especially *Aspergillus* spp.)
- Non-infectious: sequestria (bone fragments with poor blood supply), trauma to bone and foreign bodies, implants.

Treatment involves culture of infected material together with sensitivity testing in order to determine the most effective antibiotic, which should be administered for at least a month.

In addition to antibiotic therapy, surgical intervention may be required in order to remove sequestria, implants or foreign bodies associated with the osteomyelitis.

Bone tumours

There are many tumours which can affect bone. As with other tissues, tumours may be primary (arising from the tissue itself) or secondary (metastatic spread of tumours from another tissue). The most important primary bone tumours are osteoma and osteosarcoma.

Osteoma is a slow-growing, hard but benign tumour which only causes problems due to mechanical interference with function, i.e. interference with joint movement or adjacent tissues such as muscle or nerves. These tumours may occur anywhere in the axial or appendicular skeleton.

Osteosarcoma is a primary, highly malignant and usually solitary tumour with very aggressive growth characteristics. The tumour most frequently spreads to local lymph nodes and the lungs. There appears to be a greater incidence in St Bernards, Dobermanns, Irish wolfhounds and Great Danes. Dogs over 7 years old are more often affected. The most common sites involved are the proximal humerus, distal radius and ulna, and the distal femur and proximal or distal tibia.

Other primary bone tumours include:

- **Chondrosarcoma** – often involves flat bones and is slow to spread.
- **Fibrosarcoma** – rare, affects growth plates and periosteum.
- **Chondroma** – affects the skull, with local invasion to brain.
- **Osteochondroma** – affects the limbs and vertebrae and occurs most frequently during active bone growth.

Arthritis

Arthritis may be defined as inflammation of a joint. There are several different types of arthritis and consequently several different aetiologies. The classification of arthritis includes degenerative and inflammatory conditions described in Table 17.30, which also gives treatment for different types.

Exercise

It is very important that exercise in dogs or cats with osteoarthritis should not be totally restricted, as this will result in reduced joint mobility. However, it is equally important not to provide excessive exercise, as this will exacerbate the condition. Short frequent walks are more beneficial than single long walks. In other forms of arthritis a restriction on exercise may be important, especially in the early stages of therapy.

Table 17.30 Arthritis: classification and description of types

Classification	Description	Treatment

Degenerative:
Osteoarthritis
– Primary: aetiology not known.
– Secondary: hip dysplasia.
  Cruciate rupture.
Inflammatory:
Infective
– Bacterial, viral, fungal,
  Mycoplasma.
Crystals – Gout.
Immune:
Erosive
– Rheumatoid arthritis.
– Polyarthritis.
Non-erosive
– SLE
– Polymyositis
– Polyarteritis nodosa.
	(a) *Osteoarthritis*. Chronic condition, insidious in onset, leading to lameness, pain, crepitation and joint instability. Progressive; leads to thickening of joint and eventually limited joint movement.
	
	(b) *Infective or septic arthritis*. Usually occurs in single joint; results in pyrexia, joint swelling, heat and pain in joint. Severe cases may become anorexic and depressed.
	
	(c) *Immune-mediated arthritis*. Part of a systemic disease with signs involving other tissues. With regard to joints, lamenesss (single or multiple) may shift (involve different joints on different occasions). Pyrexia, stiffness, depression and associated muscle atrophy; muscle pain, pyrexia, clotting defects, renal disease, splenomegaly, anaemia, skin changes.
		Depends on underlying cause: definitive diagnosis important.
		
		Osteoarthritis: non-steroidal anti-inflammatory drugs such as phenylbutazone and piroxicam.
		
		Infective arthritis: important to determine the type of micro-organism and its antibiotic sensitivity; give for minimum of 3–4 weeks.
		
		Immune-mediated arthritis: high doses of corticosteroids such as prednisolone depress the immune response and improve overall condition.

Diet

The dietary management of every case should be carefully examined. Those on an unsatisfactory diet should be placed on one that is suitable for the animal's life stage. Animals who are obese must be placed on a reducing diet, as obesity exacerbates arthritis and reduces the long-term prognosis.

Mucocutaneous system

Various descriptive terms are used when discussing disease of the mucocutaneous system and it is important these are clearly understood. **Alopecia** is a general term used to describe a loss of hair from any site and for any reason. **Pruritus** is a sensation within the skin which produces the desire to scratch in order to relieve the irritation. **Seborrhoea** describes an abnormally copious excretion of sebum which may make the skin appear oily. **Pyoderma** describes any pyogenic skin infection most of which occur secondary to some other skin condition.

Parasitic skin disease

There are several ectoparasitic conditions which are of importance in dogs and cats (Table 17.31). Each ectoparasite has a different life cycle and host specificity which influences the clinical signs exhibited by the host and the methods of treatment employed. These signs are given in Table 17.32, along with general descriptions of each species and the appropriate treatment after diagnosis. See also Chapter 15, p. 378.

The diagnosis of ectoparasites usually depends on the collection and examination of **skin scrapings.** This is a relatively simply procedure but can lead to inaccurate results if it carried out incorrectly. The procedure is detailed in Chapter 15, Elementary mycology and parasitology, p. 381, which also describes microscopic examination of the samples for different ectoparasites.

Hormonal alopecia

There is a specific group of hormonal diseases which tend to cause bilaterally symmetrical alopecia. Hormonal alopecia

Table 17.31 A list of the most common ectoparasites found on dogs and cats together with some details of their epidemiology

Clinical signs	Live off host	Host specificity	Life cycle	Surface or deep dwelling
Cheyletiella spp.	Possible	Dog, cat, rabbit	5 weeks	Surface
Sarcoptic mange	Possible	Primary dogs	3–4 weeks	Deep
Neotrombicula spp.	Yes	Not specific	50–70 days	Surface
Otodectes spp.	Yes	Dog/cat only	3 weeks	Surface
Demodex spp.	No	Dog/cat only	–	Hair follicle
Fleas	Yes	Not specific	3 weeks/2 years	Surface
Lice	No	Specific	14–21 days	Surface
Ticks	Yes	Not specific	2 months/2 years	Surface
Notoedres spp.	No	Primary cats	–	Surface

Table 17.32 Ectoparasite species (See Table 15.1 p. 377)

Species	Clinical signs	Diagnosis	Treatment
Cheyletiella spp. Mites that live on skin and cause 'walking dandruff' on dogs, cats, rabbits and (transiently) humans.	Generalised pruritus and excessive scaling. Lesions in cats can appear like miliary dermatitis. Some remain asymptomatic.	Sellotape preparations or superficial skin scrapings.	Cases respond well to most insecticidal shampoos (pyrethrin, carbamate and organophosphorus) given weekly for 6 weeks.
Sarcoptes scabiei Primarily a burrowing mite found on dogs (human cases also occur). Extremely contagious, spread by direct or indirect contact.	Alopecia, papules and crust formation which often starts on ears, elbows, brisket and legs; sites often severely pruritic. Generalised lymphadenopathy may develop in severe cases.	Mites difficult to find; may require examination of 12–20 skin scrapings.	Clipping out coat to ensure insecticidal shampoo (Amitraz) makes good contact with skin. Treat all in-contact animals. Antiseborrhoeic shampoos also useful to remove scale and crusts (sulphur/salicylic acid).
Neotrombicula autumnalis Also called harvest mite or chigger; natural host small rodents but may cause clinical signs in dogs, cats and humans.	Seasonal, normally summer and early autumn. Pruritus generalised, or lesions restricted to feet with excessive biting and licking causing acute moist dermatitis. In cats, non-pruritic papular disease can occur.	Close examination of the animal, especially between the toes where clusters of red–orange mites will be found.	Insecticidal shampoos or sprays.
Otodectes cynotis Mite is found in dog and cat; usually lives in ear but occasionally causes lesions on neck, gluteal region and tail.	Typically associated with outer ear infection (otitis externa), resulting in alopecia next to ear canal, head shaking, pawing the ears, head tilt, and presence of thick waxy discharge. Lesions on body include crusts and papules.	Careful visual examination for white pinhead-sized mites.	Proprietary insecticidal ear preparations such as gamma BHC or Monosulfiram preparations and whole-body shampoos in some cases.
Demodex canis Obligate canine ectoparasite found in hair follicles; life cycle is poorly understood, but mite can *only* be passed from bitch to puppies during the first 3 days of life. Thereafter not contagious.	Localised form typically in puppies between 3 and 6 months of age: lesions on head, forelimbs and neck as areas of alopecia with scaling, erythema, and pigmentation. Generalised disease at any age: in young animals localised lesions may coalesce and become generalised or adult onset disease may occur. Secondary deep pyoderma and generalised lymphadenopathy common. Demodecosis does occur rarely in cats.	Deep skin scrapings, or expressing pus onto a microscope slide (usually heavily contaminated with mites).	Not required for localised lesions. Generalised cases: clip out completely, then repeated application of Amitraz shampoo. Pyoderma: culture and sensitivity of purulent material; administer suitable antibiotic, often for months, until negative scrapings obtained on three occasions. Up to 70% of adult onset disease related to an underlying disorder.
Ctenocephalides felis Most common ectoparasite of dog and cat, one of several species of flea. Causes irritation, and flea saliva may cause hypersensitivity reaction.	Seasonal in the UK. Include erythema and papule formation at location of each bite, anywhere on the animal and in particular along back, tail, head, hindlegs and ventral abdomen. Self-trauma common, may lead to alopecia and bleeding. Cats: miliary dermatitis, granulomata (eosinophilic granuloma complex) or symmetrical alopecia.	Physical examination for presence of fleas or flea dirt; positive reaction to intradermal flea antigen if hypersensitivity is suspected.	Sustained and simultaneous assault on patient and environment: *Animal*: suitable insecticidal preparation; shampoos, sprays, powders, flea collars or systemic insecticide. Pyrethrin products safest to use in young and debilitated animals. Other parasiticides include Lufenuron and Fipronil, and carbamate preparations. Regularly worm for *Dipylidium caninum*. *Bedding material*: destroy or thoroughly wash in a hot wash at the same time.

Table 17.32 (Continued)			
Species	**Clinical signs**	**Diagnosis**	**Treatment**
			House: thoroughly vacuumed; apply insecticidal spray to carpets, paying particular attention to corners and under furniture. Discard vacuum bag to prevent reinfestation. *Owner also has lesions*: advise to seek medical attention. It is often necessary to repeat this protocol at 14-day intervals until the problem is brought under control.
Trichodectes spp. and *Linognathus* spp. Lice found on dogs and cats include sucking (*Linognathus*) and biting (*Trichodectes*) spp.; life cycle 21 days, entirely on host.	Asymptomatic, or varying degrees of pruritus, alopecia (secondary to self-trauma), and in cats miliary dermatitis. In severe infestations, may become anaemic.	Close examination for evidence of adult lice or eggs (nits) attached to hairs.	Lice susceptible to almost all parasiticidal agents. Suitable insecticidal shampoo, spray or powder; repeated 14 days later to destroy hatched larvae.
Ixodes ricinus Most common tick on dogs in the UK; presence depends on geographical location and climate. Much of life cycle off host: tick only seeks host during spring or autumn, for a meal.	Factors include: Number of ticks present. Animal's individual reaction to ticks. Whether ticks are carrying any viral, bacterial, protozoal or rickettsial diseases. Owners often seek veterinary advice because suddenly observed 'cyst like' structure on skin. Individual hypersensitivity may cause local pruritus so that animal removes tick by pawing the site; mouth parts may remain in place and subsequently cause granulomatous reaction and secondary infection.	Easily made from visual examination of animal.	If required, tick can be removed after initially soaking it in alcohol: grasp firmly with forceps and remove in a twisting action. Ensure mouth parts also removed to avoid secondary infection. Insecticidal sprays prevent future problems when entering tick area.
Notoedres cati Rare mite in UK, primarily infects cats, dogs or rabbits; life cycle very similar to *Sarcoptes scabiei*.	First appear on pinna and may extend to include face, neck and forelimbs. Skin becomes crusted and thickened with areas of alopecia; intense pruritus.	Skin scrapings.	Insecticidal shampoo (selenium sulphide) or sulphur-based alternative.

is usually associated with the flanks and/or ventral abdomen and inner aspect of the hindlimbs. In advanced cases it may involve the whole body but usually spares the head and limbs. It is rarely associated with pruritus, self-trauma or inflammation. Conditions which may be included in this category are:

- Hypothyroidism.
- Hyperadrenocorticalism.
- Sertoli cell tumour.
- Canine ovarian imbalances.
- Feline symmetrical alopecia.

Hypothyroidism and hyperadrenocorticalism have already been described under diseases of the endocrine system.

Sertoli cell tumour

This is the commonest testicular tumour to induce alopecia in middle-aged to old male dogs. Cryptorchid animals are 13 times more likely to develop this tumour. Oestrogen levels may or may not be elevated.

Clinical signs, when present, are associated with hyper-oestrogenism and include bilateral non-pruritic alopecia involving the perineal region, inner aspects of the hindlimbs, ventral abdomen and flanks. Gynaecomastia, pendulous prepuce and attractiveness to other male dogs are other hallmarks of this condition. The neoplastic testicle is often enlarged while the other testicle is atrophied. In advanced cases a non-regenerative anaemia develops due to the effect of oestrogen on the bone marrow.

Diagnosis is based on clinical history and physical examination and plasma oestrogen assay. Treatment involves castration which is usually beneficial.

Canine ovarian imbalance

The aetiology of this condition is not known but may involve either an oestrogen responsive dermatosis or dermatosis induced by hyperoestrogenism.

Hyperoestrogenism (classified type I) is usually associated with cystic ovarian disease or ovarian tumour. Clinical signs include generalised bilaterally symmetrical alopecia which starts in the perineal region. There is usually vulval enlargement, abnormal oestrus cycles and secondary seborrhoea. The treatment of choice is ovariohysterectomy, although clinical signs may take up to 6 months to decline.

Oestrogen responsive dermatosis (classified as type II) is a rare condition of the bitch occurring after ovariohysterectomy. Clinical signs include perineal alopecia which spreads to the inner aspect of the hindlimbs and ventral abdomen and also juvenile vulva and nipples. The remainder of the coat becomes soft and 'puppy like' in character. Treatment involves oestrogen or testosterone replacement therapy.

Hyperoestrogenism (classified type I) is usually associated with cystic ovarian disease or ovarian tumour. Clinical signs include generalised bilaterally symmetrical alopecia which starts in the perineal region. There is usually vulval enlargement, abnormal oestrus cycles and secondary seborrhoea. The treatment of choice is ovariohysterectomy although clinical signs may take up to 6 months to decline.

Feline symmetrical alopecia

This was also called **feline hormonal alopecia** and is a condition of complex aetiology which is not clearly understood and is very rare. It is seen more commonly in neutered cats. Alopecia initially involves the perineal region but rapidly extends to the inner aspects of the hindlimbs and

---

Table 17.33 Pyodermas

(1) Surface pyodermas	(a) Acute moist dermatitis Usually occurs following self-trauma when skin becomes physically damaged, wet due to serum exudation, painful, with areas of hair loss and hair matting on skin. Most common sites include face, feet, hindquarters, tail. *Treatment*: remove underlying cause such as ear infection, impacted anal glands or harvest mites; clip hair from site and start topical cleansing with antibacterial agents such as chlorhexidine. Prevent further self-trauma by using Elizabethan collar. (b) Skin fold dermatitis Conformational problem where folds in skin occur at various sites including lip fold, vulval fold, tail fold dermatitis, most commonly in breeds such as the Pekingese and Sharpei but may affect others. Acute moist dermatitis develops within fold of skin which rapidly becomes infected. Only when fold is opened can full extent of dermatitis be seen. *Treatment*: surgical correction of skin fold and use of chlorhexidine washes or benzoyl peroxide gel (if not ulcerated).
(2) Superficial pyodermas	(a) Impetigo Also known as juvenile pustular dermatitis or puppy pyoderma. Most often observed in young growing puppies, especially on their ventral abdomen. Multiple pustules and yellow scabs. Treatment: antibacterial shampoos, i.e. benzoyl peroxide or ethyl lactate and, where extensive, systemic antibiotics such as erythromycin. (b) Folliculitis Infection of hair follicle. Formation of pustules with a hair protruding. Sometimes lesions assume ring formation, especially on the ventral abdomen. Coat may have 'moth eaten' appearance. Many underlying causes. Treatment: detect and remove the underlying cause; antibiotic therapy.
(3) Deep pyodermas	(a) Interdigital pyoderma Also known as pododermatitis; seen in short-haired breeds of dog. Paws become swollen, painful; exude pus. Areas of alopecia and in severe cases ulceration and fistulas. *Treatment*: long-term antibiotic therapy; surgical drainage of purulent material; correction of any detectable underlying cause, such as removal of foreign bodies. (b) Furunculosis Most serious form of pyoderma, often associated with demodicosis, ringworm, hypothyroidism or general debility. Pustules, discharging pus, fistulas, alopecia and pain. Lesions most often found on nose, muzzle and flanks but can extend to any area. *Treatment*: correct any underlying cause; long-term systemic antibiotic therapy; whirlpool baths beneficial as part of the treatment regime.
(4) Feline pyoderma	Bacteria such as *Pasteurella*, *Staphylococcus* and *Fusiformis* spp. commonly found in oral cavity of cats: when cat bites, its long sharp canines inoculate infection deep within skin, commonly resulting in cellulitis (diffuse infection of subcutaneous tissue). Cats exhibit signs of pyrexia, anorexia, depression, pain and swelling at site of bite wound. *Treatment*: systemic antibiotics; drainage usually successful.

Table 17.34 The prevalence of microsporum and trichophyton species in the dog and cat within the UK (% cases)

	Microsporum canis	*Trichophyton* spp.
Cats	94.5–98.5	1.5–5.0
Dogs	37.8–88.0	12.0–62.0

ventral abdomen. In some cases generalised alopecia develops. Diagnosis is based on clinical examination and is generally one of exclusion (hair regrowth will not occur when an Elizabethan collar is worn). Various treatments have been suggested including:

- Thyroid hormone replacement.
- Megoestral acetate therapy.
- Testosterone therapy in males and females.

Table 17.35 Allergies

Allergic reactions	Clinical signs	Diagnosis	Treatment
Urticaria Wide variety including drugs, vaccines, insect bites/stings.	Appear suddenly as multiple swellings or wheals on the skin where the hair becomes erect and stands out. May be pruritic.	Based on clinical signs.	Remove cause and administer corticosteroids.
Atopic dermatitis Wide variety in the environment – most common include house dust, house dust mites, fungi, danders and pollens.	*In dogs*: 1–3 years of age, often initially seasonal but in some cases rapidly become permanent. Pruritus, especially face, feet, axilla and ventral abdomen. Self-trauma may lead to secondary infection, alopecia and pigmentation of the skin. Some dogs develop ocular discharge and otitis externa. *In cats*: similar clinical picture, or atopy associated with miliary dermatitis, symmetrical alopecia, eosinophilic granuloma complex or facial pruritus.	Intradermal skin tests with multiple allergens.	Usually life-long. May involve corticosteroids, antihistamines, hyposensitisation, essential fatty acid supplements or topical shampoos such as colloidal oatmeal every 3 days.
Food hypersensitivity Individual cases reported following sensitisation to specific foods such as beef, horse meat, milk, eggs and fish.	May be associated with pruritic skin disease and occasionally gastroenteritis.	Difficult; may be achieved by feeding 'elimination diet' composed of single protein and carbohydrate source to which animal has no previous exposure. No other food (including titbits) should be permitted. Clinical signs should regress within 6 weeks but may be as long as 8 weeks, at which point single food items can be reintroduced to the diet in order to determine allergens involved.	Long-term therapy: avoid specific allergens identified by the dietary trials.
Contact dermatitis Soaps, detergents, shampoos, topical drugs, plastic, rubber, nylon and other synthetic agents.	May develop after only 4–6 weeks' exposure to allergen but usually follow a period of over 2 years. Lesions (most frequently on feet, ventral abdomen, neck and chin) are pruritic, erythematous, and often secondarily infected following self-trauma.	(a) Patch testing: suspect allergen is applied to clipped area of skin and held in place with bandage; patch is removed after 48 hours and skin examined for erythema. (b) Hospitalising animal in kennel without access to any bedding or other items from own environment: if clinical signs resolve, circumstantial evidence of contact dermatitis. Animal should now be introduced to single items from home environment until allergen(s) identified.	Avoid contact with identified allergens.

Pyoderma

Pyoderma is rare in the cat. In the dog it is usually associated with an underlying predisposing disease. The most common pathogen isolated in canine pyoderma is *Staphylococcus intermedius*. Secondary opportunist bacteria such as *Proteus, Pseudomonas, Corynebacterium* may also be isolated usually in association with *Staphylococcus*. Resident bacteria, including coagulase-negative Staphylococci, are thought to be important to normal skin defence mechanisms. The severity of the infection depends on how deep the infection penetrates the skin and this is used to classify pyodermas (Table 17.33).

Ringworm

Ringworm, also known as **dermatophytosis**, may infect the skin, nails and/or hair. It is a fungal disease caused by only two organisms of major significance in the dog and cat: *Microsporum* spp. and *Trichophyton* spp. (Table 17.34). More details of these species are given in Chapter 15, Elementary Mycology and Parasitology, p. 376.

Ringworm is not common in the dog but it is a common cause of skin disease in the cat. Infection is acquired by direct contact or through fomites. It is important to remember that ringworm is a *zoonosis* – so owners might become infected and should be advised accordingly.

Clinical signs

In dogs, clinical signs include circular areas of alopecia which may appear grey or erythematous with scaling and crusting. Lesions may be confined to specific areas such as the head or forelimbs or may be generalised. In cats, lesions may appear as circular areas of grey scaling or as miliary dermatitis, or the animal may remain asymptomatic. Details of diagnosis for ringworm are given in Chapter 13, Diagnostic Aids, p. 354 and also Chapter 15, p. 376.

Treatment

Many cases of ringworm are self-limiting and will ultimately settle without treatment. However, because this is a zoonosis and because cases can become severe, it is usual to treat clinical cases. As ringworm can survive off the host it is necessary to carry out a detailed programme as follows:

- Treat the animal with oral griseofulvin, given with a fatty meal to improve absorption of the drug. Maintain treatment until all the lesions have regressed. Griseofulvin should not be used in pregnant animals.
- Clip away the hair from lesions, especially in long-haired animals, to allow access for topical treatments.
- In dogs, apply enilconazole (Imaverol) directly to the lesions. This is particularly useful where there are only a few lesions present. In cats, apply chlorhexidine washes.
- All in-contact animals should be checked for ringworm and treated at the same time. Burn all contaminated material such as bedding. Thoroughly disinfect the premises using sodium hypochlorite, formalin or Imaverol solutions. Paint all woodwork. Advise the owner to seek medical advice if they develop skin lesions.

Allergic dermatitis

Allergic skin conditions include:

- Urticaria (uncommon).
- Atopic dermatitis (common, inherited).
- Food hypersensitivity (true incidence not known).
- Contact dermatitis (uncommon condition due to delayed hypersensitivity reaction).

Table 17.35 describes typical allergens, clinical signs, diagnosis and treatment for each group.

Intradermal skin testing

(1) Only xylazine and atropine sulphate should be used as sedatives – other drugs may interfere with the test.
(2) Lay the animal on its side.
(3) Clip the flank completely.
(4) Use a felt tip pen to label the flank for each allergen to be tested.
(5) Inject 0.05 ml of allergen intradermally together with a positive control (histamine) and negative control (sterile diluent).
(6) After 30 minutes read the test by examining each site for a wheal formation. A positive result is where the wheal is greater than half the difference of the diameter of the positive and negative control.

18

Obstetric and paediatric nursing of the dog and cat

G. C. W. England

Before breeding from a dog or cat the owner should give careful consideration to the quality of their animal as well as the availability of homes for the potential offspring.

Breeding should not be undertaken lightly; both the male and female should be carefully assessed, and should be clinically sound, free from hereditary diseases, have excellent temperaments, be good examples of the breed and should be free from infectious disease. Many animals which are used at stud do not meet these criteria.

There are both moral and legal responsibilities (under the Sale of Goods Act) for breeders of animals to ensure that the offspring are clinically healthy and have a sound temperament. There are many hereditary defects which should preclude animals from breeding including the presence of congenital cardiac disease, congenital cleft palate, bleeding disorders and disorders of other systems proven to be hereditary in nature. In the case of cryptorchidism the affected dog and both parents should be considered to be carriers and should not be used for breeding.

Breeding control schemes

Three schemes were created in collaboration with the Kennel Club and the British Veterinary Association (BVA) with the aim to control the incidence of specified hereditary diseases in pedigree dogs.

The **BVA/Kennel Club/International Sheepdog Society Eye Scheme** is designed for the control of specific known inherited conditions such as central and generalised progressive retinal atrophy, hereditary cataract, primary glaucoma, primary lens luxation, collie eye anomaly, retinal dysplasia, persistent pupillary membrane, and persistent hyperplastic primary vitreous (other conditions are under investigation). Dogs should be examined every 12 months to ensure that they remain clear from the hereditary condition. This is very important for certain diseases (such as hereditary cataracts and certain retinopathies) which are not evident at birth. However, in practice, examination generally ceases when the dog exceeds the age at which the disease is commonly identified.

The **BVA/Kennel Club Hip Dysplasia Scheme** is designed to help control hip dysplasia in pedigree dogs. Dogs are usually radiographed on one occasion after they reach 12 months of age. The radiographs are assessed on nine detailed points and are scored for abnormality; radiographically normal hips score zero (0:0) and the maximum score is 106. Breed averages are regularly published and it is hoped that breeding from animals with

scores less than the average will result in improved quality of hips in subsequent generations.

The **BVA/Kennel Club Elbow Dysplasia Scheme** is designed to help control elbow disease in pedigree dogs. Three radiographs are taken of each elbow and a score awarded according to the presence of typical dysplasia or secondary osteoarthritits. Each elbow is scored 0 to 3, and the overall score is the highest of the two elbows (the scores are not summed as in the Hip Dysplasia Scheme). The threshold level not to breed is a score 2.

Other schemes have been adopted by certain breed societies to monitor the level of specific diseases. Examples are the monitoring of cardiac disease in Boxers, and the assessment of Dobermann pinscher dogs for cervical spondylopathy. Certain breed societies have established codes of conduct which aim to control the number of litters bred per bitch and the age of first mating. The Kennel Club will not register pups born from bitches over the age of 7 years.

Potential breeders should take advice from many sources before breeding from any male or female animal.

The male

Male dogs and tom cats are sexually active throughout the year, although a minor seasonal effect may be noted in some countries. The testes are descended into the scrotum at birth in the cat, and they descend into the scrotum by 10 days after birth in the dog. Both pups and kittens may show sexual activity from several weeks of age, however, puberty does not occur until 6 to 12 months in the dog and 8 to 12 months in the cat. For both species **spermatogenesis** (the production of spermatozoa) commences at approximately 5 months of age.

It is preferable not to use a male at stud until he is at least 12 months of age, since is not possible to fully evaluate his qualities until this time, and even then the occurrence of certain hereditary diseases may not be apparent. It is advisable that the first mating attempts should be with an experienced female.

The fertile lifespan of a male varies considerably and is probably related to the longevity of that particular breed. It is certain, however, that seminal quality of male stud dogs is reduced from 7 years of age onwards.

Endocrinology

The interstitial (**Leydig**) cells are the source of testosterone production from the testes. The production of this hormone is stimulated by **luteinising hormone** (LH), a gonado-trophin hormone released from the pituitary gland. A second pituitary gonadotrophin called **follicle stimulating hormone** (FSH) appears to increase the process of sperm production (spermatogenesis) directly via the **Sertoli cells**. Testosterone has a negative feedback effect upon the release of FSH and LH which is mediated by **gonadotrophin releasing hormone** (GnRH).

Control of reproduction

The majority of male dogs do not cause problems if they remain entire. However, there are situations where control of antisocial behaviour may necessitate the control of male hormone release. The situation in the entire tom cat is rather different because the problems of territory marking, roaming and aggression are greater than the dog.

Chemical control of reproductive function can be achieved in both species on a short-term basis with hormones which suppress the normal release of testosterone. The most commonly used agents include the **progestogens** (drugs with progesterone-like activity) which may be administered daily orally (e.g. megestrol acetate) or as a depot injection (e.g. proligestone or delmadinone acetate). These drugs do not produce infertility, only a reduced libido. No single drug is commercially available as a male contraceptive agent; complicated drug regimes are required for this effect.

The commonest method for the regulation of sexual activity is **castration** which is not reversible. Castration before puberty may result in failure of development of the secondary sexual characteristics. In some males a change in metabolic rate may result in increased bodyweight. Castration after puberty and correct dietary control eliminate the majority of problems associated with castration.

Vasectomy is rarely performed in the dog or tom. It involves removal of part of the vas deferens, which prevents sperm being ejaculated. The procedure does not interfere with sexual behaviour, and since in many cases this is the primary aim, it has no advantages over castration.

Diseases of the reproductive tract

There are a variety of conditions which may affect the reproductive organs of both the tom cat and the male dog.

Endocrinological abnormalities

Primary abnormalities in the secretion of pituitary hormones may result in the poor development of gonadal tissue; a condition called **hypogonadism**. This is rare but has been reported in both species.

Diseases of the testes

An absence of the testes (**anorchia**) is very rare; in most cases the testes are retained within the abdomen. These undescended testes belong to the condition known as **cryptorchidism** which literally means 'hidden testicle'. Often the condition is unilateral with one testicle present within the scrotum and the other retained within the abdomen. These cases are often wrongly called monorchids; **monorchidism** refers to an animal with a single testicle. Some cryptorchid animals are bilaterally affected and no testes are seen within the scrotum. The treatment for all cryptorchids is removal of both testes, because of the high incidence of neoplasia within the abdominal testis and the fact that the condition is likely to be inherited.

Inflammation of the testes (**orchitis**) is rare but may follow trauma or ascending bacterial infection. In some countries (but not the UK) orchitis may be caused by the bacterium *Brucella canis* which is a venereal pathogen transmitted at coitus.

Testicular tumours are the second most common tumour affecting the male dog but are rare in the tom cat. There are three common tumour types: those affecting the Leydig cells (Leydig cell tumour), those affecting the Sertoli cells (Sertoli cell tumour) and those affecting the germ cells (Seminoma). Some of these tumours may be endocrinologically active and secrete female hormones (oestrogens) which produce signs of feminisation.

Diseases of the accessory glands

The prostate gland in the male dog is the only accessory sex gland. The tom cat has both prostate and bulbourethral glands although disease of either is rare.

Prostate abnormalities in the dog are common and include benign enlargement (**hyperplasia**), bacterial prostatitis, prostatic cysts and prostatic tumours. The clinical signs of these diseases may be similar and include difficulty urinating and defecating and the presence of blood within urine and/or semen.

Diseases of the penis and prepuce

It is common for there to be a purulent discharge from the prepuce of the male dog which should be considered normal unless it is excessive. It is not seen in the tom cat.

Phimosis is a condition where there is inability to extrude the penis due to an abnormally small preputial orifice. This may occur either congenitally or as a result of trauma or inflammation and may result in pain during erection. **Paraphimosis** is a failure to retract the penis into the prepuce and may also be due to a small preputial orifice. The penis becomes dry and necrotic, and urethral obstruction may result. Priapism refers to the persistent enlargement of the penis in the absence of sexual excitement.

Antisocial behaviour

In many cases behaviour which may be normal for a male animal is considered to be antisocial by man. These problems include territory marking, mounting inappropriate objects and aggression towards other males. These problems often necessitate treatment which may include behavioural modification therapy in conjunction with drugs which inhibit male hormone production such as progestogens. Castration may be required in certain cases.

Normal mating

The sexual behaviour of the tom cat and male dog are considerably different from each other and from other species. It is important therefore that the events of natural mating are understood so that abnormalities can be recognised whilst remembering that the modern mating environment is often artificial. On the day of mating, bitches and queens are frequently transported large distances, are introduced to the male briefly and then expected to mate immediately. This situation eliminates the normal courtship phase associated with proestrus behaviour and may result in mating problems. In addition many females are presented to the male at an inappropriate time, either because this is convenient for the owner or because of inexact assessment of the stage of the oestrous cycle. In these events sexual behaviour of both the male and female may not be optimal.

The domestic dog

The dog and bitch will normally exhibit play behaviour when first introduced. The bitch will then usually settle and stand with her tail deviated to one side to allow mating. This is not always the case and it may be necessary to steady the bitch by holding her at the head. The dog may ejaculate a small volume of clear fluid before mounting; this does not contain sperm and is termed the **first fraction** and originates from the prostate gland. It probably flushes urine and cellular debris from the urethra. After mounting, the dog commences slow thrusting movements until the penile tip enters the vulva. At this stage thrusting movements become rapid and the penis enters the vagina (**intromission**) and the dog achieves a full erection. The **second fraction** (which contains sperm) is then ejaculated, following which the dog turns through 180° and dismounts from the bitch whilst the penis is still within the vagina. The dog and bitch stand tail to tail and this is called the tie. It is associated with ejaculation of the **third fraction** of the ejaculate, the function of which is to flush sperm forwards through the cervix into the uterus. This stage may last for 20 minutes or longer in some dogs.

The domestic tom

The period of sexual introduction and play is variable in the cat depending upon the experience and aggression of the male. The normal sequence of events occurs rapidly compared with the dog. The male usually approaches the female from the side or back and grasps her neck in his mouth. Whilst maintaining this grasp he mounts the female and positions himself to align the genital regions. The queen normally lowers her chest and elevates the pelvic region whilst deviating her tail. Pelvic thrusting and ejaculation occur rapidly. During intromission the queen often emits a cry and attempts to end mating by rolling, turning and striking at the male. The female then exhibits a marked post-coital reaction consisting of violent rolling and excessive licking. She will not allow further mating at this time.

Assessment of fertility

Male fertility may be assessed by the evaluation of semen quality. Semen may be collected by stimulating the male dog to ejaculate by hand; artificial vaginas are no longer used for this purpose. Semen collection is more difficult in the tom cat, and may require general anaesthesia and electroejaculation. A special artificial vagina may be used to collect from trained tom cats. Collection equipment should be warmed before use.

Semen, once collected, should be placed into a water bath at body temperature to prevent damage to the sperm. The second fraction of the dog ejaculate and the entire cat ejaculate should be used for evaluation.

(1) The volume should be measured and the colour recorded.
(2) After gently mixing the sample, a drop should be placed upon a warmed microscope slide and a subjective assessment made of the percentage of sperm with vigorous forward progression.
(3) The spermatozoal concentration should be measured using a haemocytometer counting chamber and the total sperm output should be calculated by multiplying this value with the volume of the sample.
(4) A portion of the sample should then be stained to allow the differentiation of live and dead sperm and the assessment of spermatozoal morphology. A combination of the two stains nigrosin and eosin is suitable

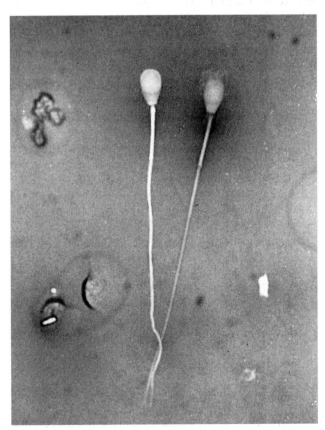

Fig. 18.1 Photomicrograph of a live normal dog spermatozoon (left) and a dead dog spermatozoon with a detached acrosome (right). The specimen has been stained with nigrosin and eosin; the dead sperm appears pink (grey in the black-and-white photograph) whilst the live sperm remains unstained (white).

Table 18.1 Mean seminal characteristics from 30 stud dogs

	Mean	Range
Motility (%)	85	42–92
Volume (ml)	1.3	0.4–3.4
Concentration (10⁶/ml)	310	50–560
Total sperm output	400	36–620
Live normal (%)	75	52–90
Dead normal (%)	10	2–26
Primary abnormal (%)	2	0–12
Secondary abnormal (%)	10	2–24

There is a wide range of normal values associated with fertility.

for this purpose. Nigrosin is a background stain and eosin is a vital stain – it only stains sperm with a damaged membrane, i.e. dead sperm (Fig. 18.1). Using nigrosin and eosin, sperm are stained either pink (these are termed dead), or are unstained (these are termed live).

The semen characteristics of fertile dogs is given in Table 18.1.

The female

The domestic bitch

Bitches generally have one or two oestrous cycles per year followed by a variable period of acyclicity. The bitch is **polytocous** (produces numerous offspring in each litter) and the oestrous periods are non-seasonal and terminate in spontaneous ovulation. The interval between each cycle can vary between 5 and 13 months although the average is 7 months.

The domestic queen

Queens have multiple oestrous cycles each year. They are **seasonally polyoestrus** and typically cycle from February to September. Ovulation is induced by coitus and the interval between each oestrous cycle varies depending upon whether the queen has ovulated, or fails to ovulate either because she is not mated or because there is insufficient hormone release at mating. Unmated queens return to oestrus at intervals of 14–21 days.

Puberty

The domestic bitch

In the bitch the onset of cyclical activity (puberty) is normally between 6 and 23 months of age, with most bitches having their first oestrus by the age of 12–14 months. Bitches that do not exhibit oestrous behaviour by the anticipated age are considered to have delayed puberty, but it should be remembered that many normal bitches will not cycle until they are 2 years old. The majority of bitches start to cycle about 6 months after they have reached adult height and weight, which may explain some of the variations exhibited between breeds.

The domestic queen

Female cats generally exhibit their first oestrus at 6–12 months of age, but this is dependent upon the **photoperiod.** Those which are born in the summer frequently commence cycling at the first spring; however, those which are born in the winter may not cycle until they are least 12 months of age.

The oestrous cycle

The domestic bitch

The stages of the oestrous cycle in the bitch are proestrus, oestrus, metoestrus (dioestrus) and anoestrus. The terms '**in season**' or '**in heat**' are used to indicate the stage of the cycle when the bitch is receptive to the male dog, i.e. oestrus.

During **proestrus** the bitch is receptive to the dog but will not allow mating. **Oestrus** commences when the bitch will accept the male and it is during this stage that the eggs are released from the ovaries – a process known as **ovulation**. Ovulation in the bitch occurs spontaneously towards the end of oestrus. Each egg is contained within a fluid-filled structure called a **follicle**. After ovulation the follicle develops into a solid structure called a **corpus luteum**. One corpus luteum forms from each follicle that has ovulated and the corpus luteum produces a hormone called **progesterone**.

In many species the phase of progesterone production (the **luteal** phase) is divided into two. The early luteal phase is termed **metoestrus** and the mature luteal phase is termed **dioestrus**. However, in the bitch the early luteal occurs during **standing oestrus** (i.e. when the bitch will stand to be mated), making this terminology difficult to adopt (since metoestrus would then be occurring during oestrus). In the bitch the terms metoestrus and dioestrus are therefore often used synonymously to reflect the luteal phase of the cycle after the end of standing oestrus. This phase is therefore characterised by the presence of the corpora lutea upon the ovaries and the presence of the hormone progesterone in the blood.

The bitch is unusual compared with other species in that the duration of the luteal phase is similar whether the bitch is pregnant or not (Fig. 18.2). This explains why the condition known as false or pseudo-pregnancy is common in the bitch (see later). The luteal phase is followed by a period of quiescence termed anoestrus.

The hormonal changes of the oestrous cycle are shown in Fig. 18.3.

Late anoestrus. During late anoestrus two hormones are released from the pituitary gland: **follicle stimulating hormone** (FSH) and **luteinising hormone** (LH). These initiate the growth of follicles within the ovaries and cause the follicles to produce the hormone **oestrogen.**

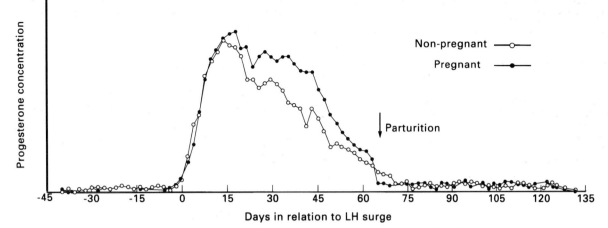

Fig. 18.2 Changes in plasma progesterone concentration in the pregnant and non-pregnant cycle of the bitch. The pregnant cycle demonstrates a more rapid decline in progesterone concentration immediately prior to parturition. Progesterone concentrations cannot be used as a method of pregnancy diagnosis in the bitch.

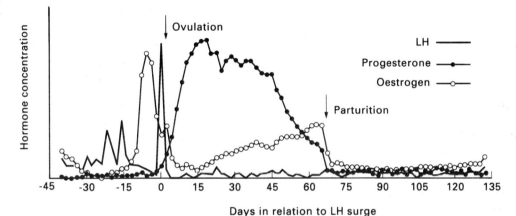

Fig. 18.3 Changes in plasma hormones during a pregnant cycle of the bitch. Oestrogen concentrations are elevated during proestrus, oestrus and late pregnancy. The LH surge stimulates ovulation which occurs within 36–48 hours of its peak. Progesterone is released before ovulation from luteinisation of follicles and subsequently from the corpora lutea.

Proestrus. Proestrus is characterised by increased plasma concentrations of oestrogen which causes swelling of the vulva and the development of a serosanguineous vulval discharge. Oestrogens also induce the release of specific pheromones which are responsible for attracting male dogs. During proestrus the bitch will not allow mating but may show increased receptivity to the male. This period lasts for approximately 7 days. Oestrogens also cause thickening of the vaginal wall and an increase in the number of epithelial cell layers. During proestrus the elevated concentrations of oestrogen have a negative feedback effect upon the release of the gonadotrophin hormones from the pituitary gland, and the concentrations of FSH and LH are reduced compared with late anoestrus.

Oestrus. During oestrus the bitch demonstrates characteristic behaviour towards the male dog including deviation of the tail and presentation of the vulva and perineum. The bitch will stand to be mated. This period lasts for approximately 7 days. The onset of oestrus is related to a decline in the concentration of plasma oestrogen and at the

same time the production of progesterone. The bitch is unusual in that progesterone is produced in low concentrations by luteinisation of the follicle, a process which occurs before ovulation. In many species progesterone is only produced after ovulation. It is this decline in the concentration of oestrogen and the slight increase in the concentration of progesterone which is responsible for stimulating a surge of both FSH and LH. This surge is the trigger for ovulation which occurs approximately 2 days later. It can therefore be seen that the hormonal stimulus for ovulation occurs during oestrus (i.e. when the bitch will stand to be mated) and that the release of eggs also occurs during this period. After ovulation corpora lutea form and produce greater amounts of progesterone. The end of standing oestrus is associated with relatively high concentrations of progesterone in the blood.

Metoestrus (dioestrus). The period of metoestrus lasts whilst the corpora lutea continue to produce progesterone and is approximately 55 days in length. In the pregnant bitch the period of metoestrus is synonymous with pregnancy, for the birth of pups occurs when progesterone secretion is terminated. In the non-pregnant bitch the corpora lutea persist for a similar period of time.

Towards the end of metoestrus another hormone called **prolactin** is released from the pituitary gland. This is responsible for the development of mammary tissue and the onset of lactation. Prolactin is produced in both the pregnant and the non-pregnant bitch, and is the reason why pseudopregnancy is a common event in the bitch.

Anoestrus. Metoestrus is followed by a period of quiescence, during which time there is effectively no hormonal activity. In the non-pregnant bitch there is no sudden decline in the concentration of progesterone but values gradually reduce and the transition to anoestrus is smooth. The situation is slightly different during pregnancy because progesterone concentrations rapidly decline and it is this event which stimulates the onset of parturition. The length of anoestrus varies considerably between bitches, but it is 4 months on average.

The domestic queen

The stages of the oestrous cycle in the queen are anoestrus, proestrus, oestrus and interoestrus. The terms 'in season' or 'in heat' are used to indicate the stage of the cycle when the cat is receptive to the male, i.e. **oestrus**. During winter there is essentially no hormone activity; the queen is in **anoestrus**. In spring time cyclical activity commences and in the unmated queen periods of sexual activity (proestrus and oestrus) are interrupted by periods of non-receptivity (**interoestrus**). If the queen is mated and ovulation is induced the queen enters **metoestrus** or pregnancy. Pregnancy follows a fertile mating; metoestrus (also called pseudopregnancy) follows a sterile mating. The duration of pseudopregnancy in the queen is shorter than that of pregnancy (Fig. 18.4), unlike the situation in the bitch.

Proestrus. Follicular development occurs during this phase due to the release of LH and FSH. This causes the secretion of oestrogen which is responsible for the develop-ment of the signs of proestrus including attraction of the male and the changes in the vaginal epithelium similar to those seen in the bitch. Proestrus in the queen is often poorly recognised unless a male is present, however, during this stage the queen will not accept mating. Proestrus lasts between 2 and 3 days.

Oestrus. The exact hormonal changes which cause the onset of standing oestrus are uncertain, although this may be associated with declining concentrations of oestrogen similar to that seen in the bitch.

The clinical signs of oestrus (also termed calling) include persistent vocalisation, rolling and rubbing against inanimate objects. In the presence of the male the queen may show persistent treading of the hind feet, lateral deviation of the tail and lordosis of the spine. Oestrus lasts between 2 and 10 days.

Interoestrus. In the absence of mating, or when mating does not result in ovulation, the signs of oestrus gradually decline and the queen enters a stage of non-receptivity. This period may last for between 3 and 14 days. After this time the queen returns to proestrus and oestrus.

Pregnancy. Ovulation in the queen is caused by the release of LH which is stimulated by mating. Each mating results in a surge of LH; however, there appears to be a threshold value below which ovulation will not be induced. Multiple matings are therefore more likely to result in ovulation than are single matings.

Ovulation is followed by an increase in the plasma concentration of progesterone released from the newly formed corpora lutea. Peak progesterone concentrations are reached approximately 1 month after mating and are maintained for the duration of pregnancy which varies between 64 and 68 days. It is not uncommon for queens to have an absence of cyclical activity during lactation. This has been called lactational anoestrus.

Metoestrus (pseudopregnancy). Non-fertile matings result in ovulation without conception. Ovulation may also

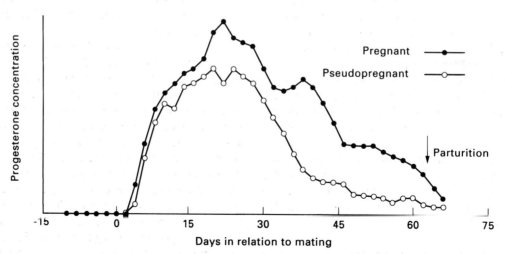

Fig. 18.4 Changes in plasma progesterone concentration in the pregnant and pseudopregnant (ovulation but without conception) cycle of the domestic queen. The pseudopregnant queen returns to cyclical activity 40–45 days after oestrus when progesterone concentrations return to basal values.

occur following stimulation of the vagina (e.g. following collection of a vaginal smear), stimulation of the perineum (which may be self-induced) or may occur spontaneously in some queens. Ovulation results in the formation of corpora lutea and the production of progesterone in a similar manner to early pregnancy. After approximately 40 days progesterone concentrations decline and the queen returns to cyclical activity. Should pseudopregnancy occur late in the year (autumn) the queen may not return to cyclical activity but may enter anoestrus.

Determination of the optimum time for mating

The domestic bitch

The determination of the time of ovulation in the bitch is important because the bitch is monoestrous and the mean interoestrus interval is 31 weeks. The clinical signs of oestrus are not always reliable indicators of the time of ovulation; in many bitches the behavioural signs do not correlate well with the changes in hormone concentration. There are, however, two natural methods which increase the likelihood of conception despite these potential problems. The first is the relatively long fertile period of eggs and the second is the relatively long survival of spermatozoa within the female reproductive tract.

There are several methods by which the optimum time for mating can be detected and these include clinical assessments, measurement of plasma hormone concentration and vaginal cytology.

Clinical assessments. The clinical signs of oestrus do not correlate well with the underlying hormonal events. The 'average bitch' ovulates 12 days after the onset of proestrus and should be mated from day 14 onwards when oocytes have matured. However, in some bitches ovulation may occur as early as day 8 or as late as day 26 after the onset of proestrus. These would be unlikely to become pregnant if mated on the 12th and 14th day which is common breeding practice.

Studies on laboratory kept dogs has shown that the LH surge often occurs around the same time as the onset of standing oestrus. Although there is some variation of this event, mating 4 days after the onset of standing oestrus may be a suitable time in many bitches.

One clinical assessment that may be useful in the bitch is the timing of vulval softening (Fig. 18.5). This often occurs during the LH surge when there is a switch from oestrogen dominance to progesterone dominance of the reproductive tract.

If only clinical assessments are available the combination of the onset of standing oestrus and the timing of distinct vulval softening may be useful in the prediction of the best mating time, since each event occurs on average 2 days before ovulation.

Measurement of plasma hormone concentration. The three relevant plasma hormones are LH, oestrogen and progesterone.

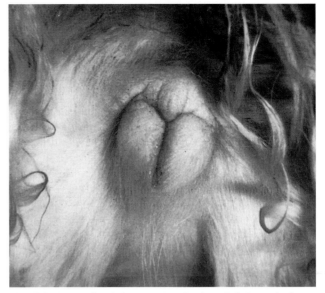

Fig. 18.5 Bitch's vulva during oestrus at the time of distinct softening. This is usually coincidental with the surge of plasma LH and therefore precedes ovulation by 2 days.

The measurement of plasma concentrations of LH would indicate impending ovulation; the fertile period is between 4 and 8 days after the LH surge. There is, however, no simple method by which plasma LH concentrations can be readily measured.

There is little value in the measurement of plasma oestrogen concentrations because the oestrogen plateau is not predictive of the timing of ovulation. Plasma progesterone concentrations are, however, very useful since this hormone is absent during proestrus and begins to increase coincidentally with the plasma surge of LH; thus detecting a rise in the concentration of plasma progesterone is predictive of ovulation. Progesterone can be easily measured in the practice laboratory within 1 hour of sample collection using a commercial enzyme linked immunosorbent assay test kit.

Vaginal cytology. The changes in the concentration of plasma hormone concentrations have a marked effect upon the vaginal mucosa.

When the bitch is not cycling, there are approximately two or three layers of cells lining the vagina. However, during oestrus, the vagina develops many cell layers in order to protect itself during mating. The cells within these layers differ from each other in their shape and size. When cells are collected from the vagina (the technique called a **vaginal smear**), only the cells on the surface of the vagina are removed. Different cell types are therefore collected at the various stages of the reproductive cycle. Staining of these cells and subsequent microscopic examination allows an assessment of the underlying hormone changes to be made. Cells can be collected either by aspirating vaginal fluid using a pipette, or using a cotton swab. Once collected, cells are placed onto a glass microscope slide, spread into a thin film and stained so that they can be individually examined (Fig. 18.6).

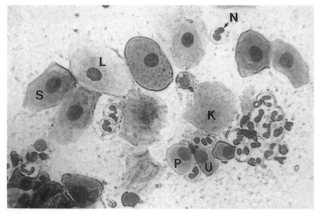

Fig. 18.6 Photomicrograph of the vaginal smear from a bitch in metoestrus demonstrating the range of epithelial cell types (P, parabasal cell; S, small intermediate cell; L, large intermediate cell; K, keratinised anuclear cell). In addition, uterine cells (U) and neutrophils (N) are present.

During anoestrus the vaginal wall is only a few cells in thickness; these cells are small and spherical in shape. Because they are positioned close to the basement membrane they are called **parabasal cells**. The anoestrus vaginal smear is characterised by the presence of these cells. There are also normally a few white blood cells (**neutrophils**) which remove cell debris and bacteria.

During proestrus the vaginal mucosa increases in thickness under the influence of oestrogen. The mucosa may be up to five or six cells thick. The cells further away from the basement membrane are larger in diameter than those nearer to the membrane. These cells have a large area of cytoplasm surrounding the cell nucleus and are called small intermediate cells. When the surface cells are collected during proestrus they are therefore predominantly these **small intermediate cells**, although there will also be a small number of the parabasal cells present. White blood cells are also present during proestrus; however, numbers are reduced compared with anoestrus. This is because the increased thickness of the vaginal mucosa prevents movement of the white blood cells into the lumen of the vagina. Red blood cells are also present in the vaginal smear during proestrus. These cells originate from the uterus and pass into the vagina via the cervix.

During oestrus the vaginal mucosa continues to thicken and the number of cell layers increases. There may be up to 12 cell layers during oestrus. Surface cells are large and irregular in shape and are called **large intermediate cells**. Cells of this size may accumulate the material keratin and are then termed **keratinised**. The nucleus of these large keratinised cells often disappears. The cells are then called **anuclear** because of the absence of the nucleus. White blood cells are not found in the vaginal smear during oestrus because the thick vaginal wall does not allow them to penetrate. Red blood cells are present in large numbers during oestrus.

During metoestrus there is sloughing of much of the vaginal mucosal epithelium. This is caused by the increasing concentrations of the hormone progesterone. The number of cell layers is reduced and the surface cells are again the small intermediate epithelial cells or parabasal cells. Several of the epithelial cells may have vacuoles within the cytoplasm giving the cell a 'foamy' appearance. **Foam cells** and epithelial cells with cytoplasmic inclusion bodies are characteristic of metoestrus. Because of the large amount of degenerate cellular material within the vaginal lumen there is a rapid influx of white blood cells as soon as the mucosa is thin enough to allow their penetration. Large numbers of white blood cells are therefore found in the metoestrus vaginal smear. Few red blood cells are present during metoestrus.

The bitch should first be mated when the percentage of anuclear cells is maximal – usually 80% or above (Fig. 18.7). There are, however, variations from the normal; some bitches may have two peaks of anuclear cells and some have a low percentage of anuclear cells during the fertile period.

The domestic queen

Unlike the bitch, in the queen ovulation is induced by coitus. After mating, assuming that a sufficient release of LH has occurred, follicles increase in size and ovulation follows 24–36 hours later. Mating is best planned during the peak of oestrus and vaginal cytology may be used to assess this time; however, collection of the smear may induce ovulation. Multiple copulations should be permitted to ensure an adequate release of LH and therefore ovulation.

Assisted reproduction

The domestic bitch

There are several techniques that may be used to assist reproduction in the bitch, the most common being **artificial insemination**. Artificial insemination is the technique of collecting semen from a male animal and placing it into the reproductive tract of the female.

Artificial insemination may involve the use of freshly collected semen, semen that has been diluted and chilled or semen which has been frozen and then thawed. Artificial insemination has several advantages over natural mating:

- It reduces the requirement to transport animals.
- It is an acceptable way of overcoming, to some extent, the quarantine restrictions that prevent the movement of animals from one country to another.
- It increases the genetic pool available to an individual breed within a country.
- It reduces the disease risk which is always present when unknown animals enter a kennel for mating. In some countries the use of artificial insemination may reduce the spread of infectious diseases.
- In certain circumstances, artificial insemination may be useful when natural mating is difficult (e.g. bitches which ovulate when they are not in standing oestrus or bitches that have hyperplasia of the vaginal floor).
- Semen may also be collected from male animals which due to age, debility, back pain or premature ejaculation are unable to achieve a natural mating.

The greatest area of interest is probably the storage of genetic material by freezing semen for insemination at a

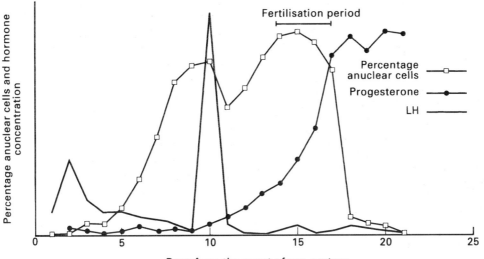

Fig. 18.7 Changes in vaginal cytology, plasma LH and plasma progesterone concentrations during proestrus, oestrus and early metoestrus of the domestic bitch. Eggs may be fertilised from 4 to 7 days after the LH peak. The fertilisation period therefore occurs during increasing concentrations of plasma progesterone whilst there are maximum numbers of anuclear epithelial cells. It is not uncommon for two well-defined peaks of anuclear cells to be identified. Regular collection of vaginal smears is important for the correct interpretation; single smears are of limited value.

future date. This may be necessary in male animals that are likely to become infertile due to castration or to medical treatments with certain hormones. The more common reason is, however, the preservation of semen from superior animals for use in future generations.

Collected semen may be deposited easily into the vagina of the bitch using a long inseminating pipette which is gently introduced near to the cervix. When semen is placed in this position spermatozoa must swim through the cervix, into the uterus and up the uterine horns. During a natural mating contractions of the vagina and uterus help in transporting semen. These contractions generally do not occur during insemination, although some may be produced by stimulating the vagina. Vaginal insemination is therefore not ideal, but usually when fresh or chilled semen is used the spermatozoa will live long enough to fertilise the eggs. However, in the case of frozen semen the spermatozoa do not live for long after thawing and so vaginal inseminations are not very satisfactory.

The chance of pregnancy can be improved if the semen is placed directly into the uterus rather than into the vagina. It is very difficult to place a catheter through the bitch's cervix into the uterus (a technique that is simple in many other animals) because the vagina is long and narrow and because the cervical opening is small and at an angle to the vagina. A special insemination pipette has been developed for this purpose. Recently some research workers have been able to catheterise the cervix using an endoscope. However, in certain countries the commonest way of performing uterine insemination is surgically via a laparotomy.

Because of the short life-span of the preserved sperm, it is most important that inseminations are accurately timed in relation to ovulation. The ideal time is between 2 and 5 days after ovulation, and this is best assessed by using the measurement of plasma progesterone concentration and the study of vaginal cytology.

In the UK, pups which are the result of artificial insemination can only be registered if the Kennel Club has given prior permission. The permission of the Kennel Club is not required before semen is imported or exported. There are, however, specific regulations set by the Ministry of Agriculture, Fisheries and Food in this country, and similar organisations in other countries, which aim to prevent the introduction of infectious diseases. Import regulations vary between countries but are particularly stringent for the UK. Import permit requirements usually include health certification before, and a set time period after, semen collection, quarantine of semen until the second health examination and various serological tests.

The domestic queen

Whilst artificial insemination has been widely practised in the domestic cat as a research model for wild cats, the technique is not commonly used in this country. Techniques used in the cat are, however, further advanced than those in the dog, and include the induction of ovulation, *in vitro* fertilisation and embryo transfer.

Control of reproduction

There have been many methods employed to control the reproductive cycle of the bitch and queen. These involve surgical methods and medical control of cyclical activity. More recently advances have been made in the induction of oestrus and the termination of pregnancy.

The domestic bitch

Surgical prevention of cyclical activity. **Ovariohysterectomy** is the removal of both ovaries and the uterus to the level of the cervix. The term **spaying** is commonly used to describe this procedure although by definition this refers to removal of the ovaries only. Ovariohysterectomy should be considered in any bitch that is not required for breeding since it has several advantages to the bitch including a reduction in the incidence of mammary tumours, elimination of the problems of false pregnancy and of pyometra as well the obvious advantages of absence of oestrous behaviour and inability to produce offspring. There are, however, several claimed adverse effects including an increased incidence of incontinence, changes in coat texture and a tendency to gain weight. Whilst little can be done regarding the former two conditions, the latter may easily be controlled by correct dietary management.

There is considerable discussion concerning the correct time to perform the procedure on a bitch. There is no doubt that surgery is technically easier and recovery is more rapid in young animals, and some veterinary surgeons perform surgery as early as 4 months of age. However, it has been suggested that when performed before puberty (the first oestrus) there is an increased tendency for under-development of the secondary sexual characteristics and there may also be effects on the closure time of the animals' growth plates. However, waiting until after the first oestrus suffers the risk of pregnancy and false pregnancy.

Medical inhibition of cyclical activity. There are a variety of compounds which may be used to inhibit cyclical activity including progesterone or progesterone-like compounds (**progestogens**), testosterone or other male hormones (**androgens**) and gonadotrophin releasing hormone agonists and antagonists. Drugs may either be administered during anoestrus to prevent the occurrence of an oestrus (the term **prevention** is used) or may be given during proestrus or oestrus to abolish the signs of that particular oestrus (the term **suppression** is used). The most commonly used compounds are the progestogens which are formulated as **depot injections** or as **oral tablets**. The depot injections may be used during anoestrus to prevent the occurrence of the next anticipated oestrus. The oral tablets may be used either during anoestrus for oestrus prevention or during proestrus to suppress the signs of that oestrus. A normal oestrus often occurs between 4 and 6 months after the administration of these hormones.

These drugs are not recommended for use before the first oestrus or in an animal that is required for breeding. The side effects of these drugs include increased appetite, weight gain, lethargy, mammary enlargement, coat and temperament changes and the risk of inducing pyometra.

Induction of oestrus. With the development of new drugs and new drug regimes it has become possible to induce an oestrous cycle in the bitch. In many cases the success rate in terms of the birth of live pups is poor and the administration of the drugs is complicated. However, these methods may be useful in those bitches which have longer than average interoestrus intervals, those which are slow to reach puberty and those which do not exhibit behavioural signs of oestrus.

The termination of pregnancy. Unwanted matings are commonly seen in general practice. The term **misalliance** is often used to describe these cases; however, by definition this means 'an unsuitable or improper marriage' in translation and is therefore best avoided. There are several treatment options should pregnancy termination be necessary. If the bitch is not required for breeding, an ovariohysterectomy may be performed early in metoestrus, approximately 2 weeks after the end of oestrus. Medical therapy using oestrogens within 5 days of mating is often successful in preventing conception but suffers the risk of induction of pyometra and the disadvantage that oestrus will be prolonged. In later pregnancy it is possible to use various drugs (e.g. cabergoline) which lower the concentration of progesterone in the blood and therefore induce resorption or abortion. These are not commonly used in the UK.

The domestic queen

Surgical prevention of cyclical activity. The indications and potential adverse effects of ovariohysterectomy in the cat are similar to those of the bitch. The procedure is usually performed when the queen is 5–6 months of age regardless of the onset of puberty; poor development of the external genitalia does not cause problems. In the UK the surgical procedure is frequently performed through a flank incision. This approach is, however, best avoided in oriental breeds where coat colour is a temperature-dependent effect and clipping the coat may result in the growth of dark-coloured hairs.

Medical inhibition of cyclical activity. The drugs available for use in the queen are similar to those described for the domestic bitch. Long-term drug therapy is, however, less commonly used because queens that are not wanted for breeding are usually surgically neutered.

The induction of oestrus and termination of pregnancy. Various drugs may be used for the induction of oestrus and the termination of pregnancy. In general the guidelines given for the bitch may be followed.

Diseases of the reproductive tract

The domestic bitch

There are several abnormalities of the reproductive tract in the domestic bitch. These may be considered under general headings of endocrinological, ovarian, uterine or external genital abnormalities.

Endocrinological abnormalities. The common endocrinological abnormalities of the bitch include:

- Delayed onset of puberty (cyclical activity is not present at 24 months of age).
- Prolonged anoestrus (failure of return to cyclical activity resulting in a prolonged interoestrus interval).
- Silent oestrous cycles (normal cyclical activity including ovulation but without the external signs of oestrus).

- Split oestrus (signs of proestrus but this does not terminate in ovulation and is followed 2–12 weeks later by a normal cycle).
- Ovulation failure (when bitches have apparently normal oestrous periods with an absence of ovulation – these bitches often return to oestrus with shorter than normal intervals).

One specific endocrinological condition frequently seen in the bitch is **pseudopregnancy** (false pregnancy, phantom pregnancy or **pseudocyesis**). The signs of the condition include anorexia, abdominal enlargement, nest making, nursing of inanimate objects, mammary development and lactation. False pregnancy should be considered normal in the bitch because the changes in plasma hormones are similar in both pregnant and non-pregnant individuals. It has been wrongly thought that pseudopregnancy is produced by either an overproduction of progesterone or abnormal persistence of the corpus luteum. The actual mechanism is related to the decline in plasma progesterone concentration during late metoestrus which is associated with an increase in plasma concentrations of prolactin. In many cases therapy is not required because the signs will gradually decline. However, in certain cases it may be necessary to use hormonal therapy to reduce the plasma concentrations of prolactin.

Diseases of the ovary. There are few abnormalities of the ovary. An absence of ovarian development (**agenesis**) may occur, which usually affects one side only but which may affect fertility. Ovarian cysts are rare and may be associated with signs of persistent oestrus. However, most cysts originate from the ovarian bursa and are not endocrinologically active. Ovarian tumours are also rare.

Occasionally bitches with both ovarian and testicular tissue are seen. These animals are termed **intersex** and may be recognised because of the appearance of their external genitalia. The vulva may be cranially positioned and an os clitoris may develop. The gonads may be found in a normal ovarian position or within the scrotum. These animals are usually sterile.

Diseases of the uterus. Developmental problems of the uterus include **aplasia** (abnormal development) or **agenesis** (failure of development); in these cases reproductive cyclicity will be normal but the bitch may fail to become pregnant. Intersex animals may have the presence of both uterine tissue and vasa deferentia.

The most common uterine disease of the bitch is **cystic endometrial hyperplasia** (CEH) which may develop into pyometra. Hyperplasia of the endometrium occurs in response to progesterone during normal metoestrus. In young animals the hyperplasia resolves at the end of the luteal phase. This is not the case in older bitches and small cystic regions develop within the glandular tissue. The uterus in this state is probably more prone to infection than the normal uterus and should bacteria enter during oestrus (when the cervix is open) they may proliferate. The accumulation of pus within the uterus (pyometra) leads to the bitch becoming unwell. Clinical signs may include the presence of a malodorous vaginal discharge, lethargy, inappetance, pyrexia, vomiting, polydipsia and polyuria. In some cases the cervix is not open and a vaginal discharge is absent; these cases are called 'closed' pyometra. In all cases of pyometra the treatment of choice is ovariohysterectomy following stabilisation of the patient using appropriate fluid therapy. Medical treatment has been advocated although the success rate is not high.

Treatment of bitches with progestogens for the prevention or suppression of oestrus, or oestrogens for the treatment of unwanted matings, may predispose to the development of pyometra.

Diseases of the vagina and vestibule. Congenital abnormalities of the caudal reproductive tract include segmental aplasia and hymenal or vestibular constrictions.

Vaginitis (inflammation of the vagina) is sometimes seen in prepubertal bitches and usually resolves after the first oestrus. Specific infectious causes of vaginitis include *Brucella canis* (not present in the UK) and herpes virus. Many bacteria are found within the vagina as normal commensal organisms including beta-haemolytic streptococci which many dog breeders wrongly consider to be venereal pathogens. There is little value in routine bacteriological swabbing of the vagina before breeding, since usually only these commensal bacteria are isolated.

Diseases of the external genitalia. Congenital abnormalities such as vulval atresia and agenesis are rare. Clitoral hypertrophy may occur associated with intersexuality.

The domestic queen

Endocrinological abnormalities. Delayed puberty may be difficult to assess in the queen since the onset of cyclical activity is related to the season of the year at birth (see above). Delayed puberty and prolonged anoestrus has, however, been seen although they are rare.

The most common abnormality is **ovulation failure** which often results from insufficient reflex release of LH at mating. The majority of queens will ovulate if 4–12 matings are allowed in a 4-hour period.

Pseudopregnancy also occurs in the queen although this condition is dissimilar to that seen in the bitch and usually follows a sterile mating (or occasionally spontaneous ovulation). After ovulation there is an increase in plasma progesterone, which does not occur in the absence of mating, and no return to oestrus for a further 35–40 days. The clinical signs are an absence of oestrus; treatment is not required (see Fig. 18.4).

Diseases of the ovary. Congenital diseases of the ovary such as ovarian agenesis and ovarian hypoplasia are rare. Ovarian cysts and neoplasms may develop similar to those seen in the bitch and are also rare.

Premature ovarian failure may be seen in queens aged 8 years and above; these animals stop cycling for an unknown reason.

Diseases of the uterus. The range of uterine abnormalities seen in the cat are similar to those of the bitch. Pyometra may be less common because in the absence of mating ovulation does not occur and the luteal phase is therefore absent. However, spontaneous ovulations or the common use of progestogens may cause the development of cystic endometrial hyperplasia and pyometra.

Diseases of the vagina, vestibule and external genitalia. Congenital abnormalities of the vagina, vestibule and external genitalia are rare but include vaginal and vulval aplasia and defects associated with intersexuality. Vaginitis is uncommon.

Pregnancy

The domestic bitch

The length of pregnancy in the bitch is relatively consistent at 64, 65 or 66 days from the preovulatory LH surge. However, the apparent length of pregnancy, assessed from the time of mating, may vary between 56 and 72 days since both early and late matings may be fertile:

- Early matings require sperm survival within the female reproductive tract until ovulation and egg maturation; such matings produce a long apparent pregnancy.
- Late matings occur when eggs are waiting to be fertilised for some time after ovulation; such matings produce a shorter pregnancy.

The clinical signs of pregnancy might include:

- Increased body weight and abdominal enlargement; however, these signs may not be obvious if the number of pups is small.
- A reduced food intake and a vaginal discharge are common approximately 1 month into the pregnancy. Enlargement and reddening of the mammary glands may be noted especially from 40 days after mating (these signs may, however, be present in bitches with pseudopregnancy).
- The production of milk is a variable finding: some bitches produce serous fluid from day 40 and milk from day 55 onwards, whilst in others this may not occur until just before parturition.

Certain physiological changes occur during pregnancy, and include the development of a normochromic, normocytic anaemia and a reduction of the packed cell volume; these changes are normal.

Food intake does not increase during the first 30 days of pregnancy. After this time the absolute requirement for carbohydrate and protein increases. During the last half of pregnancy food consumption may be doubled. Provided that diet is well balanced and contains suitable amounts of vitamins and minerals it is not necessary to provide extra supplementation although it may be necessary to provide the food divided into two or three meals during the day. Supplementation with calcium and vitamin D should be avoided since this does not prevent eclampsia and can be dangerous. See Chapter 8, p. 185.

Regular exercise should be provided throughout pregnancy, limited by the amount the bitch is willing to undertake.

For the control of ascarid infections (*Toxocara*) it is necessary to administer medication during pregnancy to reduce or prevent perinatal transmission. Various drugs (benzimidazoles) and treatment regimes have been advocated for the treatment of pregnant bitches.

It is advisable to ensure that **routine vaccination** has been performed before mating. Vaccination during pregnancy is unlikely to be damaging to the foetus and therefore may be undertaken if necessary, but no live vaccine is licensed for this purpose.

Pregnancy diagnosis

As well as observation of the clinical signs already described (noting that mammary gland development, increased weight and abdominal enlargement may be present in pseudopregnancy as well as in pregnancy), there are several methods for pregnancy diagnosis in the bitch.

Abdominal palpation. This is best performed approximately 1 month after mating when the conceptual swellings are approximately 2.0 cm in diameter. The technique can be highly accurate but may be difficult in obese or nervous animals and may be inaccurate if the bitch was mated early such that pregnancy is not as advanced as anticipated. After day 35, individual conceptuses cannot easily be palpated and diagnosis becomes more difficult.

Identification of foetal heart beats. In late pregnancy it is possible to auscultate the foetal heart beats using a stethoscope, or to record a foetal ECG. Both of these methods are diagnostic of pregnancy; foetal heart rate is more rapid than that of the dam.

Radiography. From day 30 it is possible to detect uterine enlargement with good-quality radiographs. However, this is not diagnostic of pregnancy since pyometra may have a similar appearance. Pregnancy diagnosis is not possible until after day 45 when mineralisation of the foetal skeleton is detectable radiographically. At this stage it is unlikely that there will be radiation damage to the foetus; however, sedation or anaesthesia of the dam may be required and is a potential risk. In late pregnancy the number of pups can be reliably estimated by counting the number of foetal skulls.

Hormone tests. Plasma concentrations of progesterone are not useful for the detection of pregnancy in the bitch. Measurement of the hormone relaxin is diagnostic of pregnancy; however, there is no commercial assay for this hormone in the UK.

Acute phase proteins. The rise in the concentration of acute phase proteins has been used as the basis of a commercial pregnancy test in the bitch. Concentrations of these proteins increase from approximately 30 days onwards. The test is reliable although these proteins are also released in inflammatory conditions such as pyometra.

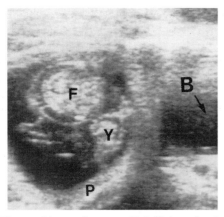

Fig. 18.8 Ultrasound image of pregnant bitch 32 days after the LH surge. A single conceptus is positioned adjacent to the bladder (B). Within the conceptus the foetus (F) can be seen in transverse section, and the collapsing yolk sac (Y) is positioned adjacent to the placenta (P).

Ultrasound examination. Diagnostic B-mode ultrasound is now commonly used for pregnancy diagnosis (Fig. 18.8). The technique is non-invasive and without risk to the pups, dam or veterinary surgeon. The bitch can be examined in the standing position with minimal restraint.

With ultrasound it is possible to diagnose pregnancy as early as 16 days after ovulation, although because in most cases this time is not known it is prudent to wait until 28 days after mating. At this time the fluid-filled conceptuses can easily be imaged and embryonic tissue can be identified. It is possible to assess the number of conceptuses; however, this can be inaccurate especially when the litter size is large. Movement of the foetal heart can be seen ultrasonographically and this confirms foetal viability. It is possible to examine the bitch at any time after day 28 to diagnose pregnancy, and to confirm foetal viability and growth. With later examinations it is less easy to estimate the number of pups.

The domestic queen

The average length of pregnancy in the queen is 65 days with a range of 64–68 days.

The clinical signs of pregnancy include increased body weight and abdominal enlargement (these signs are often apparent in all but young queens) and mammary development which is obvious from approximately day 40. These changes are usually diagnostic for pregnancy since pseudopregnancy is not common and is not usually associated with clinical signs.

During the second half of pregnancy there is an increase in food intake, and in the requirement for both carbohydrate and protein. Provided that diet is well balanced and contains suitable amounts of vitamins and minerals it is not necessary to provide extra supplementation.

Many queens continue to be active during pregnancy; the amount of exercise is best limited by the individual cat. It is advisable to ensure that routine vaccination has been performed prior to mating.

Pregnancy diagnosis

As well as observation of clinical signs (mammary development, increased weight and abdominal enlargement may be present from mid-pregnancy onwards, and it is unlikely that pseudopregnancy will produce similar signs) various methods may be used for pregnancy diagnosis of the queen.

Abdominal palpation. Conceptual swellings can be palpated from approximately 21 days after mating. These are discrete until 30 days after mating but then become more difficult to palpate from this time onwards.

Identification of foetal heart beats. In late pregnancy the foetal heart beats may be auscultated using a stethoscope; however, at this time it is usually possible to palpate the foetus in all but the most obese cats.

Radiography. From day 30 it is possible to detect uterine enlargement with good-quality radiographs. Mineralisation of the foetal skeleton is detectable radiographically from 40 days after mating.

Hormone tests. Plasma concentrations of progesterone are elevated in both pregnancy and pseudopregnancy, therefore measurement of this hormone is not diagnostic. Plasma relaxin concentrations are elevated from day 25; this hormone is diagnostic of pregnancy; however, there is no commercial assay available.

Ultrasound examination. Diagnostic B-mode ultrasound may be used for pregnancy diagnosis in the cat. The pregnancy length can be assessed from mating time unlike the bitch. Conceptuses can be imaged from 12 days after mating and embryonic tissue can usually be seen from day 14. From this time onwards it is possible to identify pregnancy, confirm foetal viability and assess foetal growth. It is more difficult to assess the number of kittens in later pregnancy.

Abnormalities of pregnancy

A great concern for owners is the risk of resorption or abortion during pregnancy. To understand the differences in these processes it is necessary to define the stages of development. In general the term embryo is used when the characteristics of the pup are not discernible. From approximately 35 days after ovulation the characteristics of the pup become obvious and the term foetus is used. Resorption refers to the resorption of the entire conceptus and occurs during the embryonic stage of development. Abortion refers to the expulsion of the foetus and the foetal membranes before term (i.e. before 58 days after ovulation). A stillbirth is the expulsion of the foetus and foetal membranes after day 58 (i.e. close to term).

The incidence of resorption or abortion of the entire litter is not known, although it is certain that up to 5% of bitches suffer isolated resorption of one or two conceptuses with continuation of the remaining pregnancy.

There are many potential causes of resorption/abortion which include infections agents, trauma, foetal defects and maternal environment. In the dog the infectious agents *Brucella canis* (not present in the UK), canine distemper virus, canine herpes virus and *Toxoplasma gondii* infection have all been implicated as causes of abortion and resorption. In the cat feline herpesvirus I, feline pan-leukopaenia virus, feline leukaemia virus, feline infections peritonitis virus and *Toxoplasma gondii* infection may produce abortion, resorption or stillbirths.

In many cases embryonic death and pregnancy loss is best assessed using real-time diagnostic B-mode ultrasound. Resorptions may be unrecognised by the owner unless it is associated with a period of illness. Abortion of foetal tissue may be obvious but may not be noticed should the dam eat the aborted material. In the face of an abortion there is little except supportive therapy that can be administered to the patient.

Pregnancy hypoglycaemia has been reported in the bitch and is associated with reduced blood glucose concentrations during late pregnancy. The clinical signs include weakness which may progress to coma.

The condition may be confused with **hypocalcaemia** which occurs at a similar time (see p. 486).

Parturition

In the last few weeks of pregnancy attempts should be made to encourage the bitch or queen to accept a nest in a suitable place — ideally a warm and clean room isolated from the rest of the household into which a whelping or kittening box may be placed.

The box should be large enough to allow the dam to stretch and have sufficient room for a large litter. The sides of the box should be high enough to prevent the pups or kittens from escaping up to about 4 weeks of age. The provision of a ledge around the box sides may be useful to prevent the dam from crushing her offspring. The bedding material should be easily removable when soiled. The environmental temperature should be approximately 25°C; however, the avoidance of draughts is most important.

Before parturition it is useful to clip the hair from around the mammary glands and the perineum; this makes the nipples more accessible and allows cleaning of the dam after parturition.

In the last week of pregnancy it is prudent to record the rectal temperature of the bitch at least twice daily. This is to detect the **prepartum hypothermia** which precedes the onset of parturition by 24–36 hours. This decline in body temperature is mediated by a sudden reduction in the plasma concentration of progesterone. The rectal temperature usually changes from approximately 39°C to below 37°C.

There are five stage of parturition:

(1) Stage of preparation.
(2) First stage of parturition (onset of contractions).
(3) Second stage parturition.
(4) Third stage parturition.
(5) Puerperium (after parturition).

The **stage of preparation** encompasses the decline in plasma progesterone concentration (and subsequent pre-partum hypothermia of the bitch) and relaxation of the vaginal and perineal tissue. This occurs in preparation for parturition; however, the dam may show few overt signs.

The first stage of parturition commences with the onset of uterine contractions. First stage parturition averages 1–12 hours in duration, although this is variable. Milk is usually present within the mammary glands or appears during this stage.

Contraction of the uterus may cause discomfort, and the dam may be restless and pant and may exhibit classical nesting behaviour. In addition anorexia, shivering and vomiting may be observed; most cats seek seclusion during this time.

The uterine contractions push the first foetus against the cervix which is starting to dilate. The allantochorion may rupture and allantoic fluid may be produced from the vulva.

The second stage of parturition is characterised by increased uterine contractions and propulsion of the foetus through the cervix into the vagina. As the first foetus enters the pelvic canal forceful abdominal straining commences. Bitches and queens are often in lateral recumbency during delivery although some bitches will remain standing.

The delivery of the foetal head is often most difficult and this may be associated with some pain; after this the foetus is usually produced rapidly.

The **amnion** (which surrounds each foetus) is often seen at the vulva during straining. This may either rupture spontaneously, be broken by the dam or is unruptured and the foetus is born within it. The dam will normally break the sac if the foetus is born within it, but this should be done quickly if she fails to do so.

The time between the onset of straining and the birth of the first foetus is variable; it may be as short as 10–30 minutes, but it may take longer in young animals. Non-productive straining for greater than 60 minutes may indicate **dystocia**.

The birth of a foetus is usually followed by the expulsion of the allantochorion (placenta) usually within 20 minutes.

The subsequent foetuses may be delivered quickly although the interval between foetuses may be up to 6 hours. The time taken from the birth of the first to the last foetus is variable and may be as long as 24–36 hours.

After the delivery of the foetus the dam usually commences vigorous licking, removing membranes and fluid away from the neonate's face and promoting respiration. If she fails to do this it may be done for her using a clean, soft towel. Usually the dam will sever the umbilical cord with her teeth, and eat the placenta when it is expelled. It is important to ensure that the dam does not excessively chew the umbilicus since this may damage the foetus. If the umbilicus is not severed this can be achieved using scissors.

Pups and kittens are best left with the dam during the remainder of delivery. If they are removed this may be distressing and may inhibit further straining.

The **third stage of parturition** *is classically associated with passage of the allantochorion (placenta).* In the bitch and queen this occurs during second stage parturition and cannot be defined as a separate period. Occasionally one or more foetuses are delivered without their placentae which are expelled at a later stage, although they may be delivered together with a subsequent foetus.

There is commonly a dark-coloured vulval discharge after parturition which contains a green-coloured pigment originating from the placenta. The discharge declines in volume but may persist for 1 week after parturition.

The **puerperium** *is the period after parturition during which the reproductive tract returns to its normal non-pregnant state.* This includes the period of uterine involution which may take 4–6 weeks. A mucoid vulvar discharge may be present during this period.

Dystocia

The term dystocia literally means difficult birth; it is used to indicate any problem that interferes with normal birth. Dystocia is rare in the queen; however, problems are not uncommon in the bitch, especially in brachycephalic breeds such as the Bulldog and Boston terrier. The two main causes of dystocia are maternal factors and foetal factors.

Maternal dystocia

Maternal dystocia may be divided into two categories – poor straining efforts by the dam and constriction of the birth canal.

Poor straining efforts of the dam. Poor straining may be the result of nervousness or pain which inhibit normal parturition, but it is more commonly the result of poor myometrial contractions, a condition that has been termed **uterine inertia**. Inertia may be primary, in which case parturition does not commence, or may be secondary to some other factor occurring during parturition.

Primary uterine inertia is rare in the cat but is seen not uncommonly in young bitches with only one or two pups, or in older overweight bitches with large litters. The cause of the condition is unknown; however, it may relate to poor condition of the uterine musculature in fat or debilitated animals, overstretching of the uterus when the litter size is large, poor stimulus for parturition when there are only a few foetuses or low plasma calcium concentrations.

The endocrinological events of parturition are usually normal; however, subsequent uterine contractions are not fully initiated and parturition does not follow. A green vulval discharge, which indicates placental separation, may be seen some days after the expected date of parturition. In some cases the owner may have observed initial weak uterine contractions or have noted the decline in body temperature. At this stage the administration of the hormone oxytocin may stimulate uterine contractions. Some cases may respond to the intravenous administration of calcium borogluconate. Repeated doses of oxytocin may be necessary but oxytocin should only be given when it is certain that there is no obstruction to the birth canal. However, it is not possible in the bitch to assess the patency of the cervix by digital palpation (the vagina of an average 20 kg bitch is 20 cm long). In certain cases Caesarean operation may be necessary.

Primary uterine inertia may be anticipated in some bitches because of a previous history of this problem or because of their age, physical condition or the number of pups. The best assessment of the bitch is to monitor the rectal temperature twice daily during the last 7–10 days of pregnancy.

Secondary uterine inertia is the cessation of uterine contractions after they have started. Most commonly this is the result of uterine exhaustion following obstructive dystocia but may occur spontaneously during second stage parturition, presumably because of factors similar to those seen with primary uterine inertia. If the cause of the dystocia can be relieved the administration of oxytocin and calcium may be suitable treatments. In some cases, however, Caesarean operation may be necessary.

Obstruction of the birth canal. Obstruction may be the result of abnormalities of the birth canal, such as:

- Deformity of the pelvic bones. These may be congenital malformations, developmental abnormalities or the result of previous trauma, commonly following a road accident.
- Soft tissue abnormalities within the pelvis which press against the reproductive tract. They might include pelvic neoplasms, although these are rare in animals of breeding age.
- Abnormality of the reproductive tract itself (e.g. torsion of the uterus) or congenital vaginal or uterine constrictions.

Foetal dystocia

Foetal oversize. Oversize of the foetus relative to the birth canal may be the result of:

- Breed conformation (dystocia may be considered almost 'normal' for certain breeds with exaggerated physical characteristics such as a large head size).
- Actual foetal oversize, when the litter size is small and large foetuses develop within the uterus.
- Foetal abnormalities, including foetal monsters, resulting in relative oversize and dystocia.

In the majority of these cases Caesarean operation is necessary for the delivery of the foetuses, whether normal or abnormal.

Abnormalities of foetal alignment. The normal presentation, position and posture of the foetus during delivery has been previously described (see also p. 482 and Fig. 18.9). Variation from the normal disposition may result in dystocia. This may be corrected in certain cases by manipulation per vaginum; however, Caesarean operation may be necessary.

ORIENTATION OF THE FOETUS

- The **presentation** of a foetus is a description of the direction of its long axis in relation to the long axis of the dam. Pups and kittens can only be delivered in longitudinal presentation (i.e. the long axis of the foetus is parallel to the long axis of the dam) but may have either anterior (foetal head delivered first) or posterior (foetus delivered backwards) presentation (see below).
- The **position** of a foetus is a description of its dorsal axis with respect to the dorsum of the dam; this describes the degree of rotation of the foetus. Most species are normally born in dorsal position, i.e. the back of the foetus is uppermost in the same orientation as the dam.
- The **posture** of a foetus is a description of the orientation of the head and legs which may be extended or flexed. For anterior presentation the head must be extended and this occurs naturally during a posterior presentation.
- A **breech birth** refers to a foetus delivered in posterior longitudinal presentation, usually in dorsal position with the hindlimbs flexed. This means that the foetus is presented 'bottom first' with its hindlegs directed towards the dam's head (Fig. 18.9). A foetus delivered in posterior presentation with the legs extended is not a breech presentation.

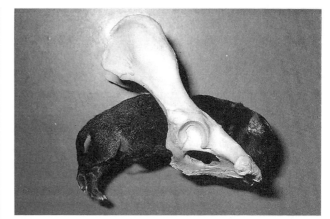

(a)

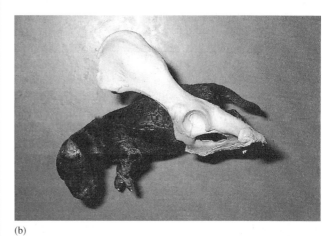

(b)

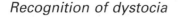

(c)

Fig. 18.9 Presentations: (a) lateral view of a pelvis demonstrating anterior longitudinal presentation of a pup in dorsal position with the head and forelegs extended (normal orientation); (b) lateral view of a pelvis demonstrating posterior longitudinal presentation of a pup in dorsal position with the hindlegs extended (normal orientation); (c) lateral view of a pelvis demonstrating posterior longitudinal presentation of a pup in dorsal position with hindlegs flexed cranially (breech orientation).

Recognition of dystocia

The normal events of parturition should be clearly understood so that recognition of dystocia can be achieved rapidly, thus allowing prompt intervention.

Collection of a relevant history is essential in the evaluation of a potential case of dystocia. This includes the estimation of the stage of pregnancy. Determining the mating date is most helpful in establishing the stage of pregnancy of the cat but this is not very useful in the bitch where pregnancy length can vary between 56 and 72 days from mating. Regular monitoring of rectal temperature is therefore essential in the bitch. It should be established whether this has been done by the owner and if so what changes were observed.

Of particular importance is the time-course of events from the onset of parturition, e.g. the onset of behavioural changes such as restlessness, nest making and panting. The time when straining first occurred and the character of the straining efforts may also be useful as an indicator of dystocia as will the times that any foetuses were produced.

It is not possible to give definite guidelines regarding potential cases of dystocia but examination of the patient is warranted in certain situations:

- A bitch that has exceeded 70 days from the last mating and has no signs of impending parturition.

- A cat has exceeded 65 days from the last mating and has no signs of impending parturition.
- The dam is unsettled and strains forcefully but infrequently.
- There are signs of straining which then cease.
- There is a black/green vulval discharge with no signs of parturition.
- There has been a decline in rectal temperature and parturition has not commenced within 48 hours.
- There has been ineffectual straining for 1 hour or more.
- Several foetuses have been produced, the last more than 2 hours ago, and the dam is restless.
- Several foetuses have been produced, the last more than 2 hours ago, and a larger litter is expected (may not be known by the owner).

Investigation of potential cases of dystocia. In most cases it is necessary to ensure that the animal is pregnant and/or that viable foetuses remain within the uterus. This can be achieved by transabdominal palpation, auscultation of foetal heart beats, real-time ultrasonography and radiography, as described earlier for pregnancy diagnosis.

Further investigation involves digital examination of the vagina to assess whether a foetus is present and to establish foetal alignment. This should only be performed after cleaning the vulvar area thoroughly with an antiseptic solution and scrubbing the hands or wearing surgical gloves. A water-soluble lubricant should be applied to the fingers, and the vestibule and vagina should be carefully examined. The presence of bone or soft tissue abnormalities of the pelvis should be noted. The presentation, position and posture of the foetus should be established before any further intervention is contemplated.

For normal presentations delivery can be assisted using the thumb and forefinger placed in a cradle manner around the foetal head (anterior presentation) or pelvis (posterior presentation). Traction should only be applied during the straining effort of the bitch; however, pressure on the roof of the vagina with a finger may be applied with the finger to stimulate straining. Sterile gauze or similar fabric may help the nurse to grip the puppy or kitten when assisting delivery. Undue force should never be applied to the feet as these are easily damaged or deformed.

Caesarean operation

There are many reasons for performing a Caesarean operation. In many cases this may be for the relief of dystocia, whilst occasionally it may be an elective procedure when there is concern over foeto-maternal disproportion.

Anaesthesia

It is important to remember that there are several marked physiological changes during pregnancy which may affect the requirements for anaesthesia. These physiological changes result in decreased minimum alveolar concentrations of anaesthetic gases, an increased oxygen requirement, and commonly hypoventilation and subsequent hypoxia and hypercarbia. In addition in cases of dystocia the animal may be debilitated and may have recently been fed.

The general aims are to:

- Ensure adequate oxygenation (intubation and oxygen administration).
- Maintain blood volume and prevent hypotension (intravenous fluid therapy).
- Minimise depression of the foetus and dam during and after surgery (reduce the dose of anaesthetic agents used).

There are many anaesthetic regimes suitable for this procedure, they include the use of volatile agents for induction and maintenance of anaesthesia and the use of rapid-acting intravenous induction agents (such as propofol) followed by maintenance of anaesthesia using a volatile inhalational anaesthetic.

Complications

There are several complications of Caesarean operation in both species. These include:

- Anaesthetic risks in the dam and the neonate.
- Risks during surgery of uterine rupture and haemorrhage resulting in hypovolaemia.
- Post-operative risks including wound infection and wound breakdown.
- Interference with the wound by neonates trying to suck.
- Problems in the dam of accepting the litter.

Some veterinary surgeons prefer to perform the operation via a flank incision to avoid the problem of wound interference when the neonates try to suck.

The problem of rejection of the litter by a young dam after a Caesarean operation may be overcome by placing the offspring with the dam as soon as possible after surgery. The mother's milk should be squeezed onto the newborn's head if rejection is a problem. The dam should be carefully observed until she is able to co-ordinate sufficiently enough to not damage them and she must not be left unattended until successful sucking has been noted.

Post-parturient care

Care and management of the neonate

The first essential steps after birth are:

(1) Establish a clear airway and stimulate respiration.
(2) Cut the umbilicus.
(3) Keep the neonate warm until active.
(4) Encourage the neonate to suck.

It is essential that a clear airway is established as soon as a foetus has been born (or delivered via a Caesarean operation). This involves removal of the surrounding foetal membranes and clearing of the mouth and nose of foetal fluid using either a dry towel or a small pipette. Gentle compression of the chest usually results in the establishment of respiratory effort. If this is not the case but the heart is beating, respiratory stimulation should continue by rubbing the thorax and removal of further fluid by gently swinging the neonate in a small arc (but this should be avoided unless absolutely necessary because of the risk of brain trauma).

In certain cases the administration of respiratory stimulant agents such as doxopram hydrochloride may be efficacious, as may the administration of oxygen. If respiration does not commence then artificial respiration can be attempted by blowing gently into the nose and mouth of the neonate. This should be done carefully to induce only slight lung expansion without overinflating the lungs. If the heart is not beating, external cardiac massage combined with artificial respiration may be attempted.

The umbilicus should be cut approximately 3 cm from the foetal abdomen; excessive bleeding can be prevented by the application of a ligature.

Once regular respiratory efforts are maintained the neonate may be placed into a prewarmed box or incubator until it is active when it may be returned to the dam and encouraged to suck. Sucking normally occurs immediately after birth and at intervals of 2–3 hours for the first few days.

Environment

Hypothermia is a major cause of neonatal mortality and so the environmental temperature is critical. Recommended temperatures (25–30°C) are only necessary for the first few days; they are often unbearable for the dam and can be safely reduced (22°C) as long as draughts are avoided. One method of reducing heat exposure of the dam is to heat only half the box.

Underfloor heating is ideal, but properly protected hot water-bottles or circulating water blankets provide good alternatives. Heat lamps suspended above the nest should be used with caution, since the environment may become too hot.

Examination

Pups and kittens should be carefully examined after birth:

● Bodyweight should be recorded. Normal neonates increase in bodyweight by 5–10% per day; a failure to achieve this rate may indicate ill health.
● The umbilicus should be clean and there should be no evidence of herniation.
● Respiration should be regular without excessive noise; the normal respiratory rate is 15–40 breaths a minute.
● There should be no discharge from the eyes or ears. The neonate should be examined for the presence of congenital diseases (described later).
● The rectal temperature need not be recorded but the normal range in the first week after birth is 32–34°C.

Neonatal characteristics

Neonatal pups and kittens are unable to stand at birth. They should, however, be quite mobile using their limbs to crawl.

Neonates should be assessed for their general strength and the weakest should be carefully observed since these do not feed adequately and may fail to thrive. Standing may be seen from 10 days from birth and most neonates should be able to walk at 3 weeks of age.

Pups and kittens are born with their eyes closed; separation of the upper and lower lids with opening of the eyes should occur by approximately 10–14 days after birth. The cornea at this stage may appear slightly cloudy although this will disappear over the first 4 weeks. Many kittens are born with strabismus which persists until they are 8 weeks old.

Care of the litter

In the first few weeks of life the dam will provide all the care of her offspring needed, provided that the environment is clean and dry. The choice of bedding material includes shredded paper, newspaper with blankets, or newspaper with synthetic rags. Materials should be washable or easily disposed of and soiled material should be removed frequently.

The dam normally licks the perineal region to stimulate defecation and urination and this is performed for the first 2–3 weeks after birth. Pups and kittens defecate and urinate voluntarily at 3 weeks of age and at this time soiling of the bedding will increase: more frequent changing is necessary. Pups and kittens should ideally be encouraged to soil an area away from the nest as early as possible to facilitate cleaning and to hasten toilet training.

Care of the dam

Immediately after parturition or surgery the perineum of the dam should be cleaned and she should be allowed to settle during suckling. She should be given the opportunity to exercise shortly afterwards. The bedding may then be cleaned and the dam can be given food. It is likely that in the first few days she may develop diarrhoea especially if the afterbirths were eaten. The bitch and queen will spend much of their time with their offspring during the first 2 weeks but should be encouraged to leave the nest as weaning is attempted.

The food intake during lactation may increase up to 3 times the normal and it is necessary to provide frequent small meals. These may be balanced diets or commercial preparations formulated for lactating animals. It is important not to change food intake dramatically since this may worsen the gastrointestinal disturbances normally seen. See Chapter 8, pp. 185 and 186.

Periparturient abnormalities

There are several conditions which may occur during late pregnancy or soon after parturition in both the domestic bitch and queen. Certain conditions are emergencies and prompt recognition of the clinical signs is essential to allow successful treatment.

Hypocalcaemia (eclampsia, puerperal tetany). Low plasma concentrations of calcium are related to calcium loss in the milk and poor dietary calcium availability. The condition is most commonly seen during late pregnancy or early lactation. It is rare in the cat. The clinical signs include restlessness, panting, increased salivation and a stiff gait, which may progress to muscle fasiculations, pyrexia and tachycardia. If untreated, tetany and death results. The slow administration of calcium borogluconate by intravenous injection produces a rapid resolution of the clinical signs. During administration, cardiac rate and rhythm should be monitored. Calcium supplementation may be then be given orally or by subcutaneous injection to prevent recurrence of the condition.

Placental retention. The retention of placental tissue is uncommon in both the bitch and the cat; however, it causes great concern for many owners. Placentae are normally delivered following each pup or kitten and may be quickly eaten by the dam. If a placenta is retained the clinical signs are a persistent green-coloured vulval discharge. This should be differentiated from the normal haemorrhagic discharge which may persist for 1 week after parturition (a mucoid discharge may be present for up to 6 weeks). If a retained placenta is diagnosed by either ultrasound examination or palpation, the administration of oxytocin is usually curative.

Post-partum metritis. Infection and inflammation of the uterus may occur following prolonged parturition, abortion, foetal and/or placental retention or obstetrical manipulation. The clinical signs commonly include a persistent purulent vulval discharge, lethargy and pyrexia. Treatment with broad-spectrum antimicrobial agents should be instituted immediately, and fluid replacement therapy may be required.

Mastitis. Inflammation of the mammary gland is not common in the bitch or queen although it may have disastrous results should the dam reject the litter because of pain on suckling. It is usually the result of bacterial infection following trauma (sucking). The mammary glands are tender, warm and firm upon palpation, and the milk may be contaminated with blood and inflammatory cells so that it becomes yellow, pink or brown in colour. The dam may become lethargic and anorexic if the condition is not treated. Bathing and massaging the gland with warm water and gently removing the infected fluid may be helpful; however, antimicrobial agents are usually required. It should be remembered, however, that these agents will be excreted in the milk and ingested by the neonates.

Artificial rearing of neonates

Hand rearing of neonates may be necessary when the dam dies or is unable to nurse the litter for some other reason. In many cases the litter may be too large or the dam may produce inadequate volumes of milk. It may be necessary to either cull some of the litter or for them to go to a foster home. A bitch in pseudopregnancy or a bitch who has lost her litter may prove to be suitable foster-mothers. If these are not acceptable alternatives the litter can be divided and

Species	Preparation	Distributor
Canine	Esbilak	PetLife
Canine	Lactol Milk Powder	Shirleys
Canine	Pedigree Instant Milk Substitute	Pedigree Petfoods
Canine	Welpi	PetLife
Feline	Cimicat	PetLife
Feline	Kitten Milk Replacer	Kruue
Feline	Lactol Milk Powder	Shirleys
Feline	Whiskas Instant Milk Substitute	Pedigree Petfoods

Table 18.2 Commercially available milk substitutes for pups and kittens

rotated between the bitch and artificial rearing. It has been suggested that some neonates should be reared entirely artificially rather than alternating the whole litter. However, all neonates should remain with the dam to ensure a normal social development.

It is essential that all neonates receive **colostrum** from the dam during the first few hours after birth to ensure an adequate uptake of maternal immunoglobulins. Should the dam have died it may still be possible to milk some colostrum from the mammary glands as long as it is not contaminated with high concentrations of drugs or toxins.

After the first day it is possible to commence **supplementary feeding**. There are several commercially available milk substitutes that are useful for feeding pups and kittens (Table 18.2). It is important that a correctly formulated diet is utilised. Neither cow's milk nor goat's milk is suitable since their compositions are markedly different to the milk of both the bitch and the queen. Whilst it is possible to use home-made milk substitutes these are often inappropriate in lactose, fat and protein concentration. The milk replacer should be warmed to body temperature (39°C) before feeding and then fed to the manufacturer's instructions, depending upon bodyweight.

Normally neonates feed every 2–4 hours for the first 5 days of life and it is best to mimic this regime with artificial feeding. The interval can be reduced to every 4 hours after day 5.

Artificial feeding is time-consuming and demanding, particularly if the litter is being reared without the dam. Milk substitutes may be administered using syringe feeders, eye droppers, sucking devices or stomach tube. In most cases it may be easiest to feed from a small syringe (2 ml) for the first 2–5 days. After this time a small bottle with a nipple may be used; this encourages normal sucking but takes the greatest time. When these devices are used the aperture should be large enough to prevent wind sucking but small enough to prevent excessive volumes being administered since this may result in aspiration.

The technique of feeding using a stomach tube (orogastric intubation) is relatively simple. It may be useful in the first few days of life for the rapid feeding of particularly sick neonates. A soft polythene tube (2 mm diameter) is measured against the neonate from the mouth to a level with the 9th rib and this distance is marked on the tube. The tube is lubricated with a small volume of water on its outside.

The head is held in the normal position and the mouth is held just open using a finger and thumb; if the head is extended or flexed, passage of the tube into the trachea is more likely. The tube is directed gently over the tongue into the back of the throat. Swallowing greatly assists passage into the oesophagus; however, this is not essential. The tube can usually be seen on the left side of the neck as it in passes down the oesophagus. There is little resistance as the tube is introduced into the stomach; the length of tube introduced is the best guide. Once in position the syringe can be attached and its contents slowly injected into the stomach. The tube is then gently removed.

Orphaned pups and kittens should be maintained at an environmental temperature of approximately 25°C. Normally the dam would lick the anogenital region after feeding to stimulate urination and defecation and in her absence this stimulation needs to be performed manually, using a moistened cloth or cotton wool, every 2 hours (4 hours during the first few days of life). See Chapter 8, p. 188.

Weaning

Pups and kittens generally receive all of their nutritional requirements from the dam until 3 weeks of age. (This must be provided artificially if they are hand reared.) Signs associated with under-nutrition include failure to gain weight, crying and inactivity.

Small volumes of meat fed on a finger can be introduced from 2.5 weeks of age and lapping of semi-solids can be encouraged from 3 weeks of age. This can be done by encouraging sucking and licking of a finger and gradually placing the finger in contact with the solution. This is the start of the weaning process which may last between 3 and 5 weeks. The volume and range of foods fed during this stage may be increased. It is common for semi-solids such as rice pudding and finely chopped meats to be used initially, although there are several proprietary brands of foods designed for this purpose. Neonates generally have twice an adult's energy and nutrient requirement per unit bodyweight.

For neonates weaned from the dam, the volume of food provided is increased and they usually receive five or six meals during the day at 5 weeks of age. As their food intake increases the dam should be removed from the nest for increasing periods of time. Usually by 5 weeks of age the dam spends very little time in the nest during the day, but returns at night. There is some discussion concerning the best time for removing the neonates from the dam. When neonates are introduced directly into a home environment weaning can be safely accomplished by 6 weeks of age.

For hand-reared neonates, the volume of bottled milk is reduced in a similar manner to weaning from the bitch. See also Chapter 8, pp. 186 and 187.

Abnormalities of the neonatal period

A number of diseases may affect pups and kittens early in life. A certain percentage of neonates may die before weaning and it has been suggested that this can be as high as 15–20%. However, with good management systems (including the avoidance of hypothermia) the number of offspring lost should not be greater than 5%.

Fading puppy and kitten syndrome

The condition known as fading puppy or kitten syndrome is a true syndrome in that there are multiple potential causes, ranging from poor maternally derived immunity, viral, bacterial and parasitic infections and genetic abnormalities. An accurate diagnosis cannot be established in all cases. The clinical signs are often unhelpful because they are similar regardless of cause; the neonates become lethargic, do not feed and usually die before 14 days of age.

Congenital abnormalities

Congenital abnormalities are those abnormalities which are present at birth. Common problems include cleft palate where there is failure of the normal fusion of the palatine arches. The defect may occur anywhere along the length of the hard or soft palate, although most commonly it arises caudal to the incisor ridge. The defect is common in certain breeds and it has been suggested that it is a trait inherited either in a recessive or polygenic manner. In most cases euthanasia of the neonate with this problem is advisable because of the problems of sucking and aspiration of milk.

The condition of hare lip (cleft lip) is also observed in brachycephalic breeds and Yorkshire Terriers and Bull Terriers. This may be associated with cleft palate although this is not often the case. The condition is known to be inherited as a simple autosomal recessive trait in the English Bulldog but the mode of inheritance in other breeds is not clear.

There are many other congenital abnormalities which may affect each organ system, such as hernias, foetal monsters, hydrocephalus, microphthalmus, flat puppies (swimmers), congenital heart disease and atresia of the terminal rectum. A thorough clinical examination of each pup after birth should allow these abnormalities to be readily detected.

Further reading

Concannon, P. W. (1991) Reproduction in the dog and cat. In *Reproduction in Domestic Animals*, 4th edn, Academic Press, New York, pp. 517–554.
England, G. C. W. (1998) *Allen's Fertility and Obstetrics in the Dog*, 2nd edn, Blackwell Scientific, Oxford.
Hoskins, J. D. (1995) *Veterinary Pediatrics: Dogs and Cats from Birth to Six Months*, 2nd edn, W. B. Saunders, Philadelphia.
Simpson, G. M., England, G. C. W. and Harvey, M. J. (1998) *Manual of Small Animal Reproduction and Neonatology*, BSAVA, Cheltenham.

19

Surgical nursing

M. R. Owen and C. May

Inflammation

Inflammation may be defined in two ways:

(1) Inflammation is the reaction of normal tissues to an irritant.
(2) Inflammation is a process which begins following injury to a tissue and ends with healing or the eventual death of the tissue.

The second definition, though more cumbersome, is useful because it emphasises the dynamic nature of inflammation by referring to it as a process.

There are many different causes of inflammation, but they can all be divided into a few basic categories (Table 19.1).

The signs that characterise inflammation are known as the **cardinal signs**. They are:

● Redness.
● Swelling.
● Heat.
● Pain.
● Loss of normal function.

The cardinal signs of inflammation have been recognised for almost 2000 years. The redness, heat and swelling are all associated with an increase in blood flow to the inflamed tissue. Swelling occurs because fluid, rich in protein and white blood cells, leaves the blood vessels and enters the tissue spaces. Sometimes inflammation is classified by the nature of this exudate (Table 19.2).

The inflammatory exudate serves a number of important functions:

● It dilutes irritating substances in the tissues.
● It delivers cells of the immune system to the tissues.

Table 19.1 Causes of inflammation

Cause	Examples
Pathogenic organisms	Viruses, bacteria, fungi, external and internal parasites.
Mechanical trauma	Blunt (direct) trauma, indirect trauma, lacerations, chemical injury.
Thermal injuries	Heat (burns), cold (frostbite), electrical burns, radiant energy (X-rays, sunburn).
Immune reactions	Serum sickness, delayed hypersensitivity, autoimmune diseases (e.g. rheumatoid arthritis, systemic lupus erythematosus).
Foreign material	Foreign bodies, tumours.

Table 19.2 Classification of inflammation by the nature of the inflammatory exudate

Type	Notes
Serous	Serum is exuded from blood vessels into the interstitial space.
Fibrinous	The exudate has a high fibrinogen content and clots spontaneously. Especially seen at mucous and serous membranes (e.g. pericardium; pleura; peritoneum).
Purulent	The exudate consists of pus. Also called suppurative.
Haemorrhagic	Large numbers of erythrocytes are present together with some, or all, of the other constituents of exudates.
Mucus	Also called catarrhal. Characterised by the presence of mucus secreted from epithelial mucosa. Therefore restricted to mucous membranes. There may also be cell debris.

● It delivers immunoglobulins and other immune substances to the tissues.
● It delivers fibrinogen to the area to commence 'walling off' the inflamed site.

The pain associated with inflammation is due to increased pressure on nerve endings because of the swelling and to a direct irritating effect of toxic products. The toxins may arise from the cause of the inflammation (e.g. a bacterium) but they are more commonly a by-product of the inflammatory process itself.

The loss of function with inflammation results from pain-induced inhibition of muscle activity ('guarding'), the mechanical effects of swelling and tissue destruction.

Inflammation may also be classified by its duration as either acute or chronic.

Acute inflammation

Acute inflammation is a process of short duration in which the cardinal signs of inflammation are usually obvious. There may also be systemic signs of illness including:

● Fever
● Increased pulse rate
● Increased circulating white blood cells, especially polymorphonuclear leucocytes (PMNL).

In most cases acute inflammation is a beneficial process leading to the elimination of the initiating factor and to

Table 19.3 Possible sequels to acute inflammation	
Sequel	**Notes**
Resolution	The acute inflammation subsides without significant tissue injury.
Healing	There is regeneration and repair of tissues damaged by the inflammatory process.
Abscessation	There is accumulation of pus which persists.
Degeneration	Damaged cells degenerate. This is most commonly seen in the liver and may be associated with fatty deposition in the cells.
Mineralisation	Mineral deposits in soft tissues are especially seen in chronic inflammation and in inflamed connective tissues.
Necrosis	Cell death occurs and the affected tissue is sloughed. Examples are seen in inflammation of the skin or intestinal lining.
Gangrene	Gangrene is cell death associated with the loss of local blood supply and putrefaction of the tissues by bacteria.
Chronic inflammation	See main text.

eventual healing. However, there are several other possible outcomes and these are summarised in Table 19.3.

Treatment of acute inflammation

There are two aims in the treatment of acute inflammation:

- Removal of the inciting cause.
- Limitation of the body's inflammatory response.

The method of removing the inciting cause depends on the particular initiating factor. For example, antibiotics may be prescribed when the initiating factor is a bacterium or injurious chemicals may be washed away by lavage.

It is not always desirable to reduce the inflammatory response of the body, but when this is appropriate it is achieved by administering inhibitory drugs. The most commonly used drugs in the treatment of acute inflammation are corticosteroids and the non-steroidal anti-inflammatory drugs such as carprofen, ketoprofen, meloxicam and phenylbutazone. These drugs have potential toxic side effects and should only be used under the direction of a veterinary surgeon.

In superficial acute inflammation caused by trauma, damage can sometimes be limited in the early stages by the application of cold compresses to the inflamed area.

Chronic inflammation

In some cases, the acute inflammatory phase fails to eliminate the inciting cause of the inflammation. Chronic

inflammation is an ongoing response to persistent irritants. It is characterised by a marked mononuclear cell reaction and by proliferation of fibroblasts. The fibroblasts are a manifestation of repair. In chronic inflammation the processes of repair and inflammation occur together.

Chronic inflammation is a notable feature of certain diseases in which the inciting agent is of low toxicity and fails to elicit a sufficiently vigorous acute response in the host. Three major categories of this type of disease can be identified:

- **Persistent infections**, e.g. by intercellular organisms and by fungi.
- **Prolonged exposure to non-degradable material**, e.g. non-absorbable suture materials or inorganic foreign bodies.
- **Autoimmune disease**, e.g. rheumatoid arthritis and systemic lupus erythematosus. In these diseases, some of the inciting factors of inflammation are the animal's own body tissues. These can obviously not be eliminated and thus give rise to a chronic inflammatory response.

It is sometimes difficult to classify a particular inflammatory response as either 'acute' or 'chronic' because there is no clear dividing line between the two and both processes may occur simultaneously.

Tissue type and inflammation

The type of tissue in which an inflammatory response occurs can affect the structural changes and the course of events that ensue. **Abscesses** and **ulcers** are good examples.

Abscessation

Tissues such as the dermis, liver and kidney may be regarded as 'solids'. The presence of a pyogenic organism within these tissues can lead to the formation of pus which can be either localised (abscess) or diffusely distributed throughout the tissue (cellulitis).

DEFINITIONS

- **Abscess:** A localised inflammatory reaction with a necrotic pus-filled centre.
- **Cellulitis:** A diffuse inflammatory reaction with pus distributed through cleavage planes and tissue spaces.
- **Pus:** An inflammatory exudate containing partially or completely liquefied dead tissue mixed with large numbers of dead or dying PMNL.

Within an abscess, several different stages of inflammation and repair can be recognised at a single moment. Adjacent to the pus-filled centre is a layer of fibrin within which there are more PMNL. Peripheral to this zone is a layer of capillary and fibroblast formation. This outermost layer represents repair and serves to 'wall off' the inflammatory process to prevent it spreading to neighbouring tissue.

Toxins may sometimes be released from the abscess causing toxaemia which is potentially life-threatening. It is therefore helpful to encourage healing of abscesses as soon as possible. Healing of an abscess only occurs once there is discharge of its content. This sometimes occurs naturally by rupture of the abscess at a point.

Treatment of abscesses. Abscesses are treated by encouraging them to discharge their contents in one of two ways:

● By the application of hot compresses.
● By perforating (lancing) the abscess to drain it.

Hot compresses are only applicable to abscesses of the skin. They encourage eruption of the abscess at the skin surface, beneath the compress. More commonly, abscesses are treated by **lancing**. The abscess cavity is then drained and can be flushed with either sterile saline or with antiseptic solutions. Following the initial incision, **drainage** is encouraged by the continued application of hot compresses or by leaving in place a surgical drain. The drained abscess collapses and heals by the deposition of scar tissue in the abscess cavity. Once drainage has been established, antibiotics may be administered to help eliminate causative bacteria.

In deep tissues, e.g. in the abdomen, it may not be possible to treat an abscess by drainage. In these circumstances the abscess may be completely excised along with a margin of normal tissue.

Chronic abscesses. A chronic abscess forms when an abscess fails to heal after it has drained. Chronic abscesses may result from incomplete drainage of the abscess at the time of discharge or from the persistence of a foreign body in the abscess.

Chronic abscesses are characterised by a thick, fibrous wall enclosing granulation tissue. A sinus tract, lined by granulation tissue, may communicate from the abscess to the skin or a mucosal surface.

Treatment of chronic abscesses relies on removing the inciting cause (e.g. by surgically removing a foreign body) and by providing adequate drainage.

Ulceration

An **ulcer** is a local excavation of the surface of an organ or tissue resulting from the sloughing of inflammatory necrotic tissue.

Ulcers particularly occur in the skin and mucous membranes, but they are also seen in other structures (e.g. the cornea of the eye). Ulcers usually result from mechanical injury, infections or damage by chemical irritants. Poor local blood supply may also contribute to their formation and they often become secondarily infected by bacteria regardless of the initial cause.

Ulcers contain inflammatory exudate within the crater and the edges are ragged after sloughing of the surface layers. In the healing phase, the base of an ulcer becomes covered with granulation tissue and there is re-epithelialisation from the edges.

Treatment of ulcers. There are three main aims during treatment of ulcers:

(1) To remove the inciting cause.
(2) To treat any secondary bacterial infections.
(3) To provide temporary protection for the healing surfaces.

Protection may be provided by dressings or by using the animal's own tissues. A good example of the latter technique is the suturing of the third eyelid over the eye in the treatment of corneal ulcers. It is not always possible to provide temporary protection of the healing surfaces. In situations (such as the mouth) where it is impractical to cover an ulcer, the surface may be kept clean with a suitable antiseptic solution until healing occurs.

Wound healing

In most cases, acute inflammation is followed by healing. The precise outcome of healing varies depending on the nature and severity of the initial injury and the tissue involved. However, a number of basic processes can be recognised:

● Removal of dead and foreign material.
● Clearance of the inflammatory response.
● Regeneration of lost tissue components if possible.
● Replacement of lost tissue components by connective tissue.

The different outcomes can be summarised in three categories:

● **Resolution** – the return of tissue to its state prior to the onset of inflammation.
● **Regeneration** – the replacement of tissue destroyed by the inflammatory process with similar functional tissue.
● **Organisation** – the replacement of tissue destroyed by the inflammatory process with connective (scar) tissue.

For **resolution** to occur, there must be no tissue destruction by the inflammatory process and this is only likely to occur in mild injuries.

Regeneration of tissues is dependent on two factors:

● The lost cells must be capable of being replaced.
● The connective tissue framework and the vascular supply on which the tissue depends must both be intact.

Cells may be classified into three basic groups, based on their ability to regenerate:

● **Labile cells** normally divide and proliferate throughout life. They are highly capable of regeneration and include all epithelial cells, blood cells and lymphoid tissue.
● **Stable cells** are normally quiescent, but are capable of increased mitosis in response to certain stimuli and may therefore regenerate in some circumstances. They include cells of the liver, kidney, endocrine glands, bone and fibrous tissue.

- **Permanent cells** normally only proliferate in foetal life and are incapable of regeneration. They include neurons and cardiac muscle cells. Skeletal muscle has limited powers of regeneration.

When tissues are unable to repair by regeneration, they will undergo **organisation**. The initial step in organisation is invasion by macrophages, fibroblasts and new capillaries. This new tissue is the **granulation tissue**. Gradually, the granulation tissue is replaced by **collagen fibres**. The blood vessels regress and there is shortening of the collagen fibres which causes the scar to contract.

This type of repair by connective tissue can be further classified into two subgroups:

- First intention healing (healing by primary union).
- Second intention healing (healing by secondary union).

First intention healing

First intention healing of tissues is seen in clean, surgical wounds when the wound edges are **coapted** (brought together) by sutures. The events in first intention healing are conveniently illustrated by considering such a wound in the skin:

- **Day 1**: The incision fills with blood clot which dries to seal the wound. There is an acute inflammatory reaction at the wound margins.
- **Day 2**: The surface of the epithelium begins to heal by regeneration. Damaged hair follicles, sebaceous glands and sweat glands may also begin to regenerate. The underlying connective tissue cells cannot regenerate, but there is hypertrophy of fibroblasts.
- **Day 3**: The inflammatory response begins to subside. Macrophages begin removal of dead tissue debris.
- **Day 5**: The tissue space below the regenerating epithelium is filled by highly vascular granulation tissue.
- **Day 7**: Epithelial regeneration is almost complete. Collagen fibrils are deposited in the underlying tissue space.
- **Week 2**: Fibroblast proliferation and collagen deposition continue. Contraction of the collagen and regression of the blood vessels begins.

Second intention healing

Second intention healing occurs when there is significant loss of the tissue, thus preventing coaptation of the wound edges. Second intention healing is a prolonged process involving the removal of dead material and the filling of a large tissue defect.

In the early stages, the base and margins of the wound are filled with granulation tissue. This process often starts whilst there is still active inflammation in the wound. As debris is gradually removed, the granulation tissue migrates in from the wound margins to fill the defect. Re-epithelialisation, by regeneration, starts at the wound margins on the bed of granulation tissue that is laid down. Fibroblasts in the granulation tissue undergo contraction and this serves to shrink the size of the wound considerably (**wound contraction**). Granulation and epithelial proliferation continue in the wound until repair is complete.

The management of wounds

Wounds are generally classified into four categories based on the degree of contamination of the wound:

- **Clean wound**: A relatively non-traumatic surgical wound, made under aseptic conditions and not entering the oropharynx or the respiratory, alimentary and urinogenital tracts. Clean wounds may be closed by suturing without drains.
- **Clean-contaminated wound**: An operative wound, made under aseptic conditions, penetrating the oropharynx, respiratory, alimentary or urinogenital tracts but without undue contamination.
- **Contaminated wound**: A fresh traumatic wound or a surgical wound with a major break in aseptic technique. Also surgical wounds which encounter acute non-purulent inflammation, such as cystitis.
- **Dirty (infected) wound**: Includes old traumatic wounds (more than 6 hours) or surgery for perforated viscera in the abdomen. The organisms which cause wound infection are already present in the field of surgery before operation. Primary closure of these wounds generally seals in infection, leading to abscessation. These wounds often require special surgical management such as the use of drains or they may be left open to allow wound debridement, control of infection and drainage.

Peri-operative management of surgical wounds

Clean wounds generally do not become infected post-operatively. The chance of post-surgical infection occurring in clean-contaminated wounds can be reduced and the severity of post-surgical infection in dirty wounds can be lessened in selected circumstances by the use of intravenous antibiotics, which should be given immediately prior to surgery.

Post-operative management of surgical wounds

Wound dehiscence (the breakdown of a wound along all or part of its length) and infection are prevented partly by attention to pre-operative preparation of the patient and by good surgical technique, but also by good post-operative care of surgical wounds. The main principles of managing a clean surgical wound are:

- Dressing the wound.
- Observation of the wound and patient.
- Prevention of self-mutilation.
- Suture removal.

Dressing of surgical wounds

The purposes of wound dressings are:

- To absorb exudate from the wound.
- To protect the wound from contamination.

Some surgical wounds require no post-operative dressings. In many other cases, a simple dressing of an absorbent pad and non-adhesive surface in contact with the wound can be held in place with adhesive tape for 24 hours, by which time a clean surgical wound forms a 'serum seal', which resists bacterial contamination. Alternatively a spray-on film dressing is preferred by some surgeons. In some cases additional padding is required by providing a thick cover of absorbent material such as cotton wool or cast padding. Particular indications for additional padding in wound dressings include:

- Over wounds at sites exposed to trauma, such as the limbs.
- Over wounds which have a heavy exudate.
- Beneath pressure bandages.

Once in place, most dressings can be left until the time of suture removal.

Observation of the wound and patient

Nurses are very well placed to detect early signs of wound complications by careful observation of the surgical wound. If a dressing is placed on the wound it may not be possible to observe the wound directly, but the skin surrounding the wound and the dressing itself can be observed. The factors to pay particular attention to are:

- **Exudate**: Note the amount, colour and type (e.g. serous, purulent). If exudate continues to leak through a dressing, the dressing should be removed to observe the wound.
- **Erythema**: Note whether limited to the vicinity of the sutures or whether it extends further. Has the erythematous area increased or decreased in size since the surgery?
- **Oedema**: Note how severe the oedema is and whether it is increasing or reducing.
- **Haematoma**: Note how severe the haematoma is and whether it is increasing or reducing.
- **Pain**: Note the severity of the pain (a subjective 1–10 scale is sometimes helpful) and whether the pain is continuous, intermittent, only present when the wound is handled or if there is no pain.
- **Odour**: Note if there is a foul odour from the wound.

In addition to monitoring the wound, good post-surgical wound care involves monitoring the patient for any signs of systemic illness which may be associated with wound complications. Both subjective and objective assessments should be performed:

- **Subjective assessments**: Note whether the animal is bright, alert and responsive or whether there has been a change in demeanour since before the surgery. Also note progressive changes in demeanour throughout the post-operative recovery phase.
- **Objective assessments**: Daily monitoring of temperature, pulse and respiration, a note of appetite, defecation and urination should constitute the minimum daily assessment of hospitalised patients in the post-operative phase. In some cases a more detailed clinical examination including other factors such as water intake or blood parameters may be indicated.

Prevention of self-mutilation

Self-mutilation at the surgical incision may lead to wound dehiscence. Some tendency to lick the wound is common in many animals post-operatively and need not necessarily give cause for concern. Persistent licking or chewing at the wound may be an indicator of wound complications. In other cases an individual animal will continuously lick or chew at the surgical site for no obvious reason.

Wounds closed under tension, or with sutures placed too tightly, are more likely to irritate the animal and lead to excessive chewing at the wound. A good post-operative

---

INSTRUCTIONS FOR OWNERS TAKING A PET HOME WITH A SURGICAL WOUND

(1) Your pet's wound needs to be carefully looked after to ensure a good result following his/her surgery. Please make sure that the wound is kept clean and dry.

(2) Do not allow your pet to lick or scratch the wound. This will cause irritation and may lead to infection.

(3) Restrict your pet to leash exercise, and avoid strenuous activities and boisterous playful activities for the next 10 days, which could disrupt the healing wound.

(4) Some redness, mild soreness and swelling is to be expected after an operation. This normally resolves over the first few days after surgery.

(5) Watch your pet for signs of increased interest in the wound, which may suggest increased soreness, and check the wound daily for signs of increased swelling, redness or discharge.

(6) The wound needs to be re-examined in 7–10 days' time, at which time the stitches may be removed.

(7) Please contact your veterinary surgeon if your pet shows any evidence of problems with the wound or signs of discomfort or general illness (dullness, lethargy or lack of appetite).

REMEMBER – IF YOU ARE WORRIED AT ANY STAGE, CONTACT YOUR VETERINARY SURGEON.

dressing will help in some measure to protect a wound from self-mutilation, but a determined animal will soon destroy most bandages.

Many devices exist for the prevention of self-mutilation and all rely on preventing the animal traumatising the wound by either chewing or scratching. The Elizabethan collar (Fig. 2.10) is one of the most useful and commonly employed devices to prevent chewing or alternatively the use of bitter tasting substances painted on the dressing. Damage by scratching can often be prevented by covering the feet with well-padded foot bandages.

When the animal is discharged, the owner should be given instructions for wound care, potential problems and how to seek advice in the event of problems. It is a good idea to explain the procedure which has been performed. Do not forget that clients do not see the surgery, they only see the wound. Wounds which are covered with specialised dressings require particular care (see later in chapter). The box above gives an example of instructions for uncomplicated wounds (e.g. following ovariohysterectomy or castration) which can be adapted as required.

Removal of sutures

The purpose of sutures is to approximate the wound edges to allow rapid first intention healing with minimal scarring. Alternatives to sutures which may be used in some cases include metal clips or staples and wound tapes.

Skin sutures should be removed as soon as there is adequate healing of the wound. In most cases this will be between the 7th and 10th post-operative day. However, in some young animals wound healing may be quicker and in old or otherwise debilitated animals it may be necessary to leave skin sutures in for longer. Some surgeons may use subcuticular sutures (placed in the dermis rather than through the epidermis and dermis) to close certain wounds. Absorbable sutures are often used for subcuticular sutures and these do not require removal. However, the wound should still be inspected at 7–10 days post-operatively to ensure that adequate healing has occurred.

Complications of surgical wounds

The main complication of surgical wound closure is **dehiscence** (the breakdown of a wound along all or part of its length). Several factors increase the chances of dehiscence:

- Infection of the wound.
- Seroma formation.
- Decreased blood supply to the wound.
- General health of the patient.
- Poor pre-operative preparation of the patient.
- Poor surgical technique.
- Poor suture technique or inappropriate suture materials.
- Poor post-operative care of the wound.

Of these, infection is by far the most common cause of wound dehiscence.

Other complications of wound healing include:

- **Sinus**: A late infective complication of surgery. A sinus is a blind-ending tract, lined by granulation tissue and usually ending in an abscess cavity. Sinuses in surgical wounds are often focused on suture material or other foreign material left in the wound at the time of surgery.
- **Fistula**: An abnormal tract connecting two epithelial surfaces or connecting an epithelial surface to the skin. This may be a complication of wound healing or, rarely, a congenital abnormality. An example of a congenital fistula is the rectovaginal fistula in which a tract connects the lumen of the rectum to that of the vagina.
- **Incisional hernia**: A late complication of abdominal surgery in which there is dehiscence of the incision in the muscle layers whilst the overlying skin remains intact. Abdominal contents will often occupy the space between the dehisced muscles.

Some specific factors which influence wound healing include:

- The site of the wound.
- Local wound factors.
- Systemic factors.
- Duration of pre-operative stay.
- Pre-operative bathing of the patient.
- Hair removal at the operation site.
- Bowel preparation.
- Operative factors.
- Wound closure technique.

The site of the wound

Surgical incisions should normally be made along lines of natural cleavage in the skin. Incisions along these lines fall naturally together and tend to heal more rapidly than incisions across the lines of natural cleavage. Another good example of how the site of incision can affect wound healing is found in limb surgery. Approaches to joints usually avoid crossing the flexor surface of the joint where there is increased risk of post-operative contracture leading to deformity and loss of function.

Local wound factors

Poor blood supply (as occurs in some areas of the body), dehydration of the wound, excessive exudation, foreign bodies, necrotic tissue, recurrent trauma and prolonged exposure to low temperatures can all delay wound healing and increase the risk of wound breakdown.

A **seroma** is a collection of serum or, more frequently, blood and serum in tissue spaces. The formation of a seroma at the wound site increases the risk of wound complications for several reasons:

- It is an excellent medium for the growth of micro-organisms.
- It increases tension on the wound.
- It can interfere with re-vascularisation, particularly in certain skin grafting techniques when it is important that the grafted skin acquires a new blood supply.

Seromas tend to develop in surgical wounds when large gaps (known as **dead spaces**) are left between the tissue layers. They are prevented by either scrupulous attention to wound closure and elimination of dead space or, where this is not possible, by the use of a drainage tube placed at the time of surgery.

When they do occur, seromas are treated by drainage under strict aseptic precautions. The seroma may be drained surgically or by aspiration with a needle and syringe.

Systemic factors

Generalised systemic disorders (such as malnutrition, haematological, cardiovascular or respiratory disease causing reduced oxygen supply to the tissues, renal disease, liver disease, chronic infection) and certain therapies (including steroids, cytotoxic drugs and radiotherapy) may all result in delayed or impoverished wound healing.

Duration of pre-operative stay

Longer stays in hospital before operations increase the risk of wound infection and breakdown. The reasons for this are not fully understood, but it may be that hospitalisation reduces general fitness and causes endogenous release of steroids through stress. Alternatively, the patient's skin may become colonised with micro-organisms other than its normal skin commensals.

Pre-operative bathing of the patient

Pre-operative bathing with non-medicated soap does not reduce the incidence of wound infection and breakdown. However, pre-operative bathing with an antiseptic solution, such as 4% w/v chlorhexidine may be of benefit in reducing the incidence of wound infection.

Hair removal at the operation site

Shaving the operative site actually increases the risk of infection in clean surgical wounds. Hair should be clipped with electric clippers in the preparation room just prior to surgery. Pre-clipping patients the night before a surgical procedure is no longer recommended since it actually increases infection rates.

Bowel preparation

The normal colon contains large numbers of micro-organisms and some of these are potential pathogens. Some form of cleansing of the bowel may be indicated before elective colonic surgery, but the requirements vary with different surgical conditions and, to some extent, with the personal preference of the surgeon. The surgeon should be consulted about the precise requirements in each case.

Operative factors

Longer operation times, greater degrees of trauma inflicted by the surgery and increased amounts of foreign material (such as sutures) left in the wound all increase the probability of subsequent wound breakdown. Preparation of the operative site by cleansing with an antiseptic solution such as chlorhexidine or povidone-iodine and the use of sterile drapes, gowns, gloves, theatre hats and masks all restrict the contamination of wounds by bacteria from the skin of the patient and the surgical team, thereby decreasing the chances of wound breakdown.

Wound closure technique

Most surgical wounds are closed by suturing. The aim is to restore functional integrity to the sutured tissues and encourage first intention wound healing with minimal scarring. Poor suture technique can lead to a wound which is more likely to break down. Examples of poor technique include:

● Overtight sutures leading to tissue necrosis below the suture material.
● Small 'bite' of tissue; larger bites generally result in stronger wounds than small bites.
● Inappropriate distance between sutures. Different wounds require different spacing of the sutures. Placing too few sutures, or placing too many sutures, can both lead to an increased risk of wound breakdown.
● Continuous sutures lead to a weaker wound than interrupted sutures.

Treatment of wound breakdown

First aid for wound dehiscence requires covering the wound with a clean, preferably sterile, dressing until definitive therapy can be instigated. In the case of abdominal wounds, dehiscence may lead to expulsion of viscera from the abdominal cavity through the wound. This clearly constitutes an emergency and the animal may require intensive therapy for shock. The exposed abdominal contents should be enclosed and supported in a clean, preferably sterile sheet until definitive treatment is available. The management of the infected or dehisced wound will be decided by the veterinary surgeon. However, the general principles of treatment are similar to those for all contaminated wounds.

The management of contaminated wounds

The basic principles of managing contaminated wounds are:

(1) Cleanse the wound of all organic debris and necrotic, devascularised tissue. Surgical debridement may be needed to achieve this.
(2) Facilitate wound drainage, either by placing drainage tubes or by treating the wound as an 'open wound' to allow second intention healing.
(3) Administer systemic antibiotics.
(4) If large areas of skin are missing, skin grafts may be used once the wound is clean and has filled with healthy granulation tissue.

Dressing contaminated wounds

Specific dressings may be of help in managing contaminated wounds. For the purposes of dressings, contaminated wound management can be considered in three stages:

(1) Cleansing and removal of necrotic debris.
(2) Granulation.
(3) Re-epithelialisation.

Cleansing and removal of necrotic debris

The dressings of use in this stage are:

● Occlusive dressings (hydrocolloids).
● Hydrogels.
● Wet packs.
● Alginate dressings.

Occlusive dressings are dressings which retain moisture in the wound, which rehydrates necrotic tissue and encourages it to slough. These dressings are usually **hydrocolloids**, which are left in place for a few days before removing. In superficial injuries, repeated hydrocolloid dressings will successfully debride the wound, leaving a healthy bed of granulation tissue. If the areas of necrosis are extensive, the hydrocolloid dressings may be combined with periodic debridement with a scalpel.

Hydrogel dressings are an alternative to hydrocolloid dressings. They contain significant amounts of water, which contributes to rehydration of necrotic tissue. Hydrogels dry if left exposed to the air and so they should always be covered with a secondary dressing that prevents moisture loss.

Hydrogels and hydrocolloids are also available in bead or gel forms which are sometimes convenient for large or particularly deep wounds. In some cases they are combined with iodine which is released into the wound and has an antibacterial effect.

A cheap but less satisfactory way of rehydrating black necrotic tissue and encouraging it to slough is by repeated application of **wet packs** made of gauze soaked in sterile saline.

Alginate dressings are especially useful for wounds with significant tissue loss which have a heavy discharge of exudate.

Granulation

The requirements for a dressing to encourage granulation are:

● To provide a moist environment.
● To provide a warm environment.
● To have reasonable absorptive capacity.

Several dressings fulfil these requirements, many of which are also used in the cleansing stage of wound healing. Alginate dressings may be used if excessive exudation persists. If there is only slight or moderate exudation, hydrocolloid or hydrogel dressings may be continued even after all dry necrotic tissue has sloughed. When granulation is to be encouraged in a clean, low exudate wound, such as

that created surgically, then a cavity foam dressing may be used as an alternative to hydrocolloids or hydrogels.

Re-epithelialisation

The requirements of a dressing to encourage re-epithelialisation are:

● To provide a moist environment.
● To be non-adherent.

There are many products available which satisfy these needs. The older types are paraffin-impregnated tulle, perforated film absorbent dressings and semi-permeable film dressings. These are still very useful general-purpose non-adherent dressings. More modern alternatives include polyurethane foams, hydrophilic materials and some other products specifically indicated for use on high exudate wounds such as burns.

Skin grafts

Superficial wounds in which there is considerable loss of skin may not heal completely or may heal unsatisfactorily, if left to re-epithelialise from the wound edges. These animals are candidates for skin graft surgery, in which a portion of skin is taken from one body area to fill the deficit in another body area on the same animal. There are many different ways of forming a skin graft, but they can all be divided into two broad categories: skin flaps (pedicle grafts) and free skin grafts.

Pedicle grafts involve moving an entire portion of skin and subcutaneous tissue complete with an intact blood supply from one body area to another. The flaps survive because of their intact circulation. They are created from areas with a well-defined blood supply which can be preserved and which have sufficiently loose skin to enable the donor site to be closed by first intention. Common donor sites for pedicle grafts include the skin over the shoulder blade and skin over the rump.

Free skin grafts lack a blood supply of their own and must initially survive by absorbing fluid from the recipient site. They will only do this successfully if the site is clean and revascularised. Free skin grafts must therefore be made on to a fresh, clean surgical wound or on to a well-established bed of granulation tissue. Free grafts can be classified in a number of ways:

● By the source of the graft.
● By the thickness of the graft.
● By the 'design' of the graft.

The graft may come from one of three sources:

● **Autogenous graft** from skin elsewhere on the same animal.
● **Allografts** from another animal of the same species.
● **Xenografts** from an animal of a different species.

Allografts and xenografts are rarely used in veterinary medicine. They may be used as a temporary cover, but permanent grafts are invariably of autogenous tissue.

Free grafts may be of either full thickness or split thickness. **Split thickness grafts** include only the epidermis and parts of the dermis, whereas **full thickness grafts** include the whole of the epidermis and dermis. Split thickness grafts are usually harvested with a special instrument designed for the purpose, called a **dermatome**, but they can be collected with a graft knife or a scalpel. The thickness can be varied so that different amounts of dermis are included in the graft. Split thickness grafts 'take' more readily than full thickness grafts, but they are not as strong and the hair growth on them is poor. They are also more likely to undergo contraction after they are placed at the recipient site.

Free grafts may be applied as one complete piece or they may be divided into various shapes before being placed in the recipient bed. Commonly used designs include:

- **Pinch grafts** – composed of small plugs of dermis and epidermis which are implanted in matching holes cut in the granulation bed.
- **Mesh grafts** – the donor sheet of skin is 'meshed' using a scalpel or a purpose-designed machine. The end result resembles a string vest and can cover quite large areas.
- **Strip grafts** – the donor graft is cut into strips which are laid on the recipient bed of granulation tissue with small gaps in between each strip.
- **Stamp grafts** – like strip grafts, but each piece approximates to the size and shape of a postage stamp.

The aim of these different graft patterns is to create open spaces between the donor tissue to allow drainage until the whole area is covered by re-epithelialisation which progresses from the margins of the donor tissue.

Drainage systems

Drainage is indicated for:

- Prophylaxis, to abolish dead-space in wounds.
- Therapeutic drainage of contaminated wounds.
- To remove fluid or air from the body cavities (e.g. the chest or bladder).

Some drains are only needed for few hours. Most wound drains are left in place for a period of 3–5 days. All drainage systems can be categorised as open or closed.

Closed drains

Closed drains can be further classified as either active or passive. **Active** drainage systems employ some form of suction device. This may be a high pressure system driven by a pump or a low pressure system. A simple low pressure, closed, active drain can be created from a plastic catheter and syringe (Fig. 19.1). Closed **passive** systems of drainage employ a simple collection bag which usually relies on gravity, rather than suction, to encourage drainage. A simple closed drainage system for the urinary bladder can be created by connecting an indwelling urinary catheter to the end of a giving set with an empty intravenous fluid bag attached.

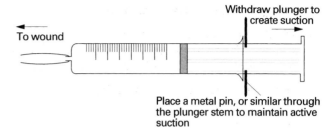

Fig. 19.1 Syringe and catheter drain.

Open drains

Open drains are most commonly used for prophylactic drainage of wounds or for therapeutic drainage of contaminated wounds. All open drains are passive. There are many different types but all are made of soft plastic materials, such as latex, which will not irritate the tissues. The Penrose drain is probably in most common usage in veterinary practice. Open drains rely on capillary action to remove fluid from a potential space in the tissues. Their ability to drain fluid is therefore directly proportional to the surface area of drain exposed to the tissues. Open, passive drains have the advantage of being cheap and simple.

Disadvantages of drains

The main disadvantages of drains are:

- They can act as retrograde conduits for secondary infections to gain access to a body cavity or wound space. This risk is greater with open drains than it is with closed drains.
- They are foreign bodies. The mere presence of a drain reduces the local resistance of local tissues to infection.
- They can cause damage to the tissues if they are made of hard materials or are incorrectly placed. Tissue damage may lead to fistulae or secondary haemorrhage because of blood vessel injury.

The management of drains

Many drains, particularly the more complex active drains, are supplied with manufacturers' instructions and these should always be read and adhered to. However, some general principles of drain management can be outlined:

- Document the volume and the nature of the fluid exuding from the drain.
- Ensure that drainage tubes are not obstructed.
- When changing bottles or bags on closed drainage systems, it is important to avoid reflux of fluid which may introduce infection to the drainage site.
- Dressings should be changed before they become soaked in exudate. Great care must be taken to maintain cleanliness around the drain and the associated wound at all times.
- Wound drain sites should be observed for leakage and signs of local wound infection. The patient should be observed for signs of systemic illness.

- Passive, open drains in wounds may be shortened to minimise the risk of accumulating infected material. The end of the drain should be anchored to the skin to prevent it being retracted into the wound.
- An Elizabethan collar, or similar device, is usually essential to prevent the animal removing the drain prematurely.
- Drains are removed using aseptic technique. The procedure is well tolerated and no sedation or anaesthesia is required.

Hypothermia

Hypothermia is an abnormally low body temperature. It occurs in warm-blooded animals whenever there is a reduction in heat production by the animal or when there is excessive loss of heat. Normal heat production occurs as a result of metabolic activity and through normal muscle activity. Animals with an abnormally low metabolic rate, such as those with malnutrition or with hypothyroidism, are more likely to be hypothermic. Similarly animals which are inactive are more likely to be hypothermic. Heat losses are increased when there is a low ambient temperature, when the skin is damp and when there is a draught. Considerable heat losses can also occur through evaporation of moisture from the respiratory tract.

Many of the conditions which lead to hypothermia are present when an animal is anaesthetised for surgery. The metabolic rate is lowered, the animal may be inactive for a prolonged period, hair is clipped from a large area of skin and the skin is soaked during routine pre-operative scrub procedures. During the surgery, much heat is lost through evaporation resulting from the externalisation of tissues and internal organs. Heat losses from the respiratory tract are greater when a non-rebreathing anaesthetic circuit is used and the animal constantly breathes cold gases.

Small animals are more prone to such heat losses than large animals because they have a relatively large ratio of body surface area to weight, giving proportionately greater heat losses. Unfortunately, it is often impossible to use rebreathing anaesthetic circuits for such animals because of the excessive resistance to breathing inherent in such devices. In very small animals, such as hamsters and budgerigars, heat loss under hypothermia is a significant risk even under the shortest anaesthetic.

The clinical signs of a hypothermic animal include:

- Shivering.
- Cold extremities.
- Pallor of the mucous membranes.
- Reduced pulse rate.
- Subnormal core temperature (rectal or oesophageal).

Prolonged or severe hypothermia leads to the death of the animal, but in many cases hypothermia is responsible for a poor or delayed recovery from anaesthesia.

Treatment of hypothermia

Treatment centres on reducing further heat losses and *slowly* restoring the animal's body temperature to normal. It is very difficult to influence heat production by the animal. The following steps are useful:

- Wrap the animal in an insulating material such as a blanket, bubble packing or a 'space blanket' (reflective foil).
- Warm all intravenous fluids to 37°C by running a coil of tubing from the giving set through a basin of warm water placed close to the animal or by using a purpose-made electric fluid warmer, if this is possible. Microwaves can also be used.
- Ensure that the animal is kept in a warm room.
- *Gently* warm the animal using hot water-bottles or a hair dryer. Care must be taken in such procedures. Hypothermic animals have a reduced peripheral circulation and are very prone to being burned by the direct application of heat. Water-bottles should be insulated in blankets and constantly checked to ensure that they are not overheating the animal's skin. Hair dryers should be used on a low setting and the direction of air flow should be constantly moved so that it does not centre on one portion of skin.
- Many hypothermic animals shiver violently during the recovery period. This markedly increases oxygen consumption and it may be necessary to provide oxygen at this time.

Prevention of hypothermia

Prevention is preferable to treatment. Many of the steps outlined above can be used as preventive measures and a few extra precautions can be taken during prolonged anaesthesia of very small animals:

- Purpose-made heating pads can be used on the operating theatre table.
- A rebreathing circuit can be used if this is practical. Alternatively a suitable humidifier can be incorporated into non-rebreathing circuits to minimise heat losses by evaporation from the airway.
- The ambient temperature of the operating room should be kept as high as possible, whilst remaining suitable for working conditions.
- During skin preparation wet the skin as little as possible and cover the animal completely with drapes. The drapes should be kept dry throughout the surgery.

It is usually necessary to continue these precautions until the animal is completely recovered from anaesthesia.

Fractures

A fracture is a complete or incomplete break of bone continuity, with or without displacement of the resulting fragments.

Fracture classification

An extensive classification system exists to describe different fracture types. Some of the more common and important terms are listed below:

- **Simple**: An uncomplicated fracture in which there is only one fracture line. Further terms are used to describe the direction of the fracture line relative to the bone. These include **transverse, oblique** and **spiral**.
- **Comminuted**: A complex fracture creating three or more fragments.
- **Open**: A fracture with an overlying open wound allowing potential contamination of the fracture with bacteria. Even pinpoint wounds are enough to justify classifying a fracture as open.
- **Closed**: A fracture which is not open.
- **Greenstick**: A fracture which is incomplete. The bone is fissured, but the fragments are not completely separated by the fracture line. Greenstick fractures are most common in immature animals.
- **Pathological**: A fracture resulting from normal use of a bone weakened by a disease process. The disease process may be generalised (e.g. a nutritional deficiency of calcium and phosphate causing weak bones) or localised (e.g. a tumour affecting the bone).
- **Avulsion**: A fracture in which a bone prominence is torn away from the rest of the bone, usually by the pull of a muscle.

Fracture sites

In dogs and cats, most fractures affect the long bones of the limbs. Various terms exist to define the site of fractures in long bones and some of the more common terms are listed below:

- **Diaphyseal**: A fracture in the diaphysis, or midshaft, of the bone.
- **Physeal**: A fracture through the growth plate of an immature animal. Sometimes called a **Salter–Harris** fracture because a system of classification of this type of fracture was described by Salter and Harris.
- **Epiphyseal**: A fracture of the epiphysis.
- **Condylar**: A fracture of the epiphysis when condyles are involved (e.g. the distal humerus or distal femur).
- **Supracondylar**: A fracture through the shaft of the humerus or femur, just above the condyles.

Other common sites of fractures include the pelvis, the mandibles and the ribs.

Causes of fractures

Except for pathological fractures, all fractures are caused by excessive trauma of the bone. Different types of trauma can cause different types of injury, so it is always important to know the cause of the injury. The type of trauma that causes a fracture is most commonly classified as either direct or indirect:

- **Direct trauma**: A physical blow to the bone causes it to break. Examples include the bumper of a car in a road traffic accident, kicks and gunshot injuries.
- **Indirect trauma**: The bone is broken by excessive leverage exerted upon it. Examples include avulsion fractures, limb bones broken if an animal puts its leg in a hole whilst running or fractures sustained as a result of twisting of the leg after a fall from a height.

In general, direct trauma is more likely to cause a complex fracture which is comminuted or open and indirect trauma is more likely to cause a simple fracture.

Clinical signs of fractures

In most fracture cases there is a history of trauma. In the initial phases a fracture is an inflammatory lesion and many of the clinical signs can be attributed to acute inflammation. The major clinical signs seen in fractures are:

- Localised heat.
- Pain localised to the affected bone.
- Local swelling.
- Bruising at the fracture site leading to discoloration of the overlying soft tissues.
- Marked loss of function.
- Visible or palpable deformity of the affected bone.
- Abnormal mobility at the fracture site.
- Crepitus when the injured part is moved.

Radiographs should always be taken to confirm the presence of a fracture before definitive treatment is given.

Fracture first aid

As described in Chapter 3, p. 56 the pain suffered by animals with fractures may cause them to bite those who offer well-meaning efforts to help them. It is essential that the animal is adequately restrained before attempting any first aid. A muzzle is often needed (see Chapter 1).

In many cases, animals with fractures have coexisting soft tissue injuries which may be more life-threatening but less obvious than the broken limb. Often, it is these soft tissue injuries which take priority in first aid. The first steps are always to ensure that there is an adequate airway, that the animal is breathing and that there is a good circulation. Shock is a major problem for fracture patients and fluid therapy may be an early requirement (see Chapter 22, p. 582).

The following specific first aid steps may be taken for the fracture itself.

(1) Cover any open wounds with a clean, preferably sterile dressing.
(2) Provide some form of immobilisation for the fracture before attempting to move the animal.
(3) Special care is needed when a spinal fracture is suspected. The entire spine should be immobilised by strapping the animal to any straight and rigid structure of suitable length.
(4) In most cases, haemorrhage is adequately controlled by firmly bandaging a sterile pad over the wound. A

tourniquet is only needed if there is pulsatile arterial bleeding which cannot be controlled by pressure pads.

(5) If a tourniquet is used, the time of its application should be noted so that it is not left in place too long (maximum 15 minutes).

(6) If possible, all drug therapies should be avoided until the patient has received a full clinical evaluation. Opiate analgesics may be given at the discretion of a veterinary surgeon. The time of administration and the dose of all drugs given in a first aid situation should be noted for later reference.

Splints in fracture first aid

This subject is covered in more detail in Chapter 3, p. 58. In an emergency, almost any rigid structure of suitable dimensions can be used to immobilise a fracture. Some splints are used for definitive treatment of fractures (external coaptation is described later). Two types of commercially available splints are useful in fracture first aid:

● **Zimmer splints** are made of malleable aluminium, backed by a foam composite. They can be shaped to conform with the limb and incorporated into a bandage to increase its rigidity. The foam backing is always placed towards the limb.
● **Gutter splints** are straight, non-malleable splints of rigid plastic, backed by a thin foam cushion. Like the Zimmer splint, they can be incorporated into a bandage to increase rigidity. They are stiffer than the Zimmer splint, but their use is limited because they are not malleable.

An alternative to splinting is the **Robert Jones** dressing described in Chapter 3, p. 57 and Chapter 2, p. 16. This is a bulky bandage applied firmly to the limb as a means of temporary stabilisation. The dressing both immobilises the injured limb and provides comfort because of its snug fit.

Fracture repair

Following successful first aid and stabilisation of any life-threatening soft tissue injuries, definitive fracture fixation is required. An understanding of fracture fixation techniques requires a knowledge of both normal anatomy and the process involved in fracture healing.

Fracture healing

The bone, its periosteum and the surrounding soft tissues are all damaged at the time of fracture. There is often considerable haemorrhage which, after 6–8 hours, coagulates to form a **haematoma** (Fig. 19.2). Some fragments of bone and connective tissues die as a result of the blood vessel damage and the dead tissues elicit an inflammatory response.

The haematoma is gradually replaced by granulation tissue and by the invasion of **stem cells** which will effect repair of the fracture. The stem cells migrate into the fracture gap, especially from the periosteum and the endosteum. Along with the stem cells there is a migration of

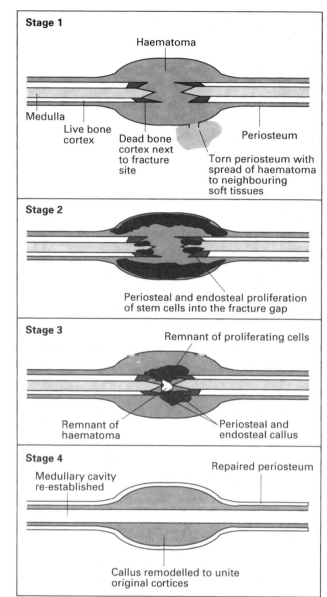

Fig. 19.2 Fracture healing stages.

new blood vessels derived from periosteal blood vessels and from blood vessels within the medullary canal of the bone.

The cells migrating into the area synthesise a tissue known as **callus**. Callus is composed of fibrous tissue, cartilage and immature bone. The callus envelops the bone ends, leading to an increase in stability at the fracture site. With time, the callus contains less fibrous tissue and more cartilage and bone. The stiffness of the callus thus increases and this further improves stability at the fracture site. Eventually the bone fragments are rigidly united by the callus. This is the point of **clinical union**.

Clinical union is followed by a prolonged period of bone remodelling. **Remodelling** is a process by which the initial callus is gradually removed and new bone is deposited. If the fracture fragments are accurately aligned, remodelling will restore the original shape of the bone. However, if the fragments are not kept in alignment during healing, the direction of the forces acting on the bone will change. The remodelling process will re-shape the bone to maximise its resistance to the new forces.

The principles of fracture fixation

The primary aim of fracture fixation is to restore the functional anatomy of the fractured bone. This is achieved by:

- Restoring continuity of the bone.
- Restoring the length of the bone.
- Restoring the functional shape of the bone.
- Maintaining essential soft tissue functions.

Essential soft tissues include the blood vessels supplying the bone, muscles acting on the bone and nerves supplying the muscles. Any techniques for fracture repair must be sympathetic to these soft tissues because without them there is no chance of restoring function to the injured limb.

Many techniques exist for successfully restoring bone continuity, length and shape. However, the same basic principles apply to all the techniques:

- **Reduction**: The fracture fragments should be brought together in correct anatomical alignment. This may be done 'closed', by traction and manipulation of the limb, or 'open', by performing surgery at which the fracture is visualised and the individual fragments manipulated back into position.
- **Fixation**: The fragments should be immobilised in correct alignment until clinical union occurs.
- **Blood supply**: The blood supply to the bone fragments must be preserved. Fractures will only heal if there is an adequate blood supply.

The rate of fracture healing

Provided that there are no complications, clinical union is usually achieved in 12–16 weeks in adult dogs and cats. Remodelling may persist for many months, or even years, after clinical union has occurred. The rate of fracture healing is assessed by clinical examination to detect the increase in stiffness and the firm swelling associated with union by callus formation. Radiographs are taken to assess the degree of callus formation and the extent of mineralisation within the callus.

Many factors influence the rate at which fractures heal and it is important to be aware of these when contemplating fracture repair:

- Fractures of immature animals heal more quickly than adult animals.
- Geriatric animals heal fractures more slowly.
- Osteomyelitis interferes with healing and is one of the most common causes of poor fracture healing after surgical fracture repair. Healing can progress once the infection is overcome.
- Debilitated animals heal fractures more slowly. Debilitation may be due to poor nutrition or systemic illness such as hormonal disorder or kidney failure.
- Fractures in cancellous bone (epiphyses of long bones) heal more quickly than fractures in cortical bone (diaphyses of long bones).

- Fractures with access to a good blood supply heal more quickly than those in areas with a poor blood supply. For example, the pelvis and scapula are covered by large muscle masses which have a good blood supply. Fractures in these bones heal well. The distal one-third of the radius and ulna has little muscle cover and a poor blood supply. Fractures at this site heal poorly, especially in very small breeds of dog.
- Oblique fractures heal more quickly than transverse fractures because there is a larger area to promote tissue re-growth.
- Poor reduction or fixation of a fracture will result in a slow rate of healing.

Complications of fracture healing

In some cases, fracture healing does not progress normally. The complications that can occur in fracture healing include:

- **Non-union**: Complete failure of the fractured ends of the bone to unite. This is usually caused by one or more of the factors which slow down the rate of fracture healing.
- **Delayed union**: Fracture healing progresses slowly. Clinical union is not achieved within the expected time.
- **Mal-union**: Fracture heals in poor alignment. This is caused by inadequate reduction or fixation.
- **Osteomyelitis**: Infection of bone. Bacterial osteomyelitis is commonly caused by inadequate asepsis during fracture repair surgery. It is more likely to occur if there is also damage to the local blood supply.
- **Short limb**: Limb shortening occurs if there is healing with inadequate reduction of overriding fracture fragments. Limb function may be severely compromised.
- **Fracture disease**: Fracture disease describes an inability to flex the joints in the limb after fracture repair. One or more joints in the affected limb may be held rigid due to scar formation within the joints or within muscles surrounding the fracture site. Fracture disease is more common after fixation by external coaptation or when there is inadequate reduction.

Fracture fixation techniques

After reduction of a fracture, the bones must be held in position until healing occurs. In some cases, such as greenstick fractures and some fractures of the pelvis, immobilisation may be unnecessary and simple restriction of activity will suffice. The indications for immobilisation at a fracture site are:

- To relieve pain.
- To prevent displacement of the fragments (loss of reduction).
- To prevent movement that might cause delayed union or non-union.

Fracture fixation techniques are broadly classified into three groups:

- External coaptation, using casts or splints.
- Internal fixation, using pins, plates, screws and other devices.
- External – internal fixation, using 'external fixators'.

External coaptation

Methods of external coaptation fall into three main groups: splints, casts and extension splints.

EXTERNAL COAPTATION TECHNIQUES

Main advantages
- They are technically simpler than some internal fixation techniques.
- They are economical.
- They are non-invasive compared with internal fixation.

Disadvantages
- They have limited applications. For example, casts are most useful below the stifle in the hindlimb or below the elbow in the forelimb.
- They do not provide sufficient stability for some fractures, particularly comminuted or severely oblique fractures.
- They are prone to cause pressure sores.
- They restrict activity of joints and muscles in the limb and are therefore prone to cause fracture disease.

Splints. The splints described for use in fracture first aid may be used as definitive fixation in some fractures, particularly those occurring below the carpus or hock in cats and small dogs.

Casts. An ideal casting material should be:

- Strong and relatively light in weight.
- Easy to mould to the desired shape.
- Simple to handle.
- Waterproof, but sufficiently porous to prevent maceration of the skin.
- Rigid but not so brittle that it will splinter in normal use.
- Radiolucent (and, perhaps, amenable to imaging by other techniques such as ultrasound).
- Cost-effective.

Plaster of Paris bandages are still a common casting material used, though recently many alternatives have been introduced. These are mainly polyurethane-based materials or thermoplastic polymers. They have the advantage of being light, waterproof and durable and have rapid drying times so that they reach full strength quickly (usually 10–30 minutes). They are also more radiolucent than plaster of Paris and less messy. However, the modern casting materials have the disadvantages of being more expensive and more difficult to apply than plaster of Paris.

Plaster of Paris

PLASTER OF PARIS

Advantages
- Safe and non-allergenic.
- Easily moulded.
- Easy to use and does not need gloves in handling.
- Cheap.

Disadvantages
- Slow to dry and to reach its full strength.
- Weakened if it becomes wet again.
- Heavy when wet (but does become lighter when dry).
- Not completely radiolucent.

INSTRUCTIONS FOR OWNERS TAKING A PET HOME WITH A BANDAGE OR CAST

(1) The success of the surgery performed on your pet may depend on good care of the dressing. Much of this care is given by you at home, but your veterinary surgeon will need to check the bandage from time to time and the bandage may need to be changed. Bandage materials are expensive and bandaging is a skilled and time-consuming job. A charge will be made for bandage changes.
(2) If the animal goes outside in wet weather, cover the end of the dressing with a plastic bag held in place by string or a loose elastic band. **Remove the bag and elastic band as soon as the animal returns to the house.**
(3) Check the dressing daily for evidence of swelling of the limb or chafing at the edges of the bandage. A small amount of talcum powder may help stop chafing. If you are worried, consult your veterinary surgeon.
(4) You should seek prompt attention from your veterinary surgeon if there is any evidence of problems with the wound or with the general well-being of your animal. This might include, staining of the bandage with discharge from the wound, a foul smell from the bandage, slipping of the bandage from its original position, excessive chewing at the bandage or other signs of discomfort, general illness in the animal such as depression, lethargy or lack of appetite.

REMEMBER – IF YOU ARE WORRIED AT ANY STAGE, CONTACT YOUR VETERINARY SURGEON

APPLICATION OF A PLASTER OF PARIS CAST

A cast should normally stabilise at least one joint proximal to the fracture and one joint distal to the fracture. Usually a cast extends from the foot to cover one joint proximal to the fracture.

(1) After reduction of the fracture, the injured limb is first covered with a tubular gauze.

(2) The tubular gauze is covered by a layer of cast padding material placed with 50% overlap at each successive turn. A provision should be made to allow 2 cm of cast padding and tubular gauze to protrude from either end of the plaster bandage.

(3) The plaster bandage is unwound by about 10 cm and the roll and the free end are immersed in water for a few seconds until air bubbles cease to rise. Cold water is used for longer setting times and hot water for shorter times.

(4) The plaster bandage is removed from the water, then squeezed *gently* to expel excessive water.

(5) The plaster bandage is applied from the distal limb working proximally. This encourages smoother application and reduces venous congestion resulting from application of the cast. At either end of the plaster bandage, 2 cm of cast padding and tubular gauze are left protruding.

(6) The overlap of plaster bandage is kept at a constant 50% or 60%. Gussets or tucks are created to keep this overlap constant at areas where the circumference of the limb changes.

(7) Once the layers of plaster bandage are in place, the cast is smoothed and moulded to fit the limb accurately. The cast padding and tubular gauze are turned back at each end of the plaster bandage to create a smooth edge. It is normal to leave the middle two toes just protruding from the cast distally.

(8) The limb is checked at regular intervals to ensure that circulation is adequate. The animal is not allowed to weight-bear until the cast has reached full strength.

Plaster of Paris setting times vary with the temperature and with the type of solution used for immersion. Low temperatures and sugar solutions slow the setting time, whilst warm temperatures and salt or borax solutions accelerate the setting time. In most cases plaster of Paris sets in a few minutes, but drying takes much longer. Often more than 24 hours is needed for complete drying of a limb cast. The cast does not reach full strength until it is completely dry.

When the animal is discharged, the owner should be given written instructions about care of the cast, potential problems with the cast and how to seek advice if problems arise. Given in the box opposite is an example of instructions which may be adapted for use in many practice situations.

Application of plaster slabs (plaster splints). The indications for plaster slabs are:

- Slabs can be used on their own as initial splinting of an injury. They are more easily applied and allow more swelling than a normal cast. However, a plastic splint incorporated into a bandage is more frequently used in this situation.
- Slabs are more often used to reinforce a normal cast, especially at weak points such as joints.

To create slabs:

(1) Unroll the plaster of Paris bandage on a dry surface.
(2) Double the plaster bandage backwards and forwards to provide a stack of suitable length.
(3) Hold the splint at both ends and immerse in water until bubbles cease to rise.
(4) Hold it vertically above the water to allow it to drain.
(5) Squeeze it dry, keeping hold of each end at all times.
(6) Stretch slab to its original shape.

The limb is prepared as for a normal cast and a single layer of circular cast applied first. Slabs are laid on the limb lengthways and may be held in place by a layer of wet cotton bandage. The cast is completed as before.

Application of modern casting materials. The basic principles of application of thermoplastic and polyurethane-based casts are similar to those for plaster of Paris casts but the immersion and application requirements of these materials may be different. The manufacturer's instructions should always be consulted. It is necessary to wear gloves when applying resin-based casts. Conformation of the cast can often be helped by wrapping it in a wet cotton bandage during the hardening period. Often, the polyurethane materials are stronger, less bulky and lighter than a plaster of Paris.

Some of the modern cast materials are amenable to the formation of a **split cast**. The cast is applied normally and allowed to set. It is then immediately removed by a single straight cut along its length which allows it to be eased off the limb if desired. When replaced it is encircled by strong adhesive bandage which holds it in place. This technique is useful when frequent inspection of the limb is needed during the healing phase. The split cast will also 'give' a little if required and so the method is useful for growing animals. The adhesive bandage is removed and replaced every 1–2 weeks, allowing the cast to expand as necessary in order to incorporate growth of the limb.

Cast removal

> **WARNING**
>
> Care must be taken not to damage the skin and other soft tissues during cast removal.

It is advantageous to have the animal sedated, and sometimes anaesthetised, when removing a cast. An assistant is often useful to hold the cast steady whilst it is being cut.

The most commonly used tools for removing casts are plaster shears and electric oscillating saws. The line of cut is chosen carefully to avoid any bony prominences. **Plaster shears** are inserted at the distal end of the cast and the cut is advanced proximally in small regular steps. As the shears approach the more fleshy proximal limb, the skin can be stretched by the assistant to minimise the risk of damage. Final cutting of the tubular gauze and cast padding can be made with scissors.

The **oscillating saw** is held so that there is no danger of coming into contact with either the skin or the electrical cable supplying the saw. Only the *plaster* is cut – the plaster padding will catch on the oscillating blade and not be cut. The circular blade gets quite hot as a result of its rapid oscillation in contact with the cast and so the saw should be gradually rotated to use a cooler part of the blade. It is often helpful to combine initial oscillating saw cuts with the use of plaster shears to remove a cast quickly and safely.

Extension splints. Extension splints (**Schroeder–Thomas splints**) have largely been superseded by internal fixation techniques and external fixators, but they are still used occasionally. Extension splints are most commonly applied to the hindlimb, but similar structures exist for use in forelimbs.

Extension splints are traction devices designed so that soft bandages act as slings to position the limb on a metal frame and counteract the pull of muscles. In this way the skeleton is immobilised. Indications for extension splints:

- Immobilisation of fractures distal to the middle of the femur in the hindlimb or the middle of the humerus in the forelimb.
- Immobilisation of joints at, or below, the level of the stifle in the hindlimb and the elbow in the forelimb.

Successful use of extension splints is completely dependent on accurate construction, tailored to the size of each individual animal and on accurate positioning of the completed splint on the limb. Failure to use the device properly may increase the risk of non-union. They are difficult to manage and require frequent adjustment to ensure that their position on the limb is maintained.

Internal fixation

Internal fixation, using pins, plates, screws and other devices has both advantages and disadvantages compared with external coaptation.

INTERNAL FIXATION TECHNIQUES

Advantages
- They are suitable for fractures in any bone.
- They are more versatile than external coaptation for handling the full range of fracture types.
- They allow accurate reduction and relatively rigid fixation when compared to casting.
- Internal fixation often allows an early return to full functional limb use – this encourages fracture healing and minimises the risk of fracture disease.

Disadvantages
- They are relatively expensive and time-consuming.
- Some internal fixation techniques are technically demanding.
- There is capital expenditure in the equipment.
- The risks of surgery (wound healing problems, infection) are inherently greater in an open reduction and fixation than in closed reduction and fixation.

In some cases, internal fixation methods may be supplemented with external coaptation or by an external fixator.

Implants used in internal fixation. The commonly used implants for internal fixation of fractures in dogs and cats are:

- Intramedullary pins (Steinmann pins, Kirschner wires, arthrodesis wires and Rush pins).
- Cerclage wire.
- Bone plates (Venables plates, compression plates).
- Screws (tapped or self-tapping).

All of these implants can be sterilised and stored in a routine manner used for any surgical steel instruments.

Other internal fixation devices exist but are less commonly used in veterinary practice. These include intramedullary nails, locking nails and absorbable implants.

Intramedullary pins. The **Steinmann pin** is perhaps the most commonly used internal fixation device for dogs and cats. Steinmann pins are straight pins with sharpened, trocar-point ends. They are driven down the medulla of a fractured bone and across the fracture gap to hold the fragments together. A range of sizes are available to suit different sizes of animal and to fit into the many different sizes of medullary cavity. Selection of the right length and diameter of pin is important for successful fracture repair.

Kirschner wires and **arthrodesis wires** are really thin versions of the Steinmann pin. Like Steinmann pins, arthrodesis wires have a trocar point, but Kirschner wires have a flattened point at one end instead. They may be used as intramedullary pins in small bones, but they also have many other applications in fracture repair.

Rush pins are specialised curved pins which are often used in pairs to anchor small epiphyseal fragments back on to the shaft of a bone. The point of the Rush pin is flattened to form a 'sledge', which is important to the way the pin functions when used in fracture repair.

Cerclage wire. Cerclage wire is malleable monofilament wire which comes in several different sizes suitable for use in different sized animals. It is often supplied on a reel. Cerclage wire is usually used in combination with pins or plates to increase the stability of a fracture. Suitable lengths of wire are cut from the reel as required and they are anchored in place by twisting them with a pair of surgical pliers.

Bone plates and screws. Bone plates are rectangular plates of surgical steel which are fastened to bone using screws. They come in a range of sizes to suit different sizes of dog and cat. Plates are used to 'bridge' fracture gaps and therefore hold fracture fragments together. Screws may also be used to fasten fracture fragments together.

A common pattern of bone plate is the **Venables plate.** These plates are held in place using 'self-tapping' screws. A hole is drilled in the bone and the screws are inserted into the holes. The screws cut their own way into the bone as they are tightened with the screwdriver, in the same way that wood screws cut their own way into wood.

A more sophisticated type of plate is the **compression plate**. These plates are more rigid than the others and are specially designed in a way which allows fracture fragments to be compressed together. This helps to improve rigidity at the fracture site. Compression plates are used in conjunction with tapped screws. Unlike self-tapping screws, the tapped screws are not designed to cut their own way into the bone as they are driven with the screwdriver. Once a hole has been drilled, a special device (the 'tap') is used to cut a thread in the bone to the same shape as that of the screw. The screw is then placed into the 'tapped' hole. The tapped screws have greater holding power in the bone than self-tapping screws. Compression plate systems are more versatile than other plate systems and are capable of handling most fracture situations. However, the equipment for compression plating is very expensive, and the method for using the system is technically demanding. Another plate called a Sherman plate can be used, however it is lightweight and less strong than the Venables plate.

Aftercare of patients following internal fixation

Immediate post-operative management of animals with internal fixation of fractures includes:

- Post-operative radiographs to check that the fracture repair is adequate.
- Monitoring carefully to ensure that the animal is maintaining airway, breathing and circulation and to ensure that it is normothermic.

- Analgesia will be required using either a non-steroidal anti-inflammatory drug (NSAID) or ideally a combination of an NSAID and an opiate analgesic (at the discretion of the veterinary surgeon in charge of the case).
- The use of antibiotics post-operatively is controversial, but most veterinary surgeons will prescribe some antibiotics pre-operatively, which may be continued post-operatively.

When the animal returns home, its owner plays a critical role in its aftercare. They have a natural tendency to be more cautious with animals that are in a cast or splint, which they can see, than with an animal after internal fixation, which they cannot see. The following advice should be given to all owners of animals after internal fixation:

- Although repaired, the fracture is a long way from healed. The animal must be restricted to the house or to a cage. Exercise periods should be on the leash and only for long enough to allow the animal to urinate and defecate (often less than 1 minute).
- Instructions for administration of any medication must be made clear.
- Regular post-operative check-ups will be necessary in the interests of the well-being of the animal and further radiographs will usually be needed. The importance of attending clinics for such check-ups must be emphasised.
- The owners should be instructed about possible complications (see below), how to recognise them and how to seek veterinary advice if these occur.
- In most cases active rehabilitation is not necessary. Some cases may benefit from passive flexion/extension exercises or from non-weightbearing exercise such as swimming once healing is under way. These exercises should only be performed under advice from the veterinary surgeon in charge of the case.
- During the recovery phase, the animal should be fed adequate amounts of a well-balanced diet. Except for certain pathological fractures, the addition of mineral or vitamin supplements is not recommended.
- Suture removal may be necessary 7–10 days after the surgery.

Complications of internal fixation

The complications of internal fixation are those associated with wound healing and with fracture healing. The two most common complications are osteomyelitis and implant failure.

Osteomyelitis. Osteomyelitis may present shortly after internal fixation as an acute inflammation in the region of the fracture. The limb will be hot, swollen and painful. The animal may become systemically ill, inappetent and feverish. In the event of suspected osteomyelitis, veterinary attention is needed to decide the best course of treatment.

Implant failure. The metal implants used for internal fixation may fail either by breaking or by coming adrift from the bones. This will result in a sudden deterioration, with instability and pain returning at the fracture site. Some implant failures are associated with osteomyelitis. Further investigations will be needed to find the cause of the failure and to plan a suitable course of treatment.

Luxations and subluxations

A **luxation** (also called **dislocation**) is a persistent and complete displacement of the opposing articular surfaces of the bones forming a joint.

A **subluxation** is an incomplete displacement of the opposing articular surfaces of the bones forming a joint.

Luxations and subluxations may be classified according to their aetiology into two types: congenital and acquired.

Congenital luxations or subluxations arise as anatomical abnormalities present at birth. The abnormality may or may not be inherited. The most common congenital luxation is that of the patella. This is usually amenable to surgery to replace the patella in its normal position. However, some congenital luxations are so severe that they cannot be corrected. Some small dogs and cats are able to cope with the permanently luxated joint, but in larger animals severe congenital luxation may be a cause of great disability.

Acquired luxations and subluxations result from some form of trauma, such as a road traffic accident. The ligaments restraining the joint in its normal position are damaged and the joint is forced out of alignment. Acquired luxations most commonly occur in the hip and elbow joints. Less commonly affected are phalangeal joints and the hock and acquired luxations of the shoulder are rare. The stifle is a common site for acquired subluxation as a result of rupture of the cranial cruciate ligament.

Treatment of luxations requires restoration of the normal anatomical relationship of the bones of the joint and stabilisation of any ligamentous injuries. Like fracture reduction, reduction of luxations may be achieved in one of two ways:

- **Closed reduction** is the reduction of the joint by manipulation of the limb. Specific manipulations, depending on the joint involved and the direction of displacement of the bones, are essential for successful closed reduction. Simple brute force is unlikely to succeed and may cause further injury.
- **Open reduction** is a surgical approach to the joint: the luxated bones are visualised and manipulated back into the joint.

Closed reduction is preferable to open reduction whenever possible. Reduction is more successful if performed early – a delay of several days results in contraction of the surrounding soft tissues which renders closed reduction difficult or impossible.

Radiographs should always be taken before any attempt is made at reduction. This allows the diagnosis to be confirmed and also determines whether there is any other damage, such as a fracture. Fractures affecting the joint surface will complicate any attempts to reduce the luxated joint.

For many luxations, *general anaesthesia* is required before reduction can be attempted. Some luxations, such as the patella, phalangeal joints and shoulder, may be reduced in conscious animals.

Post-operative care is similar after both open and closed reductions except that open luxations require the added precautions taken following all surgery. The main post-operative aim is to avoid forces that could cause a recurrence of the luxation. Support bandages or non-weightbearing slings are useful for 5–7 days to prevent overuse of the joint. Exercise should be restricted, as for fracture healing, for a period of 3–4 weeks; thereafter, the animal's exercise can be slowly increased again.

Complications that may arise following treatment of luxations include:

- Re-luxation is the most common complication, especially if activity is not sufficiently restricted or if there is other pathology in the joint, such as a fracture.
- Joint infection is a risk, especially if an open reduction has been performed.
- There may be injury to surrounding soft tissues, associated either with the original trauma or with the reduction of the joint. These injuries may not be obvious at first. They include damage to nerves in the region of the joint.

Orthopaedic instrumentation

Orthopaedic surgery is technically complex and involves a wide range of instruments in addition to the standard surgical instrumentation (see Chapter 20, p. 548). It is beyond the scope of this text to provide a fully comprehensive review of orthopaedic instruments, but a brief discussion of the more common instruments is relevant. Care of most of the instruments is routine: they can be cleaned, sterilised and stored like any other surgical instrument (see Chapter 21, p. 559). Some require special attention.

The pin introducer

This consists of a drill chuck on a handle. It is primarily used for driving intramedullary pins into bone, but may be used as a drill on some occasions. The pin introducer is sometimes (incorrectly) referred to as a **Jacob's chuck**, which is actually the part of the introducer that grips the pin. Jacob's chucks may also be found on drills.

Orthopaedic drills

Three basic types of orthopaedic drill are available:

- Hand drills.
- Air drills (driven by compressed air).
- Electric drills (with rechargeable batteries).

Hand drills and air drills can be autoclaved. The moving parts require periodic oiling and specific instructions are provided by the manufacturers for individual drills. Electric drills cannot be immersed in solutions or autoclaved; they are supplied with a cloth 'sock' (shroud) which is autoclaved and encloses the drill when it is in use.

Depth gauge

This is a calibrated instrument used to measure the depth of a drill hole so that the appropriate length of screw can be selected.

Screwdrivers, mallets, chisels and saws

These instruments are surgical steel equivalents of normal carpentry tools. Chisels have one edge of the instrument blade bevelled. This differentiates chisels from osteotomes which have both edges bevelled.

Retractors

Retractors are useful in all sorts of surgery for restraining tissues in the surgical field. Many different types are available and they can broadly be divided into two groups:

- **Hand-held** retractors are held by the surgeon or an assistant to restrain tissues.
- **Self-retaining** retractors have a scissor-like action and some form of ratchet which locks them in place. Once inserted and locked they will remain in place and restrain tissues without being held. Self-retaining retractors are especially useful for surgeons working alone.

Patterns of retractor particularly useful in orthopaedic surgery include **Langenbeck** retractors, **Hohmann** retractors (both hand-held) and **Gelpi** retractors (self-retaining).

Bone-holding forceps

Bone-holding forceps are designed to grasp bones during open reduction of fractures and to hold them in a reduced position whilst definitive fixation is applied. They all have a scissor-like action and some have a ratchet or similar device to enable them to be locked in place. There are many different patterns. The choice of instrument depends partly on the needs of the particular fracture and partly on the personal preference of the surgeon.

Bone-cutting forceps and rongeurs

Bone-cutting forceps are shearing tools designed specifically for cutting through bone. Rongeurs are scissor-action tools designed for nibbling away at bone and removing small bits.

Common surgical conditions

In addition to anatomical terminology and the pathological terms outlined above, surgery has its own extensive terminology (Table 19.4). Surgical terms with similar meanings often share a common suffix such as -otomy, -ostomy, -ectomy, -centesis, -oscopy (which each indicate a different type of surgical procedure) or -itis (which indicates inflammation).

Some of the more common surgical conditions of the dog and cat will now be considered.

Surgery of the eye

Common conditions of the eye amenable to surgery include conjunctivitis, keratitis, entropion, ectropion, distichiasis, tumours and cataracts. There are also several emergency conditions.

Conjunctivitis

Conjunctivitis is inflammation of the conjunctival membrane characterised by reddening of the conjunctiva. It is a frequent sequel to many other ocular diseases, including ocular infections, foreign bodies in the eye, entropion, ectropion and inflammatory diseases of the eyeball.

Keratitis

Keratitis is inflammation of the cornea, which may be accompanied by ulceration. The inflamed cornea is cloudy. The addition of fluorescein to the eye allows better visualisation of corneal ulcers. In severe cases, corneal ulcers may perforate causing the cornea to rupture. Ulcers are treated medically or by creating a protective flap from the conjunctiva or third eyelid. Keratitis and ulceration is often secondary to some other disease of the eye which may also require treatment.

Entropion

Entropion is inversion of the eyelid margin such that the eyelashes rub on the cornea. There is often secondary conjunctivitis and keratitis. Entropion is treated by surgery to return the eyelid margin to its normal position.

Ectropion

Ectropion is eversion of the eyelid margin. In most cases, ectropion does not require surgical attention, but in some dogs it gives rise to chronic conjunctivitis or keratitis, thus requiring surgical correction. Certain breeds of dog exhibit both ectropion and entropion at different points along the margins of one or both eyelids.

Distichiasis

Distichiasis is the most common of a group of disorders characterised by abnormal growth of hairs at the eyelid margin so that the hairs rub against the cornea. In many cases, the hairs do not cause a clinical problem, but in some cases they cause chronic keratitis requiring treatment. Several surgical techniques exist for treating distichiasis, but all centre on removal of the offending hairs.

Tumours

Tumours on the margin of the eyelid are common in dogs. They are generally treated by excising a small wedge of the eyelid margin containing the tumour.

Table 19.4 Surgical terminology

Terminology	Meaning
Temporary openings	The suffix **-otomy** denotes a procedure for temporarily opening or dividing a tissue during surgery. The tissue is closed by allowing it to heal naturally, by suturing it or, in the case of bone, by reuniting it with pins, wires, screws or plates. Many of these terms describe common surgical approaches.
Laparotomy	A temporary opening into the abdomen.
Thoracotomy	A temporary opening into the thorax.
Cystotomy	A temporary opening into the urinary bladder.
Urethrotomy	A temporary opening into the urethra.
Enterotomy	A temporary opening into the intestines.
Gastrotomy	A temporary opening into the stomach.
Arthrotomy	A temporary opening into a joint.
Rhinotomy	A temporary opening into the nasal chambers.
Osteotomy	A temporary division of a bone.
Myotomy	A temporary division of a muscle.
Tenotomy	A temporary division of a tendon.
	Some surgical approaches can be further classified by the precise way in which the procedure is performed. For example, a laparotomy may be made in a number of ways:
Midline laparotomy	By an incision through the linea alba.
Paramedian laparotomy	By an incision slightly to one side of the ventral midline.
Parapreputial laparotomy	By an incision to one side of the prepuce in male dogs.
Pararectal laparotomy	By an incision just lateral to the rectus abdominis muscle.
Paracostal laparotomy	By an incision just caudal to, and parallel with, the last rib.
Permanent openings	The suffix **-ostomy** denotes the surgical creation of an opening, or **stoma**, which has the potential to be permanent.
Urethrostomy	A permanent opening in the urethra.
Tracheostomy	A permanent opening in the trachea.
Gastrostomy	A permanent opening in the stomach.
Pharyngostomy	A permanent opening in the pharynx.
	In some cases, the stoma is left permanently open, but in others further surgery is performed at a later date to close the stoma once again. Stomata are almost always into the airway, gastrointestinal tract or urinary tract. They allow access to these structures for special reasons. For example, animals unable to chew or swallow may be fed through a pharyngostomy or gastrostomy; animals with a blocked urethra will be able to pass urine through a urethrostomy and animals with a blocked upper airway will get air into their lungs through a tracheostomy.
Removal of structures	The suffix **-ectomy** denotes the surgical removal of all or part of a structure. This is commonly performed when neutering animals.
Enterectomy	Removal of a length of bowel.
Gastrectomy	Removal of a portion of stomach.
Lung lobectomy	Removal of a lung lobe.
Ovariohysterectomy	Removal of the ovaries and uterus (spay).
Orchidectomy	Removal of the testis (castration).
Ostectomy	Removal of a portion of bone.
	Enterectomies and gastrectomies are performed to remove irreparably damaged parts of the gastrointestinal tract. When this is done, the remaining ends of the gastrointestinal tract must be sutured back together, a procedure known as **anastomosis**. Although most commonly used in any tissue where free ends can be rejoined; for example, blood vessels, nerves, ureters, urethrae, etc.
Inflammation of tissues	The suffix **-itis** denotes inflammation in a given tissue.
Oesophagitis	Inflammation of the oesophagus.
Gastritis	Inflammation of the stomach.
Enteritis	Inflammation of the small intestine.
Colitis	Inflammation of the colon.
Cystitis	Inflammation of the urinary bladder.
Hepatitis	Inflammation of the liver.
Pancreatitis	Inflammation of the pancreas.
Rhinitis	Inflammation of the nose.
Tracheitis	Inflammation of the trachea.
Dermatitis	Inflammation of the skin.
Arthritis	Inflammation of a joint or joints.
Conjunctivitis	Inflammation of the conjunctiva.
Aspiration of fluid	The suffix **-centesis** denotes the aspiration of fluid from a body cavity.
Cystocentesis	Aspiration of urine from the bladder.
Arthrocentesis	Aspiration of synovial fluid from a joint.
Pericardiocentesis	Aspiration of fluid from within the pericardium.
Thoracocentesis	Aspiration of fluid from the thoracic cavity.
	Fluid may be aspirated so that it can be analysed for diagnostic reasons or it may be aspirated for therapeutic reasons. For example, fluid is not normally present in either the pericardium or the thoracic cavity. The presence of fluid at these sites can be life-threatening and in such cases pericardiocentesis or thoracocentesis are life-saving procedures.
Endoscopic procedures	The suffix **-oscopy** denotes examination by various devices.
Endoscopy	An endoscopic examination
Gastroscopy	Endoscopic examination of the stomach.
Cytoscopy	Endoscopic examination of the urinary bladder.
Arthroscopy	Endoscopic examination of a joint.
	Endoscopy is examination by the use of a fibre-optic device, the endoscope. Endoscopes are available in many different sizes, some small enough to fit into a hip joint or up the urethra, others long enough to reach down the oesophagus, through the stomach and into the small intestine. Other examination devices include:
Bronchoscope	A device for examining the trachea and bronchi via the mouth.
Laryngoscope	A device for examining the larynx via the mouth.
Proctoscope	A device for examining the rectum and distal colon via the anus.
Auroscope	A device for examining the ear canal.
Ophthalmoscope	A device for examining the eyes.

Cataracts

A cataract is the opacification of the fibres or capsule of the lens of the eye. This can occur for many different reasons. Cataracts may be left untreated or they may be treated by surgical removal of the cataract.

OCULAR EMERGENCIES

- **Eyeball prolapse.** Complete prolapse of the eye out of its socket (proptosis of the globe) can occur, especially in brachycephalic dogs. *First aid treatment is important if there is to be any chance of saving the eye.* The eye should be kept moist with K-Y jelly or something similar and gently supported in saline-soaked swabs. Definitive surgery to replace the eye in its socket should be performed as soon as possible.
- **Glaucoma,** an acute elevation in the pressure within the eye which *can lead to permanent blindness within 24 hours if not treated.* There are several causes of glaucoma, but two of the most common are anterior uveitis and dislocation of the lens of the eye from its normal position. This is especially seen in the terrier breeds. In glaucoma, the eye is painful, the sclera is engorged and the pupil is usually dilated.
- **Ocular trauma.** Foreign bodies (including grass seeds, glass and gunshot pellets) may lodge behind the eyelids or they may penetrate the orbit itself. The eyeball may also be lacerated, e.g. by claws or teeth during fights with other animals. All these conditions are potential emergencies and require prompt veterinary attention.
- **Chemical irritation** of the eye by contact with noxious substances may also require emergency treatment. As a first aid measure, the eye should be irrigated with copious amounts of water or saline to remove as much of the offending chemical as possible.

The retina

Although not amenable to surgery in most cases (laser surgery may be used in specialist centres for retinal detachment), the retina is an important site of disease in the eye. Of particular importance are a group of inherited diseases of the retina collectively known as **progressive retinal atrophy (PRA)**. These diseases occur in certain breeds. The British Veterinary Association and the Kennel Club check for PRA by running eye examination schemes, performed by specialist ophthalmologists.

Surgery of the ear

DEFINITIONS

- **Aural haematoma:** A discrete collection of blood in the pinna (ear flap).
- **Otitis:** Inflammation of the ear.

Three subgroups of otitis are recognised:

- **Otitis externa:** Inflammation of the external auditory meatus (ear canal).
- **Otitis media:** Inflammation of the middle ear cavity.
- **Otitis interna:** Inflammation of the inner ear, affecting the organs of balance and, less commonly, hearing.

Aural haematoma

Aural haematoma is the most common injury of the dog's pinna. It is generally believed to be self-inflicted as a result of scratching or head shaking which damages a blood vessel in the pinna. It is most commonly seen on the concave surface of the pinna, but may occur on either or both sides. The injury is usually secondary to otitis, and treatment of aural haematoma must also concentrate on treating the primary cause of the otitis.

Haematomas resolve spontaneously if left alone, but the blood is a good medium for potential infection and the scar tissue that forms during resolution may lead to deformity of the pinna. For these reasons, most aural haematomas are treated by surgical drainage either by needle aspiration or by surgical incision.

After incision, sutures are often placed in the pinna to close the dead space and prevent recurrence. Buttons, quills (lengths of rubber tubing) or some similar devices may be incorporated into the sutures to increase the compression of the dead space and to prevent the sutures pulling through. Post-operative care includes treatment of the primary ear disease and, in some cases, the ears are immobilised in a figure-of-eight head bandage to prevent further damage as a result of head shaking and scratching.

Otitis externa

Otitis externa is very common in dogs and cats. Inflammation of the ear canal may occur for many reasons, including:

- Foreign bodies in the ear canal.
- Ear mites (*Otodectes*).
- Bacterial or fungal infection of the ears.
- As an extension of generalised skin disease.
- Poor ear conformation, especially in the floppy-eared breeds.
- Polyps/tumours.

Veterinary investigation is necessary so that specific treatment can be prescribed for the problem. Animals with otitis externa show irritation, and sometimes pain, centred on the ear.

EAR DROPS

Drugs for the treatment of otitis externa are often administered by ear drops. It is important that the drug carries well down into the ear canal and the veterinary nurse must be familiar with the anatomy of the ear canal so that suitable advice can be given to owners. The drops are first placed into the canal, which is then massaged to encourage distribution of the drugs. Excessive discharge can be cleared with cotton wool or tissue, but owners must be warned against probing down the ear canal with cotton buds or anything similar. If it is necessary to probe down the ear canal, either to retrieve a foreign body or to cleanse the canal thoroughly, this should be done under the direction of a veterinary surgeon as it requires a general anaesthetic.

Cases of otitis externa that do not respond to medical therapy may undergo surgery. Several different surgeries are used for the treatment of otitis externa, including:

- **Lateral wall resection** involves removing the lateral portion of the ear canal to improve drainage from the ear and to improve air circulation in the ear canal.
- **Vertical canal ablation (VCA)** involves the total removal of the vertical part of the ear canal, thus resecting the diseased tissue.
- **Total ear canal ablation (TECA)** involves resection of both the vertical and the horizontal parts of the ear canal. This procedure is more radical and technically demanding than the VCA, but it is finding favour with many surgeons because it removes all the diseased tissue. It must always be combined with currettage and drainage of diseased tissue within the osseous bulla of the middle ear (via a lateral or ventral bulla osteotomy).

Post-operative care following ear surgery is similar for all surgical procedures. The ear must be protected from self-inflicted head shaking and scratching injuries by using an Elizabethan collar, figure-of-eight head bandage or by bandaging the pinnae together as necessary. There is often discharge of blood and exudate from the ear and this needs gentle cleaning. Ear surgery can be very painful and thought should be given to analgesia in the immediate post-operative period.

Otitis media

Otitis media is frequently an extension of otitis externa when infection penetrates the ear drum. In some cases it may arise because of ascending infection via the eustachian tube, from the pharynx. Otitis media is much more difficult to treat successfully than otitis externa, and so prompt therapy of otitis externa is indicated to reduce the risk of otitis media.

Otitis interna

Otitis interna causes a loss of balance and the head tilts to one side. There are other causes of similar findings in old cats and dogs and a careful examination is necessary to tell these apart. Examination may include taking radiographs of the skull. Treatment of otitis interna may include both medical and surgical therapies.

Surgery of the gastrointestinal tract (GIT)

The GIT includes mouth, pharynx, oesophagus, stomach, small intestine, rectum and anus.

The mouth and pharynx

Common conditions of the mouth include:

- Dental disease.
- Congenital deformities.
- Labial (skin fold) dermatitis.
- Foreign bodies.
- Tumours.
- Ulcers.
- Rodent ulcers.
- Stings.

Dental disease

DEFINITIONS

- **Periodontal disease**: Disease of the tissues and structures which surround the teeth.
- **Dental plaque**: A film-like deposit on the surface of the tooth consisting of a mixture including salivary deposits, bacteria and food particles.
- **Dental calculus**: A stone-like concretion of minerals on the teeth.
- **Gingivitis**: Inflammation of the gums.

Periodontal disease, associated with the build-up of dental plaque, is perhaps the most common dental condition encountered in small animal practice. Periodontal disease presents with gingivitis, gingival bleeding, halitosis and, in advanced cases, reluctance to eat because of pain on mastication. The problem is exacerbated by the formation of dental calculus. Although gingivitis is commonly associated with dental disease, it may have a much more complex aetiology, especially in cats.

Veterinary dentistry has now developed into a speciality in its own right and many complex dental procedures are performed. However, the most common dental procedures are still measures of basic dental hygiene aimed at controlling periodontal disease, particularly by dental scaling.

DENTAL SCALING

- General anaesthesia is required. This allows a full examination of the mouth, together with radiographic examination if necessary, before scaling begins.
- Scaling should *never* be performed at the same time as other major surgery. Scaling releases bacteria from the mouth into the blood stream and leads to a high risk of infection in surgical wounds.
- The operator should wear a face mask and protective glasses as defence against aerosol bacteria and calculus liberated from the animal's mouth, particularly when ultrasonic scalers are used.
- The animal's head can be placed on a grill to keep it dry.
- Precautions should be taken to ensure that the animal does not inhale particles of calculus or any other debris released during the procedure. These precautions include: (i) the use of a close-fitting, inflated, cuffed endotracheal tube for maintenance of anaesthesia; (ii) packing the pharynx with a 2.5 cm gauze bandage to occlude the part of the pharynx not occupied by the endotracheal tube (the end of the gauze is trailed out of the mouth as a reminder that it must be removed at the end of the procedure); and (iii) recovery of the animal from anaesthesia in a 'head down' position.
- Large deposits of calculus are initially removed with dental forceps. Smaller deposits are removed with a dental scraper or, preferably, with an ultrasonic scaler. The ultrasonic scaler loosens plaque by liberation of high frequency sound waves which cause the tooth to vibrate. A spray wash helps to cool the tooth and remove the loosened debris. The tip of the scaler is moved lightly and rapidly over the tooth surface. It should not be used to scrape the tooth surface nor should it be centred in one place for prolonged periods as the build-up in heat can damage the tooth. The gingival sulcus should also be gently cleaned.
- The spray on the ultrasonic scaler may include an antiseptic (0.2% chlorhexidine is commonly used).

Dental extractions. Dental extractions are performed for severe periodontal disease and for tooth fractures. Recent advances in veterinary dentistry have led to the preservation of teeth which would previously have been extracted. However, dental extraction is still a common procedure in small animal practice.

GUIDELINES APPLIED TO DENTAL EXTRACTIONS

- The general precautions of anaesthesia and pharyngeal packing are similar to those for dental scaling.
- The tooth is thoroughly loosened using a root elevator. A number 11 scalpel blade may be used with care as an alternative in cats.
- Every effort is made to remove the roots intact and attempts should be made to remove fragments of root should they fracture during the extraction process.
- The canines, upper fourth premolar teeth and first molars of dogs have deep roots which may require reflection of the gum and alveolar bone before they can be adequately loosened.
- Teeth with multiple roots may be sectioned with a dental saw before loosening the fragments and associated roots individually.
- Only when the tooth is thoroughly loosened by root elevation should it be grasped with dental forceps for removal. Excessive force or rocking of the tooth from side to side with the forceps should not be necessary and may lead to complications.
- Haemorrhage from the alveolar socket is usually self-limiting or it can be controlled by packing the socket for a few minutes.

Complications of dental extractions include:

- Incomplete removal of a tooth root.
- Persistent haemorrhage, which may be indicative of a bleeding disorder.
- Secondary fracture of the mandible or maxilla.
- Creation of an oronasal fistula. This is seen especially in extraction of the canine from small dogs or cats.

Congenital deformities. One of the most common congenital deformities affecting the mouth is **cleft palate** and hare lip. Suckling is difficult with this deformity and there may be problems with persistent nasal discharge. Affected animals may not thrive and they are often destroyed at an early age. However, if the puppy or kitten survives to 3 months of age, anaesthesia and corrective surgery may be practical.

Owners can help to prevent the build-up of dental plaque by regularly brushing their pet's teeth, providing the animal is amenable. A 0.2% chlorhexidine solution or a proprietary pet toothpaste may be used for this procedure.

Labial dermatitis. Labial dermatitis associated with bacterial infection of the skin folds around the lips is particularly common in breeds with prominent jowls, such as the spaniels. The infection may be a source of irritation for the dog and also gives off a foul smell which some owners mistake for halitosis. Medical treatment may give temporary relief, but many affected animals require surgery to remove the fold of skin, so that there is adequate air circulation to the area.

Similar skin fold dermatitis problems may occur in any area of the skin liable to the formation of deep folds. These include facial folds in brachycephalic dogs, inguinal folds in overweight dogs and folds at the base of the tail in screwtail dogs.

Foreign bodies. Foreign bodies such as sticks, bones and fish hooks can lodge in the soft tissues of the mouth or between the teeth, or even penetrate the wall of the buccal cavity or the pharynx. All will cause pain associated with the mouth, difficulty in swallowing and excessive salivation. In some cases, radiographic or ultrasonographic examination is helpful in reaching a diagnosis.

The mouth can be examined by inserting ropes or leashes behind the canine teeth of the upper and lower jaws. The ropes are used to pull the jaws apart. Some sticks and bones can be grasped with forceps in the conscious animal and then removed. In other cases a general anaesthetic will be required.

It is important to note that the early clinical signs of **rabies** are similar to those seen with oropharyngeal foreign bodies. Although rabies is unlikely to occur in the UK, it is such a potentially dangerous zoonosis that it must be ruled out before progressing to examine an animal closely for a possible foreign body. If the animal is unknown to the practice, the owner should be questioned carefully about its past history.

Tumours. Tumours in the region of the mouth (including the tonsils) are often locally malignant. Some are amenable to resection using radical procedures which involve removing the tumour *en bloc* with a piece of mandible (**mandibulectomy**) or maxilla (**maxillectomy**). Although these procedures may seem radical at first, they are often the only way of effecting a cure. Furthermore, the cosmetic results are generally good and the quality of life following recovery from surgery is usually excellent.

Some tumours, such as the **epulis**, are benign or locally invasive. Epulides are primarily found on the gum. They can be surgically removed by simple excision, but must always be examined histopathologically since some epulides can invade bone, consequently requiring more aggressive surgery for definitive cure.

Ulcers. Ulcers in the oral cavity have many different causes, including:

● Viruses, such as the 'cat flu' infections.
● Systemic illness, such as kidney failure causing uraemia.
● Dental disease.
● Some oral tumours may ulcerate.

Treatment of the ulcer depends on recognising the underlying cause. Some ulcerative gingivitis in cats has no clear cause and can be very difficult to treat. The use of pharyngostomy or gastrostomy tubes is sometimes useful for managing animals with severe oral ulceration which refuse to eat.

Rodent ulcers are chronic, flat, ulcerated granulomatous lesions occurring on the lips of cats. The cause of rodent ulcers is unknown, but they are often associated with excessive grooming (e.g. 'flea allergic dermatitis' cases). They usually respond to corticosteroid therapy, though recurrence may occur associated with breakdown in flea control in certain cases.

Stings. The oral cavity is a frequent site for bee and wasp stings. Although usually of little significance, stings in this area can become an emergency because the associated swelling may cause obstruction of the airway, especially in brachycephalic breeds. Treatment with corticosteroids and/or antihistamines is usually sufficient to resolve the problem, but some cases may require an emergency tracheotomy to relieve their dyspnoea.

The oesophagus

The two most common conditions encountered in the oesophagus are oesophageal foreign bodies and megaoesophagus.

Oesophageal foreign bodies. Oesophageal foreign bodies are seen far more commonly in dogs than in cats. They are usually bones and most frequently lodge in the thoracic oesophagus, at the level of the base of the heart. In most cases, they can be retrieved, or pushed into the stomach, using either long forceps under fluoroscopic guidance or oesophagoscopy. In a few cases, oesophagotomy via a thoracotomy may be needed for removal. Inevitably, oesophageal foreign bodies produce an oesophagitis and, in severe cases, there may be complete penetration of the oesophageal wall. Post-operative nursing for the oesophagitis may include feeding liquidised food or the placement of a gastrostomy tube.

Megaoesophagus. Megaoesophagus, a flaccid dilatation of the oesophagus, is seen as an idiopathic condition, but also in some disease states, most commonly myasthenia gravis. The flaccidity impairs passage of food from the pharynx to the stomach. This may be eased by feeding affected animals from a height, so that they stand on their hindlegs whilst eating, or by lifting the front end of the animal into the upright position after feeding.

The stomach

Common conditions of the stomach include acute gastritis, gastric foreign bodies, gastric dilatation/volvulus (GDV) syndrome and pyloric stenosis.

Acute gastritis. Acute gastritis is common in dogs because their scavenging habits lead them to dietary indiscretions. The main sign is acute vomiting in an otherwise well dog.

There may also be diarrhoea. These findings are not characteristic for dietary-induced upsets and so persistent vomiting and/or diarrhoea should always be investigated by a veterinary surgeon. Most uncomplicated cases of dietary-induced gastritis respond to complete withdrawal of food for 24 hours followed by a gradual return to normal feeding over a period of a few days. Initially, meals should be small and consist of bland foods. The animal's normal diet is reintroduced gradually as the bland food is withdrawn. All dietary changes are made gradually to prevent recurrence. Some individuals are very prone to dietary-induced gastritis; they should be kept on a very constant diet and may require special diets to control the problem.

Foreign bodies. Foreign bodies which are swallowed and reach the stomach may cause vomiting. A gastrotomy, via a laparotomy, is usually required for their removal. Post-operatively, drinks and bland liquid feeds may be given after 12 hours though solid feeds are usually withheld for 24 hours, after which the normal diet is gradually reintroduced.

Gastric dilatation/volvulus syndrome. *GDV is important because it constitutes an emergency.* It occurs mainly in large, deep-chested dogs but is also seen in some small breeds. It frequently presents shortly after feeding, especially if the meal was large and followed by a period of exercise. Affected dogs become rapidly depressed. They make repeated but unsuccessful attempts to vomit and they salivate profusely. The abdomen swells because of food and gas (from swallowed air) in the stomach. The abdominal swelling is usually severe enough to be noticed by the owners. The swollen stomach presses on the diaphragm and compromises breathing. Once distended, the stomach tends to rotate about its own axis forming a twist (**volvulus**). The volvulus interferes with normal blood supply to the stomach wall and, sometimes, with the blood supply to the spleen. The devitalised tissues become necrotic if the condition is not treated promptly. See Chapter 3, p. 69.

WARNING

GDV has a high mortality rate and swift emergency action is essential to maximise the chances of survival. The first priorities are:

- **Decompression of the stomach**: This may be achieved by passing a stomach tube down the oesophagus, by percutaneous catheterisation of the stomach or by a keyhole laparotomy. In severe emergencies, when the animal may be dying because of respiratory distress, a wide-gauge hypodermic needle can be used to penetrate the most prominent and palpable part of the gas-distended stomach to provide relief until veterinary assistance arrives.
- **Vigorous fluid therapy**: Dogs with GDV develop shock rapidly. Fluid therapy to counter the shock is an important priority.

Once the animal is sufficiently stabilised, surgery is needed to decompress the stomach fully, to resect any devitalised tissues and to return the stomach to its normal position. Further procedures may be performed to anchor the stomach in place. Post-operatively, fluid therapy is maintained for at least 24 hours whilst all oral food and fluids are withheld. If all progresses well, small volumes of water may be given by mouth after 24 hours and then the first small amounts of liquidised food may be given provided the patient does not regurgitate.

Cardiac arrhythmias are an important complication of GDV, often occurring 12–48 hours post-operatively. Frequent routine monitoring by auscultation and by ECG should be performed over this period.

Recurrence of GDV in susceptible animals is common. Precautions to minimise this risk include:

- Surgical anchorage of the stomach (gastropexy).
- Feed several small meals daily rather than one large meal.
- Enforce rest for 1–2 hours after feeding.
- Feed only small amounts of cereal in the diet.
- Ensure biscuit meals are thoroughly pre-soaked.
- Raise food bowl to prevent aerophagia.

Pyloric stenosis. Pyloric stenosis is a congenital deficiency in the anatomy or function of the pylorus which prevents normal emptying of the stomach. Affected puppies or kittens vomit in association with feeding. Surgical correction of the condition is possible.

The small intestine

Common conditions of the small intestine include intestinal foreign bodies and intussusception.

Foreign bodies. Swallowed foreign bodies that reach the small intestine can cause either partial or complete obstruction of the bowel, which leads to vomiting. Complete obstruction rapidly leads the animal into a state of shock requiring fluid therapy before surgery. Most intestinal foreign bodies are removed by enterotomy via a laparotomy. In cases where damage to the bowel is severe, enterectomy may be indicated. Post-operative care is as for gastrotomy (see Foreign bodies above).

Intussusception. Intussusception is the telescoping of one section of the bowel into an adjoining portion. The length of an intussusception may vary from less than a centimetre to several centimetres. It is associated with abnormal intestinal motility for any reason and is especially seen in young animals. It may occur as a complication in animals with diarrhoea. In some cases, the bowel can be reduced to its normal position by gentle traction. Often, however, the affected portion is badly damaged, requiring removal by enterectomy. Recurrences are not uncommon, though the frequency of recurrence may be reduced by enteroplication. Post-operative care is as for gastrotomy.

The rectum

Common conditions of the rectum include rectal foreign bodies, rectal tumours, chronic constipation and rectal prolapse.

> ### NOTE
>
> Most routine surgical or imaging procedures of the rectum require thorough cleansing of the rectum first by withholding food for 24 hours and administering **enemas** prior to the procedure. An enema may be a proprietary brand; or it can be warm soap-and-water which is introduced using a soft enema pump inserted gently and with plenty of lubricant, such as K-Y jelly. Great care must be taken not to injure or perforate the rectal wall, especially in small dogs and in cats. In very small animals, a soft catheter attached to a syringe can substitute for the enema pump. The pump should not be forced if the animal strains against it during insertion. Once in place, the soap and warm water is *gently* flushed into the rectum: it is both dangerous and unnecessary to pump vigorously.

Rectal foreign bodies. Rectal foreign bodies are most often either sharp or impacted bones. They cause constipation and pain which is exacerbated by attempts to defecate. The diagnosis is confirmed by radiography and by digital palpation in sufficiently large patients. In most cases, the foreign body can be manipulated through the anus with the animal under general anaesthesia.

Tumours. Tumours can arise in all sections of the gastrointestinal tract, including the rectum. In the rectum, they can be visualised by proctoscopy or by contrast radiography. Cleansing of the rectum is essential for the successful application of both these techniques.

Chronic constipation. Chronic constipation is a not uncommon disorder in dogs and cats. Many cases respond adequately to the administration of an enema, but manual evacuation is needed in some. Often the constipation is secondary to some other disease problem, such as an enlarged prostate, a tumour of the rectum, perineal rupture or narrow pelvic canal associated with an old fracture of the pelvis. If possible, the inciting disease should be treated as well as giving symptomatic relief of the constipation. The addition of lactulose (a non-absorbed disaccharide) or a bulk laxative to the diet may help to prevent recurrence of constipation.

Rectal prolapse. Rectal prolapse is eversion of the wall of the rectum through the anus. It is usually secondary to chronic straining and may be associated with a rectal tumour. Successful management of rectal prolapse requires treatment of the primary disease as well as reduction of the prolapse itself.

> ### FIRST AID MEASURES FOR A PROLAPSED RECTUM
>
> ● Protect everted mucosa using a lubricant (e.g. K-Y jelly or obstetrical lubricant) and cover with saline-soaked swabs. Simple saline- or water-soaked swabs may be used if lubricants are not available.
> ● Protect the area from self-mutilation, e.g. by application of an Elizabethan collar.

The prolapse is normally reduced under general anaesthesia by manipulation or by a surgical method. A temporary purse-string suture may be placed in the anus to help retain the inflamed rectum in place, but this must be loosened frequently following surgery, to allow normal defecation.

The anus

Common conditions of the anal area include imperforate anus, anal sac disease, anal furunculosis and anal or perianal tumours.

Imperforate anus. Imperforate anus is a congenital problem in which there is failure of the anus to unite with the rectum, thus leaving a complete obstruction to the normal passage of faeces from the moment of birth. The problem can sometimes be corrected surgically.

Anal sac disease. Anal sac disease is very common in dogs. It causes irritation focused on the anal area and affected animals chew at the region or typically drag their backside along the floor. In most cases, there is simple impaction of the anal sacs, often associated with infection. Digital evacuation of the anal sac gives relief in simple cases and this may be combined with systemic or topical antibiotic therapy. Recurrence is common and some cases may develop abscessation of the anal sac. Persistent cases require surgical removal of the anal sacs. Pre-operative preparation for anal sac removal (under general anaesthesia) includes:

● Manual evacuation of the anal sacs.
● Irrigation of the sacs with saline via a fine catheter, such as a tom cat catheter.
● Some surgeons prefer to pack the anal sacs with wax or dental mould prior to surgery.
● Routine pre-operative clipping and skin preparation of the perineum.

In rare cases, the surgery is complicated by faecal incontinence. This results from damage to the nerves to the external anal sphincter during surgery and is usually only a temporary problem. Failure to regain faecal continence 4 weeks following surgery usually indicates permanent incontinence.

Anal furunculosis. This is a deep, chronic, ulcerative infection of the skin surrounding the anus of unknown aetiology. Animals with anal furunculosis may show anal irritation and often have a foul odour. Most cases occur in German shepherd dogs. Sinuses and fistulae are found in the perianal area. Treatment requires thorough surgical debridement of the area and may include cryosurgery. Recurrences are common. Recently, medical therapy using cyclosporin (an immunosuppressive drug) has shown encouraging results.

Tumours. The most common perianal tumour is the **anal adenoma**. This is a benign tumour, primarily of old male dogs. It can become quite large and ulcerate, but responds well to surgical resection. Growth of the tumour is dependent on the male sex hormones and so affected dogs are castrated at the time of tumour removal to prevent recurrence.

The **perianal adenocarcinoma** is a malignant tumour. It is much rarer than the anal adenoma and occurs in both male and female dogs.

Surgery of the respiratory tract

The respiratory tract includes the nose, larynx, trachea and lungs.

The nose

Causes of nasal discharge include:

- Intranasal foreign bodies (especially in dogs).
- Infections:
  - viral (e.g. cat 'flu; canine distemper)
  - bacterial
  - fungal (aspergillosis in dogs)
- Tumours.

In some cases, the discharge is associated with intense sneezing and nose bleeds (**epistaxis**). Epistaxis may also be seen following trauma, such as a road traffic accident. Investigation of these problems usually requires radiography under general anaesthesia and surgical exploration by a rhinotomy may be necessary.

The larynx and trachea

Laryngeal paralysis. Laryngeal paralysis is a disease of unknown cause, usually affecting older dogs. The paralysed larynx impairs breathing. The condition is irreversible, but surgery can be performed to assist air flow through the larynx and thereby help the animal's breathing.

Collapsing trachea. Collapsing trachea affects certain toy breeds of dog. The cervical part of the trachea, the thoracic part of the trachea or the entire trachea may be affected. The collapsed trachea impairs breathing. Treatment is generally medical, though in refractory cases surgery can be performed in an attempt to prevent collapse of the trachea.

Tracheostomy and tracheotomy. **Tracheostomy** is a technique for creating a permanent opening into the trachea, usually halfway down the neck, to bypass an obstruction to breathing in the upper part of the airway. Tracheostomy is rarely indicated in dogs and cats.

Tracheotomy is a potentially life-saving procedure in the event of acute upper airway obstruction: In an emergency, the veterinary nurse should be prepared to perform a tracheotomy, using only local anaesthetic (or even no anaesthetic) if necessary. If a risk of upper airway obstruction is anticipated (e.g. following surgery on the airway) the site on the ventral midline of the neck can be clipped in readiness for a tracheotomy if it proves necessary. In a peracute emergency, time should not be wasted in clipping and surgically preparing the skin. In most cases the airway is not completely blocked and oxygen, delivered by a face mask, provides some relief whilst the tracheotomy is being performed.

PROCEDURE FOR TRACHEOTOMY

- The skin incision is made in the ventral midline, over the trachea, immediately behind the larynx.
- The underlying muscles are gently separated in the midline. This exposes the ventral surface of the trachea so that the cartilaginous rings can be identified.
- A scalpel (usually a number 15 blade) is used to incise the trachea between the second or third pair of tracheal cartilages.
- The incision is kept open by insertion of a tracheotomy tube which is held in place by ties around the neck or by sutures. A stay suture placed in the tracheal ring immediately cranial and caudal to the tracheal incision facilitates easy replacement of the tracheotomy tube if necessary. Tracheotomy tubes are available in a range of sizes to suit different animals.
- In the absence of a suitable tracheotomy tube, an endotracheal tube or any other suitably sized soft tubing, such as the end of a urinary catheter, can be used.
- The end of the tracheotomy tube obstructs with mucus if left without further attention. It must be cleaned at regular intervals, usually every 2–3 hours, with saline. Some tracheotomy tubes have an inner sleeve and an outer sleeve, allowing the inner sleeve to be removed for cleaning before replacing it in the outer sleeve. If this type of tube is not available, the tracheotomy can sometimes be cleared by aspirating mucus with an intravenous catheter or a short length of fine male urinary catheter attached to a 10 or 20 ml syringe.

EMERGENCY AIRWAY

If an animal is close to death because of acute upper airway obstruction, a wide-gauge hypodermic needle pushed quickly through the ventral midline of the neck into the trachea can be life-saving until a proper tracheotomy is established.

In cats and very small dogs, a needle tracheotomy may suffice in place of an open tracheotomy if relief is only required for a short period of time.

Brachycephalic airway obstruction syndrome (BAOS). BAOS is a condition of the short-nosed (brachycephalic) dogs in which the anatomical deformities which are 'normal' for these animals cause respiratory embarrassment because of obstruction of normal airway. The deformities which make up BAOS include:

- Narrow nares.
- Narrow nasal cavity and pharynx.
- An overlong soft palate.
- An overlong tongue.
- Enlarged tonsils
- A narrow (hypoplastic) trachea.

The number and severity of the abnormalities vary between individuals. Many dogs acquire laryngeal ventricle eversion and even laryngeal collapse. Some dogs are so severely affected that they may have acute, life-threatening respiratory distress, particularly in very hot and humid conditions. In this situation, emergency first aid may be required.

FIRST AID MEASURES FOR BAOS

(1) Extend the neck and pull the tongue forwards gently to exteriorise it, deflecting it to the side.
(2) Administer oxygen by a face mask.
(3) Perform an emergency tracheotomy if necessary.
(4) If the animal is overheated, it can be gently cooled by showering with cold water.

Some of the abnormalities that make up BAOS are amenable to corrective surgery. Care is needed with anaesthesia and recovery of these animals. They must be monitored closely until they are fully recovered from surgery and advance preparations should be made in case a tracheotomy is needed. In a small number of cases, corrective surgery is impractical because the deformities may be too extreme or they may be complicated by collapse of the larynx. Tracheostomy is the only option for such animals.

The thorax

A **thoracotomy** is a temporary opening into the thorax to allow surgery on intrathoracic organs such as the oesophagus, lungs, blood vessels and pericardium. There are several different approaches to thoracotomy:

- An incision through the intercostal muscles.
- Rib resection and incision of the underlying periosteum and pleura.
- By sternotomy (splitting of the sternum).

Of these, the intercostal approach is probably the most commonly used in dogs and cats. Following thoracotomy great care is taken to ensure a leak-proof closure and the excessive free air in the pleural cavity must be removed to allow the lungs to re-inflate. **A chest drain** is used to remove the pleural air. This consists of a length of sterile tubing with one end placed in the thoracic cavity and the other end exiting the chest. The outer end may be linked to a water seal which allows continual aspiration of air or it may be occluded with a clamp and excessive air removed by periodic aspiration using a three-way tap and syringe. The tube is normally enclosed inside a chest bandage to keep it clean and prevent excessive movement. Most chest drains can be removed after only a few hours.

Surgery of the urinary tract

The urinary tract includes kidneys, ureters, bladder and urethra.

The kidneys

The kidney is not a common site for surgery. It is sometimes necessary to biopsy a kidney to help make a diagnosis. Occasionally, severe disease such as neoplasia, chronic infection or hydronephrosis requires complete removal of one kidney (**nephrectomy**). The ureter may be removed along with the kidney (**ureteronephrectomy**). The success of nephrectomy is absolutely dependent on the health of the remaining kidney, which must be able to compensate for the lost function.

The ureters

One of the most common surgical conditions of the ureters is **ureteric ectopia**. An ectopic ureter is one which inserts further down the lower urinary tract than its normal insertion in the bladder. They usually insert at the proximal urethra, but may insert as far down as the vagina in females. Ureteric ectopia is a congenital condition seen especially in golden retrievers, labrador retrievers and Skye terriers. One or both ureters may be involved. The condition causes urinary incontinence which is evident from an early age. It presents as a clinical problem in females more commonly than in males. Ureteric ectopia is usually amenable to surgery to replace the ureter at its correct anatomical site in the bladder. Postoperatively it is important for the animals to be monitored to ensure that they can urinate normally. Temporary urinary obstruction sometimes occurs because of swelling of the bladder and may require careful catheterisation. In some cases of ureteric ectopia, ureteronephrectomy is necessary because of secondary damage to the ureter and its kidney.

The bladder

The most common surgery of the bladder is a **cystotomy** to remove **urinary calculi** which can cause an obstruction and/or act as a focus for repeated bladder infections (**cystitis**). As with correction of ureteric ectopia, animals should be monitored closely post-operatively to ensure that they urinate.

The urethra

The urethra of the male is very prone to blockage with **urinary calculi** in both dogs and cats. If not relieved, the obstruction will lead to rupture of the bladder, spillage of urine into the abdominal cavity, uraemia and a rapid death.

Bladder or urethral rupture is also a common complication of pelvic fractures. Animals with pelvic fractures should be monitored extremely carefully for normal urination.

Another common reason for urethral obstruction which may lead to bladder rupture is retroflexion of the bladder into a perineal rupture. An animal with urethral obstruction strains unsuccessfully to pass urine. There may be associated pain and depression. First aid is aimed at providing temporary relief for the overdistended bladder by **cystocentesis**.

CYSTOCENTESIS

- Anaesthesia is unnecessary and sedation is only required in the most fractious of animals. Sedation is contraindicated in very uraemic patients.
- Identify the palpably distended bladder and prepare a small overlying area on the ventrolateral abdomen by clipping and surgical scrubbing.
- Use a 20 gauge (or similar) needle of suitable length for the size of animal, a large syringe and a three-way tap.
- Puncture the bladder through the prepared skin site. Aspirate urine, turn the three-way tap and expel the urine into a bowl.
- Repeat until the bladder is drained.

Surgical removal of urethral calculi can often be achieved by urethral catheterisation and the forcible injection of sterile saline (**retropulsion**). If retropulsion is not successful, the calculi may be removed via a **urethrotomy**. A **urethrostomy** may be created if the calculi cannot be removed or to minimise the risk of recurrence. The urethrostomy can be created at one of two levels, depending on the site of the obstruction:

- Scrotal urethrostomy: at the level of the scrotum (following castration and scrotal ablation). This is the optimal site for obstruction at the level of the os penis, a common site for lodgement of urinary calculi, since the risk of post-surgical complications is low.
- Perineal urethrostomy. This procedure is commonly used in cats, but is unsuitable in dogs because the urethra is deep at this point.

Post-operative care for urethrostomy patients includes:

- Prevention of self-mutilation. The sutures at the urethral stoma are frequently irritant and an Elizabethan collar or similar device is essential.
- Prevention of chafing around the urethral stoma by application of Vaseline or a similar oil-based cream.

Surgery of the genital tract

The genital tract includes testes, prostate, ovaries, uterus, vagina and vulva.

The testes

Orchidectomy is removal of one or both testes. Bilateral orchidectomy (**castration**) is most commonly performed for socialising reasons in dogs and tom cats. The greatest effects are often seen when animals are castrated at a relatively early age. Beneficial effects that may result from castration include:

- Prevention of unwanted breeding.
- Prevention of roaming.
- Prevention of territorial spraying by tom cats.
- Reduction of excessive libido.
- Reduction of aggression.

Orchidectomy may also be performed in the treatment of testicular tumours or otherwise unmanageable infections and to control testosterone-dependent diseases such as anal adenoma and prostatic disease.

The prostate

The prostate is a common site of disease in older male dogs. A range of conditions affect the prostate, including:

- Benign hyperplasia.
- Infections (prostatitis).
- Cyst formation.
- Neoplasia.

These diseases may present with constipation or pain on defecation because of prostatic enlargement or with an abnormal discharge from the prepuce. The discharge is commonly blood or pus and may be associated with urination, or independent of it. Some of these conditions are amenable to medical therapy and others require surgery. Castration is frequently indicated as part of the management of prostatic disorders.

The ovaries and uterus

Ovariectomy (surgical removal of the ovaries) and **hysterectomy** (surgical removal of the uterus) are not common procedures in dogs. Most often complete removal of both organs is performed simultaneously (**ovariohysterectomy** or spaying). Ovariohysterectomy is most commonly performed purely for neutering in females.

The advantages of ovariohysterectomy include:

- Guaranteed absence of unwanted pregnancy.
- Cessation of all oestrus activity.
- Prevention of pyometra (see below).
- Prevention of mammary carcinoma if performed at an early age.

Elective ovariohysterectomy should be avoided during oestrus, pregnancy or false pregnancy. Most surgeons prefer to perform elective ovariohysterectomy approximately 8 weeks after the end of oestrus.

Pyometra. Pyometra, the accumulation of pus in the uterus, may be an infected or a sterile condition and it is life-threatening. It occurs most commonly in middle-aged to old animals which have never had a litter. It often presents shortly after a season. Affected animals are usually depressed and polydipsic. They may have a fever and they often vomit. If the cervix is open (**open pyometra**) there is a vaginal discharge. No discharge occurs if the cervix is closed (**closed pyometra**).

Animals with pyometra frequently need intensive fluid therapy before they are fit for anaesthesia. Ovariohysterectomy is needed as a life-saving procedure as soon as the animal is stable enough for surgery. Intensive nursing is also required in the postoperative phase.

Hysterotomy. Caesarian section (hysterotomy) is performed for the relief of dystocia because of uterine inactivity or foetal obstruction. Much of the nursing associated with the procedure centres on the wellbeing of the young:

(1) Check that the neonate's airway is clear, and remove any remaining amniotic fluid by aspirating or by *carefully* swinging the animal upside down, supporting its body and head.
(2) Wrap the animal in a warmed towel and rub vigorously to dry it and to encourage breathing.
(3) Oxygen may be useful for resuscitation in some cases as are respiratory stimulants such as doxapram hydrochloride.
(4) The umbilical remnant should be ligated with a suitable material and may be treated with an antiseptic solution.
(5) Check for any obvious congenital defects such as cleft palate or imperforate anus.
(6) Keep the animal warm and encourage suckling at the earliest possible opportunity.

The vagina and vulva

Rectovaginal fistula. Rectovaginal fistula is a congenital condition which is associated with imperforate anus.

Surgery can be performed to close the fistula and restore the normal anatomy of both the rectum and vagina.

Vaginal hyperplasia. Vaginal hyperplasia, seen most commonly in brachycephalic breeds, is an exaggerated hyperplastic response of the vaginal mucosa to oestrogen. During the follicular phase of the oestrus cycle, affected bitches have excessive folds of vaginal mucosa which protrude through the vulva. Many owners are concerned that this is a tumour, but the appearance of the tissue in association with the first oestrus makes this unlikely. The exposed tissue is likely to become traumatised.

Treatment of vaginal hyperplasia includes:

(1) Temporary relief by lubricating the exposed mucosa with K-Y jelly.
(2) Surgical resection is possible, but there is a risk of recurrence.
(3) Recurrences can be prevented by ovariohysterectomy or by treatment with progestogens in early proestrus.

Vaginal prolapse. Vaginal prolapse is far less common in dogs than vaginal hyperplasia, but the same breed predispositions exist. Mild prolapses may need no treatment other than protection of the exposed mucosa. Spontaneous regression occurs during the dioestrus period. Attempts may be made to replace the everted tissue under general anaesthesia. Further procedures may be needed in recurrent cases.

Inflamed vulva. In bitches with incontinence or cystitis, the vulva frequently becomes inflamed. Nursing of these cases requires:

- Regular washing and rinsing of the vulva.
- Application of a soothing antiseptic ointment.
- Covering the area with Vaseline or other oily barrier cream.
- Prevention of excessive licking by use of an Elizabethan collar.

Veterinary attention is necessary to diagnose and treat the underlying condition.

Hernias and ruptures

As defined in Chapter 3, p. 73, a **hernia** is an abnormal protrusion of an organ or organs through a physiological opening in the lining of the cavity within which it is normally enclosed. A **rupture** is a pathological tear in the lining of the cavity, through which enclosed organs may protrude.

Most herniations and ruptures affect the abdominal cavity, but some occur elsewhere. Examples outside the abdomen include herniation of the occipital or temporal lobes of the brain under the bony tentorium cerebelli as a complication of space-occupying lesions in the CNS and rupture of the tympanic membrane in severe otitis externa.

Two groups of physiological openings are recognised through which hernias occur: normal openings which may become enlarged, such as the inguinal canals, and openings which should have closed before birth, such as the umbilicus.

Hernias and ruptures share many characteristics. However, most abdominal hernias are lined by an outpouching of the peritoneum, whereas the peritoneum is often torn along with other structures in abdominal ruptures.

Terms used to describe hernias and ruptures include:

- **Reducible**: The contents of the hernia or rupture can be replaced in their original anatomical location via the defect itself.
- **Irreducible** or **incarcerated**: The contents of the hernia or rupture cannot be replaced, usually because of the formation of adhesions in chronic cases.
- **Strangulated**: Devitalisation of the contents of a hernia or rupture because of entrapment of the blood vessels passing through the defect. Strangulation is obviously an emergency.

Hernias and ruptures are primarily described by their location. Common examples include umbilical and inguinal hernias, and diaphragmatic and perineal ruptures.

Umbilical hernias are especially seen in puppies. Small umbilical hernias are of no consequence; hernias tend not to grow with the puppy and therefore becomes less significant with time. However, large umbilical hernias should be surgically corrected to prevent the risk of incarceration of small intestine or other abdominal organs.

Inguinal hernias are more common in bitches than in dogs. In bitches the contents of the hernia may include fat in the broad ligament, the uterus, intestines or bladder. They present as a swelling in the groin extending towards the vulva. In dogs, inguinal hernias can be an emergency because of incarceration and strangulation of a loop of small intestine through the inguinal canal and into the scrotal sac.

Diaphragmatic rupture is commonly associated with violent trauma such as a road traffic accident. The loss of a functional diaphragm hinders breathing and this may be exacerbated by incarceration of abdominal organs in the thoracic cavity. Affected animals are obviously anaesthetic risks when surgery is performed for repair of the rupture or other injuries acquired in the accident.

Perineal rupture occurs almost exclusively in older male dogs. It is associated with degeneration of the muscles of the pelvic diaphragm (primarily the coccygeus and the levator ani muscles). Affected dogs have difficulty defecating and an obvious swelling of the perineum on one or both sides of the anus. Surgical correction is usually necessary and castration helps to prevent recurrence. An important complication of perineal rupture is retroflexion and incarceration of the bladder causing acute urethral obstruction. This constitutes an emergency.

Pre-operative preparation for perineal rupture surgery includes thorough emptying of the rectum by enemas, starting the day before surgery. Postoperatively, bulking agents should be added to the diet to make defecation easier and minimise straining.

Principles of treatment of hernias and ruptures

Correction of both hernias and ruptures is by reduction of the organs followed by closure of the defect. Elongation of the defect and/or breaking down of adhesions may be needed to achieve reduction. Many hernias are thought to have an inherited component and neutering is routinely recommended after hernia repairs to prevent problems in future generations.

Tumours

A tumour is an abnormal swelling of tissue with no physiological use, in which cell growth and replication is uncoordinated and exceeds that of the normal tissue cells. All unexplained lumps and bumps on an animal should be considered as potential tumours until proven otherwise. Many owners are frightened by the implications of a diagnosis of tumour, but they should be reassured that many tumours are benign and, if removed completely, they will not grow again.

Tumours may occur at any site in the body and from any tissue with the potential for growth. However some sites are more common than others and these include:

- Skin.
- The alimentary canal (mouth to anus).
- Mammary glands.
- Lymphatic system (including solid tumours of lymph nodes and, less commonly, leukaemias).
- Bones.

Tumours are broadly classified as benign or malignant.

Benign tumours usually grow quite slowly. They are discrete and encapsulated, and are often movable relative to neighbouring tissues. The suffix '-oma' is often used to describe benign tumours (although there are exceptions) and examples include:

- **Lipoma**: a benign tumour of adipose cells, very common in the subcutaneous tissue in older, overweight animals.
- **Papilloma**: a benign wart-like tumour of epithelial cells, most often seen on the skin of cats and dogs (e.g. at the lip margins, eyelid and ear); they also occur on the bladder epithelium.
- **Melanoma**: a benign skin tumour of melanocytes, but some melanomas (especially in the mucous membrane of the mouth) behave in a highly malignant manner (**malignant melanoma**).
- **Fibroma**: a benign tumour of fibrous tissue, present as firm, superficial tumours of the skin and may be difficult to differentiate from other, more malignant, types of tumour.
- **Adenoma**: a benign tumour of glandular tissue, may be quite common in older dogs (e.g. anal adenoma).

Malignant tumours. Malignant tumours may grow quickly or slowly. They have an indefinite capsule and are usually locally invasive so that they cannot be clearly delineated from neighbouring tissues and are not freely mobile.

Some malignant tumours spread (**metastasise**) very readily to affect other organs. Metastasis may occur in one, or all, of the following ways:

- In the circulation.
- In the lymphatic system.
- By direct contact of tumour cells with neighbouring organs by direct invasion (**extension**) or by exfoliation of tumour cells into a cavity such as the abdomen (**transplantation**).

The most common site for metastases is the lungs, via the circulation.

Malignant tumours are further classified on the basis of the type of tissue from which they arise:

- **Carcinoma**: a malignant tumour arising from epithelial tissues.
- **Sarcoma**: a malignant tumour arising from mesenchymal tissues (mainly connective tissues).

Common carcinomas include:

- **Squamous cell carcinoma**: commonly found in the oral cavity.
- **Transitional cell carcinoma**: in the urinary tract.
- **Adenocarcinoma**: malignant tumour of glandular tissue.

Common sarcomas include:

- **Lymphosarcoma**: commonly seen in association with feline leukaemia virus infection in cats. Also common in dogs.
- **Fibrosarcoma**: malignant tumour in fibrous tissue.
- **Osteosarcoma**: malignant tumour of osteoblasts.

In some cases histopathological examination of sarcomas and carcinomas allows the tumour to be further 'graded' in its degree of malignancy.

Mammary tumours. Mammary tumours deserve special consideration because they are the most common site of neoplasia in female dogs. They are especially seen in older entire bitches (neutering early in life significantly reduces the risk of mammary neoplasia). Mammary tumours can appear in any of the five pairs of mammary glands in bitches, but the two caudal pairs are most frequently affected. In queens, all four pairs of mammary glands are at equal risk of developing mammary tumours.

In bitches, benign tumours (**mixed mammary tumours**) are most common, comprising almost 50% of cases. Benign mixed mammary tumours are curable by complete resection. Malignant mammary tumours include adenocarcinomas and sarcomas. Metastasis via the lymphatics or blood stream is common with all malignant mammary tumours, but survival times after surgery vary dramatically with the exact type and histopathological grade of tumour.

Most mammary tumours of queens are highly malignant mammary carcinomas or adenocarcinomas which metastasise very readily.

Biopsies and prognoses

A **biopsy** is a sample of tissue or other material obtained for diagnosis, prognosis and to aid in planning therapy. A **prognosis** is a prediction of the course or outcome of a disease.

In all cases, it is important to define the type of tumour clearly. The prognosis and treatment is very different for different tumour types. Benign tumours can often be completely cured and significant steps have now been made in the treatment of many malignant tumours. Although much can be implied from the history and examination of a tumour, the only way to type the tumour exactly is to obtain a biopsy for cytological and/or histopathological examination. Several different techniques exist for obtaining biopsies including:

- Needle aspiration.
- Needle core biopsy.
- Punch biopsy (skin and superficial lesions).
- Trephine biopsy (bone).
- Incisional biopsy.
- Excisional biopsy.

Needle aspiration. Needle aspiration involves the insertion of a fine hypodermic needle into the tumour. Cells collected in the lumen of the needle are spread onto a microscope slide for cytological examination by depressing the plunger of an attached air-filled syringe. It is a useful preliminary examination technique for many lumps, but is especially used for collecting bone marrow for examination. There is a special bone marrow biopsy needle, consisting of a stiff outer core and an inner stylet. Bone marrow is usually obtained from the wing of the ilium, but may be collected from other sites. Sedation and local anaesthesia or general anaesthesia is necessary. The overlying skin is prepared as for surgery and a small stab incision made. The bone marrow biopsy needle, complete with stylet, is inserted through the incision and driven through the bone cortex. The stylet is removed, the syringe is attached and bone marrow is aspirated. Needle aspiration of superficial soft tissue tumours or lymph nodes may be performed with a 19 gauge needle and 10 ml syringe without recourse to sedation or anaesthesia.

Needle core biopsy. Needle core biopsies are small cylinders of tissue obtained with a purpose-designed instrument. Several patterns of core biopsy needle exist, but the 'true-cut' type is one of the most popular: it has a central obturator, which is notched and an outer sleeve or cannula with an attached handle. Local or general anaesthesia and aseptic preparation of the overlying skin is required. A stab incision is made and the obturator is inserted into the tumour tissue. The cannula is then advanced over the obturator so that the core of tissue is trapped in the notch in the obturator. The needle and biopsy are then withdrawn

Punch biopsy. Punch biopsies are obtained from superficial tissues using a punch which is a small, sharp circular blade a few millimetres in diameter.

Trephine biopsy. Trephine biopsies of bone are obtained with a circular cutting tool (**trephine**) a few millimetres in diameter which removes a core from the bone in much the same way that an apple corer removes the centre section of an apple.

Incisional biopsy. Incisional biopsies involve removal of a small part of the tumour, often a wedge, by a surgical incision. They have the advantage over needle biopsy techniques of obtaining a significantly larger piece of tissue, thus improving the chances of successful diagnosis from the biopsy. However, they have the disadvantage of requiring a full surgical procedure in order to obtain them.

Excisional biopsy. Excisional biopsies involve the complete removal of all identifiable tumour tissue. They are especially useful for suspected benign lesions because, if complete, they negate the need for a second surgery to treat the tumour.

PRESERVATION OF BIOPSY SPECIMENS FOR HISTOPATHOLOGY

- Specimens should be fixed in a large volume of fixative for 24–48 hours. They may then be transferred to a smaller volume of fixative for postage to a pathologist.
- For most routine histopathology, 10% formal saline is the fixative of choice.
- Thin sections of tissue (less than 5 mm) are preferred to large masses because they fix more rapidly. If possible, margins of normal tissue should be included with the suspected tumour tissue.
- For large excisional biopsies, it is helpful to send the whole specimen to a pathologist so that it can be examined to determine if all tumour tissue has been removed. Rapid fixation can be facilitated by incomplete thin sectioning of the tissue. Alternatively, a single thin slice of the tissue can be fixed separately for identification and the remainder can be fixed whole.
- Care must be taken to satisfy posting regulations for pathological specimens, as described in Chapter 13, p. 347.
- The pathologist should be sent a detailed history of the case under separate cover.
- The owner should be warned to expect a delay, usually of 1–2 weeks, before a result is obtained. Longer may be needed for bone biopsies, which must be decalcified before they are sectioned for histological examination.

Treatment of tumours

Especially when treating a tumour that is ultimately incurable, it is important to bear in mind the goal of therapy. If there is no hope for cure, the only remaining goal is preservation of an acceptable quality of life for as long as possible.

Most tumours are likely to be treated by surgical excision. **Debulking** is a procedure to remove as much tumour tissue as possible when complete excision is impractical. There are several other tumour therapies:

- **Chemotherapy** is the use of drugs to kill tumour cells selectively. Chemotherapy is a successful way of treating some tumour types.
- **Radiotherapy** is the use of radiation to selectively kill tumour cells. Although a useful mode of treatment for some tumour types, radiotherapy is limited to use in a few specialised centres.
- **Hyperthermia** is the local application of heat to tumours. It can aid selective killing of tumour cells, particularly in conjunction with radiotherapy.
- **Cryosurgery** is where tumour tissue is destroyed by the local application of extreme cold.
- **Combined modality** or **multi-modality** therapy is when more than one method of treatment is used on a single tumour. An example is the combination of hyperthermia and radiation given above, but many other combined modality therapies exist.
- **Adjunctive therapy** is important in tumour therapy as it is in many other diseases. Adjuncts to the treatment of tumours are dictated by the problems of individual patients, but may include analgesia, nursing management of open wounds and antibiotics, amongst others.

Finally, **counselling** is a crucial part of successful cancer therapy. Full, frank and sympathetic discussions with the owner are necessary at each and every stage. This is usually the responsibility of the veterinary surgeon in charge of the case, but many owners gain great comfort from a compassionate, reassuring nurse.

Further reading

References prefixed by an asterisk are texts based on human nursing. Nevertheless, the general principles apply and these books remain useful because of a dearth of similar texts on veterinary nursing.

*Crawford Adams, J. and Hamblen, D. L. (1992) *Outline of Fractures*, 10th edn, Churchill Livingstone, Edinburgh.

*Morison, M. J. (1992) *A Colour Guide to the Nursing Management of Wounds*, Wolfe Publishing, London.

Slatter, D. H. (ed.) (1993) *Textbook of Small Animal Surgery*, 2nd edn, W. B. Saunders, Philadelphia.

Stead, C. (1988) External support for small animals. *In Practice*, July edn.

Taussig, M. J. (1981) Inflammation. In: *Processes in Pathology. An Introduction for Medical Students*, Blackwell Scientific, Oxford.

*Westaby, S. (ed.) (1986) *Wound Care*, William Heinemann, London.

Theatre practice

D. McHugh

The veterinary nurse is usually given the responsibility for running the operating theatre. This involves maintenance of hygiene in the theatre; care and maintenance of instruments and equipment, preparation of theatre, the patient and the surgical team, and assistance as both scrubbed and circulating nurse.

The most important factor in successful theatre practice is the establishment and maintenance of a good **aseptic technique**, i.e. all the steps taken to prevent contact with micro-organisms.

DEFINITIONS

- **Sepsis.** The presence of pathogens or their toxic products in the blood or tissues of the patient. More commonly known as **infection**.
- **Asepsis.** Freedom from infection, i.e. exclusion of micro-organisms and spores.
- **Antisepsis.** Prevention of sepsis by destruction or inhibition of micro-organisms using an agent that may be safely applied to living tissue.
- **Sterilisation.** The destruction of all micro-organisms and spores.
- **Disinfection.** The removal of micro-organisms but not necessarily spores.
- **Disinfectant.** An agent that destroys micro-organisms – generally chemical agents applied to inanimate objects.

Factors influencing the development of infection

Infection of a clean surgical wound is always a matter of great concern to surgeons. Obviously it is far better to prevent infection than to try and treat it. The use of antibiotics should not be relied upon to protect patients from the consequences of poor asepsis.

It has been established that most surgical wound infections occur at the time of surgery, not during the postoperative period. Poor aseptic technique will undoubtedly affect the success of any surgery and in the long term the success and reputation of the practice. Strict theatre discipline is essential if high standards are to be maintained. There has to be a specific protocol that is adhered to rigidly and that everyone involved with surgery respects. This will include correct theatre attire, scrubbing-up procedures, patient preparations, draping techniques, sterilisation, organization of surgical lists, cleaning protocol and conduct during surgery.

Sources of contamination in the operating theatre include:

- Operating room and environment.
- Equipment and instruments.
- Personnel.
- Patient.

Operating room and environment

Many micro-organisms are airborne and any movement within the operating theatre will disperse them. Good ventilation is necessary as hot, humid conditions are a great threat to asepsis. Cleaning procedures should be performed first because micro-organisms from contaminated sites will remain in the air. The operating room itself must be easily cleaned and should contain as little furniture and shelving as possible.

Equipment and instruments

All equipment and instruments used in the operative site must be sterile. There must be a new set of instruments for each operation.

Personnel

The more people present in theatre, the greater the likelihood of infection. All theatre personnel should wear theatre clothing, caps, masks, scrub suits and anti-static footwear. These are only worn in the designated theatre area. In addition, those who are in the surgical team should prepare their hands aseptically and wear sterile gowns and gloves.

The patient

The patient is probably the greatest source of contamination, especially as animals are covered in hair. The source of micro-organisms may be:

- **Endogenous** – those that originate from within the body of the patient.
- **Exogenous** – those that are found on the outside, i.e. the skin and coat. This term is also used with reference to environmental sources of micro-organisms (e.g. air, equipment, etc.).

It does not necessarily follow that introduction of micro-organisms will result in an infected wound. Micro-organisms can and will enter any wound that has been exposed to air but whether infection follows depends on several variable factors, including the balance between the **virulence** (disease-producing ability) of the organism and the resistance of the patient. Other factors that influence wound infection include:

- Duration of surgery – bacterial contamination increases the longer the wound is open. Infection rate doubles for every hour of operative time.
- Surgical technique – excessive trauma to tissues and damage to vascular supply may increase the likelihood of infection.
- Impaired host resistance – this may increase the risk of infection if it is due to drugs, nutrition or underlying disease.
- Contamination of the wound – surgical wounds are classified with respect to their potential for contamination and infection.

CLASSIFICATION OF SURGICAL WOUNDS

- **Clean** – where there is no break in asepsis. The respiratory, gastrointestinal and urinary tracts are not entered and there is no break in aseptic technique.
- **Clean-contaminated** – where a contaminated area is entered but without spillage or spread of contamination (i.e. ingesta, urine, mucus). Minor break in asepsis.
- **Contaminated** – where there is spillage from a viscus or severe inflammation is encountered, but no infection present. Open fresh traumatic wounds.
- **Dirty** – infected where there is pus present or viscus perforation spilling pus. Traumatic wound containing devitalised tissue or foreign bodies.

Sterilisation

All instruments, implants and equipment which are to be used during surgery must be sterilised before use. There are several different methods of sterilisation available. Choice will depend on:

- Amount and type of equipment to be sterilised.
- Financial constraints.
- Room available.

Each method has both advantages and disadvantages. Selection is based on the requirements of the individual practice or hospital. Usually several different methods will be chosen. They must be efficient, safe and economical. Sterilisation can be divided into two types (Table 20.1).

Table 20.1 Cold and heat sterilisation

Cold sterilisation	Heat sterilisation
Ethylene oxide	Dry heat
Formaldehyde	Hot-air oven
Chemical solutions	High vacuum oven
Glutaraldehyde	Convection oven
Commercial solutions	Autoclave (steam under pressure)
Alcohol-based	Vertical
Irradiation	Horizontal
	Vacuum-assisted

Cold sterilisation

Ethylene oxide

Ethylene oxide is a highly penetrating and effective method of sterilisation. However, concerns have been expressed about its use in veterinary practice as it is toxic, irritant to tissue and a very inflammable gas. Currently its use is permitted and the danger to operators should be negligible as long as the manufacturer's recommendations are followed. COSHH Regulations may however make its use impractical in some veterinary practices. Ethylene oxide inactivates the DNA of the cells, thereby preventing cell reproduction. The technique is effective against vegetative bacteria, fungi, viruses and spores. Several factors influence the ability of ethylene oxide to destroy micro-organisms, including temperature, pressure, concentration, humidity and time of exposure. As temperature increases, the ability of ethylene oxide to penetrate increases and duration of the cycle shortens. However the only system available in the UK operates at room temperature for a period of 12 hours.

Use of the ethylene oxide steriliser. The steriliser consists of a plastic container which is fitted with a ventilation system to prevent gas entering the work area. It should be located in a clean, well-ventilated area (e.g. fume cupboard) away from working areas. The temperature of the room must be at least 20°C (68°F) during the cycle.

Individually packed items to be sterilised are placed in a polythene liner bag. A gas ampoule containing ethylene oxide liquid is placed within the liner bag which is then sealed with a metal twist tie and placed in the steriliser unit. The top of the glass vial is snapped from outside the liner bag to release the sterilant gas. The door to the steriliser unit is closed and locked, the ventilator turned on and the items left to sterilise. The sterilisation process is frequently performed overnight. At the end of the 12-hour period a pump is switched on to aerate the container. The door may be opened after 2 hours and the load removed.

The items should then be left for a further 24 hours in a well-ventilated room to allow the ethylene oxide to dissipate.

Items which may be sterilised using ethylene oxide. Ethylene oxide is effective for the sterilisation of many different types of equipment but its use is limited by the size of the container, the duration of the cycle and concerns about toxicity. Its use therefore tends to be restricted to items which are damaged by heat:

- Fibre-optic equipment.
- Plastic catheters, trays, etc.
- Anaesthetic tubing, etc.
- Plastic syringes.
- Optical instruments.
- High-speed drills/burrs.
- Battery-operated drills.

Some commercially available products are now sterilised by this method, e.g. syringes, synthetic absorbable suture materials and catheters. Avoid sterilising equipment made of polyvinylchloride (PVC) by this method as it may react with the gas.

Preparation of materials for sterilisation. Materials to be sterilised by ethylene oxide must be cleaned and dried. The presence of protein and grease will slow the sterilisation process. Water on instruments at the time of exposure may react with the gas and reduce its effectiveness.

Occlusive bungs, caps or stylets must be removed from instruments so that gas can penetrate freely. Syringes should be packaged disassembled.

Ethylene oxide penetrates materials more readily than steam so a wider variety of packaging materials may be used when preparing items for sterilisation and storage. However, nylon film designed for autoclaving should not be used as it has been shown that there is poor penetration by ethylene oxide.

Testing efficiency of ethylene oxide sterilisation

Indicator tape with yellow stripes which turn red when exposed to ethylene oxide may be used as an indicator of exposure to the gas, but they do not guarantee sterility as they give no indication that exposure was for the correct length of time. In fact, the colour change will occur after a very short period.

Chemical indicator strips which undergo a colour change when exposed to ethylene oxide for the correct time may be placed in the centre of a pack or load to test the penetration efficiency.

Spore strips placed into a load are added to a culture medium on completion of the cycle and are incubated for 72 hours. This is a useful test of the efficiency of the system but is obviously not suitable as an immediate indicator of sterility.

Formaldehyde

In the past formaldehyde gas was used in a similar way to ethylene oxide but it has been largely superseded and COSHH Regulations have limited its use.

Chemical solutions

This method should really only be considered as a means of disinfection although some manufacturers guarantee sterilisation following prolonged immersion (usually 24 hours).

It remains a useful method for surgical equipment which may not be sterilised by any other means. It has gained particular popularity for the disinfection of endoscopic and arthroscopy equipment.

Care should be taken to use the specific concentrations and time stipulated by the manufacturer. Before immersion, check with the manufacturer that the equipment will not be damaged by wet disinfection. The chemical solution and the article to be disinfected should be placed in a tray or bowl, preferably with a lid to prevent evaporation and contamination by airborne micro-organisms. Following immersion in chemical solutions, instruments should be rinsed in sterile water before use. Chemical solutions should be discarded after use and a fresh solution made up each time.

Glutaraldehyde

Until recently this was the most widely used solution for chemical disinfection. Although readily available, COSHH Regulations prevents its use in veterinary practice.

Commercially produced solutions

There are a number of chemical disinfectant solutions produced commercially. Some are ready for use, others require dilution (usually with purified water) prior to use.

Alcohol-based solutions

A variety of these have been used, e.g. ethyl alcohol and isopropyl alcohol. They work by denaturation and coagulation of proteins.

Irradiation

This form of sterilisation is a form of gamma irradiation and can only be carried out under controlled conditions within industry.

Many pre-packaged items are sterilised by this method, including suture materials and surgical gloves.

Heat sterilisation

Dry heat

Dry heat kills micro-organisms by causing oxidative destruction of bacterial protoplasm. Micro-organisms are much more resistant to dry heat than when heated in the presence of moisture and so higher temperatures are required (150–180°C). Dry heat below 140°C cannot destroy bacterial spores in less than 4–5 hours.

The range of equipment sterilised in this way is restricted: fabrics, rubber goods and plastic cannot withstand these high, dry temperatures and are easily damaged.

There are certain items for which dry heat sterilisation is the method of choice. These include glass syringes, cutting instruments, ophthalmic instruments, drill bits, glassware, powders and oils.

Table 20.2 Temperature and time ratios recommended for hot-air ovens		
Item	Temperature (°C)	Time (min)
Glassware	180	60
Non-cutting instruments		
Powders, oils	160	120
Sharp-cutting instruments	150	180

Hot-air ovens. These are heated by electrical elements (Table 20.2). They are usually small but are economical in terms of purchase and running costs. They have been largely superseded by the autoclave, which is more efficient and suitable for most types of material.

A long cooling period is needed before the items may be used. The door should be fitted with a safety device to prevent it being opened before the oven is cool. It is important to ensure that the oven is not overloaded and that items are placed so that air can flow freely.

Spore strip tests and Browne's tubes are available which are designed specifically for testing sterility in hot-air ovens.

Monitoring efficacy of sterilisation

Other types of dry heat steriliser include high vacuum assisted ovens and convection ovens, though neither type is commonly used in current veterinary practice. **High vacuum assisted ovens** are fully automatic and incorporate a vacuum system that reduces the time required for sterilisation to approximately 15 minutes for most articles. Mechanical **convection ovens** incorporate a motor blower to circulate the air and are designed to achieve a uniform temperature in all parts of the unit.

Steam under pressure (autoclave systems)

Steam under pressure is the most widely used and efficient method of sterilisation. It is also the most economical, although the initial outlay may be large. Items which may be sterilised in the autoclave include:

● Instruments.
● Drapes.
● Gowns.
● Swabs.
● Most rubber articles.
● Glassware.
● Some plastic goods.

Heat-sensitive items which may be damaged in the autoclave include fibre-optic equipment, lenses and plastics (especially those designed to be disposable, such as catheters).

The three main types of autoclave are the vertical pressure cooker, the horizontal or vertical downward displacement autoclave and the vacuum-assisted autoclave.

Vertical pressure cooker. This is a very simple machine which operates by boiling water in a closed container like a household pressure cooker. It usually has an air vent at the top which is closed once the air has been evacuated, and pressure (15 p.s.i.) is allowed to build up. As the air vent is at the top, the main disadvantage of this type of autoclave is the danger that some air will be trapped underneath the steam. The temperature in this area will be lower and sterility cannot be guaranteed. Also, as it is manually operated there is room for human error in the sterilising cycle.

Horizontal or vertical downward displacement autoclave. This type is larger and usually fully automatic. It uses an electrically operated boiler that is incorporated in the autoclave as a source of steam. Air is driven out more efficiently by downward displacement. There is an air outlet at the bottom and a steam outlet at the top.

Most of these machines are designed for loose instrument sterilisation only, rather than packs, as they have insufficient penetrating ability and drying cycles: packs may seem to be dry but they remain damp, allowing entry of micro-organisms during the storage period.

There is usually a choice of programmes on this type of autoclave with temperatures of 112, 121, 126 or 134°C.

Vacuum-assisted autoclave (porous load). This type of autoclave works on the same principle as the other two but uses a high vacuum pump to evacuate air rapidly from the chamber at the beginning of the cycle. Steam penetration after evacuation is almost instantaneous and sterilisation occurs very quickly. A second vacuum cycle rapidly withdraws moisture after sterilisation and dries the load. It is suitable for all types of instruments, drapes and equipment and there is a choice of cycles using different temperatures and pressures.

Vacuum-assisted autoclaves are fully automatic, with failsafe mechanisms (usually warning lights and alarms) which indicate whether the load is non-sterile or has been sterilised effectively. They are generally much larger and more sophisticated than other types and are invariably connected to a central boiler to supply steam. The cost of purchase and maintenance are higher, but the machine's efficiency and reliability in sterilisation far outweigh those of the smaller types.

Principles of sterilisation using steam under pressure

Although autoclaves vary in size and type the basic principle of function remains the same. When water boils at 100°C it is converted to steam and the temperature remains the same however long it is heated. Many bacteria, spores and viruses are resistant to heat, and remain unchanged even if exposed to such a temperature for a long time. By increasing the pressure, the temperature of the steam is raised and resistant micro-organisms and spores will be killed by coagulation of

Table 20.3 Autoclave temperature, pressure and time combinations		
Temperature (°C)	Pressure (p.s.i. [kg/cm²])	Time (min)
121	15 [1.2]	15
126	20 [1.4]	10
134	30 [2]	3½

It should be noted that this is only the sterilising time. The length of the whole cycle will vary from 15 to 45 minutes.

cell proteins. It is the increased temperature, not the increased pressure, that leads to this destruction of micro-organisms. The higher the temperature, the shorter the time needed to achieve sterilisation (Table 20.3).

The autoclaving process. The central sterilising chamber of the autoclave is surrounded by a steam jacket. The pressure in the jacket is raised (depending on the cycle). Steam then enters the chamber and as it does so air is displaced downwards, because steam is lighter. When all the air is evacuated, exhaust vents are closed and steam continues to enter until the desired pressure is reached. The more sophisticated types of autoclave have a vacuum prior to introduction of steam to displace air from materials to be sterilised. If any air remains in the chamber the temperature will be lower than steam at that pressure and sterility cannot be guaranteed.

Once the air had been evacuated, steam that has entered the chamber begins to condense on the colder surfaces in the chamber, i.e. instruments, etc. The steam produces heat which penetrates to the innermost layer of the pack. The moisture increases the penetrability of the heat. After the given amount of time the steam is exhausted. As the temperature drops, the pressure returns to normal. In vacuum-assisted autoclaves the instruments are then heat dried: filtered air replaces the exhausted steam. On modern machines the door cannot be opened until the end of this stage.

Effective sterilisation also depends on correct loading of packs into the autoclave. There should be adequate space between them to allow steam to circulate freely. Care should be taken to avoid overloading and blocking of the inlet and exhaust valves. Before packing for sterilisation, instruments must be free of grease and protein material to allow effective penetration of steam.

Maintenance of the autoclave. All types of autoclave should be serviced by a qualified engineer to ensure that they remain in good working order and remain electrically safe. Vacuum-assisted autoclaves with a separate boiler should be serviced every 3 months to comply with health and safety regulations. Thermocouple testing is recommended at least annually to ensure effective sterilisation is taking place.

Monitoring efficacy of sterilisation in the autoclave. **Chemical indicator strips** show colour changes when the correct temperature, pressure and time have been reached. A strip is placed inside each pack. It is important that the appropriate strip is used for each different pressure/time/temperature cycle, otherwise a false result may be given.

Browne's tubes work on the same principle, i.e. a colour change. Small glass tubes are partly filled with an orange-brown liquid which changes to green when certain temperatures have been maintained for a required period of time. Tubes are available which change at 121, 126 or 134°C. It is essential to ensure that the correct type of tube is selected for any particular temperature cycle. Browne's tubes are also available for hot-air ovens.

Bowie–Dick indicator tape is commonly used to seal instrument and drape packs. It is a beige-coloured tape which is impregnated with chemical stripes that change to dark brown when a certain temperature is reached (121°C). As with ethylene oxide indicator tape, it is not reliable as an indicator of sterility as it does not ensure that the temperature was maintained for the required time.

Spore tests are strips of paper impregnated with dried spores (usually *Bacillus stearothermophilius*). A strip is included in the load; on completion of the cycle it is placed in the culture medium provided and incubated at the appropriate temperature for up to 72 hours. If the sterilisation process has been successful, the spores will be killed and there will be no growth.

Spore systems are more accurate than chemical indicators but the delay in obtaining results is a major disadvantage. A combination of both systems is recommended: chemical indicators should be included in each pack and spore strips should be used at regular intervals.

Vacuum-assisted autoclaves will usually have visible temperature and pressure **gauges** on the front. Some systems have a paper **recording chart** which indicates the efficiency of sterilisation.

Thermocouples (electrical leads with temperature-sensitive tips) are placed in various parts of the sterilising chamber with the leads passed out through an aperture to a recording device outside. The temperature within the chamber can be constantly recorded throughout a cycle to check that required temperatures are received and held for the specified time.

Moist heat (boiling)

Boiling should no longer be considered as a method of sterilisation. It cannot be guaranteed to kill all micro-organisms and spores, because the maximum temperature of 100°C is insufficient to kill resistant spores. With far superior sterilisation methods available, the old-fashioned boiler has no place in modern veterinary surgery.

Packing supplies for sterilisation

Various materials and containers are available for packing supplies for sterilisation, each having advantages and disadvantages. Choice will depend on several factors:

- Size of autoclave/gas steriliser.
- The packaging material must be resistant to damage when handled and not damage the equipment to be sterilised.
- Steam or gas must be able to penetrate the wrapping for sterilisation to occur and must be easily exhausted from the pack once sterilisation is complete.
- Micro-organisms must not be able to penetrate from the outer surface of the wrap to the inner.
- Cost.
- Personal preference.
- Time taken to achieve sterility.

Materials and containers

Nylon film. Nylon film designed specifically for use in the autoclave is available in a variety of sizes. It has the advantages of being reusable and transparent so that items can be easily seen. Its main disadvantage is that it becomes brittle after repeated use, resulting in development of tiny unseen holes and therefore contamination of the pack. It may also be difficult to remove sterile items from packs without contaminating them on the edges of the bag. The packs are often sealed using Bowie–Dick tape.

Seal-and-peel pouches. Disposable bags, consisting of a paper back and clear plasticised front with a fold-over seal, are available in a wide variety of sizes. They may be used with ethylene oxide or the autoclave. The risk of contamination during opening is small. Double wrapping decreases the risk of damage to the instrument during storage or when opening the pack. They are most suitable for individual instruments.

Paper. Paper-based sheets are commonly used for packing instruments. The most suitable type consists of a crepe-like paper which is slightly elastic, conforming and is water-repellent. It is therefore ideal as an outer layer for packs. Although it is frequently re-used, it is intended to be disposable. It is available in large sheets which can be cut to the appropriate size.

Textile. Textile sheets, usually linen, are commonly used to wrap surgical equipment for sterilisation. They are conforming, strong and reusable but have the major disadvantage of being permeable to moisture. Usually a double layer of linen is covered by a waterproof paper-based wrap for surgical packs.

Drums. Metal drums with steam vents in the side which are closed after sterilisation are commonly used in veterinary practice, especially with the small portable autoclaves. They can be used for instruments, gowns and drapes. Their main disadvantage is that they are frequently multi-use, so that there is a degree of environmental contamination each time the lid is opened. There is also a risk of contamination of items touching the edge or outside of the drum when they are removed. Initial outlay is relatively high but they will last for years.

Boxes and cartons. A variety of boxes and cartons are available for use in the autoclave. They are useful for gown or drape packs and for specialised kits (e.g. orthopaedic kits). They are relatively inexpensive and may be re-used.

Care and sterilisation of equipment

Gowns and drapes

After use, surgical gowns and drapes should be washed, dried and inspected for damage. Gowns should then be folded correctly so that the outside surface of the gown is on the inside (Figs 20.1 and 20.2). This is so that the surgical team can put on gowns in an aseptic fashion (described later). Plain drapes may be folded concertina style (Fig. 20.3) or so that two corners are on the top surface (Fig. 20.4). Fenestrated drapes are usually folded concertina style.

Sterilisation. Both gowns and drapes may be sterilised by ethylene oxide but this method is often uneconomical in a large practice owing to the small size of the steriliser, duration of the cycle (12 hours) and the airing time of 24 hours. Autoclaving is a quicker, more efficient method but it is essential that the machine has a porous load cycle to ensure complete penetration and drying of the load. A hot air oven is unsuitable as it will lead to charring of the material.

Gowns and drapes may be sterilised in drums, boxes, bags or packs. A handtowel is usually placed with the gown when packing for sterilisation. Drapes are sometimes incorporated into the instrument pack.

Swabs

Swabs may be purchased pre-sterilised; however, they are usually purchased non-sterile because of the cost. They may already be tied in bundles of either five or ten but it is usual for the nurse to do this. Each pack should have a consistent number which is known to all surgery staff. Swabs may be incorporated into the instrument pack, supplied in drums or packed individually in packets.

Sterilisation. Swabs should be sterilised in the same way as gowns and drapes.

Urinary catheters

Although designed for single use, most urinary catheters may be re-sterilised once. The exception to this is the Foley catheter, which will usually be unfit for re-use. After use catheters should be washed, rinsed and then dried. They should be packed, without coiling if possible, in appropriate bags.

Sterilisation. Many brands of catheter may be sterilised by autoclaving but some will be damaged by heat. Ethylene oxide can be successfully used for all types of catheter. It is essential to ensure that they are aired for the recommended time before use.

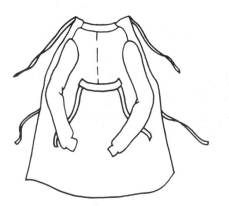

(a) Lie flat out

(b) Fold side to middle

Inside
of
gown

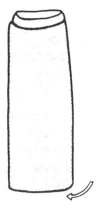

(c) Fold over other side to edge

(d) Concertina lengthways

Inside
of
gown

(e) Pick up by inside of collar
after autoclaving

Fig.20.1 Folding a gown.

Syringes

Plastic syringes are designed to be disposable. To ensure sterility after storage they must be packed individually. It is therefore rarely economical to re-sterilise small syringes but it may be profitable to re-sterilise 30 and 50 ml syringes. They should be disassembled, washed thoroughly and dried prior to sterilisation.

Sterilisation. Most plastic syringes can be autoclaved safely but some brands will be damaged. Ethylene oxide may be used effectively to sterilise syringes. The plungers should be removed from the barrel prior to this. Glass syringes may be sterilised using a hot air oven, autoclave or ethylene oxide.

Liquids

It is usual to purchase liquids pre-sterilised, although more sophisticated autoclaves have a cycle for the sterilisation of fluids. However, the risk of breakage of glass bottles is high and it is probably more economical to purchase fluids which have been commercially prepared.

Power tools

Air drills, saws and mechanical burrs are usually autoclavable but individual manufacturer's instructions should always be followed. Autoclaving can in some cases lead to jamming of the motor. Ethylene oxide can be used for all air-driven tools. Battery drills frequently have plastic casing which would melt in an autoclave but they can be sterilised by using ethylene oxide. Alternatively the unsterile drill is dropped into a sterile sleeve and a sterile chuck is then attached.

Storage after sterilisation

There should be a separate area for storage of sterile packs. It should be dust free, dry and well ventilated. Ideally all packs should be kept in closed cupboards. They should be handled as little as possible to minimise risk of damage, and

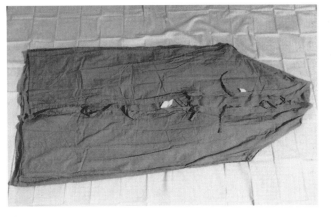

(a)

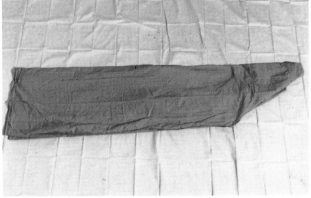

(b)

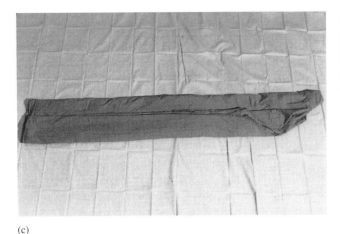

(c)

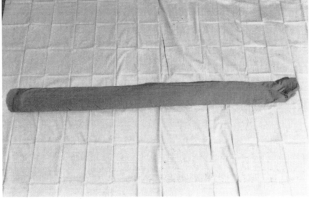

(d)

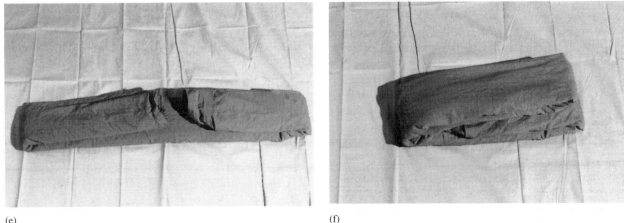

(e)

(f)

Fig. 20.2 Alternative method of folding a gown. (a) The gown is folded inside out, (b) folded in half lengthways, (c) folded in half lengthways again, (d) and again in half lengthways; (e) the top and bottom edges are folded to the middle; (f) the gown is then folded in half again.

packed loosely on shelves so that bags are not damaged. The length of time for which packs may be safely stored after sterilisation is the subject of much debate, with recommendations varying from a few weeks to 6 months. A sealed pack should remain sterile for a limitless period but it may become contaminated by excessive handling, resulting in damage to the pack, or moisture. It is therefore recommended that unused packs should be repacked and resterilised after 6–8 weeks.

The operating theatre

The design and layout of the operating theatre will rarely be within the control of the veterinary nurse. It is important, however, to have some knowledge of ideal requirements and desirable features in order to appreciate differing standards or aseptic techniques and to try and make the best of existing facilities. The operating theatre suite should ideally consist of:

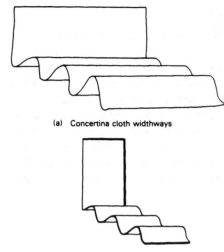

(a) Concertina cloth widthways

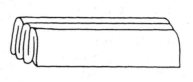

(b)

(c) Concertina lengthways

(d) Pack cloths in autoclave drum or autoclave bags sealed with indicating tape

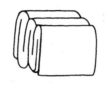

Fig. 20.3 Folding surgical drapes.

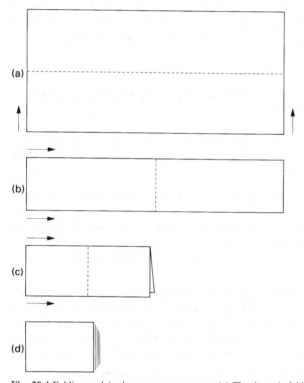

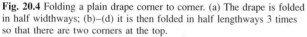

Fig. 20.4 Folding a plain drape corner to corner. (a) The drape is folded in half widthways; (b)–(d) it is then folded in half lengthways 3 times so that there are two corners at the top.

- The operating theatre.
- Anaesthetic preparation area.
- Area for washing and sterilising equipment.
- Sterile storage area.
- Scrubbing-up area.
- Changing rooms.
- Recovery room.

The operating theatre

Many practices have just one operating theatre which is used for all surgery. Larger hospitals may have theatres which are used specifically for particular types of surgery, e.g.

orthopaedic work, general surgery and 'dirty' surgery such as dental work. The size of the theatre will depend on the purpose for which it is intended. If it is to be used for simple, routine surgery it can be quite compact. However, if it is to be used for orthopaedic surgery a large amount of surgical equipment may be needed. If the theatre is too small, working conditions will be compromised and it may be difficult to maintain a high standard of asepsis. It has to be large enough to accommodate the patient, anaesthetic equipment, surgical instrument trolley, other equipment and personnel.

There are several other requirements that are essential, or at least desirable:

- The operating theatre should be an end room, not a thoroughfare to other rooms.
- It must be easily cleaned. Walls and floors must be made of impervious, non-staining materials, floors should be non-slip and hard wearing. The use of drains should be avoided where possible but should not pose a problem if maintained properly. Walls and ceiling should be painted with a light-coloured 'waterproof' paint. The corners and edges of all walls should be coved to facilitate easy cleaning.
- There should be as little shelving and furniture as possible as it will harbour dust.
- Good lighting is essential. Advantage should be taken of natural daylight. Ideally lighting should be concealed within the ceiling with additional side lights on the wall and an overhead theatre light.
- There should be a good supply of electric sockets (in waterproof casing), preferably recessed into the wall.
- Heating is an important consideration since anaesthetised animals are unable to control their own body temperature. The ambient temperature should be between 15 and 20°C. Fan heaters cause air and dust movement and should be avoided. Modern wall-mounted radiators are the most realistic method of heating. Panel heating within the walls is ideal, but expensive.
- Some system of air-conditioning and ventilation is necessary, and may become mandatory under COSHH Regulations.

- A scavenging system for anaesthetic waste gas will also be necessary.
- An X-ray viewer, preferably flush with the wall, is an important fixture in all operating theatres.
- An air supply for power tools may be needed. This should ideally be piped into the theatre from cylinders housed outside theatre. Anaesthetic gases can be delivered in the same way.
- All equipment, including the operating table, must be easily cleaned.
- A wall clock is needed for anaesthetic monitoring and timing of surgery.
- A dry-wipe board is useful for recording details such as swab numbers, suture details, blood loss, etc.
- The rooms should have double swing doors which should normally be kept closed.
- There should be no clear-glass window to the outside, as this will be distracting. Windows should not open, as this will be a threat to asepsis.
- The operating table should be adjustable to facilitate positioning of the patient and to suit the height of the surgeon. The base of the table may be static or maintained on wheels for easy moving. There is usually a hydraulically operated pump to adjust the height, and some electrically operated pumps are also available.

Anaesthetic preparation area

There should be a separate area where the induction of anaesthesia pre-operative procedures (e.g. clipping, catheterisation of the bladder and preparation of the surgical site) can be carried out. It should lead directly into the operating theatre.

Area for washing and sterilising equipment

There needs to be a room where dirty instruments are washed, packed and sterilised. It should be situated close to the operating theatre but away from the sterile storage area. It should include a washing machine and tumble drier (specifically for theatre wear, gowns and drapes), sterilisation facilities and possibly an ultrasonic instrument cleaner.

Sterile storage area

Sterile supplies should be stored in closed cupboards away from the instrument washing area, but adjacent to theatre. Here instrument trolleys can be laid out prior to surgery. Entry should be directly into the theatre.

Scrubbing-up area

There should be a separate scrub room within the theatre suite but outside the theatre itself. This should lead directly into the sterile preparation area and theatre. Swing doors which can be foot operated should separate the rooms.

Changing rooms

Changing rooms for personnel should be situated at the entrance to theatre. It is a good idea to have a red line delineating the sterile area and appropriate notices displayed to indicate these areas. Footwear for use in theatre should be placed at the entrance to theatre beyond the red line. This barrier should be adhered to at all times. The layout of rooms within the theatre suite is important for the sake of asepsis. There should be a one-way traffic system, so that the surgical team and sterile supplies enter through one door and unscrubbed personnel enter and leave through a separate doorway.

Recovery room

A room where the patient can recover following surgery may be situated near the operating theatre suite. It should be quiet and warm and contain essential equipment to deal with any post-operative emergencies which could occur.

Maintenance and cleaning of the operating theatre

A routine cleaning programme in the operating area is essential if a high standard of asepsis is to be maintained:

- At the beginning of each day, all the surfaces and all the furniture and equipment in the theatre suite should be damp-dusted using a dilute solution of disinfectant. A dry duster would simply move dust around the room.
- In between cases, the operating table should be wiped clean.
- At the end of the day, the floors in all rooms of the theatre suite should be vacuumed to remove debris and loose hair. They should then be either wet-vacuumed or washed using disinfectant. All waste material should be removed. Surfaces, equipment, lights and scrub sinks should all be washed down with disinfectant.
- Once a week there should be a more thorough cleaning session where all equipment is removed from the room and the floors and walls are scrubbed. A disinfectant with detergent properties which will remove organic matter and which is active against a wide range of bacteria, including *Pseudomonas* spp., should be used. After removing any excess solution, allow the disinfectant to dry on the surface rather than rinsing it off, for longer residual activity. All equipment should be meticulously wiped over.
- Cleaning utensils should be designated specifically for use in the theatre suite. They should be rinsed and allowed to dry after use. Buckets should always be emptied and rinsed out. Autoclavable mops are available and should be used whenever possible. Failing this, cloths and mop heads should be washed daily in a washing machine. All utensils should be stored away from the sterile area.

Preparation of the surgical team

If good surgical asepsis is to be achieved, all those involved in the surgery should change from their ordinary clothes into correct theatre attire before entering the operating theatre suite.

Theatre wear, which should be worn only within the suite, usually consists of a simple two-piece **scrub suit** or dress made of cotton or polyester. A clean suit should be worn each day, or it should be changed more frequently if it becomes soiled. Theatre **footwear** should be antistatic and traditionally has consisted of white clogs or wellingtons. These have the advantage of being easy to clean. Canvas shoes are sometimes worn but have the disadvantage of being difficult to clean on a daily basis and should be covered by waterproof overshoes. All footwear should be wiped over with a disinfectant at the end of the day. Plastic overshoes are available which fit over normal shoes, but they are not recommended since they wear through in a very short time.

Various different styles of **headwear** are available to accommodate longer hairstyles and beards. These are usually disposable and paper-based.

The purpose of **masks** is to filter expired air from the nose and mouth. Masks are effective filters for relatively short periods only and so should ideally be changed between operations.

Scrubbing up

Pre-operative scrubbing up is a systematic washing and scrubbing of the hands, arms and elbows which is performed by all members of the surgical team before each operation. As it is not possible to sterilise the skin, the aim of the scrubbing-up routine is to destroy as many micro-organisms from the surface of the arms and hands as possible, prior to donning a sterile surgical gown and gloves. Many different scrub routines have been described and no single technique is necessarily better than another. It is recommended that one of the tried and tested regimes is adopted and adhered to strictly. For example:

(1) Remove watch and jewellery.
(2) Finger nails should be cut short and any nail varnish removed.
(3) Adjust the water supply (which should be elbow or foot operated) to a suitable temperature and flow. Once the scrubbing-up routine has started, the hands should not touch the taps, sink or scrub dispenser. If they are inadvertently touched, the last stage of the procedure should be repeated.
(4) Wash the hands thoroughly using a plain soap. At this stage, clean the nails using a nail pick.
(5) Once the hands have been washed, wash the arms up to and including the elbows. Always keep the hands higher than the elbows so that water drains down towards the unscrubbed upper arms rather than the other way round (which would lead to recontamination). The purpose of this stage of the procedure is to remove organic matter and grease from the skin.

Table 20.4 Ideal properties of surgical scrub solutions

Wide spectrum of antimicrobial activity.
Ability to decrease microbial count quickly.
Quick application.
Long residual lethal effect against micro-organisms.
Remain active and effective in the presence of organic matter.
Safe to use without skin irritation or sensitisation.
Economical.
Practical for veterinary use.

Commonly used agents:
- Povidone-iodine
  Iodine combined with a detergent.
  Broad-spectrum anti-microbial activity – bactericidal, viricidal and fungicidal.
  May cause severe skin reactions and irritation in some individuals.
  Efficacy impaired by organic matter.
- Chlorhexidine
  Effective against many bacteria, including *E. coli* and *Pseudomonas* spp.
  Viricidal, fungicidal and sporicidal properties.
  Effective level of activity in the presence of organic material.
  Longer residual activity than povidone-iodine.
  Relatively low toxicity to tissue.
- Triclosan
  A newer agent, claimed to be antibacterial against both Gram-positive and Gram-negative bacteria.

---

(6) Rinse the hands and then the arms by allowing water to wash away the soap from the hands towards the elbows.
(7) Repeat this procedure using a surgical scrub solution, e.g. povidone-iodine or chlorhexidine (Table 20.4). Use only sufficient water to produce a lather, as bactericidal properties of the scrub solution are dependent on contact time with the skin. Excessive amounts of water will rinse away the scrub solution before it has achieved its aim.
(8) Rinse off the scrub solution as in stage (6).
(9) Take a sterile scrubbing brush and systematically scrub the hands. Scrub the palms of the hand, wrist and four surfaces of each finger and thumb (back, front and both sides) and the nails. Either rinse the brush and use it on the other hand or discard it and take a second brush. It is not recommended that the backs of the hand and arms are scrubbed as this may lead to excoriation, which predisposes to infection.
(10) The final stage is a repeat of stage (7). Wash the hands and arms in surgical scrub but this time the scrubbing process is not extended to include the elbow, so that there is no danger that a previously unscrubbed area is touched.
(11) Rinse the hands and arms as before.
(12) Take a sterile handtowel, holding it at arm's length. Use a different quarter to dry each hand and each arm. Then discard the handtowel.

The scrubbing procedure should take between 5 and 10 minutes.

Check the clock as you start and as you begin the final stage to ensure that you have not rushed the procedure.

Putting on a surgical gown

There are two different types of gown: back-tie and side-tie. The technique for putting on the gown is similar for both, with slight variation:

(1) The sterile gown (folded inside out) is taken from its sterile pack, held at the shoulders and allowed to fall open (Fig. 20.5a).
(2) One hand should be slipped into each sleeve (Fig. 20.5b). No attempt should be made to try and pull the sleeves over the shoulder or to readjust the gown as this will lead to contamination of the hands or outside of the gown. An unscrubbed assistant should pull the back of the gown over the shoulders (touching only the inside surface of the gown) and secure the ties at the back.
(3) With the hands retained within the sleeves, the waist ties should be picked up and held out to the sides (Fig. 20.5c).

In the case of **back-tying** gowns, the unscrubbed assistant will then take the ends of the waist ties and secure them at the back (Fig. 20.5d). The back of the gown is now unsterile and must not come into contact with sterile equipment, drapes and gowns.

In the case of the **side-tying** gown, the unscrubbed assistant takes hold of the paper tape on the longer waist tape and takes the tie around the back to the opposite side (Fig. 20.5e). The scrubbed person then pulls the tape, so that the paper tape comes away (Fig. 20.5f). The gown is tied at the waist by the scrubbed person (Fig. 20.5g). This type of gown, though uncommonly used in veterinary surgery, provides an all-round sterile field.

Putting on surgical gloves

Three methods are available: closed gloving, open gloving and the plunge method.

Closed gloving

The hands are kept inside the sleeves while gloving takes place. This technique (Fig. 20.6) has the advantage that it minimises the chances of contaminating the gloves, since the outside of the gloves do not contact the skin.

(1) Hands remain within the sleeves of the gown. The glove packet is turned so that the fingers point towards the body. (The right glove will now be on the left and vice versa.)
(2) The glove is picked up at the rim of the cuff of the glove.
(3) The hand is turned over so that the glove lies on the palm surface with fingers of the glove still pointing towards the body.
(4) The rim is picked up with the opposite hand.
(5) It is then pulled over the fingers and over the dorsal surface of the wrist.
(6) The glove is then pulled on as the fingers are pushed forwards.

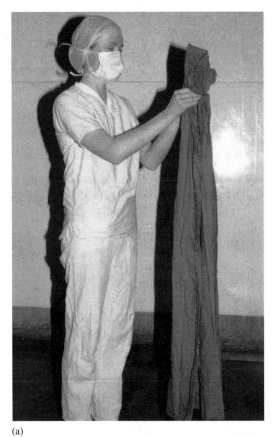

(a)

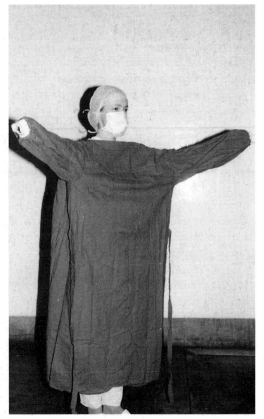

(b)

Fig. 20.5 Putting on a surgical gown.

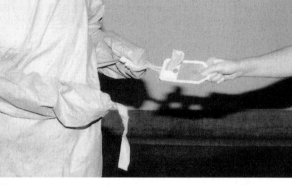

(e)

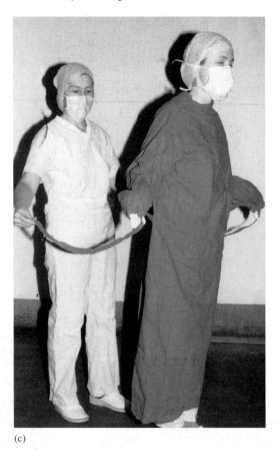

(c)

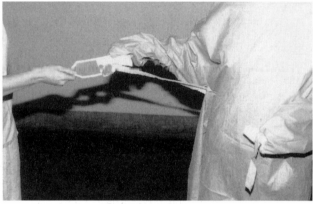

(f)

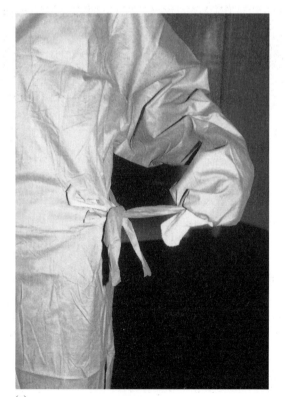

(d)

(g)

Fig. 20.5 (continued)

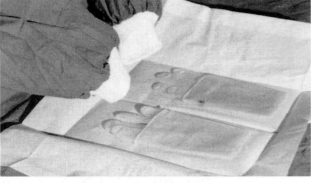

(a)

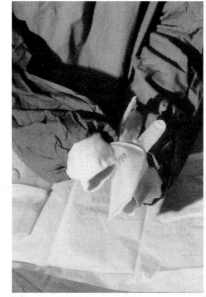

(d)

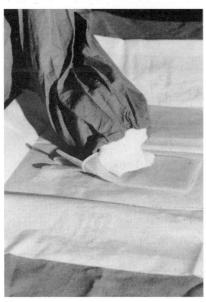

(b)

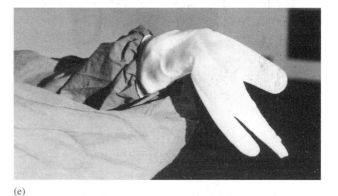

(e)

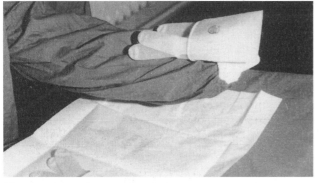

(c)

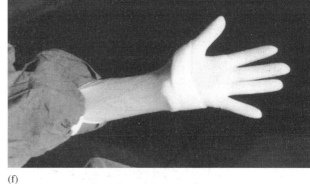

(f)

Fig. 20.6 Closed gloving technique.

Open gloving

The hands are extended out of the sleeves while gowning. This technique (Fig. 20.7) has the disadvantage that the gloves are relatively easily contaminated by skin contact.

(1) The glove pack is opened by an assistant.
(2) With the left hand, pick up the right glove by the turned down cuff, holding only the inner surface of the glove.
(3) Pull on to the right hand. Do not unfold the cuff at this stage.

(4) Place the gloved fingers of the right hand under the cuff of the left glove and pull on to the left hand holding only the outer surface of this glove.
(5) The rim of the left glove is hooked over the thumb whilst the cuff of the gown is adjusted.
(6) Pull the cuff of the left glove over the cuff of the gown using the fingers of the right hand.
(7) Repeat for the right hand.

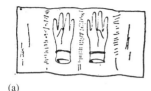

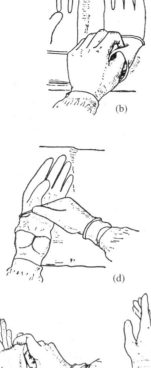

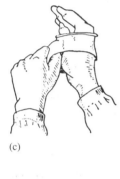

(a)

(b)

(c)

(d)

(e)

(f)

Fig. 20.7 Open gloving.

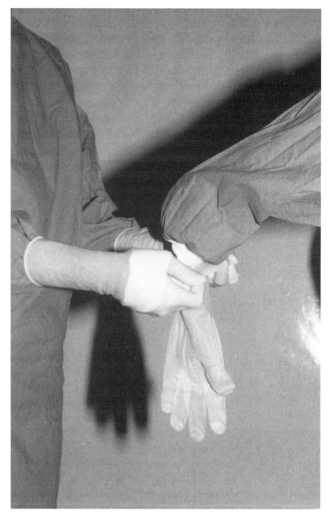

Fig. 20.8 The plunge method of gloving

Plunge method

With this method (Fig. 20.8) the sterile glove is held open by a scrubbed assistant and the hand inserted. There is a risk of contaminating both personnel involved. This technique is not commonly employed in veterinary operating theatres.

Pre-operative preparation of the patient

Surgical cases may be categorised as follows:

● **Elective and non-urgent** – the patient is usually healthy and often young (e.g. ovariohysterectomy, castration, corrective osteotomy).
● **Necessary or urgent** – not immediately life-threatening but require prompt attention (fracture repair, airway, gastrointestinal surgery).
● **Emergency surgery** – life-threatening conditions (e.g. abdominal crisis), often traumatic (e.g. chest injury).

The time between admission and surgery will depend on various factors. In the simplest elective procedures, the patient is admitted on the morning of surgery and returns home later that day. Pre-operative preparations in these

cases are minimal. In others there may be a delay before surgery is performed. Reasons for this may include:

● **Investigative procedures**, e.g. blood samples, diagnostic tests, radiographic studies, etc.
● **Fluid therapy or transfusion** – to improve the patient's physiological status before surgery.
● **Presence of other injuries** which require treatment before surgery may be undertaken (e.g. thoracic trauma associated with a limb fracture).
● **To allow reduction of swelling/debridement of wounds** – bandaging of fracture site, application of wound dressings, etc.
● **Stabilisation** of patient with concurrent metabolic disturbance (e.g. diabetes mellitus, renal disease, Cushing's syndrome).

Admission of the patient

On admission of the patient:

● All relevant details must be recorded on the case records.
● Check the reason for admission.
● Where relevant, identify the site (draw a diagram if necessary).

- Ensure that the owner understands what is to be done and how the patient will look when discharged (e.g. it will have a clipped area and may be wearing a bandage, cast, Elizabethan collar, etc.).
- Ensure that the patient is in good general health or that symptoms have not changed since last seen by a veterinary surgeon.
- Always ensure that you have a contact telephone number and that an anaesthetic consent form is signed.
- The patient should then be weighed.
- It is sensible at this stage to fit a plastic identicollar containing the patient's name/number, weight, and reason for admission to minimise the risk of mistakes occurring.

Pre-operative procedures

Starvation

Food is usually withheld for 12 hours prior to surgery. This is primarily to prevent regurgitation of food under general anaesthesia or during recovery. A full stomach could also interfere with the surgical procedure.

Clipping

Clipping the surgical site is necessary for most procedures (except intraoral). It may be carried out pre-anaesthesia or under general anaesthesia (Table 20.5). Certain considerations should be borne in mind when clipping:

- Clip a large area around the surgical site.
- Ensure that the clipping is neat. (This is what the owner will notice.)
- Ensure that clipper blades are in good order. Nicks in the skin will cause irritation, which may encourage post-operative licking and scratching at the site.
- When clipping around a wound, K-Y jelly placed in the wound and on the coat at the edges of the wound will help to prevent hair entering the wound.
- Clean clipper blades in between cases. It may be necessary to sterilise them after clipping contaminated sites, e.g. abscesses.
- Clipping should be performed away from the operating theatre to minimise contamination by hair.

- Some surgeons advocate shaving of the skin after clipping but this may lead to severe excoriation of the skin, which encourages post-operative licking, scratching and soreness.

Bathing

Ideally all patients should be bathed before surgery to decrease the risk of contamination but this is not always feasible. It should be considered in elective orthopaedic procedures such as total hip replacement.

Administration of an enema

For some surgery (e.g. rectal/colonic) it is desirable to give an evacuant enema prior to surgery. A soap-and-water enema is simplest. The patient may need bathing afterwards to remove faecal contaminants from the skin.

Preparation immediately before surgery

Some form of **premedicant** drug is usually given by intramuscular or subcutaneous injection, 15 minutes to 1 hour before induction of anaesthesia.

Antibiotic drugs are often given at the same time as the premedicant drugs to ensure effective antibiotic blood levels at the time of surgery. **Eye drops** are often applied immediately prior to ophthalmic surgery. **Catheterisation of the bladder** may be required for the following reasons:

- Monitor urine output during and after surgery.
- Minimise risk of soiling during surgery.
- Facilitate access to abdominal organs.
- Prevent risk of bladder perforation or rupture during surgery.

Other possible preparations are described in Table 20.6.

Preparation of the skin

The skin and coat are two of the greatest sources of wound contamination as it is not possible to remove all bacteria from the skin. The aim is to significantly reduce the number present without damaging the skin itself. Common skin bacteria include species of *Staphylococcus*, *Bacillus* and occasionally *Streptococcus*.

Table 20.5 Clipping: advantages and disadvantages

	Advantages	Disadvantages
Under general anaesthesia	Often takes less time. Fewer people required to restrain animal. Desirable with fractious animals or painful/inaccessible sites.	Decreases asepsis: small loose hairs are extremely difficult to remove even with a vacuum cleaner. Increases anaesthetic time.
Pre-anaesthesia	Shorter anaesthetic time. Improves asepsis: loose hairs generally shed before surgery. Improves operating theatre efficiency (more operations can be performed).	Patient may be un-cooperative. Requires two or more people. Clipping more than 12 hours before surgery may increase skin bacteria.

Table 20.6 Other preparations immediately before surgery

(1) Purse-string suture around anus to prevent contamination by faecal material during surgery in the peri-anal region. The nurse should ensure that it is removed at the end of surgery.
(2) Application of Esmarch's rubber bandage and tourniquet for a bloodless operating field during surgery on distal limbs.
(3) Introduction of a throat pack to prevent aspiration of blood, mucus, etc., during oral or nasal surgery. Usually a dampened conforming bandage is used for this purpose.
(4) Cover any additional wounds not associated with the surgery to prevent risk of further contamination.
(5) Application of a foot bandage to cover any unclipped areas where the surgery involves a limb.

As antiseptic and detergent properties are required in skin-cleansing agents, surgical scrub solutions such as chlorhexidine and povidone-iodine are ideal. An antiseptic solution (which may be water- or alcohol-based) is then usually applied to give residual bacterial activity.

Initial skin preparation should be done in the preparation room. There are several different techniques which are used commonly and one that is recommended is as follows:

(1) Surgical gloves should be worn to prevent contamination of the patient's skin from the nurse's hands. It is not necessary for the gloves to be sterile during the initial preparation.
(2) Using lint-free swabs, wash the site using a surgical scrub solution and a little warm water, beginning at the proposed incision site and working outwards. Once the edges of the clipped area are reached, discard the swab and take a new one.
(3) Continue this procedure until the area is clean, i.e. there is no discoloration on a white swab.
(4) A small amount of a 70% alcohol solution can then be sprayed over the site to remove any remaining detergent. It should not be used on open wounds or mucous membranes.
(5) Move the patient into theatre and position for surgery. For limb surgery, a tape is applied over the foot and attached to a drip stand to allow preparation around all sides of the limb.
(6) As the site is likely to have been contaminated to some extent in the transition to the theatre, the skin is given another wash in the manner previously described. This time, however, use sterile gloves, water and swabs.
(7) The final stage of preparation is carried out by the scrubbed surgical team with an antiseptic solution using sterile swabs on sterile Rampley sponge-holding forceps, which are then discarded.

Care should be taken to avoid soaking the coat as this would increase the risk of 'strike through' from the drapes and may make the patient hypothermic.

Preparation of eyes and mucous membranes

The solutions commonly used for preparation of the skin are likely to be irritant and cause damage to mucous membranes and in particular the eye. Dilute solutions of povidone-iodine (0.1–0.2%) are commonly used to irrigate the eye and may also be used on oral and other mucous membranes. Chlorhexidine solutions are shown to be more irritant to the surface of the cornea. Alcohol-based solutions should not be used on this sensitive tissue.

Some surgeons do not advocate clipping around the eye for intraocular surgery but use adhesive drapes to protect the eye from the hair and skin. Others prefer to clip a minimal amount of hair around the eye. Application of petroleum or K-Y jelly to the hair prior to clipping with a narrow fine blade will help to prevent hair being introduced into the eye. The skin around the eye is extremely thin and sensitive, and so it is important that the clippers are in good order and great care is taken when clipping. The eye should then be irrigated several times with physiological saline before irrigating with a povidone-iodine solution, as described. The skin should also be prepared with the povidone-iodine solution.

Positioning the patient for surgery

Most surgeons have individual preferences with regard to positioning of the patient for surgery, although there are some standard positions for specific operations. The veterinary nurse needs to be familiar with positioning for different surgical techniques and individual variations. When there is any doubt, the nurse should check well in advance of surgery.

Some operating tables have adjustable sides and tilting facilities which assist positioning of the patient. If not, the use of additional restraining aids such as troughs, sandbags and tapes will be necessary. Care should be taken to avoid placing heavy sandbags over the limbs or tying tapes tightly, which may occlude blood supply to the area.

Draping the patient

The reason for draping the patient is to maintain asepsis by preventing contamination of the surgical site by hair and the immediate environment. Drapes must therefore cover the entire patient and operating table, leaving only the surgical site exposed. Drapes may be disposable or reusable. The relative advantages of each type are shown in Table 20.7.

Disposable drapes are usually paper based. Many different types are available and cost tends to reflect the quality. Most of these are designed for the medical market but many are suitable for veterinary use. They are usually water-resilient and may be purchased pre-sterilised. One disadvantage is that cheap varieties tend to be non-conforming and may tear easily.

Table 20.7 Drapes: advantages and disadvantages

	Advantages	Disadvantages
Disposable	Labour saving. Less laundry. Pre-sterilised. Usually very water repellent. Always in perfect condition.	Expensive. Cheaper brands can be less conforming. Large stock needed.
Re-usable drapes	Cheaper.	Porous – all fluids leak through leading to a break in asepsis. Time-consuming – washing and folding. Danger of threads detaching and gaining access to wounds. After repeated use quality becomes poor.

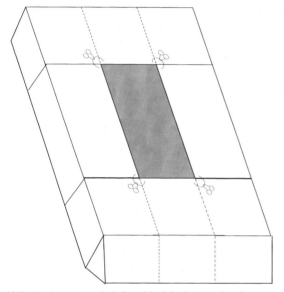

Fig. 20.9. Draping the surgical site with plain drapes, placed longitudinally on both sides of the operating table. Plain drapes are then placed over each end and secured by towel clips.

Draping systems

Plain drapes. Four rectangular drapes are used to create a 'window' (**fenestration**) for the surgical site (Fig. 20.9). The fenestration created can be of any size. The first drape should be placed between the surgeon and the nearest side of the table. Then a drape is placed over the opposite side of the patient (i.e. furthest from the surgeon). Drapes are then placed over both ends. They are then secured in place using towel clips.

Fenestrated drapes. Fenestrated drapes achieve the same effect as the plain drapes in leaving a surgery window, but the window is already formed in a single ready-made drape. Fenestrated drapes can be large enough to cover the entire animal and table top. A selection of different sized fenestrations are needed however to cater for all the different surgical sites.

Adhesive 'barrier' drapes. Sterile clear adhesive plastic sheets are sometimes placed over the surgical site. Standard drapes are then applied in the usual way. The skin incision is made through the adhesive material.

Draping limbs. There are various ways of draping limbs for surgery (Fig. 20.10). The surgeon's individual preference will govern the choice of method. Commonly, the lower limb is tied to a drip stand, using tape. A sterile drape is placed on the table top underneath the limb. Then either a sterile drape or stockinette is secured to the lower limb and the suspending tape is cut. The surgical site is then draped in a routine fashion.

Sub-draping. Additional towels are sometimes used to protect the incision site from contamination. They are applied to each side of the incision by towel clips. The towel is then folded back over the towel clips.

Surgical assistance

The theatre nurse has two main roles: one as a circulating nurse and one as a scrubbed nurse. Duties in the respective roles are shown in Table 20.8.

Guidelines for the scrubbed nurse

The role of the scrubbed nurse is an extremely important one and requires rigid adherence to a set of rules. It is very easy to make mistakes if corners are cut or changes made. Knowledge of the procedure to be performed is important so that the needs of the surgeon can be anticipated:

(1) The instrument trolley should not be prepared until just before it is needed but it must be ready by the time the patient arrives in theatre.
(2) It is essential to know exactly what instruments and equipment are on the trolley at the start and throughout surgery.
(3) All swabs, sutures, needles, etc., must be counted before surgery begins and again before the wound is closed, to prevent any items being accidentally left within a wound cavity.
(4) The nurse should watch the operation carefully in order to anticipate the surgeon's needs.
(5) Instruments should be passed to the surgeon so that they are ready to be used, i.e. not upside down.
(6) Instruments should be returned to the same place on the trolley each time so that the nurse knows exactly

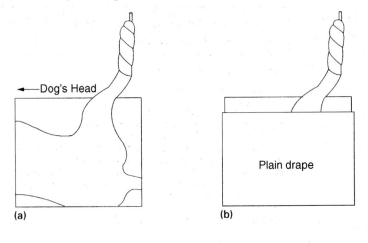

(a)

Plain drape

(b)

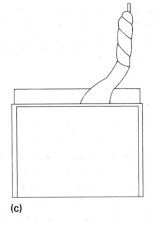

(c)

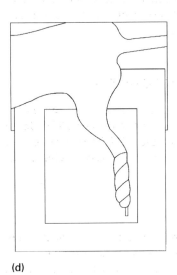

(d)

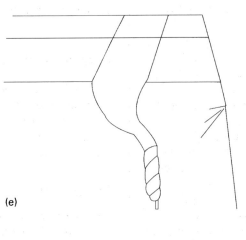

(e)

Fig. 20.10 Draping a limb for surgery. (a) The lower limb is bandaged and attached by tape to a transfusion stand. (b) A plain drape is laid over the body and the opposite limb of the patient. (c) A smaller plain drape is laid on top of this. (d) The tape is then cut and the limb lowered on to the inner drape. (e) The drape is carefully wrapped around the limb and secured with a towel clip; plain drapes or a fenestrated drape are then applied over the surgical site.

where they are. They should not be left around the surgical site, because they are likely to fall on the floor and because they will not be immediately to hand when needed.

(7) Instruments should be wiped over with a dry swab when they are returned to the trolley.

(8) Only one swab should be given to the surgeon at any time and the nurse must keep a constant check on the number of swabs.

(9) Swabs should be applied firmly to a bleeding site, without wiping across the tissue which may both damage the tissue and disturb a clot.

(10) All tissues should be handled gently to avoid trauma. Viscera in particular should be handled very carefully.

(11) One of the nurse's roles may be to irrigate the tissues with warmed saline to prevent desiccation, particularly during long operations.

(12) On completion of surgery ensure that all instruments, needles and swabs are returned to the trolley and that needles, blades and glassware are safely disposed of.

Preparing an instrument trolley

Instrument trolleys should be prepared immediately prior to use. The longer that instruments are exposed to air, the greater the chance of contamination from the environment or personnel. If there is a delay once the trolley has been laid out, then a sterile drape should be placed over the top.

GENERAL RULES FOR MAINTENANCE OF ASEPSIS

(1) Correct theatre attire to be worn at all times.

(2) There should be a minimum number of people present and movement should be kept to a minimum.

(3) There should be a new set of sterile instruments for each operation, even when dealing with a contaminated site.

(4) Plan to perform 'clean' operations first, i.e. orthopaedic operations (especially when implants are used), and contaminated surgery to be carried out last (i.e. aural and oral).

(5) Wherever possible there should be a room for 'dirty' procedures.

(6) Adopt an efficient sterilisation programme.

(7) Ensure that the theatre is maintained at an ambient temperature and the ventilation is good. Hot, humid conditions will encourage the growth of pathogens, in particular *Pseudomonas* spp.

(8) Wherever possible, clip and bath the patient before taking it to theatre.

(9) The surgical team must ensure that they do not touch any non-sterile surfaces during surgery. Any break in asepsis must be reported and rectified.

(10) Ensure that any contaminated instruments or equipment are not returned to the sterile trolley.

(11) Keep a record book of all operations so that if any sepsis problems arise the cause can be detected.

(12) Maintain a strict cleaning protocol.

Table 20.8 Duties of a circulating nurse and of the scrubbed nurse

Duties of a circulating nurse

(1) Help prepare theatre, instruments and equipment for surgery.
(2) Tie the surgical team into gowns.
(3) Help position the patient on the table.
(4) Preparation of the surgical site.
(5) Connect apparatus (diathermy, suction, airlines, etc.).
(6) Open packs of sutures/instruments, etc.
(7) Count swabs, sutures, etc., with the scrubbed nurse.
(8) Be in theatre at all times when surgery is in progress.
(9) Assist the anaesthetist.
(10) Prepare post-operative dressings.
(11) Help clear theatre at the end of surgery.

Duties of the scrubbed nurse

(1) Prepare the instrument trolley.
(2) Assist in draping the patient.
(3) Pass instruments, swabs, etc., to the surgeon.
(4) Assist with surgery: retract tissue, cut sutures, etc.
(5) Be responsible for all equipment, swabs, sutures, needles, etc.

Trolleys can be laid up by a scrubbed nurse or by using sterile Cheatle forceps. The top of the metal instrument trolley will not be sterile and it is important to cover this with a waterproof, sterile drape first to prevent bacterial strike-through from the trolley if it becomes wet.

Instrument sets may be packed in trays complete with drapes, swabs, blades, etc. In these cases the outer wrappings of the set can be unfolded to cover the base of the trolley.

Where instruments are taken from multi-use containers the trolley should be covered by a waterproof drape followed by two layers of linen cloth. Swabs, drapes and instruments are then added.

Hazards in the operating theatre

The avoidance of accidents to patients and staff in the operating theatre is of the utmost importance. The Health and Safety at Work Act and the COSHH Regulations are designed to ensure safety in the workplace, including the operating theatre.

Equipment

With the increasing use of new and sophisticated equipment, the risk of accidents has also increased. It is very important that all nursing staff are instructed in the use and maintenance of all new equipment. It is also important that all equipment is serviced regularly and tested for electrical safety to minimise risks.

Pollution from anaesthetic gases

All staff should be aware of the dangers associated with inhaling anaesthetic gases. An anaesthetic gas scavenging system must be fitted or absorptive filters used to minimise exposure to gases.

Disposal of needles/sharp instruments

Many sharp blades, needles and stylets are used in the surgical unit. The disposal of these can create a major and serious hazard. They should be placed in commercially produced sharps containers which, when full, are sealed and disposed of as 'clinical waste'.

Clinical and pathological waste

It is a requirement of the COSHH Regulations that all clinical and pathological waste is separated from ordinary refuse using colour-coded bags.

- **Clinical waste** (i.e. anything contaminated by blood, body fluids or tissue) should be placed in yellow bags, sealed and incinerated.
- **Pathological material** (i.e. infected) should be placed in red bags and sealed. This too should be disposed of by incineration.

Chemicals

In the operating theatre nursing staff will be exposed to various chemicals. Protective clothing, masks and gloves should be worn where appropriate.

Care of the patient during surgery

It is important to remember that underneath the drapes is a live patient! Care must be taken to avoid leaning on the animal's chest, which may compromise breathing in a small patient. Careful positioning of towel clips is important to avoid delicate structures such as the eye, which cannot be seen once drapes have been placed. Attention should be paid to the conservation of heat especially in the small or very young. The use of heated water beds, insulation (e.g. bubble-wrap) and warmed intravenous and irrigation fluids should be encouraged. Careful positioning of the animal on the table is also important to avoid post-operative complications.

Immediate post-operative care

Recovery from anaesthesia

The patient should not be left unattended until it is conscious and sitting up. The endotracheal tube is usually removed just before the cough reflex returns. The animal should be watched closely to ensure that an adequate airway is maintained once the tube has been removed, especially in brachycephalic breeds or following airway surgery. A source of oxygen and a means of ventilation should be available during this time in case any problems arise. Colour of the mucous membranes, presence or absence of respiratory noise and effort will be indicators of effective ventilation by the animal. The ability to maintain body temperature is lost under anaesthesia, so steps should be taken to prevent hypothermia.

Haemorrhage

During recovery the patient should be observed for signs of external haemorrhage (which is usually obvious) or internal haemorrhage (signs of shock).

Recognition of pain

It is important to be able to recognise when an animal is in pain (see Chapter 2). The nurse should obtain instructions from the veterinary surgeon regarding post-operative analgesia.

Application of dressings of casts

Many orthopaedic and some soft tissue cases will require post-operative bandages or casts. This should be done before the animal regains consciousness. Take care not to apply too tightly (especially head and ear dressings).

Comfort

Make sure that the animal has comfortable bedding, especially orthopaedic patients. Turn the animal regularly if it is disinclined or unable to do so by itself. Give opportunities for the animal to urinate, or empty the bladder manually if necessary. Do not forget to offer food and drink if this is allowed, especially in young and old patients.

Instrumentation

The cost of good-quality surgical instruments is extremely high but they will last for years if handled correctly, whereas cheaper instruments of poor quality will require early replacement.

Stainless steel is the material of choice for most surgical instruments. It combines high resistance to corrosion with great strength and it has an attractive surface finish.

Tungsten carbide inserts are often added to the tips of stainless steel instruments that are used for cutting or gripping, such as scissors and needle-holders. They are very hard and resistant to wear but tend to be expensive. Instruments with tungsten carbide inserts are often identified by their gold-coloured handles.

Chromium-plated carbon steel surgical instruments are commonly used in veterinary practice because they are lower in price. However, they will rust, pit and blister when in contact with chemicals and saline and they tend to blunt quickly.

Care and maintenance of surgical instruments

Surgical instruments should be handled carefully at all times. They should not be dropped into trays and sinks or on to trolleys. Special care should be taken of sharp edges and pointed instruments. See Chapter 21, p. 559.

Care of new instruments

Most new instruments are supplied dry without lubrication. Before use, therefore, it is recommended that they should be carefully washed and dried and their moving parts should be lubricated.

Cleaning after use

To comply with Health and Safety Legislation, the veterinary nurse must wear protective clothing (i.e. a plastic apron and rubber gloves) when dealing with surgical instruments.

Sharp items such as needles, glass vials and scalpel blades should be safely disposed of before removing other disposable items such as suture packets, swabs, etc., from the instrument trolley. Any specialised or delicate equipment should be separated from the general instruments and cleaned separately.

Instruments should be cleaned as soon as possible on completion of surgery to prevent blood, tissue debris or saline drying on them, as this will lead to pitting of the surface and subsequent corrosion. Initial soaking or rinsing in cold water is extremely effective for this. Hot water should not be used as it causes coagulation of proteins (e.g. blood). Alternatively instruments may be initially soaked in a chemical cleaning solution specifically manufactured for instrument cleaning. Where indicated, instruments should be dismantled and ratchets and box joints opened before immersion.

Instruments should then be cleaned under cool or warm running water, using a hand brush with fairly stiff bristles. Particular attention should be paid to ratchets, box joints, serrations, etc. Abrasive chemical agents or materials should never be used as they may damage the surface of the instrument.

Ordinary soap should also be avoided as it causes an insoluble alkali film to form on the surface, thus trapping bacteria and protecting them from sterilisation.

After washing, instruments should be rinsed thoroughly – preferably in distilled or deionised water – and then dried prior to packing.

Ultrasonic cleaners (see also Chapter 21, p. 560).

Bench-top ultrasonic cleaners suitable for veterinary use are readily available. They are extremely effective at removing debris from areas inaccessible to brushes (e.g. box joints). They work by the production of sinusoidal energy waves with a vibration frequency in excess of 20 000/second.

Following an initial rinsing or soaking in cold water to remove excess blood and debris the instruments are placed in the wire mesh basket of the ultrasonic cleaner. The unit is filled approximately half full with water to which a specific ultrasonic cleaning detergent has been added. The basket is placed in the solution, the lid replaced and the unit switched on. Usually a period of approximately 15 minutes is sufficient. On completion of the cycle, the basket is removed and the instruments rinsed individually under running water.

All instruments should be dried after washing, as water collecting in trapped areas may lead to corrosion. After cleaning, each instrument should be inspected for distortion, misalignment and incorrect assembly. Pivot movements should be checked.

Lubrication

Lubrication of instruments on a regular basis is recommended, particularly after using an ultrasonic cleaner. It is important to use lubricants which are recommended by the manufacturer. Mineral oils and grease must be avoided as they leave a film on the surface under which bacterial spores may be trapped, preventing adequate penetration during sterilisation. Antimicrobial water-soluble lubricants (instrument milk) are available: instruments are dipped into the solution for a short period and then removed and allowed to dry. They do not need to be rinsed.

Cleaning of compressed air machines

Compressed air machines should never be immersed in water or ultrasonic cleaners. The machine's detachable parts (drills, etc.) can be cleaned in standard fashion. The instrument itself should be detached from the air hose and wiped over thoroughly with disinfectant, paying particular attention to triggers and couplings. Use of a handbrush may be necessary. It should then be rinsed without immersing it completely. The air hose should be cleaned in the same way and then both should be dried. The machine should be lubricated, using the manufacturer's recommended lubricant, before packing for sterilisation.

General surgical instruments

There is a wide variety of different surgical instruments available. It is not expected that the veterinary nurse should be familiar with them all but a broad knowledge of general instruments can be gained by reference to manuals and catalogues to learn the names and appearance of the more common ones.

Scalpel

The scalpel is the best instrument for dividing tissue with minimal trauma. Usually scalpel blades with interchangeable disposable blades are used (Fig. 20.11). A size 3 handle is commonly used for small animal surgery with blade sizes 10, 11, 12 and 15. A size 4 handle is used for large animal surgery with blade sizes 20, 21 and 22. The primary advantage of disposable blades is consistent sharpness. A scalpel with a blade and handle as a disposable package is available, as is a small, rounded (Beaver) handle with smaller disposable blades which has gained popularity with ophthalmic surgeons.

Dissecting forceps

These are commonly referred to as thumb forceps (Fig. 20.12) and are designed to hold tissue. They have a spring action and the jaws are opposed by holding the metal blades

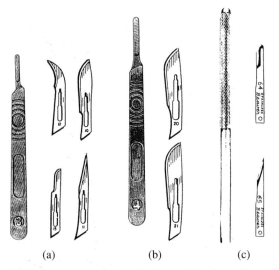

Fig. 20.11 Scalpel handles and blades. (a) Size 3 handle and sizes 10, 11, 12 and 15 blades. (b) Size 4 handle and sizes 21 and 20 blades. (c) Beaver handle with two different blades.

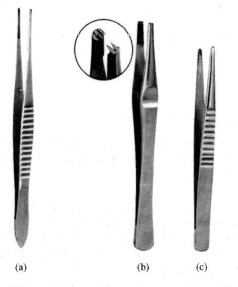

Fig. 20.12 Dissecting forceps. (a) Fine toothed. (b) Heavy-duty toothed. (c) Plain dressing forceps.

together. They may have plain or toothed ends. Generally forceps with plain ends are used for handling delicate tissues such as viscera whilst toothed forceps are used for denser tissues. Dissecting forceps should be held like a pencil.

Scissors

Operating scissors are available in various lengths and shapes (Fig. 20.13). Mayo dissecting scissors are commonly used for routine surgery; the finer, long-handled Metzenbaum scissors tend to be used for more delicate work. Special suture scissors (e.g. Carless scissors) should be used for cutting sutures to prevent unnecessary blunting of dissecting scissors. For removal of sutures, Paynes scissors are used. These are small and curved with the cutting surface of one blade hollowed out to fit under the suture easily. Scissors should be held with the ring finger and thumb inserted in the ring of the scissor and the index finger placed on the shaft to guide the scissors.

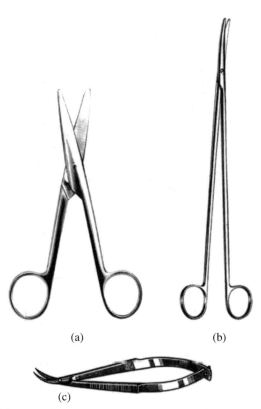

Fig. 20.13 Surgical scissors. (a) Mayo. (b) Metzenbaum. (c) Corneal.

Haemostatic or artery forceps

Artery forceps (Fig. 20.14) are designed to clamp blood vessels and thus stop bleeding. They come in several different lengths and shapes. Most have transverse striations to facilitate holding tissue. There are many different patterns of artery forceps. Some of those commonly used include the Spencer Wells, Dunhill, Crile, Cairns and Kelly. Mosquito forceps are very small artery forceps for finer blood vessels, the most common type being the Halstead forceps. Like scissors, artery forceps should be held with the ring finger and thumb using the index finger to steady the forceps.

Sponge holding forceps

These are designed to hold sponges or swabs for skin preparation prior to surgery (Fig. 20.27).

Tissue forceps

Allis tissue forceps and Babcock's forceps are the most commonly used type of tissue forceps (Fig. 20.15). They are designed to grasp tissue with minimal trauma but neither should be used to grasp and hold viscera; more specialised forceps such as Duvall's should be used for this.

Towel clips

These are used to attach drapes to the patient and instruments to the operating site (Fig. 20.16). Backhaus and Mayo forceps have a ringed handle and curved, pointed, tong-like tips. Gray's cross-action forceps, commonly used in veterinary surgery, have a strong spring-clip attachment.

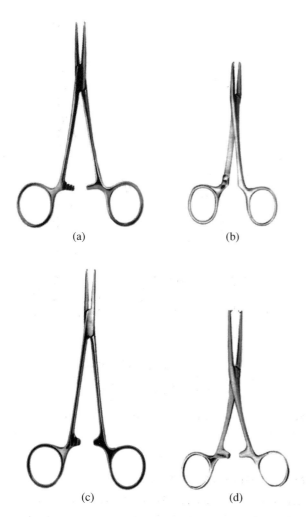

Fig. 20.14 Artery forceps. (a) Cairns, with a fine, slightly curved blade. (b) Spencer Wells, with a short, stubby blade. (c) Crile's, similar to Mayo but longer and finer. (d) Kocher's, with a toothed end and long serrated jaw.

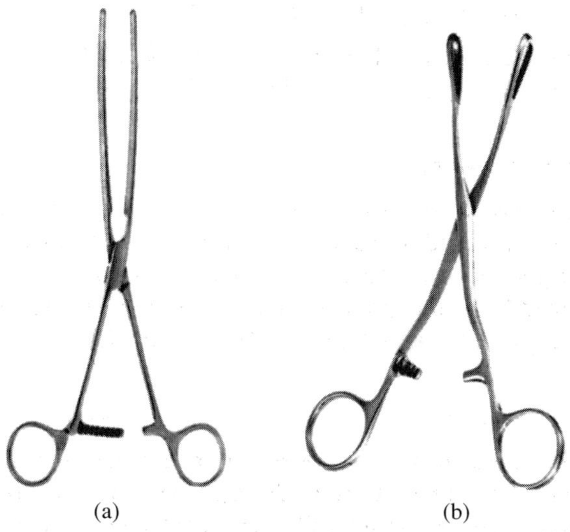

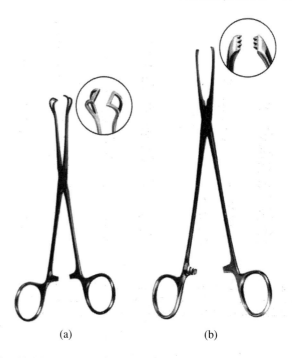

Fig. 20.16 Tissue forceps. (a) Babcock's. (b) Allis.

Needle-holders

Needle-holders are forceps that are specifically designed for holding suture needles during suturing and for knot tying (Fig. 20.18).

- Gillies needle-holders are very commonly used in veterinary surgery. They have a scissor action as well for cutting the suture ends. Their major disadvantage is that they have no ratchet, so that the needle has to be held in place by gripping the blades tightly.
- Olsen–Hegar needle-holders also have a cutting edge but have the advantage of a ratchet to hold the needle securely in place. The disadvantage of the scissor edge is that the suture material may be inadvertently cut.
- Mayo–Hegar needle-holders resemble a pair of long-handled artery forceps. They have a ratchet but no scissor action. This is one of the most popular types of needle-holder.

Fig. 20.15 (a) Doyen's bowel clamps. (b) Rampley's sponge-holding forceps.

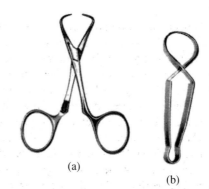

Fig. 20.17 Towel clips. (a) Backhaus. (b) Cross-action.

(a)

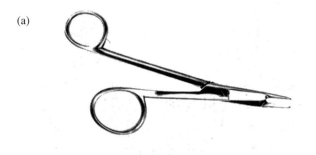

(b)

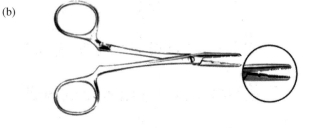

(c)

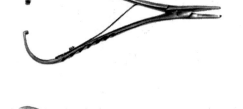

(d)

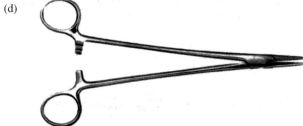
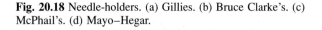

Fig. 20.18 Needle-holders. (a) Gillies. (b) Bruce Clarke's. (c) McPhail's. (d) Mayo–Hegar.

● McPhail's needle-holders traditionally have copper inserts in the tips, although those with tungsten carbide inserts are of superior quality. The handles have a spring ratchet so that by squeezing them together the jaws open and release the needle.

Retractors

These are used to facilitate exposure of the operating field (Fig. 20.19). They may be hand-held or self-retaining. Hand-held retractors include Langenbeck, Senn and Czerny; muscle and joint retractors include Gelpi, West's and Travers; examples of abdominal wall retractors are Gossett and Balfour; and Finochietto retractors are used for the chest.

Orthopaedic instruments

See also Chapter 19, p. 506.

Osteotomes, chisels and gouges

These are used to cut or shape bone or cartilage (Fig. 20.20). They are available in a wide variety of sizes. The cutting edge of the osteotome is tapered on both sides whereas the chisel is tapered on one side only. The gouge has a U-shaped edge to remove larger pieces of cartilage or soft bone.

Curettes

These have an oval-shaped cup. They scoop the surface of dense tissue to remove loose or degenerate tissue (e.g. cartilage flaps, necrotic bone). The cup has a sharp cutting edge and is available in various sizes (Fig. 20.20).

Periosteal elevators

These are used to lift periosteum and soft tissue from the surface of bone (Fig. 20.21).

Bone-holding forceps

These are designed to grip bone fragments during reduction and alignment in fracture repair (Fig. 20.22).

Bone cutters and rongeurs

Bone rongeurs (Fig. 20.23a) are used to cut out small pieces of dense tissue such as bone or cartilage. Bone cutters (Fig. 20.23b) are designed to cut larger pieces of bone.

Bone rasps

Bone rasps may be used to remove sharp edges following arthroplasty procedures.

Retractors

Standard retractors are commonly used in orthopaedic surgery but in addition hand-held Hohmann retractors are often used for retracting muscle, tendons and ligaments (Fig. 20.24).

Drills, saws and burrs

Hand, battery and air drills are commonly used in orthopaedic surgery (Fig. 20.25). Hand drills are useful around delicate structures and when only minimal drilling is required but for most major surgery a battery-operated or air

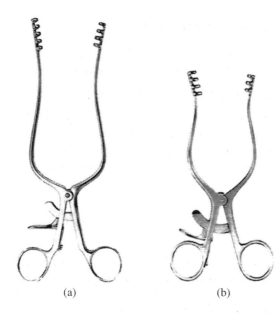

(a)

(b)

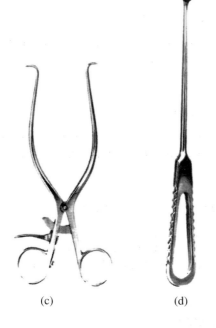

(c)

(d)

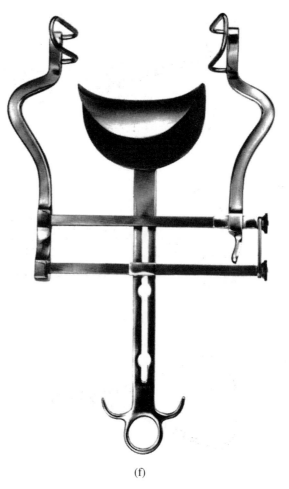

(f)

Fig. 20.19 Retractors. (a) Travers. (b) Weitlander's. (c) Gelpi. (d) Langenbeck. (e) Gossett. (f) Balfour.

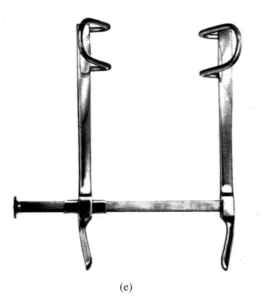

(e)

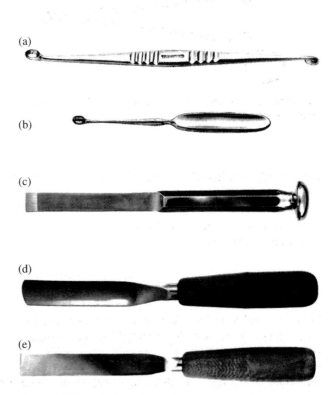

(a)

(b)

(c)

(d)

(e)

Fig. 20.20 Some basic orthopaedic instruments. (a) Volkmann's scoop. (b) Curette. (c) Chisel. (d) Gouge. (e) Osteotome.

(a)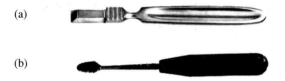

(b)

Fig. 20.21 Periosteal elevators. (a) Farabeuf's rugine. (b) Straight periosteal elevator

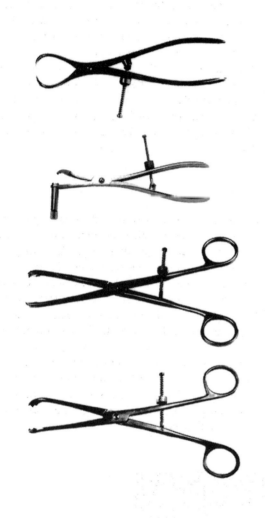

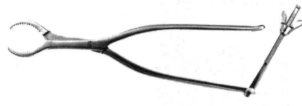

Fig. 20.22 Bone-holding forceps: self-centring forceps with speedlock fastening.

drill should be a prerequisite. These allow more speed and precision than hand drills. Battery drills tend to be slower and more cumbersome than most of the compact air drills available but they are suitable for most veterinary procedures and are less expensive. They should be recharged after each use.

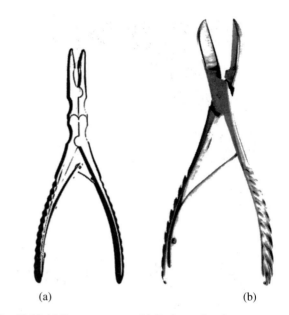

(a)   (b)

Fig. 20.23 (a) Bone rongeurs. (b) Bone-cutting forceps.

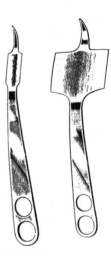

Fig. 20.24 Hohmann retractors.

Oscillating saws and mechanical burrs are either air or electrically driven. Great care should be taken when connecting attachments and during use. The power supply should not be applied until the couplings are assembled.

Wire forceps

Various wire-cutting and twisting forceps are available for applying cerclage wires and for stabilising bones with wire.

Gigli wire and handles

These are used in osteotomy techniques to saw through bone with a cheese-wire effect.

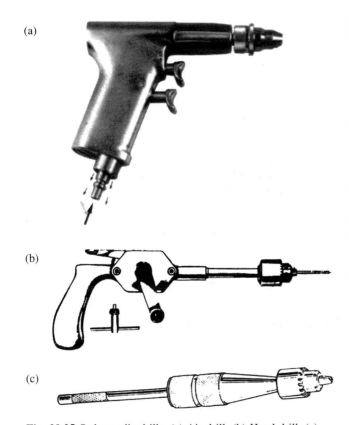

(a)

(b)

(c)

Fig. 20.25 Orthopaedic drills. (a) Air drill. (b) Hand drill. (c) Jacob's chuck.

Instrumentation for fracture repair

The instruments required for fracture repair depend on the technique which is to be used and are described in Chapter 21 (Care and Maintenance of Surgical Equipment). Materials used to repair fractures internally include Steinmann pins, orthopaedic wire, bone plates, screws and external fixator apparatus (see Fig. 20.28).

Packing a surgical set

Instrument sets are often packed together with swabs, drapes, suction tubing, etc. They are usually wrapped so that, when unfolded, the layers of wrapping will cover the base of the instrument trolley. A metal or plastic tray is usually lined with a towel or linen sheet. The instruments should then be laid out in a specific order. This is usually the order in which they are likely to be used (Fig. 20.26). Swabs, drapes, etc., are then added. A water-resistant paper wrap is then laid over the top of the trolley, followed by two layers of linen sheet. The tray is placed on this and the pack is then wrapped (Fig. 20.26). The set is secured with Bowie–Dick tape and tied with string. It should then be labelled and dated prior to sterilisation.

Instrument sets

Instrument sets are made up to suit individual requirements and they vary from one practice to another. Some practices have sets for specific procedures (e.g. bitch spay set). Others have a standard instrument set that is used for all operations, to which other instruments will be added depending on the procedure (Table 20.9). Often a smaller set will be available for minor procedures such as a cat spay. It is important that each of the standard instrument sets should contain the same number and type so that the surgical team always know what instruments they will have and so that it is easy to check that all are present at the end of the procedure. Table 20.9 lists suggested contents for various instrument sets required for surgical procedures but these are only guidelines.

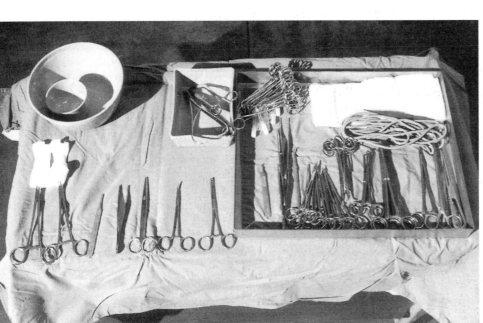

Fig. 20.26 Instruments laid out ready for use.

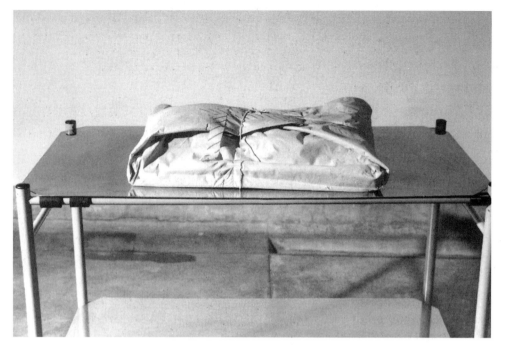

Fig. 20.27 Instrument set packed and ready for use.

Suction apparatus

A suction unit in the operating theatre is important for several reasons. It may be used for aspiration of the oropharynx and nasopharynx during or after surgery. It may be used for thoracocentesis following surgery or for suction of fluids and blood during the surgical procedure. Various suction machines are available and a size suitable for individual requirements should be chosen. It is sensible to choose a unit with two bottles so that there is always a spare when one bottle becomes full.

Suture materials

The ideal suture material should:

- Be suitable for use in any situation.
- Be readily available and inexpensive.
- Be readily sterilised by steam or ethylene oxide.
- Show high initial tensile strength, combined with small diameter material.
- Have a good knot security – it should tie easily, with no tendency to slip or loosen, and the knot should hold securely without fraying.
- Produce minimal tissue reaction – it should be inert (i.e. not cause pain or swelling or delay healing), non-allergenic, non-carcinogenic and non-electrolytic.
- Show good handling characteristics – it should be easy to handle when wet or dry and pass through tissue without friction or cutting.
- Not create an environment for bacterial growth, i.e. not show capillary or wicking of fluids (ideally monofilament).
- Be absorbed after its function has been served.

No single suture material in the wide range available possesses all of these ideal characteristics. Selection tends to depend on the surgeon's teaching and preferences. Table 20.10 gives the terms used to describe the characteristics of suture materials.

Classification of sutures

Suture materials are either absorbable or non-absorbable. They may be further classified as natural or synthetic, and as monofilament or multifilament. Examples of each category are shown in Table 20.11.

Common suture materials

Absorbable sutures

These materials are degraded within the tissues and lose their tensile strength by 60 days. The natural fibres (i.e. catgut) are removed by phagocytosis, which tends to produce some degree of tissue reaction. The synthetic absorbable materials are hydrolysed and tend to produce minimal tissue reaction. In general, absorbable suture materials are used when closing internal tissue layers or organs which do not require long-term support.

Catgut. Catgut is a derivation of the word 'kid-gut'. It is made from the submucosa of sheep small intestine or the serosa of cattle intestines. 'Plain catgut' is untreated; 'chromic catgut' is tanned with chromic salts to slow its absorption, increase its strength and decrease the tissue reaction (Table 20.12). Catgut is absorbed by phagocytosis and enzyme degradation. The rate of absorption is influenced by infection, blood supply and tissue pH.

- It loses its initial tensile strength very rapidly.
- It always causes a mild to severe inflammatory reaction.

- In contaminated sites it may act as a nidus for infection.
- It handles well; the knots are secure when dry but may loosen as it swells when it becomes wet.
- It also tends to break if pulled sharply during knot tying.

Polyglactin 910. This material is a co-polymer of lactide and glycolide and is absorbed by hydrolysis. It is available in dyed and undyed preparations, the latter causing less tissue reaction; it is coated to improve its handling characteristics and it is braided.

- It has a higher initial tensile strength than catgut.
- It loses 50% of its strength in 14 days and is totally absorbed in 60–90 days.
- There is considerable tissue drag and careful placement of knots is necessary.

Polyglycolic acid. This is an inert, non-antigenic, non-pyrogenic polyester made from hydroxyacetic acid and it is braided. It is absorbed by hydrolysis; the hydrolysed breakdown products have been found to be bacteriostatic experimentally, therefore its use has been advocated in infected sites.

- It loses approximately 30% of its strength in 7 days and 80% in 14 days.
- Tissue drag is considerable even in the coated formulation.
- It has poor knot security.

Polydioxanone. This is a monofilament absorbable suture which is absorbed by hydrolysis.

- It loses only 30% of its strength in 2 weeks and is minimally absorbed at 90 days.
- Tissue reaction is minimal.

- As it is monofilament, tissue drag is reduced.
- It is ideal in infected sites and where an absorbable material is required for a long period of time.
- Its main disadvantage is its springiness.

Polyglyconate. This is also a synthetic monofilament absorbable suture which is very similar to polydioxanone. It is slightly less springy and therefore easier to handle than polydioxanone.

Polyglecaprone 25. This is a new synthetic monofilament absorbable suture that is similar to both polydioxanone and polyglyconate, though duration of tensile strength is shorter.
- Less springy than polydioxanone and polyglyconate.
- Tissue reaction minimal.
- Tissue drag minimal.
- Broken down by hydrolysis.
- Main disadvantage is that at 14 days only 30% original strength maintained.

Non-absorbable sutures

These maintain their strength for longer than 60 days. The material is neither hydrolysed nor phagocytosed: it becomes encapsulated within fibrous tissue. Non-absorbable sutures are used where prolonged mechanical support is required. The main indications for use are:

- In skin closure, where sutures are generally removed after 10 days.
- Within slow-healing tissues.

Silk. This is available as braided or twisted strands. It is obtained from threads spun by the silkworm larvae. It may be coated with silicone or wax to minimise the capillarity which may promote infection.

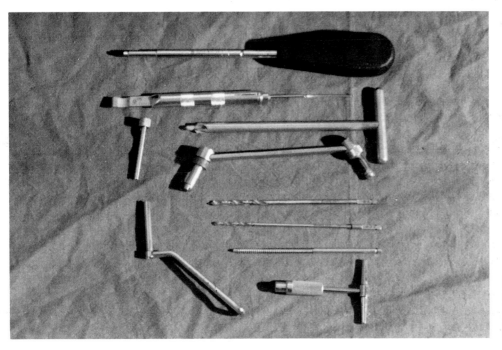

Fig. 20.28 ASIF (Association for the Study of Internal Fixation) instruments for internal fixation.

Table 20.9 Instrument sets for various surgical procedures: some suggested contents

			No. of pairs
Standard instrument set	Scalpel handle no. 3		×1
	Dissecting forceps –	rat toothed fine	×1
		rat toothed heavy duty	×1
		fine plain	×1
	Mayo scissors –	straight	×1
	Metzenbaum scissors		×1
	Artery forceps		×10
	Mosquito forceps		×5
	Allis tissue forceps		×4
	Suture scissors		×1
	Needle-holders		×1
	Langenbeck retractors		×2
	Gelpi retractor		×1
	Probe		×1
	Backhaus towel-holding forceps		×10
	Gallipot		×1
	Receiver		×1
	Suture tray		×1
	Suction tubing and tip		×1
	Electrocautery and handle		×1
	Swabs (X-ray detectable)		×10
	Scalpel blades size 10 and 15		×2

Different types of surgery may require the addition of other instruments.

Abdominal surgery	Self-retaining retractors (e.g. Gossett)
	Doyen's bowel clamps (Figure 20.27)
	Long dissecting forceps
	Long artery forceps (e.g. Roberts)
	Towels to pack abdomen

Thoracic surgery	Rib cutters
	Finochietto rib retractors
	Periosteal elevator
	Chest drain
	Suture wire ⎫
	Oscillating saw ⎭ If sternotomy approach
	Lobectomy clamps
	Long-handled artery forceps (e.g. Roberts)
	Rib raspatory

Orthopaedic surgery

General:

Osteotome	Gigli wire and handles
Chisel	Periosteal elevator
Curette	Hand drill
Gouge	
Mallet	
Hohmann retractor	
Putti rasp	
Hacksaw	
Lister's bone cutting forceps	
Bone rongeurs	

Power tools:
  Battery drill
  Air drill
  Mechanical burr
  Oscillating saw

Implants:
  Stainless steel wire
  Intramedullary pins
  Kirschner wires
  Rush pins
  Staples
  Screws
  Plates

In addition to general orthopaedic instruments:

Bone pinning:
  Jacob's chuck and key
  Pin cutters
  Steinmann pin

Wire fixation:
  Stainless steel wire
  Wire-holding forceps
  Wire-cutting forceps

Table 20.9 (Continued)

	Bone staples:
	  Bone staples
	  Staple introducer
	  Staple remover
	External fixator:
	  Steinmann pins
	  Kirschner Ehmer rods
	  Kirschner Ehmer nuts
	  Pin cutter
	  Drill or Jacob's chuck
	Bone plating or screw fixation:
	  Venables/Sherman bone plates
	  Sherman screws
	  Drill bit
	  Air/hand drill
	  Depth gauge
	  Screw driver
	  Plate bender
	ASIF technique (Figure 20.28)
	(Association for the Study of Internal Fixation)
	  Dynamic compression plates and screws
	  Bone drills: standard and overdrill
	  Bone tap and handle
	  Drill guide – neutral and loaded
	  Tap sleeve
	  Drill insert
	  Depth gauge
	  Counter sink
	  Screw driver
	  Plate bender or irons

Ophthalmic instruments	No. 3 scalpel handle Scalpel blade sizes 11, 15 or Beaver handle and blades Fine dissecting forceps Fine scissors Corneal scissors Capsule forceps Vectis Iris repositor Castroviejo needle-holders Eyelid speculum Irrigating cannula Distichiasis forceps
Dental instruments	Mouth gag Dental scalers Dental elevators Dental chisels Dental forceps Ultrasonic descaler

Silk has good handling characteristics, excellent knot security and good tensile strength. It is relatively inexpensive. Its main uses include cardiovascular and thoracic surgery, genital mucosa, and adjacent to eyes. It should not be used in infected sites, oral mucosa or hollow organs where it may act as a nidus for infection.

Linen. This is twisted from long strands of flax. It is easily sterilised, handles well and has excellent knot security. It does show capillary properties however and has been shown to contribute to sinus formation. It has been largely superseded since the advent of the synthetic absorbable materials.

Polypropylene. This is an inert, non-absorbable, monofilament material. It has high tensile strength but tends to stretch and will snap if crushed by needle-holders. The knot security is varied and a bulky knot may be formed. It is very springy but shows little tissue drag. It becomes encapsulated in a thin fibrous covering.

Polyamide. This may be either monofilament or braided. The monofilament form causes little tissue reactions, has little tissue drag and is non-capillary. Its handling characteristics are not good and knot security can be poor. It loses approximately 15% of its tensile strength each year. It can be used on fascia and muscle, but the buried ends can be irritant in serous or synovial cavities. The braided form is usually sheathed in an attempt to decrease capillarity but its use as a buried suture is not recommended. It shows more tissue drag than the monofilament variety, although it handles better.

Table 20.10 Characteristics of suture materials: terminology

Tensile strength	The breaking strength per unit area of tissue.
Knot security	Related to the surface frictional characteristics of the material. Every suture is weakest where it is tied. Often the strongest sutures have the poorest knot security.
Tissue reaction	The response of the tissue to the suture material involved.
Tissue drag	The degree of frictional force developed as the material is pulled through the tissue.
Capillarity	The extent to which tissue fluid is attracted along the suture material. Materials with high capillarity act as a wick and encourage fluids to move along them. Such materials should not be used in the presence of sepsis.
Memory	The tendency of the material to return to its original shape. A material with high memory tends to unkink during knot tying, i.e. knot security is poor with materials possessing high memory.
Chatter	The lack of smoothness as a throw of a knot is tightened down.
Stiffness and elongation	The less force required to stretch a suture, the more it will elongate before it ruptures.
Sterilisation characteristics	The ability of the material to undergo sterilisation without deteriorating. Autoclaving is satisfactory for the nylon materials. Repeated autoclaving will, however, weaken them. The natural products and synthetic absorbable materials should not be steam sterilised. Ethylene oxide sterilisation is safe for all sutures provided the packs are sufficiently aerated.

Table 20.11 Examples of suture categories

	Natural fibres	Synthetic	
Absorbable sutures	Multifilament: Catgut: plain chromic	**Monofilament** Polydioxanone Polyglyconate	[PDS II]** [Maxon]
		Multifilament Polyglecaprone 25 Polyglactin 910 Polyglycolic acid	[Monocryl] [Vicryl]** [Dexon]*
Non-absorbable sutures	Multifilament Silk Linen	**Multifilament** Braided polyamide Polyester Coated polyester	[Nuralon]** [Supramid] [Mersilene]** [Ethibond]**
		Monofilament Polyamide Polypropylene Polybutylester Polyethylene	[Ethilon]** [Prolene]** [Novafil]* [Dermalene]**
		Stainless steel	

* Trademark Davis & Geck Ltd.
** Trademark Ethicon.

Table 20.12 Catgut: approximate absorption times

Plain gut	3–7 days	Severe tissue reaction
Mild treatment	14 days	
Medium treatment	21 days	Most commonly used
Prolonged treatment	40 days	

Polyesters. Various braided polyesters are available. They are easy to handle and retain their tensile strength well. Some are coated with silicone, Teflon or polybutylate to reduce tissue drag. They tend to have poor knot-tying quality and some have shown signs of capillarity.

Stainless steel. This is available in monofilament or braided varieties. It is very strong, inert and non-capillary. It is relatively difficult to handle as the wire lacks elasticity and knots may be difficult to tie, but knot security is good. It is useful in slow-healing tissues such as bone, tendon and joint capsules, and in contaminated sites. It has become less popular in recent years as newer materials have become available.

Alternatives to sutures

Staples

Metal clips or staples for use in skin and other tissues have gained popularity in the field of veterinary surgery over the last few years. Staples designed for skin closure are packed in a gun-like applicator for rapid insertion. These instruments are intended to be disposable, although they may be safely sterilised by ethylene oxide.

The main advantage of staples is speed of insertion. They are inert and well tolerated. Re-usable staple-removing forceps are available to remove metal skin staples.

Stapling machines have also been designed for gastrointestinal anastomosis. Although designed for the human market, they are suitable for veterinary applications and are gaining popularity. They may permit resection of areas of bowel that are inaccessible to routine suturing, particularly in the equine abdomen. Their major disadvantage is cost, but their ease of use and the shortened surgery time have much to recommend them.

Metal clips are also available for use as ligatures. They come in various sizes with re-usable applicators. They are simple and quick to use.

Table 20.13 Suture materials suitable for different tissues

Skin	Monofilament nylon or polypropylene Metal staples Avoid materials with capillary action
Subcutis	Fine synthetic absorbable material with minimal tissue reaction, e.g. polydioxanone, polyglactin, polyglycolic acid
Muscle	Synthetic absorbable, non-absorbable, e.g. nylon
Fascia	Synthetic non-absorbable if prolonged suture strength required
Hollow viscus	Synthetic absorbable or polypropylene. In bladder: monofilament synthetic absorbable
Tendon	Nylon, polypropylene, stainless steel
Blood vessels	Polypropylene: least thrombogenic is silk
Eyes	Synthetic absorbable, e.g. polyglactin, polydioxanone
Nerves	Nylon or polypropylene: minimal tissue reaction

Table 20.14 Sizes of suture material

Metric	USP – non-absorbable Synthetic absorbable	Catgut
0.2	10/0	
0.3	9/0	
0.4	8/0	
0.5	7/0	8/0
0.7	6/0	7/0
1	5/0	6/0
1.5	4/0	5/0
2	3/0	4/0
3	2/0	3/0
3.5	0	2/0
4	1	0
5	2	1
6	3 & 4	2
7	5	3
8	6	4

Sutures come in either metric or USP (US Pharmacopeia) sizes

Tissue glue

There are cyanoacrylate monomers which polymerise on contact with moisture in the wound. They have been found useful by some surgeons.

Adhesive tapes

Designed for use in humans, these have been of limited use in animals as they do not adhere well to moist skin.

Suture selection

The veterinary surgeon will normally select the suture material but the veterinary nurse should have some idea of which materials may be used in different tissues (Table 20.13) and the sizes that will be required (Table 20.14).

When selecting suture sizes, small-diameter materials should be chosen. These cause less tissue reaction, form smaller knots, knot more easily and are less likely to tie too tight (because they will break). If sutures are tied too tight, they will cut through friable tissue.

Packaging of suture materials

Individual packets. Most suture materials are purchased in pre-sterilised individual packets. This guarantees a sterile suture (unless the packet is damaged) and a needle in perfect condition where one is attached. The only disadvantage is that of cost. Synthetic absorbable suture materials are only available packaged in this way.

Cassettes. Multi-use cassettes are frequently used in veterinary practice for packaging catgut, nylon and stainless steel sutures. The disadvantage of these is the likelihood of contamination of cassettes during use – they often become damaged. It is also easy to contaminate the material as it is cut from the reel and transferred to the instrument trolley.

Suture needles

Suture needles are designed to pass through tissue easily. They must be sharp enough to penetrate tissues with minimal resistance, rigid enough to prevent excessive bending and yet flexible enough to bend before breaking. They should be made from corrosion-resistant stainless steel.

Swaged needles

Swaged or atraumatic needles are attached to the suture material, i.e. they do not require threading. The advantage of this is that a needle in perfect condition is available with each strand and tissue trauma is minimised by the passage of material and needle of a comparative size. All of the pre-packed suture materials are available with a variety of different needle shapes and sizes.

Eyed needles

This type of needle requires threading. The primary indication for its use is economy of suitable material or use of speciality needles, e.g. for large animal work. The disadvantages are increased tissue trauma due to the eye size, loss of sharpness of the needle tip, bending and corrosion following repeated use. The needle shape refers to both the longitude shape of the shaft and the cross-sectional shape.

Longitudinal shape

Of the great variety of different sizes and shapes that are available, some of those used in veterinary surgery are shown in Fig. 20.29.

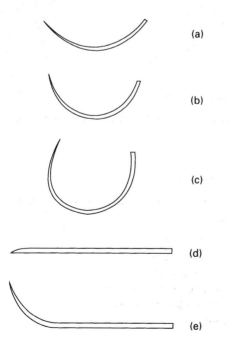

Fig. 20.29 Suture needle shapes: (a) ⅜ circle, (b) ½ circle, (c) ⅝ circle, (d) straight and (e) ½ curved.

Cross-sectional shape

Round-bodied. These are designed to separate tissue fibres rather than cut them, and are used for soft tissue or in situations where easy splitting of tissue fibres is possible.

Modified point. The **taper-cut** needle has a cutting tip on the point of the needle and a round body. This provides increased penetration of the needle without increased tissue trauma.

The **trocar-point** needle has a strong cutting head and a robust round body. This is useful in dense tissue.

Cutting needles. These are required wherever dense or tough tissue needs to be sutured. The cross-sectional appearance of the needle is usually a triangular cutting edge which extends at least half-way along the shaft. The reverse cutting needle has the cutting edge on the outside of the needle curvature to improve strength and resistance to bending.

Micro-point needles. These are very fine needles with a sharp cutting edge. They are designed for ophthalmic and micro-surgery.

Selection of needles

The use of swaged needles is to be encouraged – their advantages far outweigh those of eyed needles. Other needles should be as close as possible in diameter to that of the suture. A large needle tract invites bacteria and foreign substances to enter the wound, thus delaying healing. The needle should be of the appropriate shape and size to enable the veterinary surgeon to close the wound accurately and precisely.

The smaller and deeper the wound, the greater the curve should be. Straight needles are designed to be hand held and tend to be used in the skin. Half-curved cutting needles have been commonly used in veterinary surgery but have little to recommend their use. The tissue type will determine the necessary point of the needle. Generally speaking:

- Round-bodied needles are used for viscera, subcutaneous and friable tissue.
- Taper-tip needles are used for easily penetrated tissue, i.e. for denser tissue.
- Cutting needles are generally used in the skin.

Suture patterns

Veterinary nurses maintained on the list held by the RCVS are now legally allowed to perform minor acts of surgery, including the suturing of wounds, and it is important that they should be familiar with basic suturing techniques. The veterinary surgeon should give practical instruction and reference should be made to surgical technique textbooks.

Suture patterns (Fig. 20.30) may be interrupted or closed, and may be further classified as apposing, everting or inverting:

- **Apposing** sutures bring the tissues in direct apposition.
- **Everting** sutures tend to turn the edges of the wound outwards.
- **Inverting** sutures turn the tissue inwards (e.g. towards the lumen of a viscus).

Surgical knots

A surgical knot has three main components:

- The **loop** is the part of the suture material within the opposed or ligated tissue.
- The **knot** is composed of a number of **throws**, each throw being the linking of two strands of tissue around each other.
- The **ears** are the cut ends of the suture which prevent the knot coming untied.

Knots can be tied by hand or by an instrument. Hand ties may be single- or two-handed.

The basic surgical knot is the reef knot or square knot. A surgeon's knot has an initial double throw instead of a single throw. This reduced the risk of the first throw loosening before the second throw is placed.

Hand-tying helps to prevent slippage of the first throw, since tension can be kept on both ends of the suture throughout the procedure. However, it tends to be wasteful on suture material.

The knots of skin sutures should be pulled to one side of the incision and the suture loop should be loose. Sutures which are too tight compromise the vascular supply, enhance infection and delay healing. They are also uncomfortable and encourage the patient to interfere with the wound.

Suture material should not be crushed in the jaws of needle-holders. When tying knots, only the end of the suture material should be grasped. Needle-holders should not be clamped on to the eye of swaged needles as this will cause damage or breakage of the needle.

Interrupted sutures

The main advantage of the interrupted suture is its ability to maintain strength and tissue apposition if part of the suture line fails. Each suture is individually tied and cut distal to the knot. Its main disadvantage is the amount of suture material used and left within the tissue and the time required to suture.

Continuous sutures

These are neither knotted nor cut, except at each end of the suture line. The advantages of the continuous suture line are ease of application, use of minimal amount of suture material and ease of removal. The main disadvantage is that slippage of either the beginning or end knot is likely to cause failure of the entire suture line.

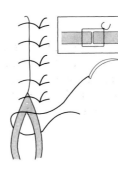
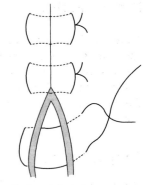

Simple interrupted   Horizontal mattress

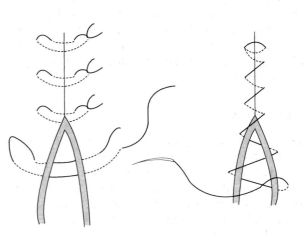

Vertical mattress   Simple continuous

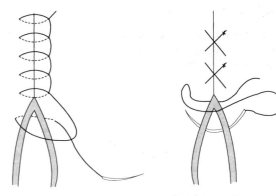

Ford interlocking   Cruciate mattress

Fig. 20.30 Common suture patterns used in the skin.

Common suture patterns

Skin. Common suture patterns used in the skin (Fig. 20.30) include:

- Simple interrupted.
- Simple continuous.
- Ford interlocking.
- Interrupted vertical mattress.
- Interrupted horizontal mattress.
- Cruciate mattress.

Skin sutures should be placed at least 5 mm from the skin edge and be placed squarely across the wound. The skin should be handled gently with fine rat-toothed forceps. The wound edges should be apposed or slightly everted with no gaping or overlapping.

Muscle and fascia
- Simple interrupted.
- Simple continuous.
- Ford interlocking.
- Cruciate mattress.
- Horizontal mattress.
- Vertical mattress.
- Mayo mattress.

Hollow organ closure
- Simple interrupted.
- Parker–Kerr.
- Purse-string.

- Connell.
- Cushing.
- Lembert.
- Gambee.
- Halstead.

Further reading

College of Animal Welfare, (1997) *Veterinary Surgical Instruments*, Butterworth-Heinemann, Oxford.

Knecht, C. D., Allen, A. R., Williams, D. J. and Johnson, J. H. (1987) *Fundamental Techniques in Veterinary Surgery*, 3rd edn, W. B. Saunders, Philadelphia.

McCurnin, D. M. (1990) *Clinical Textbook for Veterinary Technicians*, 2nd edn, W. B. Saunders, Philadelphia.

Tracey, D. *Small Animal Surgical Nursing*, Mosby, St Louis.

21

Care and maintenance of surgical equipment

K. A. Wiggins

Care and maintenance of surgical equipment is generally the responsibility of the veterinary nurse. To assist with the day-to-day running of a veterinary establishment, surgical equipment should be well maintained and frequently checked. Manufacturers' instructions for cleaning and general care should be carefully followed to maintain a consistently low level of contamination and to keep items in efficient working order but also to extend the working life of each item.

An efficient method of maintaining surgical equipment is to compile a file of maintenance manuals and to establish a checklist of the equipment, with details of the maintenance procedures required and the intervals at which maintenance should be performed.

The following information could be collated in a maintenance file for each piece of equipment:

- Name of equipment.
- Location.
- Model number and serial number.
- Name of manufacturer.
- Name and telephone number of company from which it was purchased.
- Name and telephone number of salesperson.
- Name and telephone number of person to call for servicing.
- Date of purchase.
- Period of warranty.
- Dates of routine maintenance.

This system of recording information will save time in the future should the equipment require some form of repair.

Items that should be listed for maintenance of this type include the following:

- Anaesthetic equipment.
- Monitoring devices.
- Suction equipment.
- Ventilator.
- Diathermy equipment.
- Surgical lights.
- Surgical table.
- Air-conditioning/heating system.
- Dental scaler.
- Clippers.
- Laundry equipment (washer and dryer).
- Refrigerator.
- Ultrasound machine.
- ECG machine.
- Cryosurgery equipment.
- Endoscopes.

Care and maintenance of surgical instruments

The basic rules for the care and maintenance of surgical instruments apply whether a veterinary nurse works in general practice or in a specialised institution.

Many varieties of surgical instruments feature in a wide range of instrumentation catalogues that are readily obtainable from manufacturers and wholesalers. These catalogues provide excellent descriptions of surgical equipment and are very useful for revision and training purposes.

The cost of surgical instruments may appear to be extraordinarily high but in most cases high quality is worthy of investment. Instruments of lesser quality may be cheaper to purchase but may prove to be more expensive in the long term: their performance may not meet certain needs and rapid wear or corrosion may necessitate early replacement. Good-quality stainless steel surgical instruments that are handled and cared for properly will last for years before replacement becomes necessary.

Instrument metals

Chromium-plated carbon steel surgical instruments are commonly found in veterinary hospitals. They are popular because of their low price, ease of maintenance and highly polished finish. The plated surface, however, is susceptible to attack by low pH solutions, saline and other chemicals. Early deterioration by pitting, rusting and blistering of the plated surface is a very common problem, resulting in early repair or replacement.

Better quality surgical instruments are made from **stainless steel**. Stainless steel is not a single specific material but consists primarily of iron, chromium and carbon, with other elements such as nickel combined in different proportions to achieve the desired properties.

Two major types of stainless steel are used for surgical equipment. The first is **martensitic**, a higher carbon stainless steel that provides greater hardness through heat treatment. This imparts wear resistance, which is especially important for sharp-bladed surgical instruments (e.g. scissors and ophthalmic equipment) where fine edges must be maintained and strength and durability must be exhibited. The hard martensitic steels are most commonly used in the manufacture of surgical instruments.

The second type of stainless steel is **austenitic**. This is hardened, not by heat treatment but by work: as machine-forming takes place, the material gets harder. Its use is limited to the fabrication of bowls, sinks and some types of retractor blades and speculae.

The lack of hardness exhibited by these alloys is offset somewhat by their higher resistance to corrosion. Austenitic steels are often used for screws and rivets in surgical instruments.

Tungsten carbide inserts add an extra dimension to gripping and cutting surfaces. These substances are very hard and very resistant to wear. The inserts are attached to stainless steel instruments by various means and can be removed and replaced by the manufacturer. Some manufacturers identify these better quality instruments by gold-coloured handles.

Resistance to corrosion

A stainless steel instrument attains its resistance to corrosion by passing through a series of manufacturing processes. This begins with selection of the correct material, which is then forged, descaled, machined and fitted. The new instrument is hardened by heat-treatment and then buffed and polished to a smooth surface. A highly polished finish is more resistant to spotting and discoloration, but it reflects light easily and can cause mild eye irritation. More recently a dull satin finish has become popular, one advantage of which is reduced eye strain.

The final process of corrosion resistance is passivation. This involves bathing the finished instrument in a nitric acid solution, which burns out foreign particles that may have become embedded on its surface during the manufacturing process. Additionally a thin layer of chromium oxide forms on the stainless steel, providing more corrosion resistance.

Instrument cleaning

Careful consideration should be given to the cleaning of instruments. To comply with COSHH Regulations, a veterinary nurse dealing with used surgical instruments must wear protective clothing, i.e. rubber gloves and plastic apron.

- The first task should be the safe removal and disposal of **sharps** such as scalpel blades and suture needles. The safest way to attach and remove scalpel blades is with a **haemostat**. After use, blades should be placed in a rigid clinical waste container. Bear in mind that old and worn blades can inflict serious lacerations.
- Instruments should be *separated* so that heavy pieces, especially orthopaedic equipment, are kept apart from smaller, more delicate instruments.
- All *blood and tissue debris* should be cleaned off immediately, before it dries on the instruments. Initial soaking in cold water is very effective. Hot water will cause coagulation of proteins and should not be used.
- *Saline solutions* used during surgery should be rinsed from the instruments as soon as possible. Instruments should never be soaked in saline, as this can cause pitting of the instrument surface and will lead to corrosion.
- The *washing* of instruments is carried out effectively under cool or warm running water using a hand brush with stiff plastic bristles. Particular attention should be paid to serrations, ratchets, box joints and other areas not easily exposed. A range of hand brushes for cleaning instruments is very useful. Those with long handles and round ends, used for cleaning endotracheal tubes, are very effective for instruments with tubular cavities.
- *Abrasive cleaners* should be avoided as repeated cleaning can damage the instrument surface. Ideally, a moderately alkaline low-lather *detergent* should be used or alternatively a chemical cleaner specifically manufactured for instrument cleaning. The manufacturers' recommendations for use must be followed carefully.
- Ordinary *soap* should not be used, especially with hard water, as insoluble alkali films can form on the surface of the instrument trapping bacteria and thus protecting them from sterilisation.
- *Water* plays a major role: water alone accounts for much of the solvent action that occurs during instrument cleaning. As the quality of tap water in many areas is poor, careful consideration should be given to matching water quality with the appropriate detergent. Softened demineralised or distilled water should be considered to eliminate the deposition of hard-water salts on instruments, especially during the final rinsing.

Ultrasonic cleaners

Ultrasonic cleaners (Fig. 21.1) are convenient and can be used in any veterinary establishment. These small electrical units hold a wiremesh basket or perforated tray and are used with an ultrasonic detergent cleaner, especially formulated for its cleaning abilities and its chemical effects on the instruments being cleaned. The instruments are placed in the wire basket or tray and then submerged into the cleaner. The majority of these cleaners have timers and the cleaning cycle is generally 15 minutes.

Ultrasonic cleaners are very effective for the removal of debris from areas that are inaccessible to manual brushing, such as box joints and deep grooves. They work by the production of sinusoidal energy waves, with the frequency of vibrations in excess of 20,000 per second. The effectiveness of ultrasonic cleaning is based on a process called **cavitation**. Ultrasonic energy produces minute bubbles of gas within the cleaning solution. These bubbles form on the surface of the instruments and expand until their surface becomes unstable and then collapse by **implosion** (bursting inwards). The bubbles implode as fast as they form, creating small vacuum areas. This process releases energy and breaks the bonds that hold debris to instrument surfaces. The debris is then dislodged or dissolved into the solution.

The use of an ultrasonic cleaner is as an adjunct to the initial washing procedure rather than a replacement for it. Points to bear in mind when using the cleaner are:

- Rubber gloves should be worn, as the detergent may be harmful to the skin.
- Ensure that the manufacturer's instructions for detergent dilutions are carried out correctly.
- All instruments with joints should be opened when in the basket or tray.

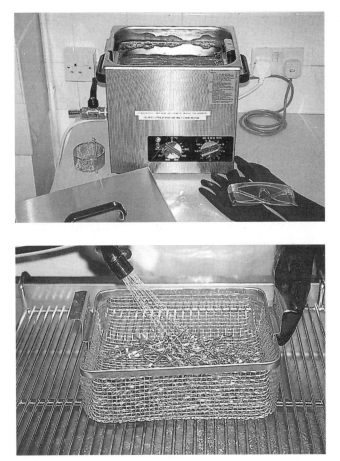

Fig. 21.1 Ultrasonic cleaner.

- Different types of metal should not be mixed. Electrolysis may occur and the instrument surfaces may be damaged.
- Instruments removed from an ultrasonic cleaner must be rinsed thoroughly to remove residual detergent.
- The use of an ultrasonic cleaner is as an adjunct to, and not a replacement for, the initial washing procedure.

Instrument lubrication

Surgical instruments with movable parts, particularly box joints, become stiff with repeated use. Instrument lubrication is commonly practised but can present problems if not properly performed. Mineral oil, machine oils and grease must be avoided: they leave an oily film on the instrument surface and can trap bacterial spores, preventing adequate penetration during steam sterilisation.

Instrument manufacturers recommend routine lubrication of instruments with an antimicrobial water-soluble lubricant (**instrument milk**). This is a water–oil emulsion that does not interfere with sterilisation. It is particularly important to lubricate instruments after cleaning with an ultrasonic cleaner, as the effective cleaning will remove all previous lubricants.

The lubricant bath should be prepared according to the manufacturer's recommendations. The instruments are submerged in the lubricant for at least 30 seconds (wearing

rubber gloves is advisable). After removal from the bath the lubricant should be allowed to drain away without rinsing or manual drying; this gives added protection against corrosion. Follow the manufacturer's instructions for the disposal of used instrument milk to comply with COSHH Regulations.

Instrument checking before packaging

Instruments should be checked regularly for distortion, misalignment and incorrect assembly. *Forceps* in particular should be checked:

- For tip alignment.
- That daylight cannot be seen through the serrations.
- That the ratchet grips are sound.

Needle-holders can be tested by lifting threads of suture material to test their grip. *Scissors* must be sharp: test them prior to packaging by checking that the tips will cut through four thicknesses of gauze swab or equivalent. It is advisable to have spare pairs of sharpened scissors sterilised separately for inclusion in the surgical pack should the veterinary surgeon discover the scissors in use are inadequately sharp for the surgical procedure.

Instrument packaging for sterilisation

Once the instruments have been cleaned and lubricated, they can be prepared for sterilisation. It is recommended that instruments that are not required on a day-to-day basis (e.g. specialised orthopaedic equipment used in elected surgical procedures) should be stored unsterilised in a clean dry environment.

There are various methods of packaging instruments prior to sterilisation. Packaging materials frequently used are textile wraps (usually cotton), paper, plastic and paper and plastic combinations.

- **Textile wraps** are commonly used for packaging instruments sets. They are easy to use, washable, flexible and long-lasting. However, they are easily contaminated by contact with moisture.
- **Double-wrapping** instrument kits with a textile wrap and a surgical paper wrap increases safe storage. The paper has a water repellency but still allows steam penetration during sterilisation.
- Double wrapping of **sterile packages** provides a margin for safety during package opening. Dust contamination that has settled on a package is thrown into the surrounding air during opening, making the contamination of contents very likely, but a second wrap greatly reduces this risk.
- **Plastic and paper wraps** and paper and plastic combinations are used extensively, especially for individual instrument packing. Packaging with peel-back openings for presentation of sterile instruments lessens the possibility of contamination.
- Plastic and cardboard boxes, available in various shapes and sizes, are also used. Again, an outer wrap increases sterility.

- **Sharp and pointed instruments** should be protected to prevent accidental penetration of the surgical packaging. Various sizes of protective covers are commercially available. As an additional measure, instruments packaged in bags should always be positioned so that the instrument handle emerges from the bag first when opened (see Figs 21.2 and 21.3).

Instrument identification

Date, label and initial all packages with a felt-tip marker, writing on the plastic side only or on the indicator tape to avoid puncturing or the bleeding through of ink.

Colour-coded plastic autoclave tape is often used for the identification of instruments, especially where different surgical kits are employed.

(a)

(b)

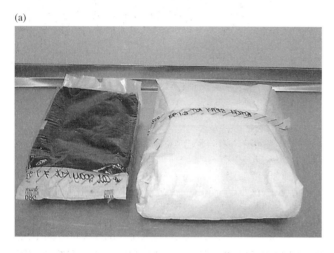

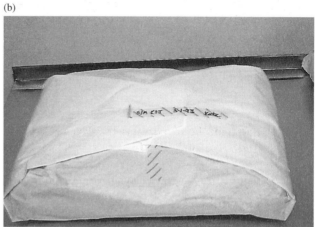

(c)

(d)

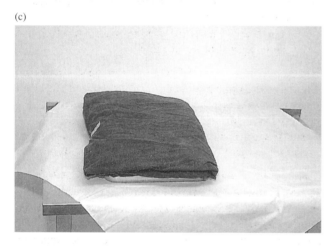

(e)

(f)

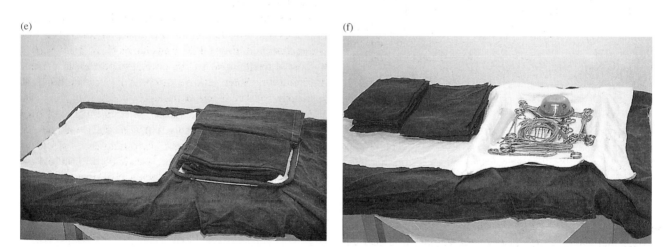

Fig. 21.2 Unpacking a small animal surgical kit. The kit has been double-wrapped to reduce contamination. Surgical drapes are sterilised with the instruments.

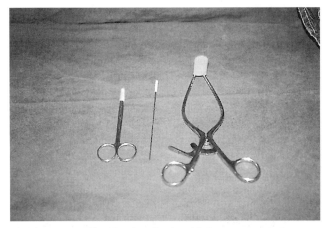

Fig. 21.3 Protecting sharp and pointed instruments to prevent accidental penetration of the surgical packaging.

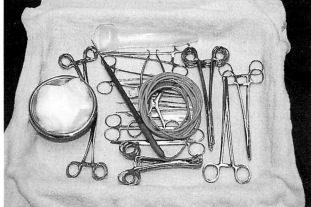

Fig. 21.4 Example of layout for a small animal surgical kit. The large empty syringe case holds the diathermy handle when not being used during the surgery.

Engraving should be avoided, as this can damage the instrument surface and predispose to staining and corrosion.

Instrument kits

Surgical instruments should be selected to suit the purpose for which they are to be used, rather than because they were convenient to use at the time. For example, artery forceps used to extract intramedullary pins may have the desired effect but will almost certainly be damaged.

The basic surgical kit generally consists of instruments for cutting, dissection, tissue-holding, retraction, haemostasis, ligation and suturing. Surgical kits can be assembled on this basis but also bear in mind the size of animal. For example, instruments used for a cat spay will vary in size to those used for a bitch spay. Most veterinary establishments develop surgical kits for various procedures. A basic kit is often employed, and then specific instruments for special procedures are packed and prepared either individually or in special procedure packs.

Chapter 20 (Theatre Practice) sets out suggestions for different instrument kits.

The laying out of instruments in a kit should be given careful thought. They should be placed in positions which relate to their actual requirement (Fig. 21.4). Every veterinary surgeon has personal preferences and through good communication, observation and anticipation, the veterinary nurse will help to ensure efficient and consistent surgical procedures.

Special equipment

Ultrasound (see also Chapter 24, p. 677)

Ultrasound is sound of frequencies higher than those audible to the human ear. Diagnostic ultrasound is a non-invasive procedure that allows the internal structures of the abdominal and thoracic cavities to be examined visually. It usually employs sound waves of frequencies between 1 and 15 MHz.

These sound waves are produced by electrical vibration of a 'piezo-electric' crystal stored in the ultrasound transducer, or probe, and they have sufficient energy to penetrate living tissue. Different structures within the body and interfaces between structures and organs impede the passage of sound to varying extents. Those sound waves that are not transmitted are reflected back towards their source of origin, where their strength can be detected and thus the degree of attenuation can be recorded electronically on an oscilloscope screen.

The ultrasound scan is recorded in images of black and white with varying shades of grey:

- Fluid is recorded as black, because the sound waves pass through it unimpeded.
- Bone, other mineral densities and also gases, reflect the sound waves totally and are recorded as white.
- Soft tissues appear as various shades of grey, depending on their proportions of fat, fibrous tissue and fluid.

There are two main types of transducer: linear and sector. **Linear transducers** have the crystals arranged in a line, each producing sound waves that form a rectangular sound beam. Superficial structures can be seen well but the transducer itself is bulky and cumbersome, which limits its use with small animals.

Sector transducers contain a single crystal which oscillates or rotates to produce a fan-shaped beam. The size and manoeuvrability of these transducers allow ready access to most of the thoracic and abdominal viscera even in small dogs and cats. Superficial structures, however, are not seen so clearly because of the shape of the beam.

Transducers are also available in a selection of frequencies. A higher frequency will penetrate far less but will provide better resolution than a lower frequency. A 5 MHz transducer provides an adequate depth of penetration for cats and small to medium-sized dogs. A 3.5 MHz transducer is required for large dogs.

Procedure

It is very important to achieve good skin contact with the transducer when scanning an animal. Hair is better clipped, although it is possible in the longer-haired dogs and cats to part the hair (this is preferable in a show animal). The skin should be clean and free from dirt and grease – surgical spirit helps to degrease it. A proprietary aqueous gel is then applied to the skin and to the transducer, to enable efficient contact. Poor contact will result in a distorted image, often with arc-shaped or horizontal white lines.

Ultrasound is generally carried out on the conscious patient and the position of the animal depends on the area to be examined. If the animal is restrained in any type of recumbency, it will usually be more relaxed and calmer on a padded table-top. For cardiac investigations, a better image of the heart is achieved by scanning from underneath an animal in lateral recumbency, because the lungs will be slightly more compressed on the recumbent side. To achieve this position efficiently, use a table-top with side cut-outs.

Applications

The clinical applications for ultrasound are extensive. The areas in which it offers the greatest imaging advances are in:

- Pregnancy diagnosis.
- Evaluation of the female reproductive tract.
- Investigation of cardiac function (echocardiography).
- Evaluation of the architecture of parenchymatous organs, such as the liver, kidneys and spleen.

Ultrasound machines work in two-dimensional 'real time': the image appears with spatial relationships that allow direct recognition of anatomical structures and it is constantly updated so that movement in the patient can be recorded. 'Hard copy' can be stored on videotape, heat-sensitive paper or medical imaging film. Cytology or histology samples can be obtained in some cases with the assistance of ultrasound; the 'real time' continual monitoring enables visual precision of the placement of a needle into the area or organ of interest. Some transducers have a biopsy guide attached.

The effects of diagnostic ultrasound on living tissue have been investigated intensively and it appears to be biologically safe and without adverse clinical effects.

Diathermy

Diathermy is a method of cutting or coagulation of tissues by means of high-frequency alternating electrical currents producing local heat within the tissues at the site of application. (This technique must not be confused with electrocautery, in which the electric current creates a red-hot probe which is then applied to the tissues.)

The conventional method for achieving haemostasis during a surgical procedure is to clamp the bleeding vessel with a haemostat and then ligate with suture material. Diathermy can be applied to:

- Control haemorrhage, allowing better visualisation of the surgical field.
- Decrease surgical time.

- Reduce the number of ligatures necessary, so that less suture material is left within the surgical site.

The nature of the waveform of the applied current used in diathermy can vary the effect from cutting to coagulating:

- Continuous waveforms are employed for cutting tissues.
- Interrupted waveforms are used for pure coagulation.
- A mixed waveform combines cutting with coagulation.

Types of coagulation

Coagulation achieved by diathermy may be described as either black or white.

Black coagulation results in the charring of the tissue surface and coagulation of the deeper tissue by the formation of an electrical arc. A cracking is often heard, with miniature explosions. Although this technique is quicker and more impressive than white coagulation, it results in greater tissue necrosis and longer wound healing.

White coagulation is the application of an electrode directly to the underlying tissues without significant arc formation. The electrical current is applied at a lower density and must be applied for longer. Heating occurs over the entire area where the electrode is in contact with the tissue and therefore the effect is more controllable and predictable than with the black method.

Applications

Diathermy currents can be applied by monopolar or bipolar electrodes.

Monopolar diathermy is the only technique that can be used for cutting and for black coagulation. The electrode for **cutting diathermy** can be a flat blade, wire or conventional scalpel blade. For **coagulation diathermy** a flat blade, ball electrode or dissection forceps can be used to grasp a vessel or area of tissue and the current can be applied by touching the instrument with the electrode.

Bipolar diathermy requires two separate electrodes which are applied across the tissue. This can be achieved using either two fixed electrodes on one handle or the two points of dissecting forceps which can be used to elevate the tissue from the surrounding area. The advantage of bipolar application is that the current allows more control over the location and depth of coagulation, but it cannot be used for cutting.

Precautions

There are several designs available for surgical use and it is important that the veterinary nurse is familiar with the specifications for the particular unit being used. Most units require the patient to be 'grounded' or 'earthed' so that the electrical current is conducted to ground. This is usually achieved by placing a special diathermy plate under and in contact with the patient. The plate is connected by a wire to the diathermy unit to enable the transfer of the current to ground. An alternative is a metal rectal probe, in the shape of a thermometer, which is grounded in the same manner as the plate.

If the patient is not properly earthed, the electrical current used for diathermy will travel along the path of least resistance, which may be through the animal or through the surgeon. Serious electrical burning of the animal can be caused by improper grounding.

Alcohol, ether or other highly flammable materials should not be present when a diathermy is used. A particular problem could arise with pooling of flammable skin preparations such as surgical spirit.

Care of the diathermy unit

Portions of the diathermy unit may be sterilised (usually the handles and attachments). The manufacturer's instructions concerning sterilisation techniques, maintenance and the operation of the unit must be followed carefully.

Cryosurgery

Cryosurgery destroys living tissue by the controlled application of extreme cold. The aim of cryosurgery is to kill cells in a diseased target area whilst simultaneously producing minimal damage to normal surrounding tissue. As a surgical agent, cryosurgery has the advantage of coagulant and destructive properties.

The fundamental principle is that living cells are at first injured and later die from the effects of freezing:

(1) The refrigerator or probe of the cryosurgical unit is placed in the target area, and heat is extracted from the surrounding tissues.
(2) Water is a major component of all living cells and is the first to be affected; therefore tissues that are relatively fluid-free are the least susceptible to freezing (e.g. bone).
(3) As the temperature of the tissue is reduced, the water in both the intracellular and extracellular spaces begins to freeze, with the formation of ice crystals.
(4) This affects the osmoregulation of the cells, leading eventually to cell dehydration, denaturation, anoxia and ultimately cell death.

A rapid freeze followed by a slow thaw is the best combination in destroying tissue, and repeat freeze–thaw cycles are recommended in order to achieve optimal lethal effects. The temperatures must fall to $-20°C$ or lower and can be monitored with thermocouples (probes that can be placed into the deeper regions of the affected tissue).

Refrigerants

Cryosurgery begins with the selection of a refrigerant (freezing medium) and a method of its application. Many gases can be converted into their liquid state to serve as a refrigerant and carbon dioxide, nitrous oxide and liquid nitrogen are readily available.

Liquid nitrogen is generally the refrigerant of choice for cryosurgery; with its lower boiling point of $-195.6°C$, it is a more effective and efficient refrigerant for destroying larger areas of tissue than the other gases. It is relatively inexpensive, readily available and non-explosive (provided that it is stored correctly). It can be stored reasonably easily in narrow-necked, large-bodied metal containers with loose-fitting stoppers (dewars) which are usually provided by the main suppliers of liquid nitrogen.

If cryosurgery is only employed occasionally by a practice, it may be sensible to approach a larger institute (veterinary, medical or research) as a local source of supply of the refrigerant. Liquid nitrogen may be collected in a domestic Thermos flask but to prevent explosion this must not be screwed shut. Some institutes may offer handling expertise.

Precautions

Liquid nitrogen is a powerful refrigerant and great care should be taken when handling it. The inexperienced should not take a casual approach to its use.

Liquid nitrogen is a harmful substance. To comply with COSHH Regulations, a Standard Operating Procedure (SOP) should be developed to prevent possible hazards when handling the substance. All persons involved in using liquid nitrogen should be trained and be aware of the SOP. General precautions are:

● Avoid splashing exposed areas of clothing in close contact with the body.
● Wear protective eye goggles, an apron or overall and thick, well-insulated gloves (the type used for handling birds are usually suitable).
● Take even greater care to avoid skin contact with metal surfaces that have been pre-cooled by liquid nitrogen. A severe cold burn will result.

First aid measures for accidental eye/skin contact:

● Immediately flush eyes thoroughly with water for at least 15 minutes.
● In case of frostbite, spray with water for at least 15 minutes.
● Apply a sterile dressing. Obtain medical assistance.

Storage containers should be clearly labelled with suitable warnings and stored in a well-ventilated safe area, i.e. where unlikely to be knocked or damaged.

The filling of vessels with liquid nitrogen can be a problem. The situation is similar to that of filling a container with hot water: steam will be produced until the container is at the same temperature as the liquid. A considerable amount of liquid nitrogen will evaporate in this way (and this should be taken into consideration when assessing the amount that is required). Once the inner surface is at liquid nitrogen temperature, evaporation losses when topping up are minimised.

Unfortunately liquid nitrogen continues to evaporate over a period of days or weeks. The evaporation rate is influenced by the size of the storage container: the losses increase as the size of the container decreases. Dipstick indicating gauges are used to estimate levels of liquid nitrogen because a constant cloud of condensate above the surface makes viewing of the level almost impossible.

Refrigerant application

There are several methods of applying the liquid nitrogen to the area to be treated. One of the simplest is to use a probe, or even a cotton bud dipped into the liquid nitrogen and then applied directly to the treatment area. Only small lesions such as warts are suitable for this type of application.

Another method is to pour liquid nitrogen on to a mass or into a cavity; however, there is not much control. Efficient application requires the use of a cryosurgical unit, which provides a direct application under pressure by spray to provide a very effective form of rapid freezing. Various sizes of orifice and hollow probe are available for use with the sprays.

Preparation

Preparation of the surgical site for cryosurgery depends on the location. Oral lesions require little or no preparation. Asepsis is not necessary for surface lesions but areas covered with hair will require clipping and cleaning to allow efficient contact and application of the liquid nitrogen. Skin antiseptics can be used for cleaning. Normal aseptic precautions must be followed when deep lesions are treated.

It is important to protect adjacent tissues, as they will be vulnerable, especially if a spray application is used. Protection can be provided by petroleum jelly or Vaseline; polystyrene from packaging material or disposable cups is also a suitable insulator.

Disadvantages of cryosurgery

Owners should be warned beforehand that postoperatively an area that has been treated cryosurgically is not an attractive sight, especially if a large region is involved.

- A slough occurs initially and this may become moist and discharge. This is not only unsightly but also in some cases smelly.
- Hair-covered areas may heal with unpigmented hair and this could be a problem in a show animal.
- Daily cleaning of the surgical area post-operatively is usually necessary.
- Immediately post-operatively there is likely to be a degree of erythema and oedema which could lead to problems, especially in the oral cavity.
- The procedure of cryosurgery is time consuming. Small warts, etc., are probably removed more easily and quickly with a pair of scissors.

Care of the equipment

Cleaning of the cryoprobes is essential, as a build-up of debris on the tips can lead to a build-up of corrosive deposits which may eventually weaken the tips and create a positive hazard. Washing in mild detergent, coupled with gentle polishing of discoloured areas, is normally adequate. Care should be taken not to use corrosive or abrasive polishes which, over a period, will result in thinning of metal components.

Sterilisation of some cryoprobes can be by autoclaving but as there are many different cryo-units and attachments it is advisable to check with the manufacturers for the cleaning and care of all equipment.

Endoscopes

Endoscopes are delicate and expensive instruments. They are used for visual examination of the interior of a body cavity or hollow organ. The word endoscopy is derived from the Greek prefix *endo*, meaning 'within', and *skopein*, meaning 'to view or observe with intent, to monitor'. Thus endoscopy is an apt term for the procedure of peering into the recesses of a living body. This is made possible by combining a light source with simple optical systems of lenses and mirrors, which have been available for centuries and which are present in every veterinary establishment in forms which range in complexity, e.g. autoscopes, proctoscopes and ophthalmoscopes.

Endoscopy was first introduced to veterinary medicine in the early 1970s. Its use has increased dramatically as veterinary surgeons have become aware of the diagnostic and therapeutic indications. It provides a non-invasive means of viewing and obtaining tissue samples from a variety of body organs.

Types of endoscope

There are two types of endoscope in common use: **flexible** and **rigid**. There are two types of flexible endoscope:

- **Fibre-optic** endoscopes use glass-fibre bundles for the transmission of images.
- **Video** endoscopes use television for the transmission of images.

The glass-fibre bundles, contained within an 'umbilical cord', have two functions:

- They transmit light from a remote source, through the instrument, to illuminate the tissues under inspection.
- They carry the image back to the observer's eye-piece.

Although the glass fibres are flexible and are protected within a stout outer cover, individually they are brittle so that even under careful working conditions occasional fractures of single strands occur. Each broken fibre ceases to transmit light. As it is not practical to replace individual fractured fibres, it can be appreciated that these delicate fibre-optic endoscopes must be handled with great care.

An air pump for insufflation is usually housed in the remote light source. A water bottle attached to the air pump assembly allows water to be flushed down the air/water channel for washing the lens.

Care of endoscopes

Endoscopes should be cleaned after use. If this is not done immediately, thorough cleaning will be much more difficult and the instrument will deteriorate due to the presence of dried mucus, blood, etc.

WARNING

Unless the endoscope is of an immersible type, it must never be immersed completely in liquid. Extensive damage will occur if liquid enters the control section or light connector plug. The endoscope should not be autoclaved or placed in a hot-air oven.

Cleaning equipment includes:

- Large bowl.
- Rubber gloves.
- Gauze swabs.
- Tap water.
- Cotton buds.
- Endoscopic cleaning brush.
- Disinfectant solution (as recommended by the manufacturer).

The endoscope should remain attached to the light source with the water bottle and suction pump also attached.

(1) Prepare approximately 1 litre of disinfectant solution in a bowl.

(2) Place the distal tip of the endoscope in the solution and aspirate disinfectant through by depressing the suction button.

(3) Unscrew the biopsy valve and clean the inside with a cotton bud; pass the cleaning brush through the biopsy channel. Follow with a clear-water rinse by suction.

(4) Disconnect the water bottle tube from the light guide connector, block the water inlet with a finger and then depress the water/air button to blow all the water out of the channel.

(5) With gauze swabs, wipe the insertion tube with the disinfectant solution. Follow with a clear-water rinse.

(6) The control section and light guide tube/plug may be wiped with gauze that has been lightly dampened in the disinfectant. Follow with a water-dampened swab to remove residual disinfectant.

(7) The ocular lens can be cleaned with a solution of 70% alcohol applied carefully with a cotton bud.

(8) Thorough drying is recommended. Hang the endoscope on a secure hook or drip-stand to enable residual fluid to run downwards away from the control and eye-piece section.

(9) Once dry, endoscopes can be stored in carrying cases or cabinets for protection. Check that the end tip is included before closing lids or doors.

Expensive injuries can be avoided and the life expectation of the equipment can be extended if routine precautions for use and care are observed.

22

Fluid therapy and shock

E. Welsh

Many medical and surgical conditions and interventions cause disturbances of body fluid, electrolyte and acid–base balance within the body. A knowledge of the homeostatic mechanisms which normally govern these physiological processes within the body is essential if disturbances are to be identified, and subsequently rectified, in a logical and effective manner. This chapter reviews briefly the physiology of body fluid, electrolyte and acid–base balance and then examines how to determine if fluid therapy is required, what the most appropriate fluids and routes of administration are and how to assess the patient's response to treatment.

Units and definitions

It is important to be familiar with the various methods of measurement of fluids and electrolytes within the body, and to understand the units which describe them.

A **solution** consists of a solute dissolved in a solvent. Saline solution is comprised of sodium chloride (a solute) dissolved in water (a solvent). In the body, water is the main solvent.

An **electrolyte** is a substance which yields ions when dissolved in water.

An **ion** is a small water-soluble particle of atomic or molecular size which carries one or more positive or negative charges. Sodium chloride (NaCl) is an electrolyte which, in solution in water, dissociates into sodium ions and chloride ions. The sodium ion loses one electron (Na^+); in contrast, the chloride ion gains an electron (Cl^-). Both sodium and chloride ions are referred to as **univalent** ions, whereas ions which lose or gain two electrons are referred to as **divalent** ions (e.g. O^{2-}, Ca^{2+}).

Cations are ions carrying one or more positive charges (e.g. Na^+, Ca^{2+}).

Anions are ions carrying one or more negative charges (e.g. Cl^-, O^{2-}).

Frequently, the strengths of biological solutions are measured in terms of their molecular, electrostatic or osmotic composition.

Molecular composition is described by the **molar concentration** measured in the number of moles per litre. However, since biological fluids are very dilute, it is more convenient to measure concentrations in millimoles per litre (mmol/l), i.e. one-thousandth of a mole (1 mmol = 1/1000 mol, or 1 mol = 1000 mmol). Molar concentration is determined as follows:

Molar concentration (mmol/l)
$$= \frac{\text{Concentration (g\%)} \times 10\ 000}{\text{Molecular weight}}$$

For example, a 0.9% solution of sodium chloride (molecular weight 58.5) contains approximately 154 mmol/l. The **equivalence** system is an older system of measurement which is still often used in physiology and in clinical practice, as it gives an indication of the ionic composition of a fluid. It is related to the molecular weight and the valence (see above).

$$\text{Equivalent weight} = \frac{\text{Molecular weight}}{\text{Valence}}$$

When the valence is 1, the equivalent concentration in milliequivalents per litre (mEq/l) is the same as the molar concentration in millimoles per litre. Where the valence is 2, the equivalent concentration is twice the molar concentration. In a solution, the sum of the equivalent weights of the cations must be balanced by the anions to ensure electroneutrality.

The **concentration of a solution** is measured by the mass of solute which is dissolved in a volume of solvent. The gram per cent (gram % or g/dl) unit describes the number of grams of solute in 100 ml of solvent. Therefore, 5% dextrose has 5 g dextrose in 100 ml of water (or 50 g/l).

Osmosis is the process by which pure solvent (water) moves from a region of low solute concentration to a region of high solute concentration when separated by a **semi-permeable membrane**, to equalise or at least minimise the difference in concentrations. Semi-permeable membranes are very common in the body and are effectively permeable to solvents but not to solutes.

The **osmotic pressure** of a solution is the pressure needed to prevent osmosis from happening and it is proportional to the **number of particles** (not the size of the particles), both in ions and undissociated molecules, in the solution.

- **Isotonic** solutions exert equal osmotic pressures to body fluid.
- **Hypertonic** solutions exert a higher osmotic pressure than body fluid.
- **Hypotonic** solutions exert a lower osmotic pressure than body fluid.

In general, when choosing fluids for parenteral administration isotonic solutions should be used, although hypertonic solutions are occasionally administered (e.g hypertonic saline; 10% glucose). When fluids are administered to an animal, by whatever route, they initially enter the extracellular fluid (ECF). If hypertonic solutions are added to the ECF, water will be drawn out of the cells into the ECF resulting in cellular dehydration. Conversely, if hypotonic solutions are added to the ECF, water may move into the cells resulting in cellular overhydration and possible lysis of the cells, although excess water is readily excreted if the kidneys are working normally.

Protein molecules contribute to the osmotic pressure of certain body fluids, because in general proteins are large molecules which cannot diffuse freely across cell membranes. In contrast, both water and salts can move freely across biological membranes by diffusion. Consequently, the proteins exert a steady osmotic pressure which is referred to as the **effective osmotic pressure** (colloid osmotic pressure or oncotic pressure). The osmotic pressure exerted by the blood protein – primarily albumin – maintains the difference between the osmotic pressure of the plasma and the interstitial fluid. This difference is important in maintaining an adequate volume of fluid within the blood vessels. Similarly, non-diffusable proteins within the cells contribute to the intracellular osmotic pressure.

Distribution of body water

It is generally accepted that, on average, the water content of the body is 60% by weight, ranging from 50% to 70% in normal healthy animals. It varies with age, sex and nutritional status. For example, the water content of the body of young animals may be as much as 70–80%, while in older animals it may be as little as 50–55% of bodyweight. Such details highlight the importance of prompt and adequate fluid therapy in neonatal and young animals suffering from excessive fluid losses, especially as their kidneys are less effective at producing concentrated urine. The body water content is also affected by the proportion of fat to lean tissue in the body, since fatty tissue contains a much smaller amount of water than do other organs and tissues. Therefore, to avoid the danger of overhydration, fluid therapy in obese animals should be based on the requirement of their ideal bodyweight as they will have a slightly lower requirement than that calculated from their actual bodyweight.

Almost two-thirds of the total body water is located inside the cells of the tissues (**intracellular fluid**, ICF), while the remaining one-third is located outside the cells (**extracellular fluid**, ECF). The ECF may be further divided into: **plasma water** (PW), which is the water contained within the vascular compartment; **interstitial fluid** (ISF), which is present in the spaces between the cells; and **transcellular fluids** (TCF), which are specialised fluids formed by active secretory mechanisms but comprising only a very small proportion of the ECF (e.g. cerebrospinal fluid, gastrointestinal secretions). The distribution of body water into its principal compartments is shown in Fig. 22.1.

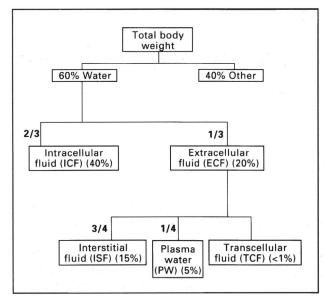

Fig. 22.1 The distribution of body water into its principal compartments.

The composition of body fluids

The intracellular and extracellular fluids differ in both composition and function; the interstitial fluid and the plasma water are similar in composition (Table 22.1). The composition of transcellular fluid reflects its specialised function and may bear no resemblance to any other body fluid.

Plasma contains sodium as the main cation, with smaller amounts of potassium (K^+), calcium (Ca^{2+}) and magnesium (Mg^{2+}). Chloride and bicarbonate (HCO_3^-) are the main anions with small amounts of phosphate (PO_4^{2-}) and protein. In all body fluids the number of positive charges must equal the number of negative charges so that an electrical gradient does not exist. Normal blood capillaries have only a limited permeability and the large protein molecules cannot pass easily through this barrier. Therefore, ISF is an **ultrafiltrate** of plasma and contains everything

Table 22.1 The approximate composition of plasma water, interstitial fluid and intracellular fluid (mmol/l)

	Plasma water	Interstitial fluid	Intracellular fluid
Cations			
Sodium	138	130	10
	4	4	110
	2.5	1.5	–
Potassium	1	1	15
Calcium	102	110	10
	27	27	10
Magnesium	17	–	50
Anions	1	1	26

found in plasma except proteins. In the ECF, sodium is the main cation with chloride and bicarbonate as its neutralising anions.

The intracellular fluid has potassium and magnesium as its main cations and relatively small amounts of sodium. The major neutralising anions are phosphate and protein. There is also some bicarbonate and chloride in the ICF.

Sodium is sometimes referred to as the 'osmotic skeleton' of the ECF, maintaining the volume of the ECF against the osmotic pull of the ICF. Protein (primarily albumin) acts in a similar manner within the vascular compartment. Blood pressure tends to force fluid out of the vascular compartment and into the ISF, while the protein within the plasma acts to pull this fluid back into the vessels.

Body water and electrolyte balance

The normal healthy animal is able to match the intake and output of water and principal electrolytes. It obtains water from two main sources:

● Ingestion (fluids and food).
● Metabolism (fats and carbohydrates).

Metabolism of ingested fats and carbohydrates provides about 10% of the animal's water requirement.

Animals lose water by four main routes:

● Kidney (this is the only route by which water loss can be regulated within certain limits by varying the urinary water content to compensate for changes in water availability).
● Gastrointestinal tract (loss of water occurs in the faeces and abnormal losses occur during vomiting and diarrhoea).
● Respiratory tract (water is lost from the respiratory tract during breathing and panting because air is humidified as it passes along the tracheobronchial tree and nasal passages).
● Skin (water is lost from the surface of the skin (pores in paws) by evaporation and this loss is influenced by ambient temperature and humidity).

The water loss via the respiratory tract and the skin is known as **inevitable** or **insensible** because it cannot be regulated by the body and continues even at times of water deprivation.

Water loss (in terms of bodyweight) over 24 hours is as follows:

● Respiratory/cutaneous losses: 20 ml/kg.
● Faecal loss (normal faeces): 10–20 ml/kg.
● Urinary loss (normal range): 20 ml/kg.

Therefore to maintain a normal water balance in a healthy dog or cat, a total of approximately 50–60 ml/kg/day of water is required. Although the inevitable water losses from the respiratory tract and skin cannot be regulated, within the body the kidneys play an important role in the regulation of not only water and electrolytes but also acid–base balance. At times of reduced intake or increased loss of water and electrolytes the osmotic concentration of the body fluids

increases and the volume of the ECF (more specifically the plasma water) is depleted. This has two effects. Firstly, the animal will become thirsty because of stimulation of thirst centres within the hypothalamus. Secondly, the increase in plasma osmotic concentration will be detected by **osmoreceptors** (cells which are sensitive to osmotic changes in the plasma water) which stimulate the release of **antidiuretic hormone (ADH)**, which is stored in the posterior pituitary. Release of ADH promotes the reabsorption of water from the renal tubules and this will increase the concentration of the urine that is voided. (Conversely, if the osmotic concentration of the plasma is reduced, less ADH will be released; therefore less water will be reabsorbed within the kidney and the urine will become more dilute.) In addition, a reduction in plasma water will be detected directly by the kidneys as a reduction in renal perfusion. This stimulates the release of a renal hormone, **renin**, which causes generation of **angiotensin** in the blood. In turn, angiotensin stimulates the release of another hormone from the adrenal cortex, **aldosterone**. Aldosterone acts on the kidney to increase the reabsorption of sodium within the distal tubule, and thence water, resulting in more concentrated urine (Fig. 22.2).

The urine **specific gravity** reflects the solute concentration and may be measured with a urinometer, refractometer or dip-stick test. The normal range for urine specific gravity is:

● Dog: 1.015–1.045.
● Cat: 1.020–1.060.

If an animal is dehydrated the specific gravity of the urine will generally increase because the urine becomes more concentrated, e.g. in the dog the specific gravity may increase to 1.060 and in the cat to 1.080.

The management of water balance is probably more important than the regulation of electrolyte status. However, electrolytes too are delicately balanced within the body, and the balance of sodium, potassium, chloride and bicarbonate is the most important. In general, conditions resulting in

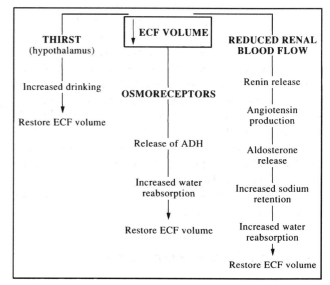

Fig. 22.2 Mechanisms involved in the restoration of extracellular fluid volume.

increased loss of water also cause loss of electrolytes. In the normal animal the daily requirement for sodium is 1 mEq/kg/day and for potassium 2 mEq/kg/day, but these requirements will change where abnormal losses or retention of body fluids are occurring.

Thus the recording of the daily intake and loss of fluid in veterinary patients is an important part of patient care, especially in animals suffering from water and electrolyte imbalances. Recording ranges from the simple monitoring of the drinking and urinary habits of elective surgical patients to the accurate observations of volumes of fluid consumed orally and administered parenterally, measurement of urine and faecal output and recording of abnormal losses. Ideally water balance should be recorded on a chart detailing route of administration, type and volume of fluid given and details of fluid losses. Each page would represent a 24-hour period and a glance at a chart would then be a useful guide to each animal's fluid status.

Disturbances of water and/or electrolyte balance

Many medical conditions and surgical interventions can disrupt the body's water and/or electrolyte status. Such conditions arise through altered intake or output of water and/or electrolytes. The term **dehydration** describes a reduction in the total body water and the signs and symptoms associated with such a loss.

Dehydration can be caused by a loss of water only which is known as **primary water depletion**. This is common where water intake is reduced or absent because of continued inevitable water losses, e.g. during excessive panting or when an animal is deprived of drinking water. In addition, certain disease states (such as diabetes insipidus) can cause a primary water depletion. More commonly, water losses are accompanied by electrolyte losses, especially sodium which is the main cation of the ECF, and this is referred to as a **mixed water electrolyte depletion**. The losses which are incurred during vomiting and diarrhoea include water, sodium, chloride and bicarbonate depletion. If diarrhoea is prolonged, potassium is also lost. In haemorrhage, protein, haemoglobin, platelets and clotting factors are lost in addition to water and electrolytes.

In conditions where urinary output has failed (e.g. blocked urethra, ruptured urinary bladder and acute renal failure), metabolites and electrolytes which are normally excreted in the urine accumulate within the body. In addition, insensible losses lead to water depletion. Therefore, the fluid imbalance which is present is very complicated and relates mainly to water loss, elevated serum potassium levels and acidosis.

Common diseases and the principal fluid disorders they cause are given in Table 22.2.

Assessing fluid requirements

It is important to assess the degree of dehydration and the state of the circulation prior to initiating fluid therapy. There

---

Table 22.2 Causes of the principal fluid abnormalities

(1) **Primary water depletion**
   Prolonged inappetence (fractured jaw, head or neck injury, etc.)
   Water unavailable (forgetful/neglectful owners)
   Unconsciousness (coma)
   Fever or excessive panting
   Diabetes insipidus
(2) **Water and electrolyte depletion**
   Vomiting
   Diarrhoea
   'Third space' losses (intestinal obstruction, peritonitis)
   Pyometra
   Wound drainage
(3) **Potassium depletion**
   Prolonged inappetence (starvation)
   Vomiting
   Prolonged diarrhoea
   Prolonged diuretic therapy
(4) **Potassium accumulation**
   Ruptured urinary bladder
   Urethral obstruction
   Acute renal failure
   Addison's disease

---

are a number of clinical and laboratory methods which may be used to establish the amount of fluid which is required by an individual animal.

History

A good history enables accurate assessment of fluid deficits. The owner should be asked questions about the animal's food and water consumption (anorexia, polydipsia), any gastrointestinal losses (vomiting, diarrhoea), urinary losses (polyuria, oliguria), abnormal discharges (open pyometra) and traumatic losses (blood loss, burns).

EXAMPLE

Consider a 20 kg dog which has been off food and water for 3 days and vomiting about 3 times daily for the last 2 days.

- 3 days' inevitable water losses (20 ml/kg/day): 1200 ml.
- 1 day's urinary water loss (20 ml/kg/day): 400 ml.
- 2 days' vomiting 3 times/day (4 ml/kg/vomit): 480 ml.

Total water deficit: 2080 ml.

Physical examination

Clinical signs are a useful, but not always accurate, means of assessing dehydration. Signs such as loss of skin elasticity, sunken eye and prolonged capillary refill time do not start to appear until the animal is 5% dehydrated, and

Table 22.3 Clinical signs associated with dehydration

Percentage dehydration	Clinical signs
<5	Not detectable
5–6	Subtle loss of skin elasticity
6–8	Marked loss of skin elasticity Slightly prolonged capillary refill time Slightly sunken eyes Dry mucous membranes
10–12	Tented skin stands in place Prolonged capillary refill time (>2 s) Sunken eyes Dry mucous membranes
12–15	Early shock Moribund Death imminent

15% dehydrated animals are moribund. When assessing the elasticity of the skin it is important to remember that it is generally reduced in cachectic animals, even when they are not dehydrated, while fat animals will lose their skin elasticity when more severely dehydrated than an animal of normal weight. Intermediate changes are described in Table 22.3.

The animal's fluid requirement is calculated by multiplying the percentage dehydration by the bodyweight in kilograms.

EXAMPLE

10% dehydration in a 20 kg dog represents a fluid deficit of 2 litres (10/100 × 20).

Laboratory analyses

There are some simple laboratory tests which can be helpful in estimating losses:

● Packed cell volume (PCV).
● Haemoglobin.
● Total plasma protein (TPP).
● Blood urea and creatinine.
● Plasma electrolytes.
● Acid–base estimations.

Packed cell volume

The PCV is an inexpensive but revealing parameter. For each 1% increase in the PCV, a fluid loss of approximately 10 ml/kg bodyweight has occurred. Rarely will the normal PCV of the patient be known, and therefore an estimate of 45% is made in dogs and 35% in cats.

EXAMPLE

If a 20 kg dog was found to have a PCV of 55%, the deficit should be calculated thus:

20 kg × 10 ml/kg/1% × (55–45%) = 2000 ml.

The equation is unreliable where pre-existing anaemia is present unless the PCV prior to fluid loss is known. Similarly acute blood loss cannot be evaluated by the PCV unless compensation has taken place or fluid has already been administered to replace the loss.

Haemoglobin

Dehydration will also result in an increase in the haemoglobin concentration of the blood but care must be taken when interpreting results from an anaemic animal.

Total plasma protein

Dehydration will cause a rise in TPP, but care must be taken because a dehydrated hypoproteinaemic animal may present with an apparently normal TPP. It is useful to assess both the TPP and PCV in an animal which has been diagnosed clinically as dehydrated because only rarely will pre-existing disease result in an elevation of both these parameters.

Blood urea and creatinine

Blood urea and creatinine levels will rise in the dehydrated animal but it is important to consider the possibility of cardiac, renal and post-renal disease, which can also result in an elevation in these two parameters.

Plasma electrolytes

Estimation of the plasma electrolyte level (e.g. Na^+, K^+, Cl^-) is possible but is frequently of limited value as recorded values are not always an accurate reflection of the total body content of the individual ion. However, determination of serum potassium concentration is of value because a marked deficit of this ion can result in severe muscle weakness and cardiac disturbances and equally an excess of this ion can result in fatal cardiac dysrhythmias.

Clinical measurement

The following measurements can be used to estimate fluid deficits but are more frequently used to monitor progress of fluid therapy and response to treatment in intensive care patients.

Bodyweight

Bodyweight is easily measured and acute losses may be due to fluid loss or catabolism. Acute increases in bodyweight are nearly always caused by increased fluid content. However, the usefulness of bodyweight in the initial estimation of fluid loss is limited by prior knowledge of the weight of the pet. However, it is always worth asking, as many owners now make an effort to weigh their pets regularly.

Central venous pressure (CVP)

The CVP is a useful means of estimating the need for fluids in any situation but especially where congestive cardiac failure is present or where circulatory overload may be a problem (acute renal failure). Following severe, acute haemorrhage, CVP is invaluable in determining the adequacy of replacement therapy. Measurement of the CVP will be discussed more fully later.

Urinary output

Measuring the urinary output is a useful means of assessing the adequacy of fluid replacement. As already discussed, urine output is low during dehydration (**oliguria**), and the return of normal urine output signifies that replacement is adequate. Urine output can be monitored casually by observation, but placing an indwelling urinary catheter allows accurate measurement. Normal urine output is 1–2 ml/kg/hour. A urine output of less than 0.5 ml/kg/hour is defined as oliguria. If fluid therapy fails to improve the urine output in an oliguric animal, the possibility of acute renal failure should be considered.

Acid–base balance

In a similar way to water and electrolyte balance, the acid–base balance is a closely guarded parameter which can be upset at times of disease. Hydrogen ions within the body are produced as a result of normal metabolic activity, and the body's acid–base status is a measure of the hydrogen ion concentration within its tissues. Hydrogen ions are measured according to the pH scale. The **pH** is defined as the negative logarithm (to the base 10) of the hydrogen ion concentration. The pH scale has a range of 1–14. A pH of 7 is regarded as neutral; a pH of greater than 7 is alkaline (bases) and a pH less than 7 is acidic (acids).

In the normal animal, blood is slightly alkaline – it has a normal range of pH 7.35–7.45. When the pH of the blood falls below 7.35 a state of **acidaemia** is said to exist, whereas when the pH of the blood is greater than 7.45 a state of **alkalaemia** is said to exist.

Acidosis and **alkalosis** describe abnormal processes and conditions which would cause acidaemia or alkalaemia respectively if there were no secondary (compensatory) changes in response to them. Acidosis and alkalosis can exist without producing acidaemia/alkalaemia because of the body's secondary compensatory mechanisms. Acidosis and alkalosis may be either **metabolic** or **respiratory** depending on their origin.

It is essential for proper cellular function that the blood pH is kept within the normal range. Large changes in pH may result in the animal becoming depressed and may ultimately lead to its death. Therefore the body has efficient mechanisms for dealing with the hydrogen ions which are produced within the body to prevent dramatic fluctuations of pH. There are three principal means of dealing with hydrogen ions, and these systems work in sequence to try to limit the effects of changes in hydrogen ion concentration. **Buffers** are the first to respond to alterations in the pH, followed by a **respiratory response** and finally a **renal response**.

Buffering

Buffers are able to react with acids and bases and reduce the extent of the pH change which they would normally produce. Buffers act by trapping the H^+ ions rather than eliminating them from the body, but are required to keep the pH within narrow limits until the H^+ ions can be delivered to either the lungs or the kidneys, where they can be removed from the body. In general, buffers are weak acids or proteins. Because weak acids do not dissociate completely in water (unlike strong acids such as hydrochloric acid, HCl) they restrict the number of H^+ ions in solution, whereas proteins (such as haemoglobin) act as anions and have many sites to which cations such as H^+ ions may bind. Most buffering that takes place within the body occurs within the cell, and proteins are among the most important intracellular buffers.

Extracellular buffers include bicarbonate and phosphate (Fig. 22.3). The reaction which converts bicarbonate (HCO_3^-) to carbonic acid (H_2CO_3) does not become saturated in the same way as the phosphate (HPO_4^{2-}) reaction because the action of the enzyme carbonic anhydrase upon the carbonic acid results in the formation of carbon dioxide and water, both of which can be expelled from the body (or in the case of water incorporated in the body water).

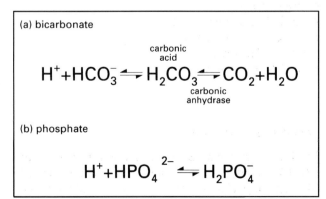

(a) bicarbonate

$$H^+ + HCO_3^- \rightleftharpoons \underset{\substack{\text{carbonic} \\ \text{acid}}}{H_2CO_3} \rightleftharpoons CO_2 + H_2O$$

carbonic anhydrase

(b) phosphate

$$H^+ + HPO_4^{2-} \rightleftharpoons H_2PO_4^-$$

Fig. 22.3 Buffers: (a) bicarbonate reaction and (b) phosphate reaction.

$$CO_2 + H_2O \rightleftharpoons H_2O_3 \rightleftharpoons H^+ + HCO_3^-$$

Fig. 22.4 Bicarbonate in kidney cells.

Respiratory system

The respiratory system controls the level of carbon dioxide within the body. The carbon dioxide is in equilibrium with the carbonic acid in solution in the body fluids which is a source of H^+ ions (see above). Increasing respiration will remove carbon dioxide from the body and therefore reduce acidity. Decreasing respiration will retain carbon dioxide and therefore increase acidity.

It has already been noted that the reaction which converts bicarbonate (HCO_3^-) to carbonic acid (H_2CO_3) does not become saturated because of a build-up of water and carbon dioxide (see above); however, the reaction may be limited by the amount of available bicarbonate.

Renal system

Bicarbonate can be generated within the cells of the kidney by a reversal of the reaction which results in the formation of water and carbon dioxide (Fig. 22.4). The bicarbonate which is generated enters the ECF pool while the H^+ ions that are generated are excreted.

Thus, it is apparent that the pH of the body fluids is dependent upon the concentration of carbon dioxide and bicarbonate ions within the body:

$$pH = [HCO_3] \div p CO_2.$$

Therefore, the pH will fall if there is an increase in the concentration of carbon dioxide within the body, a fall of bicarbonate ions within the body or if H^+ ions are added to the system. Conversely, reducing the concentration of carbon dioxide within the body, adding bicarbonate ions to the system or removing H^+ ions will cause an increase in the pH.

Acid–base abnormalities

To obtain an estimate of the acid–base balance of an animal it is necessary to obtain an arterial blood sample, although venous blood samples can provide useful information if an arterial sample cannot be taken. In dogs and cats, arterial blood is generally taken from either the main femoral artery, or a superficial branch of the femoral artery. The anti-coagulant which is used is heparin, and the sample should be drawn anaerobically. If the arterial blood is not analysed immediately, it should be stored on ice, or at 4°C, until analysis. Analysis of the blood will provide the pH of the sample, the bicarbonate ion concentration and the carbon dioxide tension (a measure of the amount of carbon dioxide within the sample), and from this information the clinician will be able to establish what deficits the animal is suffering.

Acid–base abnormalities are not uncommon during disease and Table 22.4 shows the four major disturbances

Table 22.4 Causes of acid–base abnormalities

Metabolic acidosis

Accumulation of H^+	Shock
	Ruptured bladder/blocked urethra
	Diabetic keto-acidosis
	Aspirin/ethylene glycol poisoning
Loss of base	Chronic renal failure
	Chronic diarrhoea

Metabolic alkalosis

Loss of H^+	Prepyloric vomiting
Accumulation of base	Over-administration of bicarbonate

Respiratory acidosis

Impaired ventilation	General anaesthesia
	CNS injuries (cerebral oedema)
	Severe lung damage
	Certain nerve/muscle diseases
Inspired carbon dioxide	Anaesthetic equipment
Increased carbon dioxide production	Malignant hyperthermia

Respiratory alkalosis

Overventilation	Mechanical/manual ventilation
	Apprehension/pain/fear

that can occur and the situations in which they are likely to arise. **Respiratory acidosis** arises through inadequate ventilation, or a failure of the respiratory system to respond to the increased levels of carbon dioxide which are characteristic of rebreathing or increased production. The buffers will lessen the pH disturbance but renal compensation will only occur when the condition becomes long-standing. **Respiratory alkalosis** occurs much less frequently than respiratory acidosis in veterinary practice.

Metabolic acidosis arises when acid metabolites are retained within the body or when the loss of buffer is marked. Respiratory compensation is rapid but incomplete, and ultimately the kidneys must restore the balance, either by excreting hydrogen ions or by retaining bicarbonate, or both. **Metabolic alkalosis** again occurs much less frequently.

The treatment of the various acid–base abnormalities should be directed initially at the source of the problem. Respiratory acidosis and alkalosis require therapy aimed at curing the ventilatory disturbance. Metabolic acidosis can be ameliorated by providing extra buffer in the form of sodium bicarbonate (usually 1–2 mEq/kg i.v. is adequate). Often, reduced renal perfusion is the cause of a metabolic acidosis and using fluid therapy to restore renal perfusion will be sufficient to correct the abnormality.

Objectives of fluid therapy

The purpose of fluid therapy is to replace deficits from previous losses, improve and maintain renal function and supply maintenance requirements.

The most important initial treatment is to restore an adequate circulating volume, as severely dehydrated animals may be showing signs of shock. After this, the remaining deficit can be replaced more slowly. In general, existing deficits should be replaced within the first 24 hours after admission. Thereafter it is important to remember that, while the animal is undergoing treatment, provision must be made to replace the continued inevitable and urinary losses as well as any continuing abnormal losses, e.g. diarrhoea.

Routes of administration of fluids

Oral fluid administration

If an animal is willing to drink, is not vomiting and does not have an intestinal obstruction, the oral route of fluid (and food) administration is a simple, cheap and painless method to treat an animal with mild dehydration. In addition, it is an ideal route by which to supply daily maintenance requirements after initial deficits have been replaced. Moreover, the animal does not need to be hospitalised and so the owner may take the animal home.

The intestine acts as a barrier for selective absorption of water and electrolytes, providing a wide margin of safety. However, there are a number of disadvantages and the oral route is not the route of choice if the animal is severely dehydrated. Although administering fluid orally does not require absolute sterility, only a limited range of fluids can be given (it is inappropriate for whole blood or plasma expanders such as dextrans) and it can be time-consuming.

Oral therapy is not ruled out where prehension is limited or impossible: fluid may be administered by either nasogastric tube, pharyngostomy tube or gastrostomy tube.

- A **nasogastric or naso-oesophageal tube**, lubricated with a local anaesthetic gel, may be passed via the nostril to the stomach and fluids given directly into the stomach. The tube should not remain in place if the animal is to be left unattended, and animals may resent repeated tubing.
- A **pharyngostomy tube** must be placed under anaesthesia via an incision in the skin of the neck. The tube is introduced via the pharynx into the oesophagus and stomach, allowing fluid and food to be administered.
- A **gastrostomy tube** again must be positioned under anaesthesia and is placed directly into the stomach via an incision in the left flank. Again, fluid and food may be administered through this tube. In general, pharyngostomy tubes and gastrostomy tubes are well tolerated by the animals.

Oesophagostomy, enterostomy and PEG tubes are further methods suitable for administration of enteral fluids.

Hypotonic fluids are recommended for oral administration to prevent the movement of water out of the ECF and into the bowel. However, it has been demonstrated that 120 mmol/l sodium chloride in 2% glucose will produce enhanced absorption of sodium and increased uptake of water. This can be prepared by mixing a teaspoonful of salt and a dessertspoon of glucose in 2 pints of water. There are many commercially available oral rehydration solutions available, and in general they use a similar principle to that described, although some include glycine for further promotion of electrolyte and water absorption.

Subcutaneous administration

Subcutaneous administration of fluids is practical in small animals, where the animal is only mildly dehydrated and fluids cannot be administered orally. Because absorption from this route tends to be slow, especially where peripheral vasoconstriction is present, it is unsuitable for severely dehydrated animals. Fluids given by this route should be completely absorbed within 8 hours. Only isotonic electrolyte solutions (e.g. Hartmann's) should be administered subcutaneously and only small volumes should be given at one time (no more than 10–20 ml/kg/site at a rate dictated by patient comfort). Repeated administration can be painful and in addition there is a risk of skin infection or skin slough.

Intraperitoneal administration

The intraperitoneal route of fluid administration shares many of the advantages and disadvantages of the subcutaneous route, and should only be used where the animal is mildly dehydrated and fluids cannot be administered orally. Hypotonic or isotonic electrolyte solutions may be administered intraperitoneally. The large adsorptive capacity of the peritoneum makes it a more efficient route of administration, but absorption is reduced during shock. Because of the risk of infection it is important that all manipulations are carried out aseptically. Great care must also be taken not to puncture any of the abdominal organs. Decreased ventilation after intra-peritoneal administration of fluids may also be observed.

Currently, this route of administration is least preferred in dogs and cats.

Intravenous fluid therapy

The advantages and disadvantages of intravenous administration of fluids are shown in Table 22.5.

When the intravenous route of fluid administration is going to be used, one of the first considerations is the selection of an appropriate vein. The cephalic or recurrent tarsal veins are used for short-term therapy in dogs. However, the jugular is more appropriate where long-term therapy is anticipated or where hypertonic solutions have to be given. In cats the cephalic vein is used commonly, although the jugular is often a better choice. Fluids should be warmed to 37°C prior to administration.

Table 22.5 Intravenous administration of fluids: advantages and disadvantages.

Advantages	Disadvantages
Rapid administration of fluid directly into the vascular space.	Greater risk of side effects (phlebitis, thrombophlebitis, bacteraemia, septicaemia).
Large volumes of fluid may be administered.	Specialised equipment.
Hypertonic solutions may be administered, in addition to plasma expanders and blood products.	Time-consuming.
	Animal requires constant monitoring (to ensure catheter remains within vein and fluid not being administered perivenously).
No contraindications – may be used where intravenous access is possible.	Risk of overhydration.

Needles and catheters

There are a number of different ways of administering fluids intravenously:

- **Needles** are inexpensive but are unsuitable for intravenous fluid administration. They are dislodged easily, and the sharp point can irritate the wall of the vein and can also penetrate the other side of the vein, thus delivering the fluid perivenously (extravasation).
- **Butterfly needles** (scalp vein sets) are safer because they can be secured to the limb more easily and are less likely to become dislodged. However, the sharp point of the needle may still irritate the wall of the vein.
- **Over-the-needle catheters** or cannulae are extremely useful in peripheral veins although they can also be used in the jugular vein of small dogs and cats. Catheters are plastic and may be Teflon-coated for ease of placement. They can be secured to the limb and are less likely to become dislodged than needles. Moreover, the smooth tip of the catheter is less likely to cause phlebitis than needles or butterfly needles.
- **Through-the-needle catheters** or cannulae are longer and are therefore more appropriate for use in the jugular vein. They are the only catheters suitable for monitoring central venous pressure. Unfortunately they may leave haematomas at the site of needle insertion in some animals. In other respects they are similar to over-the-needle catheters.

Drip sets and pumps

There are three main types of drip set (**giving set**) available. A normal administration set gives approximately 15–20 drops/ml. For smaller patients, a mini-drip fluid administration set (paediatric set) giving 60 drops/ml is useful because it allows more accurate administration of small volumes. A burette often is incorporated into this type of set which again is useful when only small volumes of fluid are required, helping to prevent accidental overhydration. Giving sets are supplied in sterile packaging and the number of drops per ml that they deliver is written on the packaging

---

> ### *RULES FOR REDUCING THE INCIDENCE OF THROMBOPHLEBITIS*
>
> (1) Select a suitable catheter and vein (generally the largest vein).
> (2) Prepare the site by carefully clipping and cleansing as if for surgery.
> (3) Avoid touching the barrel of the catheter or the site of insertion.
> (4) Discard any catheters which develop flared tips (after repeated attempt of cannulation).
> (5) Secure the catheter firmly to the leg so that it does not move.
> (6) Use only sterile fluid administration sets and change them daily.
> (7) Cover catheter with sterile bandage. Change at least once daily or if it becomes contaminated. Some people recommend that antibiotic or antiseptic cream should be applied to the site of insertion of the catheter.
> (8) Check the vein and monitor the animal's temperature 3–4 times daily.
> (9) Do not leave a catheter in a vein for more than 48 hours.
> (10) If fluid therapy is discontinued, flush with saline containing 5–10 IU heparin/ml and properly seal the catheter (with an injection cap or a three-way tap).

and should be checked prior to calculating the drip rate. A variety of automated infusion pumps are available for delivering a set amount of fluid over a defined period. These pumps are usually fitted with an alarm system which will alert the nurse or clinician when the fluid line is obstructed, or when the fluid bag is empty. If infusion pumps are used, it is important to remember that they are not a substitute for careful patient monitoring.

When blood is to be administered, a special blood administration set is required, which incorporates a nylon net filter to remove any aggregated red blood cells or other coagulation debris.

> ### *EXAMPLE*
>
> A 3 kg cat requires a total of 60 ml of fluid. The fluid is to be administered at 5 ml/kg/hour. A paediatric giving set which delivers 60 drops/ml is available. What flow rate (drops per minute) will be required?
>
> $$\frac{60 \text{ drops/ml}}{60 \text{ minutes}} \times 5\,\text{ml} \times 3\,\text{kg} = 15 \text{ drops/minute}$$

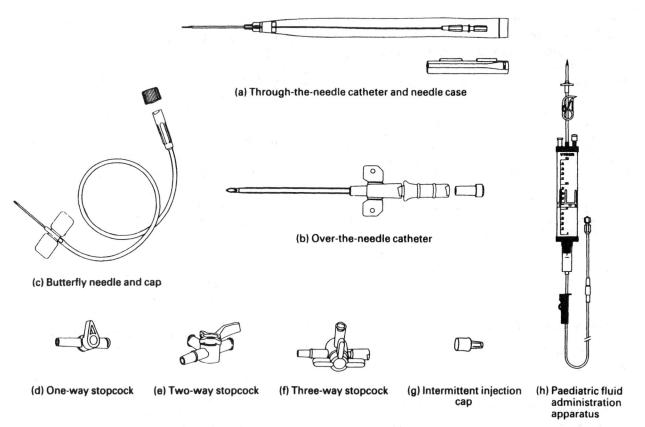

(a) Through-the-needle catheter and needle case

(b) Over-the-needle catheter

(c) Butterfly needle and cap

(d) One-way stopcock **(e) Two-way stopcock** **(f) Three-way stopcock** **(g) Intermittent injection cap** **(h) Paediatric fluid administration apparatus**

Fig. 22.5 Equipment for intravenous administration of fluids.

Various other pieces of equipment are useful when fluids are being administered via the intravenous route (Fig. 22.5). **Injection caps** and **stopcocks** are useful means of plugging catheters when fluids are not being administered, whilst allowing the catheter to be flushed periodically with heparinised saline. Simple **stylets** are also available which may be used to maintain the patency of indwelling catheters when they are not in use, and are designed to remove the requirement for periodic heparinisation to maintain patency. **Blood collection sets** containing an anticoagulant are the simplest means by which blood may be collected from a dog.

Other methods of fluid administration

Rectal administration

This route of administration should not be used if an animal is suffering from diarrhoea, nor is it suitable in severely dehydrated patients. Both isotonic and hypotonic fluids may be administered via this route. Sterility of fluids and equipment is not essential. It is important that the fluid is instilled into the colon and not into the rectum or an evacuent enema will result.

Intraosseous administration

Where it is difficult to place indwelling intravenous catheters (e.g. puppies, kittens, birds, adults with inaccessible veins due to hypotension or hypovolaemia), indwelling intraosseous catheters may be used. The inter-trochan-teric fossa of the femur, wing of the ilium, tibial tuberosity and greater tubercle of the humerus are all suitable sites for catheter placement. Fluid (including plasma, hypertonic saline and synthetic colloids) generally is administered by gravity flow. Many drugs may also be given by this route. The risk of severe infection must be considered.

Solutions commonly used in fluid therapy

Whole blood

Blood for transfusion should be collected only from fit, healthy adult animals (cats should be FeLV, FIV and Haemobartonella negative), which have not previously been transfused themselves. Approximately 10–20 ml/kg of blood may be collected from a donor dog and a total of 40 ml from a cat. Animals should not be bled more than once in every 3–4 weeks. It is important that strict asepsis is observed when collecting the blood. Blood from a donor animal may be collected in commercially available collection sets containing an anticoagulant [either acid citrate dextrose (ACD) or citrate phosphate dextrose (CPD)] to prevent the blood from clotting. However, if the blood is to be used immediately, heparin or EDTA may be used as an anticoagulant. In cats, blood is generally collected into a syringe containing anticoagulant.

Before infusion into the recipient animal, a crossmatching test should be carried out in the laboratory to ensure that the blood is compatible for transfusion. The A antigen is the most important factor in canine blood typing and ideally donor dogs should be A negative (universal canine donors are DEA 1.1, DEA 1.2 and DEA 7 negative). Three blood types are recognised, A, B and AB. Blood typing is not generally carried out in cats. However, most cats are type A and there is <40% chance of an incompatible reaction occurring if the blood is not typed prior to transfusion. Blood samples can be taken from both the donor and the recipient animal for cross-matching to ensure compatibility before obtaining a large volume of blood from the donor.

Commercially available blood collection units contain sufficient anticoagulant for 500 ml of blood, and blood may be stored in these bags in the refrigerator until required. When ACD is used as the anticoagulant the blood may be stored at 4°C for a period of 3 weeks; when CPD is used the blood may be stored for 4 weeks. Blood in which EDTA or heparin has been used as the anticoagulant should not be stored. If blood has been stored in the refrigerator, it should be warmed gently to a temperature of 37°C (and not greater than 40°C), prior to transfusion. Blood which has been stored in this manner is useful for replacement of red blood cells. However, where platelets are required (e.g. clotting abnormalities) blood must be given to the recipient immediately after collection.

Where an animal has lost only a small amount of blood, other less potentially harmful fluids may be used to restore fluid balance.

Blood products

Plasma

If fresh blood can be obtained from donors, plasma may be extracted and stored. Blood should be centrifuged immediately after collection and the plasma separated from the red blood cells. The plasma may be frozen, and can be stored for 6 months at $-20°C$. Prior to use, the plasma should be thawed and warmed. Remember to maintain sterility when transferring and decanting the plasma. Plasma is a useful replacement fluid in hypovolaemic animals and is suitable for animals which are hypoproteinaemic. Because it does not contain any red blood cells there is less risk of incompatibility reactions.

Packed red blood cells

Separated red cells may be kept in the refrigerator for 3 weeks and can be given to animals which require red cell replacement. The red cells should be resuspended in an isotonic replacement fluid which does not contain calcium (e.g. 0.9% NaCl) because calcium reacts with the citrate used to prevent clotting.

Plasma replacement fluids/colloids

When whole blood or plasma are unavailable, commercial plasma replacement fluids (colloids, plasma substitutes, plasma volume expanders) may be used. These fluids contain large molecules that will remain within the circulation, thus increasing the plasma's effective osmotic pressure and expanding plasma volume. They may be used where there has been haemorrhage (although they will not replace red blood cells), or where the plasma volume is reduced for other reasons, e.g. fluid and electrolyte depletion. The two most commonly used products are gelatins and dextrans.

Gelatins

These solutions (e.g. Haemaccel, Gelofusin) are derived from gelatin and are isotonic with plasma. They are non-antigenic and do not interfere with cross-matching tests for blood. The solution will remain in the circulation for about 5 hours and most of it will be excreted within 24 hours.

INDICATIONS FOR TRANSFUSION

- Haemorrhage (acute and chronic).
- Anaemia (acute and chronic).
- Specific deficiencies (e.g. platelets, clotting factors).

DANGERS ASSOCIATED WITH TRANSFUSION

- **Incompatibility reaction.** This usually occurs after a second transfusion of blood which has not been cross-matched and is incompatible. Mild cases show jaundice and anaemia due to haemolysis. Severe cases may show salivation, vomiting, tachycardia, muscle tremors, prostration, haemoglobinuria and bleeding. The risk of such reactions may be minimised by using universal donors, cross-matching all donors and recipients, and storing blood properly. There is currently no evidence to support routine prophylaxis of animals with antihistamines and steroids prior to transfusion.
- **Pyrogenic reactions.** Fever due to pyrogens or bacteria in the blood or transfusion equipment. It is also possible to transfer viral and other agents, especially in cats.
- **Acidosis** (metabolic) after administration of stored blood.
- **Over-administration** resulting in circulatory overload.
- **Air emboli.** This occurs infrequently when plastic blood collection bags are used, but is possible when blood is withdrawn using a syringe.

Dextrans

These solutions contain high molecular weight (MW) glucose polymers in either 0.9% NaCl or 5% dextrose. The solutions are classified by the MW of the glucose polymer, for example, the MW of dextran 70 is 70 000 and that of dextran 40 is 40 000. They remain in the circulation for times ranging from 2 to 24 hours, depending on their MW. Unfortunately, these solutions tend to interfere with the red cells: some solutions promote clumping of cells and others produce haemolysis. In addition, they interfere with the interpretation of cross-matching reactions. The raised plasma osmotic pressure caused by the dextrans tends to draw water from the cells and ISF space into the vascular compartment. Therefore crystalloids should be administered at the same time as dextrans to avoid cellular dehydration.

Oxygen carriers

Haemoglobin-based oxygen carriers manufactured from polymerised bovine haemoglobin may become available for the veterinary market in the future. These agents act as volume expanders, have minimum antigenicity and have a long half-life within the body. Their prime advantage of course is the ability to transport oxygen.

Crystalloids

In contrast to the plasma volume expanders, crystalloids are non-colloidal substances which pass readily through cell membranes. This means that they will not remain within the ECF compartment but will equilibrate with the ICF compartment, and will be excreted in the urine if renal function is normal. Table 22.6 summarises the principal constituents and some of the major indications for the most commonly used solutions in general practice, which are as follows:

- **0.9% sodium chloride (NaCl).** Useful for replacing water and electrolyte losses, especially in vomiting patients.

- **5% dextrose in water.** The dextrose in the solution is rapidly metabolised; therefore these solutions effectively provide free water which can be used to replace primary water deficits.
- **0.18% sodium chloride in 4% dextrose.** Used to replace primary water deficits, and to replace the inevitable losses of sodium and water occurring on a daily basis (maintenance requirements). Potassium will also be required during long-term administration.
- **Hartmann's solution.** Useful for replacing water and electrolyte losses, especially where the losses are post-gastric (e.g. diarrhoea).
- **Potassium chloride (KCl).** Can be used when potassium supplementation is needed. Ten millilitres 10% KCl contains 13.4 mmol. This can be added to each 500 ml of maintenance fluids to prevent further depletion. There is already adequate potassium in Hartmann's or Ringer's solution to prevent depletion. If supplementary potassium is added to a crystalloid solution, it is important that the bag is clearly labelled to avoid possible over-administration (relative or absolute).
- **Sodium bicarbonate 8.4%** Should be available to treat severe acidosis. This solution may be used intravenously as an injection but frequently it is added to intravenous infusions. However, do not add bicarbonate to any fluids which contain calcium (Table 22.6), as a precipitate will be formed. If sodium bicarbonate is added to a crystalloid solution, it is important that the bag is clearly labelled to avoid possible over-administration (relative or absolute).

Parenteral nutrition

Caloric balance is difficult to achieve by any route other than by mouth, and provision of enteral nutrition is the most effective way to provide the calories and proteins which are required by animals. However, animals that are unable to eat or drink for prolonged periods, and cannot be given enteral nutrition (gastrointestinal disease), not only require parenteral fluids but also need calories and proteins to prevent excessive breakdown of body tissues. During acute

Table 22.6 Constituents of useful replacement fluids (mmol/l)

Solution		Na+	K+	Ca2+	Cl-	Others	Indications
Haemaccel	Isotonic	143	5	3	154	Gelatins	Restore circulating volume.
Dextrans	Hypertonic	154	–	–	154	–	Restore circulating.
	Hypertonic	–	–	–	–	5% dextrose	Volume.
0.9% NaCl	Isotonic	154	–	–	154	–	Replace ECF. Gastric losses from vomiting.
Hartmann's solution (Ringer's lactate)	Isotonic	131	5	2	111	Lactate	Replace ECF. Especially from diarrhoea and post-gastric losses.
Ringer's solution	Isotonic	147	4	2.5	156	–	Replace ECF. Gastric losses from vomiting.
5% dextrose	Isotonic	–	–	–	–	5% dextrose	Primary water deficit replacement.
0.18% NaCl + 4% dextrose	Isotonic	30	–	–	30	4% dextrose	Maintenance requirements. Primary water deficit. replacement. Neonatal ECF replacement.

illness, provision of these needs is less important because the animal will be able to correct any deficits accrued in the convalescence period. However, in chronic illness, fluids containing electrolytes, amino acids and dextrose may be given parenterally in an attempt to correct some of these deficits. Requirements for replacement and maintenance are calculated in a similar manner to fluid replacement. Several commercial solutions containing amino acids and calories are now available. Fat emulsions may also be given intravenously and provide an excellent source of calories in dogs but may be dangerous in cats. These more complex fluids are not isotonic: they therefore need to be administered via a jugular catheter to ensure adequate mixing with blood and to minimise damage to the blood vessels. Manufacturers' recommendations about rates of administration should always be followed to avoid side effects associated with over-rapid administration.

Volume and rate of infusion

Volume

The replacement volume can be calculated from the history, clinical signs and simple laboratory tests described earlier. Usually, this volume can be replaced within the first 24 hours of treatment, with half of the replacement being made in the first 6–8 hours. Priority should be given to replacing the circulating blood volume and so therapy usually starts with a plasma volume expander. One-twelfth of the total

---

EXAMPLE

Consider a 20 kg dog which has been off food and water for 3 days and has been vomiting about 3 times daily for the last 2 days.

Replacement
- Inevitable water losses (20 ml/kg/day × 3 days) 1200 ml.
- Urinary water loss (20 ml/kg/day × 1 day) 400 ml.
- Vomiting 3 times/day for 2 days (4 ml/kg/vomit × 6) 480 ml.
- Total water deficit 2080 ml.
- ECF deficit (one-third of total water deficit) 693 ml.
- Plasma deficit (one-quarter of ECF, 173 ml, one-twelfth of total loss).
Replacement needed = 173 ml.

Maintenance
(50 ml/kg/day ×) 20 = 1000 ml.

Contemporary losses
Fluids should be administered to replace losses incurred due to ongoing vomiting, diarrhoea, haemorrhage, etc.

---

deficit should be replaced with a plasma substitute; the remainder of the deficit should be replaced by one of the fluids of choice. The animal also has maintenance requirements for fluids which must be met in addition to replacing existing deficits and approximately 50 ml/kg/day of 0.18% NaCl with 4% dextrose should be given to replace normal losses of sodium and water.

Because the animal in this example is suffering from a mixed water and electrolyte deficit, the fluid loss will be primarily from the ECF and a larger proportion of the total deficit will be from the plasma water. Consequently, up to one-third of the replacement fluid could be provided as plasma volume expander. This is in contrast to a primary water deficit, where fluid loss is shared between all body compartments and only one-twelfth of the total deficit should be replaced by a plasma volume expander.

During active severe haemorrhage, fluids have to be administered as rapidly as they are being lost from the circulation. Otherwise, in mild to severely dehydrated animals the **maximum** rate of infusion of crystalloids should be limited to **90 ml/kg/hour in dogs and 60 ml/kg/hour in cats**. Slower rates of **20–30 ml/kg/hour** are satisfactory in situations where dehydration is not severe or where colloidal substances are being given. It is important that **potassium** should not be given at a rate greater than **0.5 mmol/kg/hour**.

Rate of fluid replacement

The rate of fluid replacement often poses problems. A large number of factors govern how fast fluids can be given:

- Rate of loss.
- Health of patient.
- Type of fluid administered.
- Presence of ongoing losses.

Overzealous fluid administration may result in the circulatory system becoming overloaded, or the body overhydrated. This is particularly a problem in smaller cats and dogs. Typically, excess of a **colloid** leads to circulatory overload with right-sided heart failure (indicated by an elevated CVP), and ultimately congestive cardiac failure. Too much **crystalloid**, on the other hand, will initially stimulate diuresis (via inhibition of ADH release), but as the electrolyte solution moves from the circulation into the remainder of the extracellular space, signs of oedema may develop, i.e. fluid will accumulate in the ISF space. A serous nasal discharge may develop and chemosis may be noted. Most seriously, pulmonary oedema may develop which will initially impair oxygenation and can ultimately result in the death of the patient.

Overinfusion is most likely to occur with:

- Reduced cardiac output (e.g. congestive heart failure).
- Renal/urinary conditions (e.g. acute renal failure, ruptured bladder, where urine output is prevented).
- Fluid administration to normovolaemic animals (e.g. blood given in chronic anaemia).

When any of the above conditions are present, fluid should be administered slowly and the animal should be very closely monitored.

Monitoring during fluid therapy

> **MONITORING DURING FLUID ADMINISTRATION SHOULD INCLUDE:**
>
> *Cardiovascular system*
>
> - Pulse (rate, rhythm, strength).
> - Mucous membrane colour.
> - Capillary refill time.
> - Jugular distension.
> - Central venous pressure (CVP).
> - Chest auscultation (cardiac arrhythmias, pulmonary oedema).
>
> *Respiratory system*
> - Respiratory rate and depth.
> - Chest auscultation (pulmonary oedema).
> - Mean arterial blood pressure.
>
> *Temperature*
> - Core body and limb.
>
> *Urine output*
> *General checks*
> - Peripheral oedema.
> - Bodyweight.
> - Skin turgor.

Central venous pressure (CVP)

In critical patients, invasive monitoring of CVP is useful. The CVP is a measurement of the pressure in the right atrium, i.e. the chamber of the heart to which all the venous blood is returned. A long catheter is placed aseptically in a jugular vein, and advanced until the tip of the catheter lies within the chest. Note that measurements will be less sensitive if a very long catheter is used. Ideally, the catheter should lie in the right atrium itself but it is often located within the anterior vena cava, which will reflect changes in the right atrial pressure. Extension tubing is attached to the catheter (a three-way tap is helpful but not essential), and a three-way tap is attached to the other end of the tubing. A water manometer tube (marked in centimetres) and a drip set attached to a bag of crystalloids are also attached to the three-way tap (Fig. 22.6). Before the monitoring equipment is attached to the jugular catheter, the three-way tap should be adjusted to fill (a) the manometer line and (b) the extension tubing. This will prevent air emboli. To measure CVP, turn the three-way tap so that the catheter is connected directly to the manometer and read the height (cm) of the column of fluid. The zero line of the scale should be level with the right atrium, i.e. at approximately the level of the sternum when the animal is lying on its side (Fig. 22.6).

If the tip of the catheter is in the correct place, the meniscus in the manometer will fall and rise with inspiration and expiration, reflecting the changes in intrathoracic pressure that accompany respiration.

If this is not seen, either the catheter is blocked or the catheter tip is not in the chest.

> **DETERMINANTS OF CVP**
>
> - Intrathoracic pressure.
> - Intravascular volume.
> - Right ventricular function.
> - Venous tone.

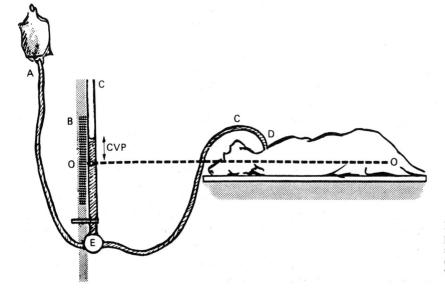

Fig. 22.6 Measurement of central venous pressure. (A) Infusion fluid and administration set. (B) Centimetre scale. (C) Extension tubing. (D) Connection to jugular catheter. (E) Three-way tap.

Blood is returned from the great veins (anterior and posterior vena cava) to the right atrium; from there it enters the right ventricle, which pumps blood to the lungs. The CVP therefore measures the filling of the great veins, which is a balance between the central blood volume, the vascular tone and the heart's contractile ability. The normal range is 3–7 cm of water. An isolated measurement of CVP may be used to indicate the need for fluids, but repeated measurements are far more useful. As fluids are administered, they will fill the vascular compartment, improve venous return and increase CVP.

● If fluids are stopped and the CVP falls, more fluids need to be administered.
● If the CVP remains elevated, fluid administration can be reduced or terminated.
● If the administration of modest amounts of fluid produce a high CVP which only declines slowly, circulatory overload or congestive cardiac failure should be suspected.

Provided that the CVP does not rise significantly during fluid administration, the infusion may be continued safely at its current rate.

RATES OF CVP

High CVP
● Occlusion of catheter.
● Over-administration of fluid.
● Right ventricular heart failure.

Low CVP
● Reduced blood volume.

Shock (acute circulatory failure)

Shock is a clinical term used to describe a clinical syndrome generally characterised by a fall in cardiac output which results in inadequate capillary perfusion of the peripheral tissues, i.e. acute circulatory failure. Insufficient capillary perfusion to meet the needs of the body tissues for oxygen and nutrients, along with inadequate removal of metabolic waste products from the tissues, results in abnormal cell function and, ultimately, tissue devitalisation. Shock is a progressive condition which may be life-threatening if it is not reversed. Its clinical signs are described in Table 22.7.

Causes of shock

Although there are many recognised causes of shock, it is frequently categorised as follows:
● Hypovolaemic.
● Vasculogenic.
  – Neurogenic.
  – Anaphylactic.
  – Endotoxic (septic).
● Cardiogenic.

Table 22.7 Clinical signs of shock

Clinical signs	Due to
(1) Weak rapid pulse.	
(2) Increased heart rate (tachycardia) with quiet heart sounds.	Poor cardiac filling.
(3) Pale mucous membranes.	Vasoconstriction.
(4) Prolonged capillary refill time (>2 s).	Vasoconstriction.
(5) Increased respiration.	Metabolic acidosis/pain.
(6) Slow jugular refill and 'poor' peripheral veins.	
(7) Hypothermia and cold extremities.	Reduced metabolic rate and vasoconstriction.
(8) Depressed level of consciousness.	Reduced blood flow to brain.
(9) Muscle weakness.	Hypoxia, vasoconstriction, etc.
(10) Reduced renal output (oliguria, anuria).	Reduced blood flow to kidneys.
(11) Low CVP and low mean arterial blood pressure.	
(12) Elevated PCV, Hb (haemoglobin), TP, urea and creatinine (a blood sample should be obtained prior to fluid administration).	

Hypovolaemic shock

Hypolovaemic shock occurs when there is an inadequate circulating blood volume, e.g. haemorrhage (external, internal), loss of plasma, severe water and electrolyte depletion (prolonged vomiting or diarrhoea which has not been treated).

Vasculogenic shock

Vasculogenic shock occurs where the blood volume is normal but the capacity of the blood vessels (primarily the veins) is increased, i.e. vasodilatation. Administration of drugs which have an effect on the capacity of the blood vessels (e.g. acetylpromazine) can induce vasculogenic shock after absolute or relative overdose.

Neurogenic shock. Neurogenic shock occurs where neurological phenomena – such as CNS trauma – result in acute vasodilatation (increased capacitance).

Anaphylactic shock. Anaphylactic shock may be classified as vasculogenic shock because many endogenous vasoactive substances (substances which affect venous capacitance and/or total peripheral resistance) are released. This occurs in association with a generalised increase in vascular permeability.

Endotoxic shock (septic shock). Endotoxic shock occurs when endotoxins, formed from the cell walls of principally Gram-negative bacteria, act to release endogenous vasoactive substances. An initial rise in cardiac output may occur, but it does not compensate for the disturbance of the distribution of blood to the tissues and the increased vascular permeability.

Cardiogenic shock

Cardiogenic shock is not common in animals. It occurs when the cardiac output is severely reduced as a result of either:

- Reduced cardiac filling (e.g. pericarditis, an accumulation of the fluid in the sac surrounding the heart).
- Reduced cardiac emptying (e.g. dilated cardiomyopathy – the heart muscle is not strong enough to force the blood out of the ventricles and round the circulatory system).

Pathophysiology of shock

Hypovolaemic shock, the most common form in veterinary practice, provides a simple model (cause, effect and result) of the course of developing shock in an animal.

Cause

Loss of blood, or effective circulating volume, ultimately reduces the venous return to the right side of the heart, and subsequently there is a fall in the output from the left side of the heart (i.e. cardiac output falls).

Effect

Pressure-sensitive baroreceptors in the aorta and carotid artery perceive the drop in blood pressure (hypotension) secondary to the fall in cardiac output. Consequently, centres within the medulla of the brain are stimulated to initiate compensatory mechanisms to restore blood pressure to normal. These compensatory mechanisms mainly involve the sympathetic nervous system and stimulation of the adrenal medulla (baroreceptor-mediated initiation of the sympathoadrenal response). Adrenaline and noradrenaline are released and cause the blood vessels of the skin, intestine, kidneys and muscles to constrict, i.e. there is an increase in peripheral vasoconstriction [increase in **total peripheral resistance (TPR)**]. This causes a direct increase in blood pressure and thus promotes increased venous return to the heart. At this stage, blood flow to the vital organs (heart and brain) is maintained. In association with these changes the heart rate increases and there is an increase in the force of contraction of the myocardium (heart muscle). *The overall result of the compensatory mechanisms so far is to increase the cardiac output.* The increased metabolic demands at this time are met in part through release of cortisol (from the adrenal cortex), which along with the catecholamines released from the adrenal medulla promote the release, mobilisation and conversion of energy substrates (e.g. gluconeogenesis).

The pressure changes within the vascular system cause a net movement of water from the ISF into the blood vessels. Release of the hormones aldosterone and ADH promote salt and water retention by the kidneys. *These mechanisms act to restore the circulating blood volume to normal.*

Result

In cases of mild shock, all of the compensatory mechanisms mentioned will come into play and often are sufficient to protect the vital organs (brain and heart) by providing an effective cardiac output. Thus, *in mild shock, homeostatic mechanisms will allow a gradual return of the circulation towards normal.*

SUMMARY

- Loss of effective circulating volume.
- Fall in cardiac output and mean arterial blood pressure.
- Sympathetic nervous system stimulation.
- Increase in TPR, heart rate, myocardial contractility.
- Increased cardiac output.
- Blood flow maintained to heart and brain.
- Blood flow reduced to gut, skin and kidney.

This occurs in association with:

(a) • Movement of fluid from ISF space to vascular space.
    • Increase in circulating volume.
(b) • Aldosterone and ADH release.
    • Water and salt (Na^+, Cl^-) retained by kidney.
    • Increase in circulating volume.

Worst case

If the haemorrhage or volume depletion is severe, then these mechanisms, which are normally life-saving, can lead to the animal's death. Prolonged vasoconstriction and low perfusion cause tissue hypoxia, anaerobic metabolism and acidosis. Consequently, the peripheral vessels dilate and become engorged with blood. Moreover, cells in the capillary wall become non-functional and fluid is lost from the capillaries into the ISF space. Both of these mechanisms act to reduce the blood returning to the heart even further. The blood soon becomes viscous and slow-moving; platelets may start to aggregate and ultimately the blood will clot within the vessels. This effectively blocks the capillaries. If it is widespread, all the clotting factors will be used up, resulting in a bleeding state known as **disseminated intravascular coagulation (DIC)**.

These changes have severe effects on the various organs of the body. Blood flow to the kidneys is reduced and urine output falls. Hypoxia causes the renal tubules to become damaged. In the gut, mucosal damage allows the invasion of bacteria and bacterial toxins are absorbed. In the lungs, although there is an initial increase in ventilation, eventually, microthrombi and other factors cause the lung to become very inefficient, and **'shock lung'** may occur during recovery. The heart is depressed by the prevailing hypoxia, acidosis and the presence of the toxins. In due course, a state of multiple organ failure develops and the animal dies.

Treatment of shock

The clinical signs of shock are given in Table 22.7. Treatments might include:

● Fluid therapy.
● General measures.
● Oxygenation.
● Corticosteroids.
● Sodium bicarbonate.
● Reduction of blood viscosity.
● Vasodilatation.
● Myocardial stimulation.
● Antibiotics.
● Other treatments.

Fluid therapy

Adequate volume replacement is the single most important measure in the treatment of peripheral circulatory failure. However, fluids should be administered with care in cardiogenic shock, which is primarily a failure of the heart to pump fluid effectively around the body rather than a volume depletion.

After clinical assessment of the animal when a 'diagnosis' of shock has been made (Table 22.7), at least one intravenous catheter should be inserted. If the peripheral veins are collapsed and difficult to catheterise, a jugular catheter should be used. To facilitate administration of large volumes of fluid over a short period of time, large-gauge catheters are required or more than one intravenous line should be established. In general, the fluid used should resemble the fluid which has been lost, e.g. whole blood would be appropriate in severe acute haemorrhage. However, the speed of fluid replacement is probably the most important factor initially. A balanced electrolyte infusion can be used in almost any circumstance of peripheral circulatory failure, while the need for other fluids is assessed by the clinician.

Blood will provide red blood cells, haemoglobin, platelets, clotting factors and proteins, whereas plasma will only provide clotting factors and protein. Blood, plasma and the plasma volume expanders will all increase the effective osmotic pressure of the plasma and so are very useful.

All fluids are given to effect. The volumes required may be very large, because of vasodilatation or because of contraction of the ISF, which also must be replaced. Frequently, fluid replacement will be the only treatment required to promote recovery.

● Dogs: 50–90 ml crystalloids/kg/hour.
● Cats: 40–60 ml crystalloids/kg/hour.

General measures

If there is an obvious source of blood loss, this should be stemmed if possible. Frequently, animals which are in shock will be (or will become) hypothermic. Although it is inadvisable to warm a hypothermic animal rapidly (because vasodilatation will occur), further loss of body heat can be prevented by ensuring a reasonable ambient temperature, avoiding draughts, lying the animal on an insulated surface, covering the animal and warming fluids to body temperature prior to administration.

Oxygenation

If hypoxia is suspected, oxygen should be provided by either face mask, nasal insufflation (via nasal catheter) or endotracheal tube. In general, animals in shock will not object to the use of a face mask, but a nasal catheter may be more suitable if the animal struggles.

Corticosteroids

The early use of corticosteroids is advocated in the treatment of shock. When they are used, it is important that they are administered in high doses and repeated at regular intervals. It is generally the aqueous soluble salts of glucocorticoids (corticosteroids) that are administered, e.g. methylprednisolone sodium succinate, dexamethasone sodium phosphate. There has been much debate about the effectiveness of corticosteroids in established shock but they still are used widely. They are *not* a substitute for adequate volume replacement but should be used in association with fluid therapy.

Sodium bicarbonate

Sodium bicarbonate should be administered intravenously to correct the metabolic acidosis. If the animal's exact requirement cannot be established, 1–2 mEq/kg of sodium bicarbonate may be administered initially (8.4% sodium bicarbonate contains 1 mEq/ml).

Reducing blood viscosity

The viscosity of blood increases in shock and reducing the viscosity of the blood will aid tissue perfusion. Fluid therapy will help to reduce the blood viscosity, but dextran 40 may be used specifically for this purpose.

Vasodilators

Once adequate volume replacement has occurred, vasodilators (e.g. acetylpromazine) may be used in an attempt to improve tissue perfusion. However, they are contraindicated in hypovolaemic shock as they will exacerbate the existing problem.

Myocardial stimulants

These agents (e.g. dopamine, dobutamine, isoprenaline) are useful in cardiogenic shock and in advanced shock where myocardial depression is possible. They are frequently administered as infusions because of their short half-lives within the circulation. Dopamine will also act to increase renal blood flow.

Antibiotics

Broad-spectrum bactericidal antibiotics are indicated because shocked animals are susceptible to infection. Antibiotics should be administered intravenously in high doses.

Other treatments

Hypertonic saline. Small volumes (4 ml/kg) of hypertonic saline (e.g. 7.0%) have been used to improve cardiac output and peripheral perfusion in shocked animals. Hypertonic saline acts by drawing water from the ICF to the ISF and PW. Its effects are rapid but transient and should be followed by definitive treatment. The use of hypertonic saline is contraindicated in renal failure, cardiogenic shock and hypernatraemia.

Anticoagulants. Heparin may be used in advanced shock where DIC (disseminated intravascular coagulation) is developing. However, care must be taken as this drug may exacerbate bleeding during subsequent surgery or where the animal has suffered trauma.

Vasoconstrictors. There is little room for the use of these agents in the treatment of shock because they will act to reduce further tissue perfusion. However, adrenaline may be used in anaphylactic shock.

Monitoring during shock

The same monitoring procedures that are used in fluid therapy also apply to animals that are in shock. Perhaps one of the most useful parameters which can be monitored is the CVP. This gives the nurse and the clinician an indication of the adequacy of fluid replacement and also serves as a useful indicator of the animal's continuing fluid requirements.

23

Anaesthesia and analgesia

D.C. Brodbelt

Introduction

Anaesthesia and the central nervous system

Anaesthesia means the elimination of sensation by the controlled, reversible suppression of nervous function with drugs. To understand anaesthesia, it is necessary to understand the nature of sensation.

Sensations like touch, pressure, temperature and pain begin with the stimulation of peripheral nerve endings in sense organs (Fig. 23.1). From these, impulses travel through sensory, or afferent, nerves to the spinal cord and then ascend to the brain, terminating in cerebrocortical projection areas dedicated to appreciating the particular sensation. Special senses like olfaction (smell) do not enter the spine: impulses travel (almost) directly to the associated projection area.

Anaesthesia occurs when sensory pathways are blocked anywhere between the peripheral sense organ and projection area. Local anaesthetics block sensation in peripheral nerves (after conduction block) or in the spinal cord (after extradural local anaesthetic injection). In contrast, general anaesthetics affect the brain, especially the particularly sensitive projection areas, and produce unconsciousness. They also reduce activity in the ascending reticular formation, a part of the neuraxis that increases cortical sensitivity to incoming stimuli.

In addition to sensation, anaesthetics depress the function of subcortical centres receiving afferent information about unconscious stimuli such as blood pressure, plasma levels of oxygen (O_2) and carbon dioxide (CO_2) and blood temperature. These 'vital centres' are relatively resistant to anaesthetics but become increasingly depressed as anaesthesia deepens; at deep levels, significant hypoventilation and hypotension occur and animals are predisposed to hypothermia.

The ways in which drugs produce anaesthesia are not fully understood but depend partly on the drug involved. Some, like the alpha-2-adrenoceptor agonists, benzodiazepines and ketamine act via specific receptors; others such as volatile agents probably act in a non-specific way on cell membranes. Some drugs acting via receptors may be antagonised.

Central analgesia: anaesthesia versus analgesia

During surgery, general anaesthetics prevent the appreciation (and subsequent memory) of pain by affecting projection areas. However, subcortical centres like the medulla and hypothalamus still respond, causing heart and respiratory rate increases, hormone release and, when anaesthesia is very 'light', limb movement. Under these conditions, anaesthesia is present but analgesia is poor.

Conversely, low concentrations of some local anaesthetics (0.25% bupivicaine) only block pain fibres, leaving other sensations 'intact'. If this formulation is used extradurally, the hindquarters become analgesic but sensitive to sensations like touch and pressure. The animal remains conscious.

Surgical anaesthesia

This is a state of insensibility which allows surgery to be performed. In addition to unconsciousness (general anaesthesia), adequate analgesia is required to suppress undesirable responses (increased blood pressure) while muscle relaxation is needed to prevent movement to facilitate surgery.

Balanced anaesthesia

Surgical anaesthesia can be produced with high doses of general anaesthetic. This may be safe in healthy animals undergoing surgery but the high doses required may jeopardise vital functions in ill patients, causing critical ventilatory and cardiovascular depression. Balanced anaesthesia describes the use of several drug types to achieve the goals of surgical anaesthesia: unconsciousness (anaesthetics/hypnotics), analgesia and muscle relaxation. By relieving general anaesthetics from the task of producing analgesia and muscle relaxation, lower doses of anaesthetics are needed and so vital centre activity is preserved.

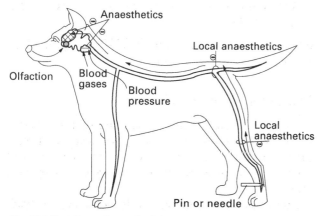

Fig. 23.1 Sensation and anaesthesia.

The objectives of anaesthesia

In veterinary practice, anaesthetics are used for several reasons:

- To permit surgery. In the UK, the 'carrying out of any operation with or without the use of instruments, involving interference with the sensitive tissues or the bone structure of an animal shall constitute an offence unless an anaesthetic is used in such as way as to prevent any pain to the animal during the operation'.
- To facilitate examination. Anxious, aggressive or painful animals may not allow examination.
- To control pain. Opioids, benzodiazepines, local and general anaesthetics are used to control pain.
- To facilitate handling. Controlling strong, aggressive animals with drugs reduces risk of injury to handlers and the need for physical restraint. Drugs for chemical restraint are chosen for potency, predictability, efficacy and speed of onset after intramuscular injection and not necessarily for safety. Drug combinations for restraint should be reserved for unmanageable cases and not regarded as anaesthetics in tractable subjects.
- To control seizures. Diazepam and pentobarbitone are used to control status epilepticus in animals.
- To perform euthanasia. Commercially available euthanasia solutions consist of concentrated anaesthetic (pentobarbitone) occasionally combined with a local anaesthetic (e.g. cinchocaine) and/or an anticonvulsant (e.g. phenytoin).

Drugs affecting central nervous function

These can be divided broadly into depressants, which reduce nervous activity, and stimulants, which increase it and oppose the effects of anaesthetics.

Depressants
- **General anaesthetics**. General anaesthetics like thiopentone and halothane eliminate sensation by causing unconsciousness; the animal is unaware of and largely unresponsive to events and is unable to remember the experience afterwards. Righting reflexes concerned with maintaining posture are lost and so animals become recumbent. Anaesthetics are classified by their physical properties: volatile liquids (halothane), gases (nitrous oxide), water-soluble (thiopentone) or water-insoluble drugs ('Saffan'). Cyclohexanones like ketamine produce a unique state in which humans would feel dissociated from the environment and be unconscious but experience vivid dreams and profound analgesia. Such drugs are known as 'dissociative' anaesthetics.
- **Sedatives**. Drugs like xylazine produce non-selective, dose-dependent central nervous depression producing drowsiness, lethargy, indifference to the environment and reduced activity. Consciousness is lost at high doses; low doses have a tranquillising effect.
- **Hypnotics**. Drugs like thiopentone produce sleep or 'hypnosis', a term synonymous with anaesthesia as hypnosis is drug-induced sleep. The 'depth' of sleep produced is dose dependent.
- **Narcotics**. Narcosis is a drug-induced stupor characterised by insensibility and paralysis. Effects are non-selective and dose-dependent. Basal narcosis is complete unconsciousness induced as a preliminary to surgical anaesthesia. Narcotics are any drugs producing these conditions and so the term includes anaesthetics, hypnotics and sedatives.
- **Tranquillisers**. Tranquillisers or ataractics, exert a quietening effect that calms aggressive animals and reduces anxiety. In high doses they cause catalepsy, a state in which the animal, though conscious, can be 'moulded'. Strong stimuli arouse tranquillised animals, whereas in sedated ones the responses, if present, are sluggish. This group is divided into 'major' or 'minor' ataractics, based on effects; major tranquillisers are also called neuroleptics.
- **Neuroleptics**. These produce neurolepsy, a state of apathy and mental detachment. Neuroleptics like acepromazine also relieve emotional distress and disturbed behaviour without clouding consciousness.
- **Neuroleptanalgesics**. Neuroleptanalgesia is a state produced by the combined effects of a neurolept and an opioid analgesic, e.g. acepromazine and morphine. Neuroleptanalgesics cause dose-dependent effects and high doses produce unconsciousness (neuroleptanaesthesia).

Stimulants. Drugs that increase nervous activity oppose the effects of anaesthetics. They are classified according to their site of action. Analeptics (medullary stimulants) are the most commonly used. Others have undesirable side-effects and, with the exception of doxapram, are not licensed for animal use. Some are controlled substances.

Drug interactions

Usually, drugs depressing central nervous function act in an additive or synergistic fashion. If a sedative drug (A) produces an effect (e), and if drug (B), which is more potent, causes an effect 2(e), then after (A) and (B) are given:

- **Additive** effects occur when the level of sedation equals 3(e).
- **Synergy** occurs when the level of sedation is greater than 3(e).
- **Antagonism** occurs if the level of sedation achieved is less than 3(e).

Inhalation anaesthetics act in an additive fashion; neurolepts and opioids act in a synergistic way.

The blood–brain barrier

In order to affect brain activity, anaesthetics must first cross the blood–brain barrier, a conceptual anatomic feature formed by 'tight' junctions between endothelial cells of capillaries and envelopment of brain capillaries by glial cells.

Drugs that are non-ionised, small, fat-soluble (or lipid-soluble) and unbound from albumen cross the blood–brain barrier rapidly. In some conditions (e.g. encephalitis), the blood–brain barrier is disrupted and the patient becomes more sensitive to anaesthetics.

Anaesthesia and the respiratory system

The respiratory and cardiovascular systems operate in concert to oxygenate blood and then deliver it to peripheral, metabolically active tissue. Here, energy-rich substrate (glucose) is oxidised (with O_2) to produce CO_2. The metabolic requirements of organs like the brain are such that diminished O_2 or glucose supplies will rapidly cause cell death.

Understanding the respiratory system during anaesthesia is important because anaesthetics depress ventilation, causing or contributing to cardiac arrest. The system also takes up and eliminates volatile anaesthetics.

Ventilation

The respiratory system must provide enough free gas to the alveoli per minute to ensure that blood is oxygenated, and 'purged' of CO_2. The volume of gas inspired per breath is the tidal volume (V_t), measured in millilitres or litres. The volume of gas inspired per minute – the 'minute volume' ($\dot{V}_m$) of ventilation – is given by:

$$\dot{V}_m = V_t \times R,$$

where R is the respiratory rate in breaths per minute.

Dead-space. Not all inspired gas reaches the alveoli and participates in gas exchange. At the end of inspiration, the last portion resides in the volume of the respiratory tree down to the level of conducting bronchioles. This does not participate in gas exchange and is called the **anatomic dead-space** volume (V_{danat}).

Anatomic dead-space is augmented by excessive equipment attached to the proximal end of the airway; overlarge masks and overlong endotracheal tubes are examples of **mechanical** (or apparatus) **dead-space** volume (V_{dmech}).

Some inspired gas reaches alveoli that are not perfused with blood and so does not contribute to gas exchange. This is known as alveolar dead-space (V_{da}). Anatomic and alveolar dead-space constitute physiological dead-space:

$$V_d = V_{danat} + V_{da} + V_{dmech}$$

The remaining volume reaching alveoli is the alveolar volume (V_A).

$$V_A = V_t - V_d,$$

and the volume of gas usefully inspired per minute, i.e. the alveolar ventilation ($\dot{V}_A$), is given by:

$$\dot{V}_A = R(V_t - V_d).$$

The importance of dead-space is now apparent: when excessive, it reduces alveolar ventilation.

The elimination of carbon dioxide (CO_2), the normal determinant of respiration, is directly proportional to $\dot{V}_A$:

$$P_aCO_2 = k \times \dot{V}CO_2/VA,$$

where $\dot{V}CO_2$ is the volume of CO_2 produced by the body per minute, k is a constant and P_aCO_2 is the partial pressure or 'level' of CO_2 in arterial blood. Consequently, under normal conditions P_aCO_2 is an indicator of the adequacy of ventilation. Normal P_aCO_2 is 5.33 kPa (40 mmHg).

Control of ventilation

The contraction of ventilatory muscles (most importantly the diaphragm and external intercostal muscles) causes lung inflation and the inspiration of tidal volume. The activity of these muscles, and therefore the level of ventilation, is driven by nerve fibres whose origin lies in the 'respiratory centre' of the medulla oblongata, located in the brain stem. Activity in these fibres is controlled by several factors such as body temperature and pain, but the most important are blood levels of CO_2 and O_2. These levels are monitored by two types of receptors known as *chemoreceptors*:

- *Central Chemoreceptors (CC).* These chemoreceptors lie in the brain stem close to the respiratory centres and are sensitive to the pH of surrounding cerebrospinal fluid (CSF). Carbon dioxide diffuses from blood into CSF, lowering its pH. The CC respond by increasing respiratory drive to the respiratory centres.
- *Peripheral chemoreceptors.* The carotid and aortic bodies are sited near the carotid bifurcation and the aortic arch, respectively, and respond primarily to falling oxygen tensions in blood. In conscious animals their activity increases dramatically when P_aO_2 falls below 8 kPa (60 mmHg). (Normal O_2 levels are 13 kPa (100 mmHg).)

Normally, P_aCO_2 levels are the major determinant of minute ventilation; when CO_2 rises, alveolar ventilation rises, restoring P_aCO_2 to normal. Blood oxygen levels only become important in driving respiration when they are critically reduced.

Hypoventilation

Hypoventilation means inadequate ventilation and causes plasma CO_2 levels to rise – a state known as **hypercapnia** (or hypercarbia). Carbon dioxide tensions in excess of 5.33 kPa (40 mmHg) indicate hypoventilation. Hypoventilation occurs when:

- Respiratory rate (R) is too low (e.g. anaesthetic overdose).
- Tidal volume (V_t) is reduced (e.g. heavy drapes on chest wall.
- Dead-space (V_d) increases (e.g. endotracheal tube projects too far from mouth, hypovolaemia reduces alveolar perfusion).
- A combination of these.

Hypercapnia can also result from increased production of CO_2. This may occur in the pyrexic animal or during malignant hyperthermia, a rare condition in companion animals but not uncommon in certain pig breeds. Carbon dioxide dissolves in blood to produce carbonic acid:

$$CO_2 + H_2O = H_2CO_3 = H^+ + HCO_3^-.$$

This increases the acidity (and lowers the pH) of blood – a state of acidosis. Because the state is caused by hypoventilation, the ensuing condition is called **respiratory acidosis**. Hypercapnia and respiratory acidosis have important effects:

- Modest levels increase heart rate and blood pressure (and bleeding at the surgical site).
- High levels depress the heart, cause arrhythmias and enhance narcosis.

Anaesthetics reduce chemoreceptor sensitivity to CO_2 and O_2 (some more than others) with the result that anaesthetised animals are usually hypercapnic.

Hyperventilation

This is an excessive level of breathing that drives off CO_2 and causes hypocapnia (or hypocarbia) and respiratory alkalosis. Pain and 'light' anaesthesia are common causes. Excessive manual or mechanical ventilation also causes hypocapnia; after periods of hyperventilation, animals usually will not breathe until $P_a CO_2$ levels rise again.

Hypoxia

Hypoxia means abnormally low oxygen tensions in arterial blood ($P_a O_2$). (Anoxia is an obsolete term meaning no oxygen.) Hypoxia is important because inadequately oxygenated haemoglobin means active tissues may become deprived of oxygen (tissue hypoxia). If the heart becomes hypoxic, cardiac arrest will occur. Lowered tissue oxygen delivery can result from several causes:

- Reduced oxygen in inspired gas (e.g. oxygen cylinder empties).
- Reduced alveolar ventilation (e.g. reduced rate, tidal volume or increased dead-space).
- Lung pathology (e.g. pneumonia).
- Insufficient haemoglobin to carry oxygen from lungs (e.g. anaemia).
- Insufficient cardiac output to deliver oxygenated blood tissue (e.g. anaesthetic overdose).
- Increased tissue demand for oxygen (e.g. increased work – the myocardium becomes hypoxic at high heart rates).

Anaesthesia and the cardiovascular system

The cardiovascular system consists of the heart, blood vessels, blood and elements of the autonomic nervous system that control its activity. The heart is considered in two parts: the right pumps unoxygenated blood to the lung, the left pumps oxygenated blood to peripheral tissue.

The goal of cardiovascular activity is **perfusion** – the movement of sufficient volumes of blood containing metabolic reagents (oxygen and glucose) through tissue capillary beds per unit time.

Anaesthetics depress many facets of cardiovascular function and, in combination with respiratory effects, may cause vital tissue to become deprived of oxygen (or glucose)

and fail. Central nervous tissue hypoxia and hypoglycaemia rapidly cause irreversible damage.

Perfusion

Blood movement through capillaries depends on three factors (Fig. 23.2):

- High upstream (arterial) pressure (blood pressure).
- Low downstream (venous) pressure.
- Low resistance through tissue (relaxation of the precapillary sphincter).

Local tissue perfusion largely depends on local requirements. When metabolic activity is high, O_2 tensions fall and CO_2 accumulates. Both local hypoxia and hypercapnia cause precapillary sphincters to relax. Provided that upstream pressure is adequate, the blood flow will increase, delivering oxygen and removing CO_2.

Cardiovascular activity aims to ensure 'adequate upstream pressure' (or arterial blood pressure) so that tissues receive blood in inverse proportion to the resistance they offer, i.e. according to their requirements. For non-vital tissue, 'whole-body' needs often override local requirements.

Systemic vascular resistance (SVR)

Arterial blood pressure is determined by cardiac output and systemic vascular resistance (Fig. 23.2): an increase in either raises blood pressure. Systemic vascular resistance is governed by the collective state of precapillary sphincters throughout the body. When these are closed, or in a state of vasoconstriction, SVR is increased and blood pressure rises. Precapillary sphincter diameter is controlled by:

- Local metabolic factors (PO_2, PCO_2).
- Tonic vasoconstrictor nerve discharge.
- Hormones and drugs: endogenous (angiotensin, adrenaline) and exogenous (drugs, e.g. acepromazine, methoxamine).

Throughout the body, SVR is controlled by tonic, vasoconstrictor discharge from nerves of the sympathetic nervous system. This activity originates from the vasomotor centre of the medulla and is of fundamental importance in maintaining blood pressure by increasing SVR. It should be appreciated that perfusion downstream from constricted precapillary arterioles is reduced. Not surprisingly, vasoconstrictor fibres project principally to blood vessels of non-vital tissue, including the gastrointestinal tract and skin, the perfusion of which is reduced when whole-body needs dictate. During haemorrhage, vasoconstrictor nerve activity increases in these tissues, preserving blood pressure and maintaining perfusion of vital tissue (brain and heart).

Vasomotor centre function is depressed by general anaesthetics, which lower SVR and therefore blood pressure. Extradural local anaesthetics block vasoconstrictor fibres leaving the spinal cord; SVR is therefore lowered in areas affected by the block.

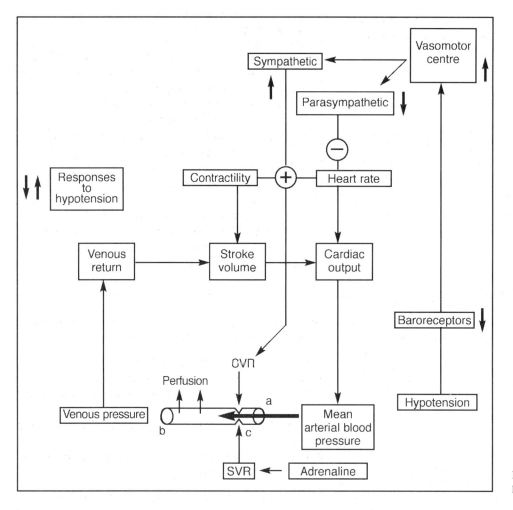

Fig. 23.2 The control of blood pressure.

Cardiac output

Cardiac output, the volume of blood ejected by the heart per minute (measured in litres per minute) is the product of stroke volume (volume of blood ejected per beat) and heart rate. Variations in either component influence cardiac output.

Heart rate is governed by relative activity in either division of the autonomic nervous system; cardiac accelerator fibres (sympathetic) increase heart rate, while vagal (parasympathetic) activity slows heart rate. The rate also increases in response to circulating adrenaline. Stroke volume is governed by myocardial contractility and venous return – the volume of blood returning to the heart. Venous return depends on several factors including the circulating blood volume. Myocardial contractility is increased by circulating adrenaline.

Rapid heart rates reduce the time available for ventricles to fill with blood and lower stroke volume. At very high heart rates, cardiac output is reduced.

Control of blood pressure

Arterial blood pressure is sensed by baroreceptors (or mechanoreceptors), which are stretch-sensitive nerve endings lying within the elastic walls of the arterial tree. The most important group lie in a dilatation of the internal carotid artery known as the carotid sinus. These stretch when exposed to high pressure, and activity in baroreceptor nerve fibres increases. These fibres project to the medulla where their activity initiates three responses:

● Reduced activity in cardiac sympathetic nerves lowers heart rate and the force of contraction.
● Increased parasympathetic (vagal) activity causes slowing of the heart.
● Vasomotor centre activity is suppressed; reduced vasoconstrictor activity causes vasodilatation in mesenteric and cutaneous vascular beds, lowering SVR and blood pressure.

During haemorrhage, blood pressure falls because venous return is reduced. Normally, this would lower baroreceptor activity, initiating an increase in heart rate and contractility, a reduction in vagal tone and increased vasoconstrictor activity and so restore blood pressure. During anaesthesia, these responses are depressed for several reasons: general anaesthetics suppress vasomotor centre sensitivity, while SVR and cardiac output are lowered by drugs.

Hypotension

Hypotension, or low blood pressure, results from:

● Reduced cardiac output. Most anaesthetics depress heart rate and contractility. Surgical haemorrhage lowers venous return.

- Reduced SVR. Volatile agents, especially isoflurane, lower blood pressure by causing vasodilatation as does acepromazine.
- Both of the above.

Hypertension

Elevated blood pressure results predictably from increased cardiac output and SVR. It occurs when animals are inadequately anaesthetised during surgery because of adrenaline release. On recovery, it indicates pain. Hypertension can follow excessive transfusion of colloids or blood, or overdosage with drugs increasing cardiac output (inotropes).

Tachycardia

Tachycardia (excessive heart rate) is caused by adrenaline release. This preserves blood pressure and is desirable when it occurs in response to physiological changes like hypotension, hypercapnia or hypoglycaemia. In response to pain, however, severe tachycardia is undesirable because cardiac output and coronary perfusion are reduced while myocardial work and oxygen consumption are elevated. Subsequent hypoxia causes arrhythmias and eventually arrest.

Bradycardia

Bradycardia means excessive slowing of the heart. Slow heart rates are not always undesirable: ventricular filling and stroke volume are increased, while cardiac work is lowered. However, very slow rates reduce output and cause hypotension.

Oxygen flux

The combined function of cardiovascular and pulmonary systems is to deliver oxygenated blood to peripheral tissue and can be expressed as oxygen flux (DO_2). This is the volume of oxygen reaching peripheral tissue per minute.

Oxygen flux (DO_2) = cardiac output (Q_t) $\times$ oxygen content of blood (C_aO_2).

$$C_aO_2 = S_aO_2 \times [\text{Hb}] \times 1.34,$$

where S_aO_2 is the percentage saturation of haemoglobin by oxygen (when PO_2 is normal this value is nearly 1.0); [Hb] is the haemoglobin concentration in blood (which is normally 12–15 g/dl). The figure 1.34 is the amount (in millilitres) of O_2 combining with each gram of Hb.

Oxygen flux is lowered by reduced cardiac output (e.g. anaesthetics) and reduced oxygen content of blood. The latter results from lowered S_aO_2 (lung disease) or Hb (e.g. anaemia).

Pre-operative assessment and preparation

Pre-operative examination may indicate that some animals are poor candidates for anaesthesia and surgery. The

---

SUMMARY

- Anaesthesia is the elimination of sensation by controlled and reversible depression of nervous function with drugs.
- The triad of anaesthesia consists of narcosis, muscle relaxation and analgesia.
- Balanced analgesia targets each of these components specifically.
- Drugs can depress or stimulate CNS function to varying degrees.
- Anaesthesia significantly affects respiratory and cardiovascular function and a knowledge of these effects is important for safe anaesthesia.

American Society of Anesthesiologists (ASA) risk assessment classifies patients into five categories:

- Class 1 – normal, healthy patient.
- Class 2 – patient with mild systemic disease.
- Class 3 – patient with severe systemic disease that is not incapacitating.
- Class 4 – patient with severe systemic disease that is a constant threat to life.
- Class 5 – moribund patient not expected to survive 24 hours with or without surgery.

In those cases which are poor anaesthetic candidates (ASA classes 3–5), particular attention to preparation is required to minimise the risk of untoward events. Other considerations that affect the degree of preparation include the type of surgery; prolonged and/or invasive procedures require more preparation than superficial operations. Whether the procedure is elective or an emergency indicates how much preparation is possible. Emergency cases requiring immediate surgery may receive only cursory preparation. Elective procedures may be postponed without compromising the animal.

Pre-operative examination

The animal's medical condition is determined by history-taking, physical examination and, when necessary, further tests.

History

Useful information is gleaned from questioning the owner. Establishing a full medical history requires additional information:

- Duration of ownership.
- Previous medical history.
- Previous anaesthetic history.
- Vaccination status.
- Current medication, including 'over-the-counter' products. The dose, dosing frequency and duration of

Table 23.1 Drugs potentially affecting anaesthesia

Antibiotics
Glucocorticoids
Non-steroidal anti-inflammatory drugs
Organophosphorus compounds, flea collars, parasiticides
Anticonvulsants
Digoxin
Frusemide and other diuretics
β-blockers or ACE-inhibitors
Endocrine supplements, e.g. thyroxin
Antihistamines
Antitussives/bronchodilators
Sex hormones

treatment should be established. Drugs of particular concern are listed in Table 23.1.

Physical examination.

This concentrates on the organ systems affected principally by anaesthesia:

- Central nervous system status involves particular attention to the state of mind and presence of depressed function.
- Cardiovascular function is assessed with inspection of mucous membrane colour and capillary refill time, palpation of peripheral pulse rate and quality, and auscultation of cardiac murmurs and dysrhythmias. Pale mucous membranes suggest hypovolaemia or anaemia, whilst cyanotic membranes indicate a sluggish circulation or poor oxygenation of arterial blood. Cool extremities can be seen during shock and reduced peripheral perfusion. Right-sided cardiovascular dysfunction is associated with pronounced jugular pulses, and peripheral oedema.
- Respiratory system examination includes observation of respiratory rate and pattern, auscultation and percussion of the chest. Auscultation of rales and crepitus suggest airway secretion and respiratory disease. Reduced sounds are associated with lung consolidation. Chest percussion with low resonance supports the presence of consolidation, whilst high resonance is consistent with pneumothorax.

Further tests

Haematology and biochemistry. A blood sample should be examined if the history or physical examination raises the suspicion of anaemia, polycythaemia, hypoproteinaemia or coagulation disorders. Metabolic and electrolyte disorders, including hypo- and hyperkalaemia, can be detected. Liver function tests and liver enzymes can alert to liver pathology whilst serum urea and creatinine are useful indicators of renal status. Urinalysis is valuable in investigating renal function if particular concern exists.

Electrocardiography. Abnormal pulse rhythms require further investigation.

Radiography. Animals involved in road traffic accidents, those with neoplastic disease and those with signs of cardiovascular or pulmonary disease should undergo radiographic examination of the thorax and possibly abdomen.

Ultrasonography. Allows thorough investigation of cardiac function.

Significance of clinical findings

Central nervous system

- Behaviour better indicates an animal's suitability for surgery than chronological age: a tail-wagging, active 15-year-old is a better risk than the depressed, small, inactive 8-month-old with a porto-systemic shunt.
- Depression increases patient sensitivity to anaesthetics and may indicate the presence of intracranial pathology (tumours, meningitis), systemic disease (pyrexia, hyperkalaemia, toxaemia) or cardiovascular problems (anaemia).
- Excitable, nervous or aggressive animals may require profound sedation.
- Epileptic animals are sensitive to anaesthetics if anticonvulsant therapy has only recently begun. In time, liver enzyme induction occurs and accelerates the metabolism of some anaesthetics.

Cardiovascular and respiratory disease

Signs of cardiac and respiratory disease (including exercise intolerance) are always important. When disease is present, the fundamental goal of preparation is to optimise the factors contributing to oxygen delivery to the tissues, i.e. cardiac output, haemoglobin and pulmonary function.

Cardiac disease is not a contraindication to anaesthesia if the effects on cardiac function and blood flow are appreciated and drugs selected accordingly. In general, 'stress', pain and volume losses are less well tolerated by animals with cardiovascular disease. Drugs used for treating cardiac disease (e.g. digoxin, beta-antagonists) may interact with anaesthetics. Cases with congestive failure may require cage-rest, sodium restricted diet and digitalisation. Pre-existing arrhythmias may require treatment.

Respiratory disease predisposes the animal to hypoxia and hypercapnia. It may contribute to secondary right ventricular changes (cor pulmonale) or polycythaemia. A common form of restrictive respiratory disease is morbid obesity. Restricted airways (e.g. nasal discharge, brachiocephalic canine anatomy) require careful attention for maintenance of an airway.

Causes of respiratory embarrassment (e.g. pneumothorax, gastric tympany) must be relieved pre-operatively. Pleural effusions should be drained pre-operatively. Excessive alveolar transudate may be cleared with diuretics and/or drugs that improve cardiac contractility and function (inotropes).

Hypovolaemia or dehydration

In dehydrated and hypovolaemic animals, tissue perfusion may become compromised during anaesthesia. Animals with chronic fluid loss (e.g. those with chronic vomiting and diarrhoea) may have electrolyte and/or pH disturbances.

Animals with nephritis cannot concentrate urine and become dehydrated if access to water is restricted. Dogs with chronic renal failure, or any disease characterised by polyuria and polydipsia, must not have water withheld pre-operatively; if necessary, parenteral fluids may be given.

When reduced, circulating blood volume must be restored pre-operatively with appropriate fluids. Oral, intravenous, intraperitoneal, intraosseous or subcutaneous routes may be used, depending on the fluid type.

Animals with unstable blood glucose levels

Diabetes mellitus causes hyperglycaemia with diuresis, fluid loss and keto-acidosis. Severe hypoglycaemia resulting from insulinomata or liver disease causes considerable neuronal damage if brain glucose supply is curtailed. Glucose levels must be controlled with soluble insulin or dextrose solutions pre-operatively.

Anaemia

Low haemoglobin levels (below 8 g/dl) caused by blood loss or renal disease must be resolved before surgery; oxygen flux may become inadequate when compensatory changes (increased cardiac output and modest hyperventilation) are depressed by anaesthetics. In elective cases, low haemoglobin levels may be raised by treating the underlying cause; otherwise blood transfusion, preferably with 'packed' cells, may be required.

Polycythaemia

Haematocrit values in excess of 55% make blood hyperviscous, causing it to 'sludge' in capillaries. They may also indicate that the animal is dehydrated or suffering from chronic hypoxia (cardiopulmonary disease). High haematocrits are lowered by the process of normovolaemic haemodilution. This involves the withdrawal of whole blood and simultaneous replacement with plasma or fluids.

Pyrexia

Pyrexia increases metabolic rate; there are rises in the consumption of O_2 and glucose and in the production of CO_2. The cause of pyrexia should be sought because, while there is little problem anaesthetising animals with superficial abscesses, there is considerable risk when pyrexia results from endocarditis or meningitis. Pyrexia is treated with antibiotics if the cause is infective.

Hypoalbuminaemia

This indicates liver or renal disease and has two consequences. First, the albumen-bound fraction of drugs normally bound (e.g. thiopentone) is lowered and so more free drug is available. Second, plasma oncotic pressure may be lowered, promoting oedema and increased diffusion distance for gases in the lung.

Coagulation problems

Clotting failure may be genetic (von Willebrand's disease in Dobermanns) or indicate liver failure. Fresh blood transfusion may be required pre-operatively.

Electrolyte and pH abnormalities

High potassium levels resulting from Addison's disease or renal failure must be lowered pre-operatively, while low serum potassium should be raised. Normal pH should be restored by treatment of conditions causing alkalosis or acidosis.

High potassium levels are lowered with sodium bicarbonate solutions, calcium gluconate, insulin–glucose solutions, or cation-exchange resins. In extreme cases, peritoneal dialysis may be required. Potassium is raised by infusing solutions at rates not greater than 0.5 mmol/kg/h. Extremes of pH are ameliorated by treating the underlying cause.

Any 'emergency' case

These are cases where surgical delay is unacceptable:

- Thoracic visceral damage.
- Airway obstruction.
- Uncontrollable haemorrhage.
- Obstetric emergencies in which neonates are at risk.

In emergencies, preparation may be limited to catheterising a vein, administering fluids and enriching inspired breath with oxygen.

Final details

Before admitting normal animals for surgery, owners must:

- Be informed of the risks and possible outcomes.
- Have signed an anaesthetic consent form.
- Be asked to withhold food the night before (water can be given).

Food and water deprivation

A full stomach reduces lung volume, limits breathing and predisposes to vomiting; this may result in fatal aspiration. If an animal scheduled for surgery has received a large meal pre-operatively, the best option is to delay surgery to allow adequate emptying of the stomach (i.e. 6 hours).

SUMMARY

- Clinical examination includes attention to patient history, physical examination findings and results of further tests.
- Careful patient evaluation identifies particular risks including cardiovascular and respiratory compromise, CNS depression, reduced liver and renal function and metabolic imbalances.
- Higher risk patients require more pre-operative preparation.
- Adequate preparation avoids unnecessary anaesthetic complications.

Sedation and premedication

Sedatives and tranquillisers can be used on their own to allow minor procedures or as premedication in preparation for general anaesthesia. Many procedures require restraint only. An ideal sedative produces:

- Stoical indifference to the surroundings.
- No hyperaesthesia.
- Analgesia, particularly if the animal is in pain.
- Recumbency if required.
- No side-effects.

Effective sedation and chemical restraint require a quiet environment without disturbance of the animal, adequate time to allow full effect, and quiet, firm and sensible handling.

Potential cardiovascular and respiratory depression can occur with the use of chemical restraint. Sedation is not always safer than general anaesthesia as often no oxygen is supplied, facility for intermittent positive pressure ventilation is not available and monitoring of the patient is frequently minimal.

Premedication is given before surgery to smooth subsequent events. The objectives of premedication are:

- To reduce anxiety. Nervous animals may resist restraint for induction, and possess undesirable catecholamine levels. Intravenous injection is easier in calm animals. For animals excited by pain, analgesics will reduce anxiety.
- To enable 'smooth' induction and recovery.

- To provide analgesia.
- To reduce induction agent dose.
- To reduce maintenance agent requirements.
- To reduce associated side-effects of the anaesthetic to be given.
- To reduce adverse effects of surgery. Some surgical procedures may cause increased vagal activity, in which case atropine or glycopyrrolate can be given beforehand.

In providing 'background' narcosis, premedication and analgesics lower the requirement for maintenance agents and consequently the incidence of associated side-effects. However, certain premedications may be more hazardous than the induction or maintenance agents themselves.

Long-acting drugs like acepromazine smooth recovery after induction with methohexitone and other drugs. Similarly, analgesics smooth recovery after painful procedures.

Disadvantages of premedication include the potential for drug interactions and side-effects, prolongation of recovery, and the need to allow sufficient time for the drugs to have full effect. Not all animals require pre-anaesthetic medication, e.g. those already depressed by toxaemia, shock or head trauma. After haemorrhage or in shocked animals, normal doses produce more profound effects.

Drugs maintaining the health status of the patient (Table 23.1) are not usually recognised as 'premedication' because most are pharmacologically unrelated to anaesthetics. Their consideration is important because they may:

(1) Have adverse pre-operative effects (e.g. digoxin may cause intraoperative arrhythmias).
(2) Interact with anaesthesia (e.g. propranolol may block pressor responses of hypercapnia).

Despite this, it is generally true that withdrawing medication pre-operatively is likely to cause more problems than are possible through adverse drug interaction. A range of drugs (Table 23.2) is used to achieve the classical goals of premedication.

The route by which pre-anaesthetic medication is given influences time to peak effect, duration of action (Table 23.3) and the incidence of side-effects.

Phenothiazines

Acepromazine

This phenothiazine neuroleptic is available for small animals as a 2 mg/ml solution, at doses of 0.01–0.05 mg/kg

Table 23.2 Range of premedicant drugs

Drug class	Type	Examples
Phenothiazines	Neurolept	Acepromazine, chlorpromazine
Butyrophenomes	Neurolept	Azaperone, fluanisone
Opioids	Narcotic analgesic	Morphine, methadone, pethidine, butorphanol, papaveretum, pentazocine, buprenorphine
Alpha-2-agonists	Sedative	Xylazine, medetomidine
Benzodiazepines	Tranquilliser	Diazepam, midazolam
Anti-muscarinics (also known as anti-cholinergics)		Atropine, glycopyrrolate

intramuscularly or intravenously. It remains a popular and useful drug despite important side-effects. At normal doses the drug is safe and produces moderate sedation. Increasing the dose does not increase the degree of sedation but extends the duration of action and increases the severity of adverse reactions.

PHENOTHIAZINES

Advantages

- Synergism: improves sedative effects of opioids.
- Antiarrhythmic: low doses exert antiarrhythmic activity.
- Antiemetic: offsets the emetic effects of some opioids.
- Safety: doses do not cause coma in overdose.
- Spasmolytic: reduces discomfort when 'colic' results from gastrointestinal spasm.
- Antihistamine: potentially useful with some histamine-releasing opioids.

Disadvantages

- Hypotension. This side-effect, which causes most concern, results from vascular smooth muscle relaxation via alpha-1-adrenergic blockade. Problems occur when high doses (above 0.15 mg/kg) are used or when normal doses are used in hypotensive (e.g. hypovolaemic) animals. It causes acute decompensation and hypotension when blood pressure relies on increased systemic vascular resistance (e.g. hypovolaemia, cardiac failure).
- Syncope. In some breeds, syncope may occur. Some breed-lines of Boxers collapse after low doses.
- Unpredictability. Failure to produce dose-dependent sedation. Aggressive dogs are often resistant. Occasionally 'release of inhibitions' is seen in aggressive dogs.
- Long-acting. Dose-dependent duration of action; clinical sedation lasts 4–6 hours.
- Slow onset. Peak effect does not occur for 10–20 minutes after intravenous and for 30 minutes after intramuscular administration.
- No analgesia.
- Hypothermia. Cutaneous vasodilatation and (hypothalamic) thermoregulatory depression cause heat loss.
- Poor muscle relaxation. The drug has no relaxant effects but reduces hypertonicity with ketamine.
- Penile prolapse may be seen in horses.

Table 23.3 Comparison of drug administration routes

Convenience	SC > IP > IM > IV
Pain on injection	IM > IP + IV > SC
Restraint needed	IV > IP > IM > SC
Animal tolerance	SC > IP > IM > IV
Onset of action	IV > IM > SC > IP
Duration of action	IP + SC > IM > IP
Predictability	IV > IM > SC > IP
Relative dose required	IP + SC > IM > IV
Risk of complications	IP > IV > IM > SC
Technical ease	SC > IM > IP > IV

SC, subcutaneous; IP, intraperitoneal; IM, intramuscular; IV, intravenous.

Butyrophenomes

These behave like phenothiazines though produce unpredictable results. There are no butyrophenomes licensed for sole use in small animals, but fluanisone and droperidol are available combined with opioids.

Neuroleptanalgesia. Phenothiazines and butyrophenomes mixed with opioids create a neuroleptanalgesic combination. The two components are synergistic; lower doses of each are needed, which lowers the incidence and severity of side-effects. Commercially available mixtures are convenient but effects are sub-optimal in about 40% of recipients.

- Small Animal Immobilon (etorphine 74 μg, methotrimeprazine 18 mg/ml).
- Hypnorm (fentanyl 0.315 mg, fluanisone 10 mg/ml).

Neuroleptanalgesics may be 'home-made: doses and drugs are modified to suit the individual case, e.g. acepromazine and buprenorphine.

BUTYROPHENOMES

Advantages

- Lower incidence of side-effects.
- Increased degree of sedation.
- Increased predictability.
- Stable cardiopulmonary performance.

Disadvantages

- Animals remain sensitive to, and are aroused by, certain stimuli (e.g. acoustic).
- Only opioid antagonism is possible. The neuroleptic is not antagonised and is the longer-acting component.
- Behavioural changes are alleged to have occurred after neuroleptanalgesia in dogs.

Alpha-2-adrenoceptor agonists

Xylazine (1–3 mg/kg, 2%) and medetomidine (5–80 μg/kg (dog), 30–100 μg/kg (cat), 1 mg/ml) are alpha-2-adrenoceptor agonists licensed for use in companion animals. Medetomidine is more potent and longer acting.

ALPHA-2-ADRENOCEPTOR AGONISTS

Advantages
- Profound dose-dependent sedation.
- High doses produce basal narcosis. Duration of action is also dose-dependent.
- Marked drug-sparing effect.
- Doses of induction and maintenance agents are considerably reduced. Circulation time is prolonged, accelerating the uptake of volatile anaesthetics. A greater lag time elapses before effects of induction agents are seen.
- Muscle relaxation.
- Relaxant effects offset muscle rigidity seen with ketamine, making alpha-2-agonist/ketamine combinations popular.
- Visceral analgesia.

Disadvantages
- Cardiovascular depression. There are dose-dependent and profound cardiovascular effects; hypertension then hypotension, reduced cardiac output and bradycardia. Antimuscarinic pre-treatment, which counteracts bradycardia is controversial. Medetomidine has only modest hypotensive effects. In dogs, xylazine sensitises the myocardium to adrenaline-induced arrhythmias during halothane anaesthesia.
- Respiratory depression. While breathing is periodic with apnoeic pauses of 45 seconds and mucous membranes turn grey, P_aO_2 and P_aCO_2 are often satisfactory.
- Emesis. Vomiting occurs in dogs and cats after xylazine and, to a lesser extent, after medetomidine.
- Diuresis. ADH inhibition and insulin suppression, causing hyperglycaemia, contribute to this effect.
- Gut motility. This is reduced or abolished and barium meal interpretation may be confused. Because aerophagia occurs, some suggest caution in use of alpha-2-adrenoceptor agonists in breeds predisposed to gastric-dilatation-volvulus
- Thermoregulation. Alpha-2-adrenoceptor agonists impair thermoregulation, allowing hypo- or hyperthermia depending on ambient temperatures.
- Personal risk. The data sheet instructs that gloves should be worn when handling medetomidine.
- Low safety. The data sheet states that medetomidine should not be used in animals 'in poor general health'.
- Muscle relaxation. Relaxation may cause problems in brachycephalics with redundant oropharyngeal tissue.

Atipamezole

Atipamezole is used to antagonise the effects of medetomidine in companion animals; the antagonist dose is the same volume as agonist injected in dogs and half the volume in cats. Its use is desirable because the prolonged effect of medetomidine predisposes recipients to hypothermia and hypostatic lung congestion. However, after painful procedures, antagonism may expose the animal, acutely, to discomfort.

Benzodiazepines

In humans, benzodiazepines like diazepam and midazolam produce anxiolysis, muscle relaxation, sedation, hypnosis and amnesia and have powerful anticonvulsant effects. Paradoxically, intravenous diazepam can cause marked stimulation in non-debilitated dogs. Diazepam is water-insoluble and its formulation causes pain on injection and thrombophlebitis. Midazolam is water-soluble and does not cause these problems. It is short-acting; it is approximately twice as potent and is more effective after intramuscular injection than diazepam. Doses of 0.1–0.2 mg/kg of both drugs are routinely used.

BENZODIAZEPINES

Advantages
- Safety. The drugs have high therapeutic indices and minimal cardiopulmonary effects.
- Drug-sparing effect. They prolong and enhance effects of other anaesthetics. Anaesthetic doses are lowered and predicted excitement (e.g. recovery after methohexitone increments) is prevented.
- Muscle relaxation. Diazepam or midazolam are used with ketamine in cats to provide heavy sedation and eliminate excitation/convulsions and associated muscle hypertonicity of ketamine administration.

Disadvantages
- Unpredictable. In animals, benzodiazepines often stimulate rather than depress but become increasingly effective as the animal's health status deteriorates. In normal, fit dogs, high intravenous doses of diazepam cause marked ataxia, no sedation and violent struggling. Eating is usually stimulated in cats.
- Formulation. Diazepam causes pain on injection and thrombophlebitis. It should not be drawn up into plastic (polyvinyl chloride) syringes unless used immediately, because the drug 'binds' to polyvinyl chloride.

Flumazenil (Ro 15–1788)

A benzodiazepine antagonist used to treat overdosage in people and accelerate recovery in outpatient anaesthesia, this drug is of little benefit in animals as the need to antagonise rarely arises.

Anticholinergic drugs

The routine use of antimuscarinic drugs like atropine (0.02–0.04 mg/kg, 600 µg/ml) and glycopyrrolate (0.01–0.02 mg/kg, 200 µg/ml) for anaesthetic premedication is controversial. In previous times, the widespread use of diethyl ether anaesthesia in humans justified this practice; diethyl ether promotes oropharyngeal secretion, bronchosecretion and bronchoconstriction. Modern volatile anaesthetics do not produce excessive secretions and most cause bronchodilatation.

SUMMARY

- Sedation may be appropriate for simple procedures.
- Where general anaesthesia is required premedication is often valuable, smoothing anaesthesia and reducing complications.
- Phenothiazines, alpha-2-adrenoceptor agonists, benzodiazepines and anticholinergics are appropriate for premedication under different circumstances.
- Neuroleptanalgesia can potentiate sedation with less cardiopulmonary depression.
- For effective sedation and premedication a quiet environment, adequate time to allow full effect and careful patient handling are required.

ATROPINE

Advantages
- Bronchodilates, reduces total airway resistance.
- Rapidly controls intra-operative vagally mediated bradycardia.
- Protects against adverse vagal effects of anticholinesterases during antagonism of neuromuscular block.

Disadvantages
- Increases metabolic rate.
- Increases heart rate, increases myocardial oxygen consumption.
- Is arrhythmogenic, causing bradyarrhythmias and/or tachyarrhythmias.
- Viscidifies bronchial secretions, promoting peripheral airway collapse.
- Causes gastrointestinal ileus.
- Pupil dilatation.

Glycopyrrolate (glycopyrronium).

This has a slower onset time, a longer duration of action and a greater antisialogogue effect than atropine. Tachyarrhythmias are said to be less likely and cardiovascular stability is better preserved.

It may be wiser to withhold antimuscarinic drugs from pre-anaesthetic medication, to monitor closely and to use them only when vagal activity (e.g. bradycardia, bradyarrhythmias and hypotension) becomes a concern.

Pain and analgesia

Analgesia is a state of reduced sensibility to pain. Painful (noxious) stimuli reach the brain in similar ways to other sensations but are amenable to interruption by a greater range of drugs. The perception of pain requires conscious awareness, whilst nociception is the transmission of impulses to lower levels within the central nervous system in response to a noxious stimuli. An animal's response to pain depends on the level of the central nervous system to which the pain message ascends (Fig. 23.3):

- Spinal responses include, for example, reflex limb withdrawal.
- Medullary responses include increased heart rate, blood pressure and respiratory rate.
- Hypothalamic responses take several forms. The hypothalamus initiates catecholamine release from the adrenal

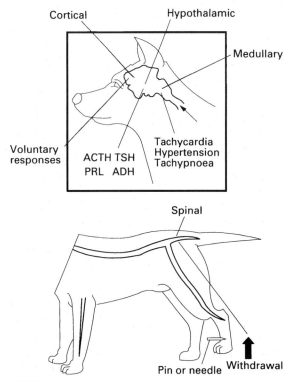

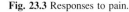

Fig. 23.3 Responses to pain.

medulla and nerve endings of the sympathetic nervous system. This further increases heart rate and blood pressure and causes pilo-erection. Less obviously, the hypothalamus secretes releasing factors which cause the pituitary gland to release 'stress' hormones such as adrenocorticotropic hormone (ACTH). Other pituitary hormones like thyroid stimulating hormone (TSH), antidiuretic hormone (ADH) and prolactin (PRL) are also released.

- Cortical responses are the most complex: they include activity like vocalisation and voluntary acts such as attempting to escape or to bite at the noxious stimulus.

Analgesics

Analgesics interrupt the ascending pain pathway at various levels (Fig. 23.4) and suppress the sensation of pain. After analgesics are given, pain responses are modified according to the level of interruption, which in turn depends on the sensitivity of that level to the analgesic. For example, general anaesthetics like halothane exert their greatest effect on the cortex. Therefore, in the halothane-anaesthetised animal, complex responses like vocalisation or escape will not occur. However, if anaesthesia is very 'light', limb withdrawal from noxious stimuli (e.g. toe-pinches) may still be seen. Several drug groups suppress pain. These include:

- Non-steroidal anti-inflammatory drugs (NSAIDs).
- Glucocorticoids.
- Local anaesthetics.
- Benzodiazepines.
- Opioids.
- General anaesthetics.

Each group operates at specific levels of the pain path. Some, like the opioids, act at several points along this path. Blocking pain at a number of sites can produce more effective analgesia; this is termed balanced analgesia.

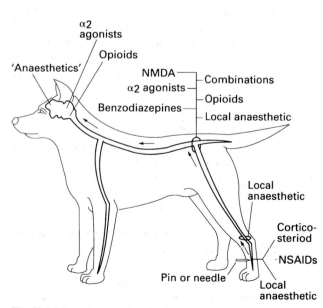

Fig. 23.4 Pain pathways and analgesia.

Peripheral nerve endings

Glucocorticoids and NSAIDs reduce nerve-ending sensitivity to pain-sensitising chemicals released from damaged tissue (autocoids). Topical local anaesthetics block nerve endings.

Peripheral nerves

Local anaesthetics block the nerve impulse in peripheral nerves. They are frequently neglected as a method of pain relief but can produce very effective analgesia. Local analgesics are discussed later.

Spinal cord

Pain can be suppressed in the cord by the extradural injection of several drug types:

- Local anaesthetics block all nerve fibre types producing anaesthesia, analgesia and muscle relaxation.
- Opioids diminish sensitivity to pain but do not eliminate sensation, proprioception or muscle function. Animals are therefore free from pain but can walk.
- Benzodiazepines, NMDA, *N*-methyl-D-aspartate receptor (involved in allowing calcium ion entry into post-synaptic ganglion) antagonists and alpha-2 agonists have analgesic effects at the spinal level although they are less frequently used.
- Combinations of drugs that are compatible *in vitro* may be injected in order to capitalise on desirable properties of each, e.g. lignocaine, bupivacaine, morphine.

Brain

Opioids, alpha-2-adrenoceptor agonists and general anaesthetics cause analgesia through effects on the brain. Consciousness need not be lost for analgesia to be present.

Administration of analgesic drugs prior to tissue trauma is suggested to reduce post-operative analgesic requirements. This concept is called pre-emptive analgesia and, although work in the human literature remains equivocal, the general consensus is that analgesia given prior to surgery combined with adequate post-operative pain relief produces the most effective analgesia. For example, pre-medication with an opioid and carprofen, followed by a local block prior to surgery and continued with regular dosing of an opioid post-operatively, will provide excellent analgesia and encourage a rapid recovery.

Opioid analgesics

Opioids are often included in premedication:

- To relieve pre-operative pain and therefore anxiety.
- To contribute to sedation.
- To provide analgesia during maintenance and on recovery.

While the properties of individual opioids differ, there are common advantages and disadvantages.

OPIOIDS

Advantages

- Profound, drug- and dose-dependent analgesia.
- Benign cardiovascular effects. With some exceptions, opioids slow heart rate. In high doses, bradycardia and bradyarrhythmias may occur. Cardiac output is usually maintained.
- Anaesthetic-sparing effect. Opioids reduce dose requirements of induction and maintenance agents.
- Sedation. Some opioids produce sedation in non-painful animals.
- Positive ventilatory effects. By reducing chest-wall pain after thoracotomy or trauma, opioids improve ventilation. This frequently offsets any respiratory depression seen.

Disadvantages

- Dysphoria. In pain-free animals, opioids may stimulate rather than sedate and cause excitation on overdosage. Central nervous effects depend on dose, species and degree of pain present. At normal analgesic doses, opioids in pain-free animals do not cause marked stimulation. Stimulation is also unlikely when neuroleptics are given concurrently.
- Respiratory depression. Probably a greater problem in people than animals, pre-anaesthetic opioids prolong apnoea after induction with thiopentone. Intra-operative alfentanil and fentanyl often depress breathing, mandating ventilatory support.
- Antitussive effects. Opioids suppress the coughing reflex, which may be useful in animals requiring analgesia and prolonged intubation. However, accumulated bronchial secretion may impair respiration.
- Gastrointestinal effects. Morphine causes vomiting in dogs. Other opioids are less likely to cause vomiting. With the exception of pethidine, opioids increase non-propulsive segmenting intestinal contractions leading to constipation with prolonged use. Opioids cause contracture of the sphincter of Oddi, and increased pressure in the biliary tree. They should not be used in pancreatitis and obstructive jaundice.
- Urinary retention. Opioids cause urinary retention which seems to be of little clinical importance. However, the urethra may need catheterisation after surgery on the bladder.

- Tolerance. The diminishing effect of constant opioid doses is unlikely to occur in animals, as prolonged administration is not practised.
- Dependence. Animals are unlikely to become 'addicted' to opioids, as long-term administration is rarely required.

Individual properties

Opioids have slightly different properties (Table 23.4) and their use in any situation is governed by several factors.

Potency. Although drugs vary in anaesthetic potency, this is of little relevance as 'weaker' opioids like pethidine are given at greater doses. The quality of analgesia is more important. Pure agonists (morphine, fentanyl) should be chosen if severe pain is anticipated.

Pharmacodynamic effect. The central nervous, autonomic, cardiopulmonary and gastrointestinal effects of individual drugs may render them useful or hazardous under different circumstances.

Pharmacokinetic factors. Onset time, duration of action and elimination pathways may be important considerations in choosing specific opioids.

Others. Personal preference, cost and controlled drug status may also influence choice.

Drug legislation

Because of their abuse potential, most opioids are controlled drugs (CD), i.e. their use is controlled by the Misuse of Drugs Act 1971.

Controlled drugs are 'scheduled' according to the degree of control applied to their use. Schedule 1 agents (e.g. LSD) are stringently controlled but unused in veterinary practice. Schedule 2 drugs like morphine, etorphine ('Immobilon'), fentanyl, alfentanil and pethidine are regulated in terms of:

- Special prescription requirements.
- Requisition requirements.
- Record keeping: acquisition and prescription must be recorded in a controlled drugs register (CDR).
- Safe custody. Schedule 2 drugs must be kept in a locked receptacle.
- Destruction of expired stocks.

Schedule 3 drugs include pentobarbitone and phenobarbitone, pentazocine and buprenorphine. These are subject to prescription and requisition requirements but transactions do not have to be recorded in the CDR. With the exception of buprenorphine, they do not have to be kept in a locked receptacle.

Table 23.4 Comparison of selected features of opioid analgesics

Drug	Controlled?	Potency	Efficacy	Duration
Morphine	Yes (Schedule 2)	1	+++++	2–4 h
Pethidine	Yes (Schedule 2)	0.1	+++	30 min–1 h
Papaveretum	Yes (Schedule 2)	0.5	++++	2–4 h
Methadone	Yes (Schedule 2)	1	++++	2–4 h
Butorphanol	No	5	++	2–4 h
Buprenorphine	Yes (Schedule 3)	5	++	3–7 h

Pure agonists: (mu-agonists)

- Morphine: Dose 0.1–0.5 mg/kg intramuscularly (dog), 0.1–0.2 mg/kg (cat). It is the gold standard analgesic, producing some sedation. However it can cause vomiting and constipation, and at higher doses morphine can cause excitement in cats.
- Methadone: Dose as for morphine. It is said to produces less vomiting, sedation, excitement and histamine release compared to morphine.
- Papaveretum: Dose 0.2–1.0 mg/kg intramuscularly. It is associated with less vomiting than morphine and greater synergy with acepromazine producing greater sedation.
- Pethidine: Dose 1–2 mg/kg intramuscularly. It rarely causes vomiting, or excitement in cats, and uniquely is spasmolytic on the intestines.

Partial agonists/mixed agonist–antagonists

These agents are weak agonists (partial agonist) or antagonists at the mu receptor and agonists at peripheral kappa receptors (mixed agonist–antagonist), giving peripheral analgesia of moderate efficacy though variable consistency. Their bell shape curve makes higher doses produce less analgesia.

- Buprenorphine: Dose 6–10 μg/kg intramuscularly or intravenously. It is a partial agonist and has a relatively slow onset (30 minutes). Tight mu receptor binding underlies the duration of action and also makes subsequent pure agonists (and vice versa) less effective.
- Butorphanol: Dose 0.1–0.5 mg/kg (cats lower end of range). It is a mixed agonist–antagonist and analgesia is of an inconsistent nature though better for visceral than somatic pain. It has antitussant properties.

Antagonists

Opioid antagonists may be beneficial to reverse some aspects of opioid activity. In veterinary medicine, naloxone is occasionally used to reverse sedation and respiratory depression, though analgesia is also reversed. Partial agonists such as buprenorphine can be used to reverse the fentanyl component of Hypnorm (Janssen Animal Health) to speed recovery without compromising analgesia.

Non-steroidal anti-inflammatory drugs (NSAIDs)

NSAIDs act peripherally as a group inhibiting cyclo-oxygenase and hence reducing the level of prostaglandins in the tissues. This reduction in prostaglandins reduces inflammation around the injured tissue. Direct analgesia is also said to occur though its mechanism is unclear. Administration prior to tissue trauma should reduce tissue inflammation more effectively. Pre-operative administration of some of the newer agents (i.e. carprofen) provides good post-operative analgesia with lower incidence of side-effects.

Due to this prostaglandin inhibition, certain side-effects can occur:

- *Gastric irritation*: Manifest as vomiting, diarrhoea and gastric haemorrhage. Prostaglandins inhibit gastric acid secretion, stimulate mucus production, maintain blood flow to the gastric mucosa and are involved in mucosal repair. Hence reduction in prostaglandins can compromise the gastric mucosa leading to ulcers.
- *Renal compromise*: Prostaglandins modulate renal haemodynamics and are involved in autoregulation of blood flow to the kidney. They are especially important in states of decreased renal perfusion, e.g. hypotension during anaesthesia, and under such circumstances, NSAIDs administration can lead to renal insufficiency. Hence as a group they are not recommended pre-operatively.
- *Blood dyscrasias and platelet dysfunction*: Thromboxane, and prostaglandins are involved in induction of aggregation of platelets. Thus NSAIDs prolong bleeding time.

Agents include:

- Aspirin: Dose 10–20 mg/kg (dog), 10 mg/kg (cat) per os. The duration of action is 12–24 hours (longer in the cat). Inhibition of platelet aggregation and gastric irritation are notable.
- Paracetamol: Dose 25–30 mg/kg (dog). Not safe in cats. The duration of action is 4–6 hours. It inhibits CNS cyclo-oxygenase and is a less effective analgesic than aspirin.
- Phenylbutazone: Dose 10 mg/kg (dog). Duration of action is 6–12 hours. It produces less gastric irritation, but notable water and sodium retention, so caution in renal and cardiac disease.

- Flunixin: Dose 1 mg/kg (dog) (cats 1 mg/kg – not licensed). It has a 4 hour half-life but is found in tissue exudate for up to 24 hours. It is a good analgesic and antiendotoxic drug. Gastrointestinal toxicity and renal papillary necrosis have been recorded.
- Ketoprofen: Dose is 1–2 mg/kg. It is a potent cyclo-oxygenase inhibitor
- Tolfenamic acid: Dose 4 mg/kg; the half-life is 6.5 hours.
- Carprofen: Dose 4 mg/kg (subcutaneously or intravenously). The duration of action is 12–24 hours. Carprofen produces poor inhibition of cyclo-oxygenase, thus is prostaglandin sparing. Less renal toxicity and gastric irritation are reported, but it has greater anti-inflammatory potency than phenylbutazone. Uniquely it is recommended for administration pre-operatively prior to tissue trauma.

Supportive therapy

Good patient nursing is essential for post-operative comfort. Bandaging and support of injured areas, e.g. Robert Jones bandage stabilises the wound and reduces pain on movement. Warmth, comfortable bedding, an empty bladder, food and water post-operatively and attentive care can significantly improve patient welfare.

SUMMARY

- Analgesia reduces post-operative morbidity and speeds recovery.
- NSAIDs, local analgesics and opioids are particularly useful.
- Balanced analgesia involves the concurrent administration of more than one type of analgesic to increase effective analgesia without increasing side-effects.
- Pre-emptive analgesia, administering the analgesic prior to surgical trauma, can produce better analgesia on recovery.
- Good nursing and supportive therapy are essential for effective analgesia.

Local anaesthesia

Local anaesthetics produce reversible block of nerve impulse conduction. Uses include:

- Superficial surgery. Some minor procedures may be done in the conscious animal using local anaesthetics alone (e.g. skin infiltration for wart removal). More invasive procedures may require moderate sedation (e.g. intravenous regional anaesthesia for toe amputation).
- Adjunct to surgical anaesthesia. Local techniques may be superimposed on light general anaesthesia for major surgery. The local technique usually does not affect cardiopulmonary function and so less general anaesthetic

is required. This preserves cardiopulmonary performance, making the combined technique useful in high-risk cases. Animals also recover consciousness rapidly and, importantly, the surgical site remains pain-free.
- Facilitate procedures. Topical anaesthetics facilitate catheterisation, endotracheal intubation and ophthalmic examination.
- Diagnosis. Local anaesthetics are used to assist lameness diagnosis in horses.
- Antiarrhythmics. Lignocaine is used to treat certain types of cardiac arrhythmia.

LOCAL ANAESTHESIA

Advantages
- Lower equipment requirement.
- Excellent anaesthesia and muscle relaxation when technique is satisfactory.
- Consciousness is retained when used alone; there is no loss of protective reflexes.
- There is little cardiopulmonary depression; techniques are relatively safe in ill animals.
- Techniques are inexpensive.
- Some techniques allow titration: the degree, duration and anatomic 'level' of block can be increased by repeat injections.

Disadvantages
- Not all procedures can be performed with local anaesthetic techniques.
- Some techniques are difficult to perform and subsequent block may be incomplete.
- Some techniques are painful to perform; animals may require sedation.
- Active animals may require physical or chemical restraint for surgery.
- Overdosage and toxicity is possible with some drugs.
- Some techniques (e.g. extradural anaesthesia) produce untoward cardiovascular effects.
- Some local anaesthetics have a short duration of action.

Mechanisms

Nerve fibres carrying different sensations (e.g. touch, cold and pain) vary in response to local anaesthetics. Because pain fibres are among the most sensitive, it is possible for local anaesthetics to eliminate pain but allow touch and other sensations to persist. When this occurs, the drug behaves as a local analgesic. If all sensation is lost, the drug is an anaesthetic. Motor fibres are most resistant to local anaesthetics but are usually blocked, resulting in muscle relaxation.

Toxicity

Toxic central nervous signs – convulsions or coma – are seen if high levels of local anaesthetic are absorbed. The former is controlled with diazepam or pentobarbitone. Over-dosing is avoided by using low concentrations (the minimum volume required to produce effect), by using regional rather than local techniques (where appropriate) and by adding vasoconstrictors to the injected solution.

Cardiovascular toxicity

Lignocaine can be used to control ventricular arrhythmias, but at toxic doses electrical activity is suppressed and cardiac arrest may occur.

Toxicity depends on:

- Route of injection – caution inadvertent intravenous injection.
- Total amount injected.
- Characteristics of the individual agent.
- The use of vasoconstrictors.

Pharmacokinetics

The speed of onset of a local anaesthetic block depends upon the agent diffusing into the nerve cell (usually the axon), where it has its effect. Factors influencing this include:

- Proximity of injection site to site of action.
- Lipid solubility of agent used.
- Concentration of agent used.
- Volume of agent used.
- Use of potentiating drugs.

The duration of action of a local anaesthetic depends upon:

- The agent used.
- Blood flow at site of action (tends to remove agent).
- Use of potentiating drugs.

Vasoconstrictors may be added to prolong the duration of block. The commonest vasoconstrictor is adrenaline, added to local anaesthetic solutions at 1:100 000 concentration (0.01 mg/ml). This retards drug absorption from the injection site and prolongs block. Solutions containing adrenaline must not be over-used in areas with poor or superficial blood flow; vasoconstriction may cause subsequent tissue ischaemia and gangrene.

The state of the tissues into which local anaesthetic is injected also has an effect upon the action of the drug. For example, if local anaesthetic is injected into inflamed tissue it will have a reduced action. This is because inflamed tissue is more acidic than normal and so the agent will be more ionised and less able to diffuse through the tissue.

Local anaesthetic drugs

Lignocaine

This is the most commonly used local anaesthetic in veterinary practice. It is available as a gel, topical cream, a spray and in injectable forms. Injections are usually 1% or 2% solutions with or without adrenaline (1:100 000). The drug has a rapid (less than 5 min) onset of action. It spreads rapidly through tissue and produces almost complete block. The normal duration of action is 50–90 minutes. Adding adrenaline retards absorption (and toxicity) and prolongs the duration of block. Lignocaine causes tissue irritation after injection.

Bupivacaine

This is about 4 times more potent than lignocaine and so is available in lower concentrations (0.25, 0.5 or 0.75%). It has a slower onset of action (up to 20 min) but may last from 3 to 7 hours. It does not irritate tissue but may cause cardiac arrest if inadvertent intravascular injection is made.

Mepivacaine

This drug is favoured for conduction blocks in the equine limb as it is less irritant than lignocaine.

Types of local anaesthesia

A number of different types of block can be performed.

Local block

Desensitisation is produced only at or near the site of application.

- Surface or topical. Anaesthetic is applied to skin/mucous membranes to give loss of sensation at the site of application, e.g. EMLA cream. Other applications are shown in Table 23.5.
- Intradermal. Anaesthetic is injected into the skin to form a desensitised weal.
- Infiltration. A primary injection of local anaesthetic is made at the surgical site, using as small a needle as possible (22–24 s.w.g.). The next injection is made through this site and the process repeated until the surgical area is 'infiltrated' with local anaesthetic. Liberal infiltration must be avoided as overdosage is possible, especially in small animals and birds. Irritant drugs like lignocaine and those containing vasoconstrictors may interfere with wound healing.
- Intrasynovial. Local anaesthetics injected into painful joints and synovial sheaths relieve pain but the effects are not long-acting.

Table 23.5 Topical local anaesthesia

Site	Drug	Description
Cornea	Proxymetacaine	'Ophthaine' lasts 15 minutes
Urethra	Lignocaine gel	Lubrication for catheterisation
Larynx	Lignocaine 10 mg	Metered spray

Regional block

Anaesthetic is used to produce desensitisation remote from the site of injection.

- Perineural. This involves drug injection in proximity to identifiable nerves, as opposed to nerve endings. The technique requires knowledge of topographical anatomy. Injection is made using sterile needles and syringes. For example, the intercostal nerve (behind each rib) is often blocked with 0.5 ml bupivacaine after thoracotomy. This relieves post-operative chest-wall pain, allowing adequate ventilation.
- Intravenous Regional Anaesthesia (IVRA). Intravenous regional anaesthesia is used for surgical procedures on limb extremities (e.g. digit removal). The limb is first exsanguinated using an Esmarch's bandage, which is then left in place as a tourniquet. Local anaesthetic (e.g. 3–7 ml lignocaine without adrenaline) is then injected into any vein distal to the tourniquet. Surgery may begin after 5 minutes. Anaesthesia persists until the tourniquet is removed.
- Spinal and epidural block. Anaesthetic is injected within the bony confines of the spinal canal.

Extradural (or epidural) anaesthesia

In this, drug is injected into the space between the dura mater (the thick fibrous outermost covering of the spinal cord) and the periosteum lining the spinal canal. Here, the drug blocks the nerves as they leave the cord. A large spinal needle is used and injection made into the L7–S1 interspace. The technique is useful for pain relief and muscle relaxation during pelvic-limb orthopaedic procedures in dogs, and less commonly in cats. In current practice, the technique is usually performed on heavily sedated or lightly anaesthetised animals. Lignocaine or bupivacaine combined with an opioid (e.g. preservative-free morphine) are commonly used. The main advantage of extradural opioids is prolonged and profound analgesia.

Spinal (subarachnoid or intrathecal) injection

This technique has never gained popularity in veterinary anaesthesia. It involves a midline injection at the L5–L6 interspace or, at a higher level, into the CSF-filled space below the arachnoid mater, lying below the dura. Lower doses produce the same effects of extradural injection but there is a slightly greater risk of overdosage.

Injectable anaesthesia

Anaesthesia can be produced in many ways because of the range of drugs and drug combinations, doses, routes of administration and techniques available. Selection of the optimum technique is based on:

- Patient species. Drugs are not equally safe in all species: 'Saffan' is unsafe in dogs although satisfactory in cats.

SUMMARY

- Local anaesthesia can be used on its own for certain simple procedures.
- As an adjunct to general anaesthesia it can produce excellent analgesia, reduce the general anaesthetic requirements and provide balanced anaesthesia.
- Commonly used drugs include lignocaine, bupivacaine and mepivacaine.
- Local blocks include surface desensitisation or dermal injection.
- Regional blocks include IVRA, spinal and epidural blocks.

- Patient individuality. Some breeds do not tolerate certain drugs (e.g. sight-hounds and barbiturates). Breed-related conditions complicating the management of anaesthesia may be present (e.g. Von Willebrand's disease in Dobermann pinschers). Also individual animals may have specific diseases, or be old and fat.
- The nature and duration of surgery. Greater risk is associated with invasive, prolonged surgery and so anaesthesia will be more complicated. Anaesthesia must also produce adequate conditions in terms of duration. In all cases, the magnitude and duration of physiological perturbation must be kept to a minimum.

The route of drug administration forms a basis for describing anaesthetics. Importantly, the route of administration affects drug activity.

- **Enteral**. The gastrointestinal tract is seldom used to administer anaesthetics or pre-anaesthetic medication because absorption is unpredictable and onset times are slow. Aggressive animals may be given oral acepromazine before presentation. Caged, aggressive animals are subdued if medetomidine (dogs) or ketamine (cats) is squirted on to the oral mucous membranes.
- **Parenteral**. Drugs can be injected or inhaled into the respiratory tree. Drugs injected may be given by intravenous (IV), intramuscular (IM), subcutaneous (SC) or intraperitoneal (IP) routes. Induction agents are usually given intravenously. In laboratory animals, intraperitoneal injections are sometimes used.

The advantages of the various routes are given in Table 23.3.

- **Intravenous**. Poor intravenous technique may damage veins and preclude later use. This route allows the most rapid drug response and so is used for emergency drug administration. It must be used for irritant drugs like thiopentone.
- **Intramuscular**. Some drugs (e.g. diazepam) are poorly absorbed after intramuscular injection. In general, up to 3 times the intravenous dose may be needed to produce the same effect. Some drugs (e.g. pethidine, ketamine) cause pain on injection.

- **Subcutaneous**. For animals in 'shock', the blood supply to the skin is poor, so that drug absorption after subcutaneous injection will be poor. In fat animals, drugs may be injected inadvertently into fat, which is a relatively avascular tissue, and so drug absorption may be severely retarded.

INJECTABLE ANAESTHETICS

Advantages
- Convenient; simple to inject.
- Inexpensive – less equipment needed.
- Intravenous injection usually causes a rapid loss of consciousness.
- No airway irritation.
- No explosion/pollution hazard.
- Rapid recovery.
- Some drugs can be antagonised.
- Endotracheal intubation is less necessary.
- Rapid deepening of anaesthesia is possible.
- Respiratory function does not influence drug behaviour.

Disadvantages
- Stressful restraint may be required.
- Myositis and pain may result from injection.
- Effects may be irreversible; for drugs without antagonists, recovery depends on cardiovascular, hepatic and renal function.
- Anaesthesia is readily deepened, but not 'lightened'.
- Wide dose-range requirements.
- Self-administration is hazardous with some drugs.
- Repeated doses may cause drug accumulation and prolonged recoveries.
- Injectable drugs have widely different side-effects.
- Airway protection is often neglected.

Pharmacology

The brain has a rich blood supply and receives a high concentration of drug shortly after IV injection. When a critical brain concentration is exceeded, unconsciousness occurs. In time, organs less well-perfused than the brain (such as skeletal muscle) begin to take up drug. Plasma levels fall and this creates a diffusion gradient which promotes movement of drug from brain to plasma. Consciousness returns when brain drug levels fall below the critical level. The duration of action of most modern injectable anaesthetics depends on 'redistribution' of drug from brain to less well-perfused tissues; this depends on factors like cardiac output and the mass of poorly perfused tissues available.

Most anaesthetics are metabolised in the liver by conversion from lipid to water-soluble molecules. These forms are more easily excreted in bile (appearing later in faeces) or urine. Only very small amounts are excreted unchanged in bile and urine as lipid-soluble drug.

The duration of action of drugs which are rapidly metabolised by the liver (e.g. 'Saffan' and methohexitone) depend on a combination of redistribution and metabolism.

Uses

- As **sole agents**. For short procedures (e.g. pharyngeal foreign body removal), a single injection of a short-acting drug is used. For prolonged procedures, long-acting drugs or combinations may be used although top-up (or incremental) doses of short-acting drugs are preferable. Alternatively, short-acting drugs may be infused. Drugs given by infusion or incremental doses must not accumulate or recovery will be prolonged.
- As **induction agents**. Injectable drugs used to induce anaesthesia before maintenance with volatile agents need only eliminate laryngeal reflexes and jaw tone for the purpose of intubation.
- As an adjunct to a mask induction.

See Chapter 10, p. 248.

Barbiturates

Barbiturates like thiopentone, methohexitone and pentobarbitone are hypnotics; they cause unconsciousness but have poor analgesic properties. Muscle relaxation is usually adequate during anaesthesia.

Thiopentone

This thiobarbiturate is available as a sulphurous-yellow powder and requires reconstitution with water. In solution it is highly alkaline and irritant if injected perivascularly. It is highly protein bound and slowly metabolised in the liver, relying primarily on redistribution away from the brain for recovery after administration. Solutions of various strengths (concentrations) may be made. A 1% solution contains 1 g or 1000 mg in 100 ml. A 1% solution, therefore, contains 10 mg/ml and a 2.5% solution of thiopentone contains 25 mg drug/ml. It is reconstituted by adding 100 ml water to 2.5 g of powder.

Thiopentone is a useful anaesthetic agent for short-duration procedures or for induction prior to maintenance with inhalation agents. Doses of 10 mg/kg (intravenously) are used following premedication. Incremental doses should be avoided as they prolong recovery and contribute to 'hang-over'.

Mild cardiovascular depression is seen, with hypotension, reduced cardiac output and tachycardia reported. Cardiac dysrhythmias may been seen. Dose-dependent respiratory depression and reduced respiratory sensitivity to CO_2 occur transiently.

The drug is safe in high-risk cases provided the factors which increase patient sensitivity are known (many of these apply to drugs other than thiopentone). Doses are reduced in: hypoalbuminaemia, acidaemia, hypovolaemia, congestive heart failure, azotaemia, toxaemia and obesity. Doses are also reduced when diazepam is injected immediately before or afterwards.

Note that a 2.5% solution has a pH of 10.4 (strongly alkaline) and causes tissue damage when injected outside of the vein. In large animals (but not in companion animal practice), 5% and 10% solutions are used.

Special precautions. Thiopentone causes prolonged recoveries in sight-hounds (e.g. whippet, greyhound, saluki) after otherwise uneventful anaesthesia.

The drug should not be used if there is difficulty in achieving venepuncture.

Methohexitone

This oxybarbiturate is available as a dry powder and is reconstituted to produce a 1% solution. Being twice as potent as thiopentone, its dose is halved to 5 mg/kg. Onset time is similar but its duration of action is shorter; extensive and rapid hepatic metabolism occurs in addition to redistribution. It is less irritant when injected outside a vein.

Cardiovascular and respiratory depression are similar to that of thiopentone. Recoveries are not always smooth, especially when pre-anaesthetic medication is withheld. The drug has been favoured in sight-hounds because it produces rapid recoveries.

Pentobarbitone

This once useful drug has been superseded by newer agents except, perhaps, in laboratory animal anaesthesia. Following injection, its onset of action is relatively slow (related to delay in crossing the blood–brain barrier) and recoveries are prolonged. In companion animal practice it is used as an anticonvulsant and for humane destruction.

Steroid anaesthetics

'Saffan'

'Saffan' is a mixture of alphaxalone (9 mg/kg) and alphadolone (3 mg/kg); the former is the major active component. Induction doses of 3–6 mg/kg (intravenously) are routinely used in the cat. Doses are always expressed in mg of total steroid. The drug has been favoured for some time in cats as it has a high therapeutic index. It produces only mild cardiovascular and respiratory depression at clinical doses. The two steroids are water insoluble and the formulation contains Cremophor EL (polyethoxylated castor oil). This agent causes histamine release in dogs and cannot be used safely in this species. In cats, it causes mild anaphylactoid reactions and swelling of the pinnae and paws. These are normally of little consequence but very infrequently there is fatal pulmonary oedema. Because the formulation contains no bacteriostat, open ampoules must be discarded.

The intravenous route is preferred because effects are less predictable after intramuscular injection. The solution is viscous but non-irritant. Frequently, large volumes must be given. The subcutaneous route is unsuitable; the rate of drug metabolism over absorption is high and so anaesthetic levels are not achieved.

Dissociative anaesthetics

Ketamine

Ketamine is described as a dissociative anaesthetic, producing a unique state of anaesthesia. Protective airway reflexes are maintained, the eyes remain open and the pupil is dilated. Cranial nerve reflexes are less depressed than with other agents although it cannot be assumed that these will remain entirely protected.

Heart rate is increased and blood pressure is normally maintained. Breathing is modestly reduced, although in overdose an apneustic pattern is seen in which the breath is held after inspiration. Salivation increases. Spontaneous muscle movement unrelated to surgery is a disconcerting feature of ketamine anaesthesia but can be suppressed by concurrently administered drugs. Ketamine is considered to provide profound somatic analgesia, but controversy exists over its role as a visceral analgesic.

Convulsions are seen in dogs when it is used alone. Intramuscular injection is painful although injection volumes are low because the drug is available as a 100 mg/ml solution. Doses of 2–5 mg/kg (intravenously) are frequently used.

Phenols

Propofol

This water-soluble phenol derivative (2,6-di-isopropylphenol) is a characteristic milky-white solution solubilised in an egg–phosphatidyl–soybean oil emulsion. The solution must not be frozen, though cooling is said to reduce the low incidence of pain on intravenous injection. The solution contains no bacteriostat and so opened ampoules must be discarded.

The drug produces dose-dependent levels of unconsciousness after intravenous injection. Good muscle relaxation is seen. Dogs require 4–6 mg/kg (intravenously), whilst cats require higher doses (6–8 mg/kg, intravenously) for anaesthesia. The drug is also longer-acting in this species, with induction doses lasting up to 20 minutes.

Cardiovascular and respiratory depression are comparable to those of thiopentone but are generally of longer duration.

Propofol has some advantages over thiopentone:

● Recovery is rapid and free from hang-over if a single dose is given. This makes it useful in sight-hounds. This advantage becomes less apparent if inhalation anaesthesia follows.
● Provided oxygen is given, anaesthesia can be maintained with top-up injections or infusions with less risk of prolonged recoveries.

Occasionally, twitching and spontaneous muscle activity occurs with propofol anaesthesia and excited recoveries have been described.

Combinations and neuroleptanalgesics

Minor surgical procedures may be performed using neuroleptanalgesia, benzodiazepine/ketamine and alpha-2-agonist/ketamine mixtures.

Ketamine mixtures

Several drugs are used with ketamine to reduce muscle hypertonicity. These include acepromazine, diazepam, midazolam, xylazine and medetomidine. Some of these also have anticonvulsant effects and render the combinations safe for use in dogs. However, some combinations have adverse physiological effects such as hypoventilation and arrhythmias.

Opioid mixtures

Opioids are commonly combined with neuroleptics such as acepromazine or droperidol to provide conditions for minor surgery. Fentanyl and alfentanil are used to lower the dose of propofol required for anaesthesia. Hypoventilation and bradycardia are serious disadvantages of such mixtures, although analgesia is profound.

Benzodiazepine and opioid mixtures (e.g. midazolam and sufentanil) are favoured in some centres for high-risk cases. The advantages of such combinations over well-administered halothane anaesthesia is often not apparent in companion animals.

Small animal immobilon

This combination injected intravenously, intramuscularly or subcutaneously produces profound and prolonged analgesia. Marked hypoventilation produces cyanosis, while severe hypotension caused by bradycardia may cause pale mucous membranes. Convulsions and renal failure have followed administration and the drug may recycle; the animal becomes depressed later after apparent restoration of consciousness with the antagonist diprenorphine. The major problem with this formulation is self-administration.

Techniques in anaesthesia

Intravenous catheterisation

Technique. Adequate physical and chemical restraint is a prerequisite. The site must receive full surgical preparation. A small skin incision over the vein facilitates catheter introduction in animals with resilient skin (e.g. male cats, dehydrated animals).

SUMMARY

- Injectable anaesthesia provides rapid onset and good conditions for intubation.
- Maintenance of anaesthesia can be achieved by top-up doses or intravenous infusions of an injectable anaesthetic.
- The intravenous route is often preferred though other routes can be used.
- The choice of agent depends on patient consideration, the procedure performed, equipment available and cost.

Inhalation anaesthesia

Inhalation, volatile or 'gaseous' anaesthesia refers to the inhalation of anaesthetic vapours or gases delivered into the respiratory tract. Anaesthesia is commonly maintained with inhalation agents although they can also be used to induce anaesthesia.

Some emergency drugs like adrenaline, lignocaine, atropine and methoxamine are given by the intratracheal route if venous access is unavailable.

Gases, vapours and inhaled anaesthetics

Inhaled anaesthetics used in animals include nitrous oxide (N_2O), halothane, methoxyflurane, enflurane, isoflurane and diethyl ether. Oxygen and carbon dioxide (CO_2) are used to optimise physiological conditions, while O_2 and N_2O are known as carrier gases because they 'carry' volatile anaesthetics.

Oxygen (O_2)

Oxygen is an odourless, reactive gas that allows combustion and, in the presence of organic material and activation energy (i.e. sparks or naked flames), explosions.

INTRAVENOUS CATHETERISATION

Advantages
- Reduces risk of extravascular injection, ensures full doses are given and prevents tissue damage with irritant drugs.
- Provides rapid intravenous access for emergency drugs.
- Allows fluids to be given rapidly.
- Allows rapid 'deepening' of anaesthesia with injectable anaesthetics.

Disadvantages
- Vein damage; poor catheterisation technique may damage the vein and preclude further access. This occurs when haematoma or thrombosis form.
- Sepsis; in immunosuppressed animals (e.g. diabetics) poor surgical preparation and management of catheters lead to phlebitis. More severe conditions like bacteraemia may follow.

INHALATION OF ANAESTHETICS

Advantages

- Recovery depends on respiratory function and is normally rapid and predictable.
- The depth of anaesthesia is readily controlled.
- Single dose rate; MAC is similar in most species.
- Concurrent oxygen delivery; volatile agents are usually 'carried' in oxygen.
- Volatile agent activity is independent of hepatic and renal function.
- Continued administration does not necessarily cause prolonged recoveries. Surgery may be prolonged without complication.
- Inhalation drugs have broadly similar effects.
- The airway is usually protected.

Disadvantages

- Recovery may be delayed by inadequate ventilation or lung pathology.
- A considerable range of equipment is required; some items are expensive.
- Intubation is usually necessary.
- Knowledge of breathing systems and anaesthetic machines is required.
- Hazards associated with compressed gas.
- Fire and explosion risks with some agents.
- Possible health risk associated with exposure to volatile agents.

Uses. The gas is given whenever the normal delivery of atmospheric oxygen to active tissue is threatened. This includes anaesthesia (even that produced with injectable agents).

Pure oxygen (100%) is usually given to animals which are anaemic, have pulmonary pathology or are hypoventilating. During inhalation anaesthesia, 100% oxygen may be used as the 'carrier gas' but it is frequently diluted to 50% or 33% concentrations by nitrous oxide.

Oxygen is also supplied during recovery until the animal is capable of maintaining haemoglobin saturation with room air (20% O_2).

Problems. Oxygen does not depress ventilation or cause toxic nervous or pulmonary changes during short periods of exposure. The major hazard is related to the support of combustion.

Carbon dioxide (CO_2)

Carbon dioxide is supplied in grey cylinders. On British anaesthetic machines, pressure gauges and flowmeters for CO_2 are similarly colour-coded.

Uses. Less commonly used now, applications include situations in which blood-gas analysis is unavailable and breathing is controlled. It is difficult to know the ventilation level required to produce normal levels of plasma CO_2 (normocapnia). This is avoided by moderately hyperventilating the animal and including 4% CO_2 in inspired gas.

Disadvantages. Excessive CO_2 causes hypercapnia and respiratory acidosis, which stimulates the cardiovascular system and increases blood pressure but at high levels causes depression and arrhythmias. Elevated CO_2 stimulates ventilation but high concentrations cause narcosis and depress ventilation.

Nitrous oxide (N_2O)

Nitrous oxide is an odourless relatively inert gas with anaesthetic properties. It is non-flammable, but supports combustion.

Nitrous oxide is often combined with oxygen as a carrier gas. It must not be used at concentrations greater than 80% as this lowers O_2 below normal levels. Usually no more than 66% is delivered.

The percentage of gas mixtures is calculated on a flow ratio basis. For example, a 50% O_2/N_2O mixture is produced when O_2 and N_2O flows are the same (e.g. 3 l/min O_2 and 3 l/min N_2O). Commonly, 66% or 2:1 N_2O/O_2 mixtures are used. These are produced when N_2O flow is exactly twice that of O_2.

Uses

- *Anaesthetic 'sparing' effect.* Nitrous oxide is less potent in animals than in humans but nevertheless lowers the concentration of volatile agent required to produce a given level of anaesthesia. For example, 66% N_2O reduces halothane requirements by about 25%. Because N_2O has minimal effects on cardiac output and ventilation, its inclusion preserves cardiopulmonary performance.
- *Second gas effect.* During induction with N_2O and a volatile agent, the rapid uptake of N_2O from alveoli causes the alveolar concentration of the volatile agent, or second gas, to rise. This accelerates uptake of the second gas and the rate of induction.
- *Disadvantages.* Hypoxia. Whenever N_2O is used, the O_2 content of inspired gas is lowered; this increases the possibility of hypoxia arising from other causes like hypoventilation. Different rates of uptake of N_2O occurs in rebreathing systems and the gas should be used with caution in circle or to-and-fro systems.
- *Gas-filled viscus.* Because N_2O is relatively insoluble in blood, it sequesters to gas-filled organs within the patient, e.g. the dilated stomach of dogs with gastric-dilatation-volvulus complex or the pleural space of animals with closed pneumothorax. Nitrous oxide compromises the animal by enlarging or increasing the pressure within such spaces.

- *Diffusion hypoxia.* When N_2O delivery is ended, its direction of diffusion reverses – from blood into the alveolar space. The volume evolved in the first few minutes after termination may dilute alveolar O_2. If this is low because the animal is breathing air, not 100% O_2, 'diffusion hypoxia' may occur. Therefore on ending N_2O administration, animals must receive 100% O_2 for at least 3 minutes.
- *Cardiopulmonary effects.* N_2O has a very modest stimulant effect on cardiac output and blood pressure. It has no effect on ventilation; when added to volatile agents, ventilation remains unchanged even though anaesthesia deepens.
- *Other effects.* Nitrous oxide crosses the placenta and neonates delivered from a mother receiving N_2O will need inspired O_2 enrichment, otherwise diffusion hypoxia will occur.

Special precautions. Nitrous oxide should not be used in animals whose arterial oxygen tensions are lowered by disease or where a gas-filled viscus is present.

POLLUTION

Nitrous oxide is relatively odourless and high atmospheric levels are difficult to detect. There is some evidence that N_2O causes toxic effects like bone-marrow depression after chronic, low-level exposure. It is not absorbed by activated charcoal and so 'canister' scavenging is useless.

Inhalation anaesthetics

These are delivered into the patient in a 'carrier gas'. This may be pure (100%) oxygen or a mixture of nitrous oxide and oxygen.

The behaviour of inhalation anaesthetics can be predicted and compared if two important features are known. These are the blood/gas solubility coefficient and the minimum alveolar concentration.

Blood/gas solubility coefficient. This value describes the solubility of agents in blood. Drugs with low solubility have low blood/gas solubility coefficients; they cause rapid induction and recovery rates, while 'swings' in levels of anaesthesia on changing vaporiser settings are more rapid. Values for modern anaesthetics with the fastest on the left are:

N_2O > Isoflurane > Enflurane > Halothane > Methoxyflurane
0.47   1.39   1.8   2.4   12.0

Minimum alveolar concentration (MAC). MAC of anaesthetics is the alveolar concentration (expressed as a percentage) that prevents responses occurring to a specified stimulus such as skin incision in 50% of patients. It is a measure of potency. Agents with low values have the greatest potency; low inspired concentrations are required for surgery. Many factors alter MAC, the most important being other drugs given during anaesthesia, for instance N_2O, analgesics and pre-anaesthetic medication.

Most potent:

Methoxyflurane > Halothane > Isoflurane > Enflurane > N_2O
0.23   0.8   1.3   2.2   188–220

Uptake and distribution of volatile anaesthetics

Volatile anaesthetics produce anaesthesia when a critical tension is exceeded in the CNS. This tension is achieved by movement of drug molecules down a series of tension gradients, beginning at the anaesthetic machine and ending at the site of action within the CNS. At equilibrium, the tension of drug in the brain mirrors that in arterial blood, which is the same as that in alveoli. Therefore, factors influencing alveolar tensions ultimately determine brain tensions.

Alveolar drug levels depend on alveolar ventilation rate and the inspired gas concentration. When these are high, induction of anaesthesia is rapid. The uptake of anaesthetic from alveoli depends on cardiac output, the lipid solubility of the agent in question and tension of anaesthetic in pulmonary venous blood. Alveolar tensions rise rapidly (and induction is rapid) when cardiac output is low (e.g. in haemorrhagic shock), when insoluble agents like N_2O are used and when the pulmonary venous tension of anaesthetic is high.

Halothane

Currently the most common volatile anaesthetic in small and large animal anaesthesia, this halogenated hydrocarbon is a sweet-smelling, clear liquid which decomposes in ultraviolet light and so is stored in amber bottles and contains an antioxidant (0.01% thymol). It readily evaporates producing a maximum concentration of 32%. For this reason it must be used from a calibrated vaporiser.

Pharmacokinetics. Halothane is a fast-acting anaesthetic. Up to 12–25% of absorbed halothane is metabolised to bromide, trifluroacetate and chloride by the liver.

Central nervous system. Halothane is a potent anaesthetic; concentrations of 1.0–3.0% may be needed after induction but adequate surgical conditions are obtained with inspired concentrations of 0.75–2.0%. Muscle relaxation is modest but analgesia is poor; adrenergic responses occur until deep levels of anaesthesia are reached.

Cardiopulmonary system. Halothane lowers blood pressure by reducing cardiac output. Heart rate remains unchanged. Halothane produces minimal reduction in systemic vascular resistance though causes vasodilatation in capillary beds of the brain, uterus and skin. As a halogenated hydrocarbon, the drug 'sensitises' the myocardium to adrenaline.

Halothane depresses ventilation in a dose-dependent manner causing decreased tidal volume, decreased rate and hypercapnia. It depresses ventilation to a lesser extent than other volatile anaesthetics with the exception of diethyl ether. It is non-irritant to respiratory mucosa and well tolerated for mask induction.

Other effects. In people, halothane-associated hepatitis occurs with repeated halothane anaesthetics. The cause is not fully understood but seems related to pre-operative enzyme induction caused by smoking and alcohol consumption, as well as intraoperative hypoxia. The condition has not been conclusively demonstrated to occur in animals during surgical anaesthesia.

Halothane lowers body temperature by inhibiting thermoregulatory mechanisms and producing cutaneous vasodilatation.

Special precautions. Halothane triggers malignant hyperthermia in sensitive pigs and this genetically determined condition also occurs in man. It has occurred in dogs, horses and cats but is rare.

Isoflurane

Isoflurane is an isomer of enflurane and a recently developed volatile agent. Although it is a halogenated ether, it has an unpleasant pungent smell. Its saturated vapour pressure is similar to halothane and the same (cleaned) precision vaporiser may be used for its administration. At room temperature, the maximum concentration possible is 31.5%. It is more expensive than halothane though when delivered via a rebreathing circuit this difference in cost is reduced.

Pharmacokinetics. Isoflurane has a low blood/gas solubility coefficient and so recoveries are rapid even after prolonged administration. Inductions are not as rapid as predicted because the agent causes breath-holding in some species. After induction, inspired concentrations of 2.5–4.5% are needed. Because it has a higher MAC value than halothane (MAC in dogs and cats is 1.28% and 1.63%, respectively), higher inspired concentrations are needed to maintain anaesthesia (1.5–2.5%).

Central nervous system. A potent anaesthetic providing good muscle relaxation and analgesia. Recoveries are rapid but may be associated with transient excitatory effects, especially after painful surgery.

Cardiovascular system. Isoflurane causes dose-dependent hypotension despite non-dose-dependent increases in heart rate. At 1.0 MAC cardiac output is maintained, whilst systemic vascular resistance is reduced. Isoflurane does not sensitise the heart to catecholamine-induced arrhythmias. Isoflurane is a potent respiratory depressant, but this is partly offset by surgery.

Special precautions. The insolubility of this drug in blood makes it a useful anaesthetic when rapid recoveries are required. The same feature means that 'swings' in level of anaesthesia are greatest with this agent.

Enflurane

Enflurane, a halogenated ether with a fruity smell, has never gained popularity in any branch of veterinary anaesthesia despite some useful features. Chemically it is very stable and contains no preservative.

Pharmacokinetics. Concentrations of 4–6% are needed for induction, with maintenance requirements of 1–3%. It is relatively expensive. Because it is highly volatile (SVP is 171.8 at 20°C) the maximum concentration achievable is 22% (at that temperature) and so the use of 'Enfluratec' is advisable.

Central nervous system. In humans, deep enflurane anaesthesia causes seizure-type electroencephalographic (EEG) activity which is exacerbated by hypercapnia. Involuntary muscle twitches are seen during anaesthesia and recovery in animals. The MAC in dogs and cats is 2.2% and 2.4%, respectively.

Cardiopulmonary system. Enflurane depresses blood pressure to the same extent as isoflurane, but less than halothane. Heart rate is increased in a dose-dependent manner. Cardiac output is reduced. It is the most potent respiratory depressant, decreasing rate and depth.

Other effects. Enflurane produces excellent muscle relaxation and markedly potentiates neuromuscular blockers.

Methoxyflurane

This fruity-smelling halogenated ether is the most potent volatile anaesthetic. It is non-reactive but decomposes slowly when exposed to soda-lime and ultraviolet light and so it contains butylated hydroxytoluene. The clear liquid changes to a yellow-amber colour in the vaporiser but this does not affect potency. Methoxyflurane evaporates poorly – no more than 3% can be delivered at room temperature.

Pharmacokinetics. It has high blood-gas (12.0) and rubber-gas (630) solubility coefficients making induction and recovery very slow. This precludes its use in large animals. Its low volatility allows its use in open or semi-open systems but the use of a calibrated 'Pentec' vaporiser is preferred. Induction requires 1.5–2.5% and maintenance 0.2–1.25%.

Central nervous system. A potent anaesthetic (its MAC value is 0.16 in humans, 0.29 in dogs, 0.23 in cats and 0.22 in horses) with good muscle relaxant and analgesic properties. Cranial nerve reflexes are lost early and the eye is said to 'centralise' at relatively light levels of anaesthesia.

Cardiopulmonary system. Cardiac output is reduced in a dose-dependent manner, causing hypotension. Heart rate tends to slow. It causes more respiratory depression than halothane.

Special precautions. In people, prolonged methoxyflurane anaesthesia causes renal tubular destruction, polyuria and dehydration lasting several days after administration. This is partly due to fluoride and oxalate ions generated from hepatic methoxyflurane metabolism. While the dog kidney is resistant to flurotoxicosis, acute renal failure has occurred in this species when flunixin has been given perioperatively.

Methoxyflurane should not be used in animals receiving NSAIDs or other potentially nephrotic drugs. Alternatively, these drugs should be withheld from animals in which methoxyflurane anaesthesia is considered desirable. Methoxyflurane is not a good choice when rapid recoveries are desired.

Ether

Rarely used now in veterinary anaesthesia, it is a pungent irritant vapour. Oxygen–ether mixtures are explosive. It is less potent than halothane (MAC 1.9%) though produces sympathetic stimulation providing cardiovascular support. Ether does not sensitise the heart to catecholamine-induced arrhythmias. It has some analgesic activity.

Desflurane

A relatively new agent. Its blood/gas partition coefficient is similar to that of nitrous oxide (i.e. 0.42) so is very insoluble and is associated with rapid induction and recovery. It requires a special temperature-controlled, pressurised vaporiser and is expensive. Its use in veterinary anaesthesia is presently experimental.

Sevoflurane

Popular in human anaesthesia in Japan, it has a low blood/gas partition coefficient (0.60) and also produces rapid induction and recovery. Cardiopulmonary effects are similar to those of isoflurane. It is unstable and degrades in the presence of soda lime producing toxic metabolites (i.e. compound A) which have been shown to produce renal pathology in rats.

Techniques in inhalational anaesthesia

Endotracheal intubation

When animals are rendered unconscious by injectable or inhalation drugs, protective airway reflexes are lost. Endotracheal intubation is one way to prevent related problems.

ENDOTRACHEAL INTUBATION

Advantages
- Airway protection from saliva and gastric contents. If cuffed tubes are not available an oropharyngeal pack – layers of moistened gauze laid in a horse-shoe pattern over the tube and 'packed' – may suffice. This is important during dental or oral surgery.
- Allows positive pressure ventilation. A leak-proof cuff allows lung inflation without gas escape; this is important if flammable agents are used.
- Reduces waste-gas pollution.
- Reduces anatomic dead-space.

Disadvantages
- Resistance. Cuffs limit the size of tube that can be introduced atraumatically. Small internal diameters critically increase resistance to breathing.
- Kinking or occlusion. Overinflated cuffs may compress the underlying tube. Severe occipito-atlantal flexion (e.g. during cisternal puncture) may cause tubes (especially red-rubber types) to kink. If tubes are inadequately cleaned, dried secretions accumulate within the lumen.
- Traumatic laryngitis. Poor intubation technique or the use of oversized tubes may physically damage the larynx and/or trachea, causing post-operative respiratory embarrassment.
- Chemical/ischaemic tracheitis. If tubes are inadequately rinsed or irritant sterilants are used, the tracheal mucosa may be irritated. For this reason, tubes must be adequately aired after ethylene oxide sterilisation.
- Overinflated cuffs left *in situ* for prolonged periods may produce an ischaemic tracheitis and cause post-operative coughing.
- Apparatus dead-space. Correctly sized endotracheal tubes reduce anatomic dead-space. However, overlong tubes extending beyond the incisor table constitute apparatus dead-space which should be minimised.
- Endobronchial intubation. Attempts to reduce apparatus dead-space by advancing the endotracheal tube down the airway may result in endobronchial intubation. In these circumstances, one lung receives no ventilation and blood deoxygenation may occur.
- False security. The presence of endotracheal tubes does not guarantee a patent airway; they may become kinked, crushed or filled with exudate.
- Interference. Conventionally placed (orotracheal) tubes interfere with some types of oral surgery. In such cases pharyngotracheal or tracheostomy placement may be required. In some species nasotracheal intubation is practised.

Tube selection. Ideally, the tube should extend from the incisor table to a point level with the spine of the scapula. Provided that the cuff lies beyond the glottis, the airway will be secure. Surplus dead-space is minimised by cutting off the projecting tube.

Intubation. The jaws must be relaxed and laryngeal reflexes suppressed before intubation is attempted. Laryngeal reflexes persist in cats to relatively 'deep' levels of anaesthesia, and laryngospasm is not uncommon following tactile stimulation of the glottis. In this species, laryngeal reflexes may be depressed with:

● Topical lignocaine by aerosol.
● Succinylcholine. (Suxamethonium).

Laryngoscopy is useful during intubation in cats, in dogs with pigmented oral mucosae or in those with surplus soft tissue in the upper airway.

Mask inductions

Masks are used to provide oxygen in comatose or recovering animals, or for the delivery of volatile anaesthetics when intubation is not performed.

Induction of anaesthesia using masks is a useful technique in high-risk cases because animals receive oxygen during induction; if crises develop, switching the vaporiser off may prove life-saving.

MASK INDUCTIONS

Advantages
● Mask inductions do not damage the airway.
● They produce smooth inductions when patients are depressed or heavily sedated.

Disadvantages
● Mask inductions are resisted and cause inelegant inductions in poorly sedated animals.
● Masks increase mechanical dead-space.
● They do not necessarily add to air-flow resistance but, because the airway is not clear, turbulence or obstruction can occur.
● Ventilation is possible with tightly applied, gas-tight masks. However, some gas inevitably enters the stomach, which inflates and limits diaphragmatic movement.
● Atmospheric pollution is greater with masks. This is reduced by using close-fitting face-masks or eliminating leaks with plasticine.

Chamber inductions

This technique is useful in laboratory animals and can be used in cats and small dogs. Sedation or depression should be present, otherwise inductions may be violent. Pollution is a problem when the chamber is opened. High inspired oxygen levels are present when consciousness is lost; indeed, the chamber usefully serves as an oxygen cage for neonates or small animals.

SUMMARY

● Inhalation anaesthesia requires more equipment than injectable anaesthesia.
● Greater control and adjustment of depth of anaesthesia exists.
● Recoveries tend to be faster after prolonged procedures.
● A provision of oxygen and IPPV is present.
● Halothane and isoflurane are most commonly used.
● Dose-dependent cardiovascular and respiratory depression are seen.
● Analgesia is rarely provided.

Equipment

Volatile and gaseous anaesthetics are used to maintain anaesthesia and, less commonly, for induction. In the past, the 'open method' was popular, consisting of the application of liquid anaesthetic to a gauze swab applied to the patient's nose. The 'semi-open' is similar but the gauze is within a mask through which all inspired gas passes. Ether, chloroform, trichloroethylene and methoxyflurane were used in these systems. Neither system is acceptable because of pollution and because the inspired gas concentration is difficult to control. The latter is particularly hazardous with anaesthetics like halothane which have high saturated vapour pressures and produce high concentrations at room temperature. Modern techniques require an anaesthetic machine and an anaesthetic breathing system or 'circuit'.

Anaesthetic equipment centres on the administration of inhalational anaesthetics. The main components include:

● Oxygen source.
● Vaporiser/source of anaesthetic gas.
● Breathing circuit.

Anaesthetic machines

The anaesthetic machine achieves the first two components, producing and delivering safe concentrations of anaesthetic vapour and providing a means of giving oxygen and imposing intermittent positive pressure ventilation (IPPV) during apnoea or cardiopulmonary arrest.

Understanding the function of anaesthetic machines is needed for the safe administration of volatile anaesthetics and oxygen and for machine maintenance; this prolongs the life of equipment, limits pollution and reduces the risk of equipment failure.

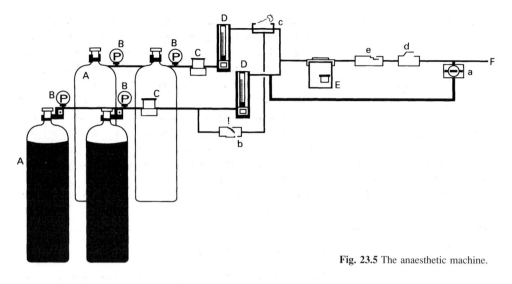

Fig. 23.5 The anaesthetic machine.

Components

The anaesthetic machine (Fig. 23.5) begins at a carrier gas source (A), passes through a pressure gauge (B), a pressure regulator (C) and flowmeter assembly (D), and ends at the common gas outlet (F), where the anaesthetic breathing system attaches. Vaporisers (E) are usually positioned downstream from the flowmeter assembly. Other features include emergency oxygen valves (a), low oxygen alarms (b), nitrous oxide cut-out devices (c), over-pressure valves (d) and emergency air-intake valves (e).

Gas supply. Cylinders, 'bottles' or 'tanks' are metal containers designed to withstand the pressure of compressed gases. Their size determines the volume of gas contained (in litres) and this is described by letters from AA (very small) to J (large). The volume of oxygen in filled cylinders at room temperature is shown in Table 23.6.

Cylinders are colour-coded as follows:

● Oxygen cylinders are black with white shoulders.
● Nitrous oxide bottles are blue.
● Carbon dioxide cylinders are grey.
● Old machines may have a facility for cyclopropane which is delivered in orange cylinders.

Cylinders are opened by anticlockwise rotation of the spindle. Before attachment to the cylinder yoke, the protective cellophane sleeve is removed from the cylinder valve and the spindle briefly opened to flush away the dust that lies in the outlet port. Once connected in the hanger yokes, spindles should be opened slowly two full turns as partially restricted valves may reduce flow when the cylinder pressure falls.

Cylinder banks. Vertically standing banks of three to five 'J' or 'G' size cylinders are used in busy practices. Two

Table 23.6 Cylinder sizes and contents

Cylinder size	E	F	G	J
Content (l)	680	1340	3400	6800

banks for each gas (oxygen and nitrous oxide) are preferable, with one being 'in use' and the other 'in reserve', gas flows to the operating room through pipes in the wall. These end in wall-mounted Schraeder-type sockets which receive probes from the anaesthetic machine. Pipes are colour-coded and the probes size-coded so that lines cannot be accidentally crossed.

Low-volume cylinders. Low-volume 'E' or 'F' cylinders attached to hanger yokes on the machine suit most practices. Machines usually hold two cylinders of O_2 and two of N_2O. The cylinder valve face has holes which correspond with pins sited within the hanger yoke. The pin and hole pattern constitutes the pin-indexing system and ensures N_2O or CO_2 cylinders cannot be connected to the O_2 yoke.

Pressure/contents gauge. The pressure gauge is indispensable for oxygen, because it indicates the gas volume in the cylinder. This is calculated using Boyle's law ($PV = k$).

An 'E' cylinder contains 680 litres when filled to 13 300 kPa (1935 p.s.i.) at 20°C. At the same temperature, a pressure gauge registering 4500 kPa (655 p.s.i.) indicates 230 litres remain:

$$\frac{(4500 \times 680)}{13\ 300} = 230\,l$$

If the calculated oxygen flow rate for the next operation is 4 l/min, then this cylinder will provide gas for 57 minutes:

$$\frac{230}{4} = 57 \text{ min}$$

The N_2O pressure gauge is less useful; the full N_2O cylinder contains liquid and gas and the gauge measures the pressure of gaseous N_2O in equilibrium with liquid. This remains constant until all liquid evaporates, after which pressure falls rapidly. Gas volume in N_2O cylinders is found by weighing the bottle and applying the following formula:

Litres N$_2$O present

$$= \frac{(net - tare)\ weight\ [\epsilon\ grams] \times 22.4}{44}$$

Cylinder tare weight is stamped on the cylinder neck.

Pressure reducing valves or regulators. These produce constant 'downstream' pressure (therefore flow) as cylinder pressure falls with use. Without them, the cylinder valve would need incremental opening to maintain constant flow. They are sited immediately downstream from the hanger yoke, and in modern machines they may be incorporated in the yoke itself and be impossible to find.

Flowmeters. Flowmeters control and measure the rate of gas passing through them. The units are litres per minute (l/min). A freely moving 'float' – either a ball or bobbin – is supported in a transparent, tapered tube by an ascending flow of gas. The flow rate is etched on the tube and read from the top of bobbins and the equator of spheres. The greater the flow, the higher the indicator rises in the glass tube. Flowmeters become inaccurate if dirt or non-vertical positioning makes the float rub against the tube. This is limited by slots machined in the rim of bobbins to encourage rotation. Flowmeters are calibrated for one gas only and so oxygen flowmeters do not accurately indicate the flow of nitrous oxide. Because of this, flowmeter control knobs are often colour-coded. Flowmeter control knobs must not be over-tightened.

Vaporisers. Vaporisers dilute the saturated vapour of volatile anaesthetics to yield a range of useful concentrations of vaporised liquid. Concentrations leaving the vaporiser depend on:

- Temperature.
- Surface area.
- Gas flow.
- The volatility of the anaesthetic.

As anaesthetic vaporises, the liquid cools due to the latent heat of vaporisation required for this process. As the temperature falls, the delivered anaesthetic concentration also falls. With increased flow rates, the delivered concentration tends to decrease. Hence insuring a constant output is not always easy. A number of compensating devices can be employed to maintain output:

- Heat source (or heat sink) – surrounds the liquid anaesthetic to prevent rapid cooling. Heat is transferred from this source to buffer the drop in chamber temperature associated with vaporisation.
- Flow splitting valve – varies the proportion of carrier gas that passes through or bypasses the vaporising chamber allowing some degree of control over percentage anaesthetic vapour delivered.
- Temperature compensating mechanism – compensates for fall in vaporising temperature and subsequent fall in

vapour concentration. Two methods are commonly employed. A bimetallic strip of two dissimilar metals placed back to back bends in proportion to a given change in temperature. When placed in the flow of the anaesthetic vapour it can alter the flow through the vaporising chamber and compensate for an increase or decrease in anaesthetic vapour pressure caused by a change in temperature. Alternatively, an ether-filled bellows can produce a linear change in anaesthetic carrier gas flow restriction in direct proportion to temperature change.

- Wicks and baffles – increase the surface area of vaporisation.

Draw over systems

Early vaporisers relied on the patient's respiratory efforts to 'draw' carrier gas (often air) over the liquid anaesthetic. They offer relatively little resistance to flow, though are subject to large variations in inspiratory flow, dependent on the ventilation characteristics of the patient. Compensation for changes in temperature are rarely employed. Consequently their output is frequently variable and they cannot be reliably calibrated. They are more commonly used when placed within the anaesthetic circuit, i.e. within a circle circuit. In this position they are termed 'in-circuit vaporisers' (IVC). Anaesthetic machines such as the Stephens machine and the Komezaroff machine incorporate VICs, and work in small animals has demonstrated that they can be safely used. However caution must be exercised when IPPV is initiated as dangerously high concentrations of anaesthetic gas can be delivered. Some models still in use include:

- Goldman halothane vaporiser – simple, small, inexpensive. It is neither temperature nor flow compensated.
- Oxford miniature vaporiser – used primarily with portable anaesthetic equipment, it is not temperature compensated, though has a heat sink (a sealed water/antifreeze compartment). It can be drained of one anaesthetic and refilled with another and detachable scales of approximate vapour percentage delivered are supplied.
- EMO (Epstein, Macintosh, Oxford) vaporiser – used for ether delivery it has a water-filled compartment as a heat sink.

Plenum systems

Plenum vaporisers are designed for use with constant flow of carrier gas and offer greater resistance to flow. Hence they are generally positioned out of the breathing circuit, i.e. out-of-circuit vaporisers (VOC). They are mostly calibrated vaporisers with compensatory devices for variations in temperature and flow and are those most commonly used in veterinary practice. Earlier models include uncalibrated types though these are infrequently seen today.

- *Uncalibrated vaporisers.* The Boyle's bottle is simple, inexpensive and easily maintained. It does not have any temperature compensation, though it does have a cowl that can be lowered toward and below the liquid anaesthetic surface to increase vapour uptake for a given control lever position. However, output concentrations are not guaranteed and they 'drift' despite constant control settings. As liquid anaesthetic cools and the flows increase, the output concentration falls. Concentrations rise when low flows are used, when the vaporiser is agitated or when temperatures rise. With age the sealing washer (usually cork or rubber) becomes brittle and allows leakage of anaesthetic vapour. The cork stopper placed in the filling orifice is normally retained with a metal chain and often the metal anchor of the chain passes through the cork. If the chain breaks, the cork can act as a sparking plug; if someone charged with static electricity touches the cork–metal top, an explosion may result.

● *Calibrated vaporisers.* Temperature and flow compensation are incorporated as well as a heat source/sink into these vaporisers. Anaesthetic concentration from 'Tec and other calibrated vaporisers is similar to that 'dialled' on the spindle, provided that the gas flow through the vaporiser and the temperature of liquid anaesthetic are within ranges specific for the model. In Mark III 'Tecs (Ohmeda), output is constant between 18 and 35°C. Dialled and delivered concentrations are similar at flows between 0.2 and 15 l/min. In the earlier 'Tec 2, vapour output is reliable from above 2–4 l/min fresh gas flow. Lower flows, as used in low flow anaesthesia, produce delivered concentration different to that displayed on the dial. They come with a performance chart that indicates the delivered vapour concentration for a given dial setting and flow rate. Though obsolete they are still frequently seen in veterinary practice.

Vaporisers are agent-specific. Filling with the wrong anaesthetic is prevented by keyed filling ports. These accept a key-ended tube which only attaches to the corresponding anaesthetic bottle. Used properly, the system also assists pollution control because vaporiser filling occurs without spillage.

Back bar

Flowmeters and vaporisers may be joined by tapered connectors and attached to a back bar, producing a series of semi-permanent fixtures. The 'Selectatec SM' manifold allows rapid attachment or removal of 'Tec 3 and 'Tec 4 vaporisers and is desirable, facilitating vaporiser removal for refilling out of theatre, servicing and rewarming. In accommodating up to three vaporisers, a range of volatile agents may be available.

Common gas outlet (F).
This connects the anaesthetic machine to breathing system connectors, ventilators or O_2 supply devices.

O_2 flush.
Also known as the bypass or purge valve, this receives O_2 from the cylinder and bypasses the vaporiser. Activation produces high flows of pure oxygen to the

common gas outlet. The device is used to provide oxygen in emergency situations and may have a 'lock-in' facility: rotating the valve 90° fixes it in the open position. It is used to flush anaesthetic from breathing systems before patient disconnection, thus lowering pollution.

Nitrous oxide cut-out devices.
These devices curtail N_2O flow and sound an alarm when oxygen runs out. The machine's system is checked by means of the following steps:

(1) Switch on both O_2 and N_2O sources.
(2) Open the flowmeters to give nominal flows of 2 and 4 l/min O_2/N_2O, respectively.
(3) Close the O_2 cylinder valve.

The N_2O and O_2 bobbins should fall simultaneously while a whistle sounds.

Over-pressure valve.
High pressures downstream from the common gas outlet open this valve and sound an alarm. The device is useful for leak-testing breathing systems; the valve's presence is confirmed by occluding the common gas outlet while pressing the oxygen bypass valve.

Emergency air intake valve.
When gas flow from the machine accidentally ceases, the patient's inspiratory effort opens an emergency valve which allows room air to enter the breathing system. The valve's opening action is accompanied by a 'whistling' sound. This valve is tested by attaching a pipe to the common gas outlet and applying suction; when sufficient vacuum is present, the valve opens and a whistle is heard.

Checking the machine before use

The anaesthetic machine should receive a major check at the beginning of each working day and a minor check between cases. To ensure that no parts of the test are omitted, a list should be attached to the machine, setting out the following steps:

● Ensure that flow control valves (at flowmeter) are 'off'.
● Ensure that cylinders are closed and fit securely on the hanger yoke.
● Press the oxygen flush valve until no gas flow is apparent from the common gas outlet.
● Check that flowmeters and pressure gauges read 'O'.
● Open the oxygen cylinder valve slowly (anticlockwise) and observe the registered pressure. On machines which carry two O_2 cylinders test the 'full' or reserve cylinder first. Open the oxygen flowmeter control valve to 2–4 l/min to ensure smooth function. Whilst this is flowing repeat the procedure for the 'full' N_2O cylinder and open the flowmeter to 2–4 l/min. The tested O_2 cylinder is then closed. As the oxygen runs out, the low oxygen alarm should sound and the N_2O cut-off device should trigger, with both bobbins dropping to zero flow. The 'full' N_2O cylinder is closed. The test is repeated for the 'in use' oxygen and nitrous oxide cylinders.

- Replace bottles that have little remaining gas.
- Open the 'in use' oxygen and nitrous oxide cylinders.
- Ensure that the vaporiser is full, with the filling port tightly closed, that spindle operation is smooth, and that the connection hoses (if appropriate) are connected to the vaporiser.
- Check over-pressure and emergency air-intake valves.

The testing of machines that receive a service supply from banked cylinders is more complicated. These machines should have an emergency oxygen cylinder attached to the machine and this should be tested as should the vaporiser as above. The back-up cylinder is then turned off. The piped source is then connected to the machine and the flowmeter opened to ensure adequate flow.

'Shutting down' the anaesthetic machine

When all surgery is finished, the content status of all cylinders is checked and empty cylinders are removed. (If present, Schraeder probes are removed from the wall sockets and the pipes neatly coiled.) The oxygen flowmeter control knob is then opened to produce flow of 2 l/min. The nitrous oxide cylinder valves are then closed. The nitrous oxide flowmeters are opened and closed once the flow indicator has fallen to 'O'. The oxygen bottles are then closed and the O_2 flush valve is activated until no pressure registers on the pressure gauge. Machine surfaces are then wiped down.

Anaesthetic breathing systems

The anaesthetic breathing circuit takes the fresh gas from the common gas outlet of the anaesthetic machine and delivers it to the patient. The functions of the circuit include:

- Removal of exhaled carbon dioxide.
- Supply of oxygen.
- Supply of anaesthetic gases.

Circuit classification varies throughout the world and can be confusing. A simple basis of classification depends on whether expired carbon dioxide is flushed from the system by high gas flow or removed by chemical reaction (e.g. with soda lime).

Rebreathing systems

Expired breath, in comparison with inspired gas, is low in O_2 and anaesthetic but contains more CO_2 and water vapour and is warm. In rebreathing systems (circle and to-and-fro) expired gas passes through soda-lime (absorbent) which removes CO_2. Warm, moist gas is then re-inspired and so rebreathing systems conserve heat and moisture. Fresh gas flow requirements are based on the O_2 and anaesthetic consumption of the patient. Because these values are low (Table 23.7) rebreathing systems are efficient.

Absorbent. This absorbs CO_2 and consists of granules of:

- 80% Sodium hydroxide [NaOH] or 'soda'.
- 18% Calcium hydroxide [Ca(OH)$_2$] or 'lime'.
- Silicates.
- pH indicators.

Carbon dioxide reacts chemically with the hydroxides to produce carbonates. The reactions require water (derived from expired breath) and produce heat in the process:

$$CO_2 + 2NaOH = Na_2CO_3 + H_2O$$

$$Na_2CO_3 + Ca(OH)_2 = 2NaOH + CaCO_3$$

Silicates used to be included in medical absorbents to increase the hardness and reduce the formation of irritant dust.

pH indicators. These change colour as soda-lime becomes exhausted. Changes depend on the dyes used. Common absorbents turn from pink or lilac to white (although, confusingly, one type turns from white to lilac). The container label describes the colour change its contents undergo and should be consulted.

When soda-lime granules are 'spent', they lose their soapy, soft texture and fail to become warm when exposed to CO_2. Opened absorbent containers must be tightly sealed otherwise atmospheric CO_2 enters and causes premature exhaustion.

Soda-lime is irritant (alkali) and gloves should be worn when refilling canisters. The dust must not be inhaled or allowed to contact the eyes.

Soda-lime is contained in canisters, the design of which depends on the circuit involved. The canister contents are approximately 50% granules and 50% air space. Efficient absorption requires an air-space volume in excess of tidal

Table 23.7 Respiratory variables in companion animals

Species	Respiratory rate[a] (breaths/min)	Tidal volume[a] (ml/kg)	Minute volume[a] (ml/kg/min)	Oxygen consumption[b] (ml/kg/min)
Dogs				
>30 kg	15–20	12–15	150–250	5.8
<30 kg	20–30	16–20	200–300	6.2
Cats	20–30	7–9	180–380	7.3

[a] During surgery, factors like pain, pyrexia, light versus deep anaesthesia will affect these.
[b] Oxygen consumption depends on factors related to metabolic rate: age, temperature, thyroid status, drugs, muscle tone, response to surgery.

volume (V_t) and so the minimum 'working' soda-lime required is at least 2 V_t. Considerably greater volumes than this are needed because the absorbent is inactivated during anaesthesia. Gas flow between the granules is turbulent and when large canisters are filled to capacity resistance to breathing is increased. However, large canisters require less frequent changing.

Soda-lime reacts with trichloroethylene (a once popular volatile agent) to produce phosgene and other toxic gases; trichloroethylene should therefore not be used in rebreathing systems.

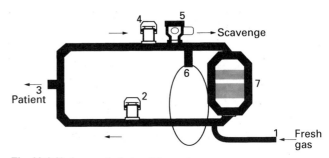

Fig. 23.6 Circle anaesthetic breathing system.

REBREATHING SYSTEMS

Advantages
- Low gas flow requirements.
- Low volatile agent consumption rate.
- 'Closed' or 'low-flow' options.
- Expired moisture and heat conserved.
- Ventilation can be altered (spontaneous to controlled) without changing system performance or efficiency.
- Low explosion risk (when explosive gases are used).
- Less pollution.

Disadvantages
- High resistance to breathing.
- Nitrous oxide must be used cautiously in rebreathing systems.
- Expensive to purchase.
- Regular soda-lime replacement required.
- Inspired gas content undetermined.
- De-nitrogenation required.
- Slow to change level of anaesthesia.
- Cumbersome.

'Closed' and 'low-flow'. Rebreathing systems are used in one of two ways. In 'closed' systems, gas inflow precisely replaces anaesthetic and O_2 taken up by the patient. Approximately 5–10 ml/kg/min is required. Under these conditions the pressure relief valve is shut. When the system is run in a 'low-flow' fashion, oxygen delivery is in excess of basal requirements (above 10 ml/kg/min) with surplus gas leaking through the partly opened pressure-relief valve. This is the easiest system to operate and therefore the most common.

Nitrous oxide. This gas can only be used safely in rebreathing systems if inspired oxygen content, arterial oxygen saturation or arterial blood-gas analysis can be performed.

De-nitrogenation. When connected to breathing systems at the onset of anaesthesia, patients expire considerable volumes of nitrogen (which is present in normal air but not in anaesthetic gas mixtures). This may lower circuit O_2 to hypoxic levels unless purged through the pressure-relief valve (de-nitrogenation). This is achieved by using high flows for the first 10–15 minutes of anaesthesia.

Otherwise, regular 'dumping' of the reservoir bag is required (every 3 minutes in the first 15 minutes and every 30 minutes thereafter).

Circle system. Circle systems (Fig. 23.6) have valves causing unidirectional gas movement through seven circuit components. These are: fresh gas inflow (1), inspiratory and expiratory unidirectional valves (2 and 4), patient 'Y' connector (3), pressure-relief valve (5), reservoir bag (6), and absorbent canister (7).

- *Fresh gas inflow (1).* This pipe connects the circuit with the common-gas outlet on the anaesthetic machine.
- *Unidirectional valves (2 and 4).* These are light transparent discs resting on knife-edge valve seats, enclosed within a transparent dome. Units should be easy to disassemble for drying and cleaning.
- *'Y' connector (3).* This connects inspiratory and expiratory limbs with endotracheal tube connectors or masks. In paediatric systems it has a septum dividing inspiratory and expiratory flows, reducing dead-space.
- *Pressure-relief valve (5).* This is opened to let surplus gas from 'low-flow' systems, during de-nitrogenation, and closed when lung inflation is imposed. In old systems it was sited at the 'Y' connector which made valve operation difficult. Relief valves should be shrouded for attachment to scavenge hoses.
- *Reservoir (rebreathing) bag (6).* This allows IPPV; its volume should be 3–6 times the animal's tidal volume. Large bags increase circuit volume, make respiratory movement less obvious and are harder to squeeze. Inadequately sized bags collapse during large breaths and over-distend during expiration. Clearly, a range is required for small animal use.
- *Absorbent canister (7).* Canisters for circle systems may have two compartments. When absorbent in one becomes exhausted, it is discarded; after refilling, the canister is replaced in the reverse direction. This allows optimal use of absorbent. Circle system canisters may have a bypass switch which excludes or incorporates absorbent from the circuit, allowing CO_2 to rise while maintaining ventilation.
- *Hoses.* These are corrugated to prevent kinking.

Circle systems for small dogs and cats are becoming more popular in the UK and modern small animal circles can be used in patients weighing greater than 5–10 kg.

CIRCLE SYSTEMS

Advantages
- High gas efficiency.
- Mechanical dead-space remains unchanged with use (unlike to-and-fro systems).
- Bronchiolitis unlikely (unlike to-and-fro systems).
- Less circuit inertia than to-and-fro systems.
- Ventilation readily controlled.

Disadvantages
- Expensive.
- Complex, cumbersome and difficult to sterilise.
- Resistance to breathing for animals less than 5–10 kg.

To-and-fro (Waters') system. In this system (Fig. 23.7) gas oscillates over absorbent in the Waters' canister. Canisters are designed for either vertical or horizontal use; only the latter are used with companion animals. Features of to-and-fro systems include:

- *Fresh gas inflow.* This is situated adjacent to the endotracheal tube connector allowing dialled concentrations of anaesthetic to be preferentially inspired and, therefore, greater control over anaesthesia.
- *Filter.* A metal gauze screen should be sited at the patient end of the canister to limit inhalation of alkali dust.
- *Scavenging shroud.* Scavenging waste gas from a to-and-fro system relies on a suitable shroud on the pressure-relief valve.
- *Canister.* Transparent canisters are desirable as they allow soda-lime colour and filling adequacy to be checked. (Canisters in horizontal to-and-fro systems must be filled to capacity, otherwise the expirate will 'channel', i.e. take the low resistance path over the absorbent, retaining CO_2.)

Non-rebreathing systems

Non-rebreathing systems rely on high fresh gas flow rates, based on multiples of minute volume, to flush expired CO_2 from the circuit so that it cannot be rebreathed at the next breath.

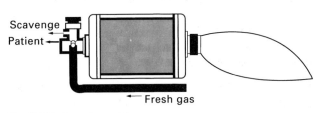

Fig. 23.7 Horizontal to-and-fro system.

TO-AND-FRO SYSTEMS

Advantages
- High gas efficiency.
- Bi-directional gas flow improves CO_2 scrubbing efficiency.
- Greater heat conservation (hyperthermia is possible in high ambient temperatures).
- Lower resistance to breathing than with circle systems (no valves and lower overall circuit length).
- Low circuit volume:
- De-nitrogenation achieved rapidly.
- Rapid changes in gas concentration.
- Simple, robust construction.
- Portable; easily moved from room to room.
- Readily sterilised.
- Inexpensive.

Disadvantages
- Valve position is inconvenient for positive-pressure ventilation.
- Mechanical dead-space increases during surgery as absorbent is exhausted.
- 'Channelling'.
- Bronchiolitis; aspiration of alkali dust from canister may cause chemical injury.
- Considerable drag. The system has much inertia and is inconvenient during head surgery.

NON-REBREATHING SYSTEMS

Advantages
- Low resistance; ideal for small animals and birds.
- Simple construction.
- Inexpensive to purchase.
- Soda-lime not required.
- Inspired gas content similar to that 'dialled' at anaesthetic machine.
- De-nitrogenation not required.
- Circuit concentration of anaesthetic can be changed rapidly, allowing more concise control over the patient's level of unconsciousness.
- Can be used with trichlorethylene.

Disadvantages
- High carrier gas flow requirements.
- High volatile agent consumption rate.
- Expired moisture and heat usually lost.
- Ventilatory modes affect system performance.
- Different types of non-rebreathing circuits behave differently, and have different flow requirements.

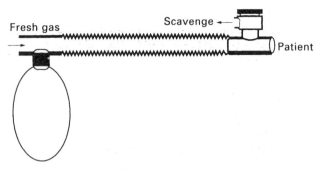

Fig. 23.8 The Magill breathing system.

The Magill system. The Magill system consists of a reservoir bag and a corrugated hose which ends at an expiratory (Heidbrink) valve (Fig. 23.8).

Rebreathing is prevented when gas flow equals or exceeds patient minute volume. When N_2O is used, its flow rate is included within this value. For example, a 15 kg dog with a V_m of 3 l receives an inspired concentration of 66% N_2O with flows of 1 l/min O_2 and 2 l/min N_2O. Similarly, 1.5 l/min O_2 and 1.5 l/min N_2O provides a 50% mixture.

MAGILL SYSTEM

Advantages
- The Magill is an efficient general-purpose circuit for most companion animal cases. The circuit is readily maintained and sterilised.

Disadvantages
- Mechanical dead-space, inertia and considerable expiratory resistance preclude its usefulness in cats, and in dogs weighing less than 10 kg. Heidbrink valve location is inconvenient for scavenging and operation, especially during surgery on the head. The behaviour of the system changes fundamentally when the reservoir bag is actively squeezed during IPPV, with late inspired gas (fresh gas) being lost through the expiratory valve and expired gas being reintroduced into the lungs rather than expelled through the valve during inspirations. Consequently, the system is best not used for prolonged positive-pressure ventilation because 'enforced rebreathing' causes hypercapnia.

The coaxial Lack system. Inconvenient valve location in Magill circuits is overcome in the coaxial version – the Lack system (Fig. 23.9). In this, a reservoir bag connects to an outer inspiratory limb; this surrounds an inner expiratory tube which ends at the expiratory valve.

The Lack system is slightly more efficient than the Magill. Expiratory resistance is also lower and so the system may be used in smaller animals.

LACK SYSTEM

Advantages
- The circuit is lightweight and exerts less drag than Magill systems. Valve position facilitates surgery on the head and scavenging. The system is 1.5 m long, allowing anaesthetic machine positioning away from surgery. Lack systems can be used in lieu of the Magill circuit.

Disadvantages
- Older versions had high expiratory (inner limb) resistance and inner hose disconnection, causing considerable rebreathing. The system is stiffer and inconvenient to use in very small animals. Because the Lack system behaves like the Magill, it should not be used for prolonged periods of controlled ventilation.

The parallel Lack system (Fig. 23.10). Problems of co-axial geometry (disconnection, fracture or kinking of the inner limb) are avoided when the inspiratory and expiratory limbs are juxtapositioned (put side by side) in a parallel configuration. The system is said to behave like a Magill circuit although it has increased drag, thus conferring little advantage in very small animal anaesthesia.

Ayre's T-piece (Fig. 23.11). Gas flows for T-piece systems must exceed double the minute volume otherwise expired gas is rebreathed ($2 \times V_m$). Rapid respiratory rates may require even higher ($3 \times V_m$) flows. Nitrous oxide is included at 50 or 66% of these levels.

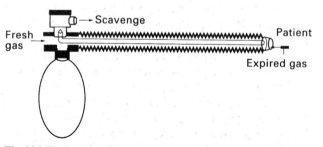

Fig. 23.9 The Lack breathing system.

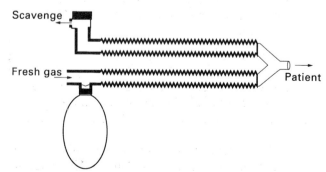

Fig. 23.10 The parallel Lack breathing system.

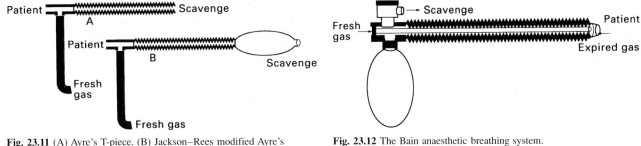

Fig. 23.11 (A) Ayre's T-piece. (B) Jackson–Rees modified Ayre's T-piece.

Fig. 23.12 The Bain anaesthetic breathing system.

AYRE'S T-PIECE

Advantages
- Minimal apparatus dead-space and resistance makes the T-piece ideal for cats, small dogs (below 5 kg), neonates and birds. It is simple, inexpensive and easy to sterilise. The system is scavenged with appropriate connectors.

Disadvantages
- Ventilation is controlled by occluding the distal end of the expiratory limb but gas flow must be increased, otherwise the duration of inspiration is prolonged and limits adequate ventilation.

Ayre's T-piece with Jackson–Rees modification.
This circuit is an Ayre's T-piece with an open-ended reservoir bag on the expiratory limb (Fig. 23.11). Flows of $2.5-3 \times V_m$ are needed.

AYRE'S T-PIECE WITH JACKSON–REES MODIFICATION

Advantages
- The bag facilitates IPPV and bag movement acts as a useful respiratory monitor. Ventilation is controlled by occluding the bag's end, allowing distension, then squeezing the contents into the patient. The end is then released. The system has the advantages of a T-piece so is used in similar circumstances. Flows need not be increased when IPPV is imposed.

Disadvantages
- Scavenging the system may be complicated; connectors tend to twist and cause rapid over-distension of the bag.

The Bain system. The Bain system is a 'co-axial' (tube within a tube) T-piece with an inner inspiratory limb surrounded by an outer expiratory hose (Fig. 23.12). The expiratory limb ends either in an open-ended tube (Mapleson E), a reservoir bag and expiratory valve (Mapleson D) or an open-ended bag (Mapleson F).

The circuit requires similar fresh gas flows to the T-piece systems.

BAIN SYSTEM

Advantages
- Bain systems without valves (Mapleson E or F) are recommended for cats and very small dogs because of lower expiratory resistance. Ventilation is controlled by occluding the expiratory limb in 'E' systems. In 'D' systems, the expiratory valve is closed and then the bag squeezed. In Mapleson F versions, the reservoir bag is used like a Jackson–Rees modification. The circuit is useful for IPPV in small dogs and cats, especially when patient access is limited. The length of the system (1.8 m) allows the anaesthetic machine to be positioned well away from surgery, improving access. Spontaneous ventilation is satisfactory in dogs over 10 kg. The system has low drag and mechanical dead-space; it is easily maintained and sterilised. It is claimed that warm expirate raises the temperature of gas flowing in the inner limb, conserving patient temperature.

Disadvantages
- Expiratory resistance with high flows reduces the system's usefulness in spontaneously breathing cats and small dogs. Rebreathing problems caused by inner limb disconnection prompted development of a parallel Bain system. However, inspiratory limb integrity is easily tested by occluding its end with a 5 ml syringe plunger; when gas is flowing the flowmeter indicator falls and/or the machine's over-pressure valve is heard.

Pollution control systems

Exposure to anaesthetic gases has been associated with the development of malignancies, neuropathy, bone marrow toxicity, a high incidence of abortions and infertility in theatre personnel and congenital abnormalities in their offspring. Though many of the studies reporting these effects have been criticised for poor methodology the risk of chronic exposure remains a serious concern to veterinary staff. Under COSHH (Control of Substances Hazardous to Health) Regulations the employer has a duty to assess the risk of exposure to anaesthetic gases to his employees and take the appropriate measures to protect their health. The Health and Safety Executive have proposed the following occupational exposure standards (OES) based on an 8-hour time-weighted average (TWA), i.e. the average level of anaesthetic gas in the environment if measured over an 8-hour period:

● Nitrous oxide   100 p.p.m.
● Halothane   10 p.p.m.
● Enflurane   50 p.p.m.
● Isoflurane   50 p.p.m.
● Ether   400 p.p.m.

For shorter periods of operation, as more commonly seen in veterinary practice, it is suggested that short-term exposure should not exceed 3 times this limit. The use of scavenging systems combined with careful anaesthetic techniques can reduce pollution by up to 90% and ensure an environment safely below these OES levels.

Scavenging systems include both passive and active methods. Generally, active methods are more efficient, though in some circumstances passive methods are adequate.

Passive scavenging

These rely on the patient's respiratory efforts to void the waste gases via a wide-bore (22 mm) tube to the outside of the building. To be effective the exit must be protected from significant air currents such that excessive subatmospheric or positive pressure could be generated within the tube and effect function. Further scavenging to the roof level would produce a back pressure due to the heavier gases pooling in the tube. Generally, a tube length of no more than 2.6 m is acceptable. A variation of this method is the active charcoal absorber that chemically absorbs hydrocarbon inhalation anaesthetics. It collects gas via a short tube from the scavenging shroud of the breathing circuit and removes the inhaled anaesthetic. However it does not absorb nitrous oxide, confirming it is not exhausted can only be performed by weighing the absorber, and it adds further resistance to the passive system.

Active-passive scavenging

Similar to the passive system a wide-bore tube scavenges exhaled gas from the expiratory valve of the circuit, but passes the gas to a forced ventilation system rather than outside. It is important to ensure this ventilation system does not dump the gas in another workplace or recirculate the gas. Further some of these gases may support combustion under certain conditions.

Active scavenging

This is the preferred method and that most likely to meet COSHH standards. It consists of three main components:

● *Transfer system.* The transfer system consists of a tube and connector (usually 30 mm) attached to the expiratory port of the circuit.
● *Receiving system.* The receiving system functions as an air break, preventing excessive positive or negative pressure reaching the breathing system. Often it consists of a simple open-ended reservoir system, allowing venting of excess positive pressure or uptake of atmospheric gas if excess negative pressure develops. Alternatively a reservoir bag and safety valves can be used.
● *Disposal system to the exterior.* The disposal system delivers the gas to the outside of the building and includes an active suction method. Frequently this consists of a fan unit or otherwise a pump system.

Good anaesthetic technique is also important to ensure minimal exposure to waste gases. Recommended procedures include:

● Check the anaesthetic machine and circuit for leaks.
● Turn on the scavenging system and connect it to the breathing circuit.
● Intubate the patient with an appropriate sized cuffed endotracheal tube and inflate the cuff.
● Avoid the use of face masks when possible.
● Turn on the anaesthetic gases (other than oxygen) only after the patient is connected to the circuit.
● Avoid disconnecting the patient during anaesthesia.
● Flush the circuit with oxygen for 30 seconds prior to disconnection at the end of procedure and empty the remaining gas in the reservoir bag into the scavenging system.
● Fill the vaporisers at the end of the day in a well-ventilated area.
● Service all equipment annually.
● Consider annual monitoring of theatre pollution.

Other anaesthetic equipment

Trouble-free anaesthesia depends on equipment being available and serviceable. Inadequate equipment care causes expensive deterioration and, more importantly, may compromise the patient.

Endotracheal tubes

These connect the patient to the anaesthetic breathing system. Most patterns have cuffs at the distal (patient) end which, when filled with air, produce a gas-tight seal. Construction materials confer different properties on the tube. Red rubber tubes have poor resistance to kinking and conform poorly to airway contours. Tubes made of polyvinyl chloride (PVC) are the softest and least irritating to the tracheal mucosa; they have little tendency to kink and they mould to the curve of the airway at body temperature.

Care, maintenance and storage depend on the material of construction. Red rubber tubes are deteriorated by oil and petroleum-based lubricants. After cleaning and sterilisation, tubes should be dried thoroughly and stored in a cool, dry environment. They should not be exposed to direct sunlight.

Before use, check the tubes for patency and establish the cuffs' ability to hold pressure. The endotracheal tube connector should be tight and fit snugly with the chosen breathing system. The tube should be an appropriate length and a range of tube diameters should be made available.

After use, ensure the tubes are rinsed in running water and leave them to soak in detergent solution. Later they should be scrubbed inside and out to remove residual mucus. Rinsing must be thorough to remove detergent.

Sterilising procedures depend on material. Red rubber tubes are deteriorated by heat sterilisation. Polysiloxane tubes can be autoclaved. While most PVC tubes are designed for single use only, they may be safely re-used after cleaning and sterilising. Ethylene oxide must be used cautiously and adequate aeration allowed afterwards (at least 48 hours). Gamma-irradiated single-use items and PVC tubes should not be sterilised with ethylene oxide.

Masks

These are used for administering oxygen and for volatile anaesthetics when an endotracheal tube is not present. Patterns made of malleable rubber can be shaped to fit the animal's face and minimise apparatus dead-space. Others are made of rigid plastic with a perforated rubber diaphragm; they have high dead-space and so require greater gas flows. However, for birds and laboratory animal species they can be constructed from syringe cases and bits of latex glove. Customised equipment should have minimum dead-space, should be affixable to the animal, should not confer resistance to respiration and should allow the animal to be seen.

Care, maintenance and storage considerations for masks are the same as those for endotracheal tubes.

Masks can be sterilised by soaking in a 0.2% chlorhexidine solution or similar.

Laryngoscopes

Laryngoscopes consist of a handle and a blade and are available in several patterns and sizes. They serve to depress the base of the tongue during intubation; in so doing, they evert the epiglottis. A bulb at the tip of the blade illuminates the oropharynx. Ideally, the bulb should only illuminate when the blade is 'fixed' in the working position.

Before use, it is important to ensure that the bulb is firmly positioned and that the batteries are charged. After use, blades should be wiped clean with a swab soaked in alcohol. Laryngoscopes must not be immersed in water.

Gags

These keep the jaw open and allow safe retraction of the tongue after induction and prior to endotracheal intubation. They are also useful during oral surgery.

Suction devices

Connected either to a central vacuum pipeline or to a portable pump unit these devices allow suction of body secretions and are particularly relevant to anaesthesia. They are probably the most important piece of resuscitation equipment and are used to clear mucus, blood and other debris from the pharynx, trachea and main bronchi. Suction is also used to clear the surgical site of blood, and allow gastrointestinal drainage, wound drainage and pleural drainage. They consist of three essential components:

- Source of vacuum.
- Reservoir or collection vessel.
- Suction tubing.

The vacuum source can be via a central vacuum pipeline or a portable unit. An electric motor or pneumatic system can drive a mechanical pump. An appropriate sized collection vessel is one that is large enough to collect the aspirated material but not too large or cumbersome. The interface between the collection vessel and the rest of the unit must be kept clean and free from damage to ensure adequate suction function. The suction tubing should be of a length and diameter not to restrict flow and the wall of the tube must be strong enough not to collapse or kink once suction is applied.

Addition optional features include:

- Cut-off valve – to prevent liquid aspirated entering the pump.
- Bacterial filter – prevents contamination of the room with aspirated bacteria.
- Vacuum control valve – allows adjustment of the degree of vacuum applied.
- Vacuum gauge – indicates the degree of suction.
- Foam prevention – foam may cause closure of the cut-off valve or contaminate the filter or pump.
- Stop valve – to occlude the suction tubing and allow build-up of vacuum.
- Two collection vessels – allowing continuous operation when one vessel is full or non-functional and to provide overflow when the first vessel is full.

Syringes and needles

Disposable plastic syringes have replaced glass. Filled syringes must be labelled. After use the needle should be removed, the syringe discarded and the needle disposed of into a rigid container. If fine (e.g. smaller than 23 s.w.g.) needles are used to withdraw drugs from multi-dose vials, they should be replaced before use because they may have become blunted.

SUMMARY

- Anaesthetic equipment is essential for inhalation anaesthesia.
- All anaesthetic machine consists of similar components
- A thorough knowledge of the use of the machine will minimise equipment-induced complications.
- A proper anaesthetic equipment check is required each day.
- Anaesthetic circuits deliver oxygen and anaesthetic gas, and remove carbon dioxide from the patient.
- Anaesthetic circuits can be divided on the basis of how they remove exhaled carbon dioxide; rebreathing circuits absorb CO_2 chemically, non-rebreathing circuits remove it with high fresh gas flow rates.
- Scavenging of waste anaesthetic gases is important.
- Other equipment relates to the specific case.

Muscle relaxants

Several types of drug produce muscle relaxation, including general anaesthetics. When absolute relaxation is required, however, neuromuscular blocker agents ('muscle relaxants') are used because they are the most effective and predictable. These drugs, derived from poisons used with blow-darts by indigenous South Americans, act on nicotinic receptors at the neuromuscular junction. They have no direct effect on smooth or cardiac muscle.

Neuromuscular blocking drugs do not cross the blood–brain barrier and so do not alter consciousness. However, they eliminate some of the obvious signs of inadequate anaesthesia – movement, ocular position and cranial nerve reflexes – so that monitoring the level of anaesthesia becomes more complicated. Because the animal cannot respond normally to inadequate anaesthesia, the anaesthetist must ensure the animal is unconscious.

The respiratory muscles (external intercostals and diaphragm) are blocked by relaxants and so ventilation stops. Therefore a means of supporting ventilation must be available, i.e. a cuffed endotracheal tube and a suitable breathing system.

There are two types of relaxant based on their mechanism of action: depolarising and non-depolarising drugs.

Depolarising drugs

Succinylcholine has a rapid onset time (seconds) and is short-acting (3–5 minutes) in horses, pigs, cats and people. It is used to facilitate endotracheal intubation in humans, pigs and cats, or induction of anaesthesia in horses.

Non-depolarising drugs

Many types of non-depolarising drug have been used in veterinary practice and some have more or less fallen out of use:

- D-tubocurarine is seldom used these days because injection causes histamine release in dogs, with vasodilatation, hypotension, tachycardia and bronchial spasm.
- Gallamine became unpopular because of tachycardia and hypertension after injection. Prolonged relaxation occurs with animals in renal failure.
- Alcuronium, a long-acting relaxant, is occasionally used nowadays.
- Pancuronium, once the most popular relaxant, with intermediate onset and long duration of action (more than 30 minutes), causes modest tachycardia after injection but remains a useful agent.
- Vecuronium, a popular drug, derived from pancuronium, has an intermediate duration of action (20–30 minutes). It has little cumulative effects after repeated doses and little, if any, cardiovascular effects. It is commonly used.
- Atracurium is another popular relaxant because of its intermediate duration of action and rapid onset time. Its duration of action is curtailed when the drug molecule spontaneously degrades and so the agent is favoured in animals with diseased elimination pathways (liver and kidneys).

Indications for neuromuscular blockade

High-risk cases

Neuromuscular blockers reduce anaesthetic requirements and so cardiopulmonary function is preserved. Positive-pressure ventilation must be imposed.

Thoracic surgery and diaphragmatic hernia repair

Positive-pressure ventilation can be imposed without neuromuscular blockade. In paralysed animals however, reduced rigidity in the thoracic cage (ribs and diaphragm) means lower inflation pressures can be used.

Laparotomies

During laparotomy, neuromuscular blockers reduce the amount of traction required to produce exposure, causing less tissue trauma on the wound margins with less post-operative inflammation and pain.

Microsurgery

Intraocular and neurological surgery (which is frequently performed under microscopes) requires guaranteed immobility.

Orthopaedics

Neuromuscular blocking drugs may facilitate anaesthetic management during surgery but whether surgery itself is facilitated is debatable.

Inefficient ventilatory pattern

Joint surgery and other procedures occasionally cause bizarre breathing patterns which are inefficient in terms of gas exchange. In these, relaxants allow positive-pressure ventilation to be imposed without the animal 'fighting the ventilator'.

Monitoring blockade

The degree of relaxation is measured using peripheral nerve stimulators. Clinical signs must be used when these are unavailable. Because diaphragmatic and respiratory muscles are relatively resistant to neuromuscular blockers, the first sign of a waning block is diaphragmatic 'twitching'.

Monitoring consciousness

Neuromuscular blockers paralyse facial skeletal muscle and eliminate normal reflexes; after paralysis, the eyelids are open and the eye is central. There are no corneal or palpebral reflexes. In animals which are paralysed but not unconscious, there may be paradoxical jaw tone and mydriasis, lacrimation, salivation, tachycardia and hypertension. When these signs are present, anaesthesia must be deepened by increasing the vaporiser setting or, preferably, by injecting intravenous anaesthetic.

Antagonism

Non-depolarising neuromuscular blockers can be antagonised using one of two combinations of anticholinesterase and antimuscarinic drugs: either edrophonium and atropine or neostigmine and glycopyrrolate.

SUMMARY

- Muscle relaxants specifically block muscle activity at the neuromuscular junction.
- Muscle relaxants include depolarising and non-depolarising neuromuscular blockers.
- Indications include ocular, abdominal and thoracic surgery.
- Adequate abililty to monitor depth of anaesthesia and ensure unconsciousness is essential for their safe use.

Monitoring

The function of important organ systems – central nervous and cardiopulmonary systems – together with body temperature should be monitored continuously and recorded every 5 minutes in order that deleterious trends may be identified and corrected. Details are recorded on an anaesthetic record.

Monitoring central nervous function

Monitoring central nervous function during anaesthesia, a major component of assessing 'depth' of anaesthesia, is an important skill. Animals should be anaesthetised to a depth that only just prevents obvious responses to surgery. This allows surgery to be performed with minimum cardiopulmonary depression. The depth required depends on:

- The procedure being performed. Laparotomy requires 'deeper' anaesthesia than cutaneous tumour removal.
- The specific activity during surgery. In orthopaedics, the level of anaesthesia adequate for skin incision may prove inadequate for fracture manipulation.
- Surgical experience. Lighter levels of anaesthesia suffice when minimal traction and force are used.

Consequently, monitoring surgical events is an important aid to monitoring the 'level' of anaesthesia. The 'signs' of anaesthesia are based on:

- Cranial nerve reflexes
  - Palpebral reflex: a 'blink' occurs when the medial canthus of the eye is stroked with a finger. If the test is repeated too frequently, the reflex becomes sluggish
  - Corneal reflex: 'blinking' also occurs when the cornea is gently touched with a moistened cotton bud.
  - Jaw tone: tension in the jaws indicates light levels of anaesthesia.
  - Tongue curl: during 'light' anaesthesia, the tongue curls when the jaws are opened.
  - Eye position: the globe may be ventromedial or central within the orbit.
  - Pupillary diameter: dilatation (mydriasis) or constriction (miosis) reflects various levels of anaesthesia.
  - Lacrimation: the eye becomes dry at deep levels of anaesthesia.
  - Salivation: profuse salivation indicates inadequate anaesthesia.
- Rate and pattern of respiration. The rate, depth and pattern of respiration are altered by the level of anaesthesia and the degree of surgical stimulation.
- Autonomic responses. Heart rate, blood pressure, pupillary diameter and capillary refill time are influenced by the interaction between anaesthetic depth and surgical stimulation.
- Skeletomuscular tone and response to toe pinch.

Stages in anaesthesia

For convenience, the 'depth' of anaesthesia has been categorised into four stages, although this is somewhat arbitrary because it is based on observations in humans anaesthetised with ether.

Stage I (stage of voluntary excitement or analgesia). This begins with induction and lasts until unconsciousness is present. The animal resists induction, shows signs of apprehension and fear but later becomes disorientated. Signs reflect a generalised sympatho-adrenal response to threat. Pulse and respiratory rates are elevated although breath-holding may occur if irritant or pungent vapours are given. The pupil is dilated. Skeletal muscle activity may be marked and hyper-reflexia present. The animal may vocalise, salivate, defecate and urinate.

Stage II (stage of involuntary excitement). This lasts from the onset of unconsciousness until rhythmic breathing is present. All cranial nerve reflexes are present and may be hyperactive. Initially the eye is wide open and the pupil dilated. Later, eyes begin to rotate to a ventromedial position. Responses to toe pinch reflexes are brisk. Breathing is irregular and gasping but later becomes regular.

Stages I and II are unpleasant for the patient and hazardous for the anaesthetist. They are likely when mask induction is attempted on non-sedated animals or when inadequate doses of injectable anaesthetic are given. An elegant induction passes through these stages rapidly. This is achieved by adequate pre-anaesthetic sedative medication and/or sufficient anaesthetic for induction.

Stage III (surgical anaesthesia). This is subdivided into three planes:

- *Plane 1.* Respiration is regular and deep. Minute volume is proportional to surgical stimulation. Spontaneous limb movement is absent but pinch reflexes are brisk. Nystagmus, the lateral oscillation of the eyeball, slows and stops by the end of Plane 1; however, it is not always present. Eyeball position in the orbit is ventromedial; opening the eye reveals mainly sclera. The third eyelid moves part way across the corneal surface. Palpebral reflexes begin to slow but the corneal reflex is brisk. Cardiovascular function is only slightly depressed. This plane is suitable for abscess lancing and superficial surgery like skin suturing and cutaneous tumour removal.
- *Plane 2.* Eye position is ventromedial and the eyelids may be partially separated. The palpebral reflex is sluggish or absent although corneal reflexes persist. The conjunctival surface is moist and the pupil constricted. Muscle relaxation is more apparent. The pedal reflex becomes sluggish and ultimately is lost. Tidal volume is decreased; rate may be increased or decreased. The heart rate and blood pressure may be modestly reduced. This plane is adequate for most surgery except some laparotomy and thoracotomy.
- *Plane 3.* The eyeball becomes central and the eyelids begin to open. The pupillary diameter increases. Respiratory rate increases; tidal volume is decreased. A pause appears between inspiration and expiration (intercostal lag). The pedal reflex is lost and abdominal muscles are relaxed. Heart rate and blood pressure are lowered. This plane is adequate for all procedures.

Stage IV (overdosage). Characterised by progressive respiratory failure, which begins when ventilation is achieved by diaphragmatic function alone; this eventually ceases. The pulse may be rapid or very slow and becomes impalpable. The eye becomes central, the eyelids open, the pupils are maximally dilated and the corneal surface is dry. Cyanosis progresses to a grey or ashen colour of the mucous membrane. Capillary refill time becomes prolonged. Accessory respiratory muscle activity, indicated by twitching in the throat, represents agonal gasping. This superficially mimics gasping, or inadequate anaesthesia.

Overdosage

Excessive levels of anaesthesia should be avoided because they contribute to prolonged recovery. They also cause unnecessary cardiopulmonary depression, which in turn limits organ perfusion, causing post-operative organ failure. Ultimately it results in cardiac arrest.

Underdosage

Underdosage is equally undesirable. In response to surgery, heart rate increases and respiration becomes rapid and shallow (tachypnoea). Blood pressure rises and increased oozing at the surgical site may be noticed. Capillary refill time may become prolonged and the mucous membranes lose colour. The pupils dilate and spontaneous cranial nerve reflex activity may be seen; lacrimation and salivation may be profuse.

Maintaining inadequate levels of anaesthesia because of inexperience or to ensure that the animals 'stays alive' must be avoided because:

- The animal may recover consciousness.
- Movement will compromise delicate surgery, or the animal may extubate itself.
- Catecholamine release may cause arrhythmias, and even cardiac arrest.
- Tachypnoea may impair gas exchange and uptake of anaesthetics. Alternatively, hyperventilation may cause alkalosis.

Monitoring cardiovascular function

Assessing cardiovascular variables continuously provides information on the adequacy of anaesthesia, on the effects of surgery (haemorrhage, inadequate anaesthesia, untoward reflexes) and on cardiovascular function itself.

Monitoring can be performed by techniques which do or do not involve invasion of the body cavity. Non-invasive methods, which include clinical observation, are simpler, less expensive and more easily applied but the received information is more subjective.

Heart rate and rhythm

- *Palpation of superficial arteries.* These include the femoral, the lingual, the nasal (in the cheek), the ulnar (medio-caudal carpus), the palmar metacarpal (palmar surface of the paw), the cranial tibial (on the dorso-lateral hock) and the plantar branch of the saphenous (plantar paw) arteries.
- *Palpation of apex beat.* Useful in very small companion animals and laboratory animals, or when hypotension makes peripheral pulses impalpable.

- *Cardiac auscultation.* Auscultation of the heart gives information on myocardial contractility and valve action as well as rate and rhythm. While heart sounds may be heard with standard (precordial) stethoscopes, these tend to fall off even when adhesive tape is used. Oesophageal stethoscopes are less prone to displacement.
- *Electrocardiography.* Electrocardiograms (ECGs) show the pattern of electrical activity in the heart and demonstrate arrhythmias. Unlike heart sounds or pulse palpation, they provide no evidence of mechanical activity or cardiac output (which is more important in terms of O_2 delivery). Heart rate meters are simplified ECGs which register the larger 'R' waves. From this, a heart rate output is generated in beats per minute and there may be an audible signal. These devices are prone to counting artefacts and occasionally count large 'T' waves, in which case the displayed rate is double the true rate.

Pulse rhythm may be regularly irregular with respiration, which is normal. Grossly irregular rhythm with pulse deficits may indicate atrial fibrillation or ventricular ectopic activity.

Pulse quality. The pulsation felt indicates the pulse pressure and is the difference between systolic and diastolic arterial blood pressure (ABP). It gives an indication of the adequacy of cardiac function and generally a strong pulse indicates good cardiac output and peripheral perfusion. Arterial pulses are felt at the sites listed above. Nurses should aim to judge pulse quality using small peripheral arteries (like the lingual artery) because pulsations in these are lost at higher pressures than those in larger vessels like the femoral artery. This gives earlier warning of developing hypotension. For this reason routine use of the femoral pulse or apex beat should be reserved for cats and very small dogs.

Arterial blood pressure

Indirect measurement. Indirect methods are based on a cuff applied around a limb/tail inflating above systolic pressure and deflating until a peripheral pulse is detected again distal to the cuff (Riva–Rocci technique). The pressure registered on a manometer connected to the cuff indicates systolic pressure when the pulse first returns distal to the cuff. Cuff width should be about 40–60% of limb circumference. Wider cuffs transmit pressure more efficiently and above an optimum width frictional resistance to blood flow means excessively low pressures are required to allow blood to flow through the once occluded segment. Wide cuffs underestimate pressure, narrow cuffs overestimate.

- *Ultrasonic Doppler/sphygmomanometry.* A Doppler ultrasound flow detector probe placed over a peripheral artery emits an ultrasonic frequency; the sound is reflected back off moving arterial red blood cells at a different frequency (the Doppler effect), which is in the audible range. When a cuff is applied proximal to the detector and occluded to above systolic pressure the detected sound ceases. Deflation to just below systolic ABP restores the audible sound; further deflation until a double swoosh sound occurs (Korotkoff sounds) indicates the diastolic ABP. It is simple, cheap, and reliable, but requires an operator.
- *Oscillometric sphygmomanometry.* This non-invasive technique involves a pneumatic cuff which encircles a limb, occluding the cuff and sensing the ABP. As the cuff is deflated and blood starts to pulse through the cuff, the cuff senses this oscillation. The point of return of pulsation is the systolic pressure: maximum oscillation corresponds to mean pressure, and continuous flow indicates diastolic pressure. They are automated and easily used, but are less reliable in hypotensive states, and are expensive.

Direct measurement. This is the gold standard method. A catheter is aseptically placed in an accessible artery (dorsal pedal, metatarsal, femoral, digital, middle auricular, facial, transverse facial). It is connected via a heparin saline column to an anaeroid manometer or to a strain-gauge pressure transducer, amplifier and oscilloscope. The former is cheap but only indicates mean ABP. The electronic system provides systolic and diastolic pressures as well and a pulse waveform. Arterial catheters also allow blood gas analysis.

Capillary refill time

Blanching the oral mucous membrane and waiting for blood to return reflects the capillary refill time (CRT). Normally, this is less than 2 seconds. Intensive vasoconstriction or hypotension delays CRT.

Mucous membrane colour

This should be pink. It becomes bright pink in hypercapnia and blue with cyanosis (desaturation of haemoglobin). When blood pressure falls and blood vessels in the mucosa constrict, it turns white.

Haemoglobin saturation

Pulse oximetry is a relatively new and readily applied non-invasive monitoring technique that measures the oxygen saturation of haemoglobin (S_pO_2). Measurement involves applying a clip to the animal's tongue or lip. Some devices illustrate the passage of blood between each side of the clip by a bar plethysmograph; the amplitude of this moving column is proportional to the pulse pressure and demonstrates cardiac mechanical activity.

Perfusion

The passage of blood through capillary beds is assessed in a number of ways.

- *Combination of vital signs.* Pulse pressure, capillary refill time and pulse oximetry.

- *Examination of the surgical site*. Bright red blood at the surgical site indicates perfusion. Darkly coloured or slowly oozing blood reflects poor perfusion.
- *Core–periphery temperature difference*. Cold ears and extremities may indicate that the animal is hypothermic or that warm blood is being retained at the 'core' and withheld from non-essential tissue like skin. This phenomenon is quantified by the simultaneous use of two calibrated thermistors placed at appropriate sites, e.g. over the base of the heart via the oesophagus and on the lip.
- *Urine output*. Catheterising the urinary bladder and weighing collected urine (1 ml urine weighs 1 g) indicates urine output. A value in excess of 1 ml/kg/h is held to represent adequate renal perfusion, and therefore vital organ perfusion.

Monitoring respiratory function

Respiration is assessed in terms of rate, depth and pattern. Rate and pattern reflect depth of anaesthesia; the combinations of rate and depth indicate alveolar ventilation. As a rule, rapid shallow respirations are inefficient for gas exchange. Preferably, breathing should be slow and deep.

Observation

Rate, rhythm and pattern are assessed visually. This is difficult when heavy draping is used but observing the excursions (range of movement) of the reservoir bag helps. Excursions are seen more easily in smaller bags.

Respiratory monitors

Most of these monitors operate on the temperature difference between inspired (cold) and expired (warm) gas. They only indicate rate and give no indication of ventilatory adequacy. They are useful when surgeons must operate without assistance. Some respiratory monitors rely on expired CO_2 (capnography). The definitive test for respiratory adequacy relies on arterial blood gas analysis.

Monitoring temperature

Rectal temperature measured with a clinical (mercury in glass) thermometer is the simplest but not the most convenient technique. Flexible thermistor probes inserted per rectum or per os (to the base of the heart) are preferable.

General management

Other activities during the maintenance period include the following.

Monitoring surgery

Stimulating events should be anticipated. Haemorrhage must be continuously assessed. Liaison with the surgeon is vital during complicated surgery, e.g. a thoracotomy.

Monitoring fluid administration

If fluids are being given, administration rates should be checked periodically. If a catheter is in place but fluids are not given, it should be flushed with heparin–saline at 15-minute intervals.

'Sighing'

'Sighing' means delivering a supramaximal lung inflation at 5-minute intervals. It:

- Prevents diffuse pulmonary microatalectasis.
- Allows appraisal of compliance (low – surgical instrument, assistants on thorax, kinking of tube; high – disconnection, cuff leak).
- Reduces hypercapnia and hypoxia.
- Provides the inexperienced with the opportunity to develop manual ventilation skills.

Monitoring the breathing system

The system must be continuously monitored for behaviour, disconnection, soda-lime, valve action, etc. The pilot balloon of the endotracheal tube must be periodically checked to ensure the cuff remains gas-tight.

Monitoring gas flows and vaporiser settings

Flowmeters may 'drift' with time and should be constantly checked. Vaporiser fluid levels, settings and temperature should also be monitored. Cylinder contents must be continuously assessed.

SUMMARY

- Careful monitoring is essential for safe anaesthesia.
- Prevention of complications and assessment of intraoperative therapy can be performed.
- Monitoring depth of anaesthesia relies primarily on assessment of indirect signs suggestive of appropriate anaesthesia.
- Monitoring of cardiovascular and respiratory function is used to ensure physiological well-being of the patient.
- Monitoring should continue into the recovery period.

Special anaesthesia

Many animals with severe physiological disturbances present for procedures requiring general anaesthesia. Each procedure carries its own individual risks; however the anaesthetic approach should be similar. Careful pre-operative assessment and stabilisation (where possible) are required. Anaesthesia should be smooth with minimal disruption of physiological function. Careful attention to the recovery period should be given.

General considerations

Pre-operative assessment

Careful patient evaluation is important. Consider cardiovascular, respiratory, liver and renal function and concurrent therapy.

Pre-operative stabilisation

Aspects include fluid therapy and electrolyte and acid–base stabilisation, oxygen therapy for hypoxaemia and blood products for anaemia, clotting defects, and protein deficits. Also analgesia, antibiosis and specific procedures may be required, e.g. stomach decompression in GDV.

General anaesthesia

The high risk patient is less able to tolerate physiological disturbance. Hence it is important to maintain normal physiological status especially cardiovascular, respiratory and thermoregulatory. Preoxygenation with a face mask prior to induction of anaesthesia may be beneficial. Anaesthetic agents have a more profound effect in the debilitated animal; reduce doses and give slowly to effect. Careful monitoring is important to alert to dangers and allow rapid correction.

Recovery

This is frequently neglected. Monitoring should be continued with fluid therapy, rewarming and analgesia when appropriate.

Anaesthesia of the neonate

Neonates are defined as immature animals less than 12 weeks of age. Significant differences exist from the mature animal. Their size often leads to overdose and immature body systems make them more sensitive to anaesthetics and less able to accommodate to alterations in their normal function. An understanding of these differences is necessary for safe anaesthetic management.

Physiological considerations

- *Respiratory system*. Oxygen consumption is 2–3 times that of the adult, minute ventilation about 3 times that of the adult, there is a greater risk of airway obstruction, and alveolar collapse is more likely. Careful IPPV may be appropriate but excessive pressure may cause damage. Neonates 4–14 weeks are allowed to ventilate spontaneously.
- *Cardiovascular system*. The myocardium is less contractile, the baroreceptors are immature, and there is a predominance of parasympathetic nervous system activity. Haemoglobin concentrations are lower and the erythrocytes have a shorter life span. Thus neonates are less able to increase force of contraction to meet changes in demand; increases in cardiac output are heart rate dependent. Hypotension is a particular problem and neonates are less able to cope with blood loss.
- *Hepatorenal function*. Enzyme systems are immature or absent. Hypoglycaemia is likely. Renal function is immature, thus there is poor concentrating function and reduced ability to tolerate dehydration. Maximum preparatory starvation of 2–3 hours is suggested. Intraoperative fluids preferably include glucose, e.g. dextrose–saline.
- *Thermoregulation*. Neonates have immature thermoregulatory control, with reduced shivering ability and reliance on non-shivering thermogenesis. A large surface area to volume ratio and less subcutaneous fat exist. Hence neonates are prone to hypothermia.
- *Pharmacokinetics*. Low albumin and a larger percentage body water, lower body fat, and reduced hepatorenal function affect the pharmacology of drugs used. Low plasma proteins increase the effect of unbound drugs and increase sensitivity to protein-bound drugs, as the active drug is the unbound portion. In general the dose of parenteral drugs needs to be reduced in the neonate.

Anaesthesia

Premedication can include anticholinergics to maintain heart rate and reduce respiratory secretion. Sedatives should be use sparingly. Benzodiazepines are useful, though often sedation is poor. Below 10 weeks, acepromazine is best avoided. Alpha-2-adrenoceptor agonists are potent sedatives and best avoided. Analgesics such as opiates are useful, though may have prolonged action and a reduced dose may be appropriate.

Induction of anaesthesia can be achieved by injectable or inhaled methods. The latter is generally more stressful. Barbiturates rely on redistribution for a significant degree of recovery from them. With less body fat and reduced metabolic function prolonged recoveries are likely in the neonate. Dissociative agents, e.g. ketamine, can be used. Propofol produces smooth induction of anaesthesia and a relatively rapid recovery and may be preferred. 'Saffan' may be useful in cats but prolonged recovery may be seen.

Maintenance with inhalation anaesthesia is recommended for all but the shortest procedures. Isoflurane with lower blood gas solubility than halothane, less reliance on metabolism in the liver, less myocardial depression and more rapid recovery is preferred over halothane. Caution is required with endotracheal intubation; the larynx is more susceptible to trauma and the tube is more liable to obstruction.

Anaesthesia of the geriatric

As for the neonate, ageing affects physiological function and anaesthesia. Age results in a reduced capacity for adaptation and reduced functional reserves of organ systems. Though not a disease itself, it is frequently accompanied by systemic disease.

General considerations

- *CNS.* There are generally reduced requirements for anaesthetics.
- *Respiratory system.* Reduced tidal volume, and efficiency of gas exchange, increase the risk of hypoxia.
- *Cardiovascular changes.* The maximum heart rate falls with age and the response to stress/catecholamines is reduced. Geriatrics are poorly tolerant of volume depletion.
- *Renal system.* Tubular function is reduced and the renin–angiotensin system less responsive. Renally excreted drugs are more slowly eliminated.
- *Hepatic system.* Clearance decreases with decreasing liver mass.
- *Thermoregulation.* Geriatrics are prone to hypothermia.
- *Pharmacokinetic considerations.* Contracted blood volume increases plasma concentration of intravenous agents. Protein binding is reduced due to reduced albumen in plasma. Protein bound drugs are more active (less bound).

Anaesthesia

There is no one ideal protocol. Attention to the amount of drug given and the effect of the drug administered is important. Administer drugs slowly to effect. Increased sensitivity to compromised renal blood flow makes them more prone to renal failure post-operatively. Monitor blood pressure, infuse fluids intraoperatively.

Avoid heavy premedication as it can significantly compromise the patient and prolong recovery. Caution with alpha-2-adrenoceptor agonists again, as they are potent sedatives, causing significant depression of cardiopulmonary function. Benzodiazepines are useful. A rapid smooth induction and calm recovery are preferred. Barbiturates may be associated with a prolonged recovery in patients with significant liver pathology. Propofol provides a good rapid recovery with extrahepatic metabolism and 'Saffan' appears acceptable in cats. The shorter the procedures the better. Attention to heat loss and fluid therapy are important. Inhalation anaesthesia with isoflurane provides a more rapid recovery, but halothane is still acceptable.

Anaesthesia for caesarean section

Anaesthesia for caesarean section is often an emergency without time for extensive preparation. Both dam and foetal viability are important considerations.

General considerations

Maternal physiology. Pregnancy alters maternal physiology:

- *CNS.* Increased sensitivity to inhalation agents occurs.
- *Respiratory system.* Increased alveolar ventilation, reduced functional residual capacity due to anterior displacement of the diaphragm and increased oxygen consumption are seen. Hence there is increased inhalation agent uptake but also the tendency to hypoxia and hypercapnia.
- *Cardiovascular system.* Aortocaval compression can occur in dorsal recumbency. Increased blood volume (30%), reduced haematocrit and plasma proteins, increased cardiac output (30–50%) and reduced total peripheral resistance occur. There are reduced cardiac reserves and relative anaemia. The dam is less tolerant of cardiovascular compromise.
- *Gastrointestinal system.* Increased gastric acidity, cranial displacement of stomach by the uterus and altered tone in the lower oesophageal sphincter make the dam more prone to regurgitation, vomiting and aspiration pneumonia.

Uteroplacental circulation and foetal viability

Reduced uterine blood flow reduces placental perfusion and induces foetal hypoxia. This is particularly seen with shock and hypovolaemia, dehydration, and after administration of drugs such as oxytocin and ergotmetrine. Stress and catecholamines release can vasoconstrict the uterus.

Foetal tissues. The umbilical vein goes to the liver and also the ductus venosus. The former metabolises much before it reaches the foetal circulation, the latter goes to vena cava diluting drugs administered. The foetal circulation attempts to protect vital tissues from exposure to sudden high concentrations of drugs.

Drugs. Most drugs are transferred rapidly across the placenta and may depress the foetus or neonate after parturition.

Pre-operative preparation

This includes clipping if not stressful, to reduce anaesthesia time. Pre-operative fluid therapy is indicated if shocked. Starvation is not always possible. Positioning in off dorsal-recumbancy reduces aortacaval compression.

Anaesthesia

The goals of anaesthesia are smooth anaesthesia with rapid recovery of the dam to consciousness to allow nursing, and delivery of viable alert neonates ready to feed. Minimal sedation if possible is preferred. Induction of anaesthesia should be smooth and rapid, with endotracheal intubation. Barbiturates inhibit foetal respiration which may be significant if delivered soon after induction. Recovery of the dam and neonate may be delayed. Propofol gives a rapid and smooth induction and recovery and is recommended. 'Saffan' in cats causes minimal respiratory depression, and is also adequate. Ketamine produces minimal foetal depression but may result in disorientated kittens. Inhalation induction is potentially stressful; if used, intubation must be rapid. For maintenance of anaesthesia, inhalation anaesthesia is recommended, and isoflurane is preferred over halothane for a more rapid recovery. A light plane of anaesthesia should minimise dose-dependent cardiorespiratory depression and reduce the potential for foetal hypoxia. It is important to maintain blood pressure to protect the foetal circulation. Post-operative pain relief should be administered.

Neonate resuscitation requires adequate help. Clean mucous from the upper airways, administer oxygen if required, stimulate the skin, prevent cooling and if bleeding clamp or tie off cord. Aim to get the neonate feeding as soon as possible.

Anaesthesia for the pyometra

The bitch with pyometritis often presents dull and depressed. Closed pyometritis in which the mucopurulent discharge accumulates in the uterus can be life-threatening. Presurgical stabilisation is important; however, complete stabilisation is often impossible prior to removal of the septic focus.

General considerations

- *Shock.* This is a major concern. Hypovolaemia develops via fluid loss to the uterus combined with losses via vomiting and the kidneys. Toxaemia can induce septic shock, see Endotoxic shock, p. 582.
- *Renal disease.* Prerenal ureamia due to hypovolaemia, glomerular disease associated with antibody–antigen complexes and tubular disease due to toxins and immune complexes all interfere with the ability to concentrate urine. Concurrent renal disease of the old bitch may be present.
- *Acid–base and electrolyte disorders.* Metabolic acidosis is common with sodium and potassium loss.
- *Bone marrow suppression and clotting disorders.* Reduced erythrocyte and platelet production occurs. Anaemia is common. Clotting disorders may occur.
- *Liver disorders.* Hepatocellular damage develops due to intrahepatic cholestasis and bile pigment retention. Damage can also be secondary to endotoxaemia, dehydration and shock.
- *Arrhythmias* may be present, induced by toxins.

Pre-operative preparation

Fluid therapy (see p. 584) is essential to restore circulating blood volume, protect renal function, and correct electrolyte and acid–base disorders. Potassium may need to be supplemented. Broad-spectrum antibiosis should be commenced. Platelet-rich plasma, whole blood or red blood cells may be required if there is thrombocytopaenia, low plasma proteins, clotting disorders or anaemia.

Anaesthesia

Premedication should cause minimal depression. Sedation is often unnecessary though benzodiazepines may be beneficial to reduce the induction agent dose required. Analgesia is recommended, e.g. morphine or buprenorphine, to reduce intra-operative and post-operative pain. Induction of anaesthesia should be smooth with minimal cardiopulmonary depression. Most injectable anaesthetics are acceptable though at a reduced dose. Maintenance with inhalation anaesthesia with isoflurane or halothane is preferred. Attention to monitoring and intra-operative fluid therapy are important. Post-operatively fluid therapy may be required as well as further analgesia with opiates.

Anaesthesia for gastrointestinal emergencies: gastric-dilatation-volvulus (GDV)

GDV is an acute emergency of the large dog with a high incidence of mortality (12–43%). Though complete stabilisation prior to surgery is often impossible, a significant degree of stabilisation dramatically reduces complications/ mortality.

General considerations

- *Respiratory compromise.* Ventilation is compromised by the dilated stomach. Endotoxic mediators can disrupt ventilation/perfusion balance compromising gas exchange in the lungs. Pulmonary oedema can occur.
- *Cardiovascular disturbances.* Compression of the caudal vena cava and portal veins, and pooling of blood in splanchnic, renal and capillary beds, reduces venous return and cardiac output. Cellular hypoxia and metabolic acidosis result. Circulating catecholamines, release of myocardial depressant factor and endotoxin, myocardial hypoxia and ischaemia, metabolic acidosis and electrolyte disturbances all predispose to arrhythmias and myocardial depression.
- *Endotoxaemia.* Ischaemic injury to the gut compromises the mucosal barrier, with increased absorption of endotoxin. Liver clearance of endotoxin is reduced. Shock can ensue with disseminated intravascular coagulation and multiple organ failure.
- *Gastric damage.* Increased intraluminal pressure and reduced gastric perfusion result in gastric ischaemia. Mucosal compromise allows leakage of plasma proteins resulting in hypoproteinaemia and oedema.

Pre-operative preparation

Shock therapy is essential prior to anaesthesia. Aggressive intravenous fluid therapy to restore circulating blood volume is required. Crystalloids, e.g. lactated Ringer's (up to 90 ml/kg/h) can be used alone or combined with colloids and hypertonic saline (7.5% 4 ml/kg). Positive inotropes for hypotension unresponsive to fluids alone may be required. Correction of acidosis and electrolyte disturbances (especially hyperkalaemia) is necessary. The administration of steroids or NSAIDs remains controversial. Gastric decompression with an orogastric tube with gastric lavage can dramatically improve cardiopulmonary function. Alternatively percutaneous trocar placement (18G needle) or a gastrotomy may be required. Oxygen therapy should be given if the patient is hypoxic. Antibiosis is appropriate as the mucosal barrier may be compromised. Antacids, e.g. ranitidine or cimetidine, have been suggested. Control of cardiac arrhythmias may be necessary.

Anaesthesia

Premedication again is rarely required. Minimal cardiovascular depression is essential during induction of anaesthesia. Arrhythmias are likely. An opioid/benzodiazepine combination is good, e.g. fentanyl 1–2 μg/kg + diazepam 0.1–0.2 mg/kg (intravenously). Alternatively a benzodiazepine followed by a reduced dose of propofol given slowly is acceptable. Maintenance of anaesthesia with isoflurane is preferred, it is less arrhythmogenic and causes less cardiovascular depression than halothane. Nitrous oxide should be avoided until the stomach is decompressed as it partitions into gas-filled bodies. Careful monitoring is essential and fluid therapy should be continued. During recovery complications are frequent. Monitoring is important. Fluid therapy for shock should be continued. Arrhythmias in the postoperative period are common and may require therapy. Anaemia may result from significant blood loss. Reperfusion injury may occur as a result of bowel mucosal ischaemia occurring due to gastric torsion, with release of oxygen free radicals and superoxide ions after reperfusion of the compromised bowel.

SUMMARY

- Careful pre-operative assessment of the patient is required.
- Pre-operative stabilisation of the systemically ill patient can reduce anaesthetic complications.
- Increased sensitivity to anaesthetic-induced cardiopulmonary depression may occur.
- Continuous monitoring is important.
- Further stabilisation and therapy may be required post-operatively.

Accidents and emergencies

Peri-operative emergencies

Accidents are generally avoidable problems, affecting patients or personnel and sometimes involving equipment. Problems may be of minor consequence individually but collectively they may create emergencies. Emergencies are crises that require rapid responses, as they quickly lead to cardiopulmonary arrest.

Cardiopulmonary arrest occurs when cardiac output fails to meet the body's requirements.

DEFINITIONS

- **Apnoea**: the arrest of breathing.
- **Hypoventilation**: reduced aveolar ventilation.
- **Tachypnoea**: excessive frequency of respiration.
- **Bradypnoea**: excessive slowness of respiration.
- **Hypoxia**: lack of oxygen.
- **Hypercapnia**: excess of carbon dioxide in lungs or blood.
- **Tachycardia**: excessive heart (and pulse) rate.
- **Bradycardia**: excessive slowness of heart (and pulse) rate.
- **Arrhythmia**: irregular heart beat (and pulse).
- **Hypotension**: low arterial blood pressure.
- **Haemorrhage**: bleeding.
- **Hypothermia**: low body temperature.

Apnoea and hypoventilation

Apnoea is a dire emergency: severe hypoxia and hypercapnia rapidly cause cardiac arrest. The circumstances in which it occurs are:

- An acute event that prevents breathing (e.g. pneumothorax, upper airway obstruction, intravenous anaesthetic overdose).
- As the end result of progressive hypoventilation.
- As a sign of cardiac arrest.

When the heart stops, breathing continues for some seconds until medullary ischaemia causes apnoea. Signs of apnoea include absence of breathing or irregular gasping with twitching neck muscles and spasmodic diaphragm contractions.

- In conscious animals the neck is extended, the mouth is wide open, the eyes are staring and the pupil is dilated. Mucous membranes are blue or dirty grey.
- In anaesthetised animals, only ineffectual breathing attempts, discoloured mucous membranes and signs of overdosage may be present.

There are three possible causes of hypoventilation and apnoea (Fig. 23.13) and elements of all three are usually present during surgery:

- Failure of the brain to respond to carbon dioxide or oxygen.
- Airway obstruction (partial or complete).
- Chest-wall fixation.

Failure of the brain to respond to gases. This occurs:

- In severe head trauma.
- When intracranial pressure is raised (e.g. by tumours or by inflammatory processes).

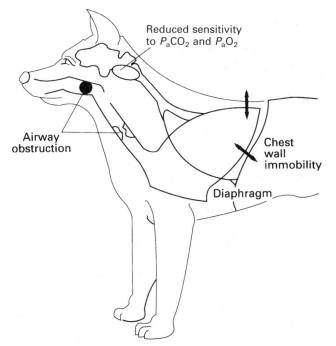

Fig. 23.13 Causes of apnoea and hypoventilation.

- In anaesthetic overdose.
- In severe hypothermia.

The most common cause of hypoventilation is profound anaesthesia, which reduces medullary sensitivity to carbon dioxide and abolishes chemoreceptor stimulation by hypoxia. The deeper the level of anaesthesia, the greater the degree of respiratory depression. Hypoventilation under anaesthesia is exacerbated by hypothermia.

Transient apnoea is common after induction with propofol and thiopentone. While spontaneous respirations resume in the course of time, lung inflations should be imposed if gross signs of overdose or mucous membrane discoloration are observed.

Bradypnoea is caused by:

- Deep anaesthesia.
- Opioids.
- Hypothermia.
- Elevated intracranial pressure.

Reduced aveolar ventilation rate results from reduced tidal volume and/or reduced respiratory rate. Conversely, very high respiratory rates with low tidal volumes (tachypnoea) also cause hypoventilation because inspired gas does not reach the alveoli. Tachypnoea results from:

- Inadequate anaesthesia.
- Pyrexia.
- Hypoxia.
- Hypercapnia.
- Restrictive lung lesions.

Airway obstruction. Airway obstruction in the non-intubated animal contributes to hypoventilation because it causes turbulent gas flow, which increases resistance to breathing. Similarly, undersized endotracheal tubes increase resistance to breathing.

Partial or total obstruction is indicated by inspiratory snoring noises and/or paradoxical thoracic wall movement during inspiration (the abdomen moves outwards and the chest wall inwards). The airway might be obstructed in several ways:

- *Soft-tissue obstruction.* This is likely in brachycephalic breeds whenever sedatives or anaesthetics depress reflex control of oropharyngeal and nasopharyngeal muscles. Sedated brachycephalics must be observed closely and endotracheal intubation performed once consciousness is lost. During recovery, the return of gag reflexes indicates the need for extubation. Thereafter, surveillance must continue because obstruction remains possible. It must be appreciated that oxygen by mask is ineffective during obstruction. Transtracheal oxygen or tracheotomy is required until the block is relieved. During recovery, sustained airway protective reflexes may be restored rapidly in cases at risk of obstruction by using drugs with little residual effect, by antagonists or analeptics.
- *Blood and debris.* Obstruction also results from mycotic or neoplastic lesions, or from blood clots after nasal and dental surgery. After surgery involving the oropharynx, nasopharynx or any part of the upper airway, surgical debris must be cleared before the animal recovers and is extubated.
- *Vomit.* Regurgitation may occur during induction or postoperatively. Rarely, passive regurgitation occurs during surgery. When there is regurgitation, the animal must be positioned head-down. If it remains conscious, its mouth is gagged and the oropharynx cleared of material. Initially, dry swabs held with towel forceps or haemostats will suffice. Later, moistened swabs may be needed. If consciousness is lost, cursory pharyngeal lavage must be followed by endotracheal intubation and positive pressure ventilation with oxygen. Endobronchial suction and lavage is then performed. After passive regurgitation in the unconscious animal, oesophageal lavage may be required because debilitating oesophageal strictures may develop later.
- *Fluid–pulmonary oedema.* A froth-filled airway indicates pulmonary oedema which results from end-stage left-heart failure or, rarely, after use of 'Saffan' in cats. Endobronchial suction should be performed, even though the prognosis is poor.
- *Bronchospasm.* Severe bronchospasm (status asthmaticus) is fortunately a rare cause of airway obstruction in companion animals but in theory could occur in response to histamine-releasing drugs, e.g. high doses of pethidine or morphine given intravenously.
- *Endotracheal tube problems.* The presence of endotracheal tubes does not guarantee an adequate airway. Overinflated cuffs may cause the lumen to collapse, or extreme neck positions may cause kinking. Unless gagged, lightly anaesthetised animals may bite the tube and close the lumen.

Chest-wall fixation. Breathing ceases when the chest wall and diaphragm are immobilised. In pneumothorax, the thorax is expanded to capacity by gas accumulation in the pleural space, resulting in apnoea. Neuromuscular blockers eliminate chest-wall and diaphragmatic activity.

Some breathing systems have expiratory valves. If these are inadvertently left closed, there is a rapid build-up in circuit pressure, preventing expiration and causing rapid death.

In very small animals, breathing may be suppressed when the chest wall is 'stiffened' by heavy drapes, when surgeons rest heavy instruments on the chest, or when the chest wall is covered by adipose tissue. Breathing is also inhibited by restrictive post-operative bandages and by pain after road traffic accidents or thoracotomy.

Treatment of apnoea or hypoventilation. If the cause of apnoea or hypoventilation is in doubt, the trachea is intubated and a breathing system is connected. The level of anaesthesia is assessed. Anaesthetic administration is ended if cranial nerve signs indicate overdosage.

The lungs are then inflated at a rate of 8–15 breaths per minute. If this is possible without high pressure being needed, the cause is probably upper airway obstruction or central nervous depression. If the lungs feel 'stiff', there is probably pneumothorax or bronchospasm.

If the animal does not breathe after 5 minutes or so, imposed hyperventilation may have caused hypocapnia. In this case the respiratory rate should be reduced.

Opioid antagonists (naloxone) or analeptics (doxapram) may be considered as a last resort. Doxapram stimulates respiration and elevates consciousness but its use is futile when respiratory embarrassment is caused by chest-wall fixation or airway obstruction. Its effects are short-lived and so the drug is only useful for 'buying time'. It can be infused for a longer effect.

Tachycardia and bradycardia

The causes and treatment of these two conditions are given in Table 23.8.

Arrhythmias

Irregularities in heart rhythm may reduce cardiac output and cause hypotension. Without treatment some rhythms may deteriorate into more dangerous forms associated with cardiac arrest (e.g. ventricular fibrillation).

Causes. Arrhythmias are caused by inadequate anaesthesia or overdosage, electrolyte and blood-gas abnormalities, certain surgical procedures and pre-existing heart disease. Certain medical conditions like gastric-dilatation-volvulus complex are associated with ventricular arrhythmias.

Treatment. This depends primarily on electrocardiography and is based on antiarrhythmic drugs. Often, ensuring an adequate level of anaesthesia and ventilation restores normal rhythm.

Table 23.8 Treating tachycardia and bradycardia

Cause	Treatment
Tachycardia	
Inadequate anaesthesia	Increase vaporiser setting or give intravenous anaesthetic.
Hypoxia	End nitrous oxide administration (if used) and ventilate with 100% oxygen.
Hypercapnia	Ventilate with 100% oxygen.
Hypotension	Begin fluid infusion at very rapid rates.
Hyperthermia	Abdominal lavage with ice-cold fluids is indicated.
Drugs	Antimuscarinics and beta-1-agonists cause tachycardia.
Bradycardia	
Anaesthetic overdose	Reduce vaporiser setting and ventilate.
Terminal hypoxia	Stop anaesthetics and ventilate with 100% oxygen. Initiate cardiopulmonary resuscitation.
Hyperkalaemia	Ventilate with oxygen and give sodium bicarbonate.
Vagal activity	Check surgeon's activity. If this is related to bradycardia then temporarily suspend surgery and give atropine or glycopyrrolate.
Drugs	Alpha-2-agonists and high doses of opioids produce bradycardia. Anti-muscarinic drugs offset the effects of opioids, but their use with alpha-2-agonist is controversial. Performing surgery with the animal at light planes of anaesthesia may increase heart rates reduced by drugs.
Hypothermia	End surgery and rewarm as soon as possible.

Hypotension

Prolonged hypotension diminishes perfusion in splanchnic and renal vasculature, ultimately causing tissue damage. When hypotension is severe or prolonged, fatal myocardial and cerebral damage occurs.

Low blood pressure results from several factors (Fig. 23.2). Inadequate cardiac output and reduced systemic vascular resistance cause hypotension. Cardiac output falls because of either extremes of heart rate or inadequate stroke volume. The latter results from poor contractility (e.g. anaesthetic overdose) or preload (hypovolaemia). Alternatively, hypotension can occur from loss of systemic vascular resistance when high doses of acepromazine are given.

Treatment. First fluid should be infused rapidly until improvement is seen. If this does not occur, inotropes (e.g. dobutamine) may be needed.

Haemorrhage

Blood loss during surgery causes hypotension and ultimately haemorrhagic or hypovolaemic shock. In healthy dogs, blood loss results in clinical signs (tachycardia, poor pulse quality, pallor) when 8–18 ml/kg blood has been lost. Blood loss is less well tolerated in cats: 6–12 ml/kg results in clinical signs.

Signs. Obvious signs of shed blood at the surgical site combined with tachycardia, pallor and a weak pulse should raise the suspicion of significant haemorrhage. Loss can be estimated by weighing swabs: 1 ml blood weighs 1.3 g. The volume of shed blood can be quantified by deducting the weight of dry swabs from those soaked in blood.

Treatment. Lost blood is replaced with either blood plasma expanders or electrolyte solutions. If blood is used, the volume required equals the volume lost. For blood losses of up to 20% of circulating volume, electrolyte solutions such as Hartmann's can be infused on a 3:1 basis (3 ml fluids are given for each 1 ml of blood lost).

Hypothermia

Hypothermia is common under anaesthesia because:

- Hypothalamic thermoregulation is impaired by anaesthetics.
- Skin blood vessels vasodilate.
- Skeletal muscle activity ceases.
- Shivering is inhibited during surgical anaesthesia.
- Visceral surfaces are exposed.
- Inspired gases are cold and dry.

Animals most at risk are those with:

- High ratios of surface area to volume (e.g. neonates, birds and small laboratory animals, e.g. mice and hamsters).
- Undeveloped or impaired thermoregulatory reflexes (the very young and old).

There are important adverse effects:

- Reduced alveolar ventilation.
- Reduced heart rate and cardiac output.
- Haemoglobin binds oxygen more strongly.
- Erythrocytes become stickier; blood viscosity increases.
- During recovery, shivering elevates O_2 consumption and plasma catecholamines.

Consequences. Prolonged recoveries result from reduced elimination of volatile agents, reduced redistribution and retarded metabolism of injectable drugs. This may result in a self-reinforcing cycle.

Cardiac arrest. Ventricular fibrillation is likely when temperatures fall below 28°C.

Prevention. Physical factors:

- Increase operating room temperature.
- Do not lay animals on cold, uninsulated surfaces.
- Do not expose to draughts.
- If possible, insulate animals with aluminium foil or bubble wrap.
- Use heated blankets, insulated hot water-bottles and radiant heat lamps.

Anaesthetic factors:

- Favour the use of short-acting anaesthetics.
- Ensure anaesthetic depth is not excessive.
- Provide adequate but not excessive ventilation.
- Use rebreathing systems where appropriate.

Surgical factors:

- During surgical preparation of high-risk animals, do not unnecessarily wet the animal, clip excessively or use volatile preparations such as alcohol.
- Minimise surgical time.
- Exposed visceral surfaces must be constantly moistened with warm irrigant fluids. Non-surgical areas must not be allowed to get wet. Incision size must be as small as possible. Viscera should be replaced in body cavities as soon as examination or surgery is completed.

Treatment. Post-operatively, the animal should be thoroughly dried using towels and hair dryers. Topical heat may then be applied judiciously using 40 W light-bulbs, radiant infrared lamps or insulated hot water-bottles. Small laboratory animals may be placed in plastic bags and their bodies immersed in warm water (they must not be allowed to get wet). If these methods fail, warm-water gastric or rectal lavage may be performed.

Cardiopulmonary arrest

Cardiopulmonary arrest occurs when cardiac output fails. Failure to initiate effective cardiopulmonary resuscitation (CPR) under these circumstances leads rapidly to death. Sometimes CPR is not appropriate: it is futile when animals with 'terminal' conditions arrest.

Factors predisposing to arrest can develop rapidly (acute arrests) or more slowly (chronic arrests). 'Acute' arrests result from single devastating events occurring in otherwise normal cases (e.g. thiopentone overdose). 'Chronic' arrests result when many derangements develop slowly and remain unnoticed until the cumulative effect is catastrophic. The latter are probably more common in veterinary practice and indicate that close monitoring and rapid treatment of even mildly deteriorating conditions are important. The axiom 'prevention is better than cure' is most important in the context of CPR.

Causes of arrest

- Myocardial hypoxia (e.g. tachycardia, bradycardia, hypotension, myocardial disease).
- Toxins (e.g. toxaemia, azotaemia, anaesthetic overdose).
- pH extremes (e.g. hypoventilation, shock, diabetic ketoacidosis).
- Electrolyte changes (e.g. hyperkalaemia, hypocalcaemia, hypokalaemia).
- Temperature extremes.

Clinical signs of cardiopulmonary arrest

- Blood at surgical site becomes dark and clots easily. Bleeding stops.
- Either 'gasping' ventilation or apnoea is seen (the former resembling 'light' anaesthesia).
- Mucous membranes may become dirty grey, blue or white.
- Capillary refill time becomes prolonged (more than 2 seconds).
- No heart sounds.
- No palpable pulse.
- Central eye position.
- Pupils dilate.
- Dry cornea.
- Cranial nerve reflexes are lost.
- Generalised muscle relaxation.
- Arrhythmias. Those normally associated with arrest include ventricular fibrillation and asystole. However, in electromechanical dissociation there is a near-normal ECG while mechanical cardiac activity is lost. This is a common cause of arrest in dogs.

Treatment

When these clinical signs are recognised, assistance must be summoned immediately. Simultaneously, preparations are made for CPR, the elements of which are remembered with the mnemonic:

- Airway.
- Breathing.
- Circulation.
- Drugs.
- Electric defibrillation.
- Follow-up.

Before these begin, the animal is laid in right lateral recumbency, positioned against a hard surface and if, possible, in a slight head-down position.

Airway. Effective CPR requires an appropriately positioned, cuffed patient endotracheal tube of suitable size. When assistance is unavailable, tracheal intubation is facilitated by laryngoscopy and is most easily accomplished with the animal in dorsal recumbency. Alternatively, a small-diameter, flexible catheter may be passed to a point proximal to the tracheal bifurcation in preparation for oxygen insufflation.

Breathing. Positive-pressure ventilation (PPV) with oxygen-enriched gas must be imposed. This can be done using any of the following:

- Expired air (containing 16% oxygen).
- An anaesthetic machine and appropriate breathing system flushed with 100% oxygen.
- Self-inflating resuscitation bags (e.g. Ambu resuscitator) which connect to endotracheal tubes and allow manual lung inflation with either air (20% oxygen) or 100% oxygen.

The lungs are inflated using sufficient volume to produce visibly supranormal chest-wall excursions. The lungs are reinflated immediately expiration is ended, but must be allowed to deflate to the normal end-expiratory position.

In single-handed resuscitation attempts, deliver two or three large lung inflations for every 15 chest-wall compressions. Alternatively, insufflate oxygen at high flow rates (5–15 l/min) into the airway.

The femoral pulse, mucous membrane colour and heart sounds should be checked within 30 seconds of beginning ventilation. Thereafter they should be monitored continuously, if assistance is available, or at half-minute intervals. Ventilation alone may restore the pulse but in most cases, circulatory support will be required.

Circulation. When the heart stops, cardiac output must be supported by either compressing the ribcage (external cardiac compression; closed chest resuscitation) or directly squeezing the surgically-exposed ventricles (internal cardiac compression; open chest resuscitation).

Cardiac output produced by either method depends on adequate venous return. This is enhanced by rapid fluid infusion, posture, abdominal compression and adrenaline.

External cardiac compression. There are two forms of external cardiac compression. The first is most suitable for cats, dogs weighing less than 20 kg, or those with narrow chests (e.g. whippets). The chest wall is compressed in the ventral third of the thorax between the 3rd and 6th rib. This is facilitated if the animal is positioned on a hard surface in right lateral recumbency. For very small dogs, cats and pups, the heart is massaged by compressing the ribs between thumb and forefinger. The compression rate is 80–100 per minute.

The second technique is suited for larger dogs weighing over 20 kg or lighter dogs with 'barrel' chests (e.g. bulldogs). The rib cage is compressed at the widest point – the junction of the dorsal and middle thirds of the 6th to 7th rib – at 60–120 times per minute. If possible, compressions should be made during peak lung inflation.

The efficiency of this second technique is increased by three manoeuvres:

- *Abdominal binding.* Applying tight bandages to the hindlimbs and then the abdomen directs blood flow (generated by external cardiac compression) towards the head.
- *Abdominal counterpulsation (interposed abdominal compression).* The abdomen is manually compressed during the diastolic or relaxation phase of chest compression to increase coronary perfusion and assists venous return.
- *Synchronous lung inflation/chest wall compression.* Cardiac output increases when the chest is compressed.

Because ventilation and cardiac compression must never be suspended, abdominal binding and counterpulsation require the presence of a third resuscitator.

The advantages of external cardiac compression are:

- Reasonably effective in certain patients.
- Requires little preparation.

- Rapidly applied.
- Few hazards.
- Can be performed by lay staff.

The disadvantage is that it is ineffective in many circumstances.

Signs of effective CPR

Early:

- Palpation of pulse during compression.
- Constriction of pupil.
- Ventromedial relocation of the eye.
- Improvement of mucous membrane colour.
- ECG changes.

Late:

- Lacrimation.
- Return of cranial nerve reflexes like blinking, gagging and coughing.
- Return of spontaneous respiratory activity. Diaphragmatic twitches and irregular breathing appear at first. Then regular deep breathing returns; this is a good prognostic sign.
- Return of special senses: response to sound
- Return of other central nervous function: vocalisation righting reflexes, purposeful movement.

If early signs are not seen within 2 minutes, two alternative options remain:

- Administer resuscitative (D)rugs and (E)xternally defibrillate (D and E of the mnemonic); or
- Perform emergency thoracotomy and internal cardiac compression.

Nurses can prepare for either eventuality by ensuring that:

- The resuscitation box is fully stocked and that drugs (Table 23.9) have not expired. (The veterinary nurse must know the drugs and equipment required during CPR and be able to reconstitute them.)
- Defibrillators are fully charged and paddles are available.

If thoracotomy is planned:

- A rapid clip of the 3rd to 6th intercostal space on the left side may be needed in long-haired dogs. (The appropriate site can be identified by flexing the forelimb so that the olecranon transects the costochondral junction; this point overlies the 5th intercostal space.) However, time must not be wasted in surgical preparation.
- Ensure that a surgical pack containing a scalpel (and blade) and rib-spreaders is available.

Accidents

Close monitoring reduces accidents but does not eliminate them. If they do occur, the veterinary nurse must respond appropriately and summon assistance if needed. The time of the accident should be noted and later a report should be entered on the patient's records.

Table 23.9 Drugs and equipment required for cardiopulmonary resuscitation

Drugs	Equipment
Adrenaline	Needles and syringes
Atropine	Urinary catheters for intratracheal
Lignocaine	drug administration
Isoprenaline	Emergency surgical pack
Methoxamine	Self-inflating resuscitator bag
Dopamine	Defibrillator
Dobutamine	Internal and external paddles
Propranolol	Intravenous catheters
Frusemide	Endotracheal tubes
Mannitol	
Methyl prednisolone	
Procainamide	
Calcium gluconate	
Sodium bicarbonate	
Edrophonium or	
neostigmine	
Verapamil	
Doxapram	
Naloxone	
Atipamezole	

A large clear chart with simple instructions for drug reconstitution should be included.

Extravascular injections

Extravascular injection of irritant drugs like thiopentone result in tissue sloughs. These are painful, take a long time to heal and leave unsightly blemishes. The risk of this is minimised by:

- Effective patient restraint (physical or chemical) before injection.
- Venous catheterisation.
- Using dilute solutions of drug (e.g. 1.25% for thiopentone) in animals with poorly accessible veins.

If extravascular injection does occur, the deposition is enthusiastically diluted with sterile saline or water. There is little advantage in using local anaesthetics or steroids. Large volumes may be safely injected under the skin and massaged. Later a record should be made of the accident.

Drug overdose

The animal must be intubated and ventilated with oxygen. When inhalation agents are responsible, vaporisers must first be switched off. If pulses are weak or absent, external cardiac compression should be imposed. Intravenous fluids and inotropes (drugs that increase contractility of cardiac muscle) may be considered if circulation fails to redistribute the drug. When available, drug antagonists may be used.

Burns

Burns occur if excess heat is applied to cold animals. This is more likely when skin blood flow is reduced, as in shock, because poorly perfused skin conducts heat less effectively.

Decubital ulcers

These sores appear when bony prominences remain in prolonged contact with hard surfaces. They are prevented by adequate bedding and frequent turning of the patient.

Hypostatic congestion

Capillaries in the dependent (lowermost) lung fill with blood and alveoli partially collapse when recoveries are prolonged and cardiac output is low. Both changes result in hypoxia. Prevention is based on frequent (2-hourly) turning.

Equipment-based accidents

Cylinders. Cylinders contain gas at high pressure (nearly 1935 p.s.i. or 13 300 kPa) and will explode if mistreated. They must not be dropped or placed in a position where they may fall or become damaged. They should not be exposed to high temperatures (including direct sunlight). They must be stored in dry conditions away from flammable materials.

When a full O_2 cylinder is exposed to elevated temperatures caused, for example, by naked flames, the pressure within it rises and may exceed the test pressure. Eventually the bottle bursts and releases O_2 that fuels further conflagration.

Explosions and fires. Explosions require a source of fuel (usually carbon-based), oxygen and activation energy (a spark or a naked flame). Once initiated, heat released from the reaction provides further activation energy and the reaction proliferates. Explosions are more likely when fuel–oxygen rather than fuel–air mixtures are present.

For these reasons, 'sticking' valves or apparatus involved with pressurised oxygen must never be lubricated or sealed with carbon- or petroleum-based lubricants.

In the past, cyclopropane and diethyl ether were commonly used for anaesthesia. They lost popularity because of their flammability and explosive properties, and their redundancy was accelerated by the introduction of thermocautery and electrical monitoring devices in the operating room. Surgical alcohol remains a possible source of fire and explosion.

Risks of fire and explosion are minimised by keeping the three 'components' separate:

- Inflammable agents must not be used when heat, sparks (from static electricity or electrical apparatus) or naked flames are present.
- If thermocautery is required, cyclopropane and ether must be avoided.
- Naked flames, carbon-based fuels and dust must be minimised.

If fires or explosions occur, the emergency services must be informed that supplies of inflammable material and compressed oxygen are within the vicinity of the accident.

Accidents to personnel

Bites and scratches. These are minimised by suitable physical and chemical restraint techniques, by equipment and by common sense precautions. Fingers should not be placed within the mouth of an ungagged, unconscious animal especially during endotracheal intubation: owners should not normally be allowed to restrain animals in case they are injected accidentally or bitten.

When an accident occurs, the appropriate report form must be completed. The injured person should report to hospital for examination and tetanus immunisation. If known, details of the animal's condition should be supplied.

Self-administration of drugs. Risks of self-administration is greatest with Immobilon preparations. There is also risk with sedatives, especially alpha-2-adrenoceptor agonists; toxicity has not yet been reported in humans although the potential is great. Absorption of these drugs across oral mucous membranes is rapid and so placing of needle-caps in mouths is especially hazardous.

Ketamine has been inadvertently self-administered, with ensuing toxic signs.

Whenever drug-based accidents occur, the data sheet or NOAH Compendium should be taken to the emergency room with the injured person. Self-administration can be avoided:

- Ensure that the animal is adequately restrained.
- Do not resheath needles but dispose of them immediately after use.
- Do not carry syringes and needles in pockets.
- Do not place syringe caps in the mouth.

When using Immobilon the manufacturer's guidelines must be followed. If drug splashes into the eye or on to skin, the site must be thoroughly irrigated with copious amounts of fresh water. If injection occurs, or if toxic signs follow 'splashing' accidents, the antagonist protocol must be followed. In any event, hospital services must be notified and the data sheet presented to attending clinicians. Many of the guidelines for the prevention of self-administration of Immobilon are appropriate for other potent injectable drugs:

- The needle used for drug withdrawal from vial should be discarded in a metal container and a new needle used for injection.
- Wear gloves.
- Do not pressurise the vial.
- Have eye and skin washes available.
- An assistant capable of giving antagonist should be present.
- The user should brief the assistant on emergency protocol and whether or not diprenorphine (which has a veterinary product licence only) constitutes part of this protocol.
- Naloxone and diprenorphine should always be available.

The recovery period

Poor attention to recovering animals contributes to post-operative mortality. Problems are probably more likely at this time because attention relaxes, the perceived high-risk periods of induction and maintenance having passed. Responsibilities during recovery include the following:

- Monitoring vital signs and keeping records.
- Keeping animals calm and dry, and surgical sites and orifices clean.
- Attending to wounds and preventing interference.
- Providing post-operative medication.
- Monitoring fluid and energy balance.
- Reporting recovery problems.

Pain

Several factors determine the magnitude of post-operative pain.

Surgical procedures

The degree of post-operative pain depends on surgery and the condition with which the animal presents. Victims of road-traffic accidents may be in severe pain but surgery, in repairing damage, represents an analgesic step. In these cases, post-operative discomfort may require treatment although the animal may, for the first time since injury, feel relatively comfortable.

Some animals experience only low-grade chronic pain on presentation (e.g. osteoarthritis) but are in considerable discomfort after surgery (femoral head arthroplasty). Aggressive treatment may be required in these cases.

Medical conditions (e.g. neoplasia or patent ductus arteriosus) cause little pre-operative discomfort but post-operative pain may be profound. After thoracotomy, special attention must be paid to the adequacy of ventilation.

Patient demeanour can be misleading. Some breeds are more hardy than others but the absence of discomfort does not exclude the presence of pain.

Poor surgical techniques characterised by slowness, indelicate tissue handling, excessive traction and poor attention to wound hydration contribute to post-operative discomfort.

Unnecessarily light anaesthesia allows muscle tonicity; greater surgical traction is then required.

Peri-operative analgesics

The efficacy of peri-operative analgesics can be affected by the type of drug, the dose used and the timing of administration.

Drugs used. Possibly because opioids produce sedation, the quality of analgesia they confer appears superior to that produced with NSAIDs. Of the opioids, pure agonists (e.g. morphine) seem to produce 'higher quality' analgesia than partial agonist drugs (e.g. buprenorphine). Some drugs are relatively short-acting; if these are not redosed frequently then analgesia will be incomplete.

Dose used. Fear of side-effects promotes a tendency to underdose opioids. As a rule, higher doses can be given with little, if any, risk to cases in which high levels of discomfort are anticipated.

Timing of first dose. Optimally, post-operative analgesics are given before surgical trauma begins because:

- The clinical impression of many is that superior quality analgesia of longer duration is achieved if analgesics are given before tissue trauma occurs. This is termed 'pre-emptive analgesia'.
- Some opioids have a slow onset of action: the onset time of morphine and buprenorphine is about 15–30 minutes.

Sequential analgesia. Problems with the side-effects of analgesics are in theory reduced by giving low doses of drugs from groups which act at different levels of the pain pathway.

Assessing post-operative discomfort

Behavioural signs of post-operative pain or inadequate analgesia depend in part on the species. 'Autonomic' signs like tachycardia are common to all species. Common signs of pain are listed in Table 23.10.

Dogs in pain have an anxious, 'hangdog', dejected or cringing appearance. The tail is held between the legs. Animals may be aggressive but are usually submissive.

Cats in pain appear depressed; ears are flattened and they adopt a 'cringing' posture. The head and neck are tucked in.

Any suspicion of post-operative pain must be reported immediately, as rapid, rather than delayed intervention is more likely to be successful.

After prolonged procedures, or when prolonged recovery period is anticipated, the urinary bladder should be catheterised to prevent the bladder from becoming distended and causing discomfort.

Prolonged recoveries

Causes. After 'analgesic' surgery, animals with painful injuries may rest comfortably for the first time since

---

Table 23.10 Common signs of pain in animals

Failure to respond to normal stimuli
Vocalisation (periodic or continuous)
Attention to surgical site
Panting
Abnormal posture (huddling)
Shivering
Disinterest in food and water
Failure to groom
Dilated pupils
Tachycardia
High or low blood pressure
Faecal and urinary incontinence or constipation and urinary retention
High temperature

presentation. These cases are recognised because cranial nerve reflexes are brisk although overt signs indicate depression. Such animals should be monitored but not unduly disturbed.

Pain is likely to stimulate rather than depress consciousness. However, depression may indicate very severe pain.

Persistent drug activity. The fact that overdose has occurred may only become apparent after review of the anaesthetic record. Acepromazine may cause slow recoveries in certain breeds of dogs (e.g. brachycephalics) and in dogs with diminished liver function. Drug retention may result from inadequate perfusion or failure of the liver or kidney. In these cases, haemodynamic support with fluids may be required. Persistent drug activity can be countered if the suspect agent has an antagonist:

Agonist	Antagonist
Opioids	Naloxone, nalbuphine
Benzodiazepines	Flumazenil
Alpha-2-agonist	Atipamezole

However, the use of antagonists cannot always be justified because endogenous pain-systems may also be antagonised.

Hypothermia causes retarded expiration of volatile agents and the redistribution and metabolism of injectable agents. The rectal temperature should be taken and recorded throughout recovery.

The fundamental approach to prolonged recovery is based on nursing (e.g. raising temperature) and creating a diffusion gradient from the drug's site of action to the organ of elimination.

Excitation. Bad recoveries characterised by excitation, hyperaesthesia, vocalisation, exaggerated responsiveness and excessive activity may result from pain, emergence, pharmacological phenomena and epilepsy/convulsion.

Pain. This responds to analgesic administration.

Emergence. Some animals recover after non-painful surgery as if in pain. Disconcerting signs are normally short-lived. The incidence is higher with certain drugs (e.g. 'Saffan') but may be reduced if sedative premedications are used and recovery occurs in a quiet environment.

Pharmacological phenomena. Cats often 'recover' poorly irrespective of the anaesthetic. In dogs it seems more common after thiopentone 'top-ups'.

Convulsions/epilepsy. Post-operative convulsions traditionally followed myelographic investigation with certain contrast media. Epileptic patients may be at increased risk of post-operative seizures.

Hypoxia. Although extubation must be performed when gagging, 'bucking' and other cranial nerve reflexes are restored, it is not safe to assume that O_2 delivery may be safely discontinued. Nor is it safe to give 5 minutes' O_2 arbitrarily after the anaesthesia ends. Hypothermia, residual anaesthetic drug activity and lung changes may combine to diminish blood oxygenation, while shivering and pain increase O_2 consumption. Oxygen (100%) should be delivered until animals can maintain satisfactory oxygenation on room air. If extubation is necessary before this time, O_2 should be given by:

- Mask.
- Intranasal catheter.
- Tracheostomy tube.
- Transtracheal catheter.

Oxygen must be given for at least 3 minutes after the discontinuation of N_2O in order to avoid diffusion hypoxia. Animals incapable of maintaining sternal recumbency should be repositioned every 2–4 hours to prevent hypostatic congestion of the lungs.

Respiratory depression caused by persistent drug activity is alleviated by antagonising drug effects under certain circumstances, enhancing drug elimination or giving analeptics.

Hypothermia. Low body temperature initiates shivering and prolongs recovery rate. Rectal temperature should be monitored at frequent intervals. Failure of temperature to rise should be countered by high ambient temperatures (25°C) supplemented with heater blankets, infra-red lamps or hot water-bottles. Evaporative and connective losses should be minimised; animals must be kept dry and in a draught-free environment. Severe depression of core temperature may necessitate more complex steps such as gastric, peritoneal or rectal lavage.

Topical heat application can have adverse consequences in addition to burns. Cutaneous blood vessel dilatation caused by topical heat may lower systemic vascular resistance and cause hypotension. This is more likely in hypovolaemic animals.

SUMMARY

- Complications are potentially numerous during anaesthesia.
- Prevention of anticipated risks is significantly more effective than treatment.
- Rapid identification and corrective measures reduce morbidity and mortality.
- During an arrest, efficient 'ABC' therapy can prevent long-term organ dysfunction (e.g. brain) whilst the underlying cause is being identified and addressed.
- Accidents involving veterinary staff should be minimised by vigilance during anaesthesia.
- The recovery period is a common time during which complications occur.
- Careful attention to the patient until it has returned to its normal state is required.

Animals which have normal body temperatures may shiver post-operatively; in humans, this is associated with halothane anaesthesia. Oxygen should be supplied.

Discharge

Animals must not be discharged before full recovery from anaesthesia and surgery. Some drugs (e.g. Small Animal Immobilon) may 're-cycle' and owners must be warned of this. The client must also be forewarned of other anaesthetic and surgery-related complications such as haemorrhage.

Acknowledgements

The author is indebted to Mr R. E. Clutton, the author of the previous edition of this chapter on which the present chapter is heavily based, and to Dr P. M. Taylor for permission to draw information from her University of Cambridge Veterinary Anaesthesia lecture notes.

Further reading

Davey, A., Moyle, J. T. B. and Ward, C. S. (1994) *Ward's Anaesthetic Equipment*, 3rd edn, W. B. Saunders, London.

Hall, L. W. and Clarke, K. W. (1991) *Veterinary Anaesthesia*, 9th edn, Ballière Tindall, London.

Hall, L. W. and Taylor, P. M. (1994) *Anaesthesia of the Cat*, Balli'ere Tindall, London.

Levick, J. R. (1996) *An Introduction to Cardiovascular Physiology*, 2nd edn, Butterworth-Heinemann, Oxford.

Thurmon, J. C., Tranquilli, W. J. and Benson, G. J. (1996) *Veterinary Anesthesia*, 3rd edn, Williams & Wilkins, Baltimore.

West, J. B. (1995) *Respiratory Physiology – The Essentials*, 5th edn, Williams & Wilkins, Baltimore.

24

Radiography

Ruth Dennis

Radiography is a fundamental part of veterinary practice and is a procedure in which most nurses become actively involved. The production of diagnostic films requires skill in the use of radiographic equipment, in patient positioning and in the processing of the films. At the same time the procedure must be carried out safely without hazard to the handlers or patient.

This chapter summarises the use of radiography in small animal practice. All parts of the veterinary nursing Part II examination syllabus are covered but it is hoped that the chapter will also prove useful for day-to-day reference.

Basic principles of radiography

X-rays are produced by X-ray machines when electricity from the mains is transformed to a high voltage current, converting some of the energy in the current to X-ray energy. The intensity and penetrating power of the emergent X-ray beam varies with the size and complexity of the apparatus, and the exposure settings used; portable X-ray machines are capable only of a relatively low output, whereas larger machines are far more powerful.

X-rays travel in straight lines and can be focused into an area called the **primary beam**, which is directed at the patient. Within the patient's tissues some of the X-rays are absorbed; the remainder pass through and are detected by photographic X-ray film producing a hidden image. When the film is processed chemically a permanent picture or radiograph is produced and the image may be viewed.

The electromagnetic spectrum

X-rays are members of the **electromagnetic spectrum**, a group of types of radiation which have some similar properties but which differ from each other in their **wavelength** and **frequency** (Fig. 24.1).

The energy in a given type of radiation is directly proportional to the frequency of the radiation and inversely proportional to its wavelength. X-rays and gamma rays are similar types of electromagnetic radiation which have high frequency, short wavelength and therefore high energy. X-rays are produced by X-ray machines and gamma rays by the decay of radioactive materials.

Members of the electromagnetic spectrum have the following common features:

- They do not require a medium for transmission and can pass through a vacuum.
- They travel in straight lines.
- They travel at the same speed – 3×10^8 m/s in a vacuum.
- They interact with matter by being absorbed or scattered.

X-rays have some additional properties which means that they can be used to produce images of the internal structures of people and animals; they are also used in engineering for detecting flaws in pipes and construction materials. Their extra properties are:

- **Penetration**. Because of their high energy they can penetrate substances which are opaque to visible ('white') light. The X-ray photons are absorbed to varying degrees depending on the nature of the substance penetrated and the power of the photons themselves and some may pass right through the patient, emerging at the other side.
- **Effect on photographic film**. X-rays have the ability to produce a hidden or latent image on photographic film which can be rendered visible by processing (film in cameras is damaged by exposure to X-radiation).
- **Fluorescence**. X-rays cause crystals of certain substances to fluoresce (emit visible light) and this property is utilised in the composition of intensifying screens which are used in the recording of the image.

X-rays also produce biological changes in living tissues by altering the structure of atoms or molecules or by causing chemical reactions. Some of these effects can be used beneficially in the radiotherapy of tumours, but they are harmful to normal tissues and constitute a safety hazard. Aspects of radiation safety are considered later in the chapter.

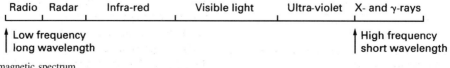

Fig 24.1 The electromagnetic spectrum.

Production of X-rays

X-ray photons or quanta are tiny packets of energy which are released whenever rapidly-moving electrons are slowed down or stopped. Electrons are present in the atoms of all elements and in order to grasp the fundamentals of simple radiation physics it is necessary to understand the structure of an atom (Fig. 24.2). Atoms contains the following particles:

- **Protons**: positively charged particles contained in the centre or nucleus of the atom.
- **Neutrons**: particles of similar size to protons which are also found in the nucleus but which carry no electrical charge.
- **Electrons**: smaller, negatively charged particles which orbit around the nucleus in different planes or 'shells'.

The number of electrons normally equals the number of protons and so the atom as a whole is electrically neutral. The number of protons and electrons is unique to the atoms of each element and is called the **atomic number**. If an atom loses one or more electrons it becomes positively charged and may be written as X^+ (where X is the symbol for that element). If an atom gains electrons it becomes negatively charged (X^-). Atoms with charges are called **ions** or are said to be ionised. **Compounds** are combinations of two or more elements and usually consist of positive ions of one element in combination with negative ions of another, e.g. silver bromide (in X-ray film emulsion) consists of silver Ag^+ and bromide Br^- ions.

In an X-ray tube head, X-ray photons are produced by collisions between fast-moving electrons and the atoms of a 'target' element. Electrons which are completely halted by the target atoms give up all of their energy to form an X-ray photon, whereas those which are merely decelerated give up smaller and variable amounts of energy, producing lower-energy X-ray photons. The X-ray beam produced therefore contains photons of a range of energies and is said to be **polychromatic**. If the number of incident electrons is increased, more X-ray photons are produced, and the intensity of the X-ray beam increases. If the incident electrons are faster-moving then they have more energy to lose and so the X-ray photons produced are more energetic; the X-ray beam's quality is therefore increased and it has greater penetrating power.

The intensity and quality of an X-ray beam can be altered by adjusting the settings on the machine, and the practical effect of this will discussed in greater detail later.

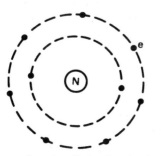

Fig. 24.2 The structure of an atom. N = nucleus (protons and neutrons); e = electron (dotted lines represent electron shells).

The X-ray tube head

The X-ray tube head is the part of the machine where the X-rays are generated. A diagram of the simplest type of X-ray tube, a **stationary** or **fixed anode** tube, is shown in Fig. 24.3.

The X-ray tube head contains two electrodes, the negatively-charged **cathode** and the positively-charged **anode**. Electrons are produced at the cathode, which is a coiled wire filament. When a small electrical current is passed through the filament it becomes hot and releases a cloud of electrons by a process called **thermionic emission**. Tungsten is used as the filament material because:

- It has a high atomic number, 74, and therefore has many electrons.
- It has a very high melting point of $3380°C$ and so can safely be heated.

The current required to heat the filament is small and so the mains current is reduced by a **step-down** or **filament transformer** which is wired into the X-ray machine (a transformer is a device for increasing or decreasing an electric current).

Next, the cloud of electrons needs to be made to travel at high speed across the short distance to the target. This is done by applying a high electrical potential difference between the filament and the target so that the filament becomes negative (and therefore repels the electrons) and the target becomes positive (and attracts them). The filament therefore becomes a cathode and the target an anode. The electrons are formed into a narrow beam by the fact that the filament sits in a nickel or molybdenum **focusing cup**, which is also at a negative potential and so repels the electrons. The electron beam constitutes a weak electric current across the tube, which is measured in **milliamperes (mA)**.

The potential difference applied between the filament and the target needs to be very high and many times the voltage of the mains supply, which is 240 volts. In fact it is measured in thousands of volts, or **kilovolts (kV)**, and is created from the mains using a **step-up** or **high tension transformer**, which is also part of the electrical circuitry of the X-ray machine.

The stream of electrons strikes the target or anode at very high speed. Tungsten or rhenium–tungsten alloy is used as the target material because its high atomic number renders it a relatively efficient producer of X-rays. Unfortunately the process is still very inefficient and more than 99% of the energy lost by the electrons is converted to heat, so the anode must be able to withstand very high temperatures without melting or cracking. Tungsten's high melting point is therefore useful in the target as well as in the filament.

In a simple type of X-ray tube as shown in Fig. 24.3 the target is a rectangle of tungsten set in a copper block. Copper is a good conductor of heat and so the heat is removed from the target by conduction along the copper stem to cooling fins radiating into the surrounding oil bath, which can absorb much heat.

The target is set at an angle of about 20° to the vertical (Fig. 24.4). This is so that the area of the target which the

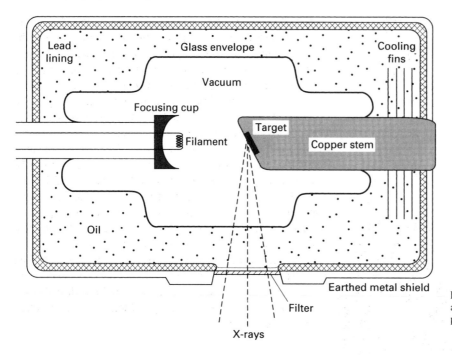

Fig. 24.3 Diagram of a stationary or fixed anode X-ray tube (reproduced with the permission of Baillière Tindall, London).

electrons strike (and therefore the area over which heat is produced) is as large as possible. This area is called the actual focal spot. At the same time the angulation of the target means that the X-ray beam appears to originate from a much smaller area and this is called the effective focal spot. The importance of having a small effective focal spot – ideally a point source – is discussed later in the chapter with regard to image definition.

Some X-ray machines allow a choice of focal spot size using two different-sized filaments at the cathode:

● The smaller filament or **fine focus** produces a narrower electron beam and hence smaller effective and actual focal spots. The emergent X-ray beam arises from a tiny area and will produce very fine radiographic definition. However, the heat generated is concentrated over a very small area of the target and so the exposure factors that can be used are limited.

● The larger filament produces a **coarse** or **broad focus** with larger effective and actual focal spot sizes. Higher exposures can be used but the image definition will be slightly poorer due to the 'penumbra effect', a blurring of margins related to the geometry of the beam (Fig. 24.5).

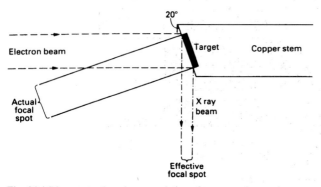

Fig. 24.4 Diagram to show how angulation of target produces a large actual focal spot and a small effective focal spot.

In practice, fine focus is selected for small parts when fine definition is required (e.g. the limbs), and coarse focus when thicker areas are to be radiographed (e.g. the chest and abdomen); these require higher exposure factors and so the heat generated at the target is higher.

The cathode, anode and part of the copper stem are enclosed in a **glass envelope**. Within the envelope is a vacuum, which prevents the moving electrons from colliding with air molecules and losing speed. The glass envelope is bathed in oil which acts both as a heat sink and as an electrical insulator, and the whole is encased in an earthed, lead-lined **metal casing**. X-rays are produced in all directions by the target but only one narrow beam of X-rays is required, and this emerges through a window in the casing, placed beneath the angled target. This beam is called the **primary** or **useful beam**. X-rays produced in other directions are absorbed by the casing.

Within the X-ray beam are some low energy or 'soft' X-ray photons which are not powerful enough to pass through the patient but which may be absorbed or scattered by the patient and therefore represent a safety hazard. They are removed from the beam by an **aluminium filter** placed across the tube window; these filters are legally required as a safety precaution and must not be removed. Old X-ray machines must be checked by an engineer to make sure that an aluminium filter is present.

In stationary anode X-ray tubes the X-ray output is limited by the amount of heat generated at the target. Overheating the target would produce melting and surface irregularity which would reduce the efficiency of the tube; however in modern machines automatic 'overload' devices prevent such high exposures from being used. Stationary anode X-ray tubes are found in low-powered, portable X-ray machines. More powerful machines require a more efficient way of removing the heat and this is accomplished using a **rotating anode** (Fig. 24.6). In such tubes the target area is the bevelled rim of a metal disc whose rim is set at

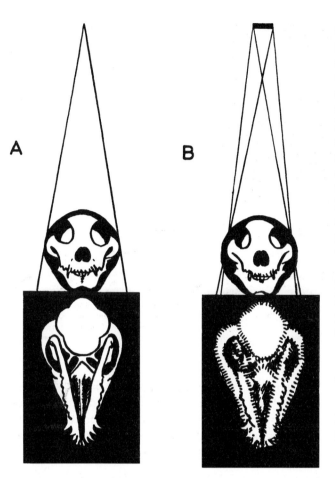

about 20°, as in a stationary anode X-ray tube. The target area is again tungsten or rhenium–tungsten. During the exposure the disc rotates rapidly so that the target area upon which the electrons impinge is constantly changing. The actual focal spot is therefore the whole circumference of the disc and so is many times greater than in a stationary anode X-ray tube. The heat generated is spread over a much bigger area allowing larger exposures to be made, whilst the effective focal spot remains the same. The disc is mounted on a molybdenum rod and is rotated at speeds of up to 10 000 r.p.m. by an induction motor at the other end of the rod. Molybdenum is used because it is a poor conductor of heat and therefore prevents the motor from overheating. Heat generated in the anode is lost by radiation through the vacuum and the glass envelope into the oil bath.

The size of the emerging X-ray beam must be controlled for safety reasons otherwise it will spread out over a very large area. This is achieved using a **collimation device**, preferably a light beam diaphragm. Methods of collimation are described later.

The X-ray control panel

X-ray machine control panels vary in their complexity, but some or all of the following controls will be present:

On/off switch

As well as switching the machine on at the mains socket there will also be an on/off switch or key on the control panel. Sometimes the line voltage compensator (see over) is

Fig. 24.5 Diagram to show the effect of focal-spot size. In (A) the spot is a pin-point and the projected image is sharp. In (B) the rays from a focal-spot of large dimensions cause a penumbra effect which blurs the projected image. (Reproduced with the permission of Baillière Tindall, London.)

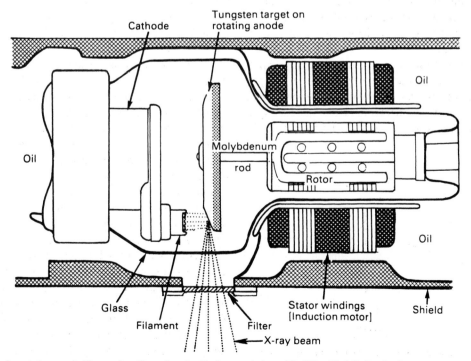

Fig. 24.6 Diagram of a rotating anode X-ray tube. (Reproduced with the permission of Baillière Tindall, London.)

incorporated into the on/off switch, which therefore performs both functions. When the machine is switched on a warning light on the control panel will indicate that it is ready to produce X-rays or, in the case of panels with digital displays, the numbers will be illuminated. In some old machines the filament is heated continually whilst the machine is on and may burn out. Such machines should always be turned off when the exposure is terminated. X-ray machines must always be switched off when not in use, so that accidental exposure cannot occur when unprotected people are in the room.

Line voltage compensator

Fluctuations in the normal mains electricity output may occur resulting in an inconsistent output of X-rays. The images produced may appear under- or over-exposed despite using normal exposure factors. In some machines these fluctuations are automatically corrected by an **auto-transformer** wired into the circuit, but in others it is controlled manually. A voltmeter dial on the control panel will indicate the incoming voltage which can be adjusted until it is satisfactory. In such machines the line voltage should be checked before each session of radiography.

Kilovoltage (kV) control

The kilovoltage control selects the kilovoltage (potential difference) which is applied across the tube during the instant of exposure. It determines the speed and energy with which the electrons bombard the target and hence the quality or penetrating power of the X-ray beam produced. Depending on the power and sophistication of the X-ray machine, the kilovoltage is controlled in various ways. Ideally it is controlled quite independently of the milliamperage, often in increments of 1 kV, and the kilovoltage meter is either a dial or a digital display.

In smaller machines the kilovoltage is linked to the milliamperage so that if a higher milliamperage is selected only lower kilovoltages can be used. Often there is a single control knob for both kilovoltage and milliamperage and as the kilovoltage is increased the milliamperage available drops. This is not ideal since, for larger patients, a high kilovoltage and high milliamperage may be required at the same time, meaning that long exposure times are needed. In very basic machines the kilovoltage and milliamperage are fixed, and only the time can be altered.

Milliamperage (mA) control

The milliamperage is a measure of the quantity of electrons crossing the tube during the exposure (the 'tube current') and is directly related to the quantity of X-rays produced. Moving electrons constitute an electrical current which is measured in amperes, but the tube current is very small and is measured in 1/1000 amperes or milliamperes (mA). Adjusting the milliamperage control alters the degree of heating of the filament and hence the number of electrons

released by thermionic emission, the tube current and the intensity of the X-ray beam.

Timer

The quantity of X-rays produced depends not only on the milliamperage but also on the length of the exposure, and so a composite term, the milliampere-seconds or mAs, is often used. A given mAs may be obtained using a high milliamperage with a short time or vice versa; the two numbers are multiplied together, e.g.

$$30\,\text{mAs} = 300\,\text{mA for } 0.1\text{ s}$$
$$\text{or} \qquad 30\,\text{mA for } 1.0\text{ s}$$

The effect on the film is the same except that the longer the exposure the more likely it is that movement blur will occur. One should always therefore use the largest milliamperage allowed by the machine for that kilovoltage setting, in order to minimise the exposure time. It will now be appreciated why the type of machine in which kilovoltage and milliamperage are inversely linked is less than ideal.

The timer is usually electronic and is another dial on the control panel, giving a choice of a wide range of exposure times up to several seconds long. However, release of the exposure button terminates the exposure even when long times have been selected. In larger machines an automatic display of the resulting mAs is also present. Some old, small X-ray machines may still be in use which rely on clockwork timers, although these should be replaced by electronic timers. The clockwork timer is a hand-set which also incorporates the exposure button. A dial is 'wound up' to an appropriate time setting and runs back to zero whilst the exposure button is depressed. The time must be reset between exposures. These timers are not only inaccurate and noisy but also they do not allow the exposure to be aborted if, for instance, a manually restrained patient moves, pulling the holder into the primary beam

Exposure button

The exposure button must be at the end of a cable which can stretch to more than 2 m to enable the radiographer to distance himself from the primary beam during the exposure. Alternatively, the button may be on the control panel itself provided that the panel is at least 2 m from the tube head or is separated from it by a lead screen. Most exposure buttons are two-stage devices; depression of the button to a halfway stage ('prepping') heats the filament and rotates the anode if a rotating anode is present; after a brief pause, depression of the button further causes application of the kilovoltage to the tube and an instantaneous exposure to be made. In some machines only a single-stage exposure button is present; in this case there is slight delay between depression of the button and exposure during which time the patient may move. In old machines with single-stage exposure buttons the filament may be constantly heated while the machine is switched on and in these there is a risk of burning out the filament.

Types of X-ray machine

X-ray machines can conveniently be divided into three broad types.

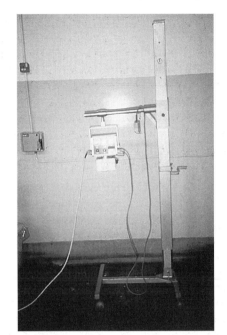

Portable machines (Fig. 24.7)

These are the commonest type of machine found in general practice. As their name suggests they are relatively easy to move from site to site for large animal radiography and many come with a special carrying case. The electrical transformers are located in the tube head and the controls may be either on a separate panel or else on the head itself. Portable machines are low powered, producing only about 20–60 mA and often less. In most the kilovoltage and milliamperage are inversely linked. Although portable machines are widely used their relatively low output means that longer exposure times are needed, and chest and abdomen radiographs of larger patients are often degraded by the effects of movement blur.

Fig. 24.7 Portable X-ray machine.

Mobile machines (Fig. 24.8)

These are larger and more powerful than portable machines but can still be moved from room to room on wheels, some having battery-operated motors. The transformers are bulkier and encased in a large box which is an integral part of the tube stand. Mobile machines usually have outputs of up to 300 mA and are likely to produce good radiographs of most small animal patients. Although they are more expensive to buy new, they can sometimes be obtained second-hand from hospitals, where they will have had relatively little use yet been well cared for, having been used mainly for bedridden patients. They are not usually suitable for equine radiography since the tube head will not reach to the floor, although special tube arm adaptors can be fitted. If used for equine radiography the horse should be restrained in stocks since the X-ray machine cannot be moved away quickly if the patient moves.

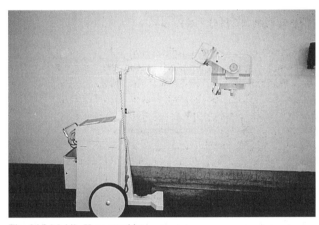

Fig. 24.8 Mobile X-ray machine.

Fixed machines (Fig. 24.9)

The most powerful X-ray machines are built into the X-ray room, being screwed to the floor or being mounted on rails or overhead gantries. The transformers are situated in cabinets some distance from the machine itself, and connected to it by high-tension cables. The largest fixed machines can produce up to 1250 mA and produce excellent radiographs of all patients, but because of the high cost of purchase, installation and maintenance they are rarely found outside veterinary institutions and large equine practices. However, several companies are now producing smaller, fixed X-ray machines especially for the veterinary market which are much more affordable. Fixed X-ray machines are often linked electronically to a floating table top and moving grid.

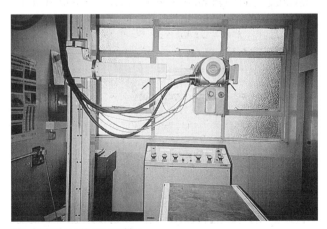

Fig. 24.9 Fixed X-ray machine.

Formation of the X-ray image

The X-ray picture is essentially a 'shadowgraph', or a picture in black, white and varying shades of grey, caused by differences in the amount of absorption of the beam by different tissues and hence in differences in the amount of radiation reaching the X-ray film and causing blackening (Fig. 24.10).

The degree of absorption by a given tissue depends on three factors:

(1) **The atomic number (Z)** of the tissue, or the average of the different atomic numbers present (the 'effective' atomic number). Bone has a higher effective atomic number than soft tissue and so absorbs more X-ray photons producing whiter areas on the radiograph. Similarly, soft tissue has a higher effective atomic number than fat.

(2) **The specific gravity of the tissue**. This is the density or mass per unit volume. Bone has a high specific gravity, soft tissue a medium specific gravity and gas a very low specific gravity, hence gas-filled areas absorb few X-rays and appear nearly black on the radiograph.

The combination of effective atomic number and specific gravity produces five characteristic shades to be seen on a radiograph:

● Gas – very dark.
● Fat – dark grey.
● Soft tissue or fluid – mid grey.
● Bone – nearly white.
● Metal – white, as all X-rays absorbed.

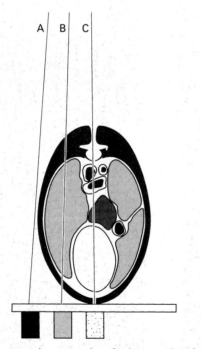

Fig. 24.10 Diagrammatic cross-section of a thorax to show formation of an X-ray shadowgraph. X-ray photons passing along path C are largely absorbed, and result in white areas on the radiograph. X-ray photons passing along path B are partly absorbed and produce intermediate shades of grey on the radiograph. (Reproduced with the permission of Baillière Tindall, London.)

Note that solid soft tissue and fluid produce the same radiographic appearance and therefore fluid within a soft tissue viscus (e.g. urine in the bladder or blood in the heart) cannot be differentiated from the tissue that surrounds it. Note also that fat is less radio-opaque (darker) than soft tissue and fluid, so fat in the abdomen is helpful in surrounding and outlining the various organs.

(3) **Thickness of the tissue**. Overlap in the ranges of grey shades on the radiograph occurs due to the fact that thicker areas of tissue absorb more X-ray photons than thinner areas, hence a very thick area of soft tissue may actually appear more radio-opaque (whiter) than a thin area of bone.

Selection of exposure factors

Kilovoltage (kV)

The kilovoltage controls the **quality**, or **penetrating power**, of the X-ray beam. A higher kilovoltage is required for tissues which have a higher atomic number or specific gravity, or which are very thick. Both the nature and depth of the tissue being X-rayed must therefore be taken into consideration when selecting the appropriate kilovoltage setting.

Milliamperage (mA)

The milliamperage setting determines the tube current and therefore the quantity of X-rays per second in the emergent beam, also known as its **intensity**. Altering the milliamperage will not affect the penetrating power of the beam but **will** change the degree of blackening of the film under the areas which are penetrated.

Time

The product of milliamperage and length of the exposure produces the mAs (milliampere-seconds) factor or total quantity of X-rays used for that particular exposure.

Increasing the kilovoltage will cause greater penetration of all tissues and hence a blacker film. Too high a kilovoltage will over-penetrate tissues resulting in a dark film with few different shades; this is called a 'flat' film or is said to be 'lacking in contrast'. Too low a kilovoltage will underpenetrate tissue (especially bone) which will appear white, on a black or dark grey background. This type of appearance is sometimes called 'soot and whitewash'; its contrast is too high. Figure 24.11 shows the effect of alterations in the kilovoltage.

Increasing the mAs will produce more X-ray photons to blacken the film, though they have no more penetrating ability. The contrast between adjacent tissues (the difference in shades of grey) will not change, but the overall picture will be darker. Figure 24.12 shows the effect of alterations in the mAs.

Although kilovoltage and mAs can be seen to govern different parameters of the X-ray beam, in the diagnostic

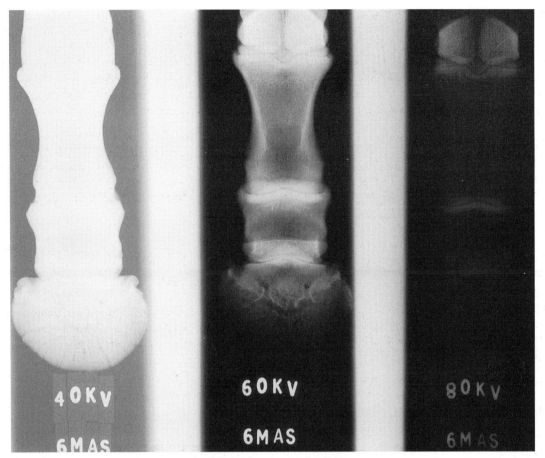

Fig. 24.11 The effect on subject penetration of altering the kilovoltage and keeping the mAs constant.

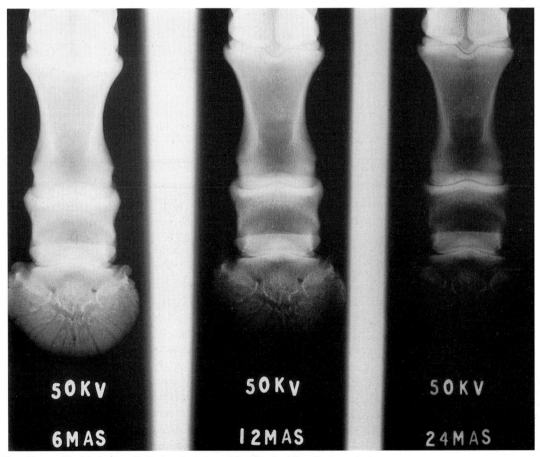

Fig. 24.12 The effect on film blackening of altering the mAs and keeping the kilovoltage constant.

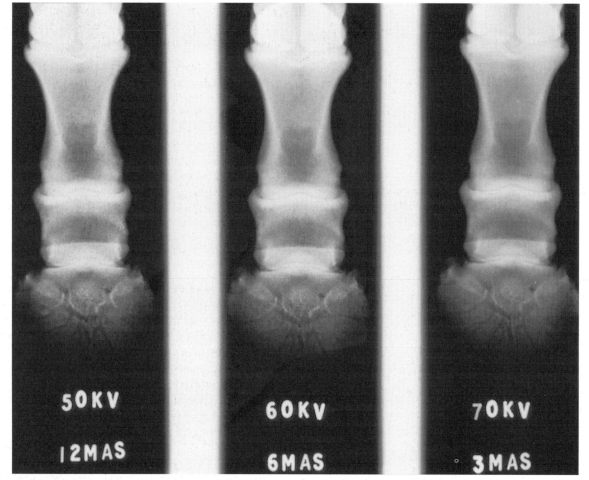

Fig. 24.13 The interplay between kilovoltage and mAs; if the kilovoltage is increased by 10 and the mAs is halved, the effect on the film is almost identical.

range of exposures they are linked, in that pictures which appear similar can be produced by raising the kilovoltage and at the same time lowering the mAs, or vice versa. A useful and simple rule is that for every 10 kV increase, the mAs can be halved (Fig. 24.13). Conversely if the mAs is doubled, the kilovoltage must be reduced by 10. In practice, the time factor is usually paramount and so it is normal to work with as high a kilovotage as possible, allowing the mAs to be kept low.

Focal–film distance (FFD)

The FFD is the total distance between the focal spot and the X-ray film. It is important because although the quality of the X-ray beam remains constant as it travels from the tube head, the intensity falls with increasing distance as the beam spreads out over a larger area. Figure 24.14 shows that if the FFD is doubled, the intensity of the beam over a given area is reduced to one-quarter and the film will appear underexposed unless the mAs is raised. Conversely, if the FFD is reduced the film will appear overexposed. The rule governing this effect is called the **Inverse Square Law**, which states that **the intensity of the primary beam projected on to an X-ray film is reduced to one-quarter by doubling the distance from the X-ray film**. Thus a long

FFD requires a higher mAs than a short FFD and the exact figure can be calculated mathematically from the equation:

$$\text{new mAs} = \text{old mAs} \times \frac{\text{new distance}^2}{\text{old distance}^2}$$

Obviously, longer FFDs require a higher mAs to be used, although image definition will be improved due to a reduction in the penumbra effect (see page 642). It is normal practice to work always at the same FFD for a given X-ray machine; a suitable distance for a portable X-ray machine is 75 cm, whilst 100 cm is normally used for more powerful X-ray machines which produce a higher milliamperage.

Exposure charts

In order to avoid wastage of film and time in repeating radiographs, it is necessary to build up an exposure chart for each machine. An exposure chart is a list of the kV and mAs required for radiography of various areas of different-sized patients. For the exposure chart to be accurate all other parameters must be kept constant (i.e. line voltage, FFD, film–screen combination, use of a grid and quality of processing). The chart may be compiled for patients of different types (e.g. cats, small, medium, large and giant

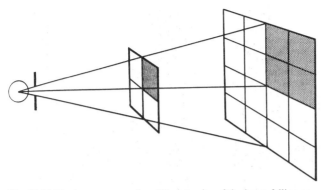

Fig. 24.14 The inverse square law. The intensity of the beam falling on a given area is reduced to one-quarter by doubling the distance from the point of source. (Reproduced with the permission of Baillière Tindall, London.)

dogs) or may be made more accurate still by measuring the thickness of the part to be X-rayed using callipers. The exposure chart can be built up over a period of time by recording all exposures made in the X-ray day book, with comments.

Exposure charts are not usually interchangeable between types of machine and may not even be accurate for other machines of the same make and model because of the varying factors listed above.

X-Ray tube rating

The maximum kV and mAs produced by an X-ray tube are determined by the amount of heat production which it can withstand. If this heat production is exceeded the tube is said to be 'overloaded' and damage may occur. The majority of X-ray machines, including all modern models, have built-in fail-safe mechanisms which prevent these limits from being exceeded and if too high an exposure combination is selected a warning light will come on and the machine will fail to expose. However in old machines this may not be the case and so care should be taken to work within the machine's capabilities by consulting the manufacturer's details of maximum safe combinations of kV, mA and time. These details are known as **ratings charts**.

Scattered radiation

Although most of the X-ray photons entering the patient during the exposure are either completely absorbed or pass straight through, a certain proportion undergo a process known as scattering. Scattering occurs when incident photons interact with the tissues, losing some of their energy and 'bouncing' off in random directions as photons of lower energy (Fig. 24.15). At lower kilovoltages and when thin areas of tissue are being radiographed, the production of **scattered** or **secondary radiation** is small and most is reabsorbed within the patient. Scatter is therefore not a problem when cats, small dogs and the skull and limbs of larger dogs are being radiographed. However, when higher kilovoltages are required in order to penetrate thicker or denser tissues, the amount and energy of the

scattered radiation increases and substantial amounts may exit from the patient's body. The problems associated with this scattered radiation are two-fold:

- Scatter is a potential hazard to the radiographers, as it travels in all directions and may also ricochet back off the table top or the floor or walls of the room. This remains a problem in the radiographic examination of equine limbs, although it should be less serious in small animal radiography where patients are usually artificially restrained and the radiographer stands further away.
- Scattered radiation will cause a uniform blackening of the X-ray film unrelated to the radiographic image, and will detract from the film's contrast and definition. The blurring which results is called fogging.

The amount of scattered radiation produced may be reduced in several ways:

- Collimation of the primary beam (i.e. restriction in the size of the primary beam using a device such as a light beam diaphragm) has a very large effect on the production of scatter. The primary beam should therefore cover only the area of interest, and tight collimation onto very small lesions (such as areas of bone pathology) will greatly improve the quality of the finished radiograph.
- Compression of a large abdomen using a broad radio-lucent compression band will reduce the thickness of tissue being radiographed and will also reduce the amount of scattered radiation produced. Compression band devices may be attached to X-ray tables but should be used with caution in animals with abdominal pathology such as uterine or bladder distension.
- Reduction of the kilovoltage factor will reduce scattered radiation and the lowest practicable kilovoltage should be selected; however this is not always feasible as in lower-powered X-ray machines the priority is usually to keep exposure time down using a low mAs factor and hence a large kilovoltage.
- Reduction of back-scatter from the table top by covering it with a 1 mm thick lead sheet.

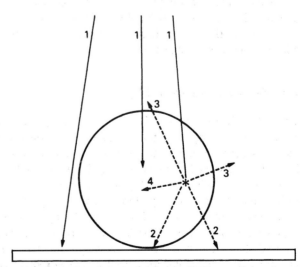

Fig. 24.15 Formation of scattered radiation. (1) Photons of the primary beam. (2) Scatter in a forward direction causing film fogging. (3) Scatter in a backwards direction which is a safety hazard. (4) Some scatter is absorbed by the patient.

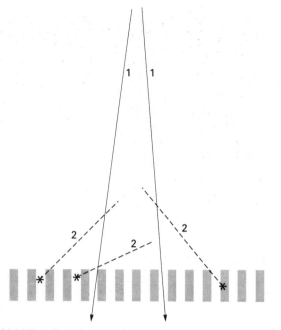

Fig. 24.16 The effect of a grid. (1) Most primary beam X-ray photons pass through the grid. (2) Obliquely-moving scattered radiation is absorbed by the strips of lead.

The use of grids

Even when the above precautions are taken, scattered radiation is still often a significant problem. However the amount of scatter reaching the film can be greatly reduced by using a device known as a grid, which is a flat plate placed between the patient and the cassette. A grid consists of a series of thin strips of lead alternating with strips of a material which allows X-rays through, such as plastic or aluminium. X-ray photons which have passed undeflected through a patient will pass through the radiolucent plastic or aluminium strips ('interspaces') but obliquely-moving scattered radiation will largely be absorbed by the lead strips (Fig. 24.16). Thus there will be a reduction in the degree of film fogging and an improvement in the image. Significant amounts of scattered radiation are produced from depths of solid tissue greater than 10 cm (or a 15 cm depth of chest, which contains much air), and so the use of a grid is usually recommended for areas thicker than this. Various types of grid are available, and there are two broad groups: **stationary** and **moving grids**.

Stationary grids

Stationary grids are either separate pieces of equipment or are built into the front of special cassettes. Various sizes are available, but it is advisable to buy a grid large enough to cover the biggest cassette used in the practice. Grids are

expensive and fragile and should be treated with care as the strips may be broken if the grid is dropped.

- *Parallel grids* – a parallel grid is the simplest and cheapest type of grid. The strips are vertical, and parallel to each other (Fig. 24.17a). This means that, since the X-ray beam is diverging from its very small source, the X-ray photons at the edge of the primary beam may also be absorbed by the lead strips, as well as scatter. There may therefore be some reduction in the quality of the film around the edges; this is called 'grid cut-off'.
- *Focused grids* – a focused grid should prevent grid cut-off as the central strips are vertical but those on either side slope gradually, to take into account the divergence of the primary beam (Fig. 24.17b). A focused grid must be used at its correct focal–film distance (which is usually written on the front of the grid), and should not be used upside down. The X-ray beam must be centred correctly over the grid and be at right angles to it. Focused grids are considerably more expensive than parallel grids.
- *Pseudo-focused grids* – a pseudo-focused grid is intermediate between a parallel and a focused grid in efficiency and price. The strips are vertical, but get progressively shorter towards the edges so reducing the amount of primary beam absorbed (Fig. 24.17c). Pseudo-focused grids should also be used at the correct focal–film distance.
- *Crossed grids* – most grids contain strips aligned only in one direction and therefore scattered radiation travelling in line with the strips will not be absorbed. Crossed grids contain strips running in both directions and so remove much more scattered radiation. The strips may either be parallel or focused. Crossed grids cost several hundred pounds and may only be used in establishments routinely X-raying equine spines, chests and pelvises.

Moving grids

The use of a stationary grid results in the presence of visible parallel lines on the radiograph. These lines may be eliminated by the use of a grid which oscillates slightly during the exposure. This requires an electronic connection between the X-ray machine and the moving grid or 'Potter–Bucky diaphragm', which is built into the X-ray table. Moving grids are used in larger veterinary institutions and moving grid tables may sometimes be available for purchase second-hand from human hospitals.

Grid parameters

- *Grid factor* – the use of a grid means that as well as scattered radiation the grid will absorb some of the

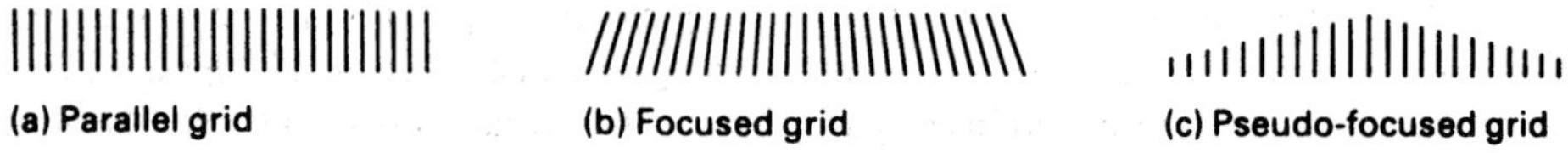

(a) Parallel grid   **(b) Focused grid**   **(c) Pseudo-focused grid**

Fig. 24.17 Types of stationary grid (diagrammatic cross-sections).

useful, primary beam. The mAs factor must therefore be increased when using a grid (to increase the number of X-ray photons in the beam) by an amount known as the grid factor. This is usually 2.5–3 times, but will be specified for each grid. In most cases it will require that a longer exposure time is used as the X-ray machine will probably be already set at its maximum mA output. The increase in time may increase the risk of movement blur on the film, and the radiographer will have to decide whether or not this is outweighed by the advantages of using a grid.

- *Lines/cm* – the greater the number of lines/cm the finer are the grid lines on the film and the less the disruption to the image; coarse grid lines may be very distracting. The usual number is about 24 lines/cm for grids used in general practice. Grids with finer lines are more expensive.
- *Grid ratio* – the grid ratio is the ratio of the height of the strips to the width of the radiolucent interspace. The larger the grid ratio the more efficient it is at absorbing scatter, but the more expensive the grid and the larger the grid factor. Practice grids usually have a ratio of 5:1 to 10:1. Grids used with more powerful machines may have a ratio of 16:1.

Recording the X-ray image

Once the X-ray beam has passed through the subject and undergone differential absorption by the tissues, it must be recorded in order to produce a visible and permanent image. This is done using X-ray film which has some properties in common with photographic film, including its sensitivity to white (visible) light. It must therefore be enclosed in a light-proof container (either a metal or plastic cassette or a thick paper envelope) and handled only in conditions of special subdued 'safe-lighting' until after processing.

Structure of X-ray film

The part of the film which is responsible for producing the image is the **emulsion**, which coats the film base on both sides in a thin, uniform layer. The emulsion gives unexposed film an apple green, fawn or mauve colour when examined in daylight (obviously an unexposed film examined in this way will then be ruined for X-ray purposes!). The emulsion consists of gelatin in which are suspended tiny grains of silver bromide. The silver bromide molecules are sensitive to X-ray photons and to visible light, both of which change their chemical structure slightly. During a radiographic exposure, X-ray photons passing through the patient will cause this invisible chemical change in the underlying film emulsion, but the picture is not visible to the naked eye and the film will still be spoilt by blackening ('fogging') if exposed to white light. The picture is therefore a hidden or 'latent' image and must be rendered visible to the eye by chemical processing or development. When the film is developed the chemical change in the emulsion continues until those silver bromide grains which were exposed lose their bromine and become grains of pure silver, appearing black when the film is viewed.

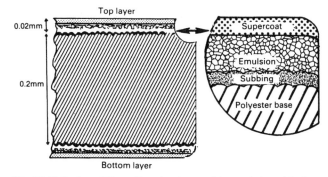

Fig. 24.18 Section of X-ray film, showing emulsion coats bound to the base by subbing layers and protected by supercoats. (Reproduced with the permission of Baillière Tindall, London.)

The emulsion layers are attached to the transparent polyester film base by a sticky 'subbing' layer and the outer surfaces are protected by a supercoat (Fig. 24.18).

Intensifying screens and cassettes

Unfortunately, X-ray film used alone requires a very large exposure to produce an image and the use of film in this way is unacceptable in most circumstances. However it was discovered many years ago that the exposure time could be greatly reduced for the same degree of blackening if some of the X-ray photons emerging from the patient were converted into visible light photons using crystals of phosphorescent material coating flat sheets held against the X-ray film. These devices are known as **intensifying screens** (because they **intensify** the effect of the X-rays on the film) and for many years the commonest phosphor used in the construction of intensifying screens was **calcium tungstate** which emits blue light when stimulated by X-rays. More recently a new group of phosphors has been used in intensifying screens; these are the **rare-earth** phosphors which produce blue, green or ultraviolet light. It is important that the X-ray film being used is sensitive primarily to the right colour of light and for this reason some film–screen combinations are incompatible. One advantage of rare earth screens is that they are more sensitive to the primary beam than are calcium tungstate screens and so exposure factors can be markedly reduced producing less scattered radiation and images with less movement blur. Additionally, they produce finer image definition.

Screens consist of a stiff plastic base covered with a white reflecting surface and then with a layer of the phosphor. Over the top is a protective supercoat layer. The screens are usually used in pairs and are enclosed in a light-proof metal or plastic box (a **cassette**; Fig. 24.19) with the film sandwiched between. Occasionally a single screen is used together with single-sided emulsion film used for human mammography; such a combination produces higher definition images but requires slightly larger exposures. These systems are especially popular for equine orthopaedic radiography. For good detail the film and screens must be in close contact and so the cassette contains a thick felt pad between the back plate and the back screen. Poor screen–

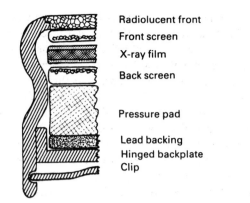

Radiolucent front
Front screen
X-ray film
Back screen

Pressure pad

Lead backing
Hinged backplate
Clip

Fig. 24.19 Exploded scene through an X-ray cassette. (Reproduced with the permission of Baillière Tindall, London.)

film contact causes blurring in that part of the film. The top of the cassette must be radiolucent (i.e. allow X-rays through), and the bottom may be lead-lined to absorb remaining X-rays and prevent back-scatter, although this is uncommon with modern cassettes. The cassette must be fully light-proof with secure fastenings and should be robust. Recently, small flexible plastic cassettes containing one or two screens have become available for small animal intra-oral radiography, to replace 13 × 18 cm size non-screen film which is no longer available (see below).

Care of intensifying screens

Intensifying screens are expensive and fairly delicate and should be treated gently. Scratches or abrasions will damage the phosphor layer permanently, resulting in white (unexposed) marks on all subsequent radiographs produced in that cassette. Screens should not be splashed with chemicals or touched with dirty or greasy fingers. Any dust particles or hairs falling on the screens when the cassette is open in the darkroom will prevent light from reaching the film and will produce fine white specks or lines on the image (even minute particles will prevent the visible light from the intensifying screens from blackening the film in that area although they will not, of course, interfere with the passage of X-rays). Screens should therefore be cleaned periodically by wiping them gently with cotton wool in a circular motion using a proprietary screen-cleaning liquid. The cassettes are then propped open in a vertical position to allow the screens to dry naturally.

Types of X-ray film

Non-screen film

Non-screen film is film designed for use without intensifying screens, i.e. the image is solely due to X-rays. This requires a very large mAs (long exposure time) but produces extremely fine image definition. The film comes wrapped in thick, light-proof paper rather than being used in a cassette. Its use is normally limited to intra-oral views especially for examination of the nasal chambers but it can also be used for extremities and small exotic animals. The

patient will be anaesthetised for this type of study so the very high exposure required is not a problem as the radiographer can retire to a safe distance and movement blur should not occur. The commonly-used size 13 × 18 cm is difficult to obtain and has been replaced by flexible plastic cassettes of the same size which can be inserted into the mouth of a dog or cat for intra-oral radiography. However, image quality is inferior to that which is obtained with non-screen film. The very small sizes of non-screen film are still available but are too small to produce meaningful images of the nasal chambers of medium and larger dogs.

Screen film

Screen film is designed for use in cassettes and is used for all other studies. The detail produced is less than with non-screen film, as the visible light produced by the phosphor crystals spreads out in all directions and will result in blackening of a larger number of silver halide grains than the initial X-ray photon would have done; an effect called 'screen unsharpness' (Fig. 24.20). **Monochromatic** or blue-sensitive film is for use with calcium tungstate or blue light emitting rare earth screens; it is sensitive only to visible light in the blue part of the spectrum. For use with green light emitting rare earth screens the sensitivity of the film emulsion is extended to include green as well as blue light; this is called **orthochromatic** film. It can therefore be appreciated that whilst green-sensitive film can be used with blue light emitting screens as well (since it is sensitive to both colours), blue-sensitive film can only be used with blue light emitting screens. Currently only one manufacturer produces ultraviolet light emitting screens which should therefore be used only with the same brand of film.

Film and screen speed

The **speed** of a film, a screen or a screen–film combination describes the exposure required for a given degree of blackening. The speed is due to the size and shape of the phosphor crystals in the screens and the silver bromide grains in the film emulsion, as well as to the thickness of the layers. Fast film–screen combinations require less exposure but produce poorer image definition (the image is more blurred) whereas slow film–screen combinations produce finer detail and are often called **high definition**. In practice, a medium speed system is usually the best compromise for keeping exposure times down and still getting reasonable quality images. Rare-earth systems give better definition at

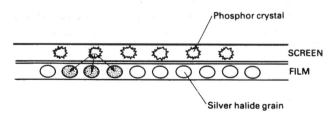

Phosphor crystal

SCREEN
FILM

Silver halide grain

Fig. 24.20 Screen unsharpness. The arrows show how visible light emitted from each phosphor crystal may affect several silver halide grains resulting in some loss of definition of the image.

the same speed. Different manufacturers describe their various films and screens with different terms which makes it difficult to make comparisons, but most produce several speeds of film and screen; e.g. slow (high detail), medium and fast. If a choice of speeds of film–screen combinations is available in the practice, then a slow, high definition combination may be used where exposure times are not a problem (e.g. for bone detail in limbs and skulls) but a faster combination should be used where it is important to keep exposure times short in order to reduce movement blur (e.g. for the chest and abdomen), especially if a grid is used.

Films, screens and cassettes come in a range of sizes from 13 × 18 to 35 × 43 cm. It is wise to have several different sizes available so as not to waste film by radiographing small areas on large plates, although multiple exposures can be made on the same film. Hangers of corresponding size must be available if the films are processed manually.

Storage of X-ray film

As has already been mentioned, unexposed X-ray film is sensitive to light and so must be stored in a light-proof container. This may be either the original film box or a light-proof hopper. Film boxes and loaded cassettes should be kept away from the X-ray area in case they are fogged by scattered radiation; they may be kept in lead-lined cupboards if stored near a source of radiation.

Films are also sensitive to certain chemical fumes and of course to chemical splashes, so good darkroom technique is essential. They may be damaged by pressure or folding so should be stored upright and handled carefully without being bent or scratched. In hot climates high temperature or humidity may be a problem and so film should be refrigerated. This is not usually necessary in the UK!

Finally, film has a finite shelf-life which varies with the type of film. It is therefore wise to date the film boxes on arrival and use them in sequence, within the expiry date shown on the box.

Processing the film

The invisible or latent image on the exposed X-ray film is rendered visible and permanent by a series of chemical reactions known as processing. As with photographic film, this must be carried out under conditions of relative darkness as the X-ray film is sensitive to blackening by white light (fogging) until processing is complete. There are five stages in the procedure of manual film processing: development, intermediate rinsing, fixing, washing and drying.

Development

The main active ingredient in the developing solution is either **phenidone-hydroquinone** or **metol-hydroquinone**. These chemicals convert the exposed crystals of silver bromide into minute grains of black, metallic silver whilst the bromide ions are released into the solution. This process is known as **reduction** and the developer acts as a **reducing agent**. The length of time for which the film is immersed in the developer (usually 3–5 minutes) is critical, since longer development times will allow some of the unexposed silver bromide crystals to be converted to black, metallic silver as well, causing uniform darkening of the film (**chemical** or **development fog**: see section on film faults). The developer must also be used at a constant and uniform temperature (usually 20°C/68°F) and ways of achieving this will be considered later. Precise times and temperatures for developing films are given in the manufacturer's instructions along with some indication of how the development time may be altered to compensate for unavoidable changes in the temperature of the solution.

Other chemicals present in the developing solution include an **accelerator** and a **buffer**, to produce and maintain the alkalinity of the solution necessary for efficient development, and a **restrainer** to reduce the amount of development fog.

X-ray developing solutions are purchased as concentrated liquids. Skin irritation may be observed after handling processing solutions. This may be due to an allergic reaction or due to the alkaline nature of the developer. Gloves should be worn when the chemicals are handled. If the problem is marked, the person's doctor should be consulted and informed of the chemicals involved.

During the development of each film a certain quantity of the developer will be absorbed into the film emulsion and so the level in the developer tank will gradually fall. On no account should the solution be topped up with water as this will cause dilution and subsequent underdevelopment of films. The original developer solution is also unsuitable for topping up, as the proportions of the different chemical constituents of the developer change with each film which is developed and the solution becomes imbalanced. Instead, special **developer replenisher** solutions should be used which take into account, and compensate for, this imbalance. Eventually, however, the developer will become exhausted as the active ingredients are used up and the solution becomes saturated with bromide ions.

Developer will also deteriorate with time by the process of **oxidation**, which will again result in underdevelopment of films. This process can be slowed by keeping the developer tank covered or by keeping the solution in dark stoppered bottles. Whether or not the developer is used it is therefore unlikely to be fit for use after 3 months, and so the general rule is to change the developer completely either every 3 months or when an equal volume of replenisher has been used, whichever is the sooner.

Rinsing

After the appropriate development time the film and hanger are removed from the solution and quickly transferred to the rinse water tank. Surplus developer should not be allowed to drain back into the developer tank because it will be saturated with bromide ions and will contribute to developer exhaustion. The film should be rinsed for about 10 seconds to remove excess developer solution and prevent carry-over into the fixer tank. Ideally the rinse tank will be situated between the developer and the fixer to prevent splashes of developer falling into the fixer.

Fixing

Following immersion in the developer, the film is still sensitive to white light and so the image must be rendered permanent by a process known as **fixing**, which removes the unexposed silver halide crystals leaving the metallic silver image which can be viewed in normal light. The fixer contains **sodium** or **ammonium thiosulphate** which dissolves the unexposed silver halide causing the emulsion to take on a milky-white appearance until the process is complete. The time taken for the removal of all of the unexposed halide is called the **clearing time** and depends on the thickness of the film emulsion, the temperature and concentration of the solution and the degree of exhaustion of the fixer. The fixer becomes exhausted as the amount of dissolved silver halide builds up within it, and exhaustion of fixer will occur more quickly than exhaustion of developer.

Fixer temperature is not critical but warm fixer will clear a film faster than cold fixer. However, above 21°C/70°F staining may occur so the fixer should not be overheated. Fixing can also be speeded up by agitating the film slightly in the fixer. After 30 seconds' immersion in the fixer it is safe to switch on the darkroom light, and the film may be viewed once the milky appearance has cleared. The total fixing time should be at least twice the clearing time, a total of about 10 minutes.

A second function of the fixer bath is to harden the film emulsion (a process known as **tanning**) to prevent the film from being scratched when handled. As well as the fixing agent (thiosulphate) and the **hardener**, the fixer solution also contains a **weak acid**, to neutralise any remaining developer, a **buffer** to maintain the acidity and a **preservative**.

Fixing solutions are normally made up from concentrated liquids by the addition of water according to manufacturer's instructions, as are developing solutions. They should be changed when the clearing time has doubled.

Washing

Following development and fixing, the film must be washed thoroughly to remove residual chemicals which would cause fading and yellow–brown staining of the film. Washing is best achieved by immersion of the film and hanger in a tank with a constant circulation of water so that the film is properly rinsed; static water tanks are much less satisfactory. Washing time should be 15–30 minutes.

Drying

Following adequate washing the films should be removed from their hangers for drying. Films left in hangers of the channel type will not dry adequately around the edges. The usual method is to clip the films to a taut line over a sink, taking care that they do not touch each other. The atmosphere should be dust-free with a good air circulation. Drying frames and warm-air drying cabinets are also available and are useful if film throughput is high.

Processing of non-screen film

As the emulsion of non-screen film is thicker than that of screen film it takes longer for the developing and fixing chemicals to penetrate the emulsion and act on the silver halide crystals. Development time should normally be increased by about 1 minute and clearing time in the fixer will be several minutes longer.

Darkroom design

Requirements

The darkroom is an important part of the radiography set-up within each practice. The following factors should be considered in its construction:

- **Size**. Ideally it should be of a reasonable size to allow for satisfactory working conditions, and should not be used for any other purpose.
- **Light-proofing**. The darkroom must be completely light-proof, and this must be checked by standing inside the darkroom for about 5 minutes until the eyes becomes dark-adapted, as small chinks of light entering may otherwise go unnoticed. The room must be lockable from the inside to prevent the door being opened inadvertently whilst films are being processed. Light-proof maze entrances or revolving cylindrical doors are used in busy hospital departments so that radiographers have free access to the darkroom.
- **Services**. There should be a supply of electricity and mains water and a drain.
- **Ventilation**. If the room is used often, some form of light-proofed ventilation is essential.
- **Walls, floor and ceiling**. The walls and ceiling should be painted white or cream (not black) so as to reflect the subdued lighting making it easier for those working inside to see what they are doing. The walls and floor should be washable and resistant to chemical splashes; it may be wise to tile any wall areas likely to be splashed.

Safe lighting

Since X-ray film is sensitive to white light until the fixing stage, illumination must be achieved using light of low intensity and a specific colour from **safe-lights**, which are boxes containing low-wattage bulbs behind brown or dark red filters. The colour of light produced must be safe for the type of film being processed as green-sensitive films require different filters to blue-sensitive films. If the wrong filter is used then the films will become uniformly fogged whilst being handled in the darkroom. The efficiency of the safe-lights may be checked by laying a pair of scissors or a bunch of keys on an unexposed film on the work bench for periods of up to two minutes and then processing it. If significant fogging is occurring the metal object will be visible on the film. It should be noted that no safe-light is completely safe if the films are exposed for too long or if the safe-light is too close to the handling area. Film manufacturers will advise on the correct filter colour needed for particular types of film.

Two types of safe-light are available: **direct safe-lights** shine directly over the working area and **indirect safe-lights** produce light upwards which is reflected from the ceiling. The number of safe-lights required varies with the size of the room but should allow efficient film handling without fumbling.

Dry and wet areas

The darkroom should be divided into two working areas, the **dry area** and the **wet area** (Fig. 24.21). If the room is large enough these areas may be separated by being on opposite sides of the room but where this is not possible they must be separated by a partition to prevent splashes from the wet area reaching the dry bench and damaging the films or contaminating the intensifying screens.

- **Dry area**. In this area the films are stored in boxes (preferably in cupboards) or in film hoppers, loaded into and out of cassettes and placed in the film hangers prior to processing. Sometimes films are also labelled at this stage. Dry film hangers should be stored on a rack above

the dry bench and there may also be a storage area for cassettes.

- **Wet area**. The processing chemicals are kept and used here. There should be a viewing box with a drip tray for initial examination of the films, a wall rack for wet hangers and some arrangement for allowing films to dry without dripping over the floor or other working areas.

Usually, the processing solutions are contained in tanks. The developer tank should have a well-fitting lid to slow down the rate of deterioration of the developer due to oxidation by the atmosphere. Ideally the intermediate rinse water is held in a separate tank situated between the developer and the fixer so as to prevent splashes of developer falling into the fixer. The rinse water should be changed frequently. The final wash tank should contain running water if possible and should be at least 4 times the size of the developer tank.

In a busy radiography unit the tanks should be housed together in a larger container filled with water and maintained at a constant temperature (usually 20°C/68°F) (Fig. 24.22). This water bath ensures that the chemicals are always at the correct, uniform temperature for processing and saves time as well as helping to avoid under-development of films. It is not essential to heat the fixer but inclusion in the water bath will prevent fixing from slowing down in very cold weather. Water bath arrangements may be purchased as special units or may be self-constructed, using an immersion heater and a thermostat.

If a water bath is not available the tanks should sit in a shallow sink to prevent wetting the floor. In this case the developer must be heated prior to use using an immersion heater with a thermostat or a thermometer (the latter requires constant checking) (Fig. 24.23). The solution must not be allowed to overheat and must be thoroughly mixed before the film is placed in the tank, as an uneven

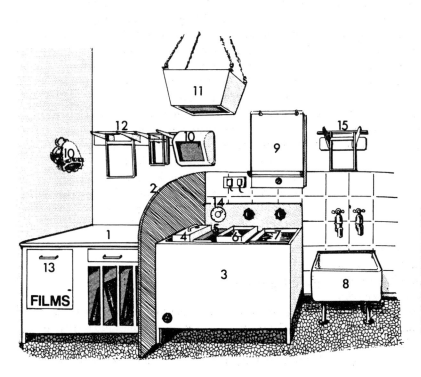

Fig. 24.21 A simple darkroom layout. (1) Dry bench. (2) High partition between dry and wet benches. (3) Wet bench – manual processing unit. (4) Developer tank with lid. (5) Rinse water tank. (6) Fixer tank. (7) Wash tank. (8) Sink. (9) Viewing box. (10) Direct safe-light. (11) Indirect/direct ceiling safe-light. (12) Film hangers on wall rack. (13) Film hopper. (14) Thermostatic control and temperature gauge for processing unit water jacket. (15) Wall rack for wet hangers. (Reproduced with the permission of Baillière Tindall, London.)

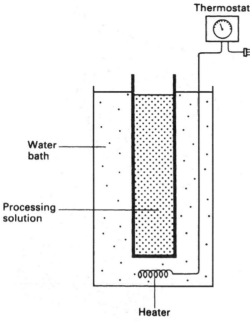

Fig. 24.22 Heating the processing solutions: water bath method.

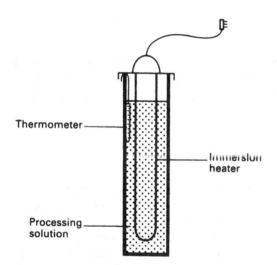

Fig. 24.23 Heating the processing solutions: immersion heater method.

temperature in the solution will result in patchy development and a mottled appearance to the film.

If few radiographs are processed, the chemicals may be kept in dark, stoppered bottles and poured into shallow dishes for use (as in photography). Unused cat litter trays make ideal processing dishes for radiographs. The correct development temperature is achieved either by heating the solution prior to use or by placing the dish on an electric heating pad. The solutions are usually discarded after use as the developer oxidises rapidly.

Other equipment

Film hangers are available in two types: **channel hangers** and **clip hangers**. Each type has its advantages and disadvantages. Channel hangers are easier to load but may result in poor development of the edges of the film. Films must be removed for drying and attached to the drying line

using clips. The hangers should be washed after the films are removed as chemicals may otherwise build up in the channels causing staining of subsequent films. Very large films may not be held securely in channel hangers. Clip hangers avoid these disadvantages but are more fragile and more cumbersome to use and they may tear the films if not used correctly.

A **timer with a bell** should be present in the darkroom so that the period of development can be timed accurately. The timer should ideally be capable of being pre-set to a given time.

A **hand towel** and a **waste-paper bin** are also useful additions to the darkroom.

General darkroom procedure

Most film faults arise during processing and often radiographs which have been carefully taken are spoilt by careless darkroom technique. Competent handling of the films during this stage is therefore vital to the success of radiography within the practice and it is a duty usually delegated to the veterinary nurse.

General care of the darkroom

The darkroom should be kept tidy, clean and uncluttered, with all the equipment in its correct place. Cleanliness is particularly important as undeveloped films handled with fingers which are dirty or contaminated with developer, fixer or water will show permanent finger prints. Splashes of liquid falling on to undeveloped films result in black (developer), grey (water) or white (fixer) patches on subsequent films due to interference with light emission.

Attention must also be paid to the maintenance of the processing solutions, as underdevelopment is the single most common film fault. They should be topped up when their levels fall and they should be changed regularly, with a record being kept of the date on which they are changed. Separate mixing rods should be used for developer and fixer and should be cleaned after use. Chemicals splashing on to the walls or the floor should be wiped up, as they produce dust when dry and they may corrode the surfaces. The chemical solutions may also stain clothing and so aprons should be worn while they are being mixed. The temperature of the solutions should be checked regularly and the heater or thermostat adjusted if necessary.

Other important points are to ensure that the cassettes are always reloaded ready for use when the previous film is removed and to ensure that a sufficient number of film hangers are always clean and dry.

X-ray film processing sequence

In order to ensure that no mistakes are made a strict protocol should be adhered to and all those involved in film processing must be familiar with it. The following steps should be carried out:

Preparation

(1) Check that the developer and fixer are at the correct level. Check that the developer is at the required temperature and is adequately stirred.
(2) Ensure that hands are clean and dry.
(3) Select a suitable film hanger and check that new films for reloading the cassette are available.
(4) Lock the door, switch on the safe-light and switch off the main light.

Unloading the cassette

Open the cassette and take hold of the film gently in one corner between finger and thumb. Shaking the cassette gently first may help to dislodge the film. Remove the film and close the cassette to prevent dirt falling into it.

Identifying the film

If labelling has not been performed during radiography, label the film using a light marker if available or by writing on the film in pencil.

Loading the hanger

Load the film into the hanger, handling it as little as possible and touching it only at the edges. With the channel type of hanger, the film is slid gently down the channels from the top, engaged in the bottom channel and then the top hinge is closed (Fig. 24.24). With the clip type of hanger, the film

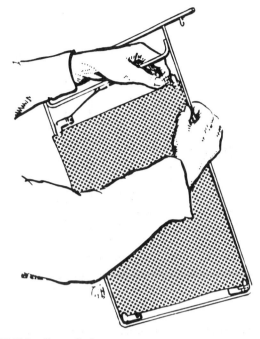

Fig. 24.25 Loading a clip hanger.

is attached to the bottom clips first with the hanger upside down, and then the hanger is placed upright and the film attached to the top clips so that it is held taut (Fig. 24.25).

Processing the film (Fig. 24.26)

(1) Remove the developer tank lid, insert the film and hanger and agitate gently to remove air bubbles from the film's surface.
(2) Close the lid and commence timing. The lid is kept on for two reasons: firstly it reduces the amount of oxidation of the developer by the atmosphere and secondly the developing film is still sensitive to fogging by prolonged exposure to the safe-light.
(3) The film may be agitated periodically during development to bring fresh developer into contact with the film surface and prevent streaking.
(4) At the end of the development period, remove the film and transfer quickly to the rinse tank.
(5) Immerse and agitate the film in the rinse water for about 10 seconds.

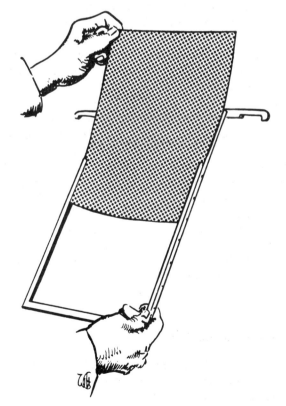

Fig. 24.24 Loading a channel hanger.

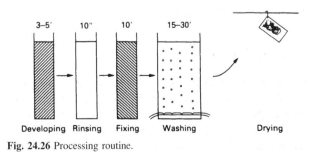

Fig. 24.26 Processing routine.

(6) Transfer the film to the fixing tank. After 30 seconds the light may be switched on or the door opened. The film may be examined briefly once the milky appearance has cleared but it should be fixed for at least 10 minutes to allow hardening to take place.

(7) Wash in running water for half an hour. (If running water is not available in the darkroom the film may be washed elsewhere.)

(8) Dry the film by hanging it on a taut wire in a dust-free atmosphere. Films in channel hangers must be removed first and hung by clips. Films must not touch each other during drying.

Reloading the cassette

This stage may be performed whilst the film is developing.

(1) Ensure hands are clean and dry.
(2) Open the cassette.
(3) Remove a new film from the film box or hopper. Handle carefully without excessive pressure or bending as unprocessed films are susceptible to damage by pressure.
(4) Lay the film in the cassette and, with a fingertip, ensure that it is seated correctly and will not be trapped when the cassette is closed.

Viewing the radiograph

Although the radiograph may be examined whilst it is still wet for technical quality, a provisional diagnosis or the need for a contrast study, the image will be somewhat blurred due to swelling of the two layers of wet emulsion. Full examination must be delayed until the film has dried, when the emulsion will have shrunk and the image is clearer. Films should be examined on clean viewing boxes (not held up to a window) in a dim area to allow the eyes to pick out detail on the film without distracting glare from elsewhere. If the film is small, the rest of the viewer may be masked off with a black card – a simple procedure that will allow very much more detail to be appreciated. Relatively over-exposed areas should be examined with a special bright light.

Automatic processing

Automatic film processing has several advantages over systems of manual film development as it saves considerable time and effort and produces a dry radiograph that is ready to interpret in a very short space of time (as low as 90 seconds with some machines). In addition, the films are processed to a consistently high standard.

Automatic processors are used in human hospitals and in veterinary institutions. They are becoming more popular in general practice, as small table-top processors are now available for about £3000. A darkroom is still required to unload and reload the cassettes, but only a dry bench is

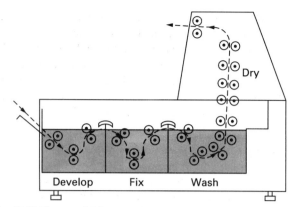

Fig. 24.27 The essential features of an automatic processor. (Reproduced with the permission of Baillière Tindall, London.)

necessary. The processor may be entirely within the darkroom, or the feed tray may pass through the darkroom wall to a processor which is located outside.

Construction of an automatic processor

An automatic processor consists of a light-proof container enclosing a series of rollers which pass the film through developer, fixer, wash water and warm air (Fig. 24.27). The intermediate rinse is omitted as excess developer is removed from the films by squeegee rollers. The chemicals are used at a higher temperature (about 28°C/82°F) to speed up the process, and the solutions are pumped in afresh for each film at a predetermined rate; there is therefore no risk of poor processing due to the use of exhausted chemicals. A considerable amount of water needs to flow through the unit for the final rinse and so there must be an adequate water supply and adequate drainage. Finally, the films are dried by a flow of warm air. If the film throughput is high, a silver recovery unit may be attached to the processor to retrieve silver from waste chemicals.

Maintenance of the automatic processor

Automatic processors usually require a warm-up period of 10–20 minutes prior to use (longer in cold weather). Films processed before the machine has reached its operating temperature will be underdeveloped. During the warm-up period an old, clean processed film may be passed through to check the correct functioning of the processor and to remove any dried-on chemicals from the rollers. At the end of the working day the machine should be switched off and the superficial rollers wiped or rinsed to remove any chemical scum. Once a week the machine may be given a more thorough clean according to the manufacturer's instructions.

The chemicals required are produced specially for automatic processors and are not usually interchangeable with solutions for manual processing as they are formulated for use at higher temperatures. Since the chemicals are pumped in afresh for each film and then discarded, there is no need for developer replenisher solution. The chemicals are made up by mixing concentrated solutions thoroughly with water; in the case of the developer there are two concentrates, one acting as a 'starter' solution.

The automatic processor should be regularly serviced by the manufacturer's engineers as breakdowns can be very inconvenient. Most engineers will also operate an emergency service but nevertheless it may be wise to have the facility to process by hand, should the occasion arise.

Disposal of waste chemicals

Ideally the silver should be removed from the fixer prior to disposal. Silver recovery is not only environmentally wise but is economically prudent. Chemicals for disposal can be stored in suitable storage containers and collected by chemical handling agents.

Film quality with automatic processing

Although automatic processing will produce films of a consistently good standard, there is always a slight loss of contrast compared with the best that can be achieved by perfect hand processing. However the latter is not often achieved and so the automatic processor is usually of great benefit to the practice and likely to increase the enthusiasm of the staff for radiography.

Assessing radiographic quality

Films must be of high technical quality if a radiographic examination is to produce maximum information about the patient. Errors can arise both during radiography and in the darkroom and the radiographer should be able to assess the film for its quality, recognise any faults and know how to correct them.

Before film faults can be recognised, it is necessary to understand the terms **density**, **contrast** and **definition**.

Density

Radiographic **density** is the degree of blackening of the film and is determined by two factors: the **exposure** used and the **processing technique**:

● **Exposure**. Film blackening is affected by the quantity of X-rays passing through the patient and reaching the film. It is influenced by both the kilovoltage and the mAs. If the patient's image is generally too dark, then the film is **overexposed** and the exposure factors should be reduced; conversely, if it is too light, then it is **underexposed** and they must be increased.
● **Processing**. Radiographic density can also be affected by processing. **Underdevelopment**, due to the use of diluted, exhausted or cold developer or development for too short a time, will cause all areas of the film to be too light, including the background. Development can be tested by performing the 'finger test', i.e. putting a finger between the film and the viewer in an area where the film was not covered by the patient and which should therefore be completely black. If the finger is visible, the

film is underdeveloped. Underdevelopment is the commonest film fault arising with manual processing, and should be corrected by topping up the developer with replenisher and not water, by changing the solution regularly and by ensuring that it is used at the correct temperature and for the correct length of time. Underdevelopment may also occur with automatic processing, if the machine is not working at the correct temperature. **Overdevelopment** may occur if the developer is too hot or if the film is inadvertently left in the solution for too long. In this case some of the *un*exposed silver halide crystals will be converted to black metallic silver leading to uniform darkening of the film or **development fog**.

Overexposure and **overdevelopment** may be hard to differentiate as both will cause an increased radiographic density. However, areas covered by metal markers during the exposure will remain white if the fault is overexposure but will darken if the film is overdeveloped.

Underexposure and **underdevelopment** can usually be easily differentiated. Underdevelopment will produce a grey background using the finger test; with underexposure the background should still be black but the area covered by the patient will be too pale.

In general, films which are too dark are to be preferred to those which are too light, as they may still yield adequate information when examined under a bright light.

Contrast

Contrast is the difference between various shades or densities seen on the radiograph. A medium contrast film with a reasonable number of grey shades as well as white and black on the image is desirable, as it will yield most information. A film that shows a white image on a black background with few intermediate grey shades has too high a contrast ('soot and whitewash') and is due to the use of too low a kilovoltage with insufficient penetrating power. A film without extremes of density showing mainly grey shades has a very low contrast and is called a 'flat' film. Poor contrast is usually due to underdevelopment, in which case the background will be grey (use the finger test). Overexposure, overdevelopment and various types of fogging will also produce a flat film but in this case the background density will be black and the remainder of the film will also be very dark.

Definition

Definition refers to the sharpness and clarity of the structures visible on a radiograph. Good definition is usually essential if the film is to be diagnostic.

Definition may be affected by a number of factors:

● *Movement blur*. This is the most common cause of poor definition on chest and abdomen radiographs and is usually due to respiration or struggling by the patient. It may also occur if the tube stand is unstable or if the cassette moves (the latter is applicable only to equine radiography). Patient movement is minimised by the use of sedation or general anaesthesia and by adequate artificial restraint using sandbags, etc. The exposure time should be kept as low as possible.

- *Scattered radiation*. Scattered radiation produced when thick or dense areas of tissue are X-rayed will produce random darkening of the film resulting in loss of definition and contrast. Its effects may be reduced by collimating the beam and by the use of a grid.
- *Fog*. Fogging is darkening of the film unrelated to the radiographic image and has a number of causes. These include scattered radiation, accidental exposure of the film to radiation or white light prior to or during processing, the use of an unsuitable safe-light filter, prolonged storage and overdevelopment. The result is a loss of definition and contrast.
- *Poor screen–film contact*. Poor contact between the intensifying screen and the film within the cassette due to shrinkage of the felt pad will cause blurring of the image in the affected area. It will be present in the same place on all films taken in that cassette.
- *Film and screen speed*. Fast film–screen combinations require a lower exposure for a given degree of film blackening than do slower combinations, but the definition of the image is poorer due to the larger size of the phosphor crystals in the intensifying screens and to the characteristics of the film emulsion.
- *Focal spot size*. Some machines allow a choice of focal spot size. **Fine focus** produces finer radiographic detail but the exposure factors available are limited. **Coarse focus** allows higher exposure factors but, since the effective focal spot is larger, some detail is lost by the penumbra effect (Fig. 24.5). The penumbra effect is reduced by keeping the object–film distance as small as possible and by using a reasonably long focus–film distance.
- *Magnification and object–film distance (OFD)*. Since the X-ray beam diverges from the focal spot, the geometry of the X-ray beam results in some degree of magnification of the image. Magnified images will usually also be

blurred because the penumbra effect increases with increasing OFD. In order to reduce this effect, the part being radiographed should always be positioned as close as possible to the film, with the focal-film distance as long as is practicable for that machine (Fig. 24.28).

The more common film faults and their remedies are summarised in Table 28.1.

Labelling of films

All radiographs should be permanently labelled with the case identification (name or number), the date, a right or left marker if appropriate and any other relevant details (e.g. time after administration of a contrast medium). Labelling of the paper sleeve or film envelope only is inadequate and liable to cause mix-ups, especially on busy days.

Films can be labelled at one of three stages:

- *Labelling of film during exposure*. Films can be identified during radiography by placing lead letters on the cassette or by writing details on special lead tape which is then stuck to the cassette. Care should be taken to ensure that the whole of the information appears on the film after processing and is neither lost on the edge of the film nor overexposed. Right or left markers should be used at this stage and not substituted for by the use of personal codes such as scissors or keys!
- *Labelling in the darkroom*. Films may also be identified by labelling in the darkroom prior to processing. The most efficient method is to use a light marker, which is a small device that prints information, written or typed on paper, on to the corner of the film, using white light. A small rectangular area in the corner of the film must therefore be protected from exposure to X-rays by the incorporation of a piece of lead in the cassette to act as a blocker and leave a space on the film on which these details may be printed
- *Labelling of the dry film*. Information may be written on the film after processing using a white 'Chinagraph' pencil, white ink or a black felt-tip pen. Such identification may not be acceptable for films used in legal cases, and so labelling after processing is not good practice.

Identification of films for the BVA/KC Hip and Elbow Dysplasia Scoring Schemes

The requirement for submission of films to the Hip and Elbow Dysplasia Scoring Schemes is that they must be identified with the dog's Kennel Club number during radiography, i.e. using lead letters or tape or by a light marker before processing. Labelling after processing is not acceptable. The date and right or left markers as appropriate must also be present.

Filing of radiographs

Radiographs may be required for retrospective study or as legal documents and so should be clearly labelled and carefully filed. Many films can accumulate within a short

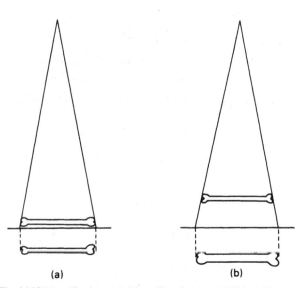

Fig. 24.28 Magnification and object–film distance. (a) Object close to film so reproduced accurately on radiograph. (b) Object not close to film so image is magnified.

(a)   (b)

Table 24.1 Common film faults and their remedies

Fault	Cause	Remedy
Film too dark	Overexposure Overdevelopment FFD too short Fogging	Reduce exposure factors Check developer temperature Time development accurately Increase FFD (see below)
Film too pale	Underexposure (background black but image too light) Underdevelopment (background pale) FFD too long	Increase exposure factors Check developer temperature; time development accurately Change developer Decrease FFD
Patch film density	Developer not stirred Film not agitated in developer	Correct development technique
Contrast too high ('soot and whitewash' film)	Kilovoltage too low	Increase kilovoltage
Contrast too low ('flat film')	Overexposure Underdevelopment Overdevelopment Fogging	Reduce exposure factors Correct development technique (see below)
Fogging	Scattered radiation from patient Scattered radiation from elsewhere Exposure to white light before fixing stage Storage fog (prolonged storage) Chemical or development fog	Collimate beam; use grid Change storage area for film/cassettes Check darkroom, film, hoppers, cassettes, safe-lights Use films before expiry date Correct development technique
Image blurring	Patient movement Tube head movement Cassette movement Scattered radiation Fogging Poor screen–Film contact Large OFD	As for causes
Extraneous marks:		
small bright marks	Dirt on intensifying screens	Clean screens
black patches	Developer splashes onto film before processing	Careful processing
white patches	Fixer splashes onto film before processing	Careful processing
grey patches	Water splashes onto film before processing Chemical splashes on intensifying screens	careful processing Clean screens
scratches	Careless handling of unprocessed film	Handle unprocessed film carefully
black crescent 'crimp' marks	Bending of unprocessed film	Handle unprocessed film carefully
fingerprints	Handling of unprocessed film with dirty hands	Wash and dry hands before processing
static electricity (branching black lines)	Static electricity	Handle unprocessed film carefully Use anti-static screen cleaner
parallel marks on film	Roller marks	Check seating and cleanliness of rollers
Chemical stains:		
yellowing or browning of film on storage	Insufficient washing	Correct washing procedure
areas of film supposed to be clear are grey and opaque	Insufficient fixing	Increase fixing time; change fixer
borders around films	Dirty channel hangers	Clean hangers
grid lines too coarse	X-ray beam not perpendicular to grid focused or pseudo-focused grid upside down	Correct alignment of beam and grid

space of time in a busy practice and the filing system must be simple and fool-proof.

Films processed manually must be completely dry before filing, otherwise they will be damaged by sticking to paper. Films may be stored in their original paper folders or in special X-ray envelopes, with case details (e.g. owner's name, patient information and date) marked clearly on the outside. These may then be kept in film boxes, filing cabinets or on shelving depending on the number of films involved. Films may be stored either chronologically or in alphabetical order of owner's name, with films from each year usually being kept separately. Films of special interest and good examples of normal anatomy should be noted for future reference. For storage of files see Chapter 6, p. 159.

Radiation protection

The dangers associated with radiography

Exposure of the human or animal body to radiation is not without hazard because of the biological effects which X-rays have on living tissues via cellular chemical reactions. X-rays have four properties which mean that the danger from them may be seriously underestimated:

- They are **invisible**.
- They are **painless**.
- The effects are **latent**, i.e. they are not evident immediately and may not manifest until some time later – even several decades in some cases.
- Their effects are **cumulative**, so that repeated very low doses may be as hazardous as a single large exposure.

Large doses are unlikely to occur in human or veterinary radiography but may be seen after nuclear accidents. It is the danger arising from repeated exposure to small amounts of radiation that concerns people working with veterinary radiography.

The adverse effects of radiation on the body may be divided into three groups: somatic, carcinogenic and genetic.

- *Somatic effects.* These are direct changes in body tissues which usually occur soon after exposure. They include changes such as skin reddening and cracking, blood disorders, baldness, cataract formation and digestive upsets. The latter cause severe dehydration which is the usual cause of death following nuclear accidents and bombs. Different tissues vary in their susceptibility to this type of damage, with the developing foetus being particularly susceptible. The somatic effect is used to advantage in the radiotherapy of tumours since tumour cells are often more sensitive to radiation damage than are normal cells.
- *Carcinogenic effects.* These are the induction of tumours in tissues that have been exposed to radiation. There may be a considerable time lag before these tumours arise, which may be as long as 20–30 years in the case of leukaemia.
- *Genetic effects.* These occur when gonads are irradiated and mutations are induced in the chromosomes of germ

cells. The mutations may give rise to inherited abnormalities in the offspring.

Despite these hazards, it is possible to perform radiography in veterinary practice with no significant risk to any of the people involved, provided that adequate precautions are taken.

Sources of radiation hazard

During an exposure, there are three potential sources of X-rays that may be hazardous to the radiographers (Fig. 24.29):

- *The tube head.* Although the tube head is lead-lined (except at the window where the primary beam emerges), older machines may have suffered cracks in the casing, which allows X-rays to escape in other directions. For this reason the tube head should never be held or touched during an exposure. Checks on the efficiency of the casing can be made by taping envelope-wrapped non-screen film to the tube head, leaving it for a few exposures and then processing it. Any cracks in the casing will cause black lines to appear on the film, where it has been exposed.
- *The primary beam.* The beam of X-rays produced at the anode is directed out of the tube head through the window. This primary beam constitutes the greatest safety hazard, since it consists of high energy X-rays. It

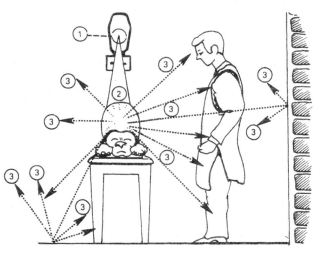

Fig. 24.29 The spread of scattered radiation. (1) The tube head. (2) The primary beam. (3) Scattered radiation. (Reproduced with the permission of Baillière Tindall, London.)

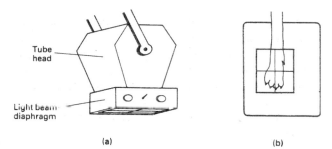

Fig. 24.30 (a) Light beam diaphragm. (b) Centring and collimating a paw.

may be visualised using a **light beam diaphragm**, a device attached to the tube head which produces a light over the area covered by the X-ray beam (Fig. 24.30). The light beam diaphragm usually contains crossed wires which produce a shadow in the illuminated area showing the position of the centre of the beam (the **central ray**). Movable metal plates operated by knobs allow the area covered to be adjusted to the size required, a procedure known as **collimation**. Collimation should always be as 'tight' as possible (i.e. to as small an area as possible) and the accuracy of the light beam diaphragm should be checked periodically. This can be done by arranging pairs of coins along the margins of the light beam with their edges touching so that one of each pair lies inside and one outside the light beam and making an exposure. After processing the image should show four coins inside the black area and the other four coins outside, if the light beam diaphragm was accurate.

An alternative but now uncommon method of collimation is to use conical or cylindrical devices or **cones** attached to the tube window to produce a circular primary beam of varying diameter. Cones are much less satisfactory than light beam diaphragms since the area covered by the primary beam is not seen. Whichever method of collimation is used, the area covered by the primary beam should be no larger than the size of the cassette, and so the borders of the beam should be visible on the processed radiograph.

No part of any handler should come within the primary beam, even if protected by lead rubber clothing. In the rare cases where animals have to be held for radiography, a light beam diaphragm **must** be used to ensure that the primary beam is safely collimated. To prevent the primary beam from passing through the table and scattering off the floor or irradiating the feet of any handlers the table-top should be covered with lead or else a lead sheet placed underneath the cassette.

The use of a horizontal X-ray beam is especially hazardous as the primary beam will pass with little attenuation through doors, windows and thin walls. This procedure should only be performed with great care, with the primary beam directed only towards a thick wall. The procedure for the use of horizontal beam radiography should be described in the Local Rules (see p. 666).

● *Secondary or scattered radiation.* Scattered radiation is produced in all directions when the primary beam strikes a solid object, and so it arises from the patient and the cassette. It is produced by the table or floor if the table-top is not lead lined and it can also bounce off walls and ceilings and travel in unexpected directions. It is, however, of much lower energy than the primary beam and is absorbed by protective clothing. Its intensity falls off rapidly with distance from the source (due to the inverse square law). The best protection against scatter is to stand as far from the X-ray machine and patient as possible.

Ways of reducing the amount of scatter produced (as already discussed in the section on scattered radiation)

include tight collimation of the primary beam, compression of large areas of soft tissue, reduction in the kilovoltage where possible and the use of lead-backed cassettes and a lead-topped table. Protection against scatter is also afforded by protective clothing. The rotation of staff involved in large animal radiography is advisable since personnel may of necessity stand closer to the primary beam. With small animal radiography and non-manual restraint, rotation of staff is less important.

Legislation

In 1985 the law governing the use of radiation and radioactive materials was revised and updated with the publication of **The Ionising Radiations Regulations (IRR) 1985**. This legal document covers all uses of radiation and radioactive materials, including veterinary radiography. As it is written in legal terms and is somewhat lengthy, a second booklet was published at the same time which attempted to explain the Regulations and is called the **Approved Code of Practice for the Protection of Persons against Ionising Radiation arising from any Work Activity**. The Code of Practice does contain some specific references to veterinary radiography but is also rather long-winded and so easy-to-read guidance notes explaining the law as it applies to veterinary radiography were published by HMSO in July 1988 (**Guidance Notes for the Protection of Persons against Ionising Radiations arising from Veterinary Use**). These cover premises, equipment, personnel and procedures and aim to minimise radiation doses received by veterinary staff. A summary of the 1985 legislation is given in the following paragraphs. The IRR are currently under revision (with consultation with relevant bodies, including the RCVS and the BVA) but no major changes are expected.

Principles of radiographic protection

Protection follows three basic principles:

(1) Radiography should only be undertaken if there is definite clinical justification for the use of the procedure.
(2) Any exposure of personnel should be kept to a minimum.
(3) No dose limit should be exceeded.

The aim is to avoid exposure at all times, but failing this a high standard of protection will exist if the advice contained in the Guidance Notes is followed.

Notification of the Health and Safety Executive (HSE)

All practices using X-ray machines must notify the HSE that they are doing so, by filling in Form F2522 9/85. They may then be subject to periodic visits by HSE inspectors to ensure that they are complying with the law.

Practices which are failing to do so may be served with compulsory improvement orders or even prosecuted.

Radiation Protection Supervisor (RPS)

An RPS must be appointed within the practice and will usually be the principal or a senior partner, although may be the Head Nurse in some practices. The RPS is responsible for ensuring that radiography is carried out safely and in accordance with the Regulations, and that the Local Rules (see p. 666) are obeyed, but need not be present at every radiographic examination.

Radiation Protection Adviser (RPA)

Most practices also need to appoint an external RPA. The qualifications necessary to act as an RPA are laid down in the Approved Code of Practice and include veterinary surgeons who hold the Diploma in Veterinary Radiology and who have a knowledge of radiation physics, and medical physicists with an interest in veterinary radiography. The RPA will give advice on all aspects of radiation protection, the demarcation of the controlled area and will draw up the Local Rules and Written Systems of Work.

The controlled area

A specific room should be identified for small animal radiography and should have sufficiently thick walls that no part of the controlled area extends outside it (single brick is usually adequate; thin walls may be reinforced with lead ply or barium plaster). The room should be large enough to allow people remaining in the room to stand at least 2 m from the primary beam. If this is not possible, a protective lead screen should be provided, unless the radiographer can routinely step outside the room and stand behind a brick wall during the exposure. Unshielded doors and windows may be acceptable if the work load is low and the room is large enough. Special recommendations are made for flooring in rare cases where there may be an occupied area below the radiography room.

Technically, the **controlled area** is the area around the primary beam within which the average dose rate of exposure exceeds a given limit (laid down in the Regulations). The controlled area for a typical practice is within a 2 m radius from the beam but usually needs to be defined by the RPA. Since the controlled area must be physically demarcated and clearly labelled, it is usually simpler to designate the whole X-ray room as a controlled area and to place warning notices on its doors to exclude people not involved in radiography. When the radiographic examination is completed the X-ray machine must be disconnected from the power supply; the room then ceases to be a controlled area and may be entered freely.

A warning sign should be placed at the entrance to the X-ray room, consisting of the radiation warning symbol and a simple legend (Fig. 24.31). For permanently installed equipment there should also be an automatic signal at the

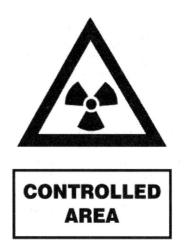

Fig. 24.31 Radiation warning signs.

room entrance indicating when the X-ray machine is in a state of readiness to produce X-rays. This signal usually takes the form of a red light or an illuminated sign. Whilst not a legal requirement for portable and mobile X-ray machines (which comprise the majority of practice X-ray machines), many practitioners have installed red lights outside their radiography rooms to warn when radiography is in progress and prevent accidental entry, and this is to be recommended.

In addition, all X-ray machines should have lights visible from the control panel indicating:

- When they are switched on at the mains.
- When exposure is taking place.

X-ray equipment

Radiation safety features of the X-ray machine should be regularly checked by a qualified engineer. Leakage radiation from the tube housing must not exceed a certain level and the beam filtration must be equivalent to not less than 2.5 mm aluminium. All machines must be fitted with a collimation device, preferably a light beam diaphragm. The exposure button must allow the radiographer to stand at least 2 m from the primary beam which means either that it must be at the end of a sufficiently long cable or else that it should be on the control panel which is placed well away from the tube head. The timer should be electronic rather than clockwork as exposures cannot usually be aborted with the latter, should the patient move.

Suppliers of X-ray machines have a responsibility to ensure that they are safe and functioning correctly, and they should provide a report to this effect when installing the equipment. Servicing of X-ray machines is a legal requirement and should be carried out at least once a year.

The X-ray table must be lead-lined, or else a sheet of lead 1 mm thick and larger than the maximum size of the beam should be placed on the table and beneath the cassette to absorb the residual primary beam and reduce scatter. Many practices now use purpose-built X-ray tables which are not only lead-lined but also fitted with hooks to aid in patient positioning.

Practices performing equine radiography also require cassette holders with long handles for supporting cassettes during limb radiography and various types of wooden blocks for positioning the lower limbs with the minimum of manual restraint.

Film and film processing

The Regulations recommend the use of fast film–screen combinations in order to reduce exposure times. They stress the importance of correct processing techniques in order to minimise the number of non-diagnostic films and avoid the need for repeat exposures.

Protective clothing

Protective clothing consists of aprons, gloves and sleeves and is usually made of plastic or rubber impregnated with lead. The thickness and efficiency of the garment is described in millimetres of lead equivalent (LE), i.e. the thickness of pure lead which would afford the same protection. It is important to remember that **protective clothing is only effective against scatter and does not protect against the primary beam.**

Lead aprons should be worn by any person who needs to be present in the X-ray room during the exposure. They are designed to cover the trunk (especially the gonads) and should reach at least to mid-thigh level. Their thickness should be at least 0.25 mm LE; many are 0.35 or even 0.5 mm LE although the latter are rather heavy to wear. Single-sided aprons covering the front of the body but with straps at the back are cheaper but provide less protection than double-sided aprons covering both front and back and are also less comfortable to wear for long periods. Aprons are expensive items and should be handled carefully; when

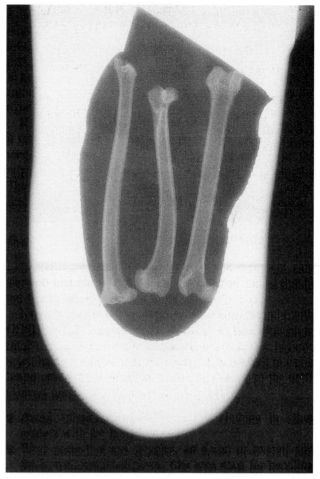

Fig. 24.33 Radiograph of bones covered by a single thickness of lead rubber; compare with the edge where there are two layers of lead rubber.

not in use they should be stored on coat hangers or on rails and they must never be folded as this can lead to undetected cracking of the material (Fig. 24.32).

Lead gloves and hand shields must be available for use in those cases where manual restraint of the patient is unavoidable. They are also required for equine radiography when a limb or a cassette holder may need to be held. Lead sleeves are tubes of lead rubber into which the hands and forearms may be inserted as an alternative to gloves. Single sheets of lead rubber draped over the hands are not adequate as they do not protect against back-scatter. Lead rubber neck guards for protection of the thyroid gland may also be used. Gloves, hand shields and sleeves should be at least 0.35 mm LE and must never appear in the primary beam since they offer inadequate protection against high energy X-rays. It is important to remember that, although a lead glove may appear completely opaque on a radiograph, the film is being protected by two layers of lead rubber but the hand by only one (Fig. 24.33).

All items of protective clothing should be checked frequently for signs of cracking. A small defect may not allow many X-rays through but will always be over the same area of skin. If in doubt, the garment may be X-rayed to check for cracks (Fig. 24.34).

Mobile lead screens with lead glass windows are also useful as the radiographer can stand behind them during the

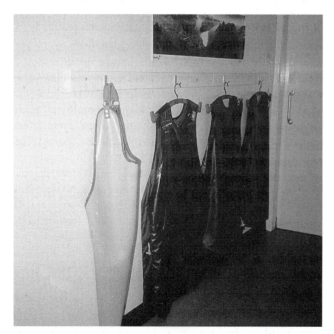

Fig. 24.32 Correct and incorrect storage of lead aprons. (Reproduced with the permission of Baillière Tindall, London.)

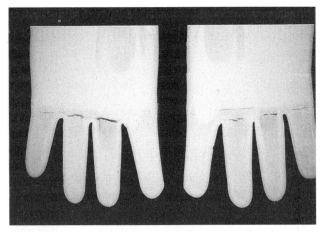

Fig. 24.34 Cracking of the lead rubber at the usual site – the base of the fingers. (Reproduced with the permission of Baillière Tindall, London.)

exposure and still see the patient. Unfortunately they are very expensive.

Dosimetry

All persons who are involved in radiography should wear small monitoring devices or **dosemeters** to record any radiation to which they are exposed. Dosemeters should be worn on the trunk beneath the lead apron, though an extra dosemeter may be worn on the collar or sleeve to monitor the levels of radiation received by unprotected parts of the body. Each dosemeter should be worn only by the person to whom it is issued and it must neither be left in the X-ray room whilst not being worn nor exposed to heat or sunlight. Two types of dosemeter are available:

- **Film badges** contain small pieces of X-ray film and are usually blue.
- **Thermoluminescent dosemeters** (TLDs) contain radiation-sensitive crystals and are usually orange.

They are obtained from dosimetry services such as the National Radiological Protection Board (RPA) and they should be sent off for reading every 1–3 months, depending on the radiographic caseload. If animals are likely to be held for radiography (e.g. equine work), special finger badges may also be worn inside the lead gloves to monitor the dose to the hands.

Dosemeters may also be used to monitor radiation levels in the X-ray room or in adjacent rooms by mounting them on the wall. They can be used to check the adequacy of protection offered by internal walls and doors. The exact arrangement for dosimetry in the practice will be made in consultation with the RPA.

Maximum permissible dose (MPD)

Maximum permissible doses are amounts of radiation which are thought not to constitute a greater risk to health than that encountered in everyday life. Legal limits have

been laid down for various categories of person and for different parts of the body. MPDs are laid down for the whole body, for individual organs, for the lens of the eye and for pregnancy. 'Classified' persons are those working with radiation who are likely to receive more than 30% of any relevant MPD. However, in veterinary practice these levels should not be reached and so veterinary workers rarely need to be designated as classified persons, provided that they are working under a Written System of Work (see below).

Staff involved in radiography

The Local Rules will include a list of names of designated persons authorised to carry out exposures. It should be remembered that nurses and other lay staff aged 16 or 17 have a lower MPD than do adults aged 18 or over and therefore their involvement in radiography should be limited. Young people under 16 years of age should not be present during radiography under any circumstances. Owners should not routinely be present as they are members of the general public and are neither trained in radiography nor wearing dosemeters, although it may be necessary in emergency situations. The Local Rules should ensure that doses to pregnant women are also well within the legal limit, but nevertheless it is wise to avoid the involvement of pregnant women in radiography whenever possible.

The general rule is that the minimum number of people should be present during radiography. When, as is usual, the patient is artificially restrained only the person making the exposure need be present, and this should be the case in the majority of radiographic studies. Often the radiographer will be able to stand outside the room during the exposure.

Local Rules and Written Systems of Work

The **Local Rules** are a set of instructions drawn up by the practice's RPA which set down details of equipment, procedures and restriction of access to the controlled area for that practice. They include the method of restraint of patients for radiography and the precautions to be taken should manual restraint be necessary. They contain an assessment of the maximum dose of radiation likely to be received by people in the practice, and this will normally be zero. A copy of the Local Rules should be given to anyone involved in radiography (including the nurses) and should also be displayed in the X-ray room.

The Local Rules include a subsection, the **Written System of Work**, which describes the step-by-step procedure to be followed for radiography.

Radiographic procedures and restraint

Whenever possible, the beam should be directed vertically downwards on to an X-ray table. The minimum number of people should remain in the room and they should either stand behind lead screens or wear protective clothing. All those present must obey the instructions given by the person operating the X-ray machine. The beam must be collimated to the smallest size practicable, and must be entirely within the borders of the film. Grids should only be used when the part being X-rayed is more than 10 cm thick, as their use necessitates an increase in the exposure.

The method of restraint of the patient is of paramount importance. Many practices previously held all their patients for radiography but this should now be discontinued as it is not only dangerous but also illegal. The Approved Code of Practice states that 'only in exceptional circumstances should a patient or animal undergoing a diagnostic examination be supported or manipulated by hand'. These exceptional circumstances may include severely ill or injured animals for whom a diagnosis requires radiography but for whom sedation, anaesthesia or restraint with sandbags is dangerous (e.g. congestive heart failure; ruptured diaphragm or other severe traumatic injuries). In these cases the animal may be held, provided that those restraining it are fully protected and provided that no part of their hands (even in gloves) enters the primary beam. A light beam diaphragm is essential for manual restraint. The majority of patients may be positioned and restrained artificially under varying degrees of sedation or general anaesthesia, and sometimes with no chemical restraint at all.

Large animal radiography

Special consideration is given to large animal radiography using a horizontal beam. The investigation may need to be undertaken outside the X-ray room, when it should preferably take place in a walled or fenced area with the primary beam directed at a wall of double brick. The extent of the controlled area should be identified using portable warning signs, in order to prevent people not involved from being accidentally irradiated. Everyone taking part in radiography must wear protective clothing and dosemeters. The extra hazards posed by the use of a horizontal beam must be remembered and care must be taken not to irradiate the legs of anyone assisting in the procedure. Collimation must be tight and accurate, especially if a limb or cassette holder is being held by a gloved hand close to the primary beam.

Contrast studies

Although much information about soft tissues can be gained from good-quality radiographs, certain structures may be unclear either because they are radiolucent or because they are masked by other structures. In addition, the inner lining (the mucosal surface) of hollow, fluid-filled organs cannot be assessed because it is of the same radiographic density as the fluid contained within the organ. A good example is the urinary bladder, which appears simply as a homogeneous pear-shaped structure of soft tissue/fluid density.

Contrast studies aim to render these structures and organs more apparent and to outline the mucosal surface where appropriate, either by changing the radio-opacity of the structure itself or by altering that of the surrounding tissue. Both procedures increase the contrast between the structure of interest and the surrounding tissues, allowing assessment of its **position, size** and **shape**. If serial films are taken over a period, it may also be possible to gain some idea of the **function** of the organ (e.g. rate of stomach emptying).

Many contrast techniques are possible, but only those of most relevance to veterinary radiography will be discussed.

Types of contrast media

Two broad groups of contrast media exist: positive and negative.

Positive contrast agents contain elements of high atomic number which absorb a large proportion of the X-ray beam and are therefore relatively radio-opaque, appearing whiter on radiographs than do normal tissues. They are said to provide **positive contrast** with soft tissues. The agents most commonly used are components of barium (atomic number 56) and iodine (atomic number 53).

- **Barium sulphate preparations**. Barium sulphate is a white, chalky material which may be mixed with water to produce a fine colloidal suspension. It is available as a liquid, a paste or a powder which is made up to the desired thickness by the addition of water. It is used almost exclusively in the gut and is not suitable for injection into blood vessels. Being inert, it is non-toxic and well-tolerated by the patient and it produces excellent contrast. Its main disadvantages are that if it is aspirated it may cause pneumonia and if it leaks through a perforated area of gut into the thoracic or abdominal cavities it may provoke the formation of granulomas or adhesions.
- **Water-soluble iodine preparations**. The iodine compounds are water-soluble and may therefore be safely injected into blood vessels. They are then excreted by the kidney and outline the upper urinary tract. They are also safe to use in many other parts of the body. Intravascular injection of these media usually causes nausea and retching and so the patient must be heavily sedated or anaesthetised. Despite being radio-opaque, they appear clear to the eye (unlike barium).

Being water-soluble, the iodine preparations are absorbed by the body and so should be used in the gut in preference to barium if there is a possibility of perforation. However, due to their high osmotic pressure they absorb fluid during their passage through the gut with the result that they become progressively diluted, so that the pictures they produce have much less contrast than those obtained using barium and there is a risk of collapse in a dehydrated patient. They are therefore not routinely used for gut studies.

Many different water-soluble iodine preparations are available but most contain diatrizoate, metrizoate or iothalamate as the active ingredients. For myelography special iodine media with lower osmotic pressures must be used to avoid irritation of the spinal cord and these are iohexol and iopamidol.

Negative contrast agents are gases which, because of their low density, appear relatively radiolucent or black on radiographs, providing **negative contrast** with soft tissues. Room air is usually used in veterinary radiography.

Studies on hollow organs may utilise both a positive and a negative agent in a **double-contrast study**. In these cases a small amount of positive contrast agent is used to coat the inner lining of the organ, which is then distended with gas. This provides excellent mucosal detail and prevents the obliteration of small filling defects, such as calculi, by large volumes of positive contrast. Examples of commonly performed studies are double-contrast cystography (bladder) and double-contrast gastrography (stomach).

Patient preparation

Adequate patient preparation is essential before many of the contrast studies. Prior to a barium study of the stomach or small intestine, the animal must be starved for at least 24 hours to empty the gut of residual ingesta. If food remains in the gut it will mix with the barium, mimicking pathology. Patients should also be starved prior to studies on the kidneys, as a full stomach may obscure the renal shadows. However, most patients are anaesthetised for these studies and so will have been starved anyway.

The presence of faeces in the colon will also obscure much abdominal detail and so an enema is often required prior to the contrast study. This is particularly important before investigations of the urinary tract as faeces may obscure or distort the kidneys, ureters, bladder or urethra. The colon must be completely empty of faeces if a barium enema is to be performed as even a small amount of faecal material will produce filling defects, giving the appearance of severe pathology. The patient should therefore be starved for 24 hours and the colon must be thoroughly washed out with tepid saline or water.

Plain films must **always** be taken and examined before the contrast study commences. They are assessed for the following factors:

- Any pathology previously overlooked.
- Correct exposure factors, to avoid the need to repeat films after the contrast study has begun.
- Adequacy of patient preparation.
- Assessment of the amount of contrast medium required.
- Comparison with subsequent films (to show whether any shadows on the radiographs are due to contrast media or were already present).

A brief description of common contrast studies is given below. More detailed information can be found in Chapter 13 of *Principles of Veterinary Radiography* and in Chapter 7 of the *Manual of Small Animal Diagnostic Imaging* produced by BSAVA (details given in Further Reading at the end of this chapter).

Gastrointestinal tract

Oesophagus (barium swallow)

Indications	Regurgitation, retching, dysphagia (difficulty in swallowing).
Preparation	No patient preparation required; plain films.
Equipment	Barium paste is usually preferred since it is sticky and adheres to the oesophageal mucosa for several minutes. Barium liquid may be used if paste is not available (5–50 ml depending on patient size). Oral water-soluble iodine preparations should be used if a perforation is suspected. Liquid barium mixed with tinned meat should be used if a megaoesophagus is suspected on plain films, as paste or liquid alone may fail to demonstrate the full extent of the oesophagus.
Restraint	Moderate sedation; heavy sedation or general anaesthesia is contraindicated because of the possibility of regurgitation and aspiration.
Technique	Barium paste is deposited on the back of the tongue. Barium or iodine liquids should be given slowly by syringe, into the buccal pouch, allowing the patient to swallow a small amount at a time to avoid aspiration. Barium/meat mixture is usually eaten voluntarily as animals with megaoesophagus tend to be hungry.

Radiographs are taken immediately after administration of the contrast medium. Lateral views are usually sufficient but ventrodorsal views may also occasionally be indicated. Two separate radiographs may be needed to cover the cervical and thoracic areas of the oesophagus.

Stomach (gastrogram)

Two techniques are used: barium only or barium and air (double-contrast gastrogram). The latter gives better mucosal detail.

Indications	Persistent vomiting, haematemesis, displacement of stomach, assessment of liver size.
Preparation	24 hours of starvation; enema if necessary; plain films.
Equipment	Barium liquid (20–100 ml depending on patient size). NB: Barium paste and barium/meat mixtures are not suitable and oral water-soluble iodine preparations should be used if a perforation is suspected. Syringe or stomach tube plus three-way tap.
Restraint	Moderate sedation (to allow positioning); acepromazine has least effect on gut.
Technique	(i) *Barium only.* Administer the required dose of barium liquid by syringe or stomach tube. Roll the patient to coat the gastric mucosa. Take four radiographs; DV, VD, left and right lateral recumbency (see section on nomenclature, p. 673). Take further films as indicated, e.g. to follow stomach emptying.

(ii) *Double-contrast gastrogram.* Stomach tube the patient. Give liquid barium, using the syringe and three-way tap, roll the patient (with the stomach tube still in place) and then distend the stomach with room air. Remove the stomach tube and immediately take four views of the stomach as above.

Method (ii) is preferred if a definite gastric lesion is suspected, but follow-up films of the small intestine may be hard to interpret because of the presence of the air.

Small intestine (barium series)

Indications   Persistent vomiting, haematemesis, abdominal masses, weight loss, malabsorption, intestinal dilatation (usually unrewarding in cases of chronic diarrhoea).

Preparation   As stomach.

Equipment   As stomach.

Restraint   As stomach.

Technique   Administer liquid barium by syringe or stomach tube. Take serial lateral and VD radiographs to follow the passage of barium through the small intestine (usually at intervals of 15–60 minutes, plus a 24-hour film) depending on pathology seen.

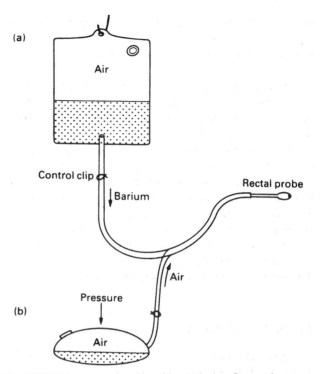

Fig. 24.35 Barium enema bag. In position (a) barium flows under gravity into the colon. In position (b) barium empties from the colon into the bag and then pressure on the bag will distend the colon with air for the double-contrast effect.

Large intestine

Three techniques are used: air only (pneumocolon), barium only (barium enema) and barium and air (double-contrast enema). A pneumocolon will outline soft tissue masses within the colon and the use of barium alone will demonstrate displacement or compression of the colon; but for most purposes a double-contrast enema is indicated as it yields maximum information about the colonic mucosa.

Indications   Tenesmus, melaena, colitis, identification of certain abdominal masses.

Preparation   24 hours' starvation; thorough enema, using tepid water or saline until no faecal matter returns; plain films.

Equipment   Cuffed rectal catheter or Foley catheter. For pneumocolon: three-way tap and large syringe. For barium and double-contrast enemas: gravity feed can and hose or a proprietary barium enema bag; barium sulphate liquid diluted 1:1 with warm water.

Restraint   Moderate to deep sedation (to allow positioning) or general anaesthesia.

Technique   (i) *Pneumocolon.* Position the rectal catheter and inflate the colon with room air, using the syringe and three-way tap, until air leaks out around the catheter. Take lateral and VD radiographs without removing the catheter.

(ii) *Barium enema.* Position the rectal catheter and allow barium to flow into the colon under gravity, until it just begins to leak out around the catheter (usually 10–20 ml/kg is required). Take lateral and VD radiographs without removing the catheter.

(iii) *Double-contrast enema.* As (ii) for initial radiographs.

Then allow excess barium to drain out and re-inflate with air. This can be a very messy procedure unless a special barium enema bag is used; when the bag is lowered to the floor the barium drains back down the tube into the bag. If the bag is then compressed, the air within it will inflate the colon (Fig. 24.35). Repeat the lateral and VD radiographs after the introduction of the air.

Urogenital tract

Kidneys and ureters (intravenous urography (IVU), excretion urography)

Contrast radiography of the upper urinary tract involves the intravenous injection of a water-soluble iodine preparation which is subsequently excreted by, and opacifies, the kidneys and ureters. Two methods are used: rapid injection of a small volume of a very concentrated solution (**bolus intravenous urogram**) and a slow infusion of a large volume of a weaker solution (**infusion intravenous urogram**). The bolus IVU produces excellent opacification of the kidneys. The infusion IVU is preferred for investigation of the ureters, as it produces more ureteric distension by inducing a greater degree of osmotic diuresis.

Indications Identification of kidney size, shape and position, haematuria, urinary incontinence.

Preparation 24 hours' starvation; enema; plain films.

Equipment Intravenous catheter (perivascular leakage of contrast medium is irritant).

For bolus IVU: syringe and three-way tap; concentrated contrast medium (300–400 mg iodine/ml) at a dose of up to 850 mg iodine/kg bodyweight, i.e. about 50 ml for a 25 kg dog.

For infusion IVU: drip giving set; weaker contrast medium (150–200 mg iodine/ml) at a dose rate of up to 1200 mg of iodine per kg bodyweight, i.e. about 200 ml for a 25 kg dog. Concentrated solutions may be diluted with saline for this study if necessary.

Restraint General anaesthesia to prevent patient nausea and allow positioning.

Technique (i) *Bolus IVU*. Warm the contrast medium to body temperature to reduce its viscosity and make it easier to inject. Inject the whole amount as quickly as possible. Take lateral and VD films immediately and at 2, 5, 10 minutes and so on as indicated by the initial pictures.

(ii) *Infusion IVU*. If the patient has urinary incontinence and the position of the ureteric endings is being assessed, a pneumocystogram should be performed first to produce a radiolucent background. Infuse the total dose over 10–15 minutes. Take lateral and VD films once most of the contrast medium has run in. Oblique films are also useful for ureteric endings.

Bladder (cystography)

Direct or retrograde cystography may be performed in three ways: using negative contrast (**pneumocystogram**), positive contrast (**positive contrast cystogram**) or a combination of the two (**double-contrast cystogram**). Pneumocystography is quick and easy but gives poor mucosal detail and will fail to demonstrate small bladder tears, as air leaking out will resemble intestinal gas. Positive contrast cystography is ideal for the detection of bladder ruptures but will mask small lesions and calculi. Double-contrast cystography is usually the method of choice as it produces excellent mucosal detail and will demonstrate all types of calculi. A positive contrast cystogram will also be seen following an IVU, if the patient cannot be catheterised for any reason. Excreted contrast should be mixed with urine already present in the bladder by rolling the animal. This type of cystogram is not ideal as an adequate bladder distension cannot be ensured.

Indications Haematuria, dysuria, urinary incontinence, urinary retention, suspected bladder rupture, identification of bladder if not visible on plain film, assessment of prostatic size.

Preparation Enema, if faeces are present; plain films.

Equipment Appropriate urinary catheter; syringe and three-way tap; dilute water-soluble iodine contrast medium for positive and double-contrast cystogram.

Restraint Sedation or general anaesthesia to allow catheterisation and positioning.

Technique Catheterise bladder and drain completely of urine (obtaining sterile urine sample if required).

(i) *Pneumocystogram*. Inflate bladder slowly with room air, using syringe and three-way tap. The bladder should be inflated until it is felt to be moderately firm by abdominal palpation (usually requires 30–300 ml air depending on patient size).

(ii) *Positive contrast cystogram*. As for (i), but using diluted iodine contrast medium instead of air. However, for detection of bladder rupture, a much smaller quantity is required.

(iii) *Double-contrast cystogram*. Inject 2–15 ml iodine contrast medium at a concentration of about 150 mg iodine/ml into the empty bladder via the catheter. Palpate the abdomen or roll the patient to coat the bladder mucosa. Inflate the air until taut. The bladder wall will be lightly coated with positive contrast, and residual contrast will pool in the centre of the bladder shadow, highlighting calculi and other filling defects. Lateral radiographs are usually more informative, but VD and oblique views may be taken if required.

Urethra (retrograde urethrography – dogs; retrograde vaginourethrography – bitches)

Indications Haematuria, dysuria, urinary incontinence, urinary retention, prostatic disease, vaginal disease.

Preparation Enema, if faeces likely to obscure urethra on either view; plain films.

Equipment Appropriate urinary catheter; syringe; dilute iodine contrast medium (150 mg iodine/ml) (may be mixed with equal amount of K-Y jelly for studies on male dogs, to increase urethral distension); gentle bowel clamp (for bitches).

Restraint Sedation (dogs) or general anaesthesia (bitches).

Technique (i) *Retrograde urethrography (males)*. Insert the urinary catheter into the penile urethra. Occlude the urethral opening manually, to prevent leakage of contrast. Inject 5–15 ml contrast or contrast/K-Y jelly mixture slowly. Release the urethral occlusion and stand back prior to exposure. Lateral views are most useful and should be taken with the hindlegs pulled forwards for the ischial arch and backwards for the penile urethra.

(ii) *Retrograde vaginourethrography (females)*. Snip off the tip of a Foley catheter, distal to the bulb. Insert the catheter just inside the vulval lips, inflate the bulb and clamp the vulval lips together with the bowel clamp to hold the catheter in place. Inject up to 1 ml/kg bodyweight of iodine contrast medium carefully (vaginal rupture has been reported). Lateral views are most informative, and demonstrate filling of the vagina and urethra.

In cats these studies are rarely performed, but may be carried out using simple cat catheters.

Spine (myelography)

A narrow gap surrounds the spinal cord as it runs along the vertebral column; this is called the **subarachnoid space** and it contains **cerebrospinal fluid (CSF)**. It may be opacified by the injection of positive contrast medium and will then demonstrate the spinal cord, showing areas of cord swelling (e.g. tumours) or cord compression) (e.g. prolapsed intervertebral discs) not evident on plain films. This technique, which is called **myelography**, requires the use of special water-soluble iodine preparations which have lower osmotic pressures than do the other iodine media and which are therefore less irritant to nervous tissue. The two low osmolar contrast media currently in use in human and veterinary myelography are iohexol and iopamidol.

Two approaches may be made to the subarachnoid space: the one most commonly used in veterinary radiology is the **cisternal puncture**, where the needle is inserted into the cisterna magna – the cranial end of the subarachnoid space just behind the skull. Myelography may also be performed by injection in the lumbar area via a **lumbar puncture**, which is more commonly used in humans. Lumbar myelography involves passing the needle through the spinal cord and injecting into the ventral subarachnoid space. Both techniques involve practice and skill and the patient must be anaesthetised to prevent movement during needle placement or injection.

Indications	Spinal pain, spinal neurological signs (ataxia, paralysis), identification of prolapsed intervertebral discs prior to surgery.
Preparation	Clip relevant area, i.e. caudal to skull or over lumbar spine.
Equipment	Spinal needle of suitable length depending on patient size; contrast medium, warmed to body temperature to reduce viscosity and ease injection (dose rate 0.3–0.45 ml/kg of 200–300 mg iodine/ml solution – dose administered depends on size of patient and expected site of lesion); syringe; sample bottles for CSF if required for analysis; some means of elevating the head end of the table for cisternal punctures, to aid flow of contrast along the spine.
Restraint	General anaesthesia.

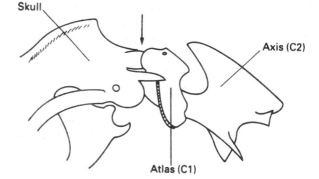

Fig. 24.36 Myelography: site for cisternal puncture.

Technique	(i) *Cisternal puncture*. Elevate table to about 10° tilt with head at the raised end. Clip and cleanse injection site. Flex head to 90° angle with neck. Insert needle carefully into cisterna magna, between skull and atlas (Fig. 24.36), advancing the needle slowly until CSF drips out of the hub. Collect several millilitres of CSF. Inject warmed contrast medium slowly. Remove needle and extend head again. Take several lateral radiographs until contrast reaches lesion, when VD and oblique films may also be taken.

(ii) *Lumbar puncture*. Clip and cleanse injection site. Flex the vertebral column by pulling the hindlimbs forwards. Insert the needle carefully (usually at L5–6); as it passes through the cord the animal's hindlegs and anus will twitch slightly. Little or no CSF may appear from this site and if this is the case a small test injection is required to check needle placement. Inject contrast medium. Remove the needle, extend the spine and take radiographs as above.

N.B. Keep the head raised during the recovery period.

Other contrast techniques

Some other contrast techniques occasionally performed in veterinary practice are described briefly.

Angiocardiography

Angiocardiography is used to demonstrate both congenital and acquired cardiac disease. It involves the opacification of the heart chambers and major vessels by the injection of a bolus of concentrated water-soluble iodine contrast medium. The procedure requires general anaesthesia to prevent patient discomfort or movement. The contrast medium may be injected into the jugular or cephalic vein (**non-selective angiocardiography**) or deposited directly into the heart chambers and major vessels via catheters inserted surgically into the jugular vein and carotid or femoral arteries (**selective angiocardiography**). The latter will also allow blood pressure and blood-gas measurements to be made if the appropriate high-technology equipment is available.

Although a single film may provide a diagnosis, it is desirable to obtain a number of radiographs taken over a very short space of time in order to follow the bolus of contrast around the heart and lungs. This is best performed using a special rapid film changing angiography table, but can also be achieved using a home-made cassette tunnel with several cassettes lined up on a piece of wood and pushed through the tunnel at the appropriate speed.

Angiocardiography is performed much less often than it used to be, since similar information can be obtained by cardiac ultrasound, which is safe and non-invasive.

Portal venography

Portal venography is used to diagnose certain types of liver disease (e.g. congenital porto-systemic shunts, cirrhosis) by demonstration of the vascular system within the liver parenchyma. Under general anaesthesia a laparotomy is performed and a splenic or mesenteric vein catheterised. A small quantity of concentrated iodine contrast medium is injected as a bolus and a single film taken at the end of the injection. The contrast medium enters the liver via the hepatic portal vein and in the normal animal shows branching and tapering portal vessels throughout the liver.

Bronchography

Bronchography is opacification of part of the bronchial tree using specially prepared iodine-containing medium, propyliodone. This medium is rather thicker than the other iodine media, to prevent alveolar flooding. Each study may only demonstrate the left or the right bronchial tree; if both sides are to be investigated then two studies must be performed several days apart. The patient is anaesthetised and placed in lateral recumbency with the side to be investigated down. The contrast medium is injected down the endotracheal tube via a dog urinary catheter. The patient is manipulated to ensure that the contrast has entered all of the bronchi on the side of interest and several films are taken over about 10 minutes.

Bronchography may demonstrate bronchial foreign bodies, *Oslerus osleri* nodules, bronchial tumours, lung lobe torsion and bronchiectasis. It has, however, been largely superseded by bronchoscopy.

Arthrography

Arthrography is the demonstration of a joint space using negative contrast (air), positive contrast (iodine) or double-contrast techniques injected under sterile conditions. The joints most amenable to arthrography in small animals are the shoulder and stifle. General anaesthesia is required as the procedure is uncomfortable. Arthrography will demonstrate joint capsule distension or rupture and defects in the articular cartilage, which is normally radiolucent.

Fistulography

Fistulography is the opacification of sinus tracts and fistulae using water-soluble or oily iodine contrast media. Fistulography will demonstrate the extent and course of these lesions and may outline radiolucent foreign bodies such as pieces of wood.

Positioning

In order to produce radiographs of maximum diagnostic value it is necessary to position the patient carefully and to centre and collimate the beam accurately. Poor positioning, with rotation or obliquity of the area being radiographed, will result in a film that is hard to interpret or misleading or that fails to demonstrate the lesion.

There are several general rules that should be adhered to when positioning the patient:

- Place the area of interest as close to the film as possible in order to minimise magnification and blurring and to produce an accurate image.
- Centre over the area of interest, especially if it is a joint or a disc space.
- Ensure that the central ray of the primary beam is perpendicular to the film otherwise distortion and non-uniform exposure of the structures will result. If a grid is being used, accurate alignment of the primary beam is essential to prevent grid faults.
- Collimate the beam to as small an area as possible, to reduce the amount of scattered radiation produced.
- Since a radiograph is a two-dimensional image of a three-dimensional structure, it is usually necessary to take two radiographs at right angles to each other in order to visualise the area fully.

Oblique views may then be taken to highlight lesions seen on the initial films if appropriate.

Restraint

Small animals should be held for radiography **only in exceptional circumstances**, when a radiograph is essential for a diagnosis but their condition renders other means of restraint unsafe. In practice, patients rarely need to be held and most views may be achieved using a combination of chemical restraint and positioning aids.

Simple lateral views of chest, abdomen and limbs may be possible on placid animals without any form of sedation. Other views require varying degrees of sedation or general anaesthesia and the positioning requirements and the temperament of the patient must be taken into consideration when assessing the depth of sedation required. It is also important to handle patients gently, calmly and firmly during radiography, and to reassure them with touch and voice.

Positioning aids

With the skilful use of positioning aids and the correct degree of sedation, almost any radiographic view may be achieved. The following positioning aids should be present in the practice:

- *Troughs*. Radiolucent plastic or foam-filled troughs are essential for restraining animals on their backs. They are available in a variety of sizes.
- *Foam wedges*. When lateral views are required, these are placed under the chest, skull or spine to prevent rotation and to ensure that a true lateral view is achieved. They are also useful for accurate limb positioning. They are radiolucent and may therefore be used in the primary beam. It is useful to have several, in different shapes and sizes, and to cover them with plastic for easy cleaning.
- *Sandbags*. Long, thin sandbags of various sizes may be wrapped around limbs or placed over the neck for restraint. They should only be loosely filled with sand, so that they can be bent and twisted. As they are radio-opaque they should not be used in the primary beam. They should be plastic-covered for easy cleaning.
- *Tapes*. Cotton tapes are looped around limbs and may then be tied to hooks on the edge of the table or wrapped around sandbags, for positioning of the limbs. Sticky tape may also be useful at times.
- *Wooden blocks*. Wooden blocks are used to raise the cassette to the area of interest, for certain views (e.g. dorsoventral skull). They are radio-opaque and so should not be placed between the patient and the film.

Nomenclature

Each radiographic projection is named by a composite term describing first the point of entry and then the point of exit of the beam, e.g. a **dorsoventral (DV)** view of the chest involves the X-ray beam entering through the spine (**dorsally**) and emerging through the sternum (**ventrally**). An exception is the lateromedial or mediolateral view, which is commonly just called the **lateral** view. A standardised nomenclature has been devised for veterinary radiology and the naming of the various body regions is shown in Fig. 24.37. Note that the terms 'anterior' and 'posterior' are no longer used in veterinary radiology as they are not appropriate to four-legged creatures. Instead, anteroposterior (AP) and postero-anterior (PA) views of the limbs are called **craniocaudal (CrCd)** or **caudocranial (CdCr)** above the radiocarpal and tibiotarsal joints, and **dorsopalmar (DPa)/palmarodorsal (PaD)** or **dorsoplantar (DPl)/plantarodorsal (PlD)** below. The correct terminology will be used throughout this section. **Dorsal recumbency** describes an animal lying on its back and **sternal recumbency** describes the crouching position.

Positions for common views

The following notes describe in brief the positioning for the more common views performed in veterinary practice. Further details are found in *Principles of Veterinary Radiography* (see Further reading). Anatomy texts and radiological atlases should be consulted for identification of normal anatomical structures.

Thorax

Lateral view (Fig. 24.38). The right lateral recumbent position is usual as the heart outline is more consistent in shape. When assessing the lungs it is useful to perform the left lateral view too, as the uppermost lung field is better aerated and is therefore more likely to show pathology.

Place a foam pad under the sternum to raise it to the same height above table-top as the spine. Draw the forelimbs forwards with tapes or sandbags to prevent them from obscuring the cranial thorax. Restrain the hindlimbs with a sandbag and place a further sandbag carefully over the neck. Centre on the middle of the fifth rib and level with the caudal border of the scapula. Collimate to include lung fields and expose on inspiration for maximum aeration.

Identify the trachea, heart, aorta, caudal vena cava, diaphragm, bronchovascular lung markings and skeletal structures. The oesophagus is not normally visible on plain films.

Dorsoventral view (DV) (Fig. 24.39). The dorsoventral view and not the ventrodorsal must be used for assessment of the heart because in the latter position the heart may tip to one side. Position the patient in sternal recumbency, crouching symmetrically. Push the elbows laterally to 'prop' up the dog or cat. Drape a sandbag over the neck to keep the head down, shaking the sand into either end to produce a sparsely-filled area in the middle of the sandbag. It may be useful to rest the patient's chin on a foam pad or wooden block. Centre in the midline between the tips of the scapulae. Collimate to include the lung fields and expose on inspiration.

Identify the structures visible on the lateral view.

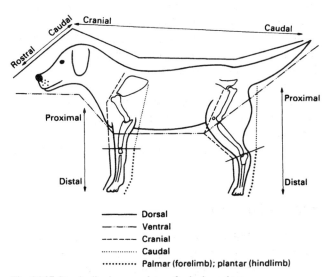

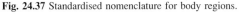
Dorsal
Ventral
Cranial
Caudal
Palmar (forelimb); plantar (hindlimb)

Fig. 24.37 Standardised nomenclature for body regions.

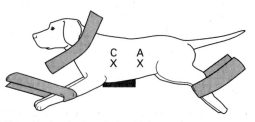

Fig. 24.38 Positioning for lateral chest/abdomen views.

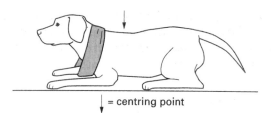

= centring point

Fig. 24.39 Positioning for dorsoventral chest view.

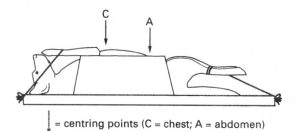

= centring points (C = chest; A = abdomen)

Fig. 24.40 Positioning for ventrodorsal chest/abdomen.

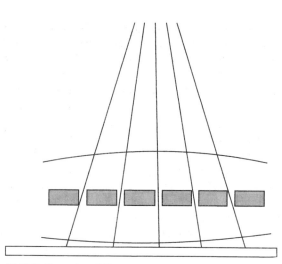

Fig. 24.41 Radiography of disc spaces.

Ventrodorsal view (VD) (Fig. 24.40). Patients must never be placed on their backs if pleural fluid, pneumothorax or a ruptured diaphragm is suspected as this may cause respiratory embarrassment.

Position in dorsal recumbency using a radiolucent trough or sandbags around the hind end. Ensure that the patient is lying straight and not tipped to one side. Draw the forelimbs forwards with tapes or by placing a sandbag gently over them. Secure the hindlimbs too if necessary. Centre on the mid-point of the sternum, collimate to the lung field and expose on inspiration.

Identify the same structures as on the lateral and DV views.

Abdomen

Lateral view (Fig. 24.38). Position the patient in lateral recumbency and pad up the sternum if necessary. Restrain the fore- and hindlimbs with sandbags, ensuring that the hindlimbs are pulled well back so that they do not obscure the caudal abdomen. Place a further sandbag over the neck (sometimes one end of the sandbag placed around the forelimbs can be used for this). Centre over the area of interest and collimate as necessary. Expose on exspiration to give a more 'spread out' view of the abdominal viscera.

Identify the liver, spleen, kidneys, bladder, stomach, small and large intestine and skeletal structures.

Ventrodorsal view (VD) (Fig. 24.40). Position in dorsal recumbency using a trough, or by placing sandbags on either side of the chest. Sandbag or tape the fore- and hindlimbs if necessary. Centre and collimate as required and expose on exspiration. **Dorsoventral** views of the abdomen are rarely performed as the viscera are usually compressed and distorted but may be all that is possible if the patient is dyspnoeic and cannot be placed on its back.

Identify the same structures as on the lateral view.

Skull

Skull views generally require general anaesthesia.

Lateral view. Position the animal in lateral recumbency, using foam wedges under the nose and mandible to ensure that the line between the eyes is vertical and that the midline is horizontal and parallel to the table. The degree of padding depends on the shape of the patient's skull. It may also be necessary to pad the neck and sternum. Centre and collimate as required.

Identify the cranium, frontal sinuses, nasal chambers, teeth, mandibles and tympanic bullae.

Dorsoventral view (DV). Place the animal in a crouching position, with the chin resting on a wooden or foam block, on which is placed the cassette. Secure the head with a sandbag over the neck if necessary. Ensure that the line between the eyes is horizontal. Centre and collimate as required. If an endotracheal tube is being used, it may require removal before exposure so as not to obscure any structures in the midline.

Ventrodorsal view (VD). Place the animal in dorsal recumbency in a trough, with the head and neck extended. Put foam pads under the neck and nose. Hold the nose down using a tape placed behind the upper canine teeth, or using sticky tape.

Oblique view for tympanic bullae. Place the animal in lateral recumbency with the side to be radiographed down. Using foam pads, rotate the skull about 20° around its long axis, towards the VD position (this will skyline the tympanic bulla nearest the table). Centre and collimate by palpation of the bulla. It is usually necessary to repeat the procedure for the other bulla, either to give a normal for comparison or to check if it is also affected. Care should be taken to ensure that the positioning is the same for the two sides.

Intra-oral DV (occlusal) view for nasal chambers.
This view always requires general anaesthesia. Place the
animal in sternal recumbency with the chin resting on a
wooden or foam block. Insert a non-screen film or flexible
plastic cassette into the mouth above the tongue, placing it
corner first so as to get it as far back in the mouth as
possible. Ensure that the head is level. Centre and collimate
over the nasal chambers.

Many other views of the skull are possible but their
description is beyond the scope of this chapter. They include
the intra-oral VD for the mandibles, special obliques for
temporomandibular joints, obliques for dental arcades and
the frontal sinuses, skyline views of the frontal sinuses and
cranium and the open-mouth view for tympanic bullae and
the odontoid peg of C2.

Vertebral column

Spinal pathology is often undramatic and therefore requires
particularly careful positioning, especially if disc spaces are
under scrutiny. General anaesthesia is usually required in
order to obtain diagnostic films. It is not possible to get an
accurate picture of the entire spine on one film, since the
X-ray beam is diverging and will not equally penetrate all
disc spaces, and so it is usually necessary to take serial
radiographs of small areas. In medium and large dogs, up to
six films may be required for a spinal survey as follows:

● Cervical C1–C6.
● Cervico-thoracic C6–T3.
● Thoracic T3–T11.
● Thoraco-lumbar T11–L3.
● Lumbar L1–L7.
● Sacral and caudal (coccygeal) L6–Cd4.

Once a lesion is suspected, collimated views taken over the
area of interest should be made. For disc disease, only the
few disc spaces in the centre of the film are fully assessable
(Fig. 24.41).

Lateral views. Ample use of foam pads is required to
prevent the spine sagging or rotating (Fig. 24.42) and to
ensure that it forms a straight line parallel to the table top.
Centre and collimate to the area of interest by the palpation
of bony landmarks (in obese animals the spine may be some
distance below the skin surface).

Ventrodorsal views (VD). The patient is positioned in
symmetrical dorsal recumbency using a trough or sandbags.
The limbs are secured as appropriate. Centre and collimate
over the area of interest. For VD views of the cervical spine
and cervicothoracic junction, the X-ray beam must be
angled 15° to 20° towards the patient's head in order to pass
through the disc spaces.

The forelimb

Lateral scapula. Lie the animal on the side to be
radiographed. Pull the lower limb caudally and the upper
limb cranially, flexing it towards the head and securing it
with a tape. Centre and collimate to the lower scapula by
palpation.

Caudocranial scapula (CdCr) Lie the animal on its back
in a trough, tipping it slightly over to the side not under
investigation. Draw the limb cranially and secure in
maximum extension with a tape. Centre and collimate by
palpation.

Lateral shoulder (Fig. 24.43). Lie the animal on the side
to be radiographed. Draw the lower limb cranially and
secure it; pull the upper limb well back out of the way.
Extend the head and neck. Centre and collimate to the
shoulder joint by palpation.

Caudocranial shoulder (CdCr). As for caudocranial
scapula but centre on the shoulder joint.

Lateral humerus (Fig. 24.43). As for the lateral shoulder but centre on the humerus.

Caudocranial humerus (CdCr). As for the caudocranial
scapula but centre on the humerus.

Craniocaudal humerus (CrCd). An alternative view.
Lie the animal on its back and pull the affected limb
caudally, securing with a tape. The humerus should lie
parallel to the film. It may not be possible to use a trough for
this view.

Lateral elbow. **Extended view**: as for lateral shoulder but
centre on the elbow (Fig. 24.43).

Flexed view (more useful for assessing degenerative joint
disease): as for lateral shoulder but flex the lower limb at the

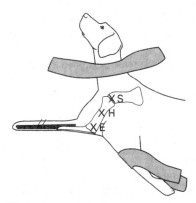
Fig. 24.43 Positioning for lateral forelimb views. X = centring points; S
= shoulder; H = humerus; E = elbow.

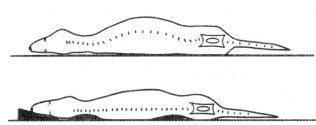
Fig. 24.42 Use of foam pads for spinal radiography.

(a)

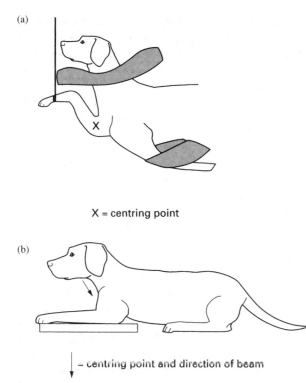

X = centring point

(b)

— centring point and direction of beam

Fig. 24.44 (a) Positioning for flexed lateral elbow. (b) Positioning for craniocaudal elbow view.

elbow so that the paw comes up to the patient's chin. Secure with a tape or sandbag (Fig. 24.44a).

Craniocaudal elbow (CrCd). Position the elbow in sternal recumbency with both forelimbs extended and pulled cranially. Turn the head and neck to the non-affected side and restrain by draping a sandbag over the neck. Take care that the affected elbow does not slide sideways. Centre on the elbow joint, angling the beam about 10° to the patient's tail (Fig. 24.44b).

Caudocranial elbow (CdCr). An alternative view. As for caudocranial shoulder but centre on the elbow joint.

Lateral forearm (radius and ulna), carpus and paw (Fig. 24.43). Lie the animal on the affected side, drawing the lower limb cranially and the upper limb caudally out of the way. Ensure that a lateral position is achieved using foam pads or sticky tape. Centre and collimate to the appropriate area.

For individual toes, it may be useful to separate them by drawing the affected one forwards and the others backwards with tapes.

Craniocaudal forearm (CrCd) and dorsopalmar carpus and paw (DPa). As for craniocaudal elbow, but centre and collimate to the appropriate area and use a vertical beam.

The hindlimbs

Lateral pelvis. Position the patient on its side, using foam pads under the spine and sternum to achieve a true lateral position. Centre on the hip joints.

Ventrodorsal pelvis (VD). **Extended hip position**: this position is described in some detail as it is required for official assessment of hip dysplasia in dogs. It requires general anaesthesia or a reasonable degree of sedation.

Place the patient on its back in a trough, ensuring that it is perfectly upright and not tipped to either side. Extend the forelimbs cranially and secure them with tapes; a sandbag may also be draped over the sternum, taking care not to impair respiration. Extend the hindlimbs caudally using tapes looped just above the hocks and tied to hooks on the edge of the table. The femora should be parallel to each other and to the table-top, and the stifles should be rotated inwards by means of a further tape tied firmly around them (Fig. 24.45). Centre on the pubic symphysis. Perfect positioning may be achieved in this way without the need for manual restraint.

For submission to the BVA/Kennel Club Hip Dysplasia Scoring Scheme the film must be permanently identified with the patient's Kennel Club number, the date and a right or left marker before processing. Films labelled after processing will not be accepted by the scheme.

Identify the various anatomical areas of the hip joint assessed under the scoring scheme.

Flexed or frog-legged view: this view allows some assessment of the hips but is not as satisfactory as the extended view. The hindlimbs are flexed and allowed to fall to either side. Sandbags may be used to steady the hindpaws.

Lateral femur. Two methods are used, both requiring the patient to lie on the affected side. In the first method the uppermost limb is pulled upwards so that it is roughly vertical, and secured with tapes or sandbags. It may be difficult to prevent superimposition of part of this limb over the femur under investigation and so an alternative is to pull the lower hindlimb cranially and the upper hindlimb back. In this case the lower femur is radiographed through the soft tissues of the abdomen.

Craniocaudal femur (CrCd). As for the extended view of the hips, but centring and collimating to the femur. It may help to tilt the patient slightly away from the side being radiographed.

Lateral stifle (Fig. 24.46). Position the animal with the affected side down. Move the other hindlimb upwards or caudally so that it is not superimposed over the lower stifle. Ensure that a true lateral projection is obtained by placing a small pad under the hock. In obese animals, the mammary tissue or sheath may obscure the stifle joint; this may be

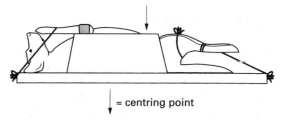

— = centring point

Fig. 24.45 Positioning for assessment of hip dysplasia.

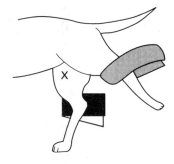

X = centring point

Fig. 24.46 Positioning for lateral stifle view.

prevented by tying a tape around the caudal abdomen to act like a corset. Centre and collimate on the stifle by palpation.

Craniocaudal stifle (CrCd). Similar to ventrodorsal pelvis (extended view) by positioning in dorsal recumbency and extending the affected limb. The other hindlimb may be left free. It may be useful to tilt the patient slightly away from the affected side to ensure a true craniocaudal view.

Caudocranial stifle (CdCr). An alternative view. Position in sternal recumbency and extend the affected limb caudally.

Lateral tibia, hock and paw. Lie the patient with the affected side down. Draw the upper limb cranially or caudally to prevent superimposition. Use sandbags to achieve a true lateral position if necessary. Centre and collimate to the required area.

Craniocaudal tibia (CrCd) and dorsoplantar hock (DPl). As for craniocaudal stifle, but centre and collimate to the appropriate area. For the hock, the tape is looped around the paw. To reduce the object–film distance for the hock view, it may be necessary to raise the cassette from the table with a wooden block.

Dorsoplantar paw (DPl). Two methods are available. Firstly, the patient may be positioned as for craniocaudal stifle, but with the paw held down to the cassette with strong radiolucent tape. Alternatively, the animal may crouch, with the affected paw pulled slightly outwards and resting on the cassette.

Other imaging techniques

Diagnostic ultrasound

Diagnostic ultrasound is being increasingly used in small animal practice as a complementary imaging tool to radiography. Ultrasound has the advantage that it is painless and safe to both patient and operators and can therefore be used in the conscious patient without the need for sedation or anaesthesia (Fig. 24.47). It can differentiate between soft

tissue and fluid, which radiography cannot, and it produces a 'real-time' or moving picture which is invaluable in the assessment of cardiac function and of peristalsis. Its main disadvantage is that it does not penetrate bone or air so it cannot be used for investigations of the skeletal system or lungs. Bone reflects all of the incident ultrasound, resulting in 'acoustic shadows' or radiating black streaks in deeper tissues (Fig. 24.48).

Ultrasonography is a difficult technique to master since experience is required both to obtain and interpret the images. However, some simple diagnoses may be made even by inexperienced operators, such as pregnancy diagnoses.

Ultrasound is sound energy at a higher frequency than can be detected by the human ear. In the diagnostic range, the frequencies used range from about 2.5 to 15 megahertz (MHz). In an ultrasound machine the sound waves are created by the vibrations of special crystals in the probe or transducer which alter their shape when an electrical current is applied to them. This is known as the 'piezo-electric effect'. When the probe is applied to the patient's skin the sound waves are passed through the patient's soft tissues as pressure waves, and at interfaces between organs or between clusters of different cells within an organ a certain percentage of the sound waves are reflected and may return

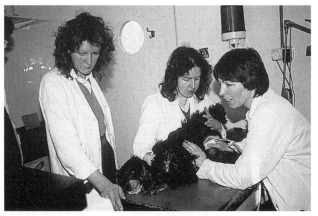

Fig. 24.47 Ultrasonography of a conscious patient.

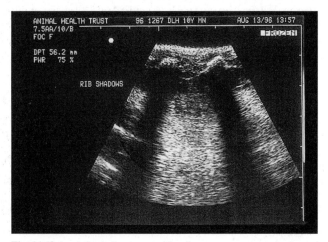

Fig. 24.48 Acoustic shadows created by ribs.

to the transducer. Returning sound waves in turn create a vibration of the tissues and of the crystals in the probe and this is converted back into electrical impulses which are quickly converted by a computer into an image. The image is basically built of many tiny dots of different brightnesses depending on the strength of the returning pulses of ultrasound and the location in the body from which they have been reflected. It is a cross-sectional picture of the internal architecture of the tissues under investigation. The basic principle of ultrasound is shown in Fig. 24.49.

Ultrasound equipment consists of one or more transducers, a TV monitor and a control panel (Figs 24.50 and 24.51). There is also likely to be some sort of printer for recording the images. Ultrasound transducers are of two main types. In linear array transducers, the piezo-electric crystals are arranged in a line and the image is rectangular (Fig. 24.52). Although a wide image of the tissues close to the transducer is obtained, linear array transducers need a long contact area with the patient which is hard to achieve in small animals (remember that ultrasound does not pass

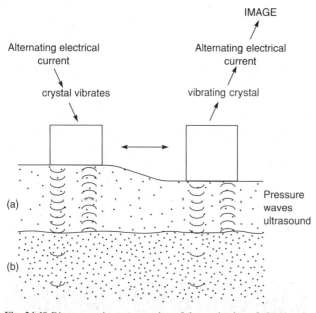

Fig. 24.49 Diagrammatic representation of the production of ultrasound waves by the transducer and the detection of returning sound waves.

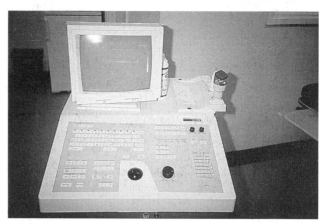

Fig. 24.51 Ultrasound TV monitor and control panel.

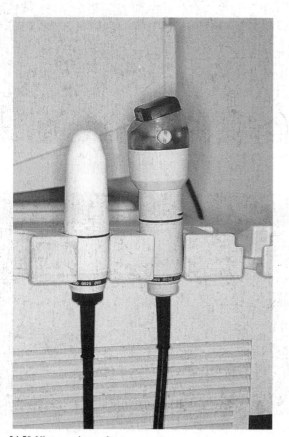

Fig. 24.50 Ultrasound transducers.

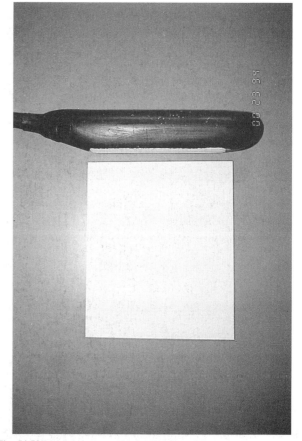

Fig. 24.52 Linear array transducer and image field.

through air). Linear array transducers are mainly used for rectal investigations in large animals. Sector scanning transducers are much more suitable for small animal work since the crystals are arranged close together so that only a small area of contact with the patient is required (Fig. 24.53). The ultrasound beam fans out to produce a triangular image which shows as much of the deeper tissues as possible. The image can be altered in depth, brightness and contrast using the ultrasound machine's controls, and measurements can be made on a frozen image. In dogs and cats the fur must be usually be clipped to allow good contact between the transducer and the skin, since small air bubbles trapped in hair will greatly degrade the image. A special coupling gel is then applied to improve contact further (Fig. 24.54).

Most ultrasound performed uses B-mode ('brightness' mode ultrasound) as described above, to create a two-dimensional image of the tissues. Small sound reflections within tissues create a fine, granular pattern to organs, with different organs producing different brightnesses on the image (Fig. 24.55). Pathology within an organ can often be recognised as a change in the overall brightness or **echogenicity** of the organ or a mottled appearance disrupting normal architecture (Fig. 24.56). Fluid is usually seen as

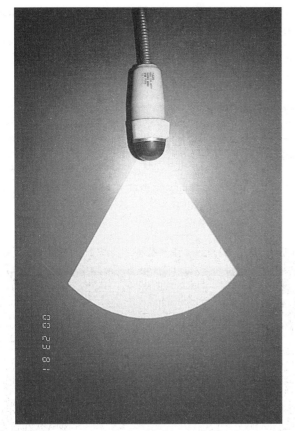

Fig. 24.53 Sector scanner transducer and image field.

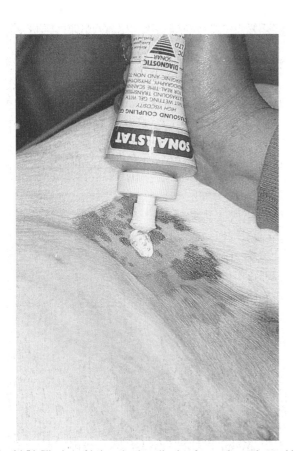

Fig. 24.54 Clipping of hair and gel application for good transducer–skin contact.

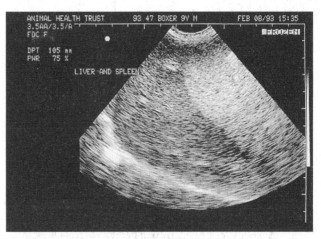

Fig. 24.55 Normal ultrasound image of liver and spleen.

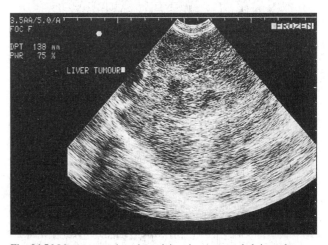

Fig. 24.56 Liver tumour in a dog, giving rise to a mottled, irregular pattern to the liver.

a much darker area because it gives rise to very few ultrasound reflections. Thus, free abdominal fluid can be seen as a black background surrounding abdominal organs (Fig. 24.57). One of the main advantages of ultrasound is that it allows examination of the abdominal structures when free fluid renders radiography unhelpful by obscuring the organs.

Ultrasound is increasingly used for biopsy or fine needle aspiration of small diseased areas within organs. Since the internal organ architecture and the needle can both be seen, the needle can be guided into the affected area without damaging other structures (Fig. 24.58). This technique can often be performed with the patient conscious and avoids the need for surgical biopsy.

A further refinement of ultrasound is the use of M-mode ('movement' mode) to quantify heart motion. First, a B-mode image is obtained and a cursor (line of dots) is placed on it and moved right or left until it passes through the heart in the required position. At the touch of a button the ultrasound beam produced by the transducer is converted into a thin line which produces a vertical band of dots

indicating reflections at tissue interfaces along that line. This is rapidly updated with the movement of the heart and the image scrolled along a horizontal axis with time. The resultant image shows the degree of heart motion and can be frozen to allow measurements of the heart chambers and walls in systole and diastole. Figure 24.59 shows a combined B-mode and M-mode image of a heart.

Computed tomography (CT scanning)

CT involves the production of a highly-detailed cross-sectional radiograph of the patient's tissues. The CT scanner is a large piece of apparatus with a central orifice, the X-ray tube head moves quickly around the circumference during the exposure. The patient lies on a movable table-top which is advanced a few millimetres between exposures so that each image shows a different 'slice' of the tissues. Naturally, veterinary patients must be anaesthetised for CT scanning because of the very high doses of radiation involved (Fig. 24.60).

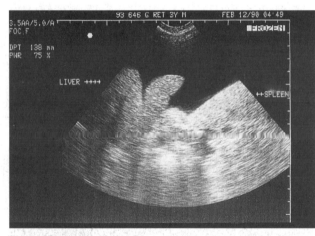

Fig. 24.57 Free abdominal fluid seen as a black area, outlining abdominal organs.

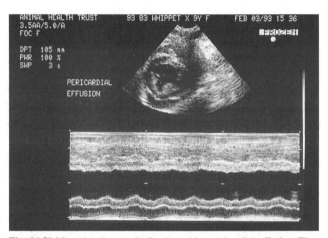

Fig. 24.59 M-mode ultrasound of a dog with a pericardial effusion. The top image is a B-mode image of the heart and the line of dots indicates the position of the fine ultrasound beam used for the M-mode study. The lower image shows the M-mode image with time along the horizontal axis. Blood in the left ventricle and pericardial fluid are seen as black areas on both images.

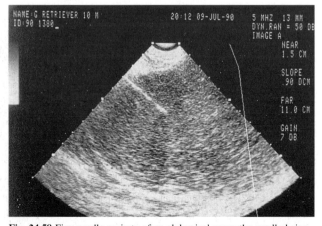

Fig. 24.58 Fine needle aspirate of an abdominal mass, the needle being seen as a bright line entering the mass.

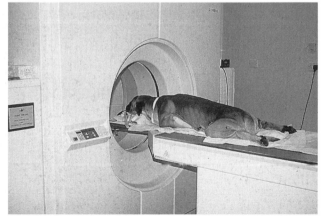

Fig. 24.60 CT scanner and patient.

Although essentially a radiographic technique, CT images produce much more tissue definition than radiography and will differentiate between different types of soft tissue and between fluid and soft tissue. CT is especially valuable for imaging the skeletal system (Fig. 24.61). The images can be manipulated on a computer after acquisition to enhance detail, a procedure known as 'post processing'. Radiographic contrast media can be given intravenously or into the subarachnoid space to enhance the images further.

Magnetic resonance imaging (MRI scanning)

MRI is the newest diagnostic imaging technique and involves completely different physical principles, combining magnetism and radio energy. Because it does not use ionising radiation (unlike radiography and CT) it is thought to be completely safe, although veterinary patients must still be anaesthetised to keep them still during the long scanning time, which may be up to an hour. The scanner itself is a very powerful magnet, which is usually long and cylindrical, with the patient lying in the centre of the magnet's bore (Fig. 24.62). The tissues within the magnet become magnetised, which has an effect on the protons of the hydrogen atoms in the body. The patient is then subjected to a series of radio waves, each lasting for several minutes; these have the effect of disorientating the protons so that they emit tiny radio signals themselves. The emitted signals are detected and converted to an image by a computer.

As with CT, the images are cross-sectional slices through the patient's tissues, but the soft tissue information produced is even greater and the images yield fantastic detail about the tissues. MRI is used particularly in the diagnosis of brain diseases in small animals (Fig. 24.63) but it can also be used to investigate many other disease processes, especially neoplasia. The use of MRI and to a lesser extent CT have meant that surgery and radiotherapy of brain tumours in cats and dogs can now be performed successfully. MRI and CT are becoming increasingly used in veterinary diagnostic imaging as referral centres gain access to human scanners or even obtain their own machines.

Nuclear medicine (scintigraphy)

Scintigraphy is used mainly in horses for the diagnosis of orthopaedic problems. A radioactive substance which will

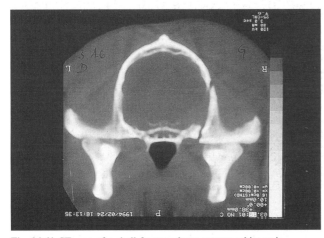

Fig. 24.61 CT scan of a skull fracture; bone appears white as in radiography. This image has been processed by the computer to 'flatten' the soft tissues into a single grey shade to emphasise bone better.

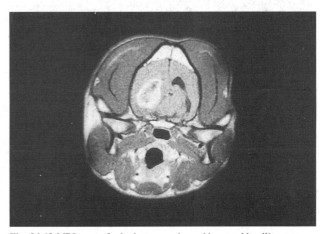

Fig. 24.63 MRI scan of a brain tumour in an 11-year-old collie cross. The brain is the central light grey area and the tumour is the ring-like bright structure within the brain. Head muscle is dark grey and bones are black (cortical bone) and white (bone marrow). This tumour responded well to radiotherapy.

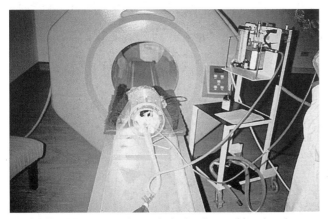

Fig. 24.62 MRI scanner and anaesthetised patient positioned ready to slide into the bore of the scanner.

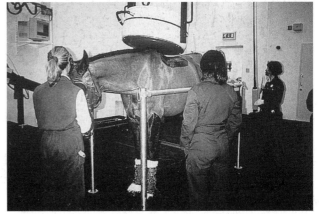

Fig. 24.64 A sedated horse and gamma camera during scintigraphy.

be taken up by the tissue under investigation (usually bone) is injected into the blood stream under conditions which protect the handler from irradiation. Several hours later the radioactivity will have become concentrated in areas of increased bone turnover creating 'hot spots', which are emitting more gamma radiation than are the surrounding tissues. The emitted photons can be detected either by a hand-held radioactivity counter or by a large detector known as a gamma camera (Fig. 24.64). A pattern of emitted radioactivity is produced which allows the source of the lameness to be diagnosed. Although the 'image' itself is rather crude, this technique is very sensitive to early bone changes which cannot be seen with radiography.

Acknowledgement

The author would like to thank Tim Donovan DCR, radiographer in the Centre for Equine Studies at the Animal Health Trust, for his assistance with aspects of this chapter.

Further reading

Dennis, R. (1992) Practice tip – choosing an X-ray machine. *In Practice*, vol. 14, pp. 181–184.

Dennis, R. (1997) Veterinary diagnostic imaging – into a new era. *The Veterinary Nursing Journal*, vol. 12, pp. 43–52.

Douglas, S. W., Herrtage, M. E. and Williamson, H. D. (1987) *Principles of Veterinary Radiography*, 4th edn, Baillière Tindall, London.

HMSO (1988) *Guidance Notes for the Protection of Persons against Ionising Radiations arising from Veterinary Use*, HMSO, London. ISBN 0 85951 300 9.

Lee, R. (1995) *Manual of Small Animal Diagnostic Imaging*, BSAVA, Cheltenham.

Ryan, G. D. *Radiographic Positioning of Small Animals*, Ballière Tindall, London.

Ticer, J. W. *Radiographic Technique in Small Animal Practice*, W. B. Saunders, Philadelphia.

25

Behaviour problems and their management

D. S. Mills and C. B. Mills

Problem behaviour

A behaviour problem may be defined as any behaviour which causes concern to an owner, for which they do not suspect a medical cause. The owner's perception of the situation is therefore critical to the definition. The behaviour is not the diagnosis but a sign of the problem and may be normal or a genuine behaviour disorder. There are therefore two fundamental considerations to behaviour problem management (Fig. 25.1):

- The owner's views and beliefs.
- The animal's behaviour.

For example, the entire male puppy which is chewing the furniture when it has never been trained to chew on specific toys is behaving perfectly normally. Successful treatment will involve educating the client about the normal behaviour of puppies and how to train their puppy to chew on toys in preference to anything else. On the other hand, the dog which appears to be easily spooked by people approaching may in fact have a disease of the eyes which results in tunnel vision, or be deaf. In these cases there may be no treatment directed at the animal but advice can be given to the owners on how to manage their pet more effectively and safely.

Accepting and admitting that a pet has a behaviour problem is often very difficult and stressful for clients. They may feel like failed parents and so may be very sensitive to whatever advice you give them and how it is given. Clients should never be criticised or made to feel stupid because they do not understand their pet's behaviour. They should always be regarded with respect and consideration and time taken to explain the situation in a non-judgemental way.

The behaviour of animals is affected by a number of factors, including:

- The genetic make-up of the individual – **genotype**.
- The current **physiological state** of the animal, e.g. hormone and metabolite levels.
- The current **external environment**.
- **Previous experience and learning**.

Genetic factors

These may determine and affect the behaviour of the species, the breed or the individual:

- It is essential to be well versed in the normal behaviours of the species in order to appreciate if something is genuinely abnormal (e.g. an owner thinking that the cat in oestrus, rolling on the floor, is abnormal or in pain).
- A good knowledge of breed characteristics will also help in the appreciation of what is normal (e.g. vocalisation of the Siamese). Breed behaviour tendencies may indicate what problems may be likely in a given breed (e.g. noise phobias in bearded collies). An understanding of the breed is also important when trying to advise a potential owner about a new pet.
- Individual behaviour is seen in the animal's character and temperament.

Physiological state

Some behaviours are more frequent or only occur in one sex. For example, some forms of aggression seen during false pregnancy are intimately associated with the hormonal changes in the bitch at this time. In other cases, e.g. urine spraying in cats, it is more common in males but neutering usually helps in both the prevention and the treatment of the problem in either sex. It is important to realise that not all aggressive behaviours are driven by male hormones; castration should not be recommended in all these individuals as it may in fact be contraindicated.

The physiology of an animal also changes with disease and this may result in an apparent behaviour problem, e.g. aggression in the hyperthyroid cat or rabid animal. Chronic lead poisoning may be seen as a result of animals licking or chewing items treated with old-fashioned lead paints; in the dog this can present as anxiety and/or a reduction in the working dog's obedience.

Drug therapy also affects an animal's physiological state, since drugs may alter the release of nerve transmitters or interfere with receptor sites in the body. Whilst there are some drugs like the antidepressants and anxioloytics which are specifically designed for this purpose, other drugs may produce behaviour changes as a secondary effect, e.g.

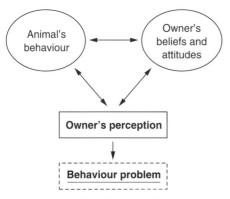

Fig. 25.1. The components of a behaviour problem and their interaction. All of these factors must be addressed when considering treatment.

phenylpropanolamine is used to control urinary incontinence in dogs but may also cause aggression in some cases, probably as a result of a change in blood pressure associated with its mode of action.

WARNING

As behaviour problems may be caused by disease and/or require medical therapy, it is essential that any case requiring more than obedience training is given a thorough clinical examination by a veterinary surgeon. By law the veterinary surgeon has responsibility for the case. The need to consult a veterinary surgeon should be explained by the veterinary nurse to any clients seeking advice and those considering referrals to behaviour experts.

The external environment

A problem may arise with an animal's behaviour because of the situation in which it finds itself. In these cases, altering the environment may eliminate the problem. Such measures include the re-homing of a dog with separation-related problems to a family where it will not be left on its own. Whilst this may resolve the situation, and save the animal's life, it is important to realise that the problem still exists but is no longer expressed. Alternatively, the environment can be temporarily changed, by bringing in a dog-sitter so that the problem does not arise, whilst the behaviour is modified through careful training and behaviour therapy.

Previous experience

In early life, dogs and cats have 'sensitive phases' when they learn more readily or form impressions which will affect their behaviour and temperament.

The **socialisation period** largely determines how an animal will react to other individuals (of the same and different species), groups and the surrounding environment for the rest of its life. This period appears to be between the 4th and 10th week of age in the puppy and between the 2nd and 7th week in the kitten. It is vital that pets receive pleasant experiences at this time, associated with things that are to be accepted later. For example, they should be handled gently by a range of handlers old and young so they do not shy away from people later in life. Overstressing, e.g. by early weaning, should be avoided as this interferes with the animal's learning ability and appears to result in fundamental emotional changes. This is the time that most temperament problems are developed: damage done at this time is much harder to undo later.

During the **juvenile period**, the animal matures sexually. Cats and dogs are still capable of forming strong attachments to new owners at this time if they have been socialised to people previously.

Many problems arise because the animal has not been properly socialised or trained when young. It is far easier to teach the appropriate behaviour from the outset than it is to correct problems later. The veterinary nurse has an important role in this aspect of preventative medicine:

● Advice should be given to breeders and potential new owners on suitable weaning, handling and exposure procedures. An outline programme for the first 6 weeks is given in Fig. 25.2.
● Practices should run 'puppy classes'. These classes combine basic obedience training with socialisation, plenty of handling and lots of novel stimuli, provided in a controlled and pleasant environment. Puppies are taught what is acceptable and what is not (e.g. biting). All vaccinated puppies can be invited to the classes and given the opportunity to mix with puppies their own age and new people. A recommended 4-week programme is given below. These are not only an important service, but excellent PR for the practice as well as a lot of fun for all involved.

Four-week puppy class programme

The whole family should be encouraged to attend the classes and take part in the exercises. The principles of training (see later) should also be described as part of the course, so owners understand not only what they should do but also why.

Each week new skills are taught and established ones are reinforced. It is important to explain the principles behind the tasks and to provide handouts, since the owners will inevitably be distracted by their puppies some of the time. The techniques described are just as applicable to training older animals but adults should not be mixed with puppies during these group classes.

Week   Exercises
1   *Sit:* With the puppy standing, move a small food treat back over its head and then slightly lower it. The nose should follow the treat and the backlegs naturally fold underneath as the treat is lowered. Try to avoid putting pressure on the hindquarters.
         Stand: Move the food lure slightly up and forward in front of the sitting puppy.
         Down: Move the food to the floor just in front of the puppy and keep it there.
         Recalls: Take the puppy away from the owners and get them to encourage it towards them. Make sure there are no distractions for the puppy when you do this the first time and tell the owners to always be pleased to see the puppy and bend down to greet it.
         Chew control: Select a range of toys for the puppy and either smear an edible reward onto them, like peanut butter, or load a hollow toy with treats which fall out as the puppy chews on them.
         Bite control: Whilst playing calmly with the puppy, slip your hand into its mouth; as its teeth make contact with your skin and well before the bite hurts, let out a scream, withdraw your hand and walk

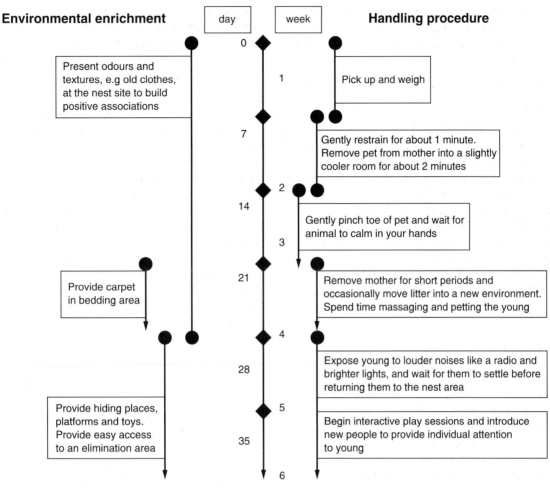

Fig. 25.2. Behaviour development programme for breeders.

away. After a short time repeat the exercise. Soon the puppy will learn to inhibit its bite around people. This is one of the most important lessons a dog can learn.

Handling exercises: Ask someone to reward the puppy with gentle praise and small treats as the dog is handled all over. Make sure you include an examination of the ears, under the tail, between the toes and in the mouth. At first, this will need to be done in stages.

Off and take it: Show the puppy some food in your hand and say 'off' loudly to interrupt its investigation. If the puppy persists then close your hand around the treat and repeat the command even louder. When the puppy stops trying to get it, ask it to take it and give the reward.

Stay: Steadily increase the time the puppy has to wait for a reward once the command word has been given.

Recall from play: Ask all the owners other than the one who gives the recall command to gather up their dogs when the owner calls their dog. The dog should be given lots of praise as it approaches the owner.

Off lead heel: Hold a treat (toy or favourite food) by your side at about the level of the puppy's head. Encourage the puppy to heel as you move forward

just a few steps. As you stop, ask the puppy to sit. When you turn for the first time, turn towards the puppy so your leg will guide him round if necessary.

Food bowl exercises: Remove the food bowl from the puppy and offer him a preferred treat before returning it with an added tit-bit.

Relax: Quietly and gently reassure the puppy as a suitable command word like 'time out' is softly repeated. Keep going until the puppy is totally relaxed.

Heeling on lead: If enough off lead practice has been given, you only need to add the lead to have a dog that heels without pulling.

Greeting people: Whilst walking the dogs on lead, stop as you meet other owners. Each owner then gives the other person's dog a 'sit' command, bends down, and gives the puppy a treat. Children must also learn how to behave around dogs. They should not encourage mouthing, chasing or clothes chewing, but should give treats when the puppy is well behaved.

Socialisation: Encourage owners to get out and about with their puppies. The idea is to expose the puppy to every situation we may want it to accept in its adult life, without getting it overexcited, scared or overtired. So do not let owners do too much in one go.

4   *Tricks:* The principles of learning are explained earlier in the course and all owners asked to teach their dog a trick in preparation for this week. This helps them demonstrate their understanding of training. Certificates can be given to all making it this far. These might include a picture of the puppy taken earlier in the course and make a great souvenir.

All visits to the practice at this time should be made as pleasant as possible. When injections need to be given, as for vaccination, distract the animal during the procedure and then reward it afterwards. Overindulging the crying animal will make it more fearful.

Behaviour problem treatment

There are two important elements to behaviour problem treatment, beyond the skills of good communication and counselling:

- The techniques to be used, i.e. what is to be done.
- The treatment strategy, i.e. how the goal is achieved.

Both need to be considered before treatment commences.

Techniques

There are four techniques available for the management of animal behaviour:

(1) *Training and psychotherapy*. This is described in more detail below.
(2) *Environmental manipulation*. This involves changing the environment in such a way as to alter the animal's behaviour, e.g. providing scratch posts for cats which are clawing the furniture, using a commercial preparation of feline facial pheromones in the home to calm the anxious cat or a muzzle on an aggressive dog.
(3) *Medical therapy*. This involves the prescription of drugs, which may only be done by a veterinary surgeon. There are a number of antidepressants (clomipramine and selegeline) and other drugs which modify behaviour (e.g. progestogens) now licensed for use in animals.
(4) *Surgery*. This would include castration of the urine-marking cat or dog.

Principles of animal training and psychotherapy

Definitions

- **Stimulus** – any event that causes a behavioural or physiological reaction in an animal.
- **Conditioning** – the learning of association between stimuli and between a stimulus and a response.

- **Reinforcement** – Any process which increases the likelihood of an associated behaviour recurring in similar circumstances. Two types of reinforcement are commonly referred to: positive reinforcement and negative reinforcement. With positive reinforcement it is the presentation of a pleasant stimulus (e.g. food) which reinforces the behaviour, whereas in negative reinforcement it is the removal of an unpleasant stimulus (e.g. the pressure from a choke chain) which has this effect.
- **Punishment** – Any process which decreases the likelihood of an associated behaviour recurring in similar circumstances.

NB: Reinforcement and punishment are defined by their effect on a behaviour *not* by the intentions of the handler. If a dog is whining for attention and the owner tells it to be quiet, they are probably going to reinforce the behaviour as they have inadvertently allowed the behaviour to achieve its goal, i.e. attention from the owner.

Training requirements

Training or retraining an animal often requires a vivid imagination and a flexible approach by the trainer. What may be suitable for one client and their pet may not be appropriate for another with the same problem. It is important to consider not only the pet but also the nature of the relationship between the pet and its owner. Communication and a good client manner are essential. Owners are often uncomfortable about the need to seek professional advice in dealing with the problem and will often approach the veterinary nurse in the first instance with some trivial remark. It is important not to dismiss this, but to let them know that you understand and wish to help them. This will often mean scheduling a special session when they can talk at length about the problem. It should be carefully explained that by booking them into a special session that you are not trying to put them off, but recognising the importance of the situation.

The problem must be fully defined (not only what is happening but where, when, with whom and why). Some owners will hold back information either because they think it is not important or because they feel guilty about some action. It is essential to build up trust and to listen patiently without making judgements about a situation. Both the trainer and the client must be relaxed. When talking about any treatment, talk about what 'we' will do, rather than telling the owner what 'they' should do.

Training approaches

The situation should be viewed and explained from the animal's point of view. Learning is greatest when motivation is highest, therefore the nature of the bond between owner and pet should be considered and modified accordingly. The owner should be in control but force is not necessary to establish this.

Rather than criticise an owner for using an ineffectual technique, suggest that it may be better to try an alternative method, explaining what the chosen method is expected to achieve and why. Do not let the client expect too much too soon, as unrealistic expectations often lead to abandonment of the plan when these goals are not reached. The requirements set must also be realistic for the owners in question, as they will not commit themselves to something that they do not really believe is possible.

It is often helpful to suggest an initial period of a week or two to try to crack a problem with quite intense treatment. The thought that it is only a temporary measure motivates the owner more to break previous habits or to follow what may be an inconvenient plan of action. Once this has been done it is much easier to continue.

Training techniques

When training an animal the following points should be noted:

- The subject must be attentive to the trainer. This may require the use of a whistle or other aids to interrupt the animal's current activity. It is also important not to exceed the animal's attention span.
- In order to encourage an animal to comply, any reward must be truly rewarding compared with available alternatives. There is no point in offering a food reward just after the animal's main meal.
- Initially, do not give commands that cannot be enforced. This may mean leaving a long training lead or lead and head-collar attached if it is safe to do so.
- Training sessions should always finish on a positive note, even if it means returning to a basic command.

The use of positive reinforcement and reward-based training

This involves encouraging an animal to perform a desired behaviour by means of pleasant lures and rewards. **Positive reinforcement** should always be used if appropriate since it trains the animal precisely what is required, is relatively easy to apply, humane and helps to strengthen the trainer – animal bond and social stability. Social stability is particularly important to dogs and many problems in this species would not occur if the dog respected the owner; therefore the teaching of basic obedience, if not already present in the problem dog, is to be recommended. Applications of positive reinforcement are:

- To teach obedience commands and build up sequences of action through **behaviour changing.** Each behaviour is taught with a command word in the normal way. A new command word is then introduced before the old instructions are given in a set order. Soon the dog will learn, through a process known as **classical conditioning**, that the first command is always followed by the set sequence and so will perform the whole act without the need for the individual commands.
- To teach a whole new action (e.g. a dog is taught to sit to greet rather than jumping up). In **counter-conditioning** a new behaviour is taught separately which is incompatible with the problem behaviour. When the behaviour has become firmly established, it is used when the problem would normally arise. So long as the association with the new acceptable behaviour is stronger than the motivation to engage in the problem behaviour, the new behaviour will be expressed at the expense of the problem.
- To put **an existing behaviour on a cue**, i.e. build an association between a behaviour and a new command. The expression of the behaviour can then be limited by restricting the use of the command word. This is useful in controlling certain types of barking.
- To **shape an existing behaviour pattern** towards another (more desirable) behaviour pattern, e.g. the training of complex activities and during systematic desensitisation (see below).

Positive reinforcement may be:

- **Continuous**, when every response is rewarded. This is often used in the early stages to lure the animal into the correct response or to explain to it what is required. The reward soon becomes predictable and so does not motivate the animal to the same degree once the behaviour has been established.
- **Variable**, when the reward is sometimes given and other times not. This is useful in shaping a behaviour – only those behaviours which are nearest to that which is desired are rewarded.
- **Differential**, when both the size and the frequency of the rewards are varied. This is used once a new response has become established in order to keep the animal keen to respond – the unpredictable nature makes the training actively addictive.

Systematic desensitisation is used to reduce an animal's excitement or fear in response to a given situation. This situation is broken down into component stimuli which do not produce a response on their own. For example, in the case of an animal that is scared of the vet, it may be possible to safely expose the animal to people in white coats or the disinfectant used in the clinic off site, the vet in different overalls on site and so forth. Acceptance can be improved if the animal is distracted during the process. It is rewarded as long as it does not show an inappropriate response. The process is then repeated and the stimuli gradually made more similar to the final goal. It is essential not to rush this process but to do it at a pace that the animal can accept.

If a response is inappropriate to a given situation then the technique known as **flooding** may be used. This depends on the process of **extinction** as well as it being safe and humane to allow the animal to express the full behaviour. The response is neither rewarded nor punished but allowed to run its course, in the hope that it will pass away. This technique may be used to treat certain attention-seeking behaviour problems. In such cases no attention should be given to the animal when it tries to solicit it from its owner, since any attention (good or bad) rewards and reinforces the behaviour. Physical punishment is contraindicated as this is still a form of attention. Doing nothing is not necessarily very easy, especially if an owner enjoys stroking the pet. Owners should also be warned that the behaviour will become more intense before it disappears. It is critical that they do not give in at this time otherwise they will make matters worse, having just reinforced a more extreme form of the behaviour.

Punishment

The use of **punishment is associated with many problems** and its misuse is an abuse. Punishment does not teach an animal what it should be doing, punishment only signals that what the animal is doing is wrong. It is therefore a much less efficient training tool than reinforcement. The overuse of punishment by owners may not only result in a dog which is fearful towards them, but possibly people in general. It also creates an animal that is less responsive and able to learn. If an animal is fearful or nervous, punishment must *never* be used as it reinforces the fear, i.e. it signals to the animal that it was right to be scared of what was going on. However, punishment may be useful and necessary in certain circumstances to eliminate a behaviour. In these situations an alternative acceptable behaviour which can be expressed by the animal must be identified and encouraged with positive reinforcement at the same time. If punishment seems to be needed a lot of the time, the trainer should always ask: 'Where have I gone wrong?'.

Punishment is most effective if it is associated with the problem behaviour rather than a given person. For this reason, remote punishments like booby traps are preferable to ones which are obviously delivered by the trainer. One of the most widely used booby traps is a drinks can with a few coins inside. When the animal starts to misbehave, this is thrown close to (but not directly) at the dog, without warning and without attracting attention to the trainer. The animal then learns that this behaviour has this unpleasant consequence. For example, the dog that tries to chase people passing by when on the lead, can have the behaviour interrupted in this way. As soon as the can lands, the owners should encourage the dog to come towards them and reward it for doing so. If a booby trap is used in the home, like a noise alarm linked to an out of bounds area, it is worth using a discriminatory stimulus, like a drop of essential oil on the threshold of the area to warn the animal. In this way the animal will soon learn to avoid wherever the scent is placed. Avoidance of these areas is then reinforced by negative reinforcement, so the booby traps can be removed.

Treatment strategies

There are usually several ways in which a problem behaviour may be managed. These can be divided into four broad strategies, the application of which is only limited by the trainer's skill and knowledge. The goal of treatment is to apply those which are most likely to bring success with the minimum of discomfort to both the pet and owner.

(1) You can prevent the expression of the problem behaviour. For example, a dog can be prevented from biting by muzzling it.
(2) The causal factors may be addressed. These may be eliminated or their perception altered. For example,

when one dog is re-homed in a case of inter-dog rivalry in the house or the thyroid removed from an aggressive, hyperthyroid cat, the causes of the problem have been removed. Alternatively the phobic dog may be desensitised or prescribed anxiolytics (anti-anxiety medication). This alters its view of the causes of the problem.
(3) The behaviour may be redirected onto something which does not cause a problem. For example, the cat which scratches the furniture may be trained to scratch on a scratching post instead.
(4) Another behaviour may be introduced which competes with the problem behaviour. This is the principle behind counter-conditioning and the use of toys to prevent problems associated with boredom.

Some common behaviour problems

The most widespread condition is lack of obedience. Other major problems are aggression, house-soiling and house destruction.

Aggression

Aggression in the dog is a serious concern for all involved. The owners of aggressive animals must be informed of their special responsibility to prevent injury to others. For this reason, aggressive behaviour problems should only be tackled by skilled handlers. Until professional intervention is possible the veterinary nurse should encourage the owner to avoid situations which are likely to exacerbate the condition. This may include identifiable trigger stimuli, like other dogs, children, etc., and/or incidences of competition, uncertainty or fearful situations. The dog should not be approached when it has no opportunity to retreat. If it is safe to do so, the **owner should be encouraged to muzzle train their pet away from arousing or dangerous environments.** A basket muzzle is preferable to a nylon one for this, as it allows the dog to pant and drink but not bite while it is on. Training involves introducing the muzzle to the dog for literally a few seconds and rewarding the dog. When it accepts the muzzle being slid on and off, the muzzle may be held on for a little while by hand and a reward given when it is removed. With time the dog will soon accept the muzzle for longer periods, at which time it can start to be fastened. The most common problem with muzzles is that they are only used when the dog is already showing aggression and will resent restraint. This is why training should begin away from distractions and the trained dog should be muzzled before a problem arises. Castration is not to be recommended as a routine procedure for aggressive dogs as it may exacerbate the condition in some circumstances.

House-soiling

When asked about a house-soiling problem it is important to check that the animal has been properly housetrained in the first place. It is then important to establish whether the animal is scent marking (spraying in the cat or spot marking in the dog) as these represent fundamentally different behaviours. They may also occur in either sex or neutered animals.

Feline urine spraying, which is not due to cystitis, is most effectively treated with a commercial preparation of the feline facial pheromone. *A **pheromone** is a chemical signal produced by one animal and released into the environment, where it has its effect either on the same or other animals.* Marked areas are cleaned with water and wiped dry with paper towels. The chemical is then applied over the marked areas daily until the cat is seen to face rub the area or stops urine marking altogether. It is recommended to treat at least half a dozen places in the house even if there are fewer marked areas. Cats which have been urine marking for some time may also stop using the litter box. Other reasons for indiscriminate elimination include lower urinary tract disease, litter box and litter aversions, an emotional problem or a substrate preference. It should be checked that the litter box is in a quiet, secluded area where the cat cannot be disturbed, that the box is cleaned regularly and completely and that there have been no changes to the normal routine, e.g. change of litter, etc. Bleach, ammonia-based disinfectants or strong-smelling cleaners are not recommended as the smell may be aversive to the cat. If the cause is not readily identifiable and the animal is healthy, then expert advice should be sought.

In the dog, house-soiling is most commonly a result of a loss of housetraining, scent marking, excitement, disease, fear or separation distress. Any disease must be recognised promptly, but in all cases the pet will need retraining. This is most effective by ensuring that the dog is taken out regularly to a particular toilet area and returned if it does not eliminate. When it does, it should be given lots of praise and a treat. This might be a longer walk or titbit. Owners should always clear up after their pet. The recommended treatment for scent marking is chemical (steroidal) or surgical neutering as this will eliminate the problem in the majority of cases. Dogs may eliminate when they feel threatened; this is a normal appeasement gesture. Owners often get annoyed at this reaction and so may make matters worse by telling the dog off. Eye contact alone may be sufficient to set off this submissive behaviour in some dogs. Owners must be encouraged not to appear threatening in any way towards their pet but should jolly it along with praise and without eye contact. Confidence-building exercises and possibly psychopharmacy may be necessary to allow these animals to lead a normal life. Dogs also eliminate when they are scared, e.g during thunderstorms, or distressed in some other way. Some dogs become over-attached to their owner and cannot cope when they are separated. In these cases, the drug clomipramine may be useful in treatment, but behaviour modification advice is essential to the long-term success of the case. This involves training the animal to getting used to being left alone and cooling the relationship between the owners and their pet. Predictable cues of the owners' departure should be removed and the dog should not be allowed to follow them around the house the whole time when they are at home. Other measures may also be necessary. Dogs with such separation-related problems may also be extremely destructive at this time and this may be the main presenting complaint.

House destruction

Dogs that destroy when left alone may be doing so because of distress at the owners' absence (see above) or because of a lack of stimulation at this time. It is essential that they have plenty of stimulating toys available for them when left alone for long periods of time. These can be made more attractive at the time of leaving by smearing them with food paste or filling them with food. They should also be taken up when the owner returns so access is limited and their value to the dog increased. Dogs should be trained to chew on appropriate items when left alone and it should not be assumed that they will naturally stop chewing on things when they stop teething. Further advice on this and other behaviour problems is given in the reading list below.

All problems of behaviour in the dog and cat reported to the veterinary nurse should be considered seriously and, if necessary, referred to a more experienced colleague.

Further reading

Askew, H. R. (1996) *Treatment of Behavior Problems in Dogs and Cats*, Blackwell Scientific, Oxford.

Landsberg, G., Hunthausen, W. and Ackerman, L. (1997) *Handbook of Behaviour Problems of the Dog and Cat*, Butterworth-Heinemann, Oxford.

Overall, K. L. (1997) *Clinical Behavioral Medicine for Small Animals*, Mosby, St Louis.

26

Bereavement counselling

D. S. Mills and C. B. Mills

Coping with the grieving or anxious client

The loss of a loved pet will always be a painful experience for an owner and may result in considerable disturbance within a veterinary practice. There is, however, much that a veterinary nurse can do to help both the client and the practice during this time. It is essential that the veterinary nurse should be mentally prepared to cope with this emotionally charged situation. There are three key areas of attention at this time:

- **The environment**. Plan ahead wherever possible.
- **Communication**. This should be clear, thoughtful and compassionate.
- **Receptiveness**. Be aware of what is happening and be prepared to respond to the unforeseen.

All staff must appear sincere and interested in anything that causes a client distress. This is achieved by making eye contact, listening carefully to what the owner has to say and letting them know that you are concerned and will take the appropriate action. When talking to owners, make sure that the pet's name is correct, identify the pet's sex with the accurate use of he or she (never 'it') and try to avoid technical jargon. There should be as few interruptions as possible. Any laughter from an adjacent room will cause suspicion in an owner about the sincerity of the practice.

A client is often more impressed by a sympathetic approach by the nurse in a stressful situation than by the best treatment a veterinary practice can offer.

Handling the situation for animal euthanasia

This situation is critical to the owner and it should never be seen to be rushed. The decision to end a pet's life is ultimately the decision of the owners. They accept the recommendation of the veterinary surgeon and the responsibility that goes with it, whilst perhaps not fully understanding the medical situation. Any uncertainty about what is happening is likely to increase the intensity of the grief process, and so it is important to take time to listen and answer any questions the client may ask. In some instances only the veterinary surgeon may be able to answer these, but communication is essential. The clients should appreciate that the recommendation is made in the best interests of their pet. They should not be blinded by scientific terminology.

It is essential that the client is given consistent information from every person they respect in a practice. Where there are several veterinary surgeons who have dealt recently with the animal, the nurse may be the most consistent feature throughout a course of treatment and the owners will turn to the nurse when a decision on euthanasia becomes necessary. A casual or ill-chosen comment may have long-lasting or devastating effects and this will affect their ability to cope with the situation. Comments such as 'I understand how you feel' or 'I can appreciate that this is a very painful decision/sad moment' will help to support the owner emotionally. In some instances the nurse may be able to refer to the loss of their own animal and a mutual understanding develop. The stress of a consultation involving a euthanasia may be reduced if the nurse prepares for it in advance:

- Make ready and complete as far as possible all documentation before the event. Where necessary, give assistance in the completion of consent forms. Details for cremation will need to be known and an explanation of the facilities available should be given. The payment for treatment should be discussed in advance if possible. If a bill has to be sent on later, it should be made clear that all services have to be paid for. The phrase 'veterinary services' is preferable to words such as 'euthanase and dispose' when charging a client.
- Avoid using the words 'put to sleep', as an owner might think an anaesthetic is about to be given to treat a particularly painful condition. If children are present, these words can be particularly confusing and cause distress or anxiety later. Considerable psychological problems have been reported in some children as a result of the same words being used at a later stage in a different context (e.g to go to bed or to have a general anaesthetic in hospital).
- Try to book an appointment at a quiet time of day, when staff will have time to spend with the client and there will be a minimal number of onlookers or little chance of distraction.
- Do not keep clients waiting unnecessarily when they arrive. If any delay is likely, explain this to the owner. They may appreciate conversation about other issues like their family, to take their mind off the event, but they may equally prefer to be left alone. Be sensitive to a client's needs.
- Do not jump to conclusions: agitation or the smell of alcohol on the owner's breath may show that the person has, until then, lacked the courage to bring in a terminally ill animal. There may be other reasons for euthanasia of a pet that the nurse may not be aware of.

- When it comes to the time for the euthanasia injection, find out if the owners want to be present. Find out their wishes: some may like to hand over the animal to the veterinary surgeon and nurse, whilst others may like to return after the euthanasia injection to see their dead animal for the last time. If an owner wishes to remain with the body or take it home, explain that even if the animal is no longer alive (i.e. its heart has stopped and there is no brain activity) it is still possible for muscles to twitch which may appear like gasping actions. Be prepared for the bladder to empty after death by arranging suitable absorbent material.
- If the patient is already hospitalised and it seems likely that the parting with the owner present is likely to be difficult, arrange for a preplaced cannula to be in the vein. Sedation before the euthanasia may help but sometimes the owners wish their animals to recognise them and respond to their voice.
- A plentiful supply of tissues, seating close at hand and a glass of water may all be needed. Tears should be anticipated and often crying is the best immediate response to death. Owners should have time to recover before appearing in public or having to drive themselves home. If necessary arrange for a taxi to take them back.
- When discussing the arrangements for the aftercare of the body (cremation, burial, etc.), it may help to retain the body for a short time on the surgery premises until the owner has come to a decision, as other members of the family may have to be asked. If a client asks the nurse about what happens to the bodies at the surgery, you must be honest but diplomatic. Saying that 'the bodies are all cremated together' is preferable to saying 'they're all incinerated'. Individual cremation with the return of the ashes is an option which should be offered as a service.
- When moving a body in' the owner's presence, do not appear immediately with a black plastic bag. If the owner wishes to remove a pet for burial, they may use their own basket or a cloth wrapping. The risk of soiling from faeces or urine should be assessed and sometimes the rear end of the body can be placed in the bag if you explain the reason for this first.
- Where possible, escort the owners out of the surgery by a route that gives as much privacy to their grief as possible. Some may need help, especially if they have come to a surgery on their own.
- It is often better to say nothing if you are not sure of a situation. Saying the wrong thing may create a long-lasting adverse impression. A friendly touch of the arm and the offer of help or suggesting a friend the owner can talk to about their pet is often very consoling if made in a sincere manner. Suitable leaflets can be given out for the owner to read as they are often too embarrassed at the event to ask all the questions.
- Finally, make sure the medical records are amended so an owner is not sent booster reminders or other communications about a deceased animal. Being active after an unpleasant experience is the best antidote to the veterinary nurse becoming over-involved in a death of an animal.

Bereavement and the grief sequence

Whilst there is obviously a lot of variation in how people react and cope with grief, there are five well-recognised stages in a grieving process:

- Shock/denial.
- Anger.
- Bargaining.
- Depression.
- Acceptance.

It should be noted that not all these events occur as distinct episodes. They often overlap so the client feels more than one emotion at the same time. The stages may be interchanged or displayed in a different sequence, or some stages may not be seen at all. Some people progress through the stages quickly; others become permanently halted at any time. They will often start before the death of the pet unless the death has been particularly sudden.

Shock

The signs in a grieving owner are a refusal to accept the death or disbelieve a grave prognosis. Watch for responses such as: 'Surely not!', 'It can't be true' or 'You can't be serious about it!'. Owners may demand a second opinion before accepting that a pet is in the terminal stages or ask about alternative treatments long after help of this nature will be of benefit. When describing an animal's illness, they may focus on minor ailments in order to try and block the reality of the situation (e.g. asking about overgrown toe-nails or the presence of a small wart).

The shocked person may look pale, dazed or confused and tearful when they realise that euthanasia may be the only outcome of the consultation. An owner might even arrive at the surgery with an obviously dead animal, refusing to believe that death has occurred and asking the veterinary surgeon or nurse to do something to save it.

This phase of shock is often brief and should not last more than a day.

Nurse's action

When clients express disbelief at the situation, do not contradict them directly. Sympathise with their shock but be direct about the situation. Phrases such as 'I know it is hard to believe but . . .' are helpful in communicating effectively at this time.

If a client wishes to seek a second opinion, this should not be refused, but a journey may not be in the best interests of the shocked client or the dying pet. Another veterinary surgeon in the same practice who knows the client and the pet may be the best person to advise the client at this time.

Anger

This is commonly directed at the practice, as the owner feels an injustice. The anger may be directed at individual members of staff or the procedures used to determine the diagnosis. Questions such as 'Why don't you . . .' and complaints such as 'You should have . . .' may be raised. This can be difficult for staff to accept, especially when they have acted in good faith and tried to avoid needless expense for the client. If owners direct the anger at themselves, it will result in feelings of guilt.

Nurse's action

Do not take a verbal attack by a client personally but stay calm. Always be courteous and do not aggravate a situation or be too defensive. It does not help an angry client to have their own faults and previous wrongdoings pointed out. The nurse should be understanding but firm in support of the practice.

An expression such as 'I can understand that you are very upset by what has happened but I can assure you this is a normal procedure' may defuse a situation before explaining (or offering to find someone in a better position to explain) the reasons for any procedure. The veterinary surgeon is better equipped to answer any accusations. When asking a veterinary surgeon to come to explain, make sure that he or she is properly briefed before they speak to the client and that the case records are available. If a client complains about someone, that person should not comment out of turn or walk away from the situation in protest.

Avoid making any statement that could be interpreted as an admission of carelessness, neglect or error.

Bargaining

At this stage of the grieving process, some clients may offer something in exchange for a more favourable situation. The nurse may even receive a small gift, which should be accepted gracefully. Clients may also express a revival or emergence of religious beliefs not previously experienced.

Nurse's action

It is important to be the guardian of the pet's welfare and to support whatever recommendations have already been made by the veterinary surgeon. Do not take advantage of the owner in this situation. Do not be tempted to advise or suggest treatments for a pet which may be expensive and have little chance of success.

Depression

Most clients will feel sad about a situation but the intensity varies with individuals and the degree of attachment to a pet (the pet may have been a substitute for a child or a close friend). Emotions associated with the owner's current concerns at work and at home may all be imposed on the feelings associated with the death of a pet. Alternatively, feelings linked to the death of a close associate in the past may be aroused all over again.

In depression, a person may become physically ill, be unable to eat or sleep properly and lose interest in their normal daily routine. Bereaved animal owners sometimes appear confused about events and easily distracted or imagine that they can still sense their pet's presence in the home. They may experience periods of unaccountable crying or 'grief pangs'. These are all normal signs of depression and may be seen a few hours or a few days after the event, often reaching a peak of intensity about 2 weeks later.

Nurse's action

Sometimes a client telephones the surgery but often the depression is only heard about when a third party contacts the surgery for help. If the client does not appear to know anyone who can appreciate their loss, the practice staff are in the best position to provide initial support as they will have known the pet as well as the client. If asked, the nurse should try to make discreet enquiries and be prepared to provide support (often by discussion over the telephone). Talking things over with a depressed person may alleviate some of the suffering but often being a good listener whilst making supportive comments can be very valuable. It is important to establish effective communication with a grieving client, who should be reassured that there is nothing unusual about the feeling of depression or the disruption in interests and normal routine. It may help to encourage the client to make a memorial gesture, e.g. give a donation to a charity, plant a tree, or a similar act to remember the lost pet, as this helps the grieving process.

Sometimes a client needs to be directed to a suitable support group, who will be far more skilled in handling the situation. A pet loss befriender service is jointly operated by the Society for Companion Animal Studies (SCAS) and the Blue Cross. Details are available from SCAS on 01877 330996 or your local Blue Cross Centre. It is important for the practice be aware of these services and to recommend them when necessary. The client should not be left to fend for themselves on this point. SCAS also produce a number of publications to support owners at this time which can be offered to the client at the time of their pet's death or shortly afterwards. Details are given at the end of the chapter. Clients will often associate a lack of information from the practice with a lack of care.

If the depression is very intense or it continues for more than 3 weeks or there are any suicidal overtones, professional medical advice should be advised immediately.

Acceptance

This is a recovery stage as the client can again talk about the pet without the distress shown before. They will be more objective about their assessment of the circumstances of the pet's death. Any new pet or other interest is accepted on its own merits.

Nurse's action

Until this time, any new pet is likely to form an association with the loss and may prolong the grieving process or inhibit acceptance. It is best not to encourage a client to obtain a replacement before this stage has been reached. The premature suggestion of a replacement may be viewed as disrespectful to the lost pet or as a failure of others to appreciate the special relationship that existed between that pet and its owner.

An offer to help in choosing a new addition to the household at this time is often appreciated, even if it is not accepted. A dog or cat from a 'rescue' centre may help the bereaved person feel that they are now able to help others again, by offering a home to a less fortunate animal in circumstances that their former pet enjoyed.

Guilt

Many clients feel some guilt after the death of a pet, for many reasons. As already mentioned this is often the result of anger turned inwards. They may feel guilty about something they did or failed to do that contributed to the pet's death (perhaps they left the gate open that led to a road accident). Sometimes these feelings are unfounded, e.g. no one would know that the first yelp of pain was a sign of a terminal illness and contacting the practice immediately may not have altered the outcome. They may blame themselves for previous episodes of punishment or minor neglect. It is important not to intensify these feelings with ill-chosen comments such as 'If only we had seen him two weeks earlier'. Equally, a well-meaning remark ('You always did your best for . . .') may trigger these episodes as the owner then remembers the times when they put their pet second. If an owner expresses guilt feelings to the nurse in conversation, give reassurance that this is a normal reaction for someone who has lost a friend in such tragic circumstances and that it is an expression of an inner desire to undo what has happened.

The greatest need for clients at this time is a reassurance that what they feel is normal.

Assessing your own and the client's needs

Every situation will be different and difficult before much experience is built up. It is normal to be a bit scared or anxious about the situation initially. These fears usually relate to a lack of confidence and uncertainty about the situation. Will I be able to cope? Will I say or do the wrong thing? Will I do something to make matters worse? These are all common thoughts amongst carers at this time. Like the grieving client, the new nurse or trainee is likely to need support and a structure to their activities in order to help them cope at this traumatic time. It is important to discuss your feelings with colleagues who can reassure you that this is normal. Preparation and organisation also help to build confidence. If you identify a client who is less likely to be able to cope, or a particularly difficult situation for yourself, then the matter should be brought to the notice of a more senior member of staff. Preparation can then be made for any extra support that may be needed.

Some of the factors that suggest an owner is at risk of coping less well with pet loss can be identified quite easily. These clients are likely to require most assistance:

- Owners who have not had time to prepare for the event or are unlikely to get the time to come to terms with it afterwards, e.g owners who are busy with young children or caring for others.
- The owner who lives alone and has few close friends. These clients lack access to the support required to help them cope.
- It is the owner's only pet, has been nursed through a period of intensive care or is a symbol of some other intense feeling or relationship, e.g. it was the deceased husband's favourite. In which case the bond is likely to be more intense.
- The owner is experiencing relationship difficulties at home or at work. The loss of the pet may then represent the loss of the owner's normal social support mechanism.
- The owner is undergoing a change of status or financial hardship. In these cases they may be electing for euthanasia when they would otherwise have preferred further treatment. Whether or not this is likely to have been successful is irrelevant to their feelings at the time.
- Owners who find it difficult to make decisions. In these cases there are likely to be intensive guilt feelings about the situation.
- Owners who have experienced difficulty in the past.

All clients who appear to be at risk should be contacted or visited a few days after the pet's death. A reason may be found for the nurse to phone or call at the home. Any contact should be sincere, provide reassurance to the client and at the same time try to establish the stage or depth of any grief shown. Solicitous enquiries about health or sleeping patterns may indicate if there is any deep depression and support can then be suggested. If the client appears to be in danger of developing a pathological depression, medical help is necessary but a further call after a few weeks may be helpful to find out how the situation has developed. Some people will feel embarrassed at the suggestion that they need additional help, such as a trained counsellor or a support group, but often they can be persuaded to see their own doctor if they are not sleeping or eating properly. They will need extra reassurance that their condition is not unusual and that help is available. If they refuse help, do not be forceful but the client can be told you are always available to talk – they may change their mind later about asking for assistance.

The euthanasia of a pet can be a very stressful occasion for all the staff involved. Some may be more abrupt than normal, whilst others may appear preoccupied or quiet. Some may not appear to care, but this is probably just their way of coping. A kind word or an opportunity to talk about why an animal had to die may relieve anxiety too. It is important not to take things personally at this time and for the team to support each other as well as the client.

Further reading and support material

A Kind Goodbye, SCAS video.
Death of An Animal Friend, SCAS Booklet.
Pet Loss Poster & Leaflet detailing the Befriender Service.
When A Pet Dies – Learning pack for people who want to support owners.
The above are all available from SCAS, 10b Leny Road, Callander, Perthshire, Scotland FK17 8BA.

Lee, L. and Lee, M. (1991) *Absent Friend: Coping with the Loss of a Treasured Pet*, Henston, High Wycombe.
Stewart, M. (1999) *Companion Animal Death: A Comprehensive Guide for the Veterinary Practice*, Butterworth-Heinemann, Oxford.

Index